Clinical Nutrition in Gastrointestinal Disease

Clinical Nutrition in Gastrointestinal Disease

Edited by

Alan L. Buchman, MD, MSPH
Associate Professor of Medicine
Associate Professor of Surgery
DIrector, Northwestern IBD Center
Medical Director, Northwestern Intestinal Rehabilitation Center
Division of Gastroenterology
Feinberg School of Medicine
Northwestern University
Chicago, Illinois

SLACK®
INCORPORATED
Delivering the best in health care information and education worldwide

www.slackbooks.com

ISBN 10: 1-55642-697-6
ISBN 13: 9781556426971

The procedures and practices described in this book should be implemented in a manner consistent with the professional standards set for the circumstances that apply in each specific situation. Every effort has been made to confirm the accuracy of the information presented and to correctly relate generally accepted practices. The authors, editor, and publisher cannot accept responsibility for errors or exclusions or for the outcome of the material presented herein. There is no expressed or implied warranty of this book or information imparted by it. Care has been taken to ensure that drug selection and dosages are in accordance with currently accepted/recommended practice. Due to continuing research, changes in government policy and regulations, and various effects of drug reactions and interactions, it is recommended that the reader carefully review all materials and literature provided for each drug, especially those that are new or not frequently used. Any review or mention of specific companies or products is not intended as an endorsement by the author or publisher.

SLACK Incorporated uses a review process to evaluate submitted material. Prior to publication, educators or clinicians provide important feedback on the content that we publish. We welcome feedback on this work.

Published by: SLACK Incorporated
6900 Grove Road
Thorofare, NJ 08086 USA
Telephone: 856-848-1000
Fax: 856-853-5991
www.slackbooks.com

Contact SLACK Incorporated for more information about other books in this field or about the availability of our books from distributors outside the United States.

Library of Congress Cataloging-in-Publication Data

Clinical nutrition in gastrointestinal disease / [edited by] Alan Buchman.
p. ; cm.
Includes bibliographical references and index.
ISBN-13: 978-1-55642-697-1 (alk. paper)
ISBN-10: 1-55642-697-6 (alk. paper)
1. Gastrointestinal system--Diseases--Nutritional aspects. 2. Gastrointestinal system--Diseases--Diet therapy. 3. Diet therapy. [DNLM: 1. Gastrointestinal Diseases--diet therapy. 2. Nutrition Disorders--diet therapy. 3. Gastrointestinal Diseases--complications. 4. Nutrition Therapy--methods. WD 100 C641 2006] I. Buchman, Alan.

RC802.C576 2006
616.3'30654--dc22

2005028646

Printed in the United States of America

Last digit is print number: 10 9 8 7 6 5 4 3 2 1

Dedication

This book is dedicated to improving education among gastroenterologists, endocrinologists, surgeons, primary care physicians, and allied health professionals, including pharmacists, dietitians, and nurses and others so that nutritional care of their patients may improve.

Contents

Section III: Nutrition in Gastrointestinal Disease

Section IV: Nutrition in the Critical Care Environment

Section V: Management of Intestinal Failure

Section VI: Nutritional Support

Acknowledgments

I wish to acknowledge the tremendous assistance of my copy editor Carie Lambert, who had a unique ability to supply order to the style of the various contributors and was able to take this text to its currently concise format. Carrie Kotlar, my Acquisitions Editor from SLACK Incorporated, shared my vision of this text and understood its importance. She helped transform it to a reality. I also want to thank all the authors whose contributions made the book what it is.

About the Editor

Alan L. Buchman, MD, MSPH is a graduate of Northwestern University and The Chicago Medical School. He completed his residency in internal medicine at Cedars Sinai Medical Center. He began his training in nutrition and gastroenterology under his mentor Dr. Marvin Ament at UCLA, where he completed his master's degree in nutrition and a fellowship in clinical nutrition. Following his gastroenterology fellowship at Emory University, Dr. Buchman served on the faculties of the Baylor College of Medicine and the University of Texas Houston Medical School prior to moving to Northwestern, where he is the Medical Director of the Northwestern Inflammatory Bowel Disease and the Northwestern Intestinal Rehabilitation Centers. He is recognized as an international authority on intestinal failure, inflammatory bowel disease, and nutrition in gastrointestinal disease.

Dr. Buchman's nearly 200 contributions to the medical literature have served to advance the field in these arenas. He has served on many peer-reviewed journal editorial boards, and has had leadership positions on numerous national committees, including the American Gastroenterological Association, the American Society for Parenteral and Enteral Nutrition, the American Federation for Clinical Research, and the United States Food and Drug Administration.

About the Contributors

Marvin Ament, MD
UCLA School of Medicine
Pediatrics Department
Los Angeles, CA

Jaime Aranda-Michel, MD
Mayo Clinic Transplant Center
Jacksonville, FL

Gavin Arteel, PhD
Assistant Professor of Pharmacology and Toxicology
University of Louisville Medical Center
Louisville, KY

Christopher C. Ashley, MD, MPH
Albany Medical College
Gastroenterology Group
Albany, NY

Albert Barrocas, MD, FACS
Clinical Professor of Surgery
Tulane University School of Medicine
New Orleans, LA

Gerard T. Berry, MD
Thomas Jefferson University
Philadelphia, PA

Charles J. Billington, MD
University of Minnesota
St. Paul, MN

Stephan C. Bischoff, MD
Professor
Lehrstuhl Ernährungsmedizin/Prävention
Universität Hohenheim
Stuttgart, Germany

Barbara B. Bivona, RN, BSN
Director of Home Healthcare
Methodist Hospital
New Orleans, LA

Alice Buchanan, MS, RD
Dietition
Vanderbilt Center for Human Nutrition
Vanderbilt University Medical Center
Nashville, TN

Eduard Cabré, MD
Department of Gastroenterology and Hepatology
Hospital Universitari Germans Trias I Pujol
Badalona, Spain

William Cameron Chumlea, PhD
Wright State University School of Medicine
Departments of Pediatrics and Community Health
Lifespan Health Research Center
Kettering, OH

Brian M. Chung, PhD
Food Science & Human Nutrition
University of Illinois
Urbana, IL, 61801

Robert Craig, MD
Northwestern Medical School
Chicago, IL

Sheila E. Crowe, MD
Division of Gastroenterology and Hepatology
University of Virginia
Charlottesville, VA

Mark H. DeLegge, MD
Medical University of South Carolina
Charleston, SC

David F. Driscoll, PhD
Senior Researcher
Department of Medicine
Boston, MA

Gerald W. Dryden, Jr. MD, MSPH
Assistant Professor of Internal Medicine
Department of Internal Medicine
University of Louisville Medical Center
Louisville, KY

Johanna T. Dwyer, DSc, RD
Professor of Medicine and Community Health
Friedman School of Nutrition Science and Policy
and School of Medicine, Tufts University
Director, Frances Stern Nutrition Center
Tufts-New England Medical Center
Boston, MA

Brintha Enestvedt, MD
Oregon Health & Science University
Department of Medicine
Portland, OR

William B. Evans, MD
Fellow, Division of GI/Hepatology
Department of Medicine
University of Louisville
Louisville, KY

Martin H. Floch, MS, MD, MACG
Clinical Professor of Medicine
Yale University
Norwalk, CT

Jonathan Fryer, MD
Northwestern Memorial Hospital
Chicago, IL

Miguel Gassull, MD, PhD
Head of the Department of Gastroenterology and Hepatology
Hospital Universitari Germans Trias I Pujol
Badalona, Spain

Marwan Ghabril, MD
Mayo Clinic Transplant Center
Jacksonville, FL

Michele M. Gottschlich, PhD, RD
Shriners Hospital
Cincinnati, OH

Sandeep Gupta, MD
Cleveland Clinic
Cleveland, OH

Lyn Howard, MD, FRCP
Emeritus Professor of Medicine
Associate Professor of Pediatrics
The Oley Foundation
Albany Medical College
Albany, NY

Daniel Hurley, MD
Division of Endocrinology
Mayo Clinic
Rochester, MN

Kishore Iyer, MBBS, FRCS(Eng), FACS
Children's Memorial Hospital
Chicago, IL

Khursheed N. Jeejeebhoy, MBBS, PhD, FRCPC
St. Michael's Hospital
Toronto, ON Canada

Gordon L. Jensen, MD, PhD
Director, Vanderbilt Center for Human Nutrition
Professor of Medicine
Vanderbilt University Medical Center
Nashville, TN

Palle Bekker Jeppesen, MD, PhD
Department of Medical Gastroenterology
University Hospital of Copenhagen
Copenhagen, Denmark

Darlene Kelly, MD, PhD
Division of Gastroenterology
Mayo Clinic
Rochester, MN

Asim S. Khokhar, MD
Department of Gastroenterology and Hepatology
Beth Israel Deaconess Medical Center
Harvard Medical School
Boston, MA

Young-In Kim, MD, FRCP(C)
University of Toronto
Toronto, Ontario, Canada

Ronald L. Koretz, MD
Olive View-UCLA Medical Center
Department of Medicine
Sylmar, CA

Catherine M. Kotz, PhD
University of Minnesota
St. Paul, MN

Robert F. Kushner, MD
Professor of Medicine
Northwestern University Feinberg School of Medicine
Medical Director, Wellness Institute
Northwestern Memorial Hospital
Chicago, IL

Allen S. Levine, PhD
Professor and Head Director, Minnesota Obesity Center
Department of Food Science & Nutrition
University of Minnesota
St. Paul, MN

Charles S. Lieber, MD, MACP, FACG
Bronx V.A. Medical Center
Bronx, NY

Timothy O. Lipman, MD
Chief, GI-Hepatology-Nutrition Section
Veterans Affairs Medical Center
Washington, DC

Henry C. Lin, MD
Division of Gastrointestinal and Liver Diseases
Keck School of Medicine
University of Southern California
Los Angeles, CA

Clifford Lo, MD, MPH, ScD
Nutrition Division
Children's Hospital
Boston, MA

Stephen F. Lowry, MD
Chairman, Department of Surgery
UMDNJ-Robert Wood Johnson Medical School
New Brunswick, NJ

Elisabeth Luder, PhD
Department of Pediatrics
Mount Sinai School of Medicine
New York, NY

Joel B. Mason, MD
Gastroenterology Division
New England Medical Center
Boston, MA

Laura E. Matarese, MS, RD, LDN, FADA, CNSD
Director of Nutrition
Thomas E. Starzl Transplantation Institute
University of Pittsburgh Medical Center
Pittsburgh, PA

Craig J. McClain, MD
Vice Chair for Research, Department of Internal Medicine
Professor of Internal Medicine, Pharmacology and Toxicology
Jewish Hospital Endowed Chair in Hepatology
University of Louisville Medical Center
Louisville, KY

Stephen A. McClave, MD
Division of Gastro/Hepatology
Department of Medicine
University of Louisville
Louisville, KY

M. Molly McMahon, MD
Division of Endocrinology
Mayo Clinic
Rochester, MN

Adib Moukarzel, MD, FAAP, FACN, CNSP
Imm. A Khoury
Beirut, Lebanon

Alexander P. Nagle, MD
Northwestern University
Chicago, IL

Lisa M. Neff, MD
Tufts University
Boston, MA

Vandana Nehra, MD
Mayo Clinic
Rochester, MN

Stephen J.D. O'Keefe, MD, MSc, FRCP
University of Pittsburgh
Presbyterian Hospital
Pittsburgh, PA

Pawel K. Olszewski, PhD
University of Minnesota
St. Paul, MN

John E. Pandolfino, MD
Assistant Professor of Medicine
Division of Gastroenterology
Northwestern University
Feinberg School of Medicine
Chicago, IL

Michelle Papaconstandinou
Division of Endocrinology
Mayo Clinic
Rochester, MN

J. Martin Perez, MD
UMDNJ-Robert Wood Johnson Medical School
New Brunswick, NJ

Carol Porter, PhD, RD, FADA
University of California–San Francisco Medical Center
Deptartment of Pediatrics
San Francisco, CA

Jay Prystowsky, MD
Department of Gastrointestinal Surgery
Northwestern Memorial Hospital
Chicago, IL

Mark Sands, MD
Department of Interventional Radiology
Cleveland Clinic
Cleveland, OH

Denise Baird Schwartz, MS, RD, FADA, CNSD
Providence Health System
St. Joseph MC

James S. Scolapio, MD
Mayo Clinic
Division of Gastoenterology
Jacksonville, FL

Cynthia Sears, MD
Divisions of Infectious Diseases and Gastroenterology
Johns Hopkins School of Medicine
Baltimore, MD

Douglas L. Seidner, MD, FACG
Director, Nutrition Support and Vascular Access Department
Program Director, Fellowship in Clinical Nutrition
Digestive Disease Center
Cleveland Clinic Foundation
Cleveland, OH

Timothy Sentongo, MD
Childrens Memorial Medical Center
Chicago, IL

Scott A. Shikora, MD, FACS
New England Medical Center
Boston, MA

Ezra Steiger, MD
Cleveland Clinic
Deptartment of General Surgery
Cleveland, OH

Neil J. Stone, MD
Feinberg School of Medicine
Northwestern University
Chicago, IL

Le-Chu Su, MD, PhD
Cleveland Clinic Foundation
Westlake, OH

Robert Suskind, MD
Professor of Pediatrics
Rosalind Franklin University of Medicine and Science
North Chicago, IL

Kelly A. Tappenden, PhD, RD
Associate Professor of Nutrition and GI Physiology
University of Illinois
Department of Food Science and Human Nutrition
Urbana, IL

Phyllis Thomason, MS, RD, LDN
Tufts-New England Medical Center
Boston, MA

Andrew Ukleja, MD
Department of Gastroenterology
Cleveland Clinic
Weston, FL

Gregg W. Van Citters, PhD
Research Fellow, Gonda Diabetes Research Center
Department of Gene Regulation & Drug Discovery
Division of Molecular Medicine
City of Hope National Medical Center/Beckman Research Institute
Duarte, CA

Charles P. Venditti, MD, PhD
National Human Genome Research Institute
National Institutes of Health
Bethesda, MD

David Ziring, MD
UCLA School of Medicine
Pediatrics Department
Los Angeles, CA

Preface

Clinical Nutrition in Gastrointestinal Disease is a compilation of the most currently available data, clinical experience, and research on the role of nutrition in the management of patients with disorders of the stomach, intestines, liver, pancreas, and colon, as well as other diseases that affect the gastrointestinal tract. Nutrition begins in the gastrointestinal system when food enters the body. This book represents a vision I had for improving knowledge on nutritional concepts in the training of gastroenterologists. This vision expanded to encompass not only the entire gastroenterology community, but those who participate in the nutritional care of patients, some perhaps even unknowingly. It is my hope that this reference text will be but one aid in the improvement in nutritional care of our patients through an understanding of how disease processes affect nutritional status, how nutritional status affects disease processes, and how the most appropriate nutritional interventions may lead to improved outcomes with minimization of complications.

Clinical Nutrition in Gastrointestinal Disease begins with the nutritional assessment. One cannot intervene until the problem is recognized. Nutrient deficiencies and their clinical consequences are covered. Contemporary nutrition as it relates to the gastrointestinal system is described. This includes chapters on absorption and malabsorption, recommended dietary intakes, pro- and prebiotics, fiber, alternative medicine, and food safety. Nutritional consequences and interventions in various disease states are discussed, including diabetes, alcoholism, obesity, inflammatory bowel disease, celiac disease, pancreatitis, motility disorders, gastrointestinal malignancy, liver disease, and intestinal failure. Particular metabolic and nutritional concerns in the critically ill patient are discussed. Both parenteral and enteral nutritional support and prevention of their complications are covered in detail. Surgical issues in gastrointestinal nutrition are covered including bariatric surgery, the consequences and remedies of extensive intestinal resection, and intestinal transplantation. The legal and ethical ramifications of nutritional therapy are disccussed. The authors have made use of figures, diagrams, tables, photos, and many seminal references. Our goal is one small step in the improved education of clinicians in the consequences of malnutrition and the appropriate preventative and treatment interventions.

Section I

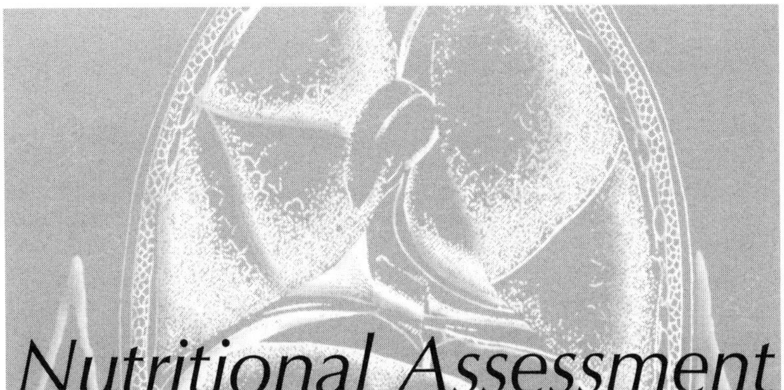

Nutritional Assessment

Chapter 1

The Practical Nutritional Assessment

Khursheed N. Jeejeebhoy, MBBS, PhD, FRCPC

Introduction

Nutritional health is maintained by a state of equilibrium in which nutrient intake and requirements balance. Malnutrition occurs when net nutrient intake is less than requirements. Malnutrition leads to a succession of metabolic abnormalities, physiological changes, reduced organ and tissue function, and loss of body mass (Figure 1-1). Concurrent stress such as trauma, sepsis, inflammation, and burns accelerates loss of function and body mass leading to losses that leave the individual's body function and mass insufficient to maintain health and life.

Clinically important evaluation of nutritional status should be able to predict whether the individual would have increased morbidity and mortality in the absence of nutritional support. In short, it can predict the occurrence of nutrition-associated complications and thus predict outcome. Unfortunately, disease and nutrition interact so that disease in turn may cause secondary malnutrition or malnutrition may adversely influence the underlying disease.

Traditional nutritional science was first developed in the field of agriculture in which the effect of nutrition was entirely judged by the amount of meat on the carcass of an animal and by the production of proteins by the animal's liver. This approach was embodied in the initial attempts to assess nutritional status in humans, as discussed below. These techniques lacked the ability to predict outcomes and to detect early changes in function that occur with nutritional support.

This chapter will address nutritional assessment, and Chapter 44 discusses pediatric parenteral feeding and addresses assessment specific to pediatric patients.

Traditional Nutritional Assessment Indices

Nutritional status has been traditionally defined by body composition, plasma protein concentrations, immune competence, and multivariate analysis.[1,2] Assessment of nutritional status based on body composition involves relating the values in a given patient to normal standards. These measurements are affected by the reproducibility and error in the measurements themselves, and the interpretation by the normal range of values. A person who begins at the upper end of the normal range and loses a lot of weight may be classified as "normal" because, despite losses, his or her measurements remain within the normal range. Therefore, it is possible for a person to be in a negative nutritional state for a long time before anthropometric measurements fall below normal.

Body Weight and Weight Loss

Body weight is a total body of components and, therefore, has to be related to the stature of the person calculated by the Body Mass Index (BMI). The BMI is calculated as weight in kilograms divided by height in meters squared. The interpretation of different BMIs can be found in Table 1-1.[3] A BMI of 14-15 is associated with significant mortality. However, measurements of body weight in patients in hospitals and intensive care units and those with liver disease, cancer, and renal failure are confounded by changes in body water due to dehydration, edema, and ascites.

Changes in body weight may provide some useful information in the clinical setting. Changes in body

TABLE 1-1.

Classifications Used for the Body Mass Index

BMI	Interpretation
<20	May be associated with health problems for some individuals
20-25	Ideal index range associated with the lowest risk of illness for most people
25-27	May be associated with health problems for some people
>27	Associated with increased risk of health problems such as heart disease, high blood pressure, and diabetes

Reprinted from Health and Welfare Canada. Classifications Used for the Body Mass Index, Table 10.7 Promoting Healthy Weights: A Discussion Paper. Health Services and Promotion Branch, Health and Welfare Canada, Ottawa, Ontario, 1988.

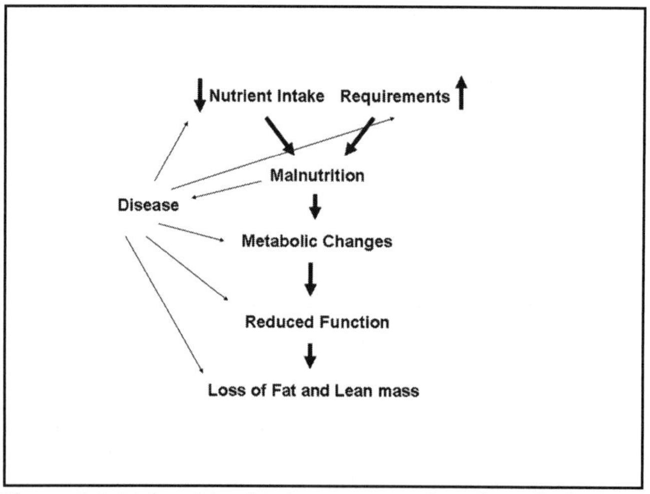

Figure 1-1. Malnutrition leads to a succession of metabolic abnormalities, physiological changes, reduced organ and tissue function, and loss of body mass.

weight can be expressed as percent of usual weight, percentage of weight loss, and rate of weight loss. Unintentional weight loss greater than 10% is often associated with a poor clinical outcome.[4,5] However, it may be difficult to determine true weight loss. Morgan et al[6] have shown that the accuracy of determining weight loss by history was only 0.67 and the predictive power was 0.75. Hence, 33% of patients with weight loss would be missed and 25% of those who have been weight stable would be diagnosed as having lost weight. Furthermore, the nutritional significance of changes in body weight can again be confounded by changes in hydrational status, presence of ascites, edema, or massive tumor growth.

ANTHROPOMETRY

Triceps and subscapular skinfold thicknesses provide an index of body fat, and midarm muscle circumference provides a measure of muscle mass. Although these measurements seem to be useful in population studies, their reliability in individual patients is less clear. The most commonly used standards for triceps skinfold thickness and midarm muscle circumference are on measurements of European male military personnel and low-income American women and those based on measurements of white males and females participating in the 1971-1974 (United States) National Health and Nutrition Examination Survey. The use of these standards to identify malnutrition in many patients is problematic because of the restricted database and the absence of correction factors for age, the effects of hydrational status, and physical activity on anthropometric parameters. Several studies have demonstrated that 20% to 30% of healthy control subjects would be considered malnourished based on these standards.[7,8] The validity of standards have been questioned and interpretation of the data may be limited by interrater variation. For example, Hall et al[9] showed that the coefficient of variation of anthropometric measurements performed by three different observers was 4.7% for arm circumference and 22.6% for triceps skinfold thickness. Therefore, a change in arm muscle circumference (arm circumference minus triceps skinfold thickness) of at least 2.68 cm was needed to demonstrate a true change in a given patient, making the measurement very insensitive to nutritional changes.

CREATININE-HEIGHT INDEX

Creatinine-height index (CHI) is the 24-hour creatinine excretion normalized for height. It is often an unreliable measurement because it is dependent upon complete 24-hour urine collections, and urinary losses or oliguria may result in an inappropriate diagnosis of malnutrition. Patients on diuretics—those with cardiac and liver failure and those with renal disease—are especially likely to have low excretions of creatinine.

SERUM ALBUMIN

Several studies have demonstrated that a low serum-albumin concentration correlates with an increased incidence of medical complications.[10-12]

In practice, it is not an index of malnutrition as exemplified by the fact that prolonged protein-calorie restriction induced experimentally in human volunteers[13] or observed clinically in patients with anorexia nervosa[14] causes marked reductions in body weight but little change in plasma albumin concentration. A protein-deficient diet with adequate calories in elderly persons causes a decrease in lean body mass and muscle function without a change in plasma albumin concentration.[15]

Prealbumin

Prealbumin is a transport protein for thyroid hormones, and it exists in the circulation as a retinol-binding prealbumin complex. The turnover rate of this protein is rapid, with a half-life of 2 to 3 days. It is synthesized by the liver and is catabolized partly in the kidneys. Protein-energy malnutrition reduces the levels of prealbumin and refeeding restores levels. However, prealbumin levels fall without malnutrition in infections[16,17] and renal failure increases,[18] while liver failure may cause decreased levels. Although prealbumin is responsive to nutritional changes, it is influenced by several disease-related factors, making it unreliable as an index of nutritional status in patients.

Immune Competence

Immune competence, as measured by delayed cutaneous hypersensitivity (DCH), is affected by severe malnutrition. While it is true that immune competence as measured by DCH is reduced in malnutrition, several diseases[19] and drugs influence this measurement, making it a poor predictor of malnutrition in sick patients. The following factors nonspecifically alter DCH in the absence of malnutrition: 1) infections (viral, bacterial, and granulomatous); 2) uremia, cirrhosis, hepatitis, trauma, burns, and hemorrhage; 3) steroids, immunosuppressants, cimetidine, warfarin, and perhaps aspirin; and 4) general anesthesia and surgery. Immunity is therefore neither a specific indicator of malnutrition nor is it easily studied.[20]

Serum Cholesterol

Low levels of cholesterol are seen in malnourished patients. However, very low levels are seen in patients with liver disease, renal disease, and malabsorption. In addition, low levels of cholesterol have been correlated with mortality.[21,22] Because of these factors that affect levels, serum cholesterol is not always a true indicator of malnourishment.

Clinical Assessment of Nutritional Status

The clinical assessment of nutritional status, described below as Subjective Global Assessment (SGA), attempts to identify the initial nutritional state and the interplay of the factors influencing the progression or regression of nutritional abnormalities. Therefore, a clinical nutritional assessment is a dynamic process that is not limited to a single "snapshot" at the moment of measurement but provides a picture of current nutritional status and insight into the patient's future status. The clinical assessment of nutritional status involves a focused history and physical examination. The information can be strengthened with selected laboratory tests aimed at detecting specific nutrient.

Subjective Global Assessment

A clinical method for evaluating nutritional status, termed SGA, encompasses historical, symptomatic, and physical parameters.[23,24] This approach defines malnourished patients as those who are at increased risk for medical complications and who will presumably benefit from nutritional therapy. The basis of this assessment is to determine whether nutrient assimilation has been restricted because of decreased food intake, maldigestion, or malabsorption; whether any effects of malnutrition on organ function and body composition have occurred; and whether the patient's disease process influences nutrient requirements. The specific features of the history and physical examination used in the SGA are listed in Table 1-2.

The history used in the SGA focuses on five areas: body-weight loss, pattern of loss, dietary intake, presence of gastrointestinal (GI) symptoms, and metabolic demands of the patient's disease state. The percentage of body weight lost in the previous 6 months is characterized as mild (<5%), moderate (5%-10%), and severe (>10%). The pattern of loss is also important: it is possible for a patient to have significant weight loss but still be considered well-nourished if body weight (without edema or ascites) recently increased. For example, a patient who had a 10% body-weight loss but regained 3% of that weight over the past month would be considered well-nourished. Dietary intake is classified as normal or abnormal as judged by a change in intake and whether the current diet is nutritionally adequate. The presence of persistent GI symptoms—such as anorexia, nausea, vomiting, diarrhea, and abdominal pain—that have occurred almost daily for at least 2 weeks is recorded. The patient's functional capacity is defined as bedridden, suboptimally active, or full capacity. The last feature of the history concerns the metabolic demands of the patient's underlying disease state. Examples of high-stress illnesses are burns, major trauma, and severe inflammation, such as acute colitis. Moderate-stress diseases might be a mild infection or limited malignant tumor.

The features of the physical examination are noted as normal, mild, moderate, or severe alterations. The loss of subcutaneous fat is measured in the triceps region and the midaxillary line at the level of the lower ribs. These measurements are not precise but give a subjective impression of the degree of subcutaneous tissue loss. The second feature is muscle wasting in the temporal areas and in the deltoids and quadriceps, as determined by loss of bulk and tone detectable by palpation. A neurologic deficit will interfere with this assessment. The presence of edema in the ankle and sacral regions and the presence of ascites are noted. Co-existing diseases, such as renal or congestive failure, will modify the weight placed on the finding of edema. Mucosal and cutaneous lesions are recorded, as are color and appearance of the patient's hair.

The findings of the history and physical examination are used to categorize patients as being well nourished (category A), having moderate or suspected malnutrition (category B), or having severe malnutrition (category C).

Table 1-2.

Features of a Subjective Global Assessment

A. History

1. Weight change
   Overall loss in past 6 months: amount = # _____ kg
   Change in past 2 weeks:
   _____ increase
   _____ no change
   _____ decrease
2. Dietary intake change (relative to normal)
   _____ no change
   _____ change: duration = # _____ weeks
   Type _____ suboptimal solid diet _____ full liquid diet
   _____ hypocaloric liquids _____ starvation
3. GI symptoms that persisted > 2 weeks)
   _____ none _____ anorexia _____ nausea _____ vomiting _____ diarrhea
4. Functional capacity
   _____ no dysfunction (eg, full capacity)
   _____ dysfunction: duration = # _____ weeks
   _____ working suboptimally
   _____ ambulatory
   _____ bedridden
5. Disease and its relation to nutritional requirements
   Primary diagnosis (specify) ____
   Metabolic demand (stress) _____ None _____ Low _____ Moderate _____ High

B. Physical (for each trait specify 0=normal, 1+=mild, 2+=moderate, 3+=severe)
   # _________ Loss of subcutaneous fat (triceps, chest)
   # _________ Muscle wasting (quadriceps, deltoids, temporals)
   # _________ Ankle edema, sacral edema
   # _________ Ascites
   # _________ Tongue or skin lesions suggesting nutrient deficiency

C. SGA rating (select one)
   _____ A = Well nourished (minimal or no restriction of food intake or absorption, minimal change in function, weight stable or increasing)
   _____ B = Moderately malnourished (food restriction, some function changes, little or no change in body mass)
   _____ C = Severely malnourished (definitely decreased intake, function, and body mass)

Adapted from Detsky AS, McLaughlin JR, Baker JP, Johnston N, Whittaker S, Mendelson RA, Jeejeebhoy KN. What is subjective global assessment of nutritional status? *JPEN*. 1987;11:8.

The rank is assigned based on subjective weighting of data gathered in the interview and examination of the patient. Equivocal information is given less weight than definitive data. Fluid shifts related to onset or treatment of edema or ascites must be considered when interpreting changes in body weight. In general, a patient who has experienced weight loss and muscle wasting but is currently eating well and is gaining weight is classified as well nourished. A patient who has experienced moderate weight loss, continued compromised food intake, continued weight loss, and progressive functional impairment, and has a "moderate-stress" illness is classified as moderately malnourished. A patient who has experienced severe weight loss and who continues to have poor nutrient intake, progressive functional impairment, and muscle wasting is classified as severely malnourished independent of disease stress. Baker et al[23] and Detsky et al[24] found that the use of SGA in evaluating hospitalized patients gives reproducible results, and there was more than an 80% agreement when two blinded observers assessed the same patient. While these studies support the SGA as a valuable tool, the test has not been scientifically validated in critically ill patients.

Illustrative Cases

Case 1

A 60-year-old female was admitted to the hospital for elective resection of a colon carcinoma. She had lost 10% of her initial weight over 8 months before admission. However, she recently gained weight after therapy with nutritional supplements was initiated. She continued to work and was active. On physical examination, there was no loss of muscle or fat. She is SGA A.

Case 2

A 40-year-old male with an acute exacerbation of Crohn's disease had lost 10% of his body weight within the previous 2 weeks and was ingesting mostly liquids to avoid GI discomfort. He was ambulatory but was not going to work. On physical examination, he had slight loss of subcutaneous tissue manifested by a reduced buccal fat pad and loose skinfolds over the arms. He is SGA B.

Case 3

A 67-year-old male with esophageal cancer had minimal food intake for almost 3 months. He lost 15% of his body weight during the previous 4 months and is continuing to lose weight. He was able to move around the house but had marked muscle weakness and fatigue and did not walk outdoors. On physical examination, he lacked subcutaneous tissue and had hollow temples, deltoid wasting, and mild pitting edema. He is SGA C.

SGA Versus Other Traditional Methods

Comparison of SGA and the traditional methods described above illustrates the effectiveness of SGA as an assessment tool. To make a meaningful comparison, Detsky et al[25] compared the predictive accuracy of the different techniques done on the same individuals in a prospective analysis of 59 surgical patients. In this study, preoperative SGA was a better predictor of postoperative infectious complications than were serum albumin, serum transferrin, delayed cutaneous, hypersensitivity, anthropometry, CHI, and the prognostic nutritional index. Combining SGA with some of the "traditional" markers of nutritional status increased the provider's ability to identify patients who developed complications (from 82% to 90%) but also increased the percentage of patients identified as "malnourished" but who did not develop postoperative complications (from 25% to 30%). Therefore, increasing assessment sensitivity also increases the number of patients who might receive unnecessary nutrition support.

SGA as a Predictor of Complications

Several studies have reported successful use of the SGA to predict complications in general surgical patients,[26] patients on dialysis,[27-29] and liver transplant patients.[30,31] While SGA predicts complications, it may not identify patients who would benefit from nutritional support. In short, it does identify patients in whom the SGA is reduced mainly because of reduced intake and not because of disease-related factors. No prospective controlled clinical trials have demonstrated that providing nutrition support to patients judged to be malnourished influences clinical outcome. However, a retrospective subgroup analysis of a large multicenter trial found that parenteral nutrition given preoperatively to patients diagnosed as severely malnourished by SGA or a nutritional risk index (based on serum albumin and body weight change) decreased postoperative complications.[32]

Nutritional assessment should involve a careful clinical evaluation with additional laboratory studies as needed to help the healthcare provider determine specific nutrient deficiencies or severity of illness. This information should be used in a prognostic fashion to decide which patients might benefit from nutritional therapy.

Measurement of Body Composition

The human body consists of compartments or components. There are over 35 well-recognized components, and these are organized into five levels of increasing complexity: atomic, molecular, cellular, tissue-system, and whole body. In healthy, weight-stable subjects, there are relatively constant relationships between these components, which are correlated with each other. For example, the atomic level component nitrogen is 16% of the molecular level component protein.

There are numerous methods to calculate body composition, including isotope dilution, bioelectrical impedance analysis (BIA) and spectroscopy (BIS), dual-energy x-ray absorptiometry, whole-body counting (or neutron-activation analysis), computerized axial tomography, and magnetic resonance imaging. While body-composition analysis is important to determine the mass and obesity classification of an individual, these measurements are also important in the assessment of predicted risks for the patients.

Although the aforementioned methods for evaluating body composition can accurately assess different components, they are difficult to apply in the clinical setting except in specialized units. The only methods that can be available for wide clinical application in nutritional assessment are BIA and BIS. Both of these techniques have shown that reduced fat-free mass increases LOS in hospital patients. However, unlike SGA, both BIA and BIS do not predict complications except in cancer patients.[33] These methods are discussed at length in Chapter 2 of this book.

The Future of Nutritional Assessment

Functional Changes

Malnutrition is associated with changes in muscle performance. Klidjian et al showed that reduced grip strength was predictive of postoperative complications.[34] Russell et al showed a direct relationship of hypocaloric feeding to muscle function before change in body composition.[35] As well, in anorexic-wasted patients, there is as restitution of function before a significant rise in body mass occurs.[36] Hence, functional changes may be more sensitive markers of malnutrition and also show the benefits of refeeding.

In addition, muscle function predicts the occurrence of surgical complications.[37] However, muscle function is difficult to assess at the bedside and such evaluation requires patient cooperation and participation. 31P-NMR studies have correlated changes in muscle function with altered rates of Adenosine Triphosphate synthesis,[38] indicating an abnormality of the mitochondria. Recent research in human subjects shows that mitochondrial complex I activity in peripheral blood lymphocytes is reduced in malnutrition, not altered by inflammation, and is restored before body mass is after short-term refeeding,[39] with further improvement after a month of refeeding. These findings may lead to the development of an objective and specific method for assessing malnutrition and effects of nutritional support.

Conclusions

The term malnutrition is a continuum that starts when the patient fails to eat enough to meet the body's needs and progresses through a series of functional changes that precede any alterations in body composition that are related to the duration of reduced intake and its severity. To base the definition of malnutrition on any one of these changes is inappropriate: only by recognizing the different facets of malnutrition can we define its various manifestations in relation to our clinical objectives. Currently, SGA, combined with selected objective parameters, provides the best clinical way of meeting these objectives. Muscle function; mitochondrial complex activity; and techniques such a BIA, DEXA, and MRI, combined with spectroscopy, may provide powerful tools in the future.

References

1. Blackburn GL, Bistrian BR, Maini BS, Schlamm HT, Smith MF. Nutritional and metabolic assessment of the hospitalized patient. *JPEN.* 1977;1:11.
2. Detsky AS, Baker JP, Mendelson RA, Wolman SL, Wesson DA, Jeejeebhoy KN. Evaluating the accuracy of nutritional assessment techniques applied to hospitalized patients: methodology and comparisons. *JPEN.* 1984;8:153.
3. Health and Welfare Canada. Classifications Used for the Body Mass Index, Table 10.7 Promoting Healthy Weights: A Discussion Paper. Health Services and Promotion Branch, Health and Welfare Canada, Ottawa, Ontario, 1988.
4. Stanley KE. Prognostic factors for survival in patients with inoperable lung cancer. *J Natl Cancer Inst.* 1980;65:25.
5. DeWys WD, Begg C, Lavin PT, et al. Prognostic effect of weight loss prior to chemotherapy in cancer patients. *Am J Med.* 1980;69:491.
6. Morgan DB, Hill GL, Burkinshaw L. The assessment of weight loss from a single measurement of body weight: the problems and limitations. *Am J Clin Nutr.* 1980;33:2101.
7. Harries AD, Jones LA, Heatley RV, Rhodes J. Malnutrition in inflammatory bowel disease: an anthropometric study. *Human Nutrition Clinical Nutrition.* 1982;36C:307.
8. Thuluvath PJ, Triger DR. How valid are our reference standards of nutrition? *Nutrition.* 1995;11:731.
9. Hall JCH, O'Quigley J, Giles GR, Appleton N, Stocks H. Upper limb anthropometry: the value of measurement variance studies. *Am J Clin Nutr.* 1980;33:1846.
10. Anderson CF, Wochos DN. The utility of serum albumin values in the nutritional assessment of hospitalized patients. *Mayo Clin Proc.* 1982;57:181.
11. Reinhardt GF, Myscofski JW, Wilkens DB, Dobrin PB, Mangan JE Jr, Stannard RT. Incidence and mortality of hypoalbuminemic patients in hospitalized veterans. *J Parenteral Enteral Nutr.* 1980;4:357.
12. Apelgren KN, Rombeau JL, Twomey PL, Miller RA. Comparison of nutritional indices and outcome in critically ill patients. *Crit Care Med.* 1982;10:305.
13. Keys A, Brozek J, Henschel A, Mickelsen O, Taylor HL. *The Biology of Human Starvation.* Minneapolis: University of Minnesota Press; 1950.
14. Russell DR, Prendergast PJ, Darby PL, Garfinkel J, Whitwell J, Jeejeebhoy KN. A comparison between muscle function and body composition in anorexia nervosa: the effect of refeeding. *Am J Clin Nutr.* 1983;38:229-237.
15. Castenada C, Charnley JM, Evans WJ, Crim MC. Elderly women accomodate to a low-protein diet with losses of body cell mass, muscle function, and immune response. *Am J Clin Nutr.* 1995;62:30.
16. Hedlund JU, Hansson LO, Ortqvist AB. Hypoalbuminemia in hospitalized patients with community-acquired pneumonia. *Arch Intern Med.* 1995;155:1438.
17. Feitelson M, Winkler MS, Gerrior SA, et al. Use of retinol-binding protein and pre-albumin as indicators of response to nutrition therapy. *JADA.* 1989;89:684-687.
18. Cano N, Costanzo-Dufetel J, Calaf R, et al. Pre-albumin retinol binding protein-retinol complex in hemodialysis patients. *Am J Clin Nutr.* 1988;47:664-667.
19. Dowd PS, Heatley RV. The influence of undernutrition on immunity. *Clin Sci Mol Med.* 1984;66:241-248.
20. Dominioni L, Diogini R. Immunological function and nutritional assessment. *J Parenter Enteral Nutr.* 1987;11(5 Suppl): 70S-72S.
21. Degoulet P, Legrain M, Reach I, et al. Mortality risk factors in patients treated by hemodialysis. *Nephron.* 1983;31:103-110.
22. Lowrie EG, Lew N. Death risk in hemodialysis patients: the predictive value of commonly measured variables and the evaluation of death rate differences between facilities. *Am J Kidney Dis.* 1990;15:458-482.
23. Baker JP, Detsky AS, Wesson DE, Wolman SL, Stewart S, Whitwell J, Langer B, Jeejeebhoy KN. Nutritional assessment: a comparison of clinical judgment and objective measurements. *N Engl J Med.* 1982;306:969.
24. Detsky AS, McLaughlin JR, Baker JP, Johnston N, Whittaker S, Mendelson RA, Jeejeebhoy KN. What is subjective global assessment of nutritional status? *JPEN.* 1987;11:8.
25. Detsky AS, Baker JP, Mendelson RA, Wolman SL, Wesson DE, Jeejeebhoy KN. Evaluating the accuracy of nutritional assessment techniques applied to hospitalized patients: methodology and comparisons. *JPEN.* 1984;8:153-159.
26. Hirsch S, de Obaldia N, Petermann M, Rojo P, Barrientos C, Iturriaga H, Bunout D. Subjective global assessment of nutritional status: further validation. *Nutrition.* 1991;7:35-37.
27. Fenton SSA, Johnston N, Delmore T, et al. Nutritional assessment of continuous ambulatory peritoneal dialysis patients. *Trans Am Soc Artif Organs.* 1987;23:650-653.
28. Yong GA, Kopple JD, Lindholm B, et al. Nutritional assessment of continuous ambulatory peritoneal dialysis patients: an international study. *Am J Kidney Dis.* 1990;17:462-471.
29. Enia G, Sicuso C, Alati G, Zoccali C. Subjective global assessment of nutrition in dialysis patients. *Nephrol Dial Transplant.* 1993;8:1094-1098.
30. Hasse J, Strong S, Gorman MA, Liepa G. Subjective global assessment: alternative nutrition-assessment technique for liver-transplant candidates. *Nutrition.* 1993;9:339-343.
31. Pikul J, Sharpe MD, Lowndes R, Ghent CN. Degree of preoperative malnutrition is predictive of postoperative morbidity and mortality in liver transplant recipients. *Transplantation.* 1994;57:469-472.
32. The Veterans Affairs total parenteral nutrition cooperative study group. Perioperative total parenteral nutrition in surgical patients. *N Engl J Med.* 1991;325:525-532.

33. Fritz T, Hollwarth I, Romaschow M, Schlag P. The predictive role of bioelectrical impedance analysis (BIA) in postoperative complications of cancer patients. *Eur J Surg Oncol.* 1990;16:326-331.
34. Klidjian AM, Foster KJ, Kammerling RM, Cooper A, Karran SJ. Relation of anthropometric and dynamometric variables to serious post-operative complications. *Br Med J.* 1980;2:899-901.
35. Russell DM, Leiter LA, Whitwell J, Marliss EB, Jeejeebhoy KN. Skeletal muscle function during hypocaloric diets and fasting: a comparison with standard nutritional assessment parameters. *Am J Clin Nutr.* 1983;38:229-237.
36. Rigaud D, Moukaddem M, Cohen B, Malon D, Reveillard V, Mignon M. Refeeding improves muscle performance without normalization of muscle mass and oxygen consumption in anorexia nervosa patients. *Am J Clin Nutr.* 1997;65:1845-1851.
37. Windsor JA, Hill GL. Weight loss with physiologic impairment: a basic indicator of surgical risk. *Ann Surg.* 1988;207:290.
38. Mijan de la Torre A, Madapallimattam A, Cross A, Armstrong RL, Jeejeebhoy KN. Effect of fasting, hypocaloric feeding, and refeeding on the energetics of stimulated rat muscle as assessed by nuclear magnetic resonance spectroscopy. *J Clin Invest.* 1993;92: 114-121.
39. Briet F, Twomey C, Jeejeebhoy KN. Effect of malnutrition and short period of refeeding on human peripheral blood mononuclear cell mitochondrial complex I activity. *Am J Clin Nutr.* 2003;77:1304-1311.

Chapter 2

Body Composition Analysis

William Cameron Chumlea, PhD, and
Khursheed N. Jeejeebhoy, MBBS, PhD, FRC

Introduction

Overweight and obesity are major health problems, with a prevalence of between 20% and 50% reported for adult populations in Europe, the United States, and urban areas of lesser developed countries.[1] In the United States, overweight and obesity are significant health problems for children also. Variation in the prevalence of overweight and obesity is affected by ethnicity, health and socioeconomic status, the definitions of overweight and obesity (Chapter 47), and body composition analysis methodology. There are always sound clinical reasons for a body-composition analysis or assessment, but the current obesity epidemic and its relationship with cardiovascular disease, type 2 diabetes mellitus, and the metabolic syndrome highlight this increased need. The World Health Organization (WHO)[1] recommends the development and validation of new and improvement in existing body-composition methodology because present analysis is not applicable among many who are overweight or obese. In this chapter, the clinical application of current body-composition analysis is reviewed.

Levels of Body Composition

The human body is quantifiable at several levels, depending on clinical concerns. Body composition can be assessed at the atomic level with the basic elements of carbon, calcium, potassium, and hydrogen; at the molecular level by amounts of water, protein, and fat; at the cellular level with extracellular fluid and the body cell mass; and at the tissue level for amounts and distributions of adipose, skeletal, and muscle tissues.

Analysis from the atomic through the cellular levels is with direct body-composition methods like neutron activation, isotope dilution, and total body counting. Criterion methods measure a property of the body, such as its density, or describe amounts and distributions of skeletal, muscle, and adipose tissues via x-ray or magnetic imaging techniques. Criterion methods include densitometry, computed x-ray tomography (CT), magnetic resonance imaging (MRI), and dual-energy x-ray absorptiometry (DEXA). Indirect methods, which include anthropometry and bioelectrical impedance analysis (BIA), provide estimates or indices of body composition based on results from direct or criterion methods. Indirect methods depend on biological interrelationships among direct or criterion measured body components and tissues and their distribution among normal individuals. Indirect methods have large errors, and the results are affected by sample specificity and disease conditions.

Direct, criterion, and indirect methods are applicable to children and adults except to some elderly and to some children who are younger than 8 to 10 years. The method limitations are the patient's inability to perform or undergo the requirements for a specific method or the unavailability of suitable reference data. Direct and criterion methods can detect body-composition changes over at least a 6-month period, but some indirect methods cannot. An interpretation of the results of a body-composition assessment, regardless of the method, must be considered in light of current population variability.

Most direct and some criterion analysis methods are impractical for most clinical examinations or studies because of the scarcity of equipment and testing centers. Neutron activation requires the use of powerful generators, and total body counting requires testing behind pre-World War II steel plating. CT and MRI are used to image the total body or specific body parts for the presence of pathology, disease, or injury. These methods can be used to quantify body-fat and lean-tissue amounts with multiple exposures and specific software. However, this use is frequently limited because of other clinical needs for these instruments.

The following descriptions are for a variety of body-composition–analysis methods, with mention of those that are applicable in many clinical settings. Many of the clinically available methods use proprietary technology and software. While a basic understanding of the underlying biological and physical principles of this technology is important, it is more important to understand equipment accuracy and reliability, which are frequently available only from the manufacturer and should be critically evaluated.

Direct Methods

Whole-Body Counting and Neutron Activation

Potassium, nitrogen, phosphorus, hydrogen, oxygen, carbon, sodium, chloride, and calcium are measured with a group of techniques referred to as whole-body counting and in-vivo neutron-activation analysis. Shielded whole-body counters count the gamma-ray decay of naturally occurring 40K but only a few such instruments are available in the US. The 40K counts are used to estimate total-body potassium (TBK), which, in turn, is used to calculate body cell mass and fat-free body mass (FFM). This passive method is safe in children and pregnant women.

Prompt gamma-neutron–activation analysis is used to measure total-body nitrogen (TBN) and total-body hydrogen. Nitrogen is used to calculate total body protein. Delayed gamma-neutron activation measures total-body calcium, sodium, chloride, and phosphorus. These elements are used to calculate bone-mineral mass and extracellular-fluid volume. Lastly, inelastic neutron-scattering methods measure total-body oxygen and carbon. Carbon is useful in models designed to quantify total-body fat.

Whole-body counting and neutron-activation methods provide estimates all major chemical components in vivo. These methods are considered the standard for evaluating the body-composition components of nutritional interest, including body cell mass, fat, fat-free body mass (FFM), skeletal muscle mass, and various fluid volumes.

Isotope Dilution

Water is the most abundant molecule in the body, and total body water (TBW) volume is measured by isotope dilution. Water maintains a relatively stable relationship to FFM; therefore, measured water/isotope-dilution volumes allow prediction of FFM and fat (ie, body weight minus FFM) in normal weight individuals. The relationship between TBW and other body-composition components may change with disease as a function of the amount and proportion of extracellular fluid; this should be considered in the interpretation of data from hospitalized or chronically ill patients.

The usual approach to calculate TBW is to measure a dilution volume using one of three isotopes: tritium, deuterium, or ^{18}O-labeled water. This first step allows estimation of a dilution volume of one of these three isotopes. In the second step, with the assumption that the proportion of FFM as water is approximately 0.732, the FFM and fat are calculated. (While the calculation is made based on the average proportion of 73% of TBW in FFM, the range is actually 67% to 80%.[2])

Body fatness is another important factor in describing TBW content among individuals, and its effects on changes in TBW with age can affect the clinical management of TBW.[3] TBW is potentially applicable to the obese, but a measure of extracellular space is necessary to correct the amount of FFM in the obese because the proportion of TBW in extracellular fluid increases with the degree of adiposity.

Extracellular-fluid volume is estimated by chemical dilution using bromide as NaBr[96] or other chemical elements similar to chloride.[4,5] This method measures the volume of chloride space that is all extracellular. A dose of NaBr is administered and bromide concentration in plasma is measured by high-pressure–liquid chromatography. It is generally not necessary to measure natural abundance of bromide in the body; however, this knowledge increases the accuracy of the results.

An estimate of TBW is needed to prescribe and monitor treatment in renal disease.[6] TBW volume (V) reflects urea distribution and is used in calculating the amount of dialysis from the formula Kt/V, in which "K" is urea clearance and "t" is the duration of dialysis.[7,8] In routine clinical practice, V is predicted from anthropometric equations for TBW or estimated as a fixed percentage of body weight.[9]

The concentration of the three isotopes in urine, saliva, or plasma can be quantified accurately with mass spectrometry, infrared spectrometry, or nuclear magnetic resonance.[10,11] Comparative studies report good levels of agreement in TBW estimates among subjects, isotopes, specimens, and laboratory methods, but some differences for individuals are as much as 2 to 3 L. These differences are within the range expected between comparisons of body-composition methods. The accepted equilibration time for isotope dilution is 2 to 3 hours, but it is not adequately documented and the variation in equilibration times with body size are also not well known. TBW measures need to be corrected for natural abundance and isotope exchange,[12] especially for deuterium, which is a naturally occurring isotope.

Criterion Methods

Body Density

Body density is calculated from measures of body weight and body volume corrected for residual lung volume. The technique is termed "densitometry." Body volume is calculated from measures of underwater weight or air displacement[13,14] and residual lung volume from computerized spirometry. Underwater weighing requires a large tank of water sufficient for an adult to completely submerge and have his or her weight recorded at full expiration while under water. Air displacement measures the change in the volume of air created by the presence of the body within a closed container of known volume. Accurate and reliable measures of underwater weight and air displacement are hampered by the problem of subject performance and potentially faulty assumptions.[15]

Body density is converted to the percentage of body weight as fat using models based on two or more body compartments of which there are several.[2,16] Two-compartment models divide the body into fat and FFM based on densities of 0.9 g/ml and 1.10 g/ml, respectively. The density of fat has little inter-individual variation across age; however, the density of FFM varies substantially, depending on the relative proportions of water, protein, and osseous and non-osseous minerals to the gender, race, and age of the person.[17] Two-compartment models are not gender- and race-specific; therefore, a variation of only 0.02 g/ml in the density of FFM can produce an error of 5% body fat. Multicompartment models combine body density with measures of bone density from DEXA and TBW volume to calculate body fatness.[18] Multicompartment models estimate body composition more accurately than do two-compartment models because they include measures of bone mineral and water that better reflect between-individual variance in body-composition estimates across age, race, and gender.

TABLE 2-1.

BMI Values, Classifications of Obesity, and Risk of Comorbidity From the World Health Organization

BMI Ranges	Obesity Classification	Risk of Comorbidity
18.5 to 24.9	Normal	Average
25.0 to 29.9	Overweight	Increased
30.0 to 34.9	Obese class I	Moderate
35.0 to 39.9	Obese class II	Severe
≥40.0	Obese class III	Very severe

Computed Axial Tomography and Magnetic Resonance Imaging

CT and MRI measure components at the tissue-system level of body composition, including skeletal muscle, adipose tissue, visceral organs, and brain. CT systems measure x-ray attenuation as the source and detector rotate in a perpendicular plane around the subject. MRI systems measure relaxation times from the nuclei of atoms whose magnetic moments are aligned within a powerful magnetic field. Clinical systems are based on hydrogen, although it is possible to create images and spectrographs from phosphorus, sodium, and carbon. The collected data is transformed into high-resolution images, which allow the quantification of whole or regional body composition. A large number of studies in phantoms, cadavers, and in vivo validate these methods. There are no studies of imaging methods in relation to outcome.

Dual-Energy X-ray Absorptiometry

DEXA quantifies total body and regional amounts of fat, lean, and skeletal tissues in children and adults. The two low-energy levels used in DEXA and their differential attenuation through the body allow the discrimination of total body adipose and soft tissue, in addition to bone-mineral content (BMC) and bone-mineral density (BMD). A typical whole-body scan takes 10 to 20 minutes and exposes the subject to ~1 mrem of radiation. Mathematical algorithms allow calculation of the separation components using various physical and biological models. A computer printout provides the DEXA body-composition analysis for body segments and the total body. Pediatric software is available from some manufacturers for DEXA body-composition estimates of infants and children.

The estimation of fat and lean tissue from DEXA software is based on inherent assumptions regarding levels of hydration, potassium content, or tissue density. DEXA body-composition estimates are also affected by differences among manufacturers in the assumptions related to these levels[19,20] as well as in differences related to technology, models, and used software. Additionally, DEXA-related technology changes frequently. Inter-machine and inter-method comparisons of DEXA body-composition estimates should be made cautiously.

Using DEXA, the weight of adipose (fat) tissue is given, and total-body FFM is calculated as the sum of the weights of soft tissue and BMC. This sum should approximate measured body weight within less than 2.0 kg. If the difference is greater, then concern should be raised for measurement and machine accuracy.

The primary use of DEXA is to measure BMC and BMD of the hip and spine in the diagnosis of osteoporosis. The method provides the first accurate and practical means of measuring bone mineral mass and offers a new opportunity to study appendicular muscle mass. However, currently, research is limited in that no data exists that supports DEXA's ability to predict outcome in hospital patients unrelated to treatment.

There are also limitations on performing DEXA. For adults, there are limitations due to body weight, length, thickness, and width as a function of the available scan-table area with each manufacturer and type of DEXA machine (ie, pencil or fan beam). For a total-body scan, the subject is supine on the table, but many overweight and obese individuals are too wide and too thick to receive a whole-body DEXA scan with current machines, although some innovative adaptations have been proposed.[21] Nevertheless, DEXA is a convenient and accurate method recommended for measuring body composition in the majority of the population.

INDIRECT METHODS

Anthropometry

Anthropometric measurements describe growth, body size, shape, and levels of fatness and leanness, and they also give information about the body at the tissue level. Such measurements are informative if body systems are homeostatic, but they are affected by changes in body size, shape, and composition that occur with maturation, aging, and disease. Anthropometric data are also covariables that account for additional variance in statistical models of body composition.[22]

The use of standardized anthropometric techniques is important for a clinical examination, and these standardized techniques are well documented in print and video. These measurements are most frequently used to assess child growth. Measures of weight, recumbent length, and head circumference from children younger than 3 years of age and weight and stature from older children document the growth of a child. These measurements are informative when plotted on growth charts. Weight and stature describe overall body size. Both increase during growth and are excellent indicators of child health and nutritional status. Most persons with high body weights tend to have high amounts of body fat, regardless of age. A loss of weight in children or in adults with chronic disease is an indicator of potential health problems (Table 2-1).

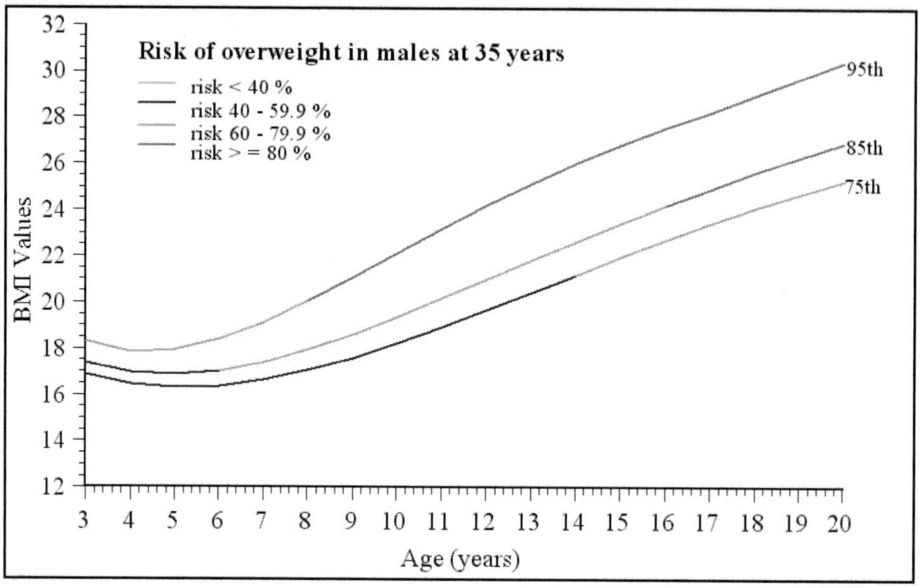

Figure 2-1. Selected percentiles for BMI in males from the Center for Disease Control (CDC) growth charts for BMI-for-age. Segments of the 75th, 85th, and 95th percentile lines are differentially shaded to indicate differences in the probability that BMI at 35 years will be ≥25 kg/m^2.

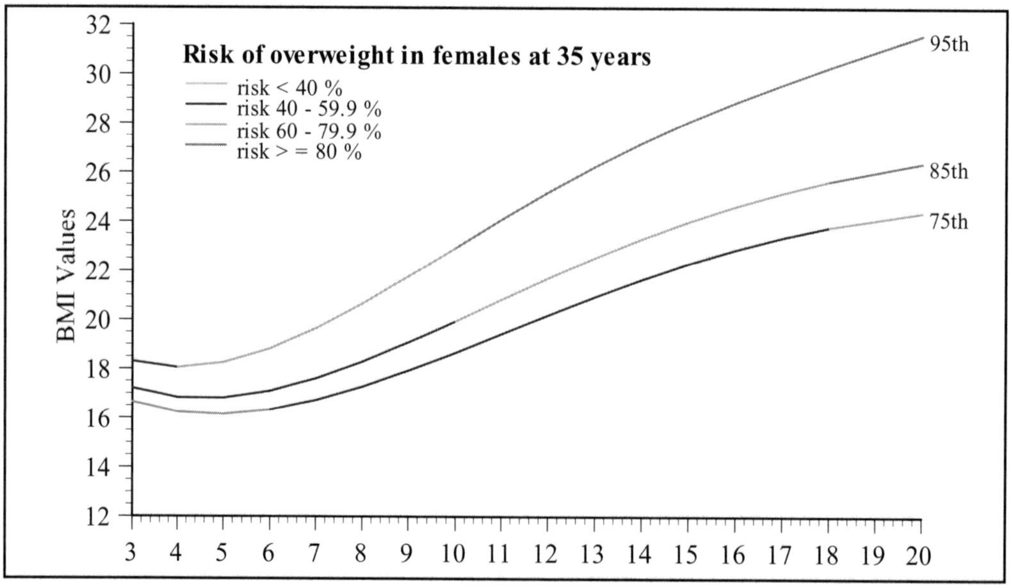

Figure 2-2. Selected percentiles for BMI in females from the CDC growth charts for BMI-for-age. Segments of the 75th, 85th, and 95th percentile lines are differentially shaded to indicate differences in the probability that BMI at 35 years will be ≥25 kg/m^2.

BMI

The body mass index (BMI) is weight (in kilograms) divided by stature (in meters squared) and is an index of overweight and obesity. The WHO classifies overweight and obesity (see Table 2-1), based on grades of BMI values related to increasing risk of comorbidity. Adults with BMI levels below 18 and above 25 are at risk for increased morbidity and mortality. A BMI of 25 to 29 is defined as overweight, and a BMI of 30 or greater is accepted as a definition of obesity. BMI values less than 19 are potential indicators of wasting. The available national and epidemiological prevalence data on overweight and obesity are not based on actual measures of body fatness because of the difficulty of collecting such data from large groups.

Weight and BMI are used to monitor treatment of overweight and obesity; however, a weight change of 3.5 kg produces a unit change in BMI. BMI in adults has established risk relationships with levels of body fatness, morbidity, and mortality, and it is highly predictive of future risk for overweight.

BMI is also used with children and the elderly. Risk relationships between a high BMI in childhood and morbidity have not been determined. However, high BMI percentile levels in childhood are linked to significant levels of future risk for overweight and obesity in adulthood.[23] As shown in Figures 2-1 and 2-2, boys and girls at age 12 years with BMI at the 85th percentile have a risk of 60% to 80% of having a BMI at that same level at 35 years of age, and for a BMI at the 95th percentile, the corresponding adult risk is greater than 80%. Figures 2-3 and 2-4 for boys and girls present the adult risks for obesity at age 35 years, based upon BMI percentiles in childhood.

If BMI is used to assess elderly individuals, it should be noted that BMI is influenced by declining bone mass and amount of FFM with age. The extreme loss of muscle mass, known as sarcopenia, can cause an elderly person of normal weight and BMI to become obese because of an increased high percentage of body fat. However, moderate overweight at older ages is associated with lower mortality, and a loss of

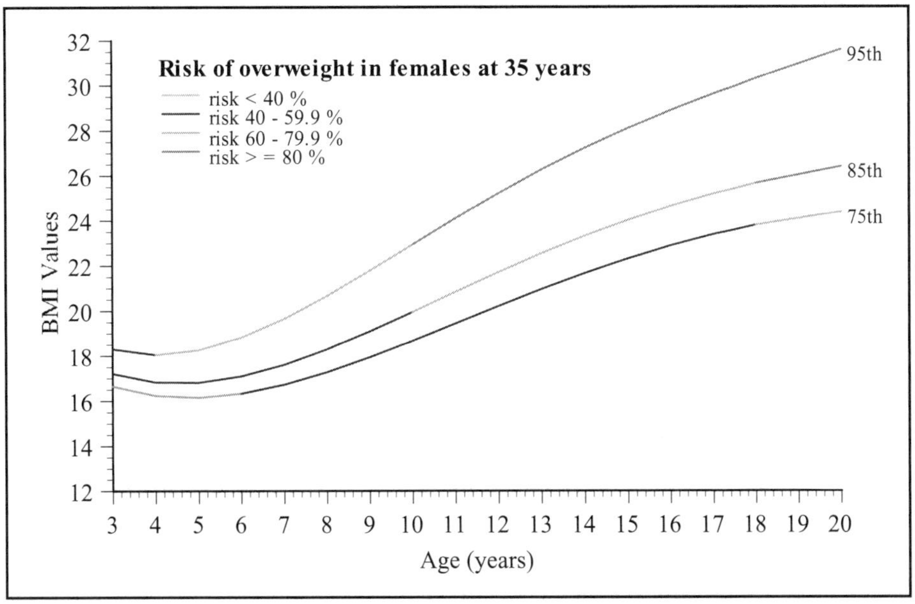

Figure 2-3. Selected percentiles for BMI in males from the CDC growth charts for BMI-for-age. Segments of the 75th, 85th, and 95th percentile lines are differentially shaded to indicate differences in the probability that BMI at 35 years will be ≥30 kg/m^2.

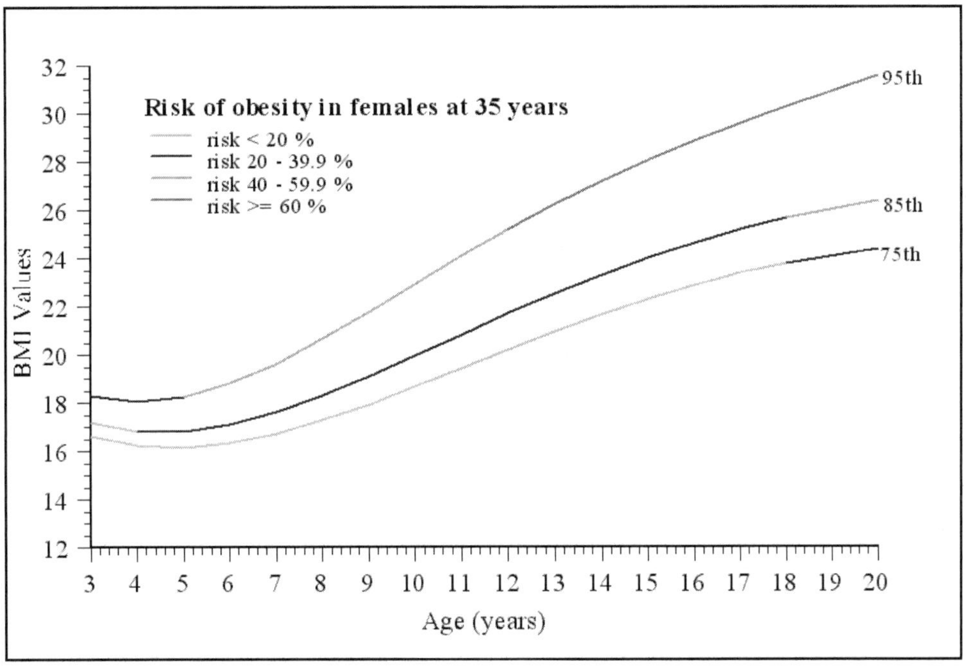

Figure 2-4. Selected percentiles for BMI in females from the CDC growth charts for BMI-for-age. Segments of the 75th, 85th, and 95th percentile lines are differentially shaded to indicate differences in the probability that BMI at 35 years will be ≥30 kg/m^2.

weight is associated with increased mortality.[24] This paradox of a high BMI associated with a high risk of mortality in middle age is characterized by a U-shaped curve, but a low weight associated with a high mortality some 20 years later in old age[25] is a result of worsening health conditions in those persons who tend to have the greatest weight in middle age.

While BMI measurements are not perfect and do not consider individualized physical characteristics, the method gives the physician an idea of the patient's overall body composition. The method allows easy calculation and is recognized by physician in all specialties.

Skinfold Measurements

Skinfolds measure subcutaneous fat thickness and are useful in all children, including most who are overweight and obese, but not in all adults. Most skinfold calipers have an upper measurement limit of 45 to 55 mm but some skinfold calipers can take larger measurements. This is not an improvement because of the difficulty of grasping a very large skinfold on an overweight or obese adult. There are several skinfold sites on the body, but reference data are generally available at only the triceps and subscapular locations. Skinfolds can effectively monitor changes in subcutaneous fatness in children where the majority of body fat is subcutaneous even in obese children.[26] However, the statistical relationships of skinfolds with percent and total body fat are not as strong as that of BMI in both children and adults.[27]

Skinfolds on the limbs are not informative in many healthy elderly because of changes in their fat distribution. Adipose tissue decrease on the arms and legs in the elderly, but subcutaneous and internal adipose tissues on the trunk increase with age. Limb circumferences are informative of changes in muscle mass in the healthy, sick, and frail elderly.[28,29] A negative correlation between calf circumference and age in the elderly is due to a general loss of muscle in response to the reduced physical activity among the elderly.

This method of measurement is not ideal, as standards must be adjusted to consider the patient's age and body build; however, the equipment is easy to access and maintain in the practitioner's office. Measurements are in standard format.

Trunk Circumference

Circumferences of the trunk provide information regarding stores of body fat and risk factors for cardiovascular disease, type 2 diabetes, and the metabolic syndrome from young adults to the elderly. Circumferences are indices of truncal adiposity. Equipment is easy to access—a simple tape measure will suffice—and measurements are in standard units.

Waist or abdominal and hip circumferences are used in the waist-to-hip ratio (WHR) as an index of central adipose tissue distribution. Men with a WHR ≥0.85 are at increased risk for cardiovascular disease, type 2 diabetes, and hormone-related cancers.[30] Central fat distribution is associated with increased intra-abdominal adipose tissue, but subcutaneous abdominal adiposity is also involved. The association between waist or abdominal circumference and internal adipose deposits has been confirmed by imaging methods,[31,32] and an abdominal circumference of ≥95 cm in males and ≥80 cm in females is a risk factor for cardiovascular disease and the metabolic syndrome.[33] Upper body, centripetal, or masculine type of adipose-tissue deposition is the major contributor to the risk of overweight or obesity. With weight reduction and corresponding decreases in the amounts of internal adipose tissue, the risk for cardiovascular disease is reduced.

Bioelectric Impedance Analysis

BIA estimates amounts of TBW, FFM, and body fatness from measures of the impedance of the body to a small alternating electric current (at 500 to 800 mA)[34] at one or more frequencies. The conductor is the body's water content, and a BIA analyzer measures the impedance of this fluid conductor. Impedance (Z) is the vector relationship between resistance (R) and reactance (Xc) measured at a current frequency, according to the equation $Z^2 = R^2 + Xc^2$. Resistance is the opposition of the conductor to the alternating current, and reactance is the dielectric component of impedance. Resistance in the body is the same as in nonbiological conductors, and reactance is from the capacitant effect of cell membranes, tissue interfaces, and non-ionic tissues.[35] According to Ohm's Law, the volume of a conductor is proportional to the length of the conductor squared divided by its resistance. BIA utilizes this relationship in the body where stature (S) squared is divided by resistance, S^2/R, as an index of body volume. At a frequency, the impedance index, S^2/R, is directly related to the volume of TBW. However, the use of the impedance index to estimate FFM and body fatness is based upon the fraction of 73% of TBW in FFM. Because the hydration fraction of FFM is not constant, S^2/R is combined with anthropometric data to predict body composition based upon direct of criterion methods.

Single-frequency BIA machines almost all operate at a current frequency of 50 kHz, and the term "single frequency" generally implies a measure of impedance at 50 kHz. BIA at 50 kHz cannot reliably distinguish the proportion of extracellular fluid, and the use of BIA at 50 kHz to estimate TBW is not recommended clinically.[36] Multifrequency BIA, also referred to as bioelectrical impedance spectroscopy (BIS), expands the use of impedance to quantify the distribution of TBW and body composition in clinical and nutritional studies. Multifrequency BIA has not improved body composition estimates over the use of single-frequency impedance; however, it provides more accurate and precise estimates of TBW. Multifrequency BIA is used primarily in research and clinical settings, especially in the area of end-stage renal disease and dialysis prescription.

The tetra-polar method is the most common way to measure single- and multifrequency BIA. Early measures of impedance were taken with the subject supine and the electrodes were connected to the right hand-wrist and right ankle-foot. Based in part on the use of segmental and multi-frequency BIA, measurements now depend on the model and manufacturer of the BIA analyzer.

BIA is used clinically where water distribution is disturbed. BIA is useful in the prescription and monitoring of dialysis based on urea kinetic modeling, and it also can serve to improve interpretation of drug pharmacokinetics. BIA is of value in cancer and human immunodeficiency virus to assess nutritional status.[37-39] Multi-frequency BIA has promise in assessing TBW volume in end-stage renal disease; this is an area of continued developing research.[40,41] Pairs and ratios of low to high frequency impedance values have been used to explore variations in levels of hydration and to differentiate disease conditions.[42-45]

BIA is not responsive to changes in FFM that reflect protein accretion parenteral and enteral nutrition. Also acute weight changes due to dieting or to protein calorie malnutrition are not reliably detected by BIA. BIA is useful in describing body composition status but cannot describe changes in body composition accurately or reliably.

There are numerous published equations to estimate body composition for single and multifrequency BIA, and there are several sets of equations resident in commercial single frequency impedance analyzers. These resident equations are not recommended unless sufficient information is provided by the manufacturer regarding the predictive accuracy and errors of the equations. Overall, BIA prediction equations are reasonably accurate body composition estimates for groups but their accuracy for individuals depends on factors specific to the construction of the equations, such as a narrow age range and the racial and ethnic makeup of the samples used. Many of the equations are for whites only, but there are a limited number for Native-American and African-American samples.[46,47] TBW and FFM BIA prediction equations using a multi-component body composition model are available for children and adults.[18] These equations provided reasonable prediction for individuals at the extremes of the distribution with only a slight tendency to over-predict at the lower end of the distribution and to under-predict at the upper end of the distributions.

BIA is useful in describing body composition for groups, but large errors for individuals continue to limit its clinical application. This is especially true when persons receiving treatment for obesity are monitored repeatedly. The predictive errors with BIA for an individual are large so that small improvements in response to treatment cannot be detected accurately and reliably.

Statistical Models of Body Composition

Statistical models use indirect measures to predict body composition for groups or individuals.[48] This requires a regression equation with indirect measures as predictor variables and some direct or criterion body composition measure as a dependent or outcome variable. The use of indirect methods as predictors depends on their biological and statistical relationships to the outcome variable. A predictor variable, or set of variables, need to have a biological and statistical relationship to the outcome variable because the strength of the relationship affects the accuracy or precision of the prediction equation.

Several regression methods are available, such as forward selection and stepwise and backward elimination regression. These are used if there is no multicolinearity among the predictor variables; however, the predictor variables are frequently interrelated, which inflates the variance of the regression coefficients and reduces the precision and accuracy of the predictions. In such cases, a maximum R^2 or an all-possible subset of regression procedure is an appropriate analytical choices.

Regression analysis assumes the bivariate relationships between dependent and predictor variables are linear; otherwise, the prediction equations will have large errors and poor performance. Another assumption is homogeneity, or the variance of the dependent variable is constant for all values of the predictor variables. It is assumed that the dependent variable is normally distributed to allow statistical inferences about the significance of the regression parameters.

A large sample results in more precise and accurate prediction equations than does a small sample, but the necessary sample size is a function of the correlation between the outcome variable and predictor variables. The sample size required to achieve accuracy on cross-validation depends on the number of predictor variables, the bivariate relationships among the dependent variable and the predictor variables, and the variance of the dependent variable in the cross-validation sample.

Available Reference Data

Body-composition references are available from national survey data collected by the National Center for Health Statistics, Centers for Disease Control and Prevention. These surveys are recognized for their multiple methods of data collection including interviews, physical examinations, physiological testing, and biochemical assessments from large, representative samples of the US population. Mean values and distribution statistics for stature, weight, selected body circumferences, breadths, and skinfold thicknesses and plots of means for TBW, FFM total, and percent body fat of children and adults (Figures 2-5 through 2-8) from the third National Health and Nutrition Examination Survey (also called the NHANES III) are available by gender and race.[48] These body-composition measurements follow techniques for corresponding measurements in the *Anthropometric Standardization Reference Manual*[49] and are similar across other national surveys. These data are selected to monitor the health and nutritional status of infants, children, adults, and the elderly rather than a desired health goal (see Figures 2-5 through 2-8).

Reference data for body measurements in infants and children are widely distributed as growth charts where the measured values for a child can be compared to percentiles plotted against age.[50] There are similar charts available for the elderly where decreases in body size occur with age. For young and middle-aged adults, there are only limited publications documenting means and standard deviations.

Conclusion

The ability to diagnosis, monitor, and treat acute and chronic health conditions is limited, in part, by the ability to assess body composition. There is no universally accepted method of measuring body fatness or quantifying overweight and obesity clearly. Current body-composition analysis is plagued with problems of non-universal assumptions, limited by application of methodology or affected by aspects of chronic disease or subject size and performance. It is important in interpreting results from any body composition analysis to recognize the limitations of the methods used. Direct body-composition methods at best have an error of 2% to 3% body fat when compared with corresponding results from other direct methods. With less direct methods, an error of 5% body fat is the best to expect, and an error of between 5% and 10% is more realistic for predicted body composition.

A person classified as overweight or obese can have associated concurrent metabolic and hormonal disruptions beyond that of a normal or overweight person. These associations together with comorbid conditions accompanying obesity can profoundly alter the relationship and assumptions underlying the validity and associations between indirect and direct methods. Furthermore, direct and indirect body-composition methods frequently have a limited application in the measurement and treatment of overweight and obese individuals. Many times, obese adults cannot be measured because their bodies are too large for the equipment available to assess body composition (eg, a patient who is too large for the opening in the magnet for MRI data collection). Of the direct methods, neutron activation is the easiest to use for the obese, but there are only a few locations in the US that have this capability. Hopefully, the technological advancements in many of the methods discussed will continue so as to clarify our perspective on the prevalence of overweight and obesity through improved measurement capabilities.

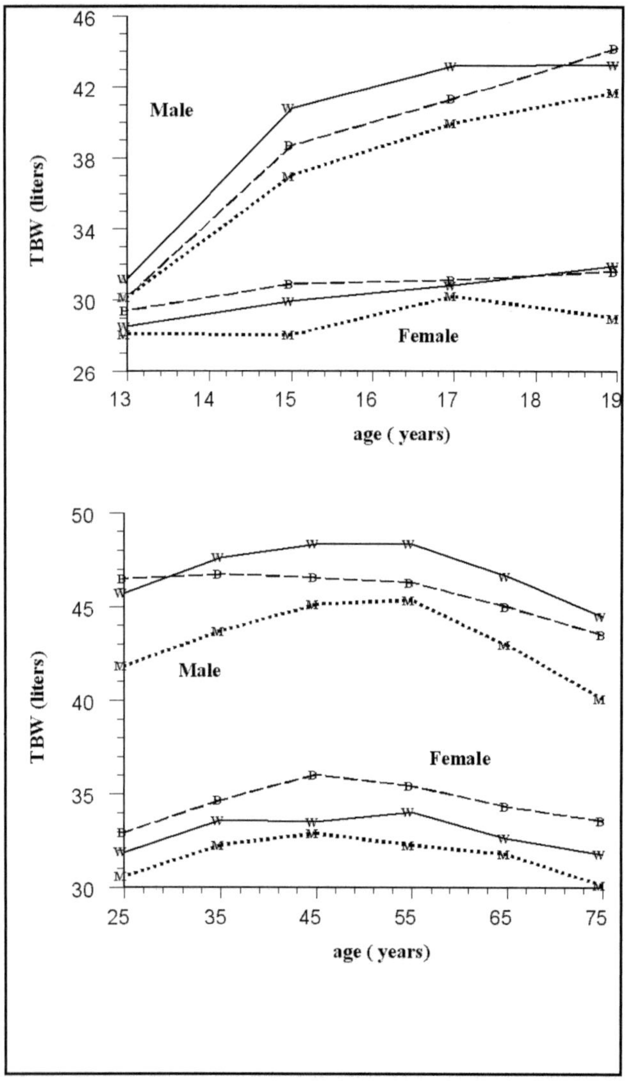

Figure 2-5. Estimated means for total TBW by 2-year age groups from 12 to 20 years and by 10-year age groups from 20 to 80 years for non-Hispanic white (W), non-Hispanic black (B), and Mexican-American (M) males and females from NHANES III.

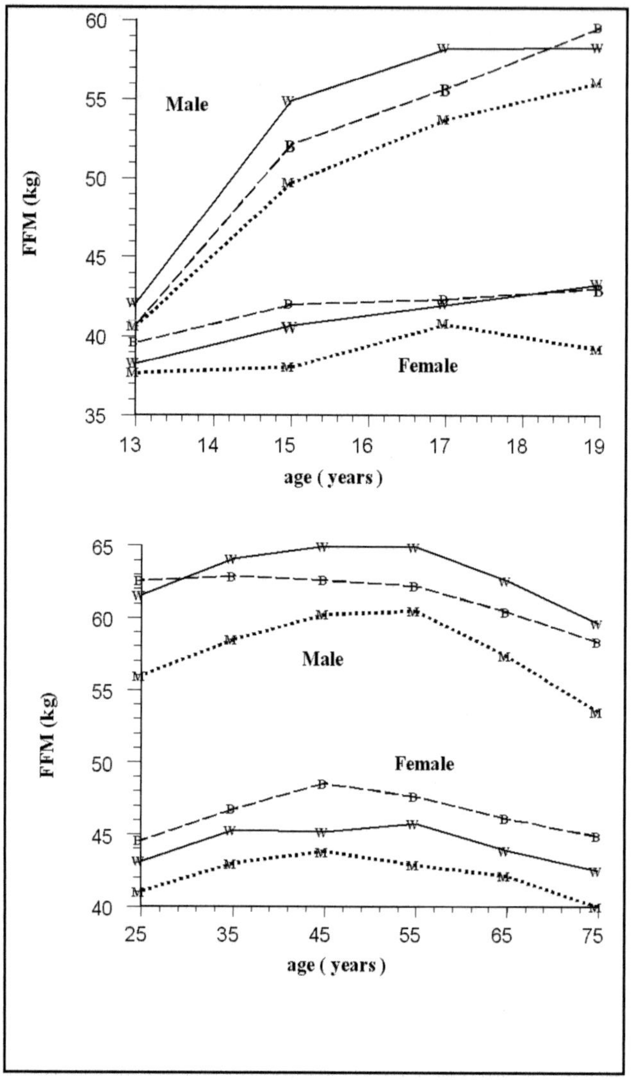

Figure 2-6. Estimated means for FFM by 2-year age groups from 12 to 20 years and by 10-year age groups from 20 to 80 years for non-Hispanic white (W), non-Hispanic black (B) and Mexican-American (M) males and females from NHANES III.

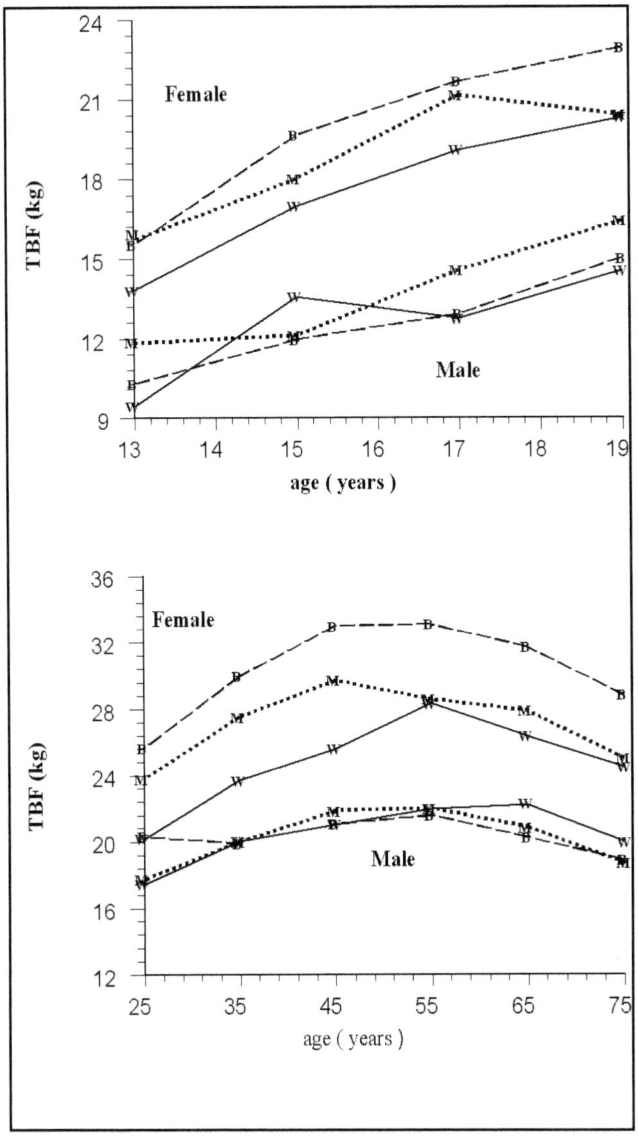

Figure 2-7. Estimated means for total body fat (TBF) by 2-year age groups from 12 to 20 years and by 10-year age groups from 20 to 80 years for non-Hispanic white (W), non-Hispanic black (B) and Mexican-American (M) males and females from NHANES III.

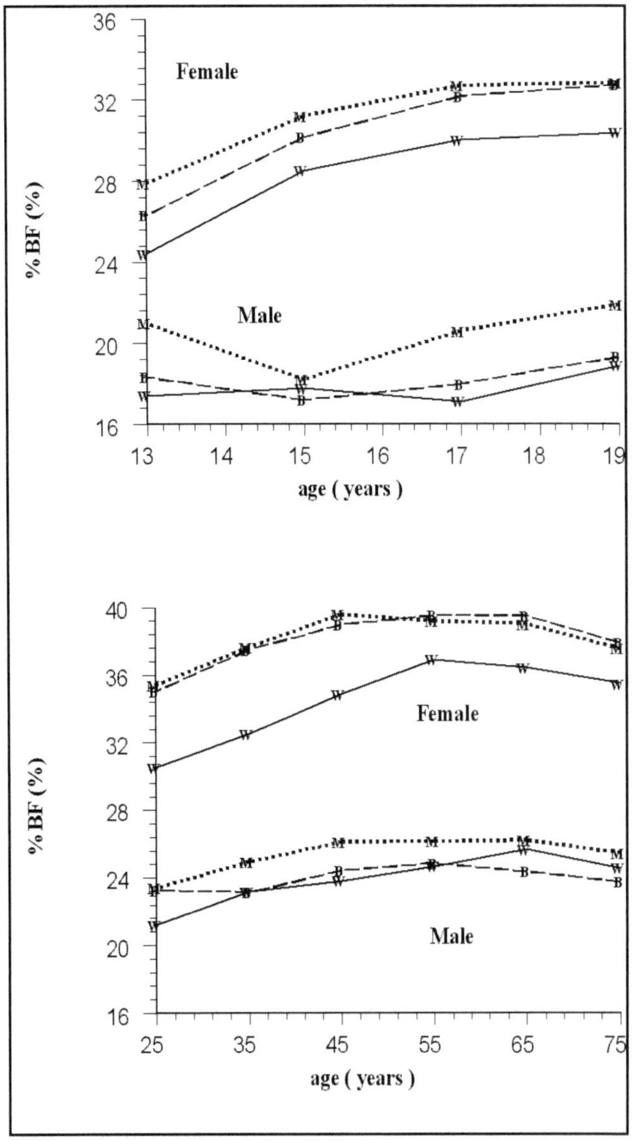

Figure 2-8. Estimated means for percent body fat (% BF) by 2-year age groups from 12 to 20 years and by 10-year age groups from 20 to 80 years for non-Hispanic white (W), non-Hispanic black (B) and Mexican-American (M) males and females from NHANES III.

Acknowledgments

This work was supported in part by grants HL-72838 and HD-12252 from the National Institute of Health, Bethesda, MD.

References

1. World Health Organization. *Physical status: the use and interpretation of anthropometry.* Geneva: Author; 1995.
2. Siri W. Body composition from fluid spaces and density analysis of methods. In: Brozek J, Henshcel A, eds. *Techniques for measuring body composition.* Vol 61. Washington, DC: National Academy Press; 1961:223-244.
3. Steen B. Body water in the elderly—a review. *J Nutr Health Aging.* 1997;1(3):142-145.
4. Cheek D. Extra-cellular volume: its structure and measurement and influence of age and disease. *J Ped.* 1961;58:103-125.
5. Vaisman N, Pencharz P, Koren G, Johnson J. Comparison of oral and intravenous administration of sodium bromide for extra-cellular water measurements. *Am J Clin Nutr.* 1987;46:1-4.
6. Chertow GM, Lazarus JM, Lew NL, Ma L, Lowrie EG. Development of a population-specific regression equation to estimate total body water in hemodialysis patients. *Kidney International.* 1997;51:1578-1582.
7. Depner TA. Quantifying hemodialysis. *Am J Nephrol.* 1996;16(1):17-28.
8. Woodrow G, Oldroyd B, Turney JH, Davies PSW, Day JME, Smith MA. Measurement of total body water and urea kinetic modelling iin peritoneal dialysis. *Clin Nephrol.* 1997;47(1):52-57.
9. Chumlea WC, Guo SS, Zeller CM, et al. Total body water reference values and prediction equations for adults. *Kidney International.* 2001;59(6):2250-2258.
10. Khaled MA, Lukaski HC, Watkins CL. Determination of total body water by deuterium NMR. *Am J Clin Nutr.* 1987;45:1-6.
11. Rebouche C, Pearson G, Serfass R, Roth C, Finley J. Evaluation of nuclear magnetic resonance spectroscopy for determination of deuterium in body fluids: application to measurement of total body water in human infants. *Am J Clin Nutr.* 1987;45:373-380.
12. Schoeller DA. Hydrometry. In: Roche AF, Heymsfield SB, Lohman TG, eds. *Human Body Composition.* Champaign, IL: Human Kinetics Books; 1996: 25-43.
13. Dempster P, Aitkens S. A new air displacement method for the determination of body composition. *Med Sci Sports Exerc.* 1995;27:1692-1697.
14. McCrory M, Gomez T, Bernauer E, Mole P. Evaluation of a new air displacement plethysmograph for measuring human body composition. *Med Sci Sports Exerc.* 1995;27:1686-1691.
15. Demerath EW, Guo SS, Chumlea WC, Towne B, Roche AF, Siervogel RM. Comparison of percent body fat estimates using air displacement plethysmography and hydrodensitometry in adults and children. *Int J Obes Relat Metab Disord.* 2002;26:389-397.
16. Brozek J, Grande F, Anderson J, Keys A. Densitometric analysis of body composition: revision of some quantitative assumptions. *Ann NY Acad Sci.* 1963;110:113-140.
17. Lohman T. Applicability of body composition techniques and constants for children and youths. *Exercise and Sports Science Review.* 1986;14:325-357.
18. Sun SS, Chumlea WC, Heymsfield SB, et al. Development of bioelectrical impedance analysis prediction equations for body composition with the use of a multicomponent model for use in epidemiological surveys. *Am J Clin Nutr.* 2003;77:331-340.
19. Roubenoff R, Kehayias J, Dawsonhughes B, Heymsfield S. Use of dual-energy x-ray absorptiometry in body-composition studies —not yet a gold standard. *Am J Clin Nutr.* 1993;58(5):589-591.
20. Kohrt WM. Body composition by DXA: tried and true? *Med Sci Sports Exerc.* 1995;27(10):1349-1353.
21. Tataranni PA, Ravussin E. Use of dual-energy X-ray absorptiometry in obese individuals. *Am J Clin Nutr.* 1995;62(4):730-734.
22. Guo SS, Chumlea WC. Statistical methods for the development and testing of predictive equations. In: Roche AF, Heymsfield SB, Lohman TG, eds. *Human Body Composition: Methods and Findings.* Champaign, IL: Human Kinetic Press; 1996:191-202.
23. Sun SS, Wu W, Chumlea WC, Roche AF. Predicting overweight and obesity in adulthood from body mass index values in childhood and adolescence. *Am J Clin Nutr.* 2002;76:653-658.
24. Andres R, Muller D, Sorkin J. Long-term effects of change in body weight on all-cause mortality—a review. *Ann Intern Med.* 1993;119(7 Part 2):737-743.
25. Losonczy KG, Harris TB, Cornoni-Huntley J, et al. Does weight loss from middle age to old age explain the inverse weight mortality relation in old age? *Am J Epid.* 1995;141:312-321.
26. Goran MI, Gower BA. Relation between visceral fat and disease risk in children and adolescents. *Am J Clin Nutr.* 1999;70(1):149S-156S.
27. Roche AF, Siervogel RM, Chumlea WC, Webb P. Grading of body fatness from limited anthropometric data. *Am J Clin Nutr.* 1981;34:2831-2838.
28. Chumlea WC, Roche AF, Webb P. Body size, subcutaneous fatness and total body fat in the elderly. *Int J Obes Relat Metab Disord.* 1984;8:311-318.
29. Chumlea WC, Baumgartner RN, Garry PJ, Rhyne RL, Nicholson C, Wayne S. Fat distribution and blood lipids in a sample of healthy elderly people. *Int J Obes Relat Metab Disord.* 1992;16:125-133.
30. Despres J, Prudhomme D, Pouliot M, Tremblay A, Bouchard C. Estimation of deep abdominal adipose-tissue accumulation from simple anthropometric measurements in men. *Am J Clin Nutr.* 1991;54(3):471-477.
31. Seidell JC, Oosterlee A, Thijssen MAO, et al. Assessment of intra-abdominal and subcutaneous abdominal fat: Relation between anthropometry and computed tomography. *Am J Clin Nutr.* 1987;45:7-13.
32. Baumgartner RN, Rhyne RL, Garry PJ, Chumlea WC. Body composition in the elderly from MRI: Associations with cardiovascular disease risk factors. In: Ellis KJ, Eastman JD, eds. *Human Body Composition: In Vivo Methods, Models and Assessment.* New York: Plenum Press; 1993:35-38.
33. National Institutes of Health. Third report of the national cholesterol education program expertpanel on detection, evaluation, and treatment of high blood cholesterol in adults (Adult Treatment panel III). NIH Publication. 2001;01:3670.
34. Lukaski HC, Johnson PE, Bolonchuk WW, Lykken GI. Assessment of fat-free mass using bioelectrical impedance measurements of the human body. *Am J Clin Nutr.* 1985;41:810-7.
35. Chumlea WC, Guo SS. Bioelectrical impedance and body composition: Present status and future directions. *Nutrition Reviews.* 1994;52:123-131.
36. National Institutes of Health. Bioelectrical impedance analysis in body composition measurement: NIH Technol Assess Statement; December 12-14, 1994.
37. Schwenk A, Breuer P, Kremer G, Ward L. Clinical assessment of HIV-associated lipodystrophy syndrome: bioelectrical impedance analysis, anthropometry and clinical scores. *Clin Nutr.* 2001;20(3):243-249.
38. Bauer J, Capra S, Davies PS, Ash S, Davidson W. Estimation of total body water from bioelectrical impedance analysis in patients with pancreatic cancer. *J Human Nutr.* 2002;15(3):185-188.

39. Horlick M, Arpadi SM, Bethel J, et al. Bioelectrical impedance analysis models for prediction of total body water and fat-free mass in healthy and HIV-infected children and adolescents. *Am J Clin Nutr.* 2002;76(5):991-999.
40. Lee SW, Song JH, Kim GA, Lee KJ, Kim MJ. Assessment of total body water from anthropometry-based equations using bioelectrical impedance as reference in Korean adult control and haemodialysis subjects. *Nephrol Dial Transplant.* 2001;16(1):91-97.
41. Konings CJ, Kooman JP, Schonck M, et al. Influence of fluid status on techniques used to assess body composition in peritoneal dialysis patients. *Peritoneal Dialysis International.* 2003;23(2):184-190.
42. Jenin P, Lenoir J, Roullet C, Thomasset A, Ducrot H. Determination of body fluid compartments by electrical impedance measurements. *Aviation Space Environ Med.* 1975;46:152-155.
43. Ducrot H, Thomasset A, Joly R, Jungers P, Eyraud C, Lenoir J. Determination of extracellular fluid volume in man. *La Presse Medicale.* 1970;78:2269-2272.
44. Fredrix E, Saris W, Soeters P, et al. Estimation of body composition by bioelectrical impedance in cancer patients. *Eur J Clin Nutr.* 1990;44:749-752.
45. Schols A, Wouters E, Soeters P, Westerterp K. Body composition by bioelectrical-impedance analysis compared with deuterium dilution and skinfold anthropometry in patients with chronic obstructive pulmonary disease. *Am J Clin Nutr.* 1991;53:421-424.
46. Lohman TG, Caballero B, Himes JH, et al. Estimation of body fat from anthropometry and bioelectrical impedance in Native American children. *Int J Obes Relat Metab Disord.* 2000;24(8):82-88.
47. Wagner DR, Heyward VH, Kocina PS, Stolarczyk L, Wilson WL. Predictive accuracy of BIA equations for estimating fat-free mass of black men. *Med Sci Sports Exerc.* 1997;29(7):69-74.
48. Chumlea WC, Guo SS, Kuczmarski RJ, et al. Body composition estimates from NHANES III bioelectrical impedance data. *Int J Obes Relat Metab Disord.* 2002:1596-1609.
49. Lohman T, Martorell R, Roche AF. *Anthropometric Standardization Reference Manual.* Champaign, IL: Human Kinetics; 1988.
50. Kuczmarski RJ, Ogden CL, Grummer-Strawn LM, et al. CDC Growth Charts: United States. *Advance Data.* 2000;314:1-28.

Chapter 3

Micronutrient Deficiencies

Clifford Lo, MD, MPH, ScD

Introduction

Vitamins are a diverse group of chemical substances that may function as coenzymes or prohormones. They are essential for human life in small quantities (as opposed to macronutrients, which are primarily used for energy) and cannot be synthesized by humans, so they must be provided in the diet. The term "vitamin" was coined by Casimir Funk from "vita-," or "life," and "amine," because they were initially mistakenly assumed to be amines. Later, McCollum separated extracts of the growth factors into fat soluble A and water soluble B, which were then further separated into many individual factors. Research on vitamins in early part of the 20th century by Sir Frederick Gowland Hopkins and others led to many subsequent Nobel Prizes (Table 3-1).[1]

Many of the classic epidemic vitamin-deficiency diseases—such as rickets (vitamin D), scurvy (vitamin C), beriberi (thiamin), and pellagra (niacin)—have been almost completely eliminated in developed countries, but subclinical deficiencies may exist in susceptible patients with chronic diseases such as intestinal malabsorption or alcoholism. However, many mineral deficiencies, such as iron deficiency, remain quite common in individuals in the United States as well as those throughout the rest of the world (Table 3-2).

Vitamin and mineral deficiencies can occur because of reduced dietary intake, intestinal malabsorption, increased physiological requirements, inadequate utilization, or increased excretion. Patients with dietary malnutrition, intestinal malabsorption syndromes, liver disease, renal disease, burns, and surgery, or those on prolonged parenteral nutrition (PN) are therefore most at risk. The fat-soluble vitamins (A, D, E, and K) are more likely to be problematic in terms of absorption, but body stores in the liver mean that deficiency takes longer to develop. Actually, the relatively low percentage absorption of minerals, especially iron and calcium, makes deficiency of these elements much more common than that of most vitamins.

Great interest and controversy continues into whether vitamin and mineral supplementation can prevent cancer, heart disease, upper respiratory infections, and other common diseases. Recent supplementation of folate into the grain supply in the United States followed demonstration that it was epidemiologically linked to reduction of risk of neural tube defects. Folate supplementation higher than could reasonably expected in usual diets was necessary in the first few weeks of pregnancy, before most women knew they were pregnant. Folate supplementation to the whole population had additional benefits in that it reduced homocysteine levels, which are related to increased risk of cardiovascular disease. Supplementation of antioxidants—such as carotene, vitamin E, selenium, and vitamin C—are somewhat more controversial, especially because a number of large controlled trials[2,3] show that beta-carotene supplementation might actually increase risk of developing lung cancer in some populations.

Most water-soluble vitamins have little toxicity as excess doses are readily excreted in the urine, but vitamin A, a fat-soluble vitamin, can produce toxicity at levels not far above the recommended intake if taken over a long period. Likewise, vitamin D toxicity, producing hypercalcemia, can occur if large supplements are taken. Many minerals, especially the heavy metals, can cause toxicity if deposited in the bones or central nervous system.

At least 20 minerals out of more than 115 elements have an essential role in human physiology. Many minerals are essential for human life, as part of enzymes

TABLE 3-1.

Nobel Prizes for Vitamins and Minerals

Year	Recipients	Discovery or Development
1929	Christiaan Eijkman	Antineuritic vitamin (thiamin)
1929	Sir Frederick Gowland Hopkins	Discovery of growth-stimulating vitamins
1931	Otto Warburg	Cellular respiratory enzymes (niacin)
1934	George Minot, William Murphy, and George Whipple	Liver treatment for anemia (vitamin B12)
1937	Albert Szent-Gyorgyi	Biological combustion (vitamin C)
1937	Sir Norman Haworth	Vitamin C and carbohydrates
1937	Paul Karrer	Carotenoids, flavins, and vitamins
1938	Richard Kuhn	Carotenoids and vitamins
1943	Henrik Dam and Edward Doisy	Discovery of vitamin K
1953	Sir Hans Krebs and Fritz Lipmann	Coenzyme A TCA cycle
1967	George Wald	Vision and vitamin A
1997	Paul Boyer and John Walker	ATP, phosphate

TABLE 3-2.

Micronutrient Deficiency States and Their Detection

Micronutrients (Chemical Name)	Role	Deficiency State	Measurement
Biotin*	Coenzyme in carboxylation; pyruvate	Dermatitis; alopecia; depression; muscle pain; paresthesias	24-h urine biotin
Calcium	Bone; cell communication	Osteoporosis; seizures	Serum ionized calcium
Carnitine	Transport of long chain triglycerides across the inner mitochondrial membrane	Cardiomyopathy; myopathy	Serum carnitine
Choline		Visual, verbal memory abnormalities; hemorrhagic nephritis§; growth retardation§	Plasma free choline
Chromium‡	Co-factor for insulin	Impaired glucose tolerance||; elevated serum lipids||; peripheral neuropathy	Serum chromium
Cobalt‡	Cobalamin	Pernicious anemia	B12, methylmalonic acid
Copper‡	Metalloenzymes	Microcytic anemia; leucopenia; neutropenia; osteoporosis; neuropathy; testicular failure; hair/skin depigmentation; poor connective tissue	Serum Cu, ceruloplasmin
Fluoride‡		Caries; osteoporosis||	
Folic acid*	Coenzyme in amino acid metabolism and DNA synthesis	Megoblastic anemia; stomatitis; diarrhea	RBC folate; homocystein
Iodine‡	Thyroxine	Thyroid disease (goiter, hypothyroidism, cretinism)	
Iron‡	Hemoglobin	Microcytic anemia	
Magnesium	Enzyme cofactor	Arrhythmias, muscle cramping	
Manganese‡	Metalloenzymes	Growth retardation§; bone deformities§; b-cell degeneration§; transient dermatitis§	
Molybdenum‡	Metalloenzymes	Growth retardation§; impaired methionine metabolism§; impaired uric acid metabolism§	
Niacin*	Constituent of the coenzymes NAD and NADP involved in hydrogen transport, glycolysis; NADH	Pellagra (dementia, diarrhea, dermatitis); scarlet	RBC or urine NAD:NADP ratio

continued

TABLE 3-2. CONTINUED

Micronutrients (Chemical Name)	Role	Deficiency State	Measurement
Nickel‡		Growth retardation§; impaired lipid metabolism§	
Pantothenic acid or panthothenate*	Acetyle CoA; precursor of coenzyme A involved in synthesis of fatty acids, steroids hormones	"Burning feet" syndrome; fatigue; leg cramps; paresthesias	
Phosphorus	ATP	Respiratory muscle dysfunction, hemolysis	Serum phosphate
Selenium‡	Selenoproteins	Cardiomyopathy; neuropathy; pseudo-albinism; macrocytosis; myositis; cancer||; infection||	Serum or whole blood Se
Silicon‡		Growth retardation§; skeletal deformities§; defective connective tissue formation§	
Taurine		Retinal abnormalities; liver disease||	
Vanadium‡		Growth depression§; impaired lipid metabolism§	
Vitamin A (retinol)†	Retinal pigment formation	Xerophthalmia; keratomalacia; night blindness; delayed wound healing; sterility (males)	Serum vitamin A
Vitamin B1 (thiamine)*	Coenzyme in oxidative decarboxylation reactions; pyruvate dehydrogenase	Beriberi (weth cardiomyopathy); peripheral neuropathy; encephalopathy	Erythrocyte transketolase
Vitamin B2 (riboflavin)*	Coenzyme of flavoproteins (FMN, FAD, FADH) involved in electron transport, tissue oxidation	Angular stomatitis; glosssitis; cheilosis; photophobia; seborrheic dermatitis (nasolabial fold and scrotum)	FAD-dep RBS; glutathione reductase activity; 24-h urine riboflavin; RBC riboflavin
Vitamin B6 (pyridoxine)*	Coenzyme involved in amino acid metabolism and DNA synthesis; transamination	Anemia; peripheral neuropathy; convulsions; glossitis; cheilosis; seborrheic dermatitis (eyes, nose, mouth areas)	Plasma pyridoxyl phosphate
Vitamin B12 (cobalamine)*	Coenzyme in amino acid metabolism and DNA synthesis	Pernicious anemia; neuropathy; paresthesias; glossitis	Serum B12; methylmalonic acid
Vitamin C (ascorbate)*	Antioxidant; collagen synthesis	Delayed wound healing; petechia; scurvy	Vitamin C plasma, WBC
Vitamin D (calciferol)†	Calcium, phosphate homeostasis	Osteomalacia (rickets)	Serum 25-OH vitamin D3
Vitamin E (tocopherol)†	Antioxidant	Hemolytic anemia; neuropathy (paresis of gaze, gait disturbance, decreased proprioception)	Serum vitamin E :total lipid ratio
Vitamin K (phylloquinone)†	Synthesis of prothrombin factors II, VII, IX, and X	Hemorrhage	Prothrombin time
Zinc‡	Metalloenzymes; growth	Anorexia; growth retardation; acrodermatitis enteropathica; hypoguesia; alopecia; diarrhea; impaired wound healing; immune suppression; night blindness; hypogonadism	

* water soluble vitamins
† fat soluble vitamins
‡ trace materials
§ findings for deficiency in animals
|| suggested findings yet still questionable

(metalloenzymes) and for structure (calcium, phosphorus) or cellular processes. Absorption of many of the minerals requires complex transport channels or transport proteins that are the subject of recent research, and some mineral deficiencies (such as that of iron, iodine, and calcium) are much more common than are vitamin deficiencies.

Every 10 years, the National Research Council and Institute of Medicine convene several committees of nutrition scientists to review the scientific literature and recommend levels of daily dietary nutrients that would keep 95% to 98% of the population from developing deficiencies. Typically, studies involve small numbers of animal or human subjects being observed for periods of 10 days to several months with a detailed and exhaustive record of dietary intake and excretion. These allowed inferences of how much of each nutrient was absorbed and how much was retained in the body. Instead of specifying only Recommended Dietary Allowances, the latest 10th edition has been set in terms of Dietary Reference Intakes (DRIs), delineating Adequate Intakes (AI), Estimated Average Intakes (EAR) for groups, and tolerable Upper Limits (UL) for each nutrient.[4-7]

Vitamin A (Retinol and Carotene)

Although probably uncommon in the United States, vitamin A deficiency is a leading cause of morbidity and mortality worldwide. Not only is it a leading cause of blindness, but vitamin A deficiency is associated with immunodeficiencies that increase susceptibility to measles and other infections to deadly levels, especially in young children in Africa and Southeast Asia. It is estimated that 42 million children under the age of 6 years have mild or moderate eye disease from vitamin A deficiency, of which 250,000 to 500,000 go blind, and 1.3 to 2.5 million childhood deaths a year might be prevented from eliminating vitamin A deficiency.[8] Supplementation trials in Africa with periodic injections of 50,000 IU vitamin A have reduced morbidity and mortality, especially to measles in young children.[9] Patients with fat malabsorption syndromes such as cystic fibrosis or liver disease may also develop biochemical vitamin A deficiency and occasionally night blindness.

Retinol, retinal (retinaldehyde), retinoic acid, and some carotenoids all have vitamin A activity. Retinyl esters are stored in the liver and transported by retinol binding protein in association with prealbumin and thyroxine. Retinal forms part of the pigment rhodopsin mainly in the rods of the visual photoepithelium in the retina. Isomerization from 11-cis-retinal to all trans retinal and dissociation from opsin in the visual cycle allows visual signals to be sent through the optic nerve to the visual cortex of the brain.

Dietary vitamin A deficiency is usually due to monotonous cereal diets low in animal fat and yellow-green vegetables, plus depletion during repeated infections. Although a fat-soluble vitamin primarily found in animal products (meat, dairy, and fish), vitamin A activity can also be provided by adequate intake of carotene in yellow and green vegetables. Carotene is essentially two retinol molecules joined together, which can dissociate to vitamin A but does not cause vitamin A toxicity during times of excess. However, large amounts of dietary carotene can cause a distinctive yellow skin pigmentation known as carotenemia.

Vitamin A deficiency leads first to night blindness (nyctalopia) as the rods in the periphery of the retina lose their sensitivity to light stimuli. However, vitamin A is also important for epithelial differentiation, and dryness (xerosis) of the conjunctiva and corneal epithelium (xerophthalmia) can cause Bitot's spots, keratomalacia, and ulceration, which can lead to permanent damage and blindness.

Serum retinol is the usual means of assessing vitamin A status. Occasionally, liver disease may result in decreased synthesis of retinol binding protein, resulting in clinical vitamin A deficiency despite adequate vitamin A liver stores, so serum retinol binding protein might be obtained. Night vision or dark adaptation testing may be more sensitive but may be difficult to arrange. Ophthalmologic slit lamp examination may detect Bitot's spots or corneal xerosis before scarring or keratomalacia occurs.

DRIs for vitamin A have been set at 700 mcg/day for adult females, 900 mcg/day for adult males, 300-600 mcg/day for children, 770 mcg/day during pregnancy, and 1300 mcg/day during lactation, with 1 mcg retinol equal to 1 retinol activity equivalents (RAE), 3.3 IU vitamin A activity, and 12 mcg carotene. Vitamin A toxicity may occur at levels not much above recommended intakes or more than 20,000 IU daily for extended periods and may be manifested by muscle and joint pains, headache, pseudotumor cerebri, eczema, alopecia, stomatitis, liver dysfunction, and bone problems. Excessive vitamin A supplementation should be avoided, especially in pregnancy because of concerns of teratogenicity.

Vitamin D

Vitamin D can be converted in the skin from 7-dehydrocholesterol by ultraviolet sunlight; thus, technically, it is not completely essential in the diet. However, vitamin D stores can be depleted, especially in the winter and spring when ultraviolet sunlight frequencies are largely filtered out by earth's atmosphere.[10,11] Numerous cases of rickets were reported in Asians in Britain recently, and contributing factors included dark skin pigmentation, northern climates, lack of vitamin D supplementation, and/or binding of vitamin D by dietary factors such as chapattis. Similarly, elderly patients and children, especially in Boston[12-15] and other northern climates, are at risk for developing vitamin D deficiency, with 24% to 57% of these subjects having low serum vitamin D and high serum parathyroid hormone levels in the winter and spring. Because vitamin D is a major regulator of blood ionized calcium levels, vitamin D deficiency can result in hypocalcemia, tetany, and seizures. EKG changes (prolonged QT intervals), Chvostek's (facial contractions) and Trousseau's signs, and carpopedal spasms may be elicited.

Chronic vitamin D deficiency can cause rickets in growing children as epiphyses widen, causing a characteristic bowed-leg appearance. A rachitic "rosary" may be noted of bony protuberances at the costochondral junctions of the rib cage. Osteomalacia occurs in adults whose epiphyseal growth plates have already fused.

Vitamin D is actually a prohormone that must be converted in the liver to 25 hydroxyvitamin D [25(OH)D] and then in the kidney to the active form 1,25-dihydroxyvitamin D [1,25 diOH D], which helps regulate serum calcium levels by increasing intestinal calcium absorption and bone calcium resorption. Therefore, patients with kidney disease or liver disease may also be susceptible to vitamin D deficiency, because of malabsorption of fat and vitamin D, possible effects on storage of vitamin D, or conversion of vitamin D to 25(OH)D or 1,25 diOH 2D. Vitamin D also has a role in epithelial differentiation and immune function, and there are vitamin D receptors throughout the body, so vitamin D deficiency may be found to affect many other diseases such as cancer, skin diseases, and infections.

Measurement of serum 25(OH)D is the best assessment of vitamin D stores, and normal values should probably be at least above 15 to 20 ng/dL. Parathyroid hormone levels will usually be high to compensate in vitamin D deficiency and will also affect 24-hour urinary phosphate excretion.

Although vitamin D can be produced in the skin, recommended dietary intakes to prevent rickets or osteomalacia are 5 to 15 mcg/day, equivalent to 200 to 600 IU, since 1 mcg/day cholecalciferol equals 40 IU of vitamin D. Milk has about 300 mg of calcium and in the United States is fortified with about 100 IU of vitamin D per 8 ounces (240 ml). Fortification of vitamin D in milk probably reduces the incidence of rickets in the United States to below that in Europe or other areas where there is no fortification, but as vitamin D is fat-soluble, the distribution and concentration is quite uneven. Breast milk does not have large quantities of vitamin D, and the American Academy of Pediatrics has recently reemphasized its recommendation to supplement breast-fed infants with vitamin D.[16]

Vitamin E (Tocopherol)

Vitamin E has been the subject of the much study because of its role in antioxidant function. Everyday exposure to cosmic radiation from the sun, aging, infection, and inflammation causes frequent nuclear and mitochondrial DNA damage that require constant repair mechanisms. Vitamin E can serve as a scavenger of free radicals and singlet oxygen to prevent lipid peroxidation and cell damage.

Vitamin E activity is actually shown by a family of compounds, tocopherols, and trienols, each in α, β, γ, and δ forms. Because bioactivity of the various compounds varies slightly, tocopherol equivalents are also expressed as international units (IU). For example, 1 mg of d-alpha-tocopherol (the most common natural form) is 1 tocopherol equivalent or 1.49 IU. The DRI is 15 mg/day of vitamin E for adults and 4 to 11 mg/day for children. Vitamin E requirements are affected by the level of polyunsaturated fat intake, as these may form lipid peroxides.

There are many vitamin E deficiency diseases known in animals, including necrotizing myopathy, neuromuscular degeneration, hemolytic anemia, hepatic necrosis, cardiomyopathy, and infertility. However, specific vitamin E deficiency syndromes were not known to occur in humans until the 1960s, when hemolytic anemia in preterm newborns was described by Oski and Barness. Possible vitamin E deficiency in patients might be suspected in patients with fat malabsorption syndromes, such as cystic fibrosis and liver disease, and may involve neurologic problems, cerebellar ataxia, skeletal myopathy, and pigmented retinopathy.

Serum tocopherol levels are usually used for assessment of vitamin E status and may be performed by high-performance liquid chromatography. Often, they are expressed as a ratio of serum vitamin E to total serum lipids in cases of hyperlipidemia. A functional test of vitamin E antioxidant activity is the red blood cell osmotic fragility test. Supplements of vitamin E may reduce risk of developing heart disease, cancer, Alzheimer's disease, and many other diseases; epidemiologic studies and controlled trials have found mixed results.[2,3,18-21]

Vitamin K (Phylloquinone)

Dietary deficiency of vitamin K is rare, but vitamin K deficiency is often iatrogenic because of the widespread use of anticoagulants warfarin or Coumadin as well as other antagonists such as antibiotics.[22-26] Vitamin K was found to work by post-translational gamma-carboxylation of glutamic acid residues in certain proteins such as prothrombin; osteocalcin; clotting factors VII, IX, and X; and proteins C and S. Warfarin and Coumadin block the recycling of vitamin K epoxide, which is formed during the gamma-carboxylation of glutamate.[22,23]

Phylloquinones from plants, menadiones, and menaquinones from intestinal bacteria all have vitamin K activity. Only a very small amount of vitamin K (1 mcg per kg body weight per day) is usually enough to prevent deficiency, and it takes months to deplete vitamin K stores even if there is no dietary intake. The DRI is 120 mcg/day for adult males, 90 mcg/day for adult females, and 2 to 75 mcg/day for children.

Many think that intestinal bacteria produce enough vitamin K to prevent depletion, although there is some question of whether this is absorbed from the large intestine.[24] Patients with liver disease may be susceptible to vitamin K deficiency, from fat malabsorption, lack of protein synthesis, or antagonism, but this is usually remedied by a large dose (1 mg) of vitamin K intramuscularly. Hemorrhagic disease of the newborn, which once caused devastating bleeding problems in some neonates, has been all but eliminated by routine intramuscular vitamin K injections given to all newborns shortly after birth.

Vitamin C (Ascorbate)

Scurvy—meaning "ulcerated, swollen mouth"—is one of the oldest diseases documented; it has caused epidemics throughout history, especially among soldiers and sailors.[27] Lind's classic "Treatise on the Scurvy"[28] described one of the first clinical trials of various remedies in 12 sailors with advanced scurvy; only the two sailors given citrus fruits showed recovery. Albert Szent-Gyorgyi and W. N. Haworth were awarded the 1937 Nobel Prize for the isolation and structural analysis of ascorbic acid. More recently, Linus Pauling created considerable controversy by claiming that megadoses of vitamin C are useful in treating various diseases from cancer to the common cold,[29-32] claims that have not been borne out in subsequent clinical trials.[33,34]

Overt clinical scurvy—with hemorrhage, petechiae, ecchymosis, bleeding gums, follicular hyperkeratosis, hemolytic anemia, and mental illness—is rare in the United States. Nevertheless, symptoms of mild vitamin deficiency, including fatigue and depression, are so common and nonspecific that a dietary history for fruit, vegetable, and vitamin supplement intake is warranted, especially in the elderly.

Vitamin C has a number of biological functions, including as an antioxidant, in prostaglandin metabolism, and in hydroxylation of proline and lysine in collagen synthesis. Ascorbate itself can be synthesized from glucose in most animals except humans, who lack an enzyme gulonolactone oxidase, which appears to be partially present but defectively coded in the human genome. The DRI for vitamin C was set at 90 mg/day for adult males, 75 mg/day for adult females, and 15 to 75 mg/day for children, a level sufficient to prevent scurvy but much lower than megadoses found in some supplements. Vitamin C supplements are relatively nontoxic, although megadoses of 5 g or more daily have raised some question of increased risk of kidney stones.

Vitamin B1 (Thiamin)

Christiaan Eijkman in Indonesia in 1906 first noted that chickens developed polyneuritis on a diet of polished white rice and recovered soon after being fed unpolished brown rice.[35] Similar results were then observed in humans, and thiamin was later found to be the antineuritic factor.[1] The classic syndrome associated with thiamin deficiency is beriberi, which may be manifested as cardiomyopathy or polyneuritis and muscle weakness. Beriberi was seen especially in Southeast Asia, manifested as polyneuropathy and muscle weakness (dry beriberi) or cardiomyopathy (wet beriberi). However, full-blown cases of beriberi are now relatively rare in developed countries. The most common cause of thiamin deficiency in developed countries is alcohol abuse. This may result from poor dietary intake, malabsorption, or liver disease. It may lead to Wernicke's encephalopathy and/or Korsakoff psychosis, which is characterized by altered mentation, eye muscle paralysis, weakness, and ataxia.[36-39] Alcoholics suffering from acute withdrawal syndromes, altered consciousness, or Wernicke's encephalopathy often are given intramuscular or intravenous injections of thiamin (25 mg) immediately and twice a day to prevent permanent neurologic deficits.[40,41] A recent nationwide PN vitamin additive shortage may have led to several deaths from lactic acidosis or a beriberi-like syndrome in patients dependent upon PN.[42,43]

Thiamin pyrophosphate is a cofactor in the pyruvate dehydrogenase reaction, which converts pyruvate to acetyl CoA, along with calcium, phosphorus (ATP), niacin (NAD), riboflavin (FAD), lipoic acid, and pantothenic acid. This is a key intermediate step between glycolysis and the Krebs tricarboxylic acid cycle in the mitochondria. Thiamin is also a cofactor in conversion of alpha ketoglutarate to succinyl CoA in the Krebs cycle, and between conversion of ketoacids to corresponding acyl CoAs in branched-chain amino acid metabolism.

Thiamin requirements are related to energy consumption: 0.5 mg/1000 kcal. Recommended daily intakes are 0.2-1.0 mg for children, 1.2 mg for adult men, 1.1 mg for adult women, and 1.4 mg during pregnancy and lactation. The best dietary sources are whole cereal grains from the layer between the germ and endosperm.

Laboratory diagnosis of thiamin deficiency can readily be obtained by an erythrocyte thiamin transketolase activity, blood thiamin concentrations, or urinary thiamin excretion after a 5-mg thiamin load.[44]

Large oral doses of up to 100-150 mg/day of thiamin are often given to patients with rare inherited metabolic defects such as maple syrup urine disease, lactic acidosis, Leigh's subacute necrotizing encephalomyelopathy, and thiamin-sensitive megaloblastic anemia. Like most other water-soluble vitamins, thiamin, even in large doses, is not toxic to humans, although it may cause gastric upset or allergic reactions in some individuals. Most of the approximately 30 mg of thiamin in the body is contained in the liver, heart, kidney, and red cells. Any excess is rapidly excreted in the urine, with a half-life of 9.5 to 18.5 days.

Vitamin B2 (Riboflavin)

The original water-soluble vitamin B complex was separated into heat-labile vitamin B1 and heat-stable vitamin B2 components. Extracts of a coenzyme with yellow fluorescence were identified as flavins, which are necessary for oxidation of glucose-6-phosphate during glycolysis. Riboflavin is the precursor of flavin adenine dinucleotide (FAD) or flavin mononucleotide (FMN), which carry high energy compounds from glycolysis and the Krebs cycle to the electron transport chain in the mitochondria.

Riboflavin deficiency may cause growth failure and skin changes in many animals, but isolated overt riboflavin toxicity is rarely seen in humans. Patients with hypothyroidism, diabetes mellitus, congenital heart disease, biliary atresia, and chronic alcoholism and those undergoing dialysis for kidney failure may be more at risk. Nonspecific cheilosis or angular stomatitis, dermatitis, weakness, fatigue, and mouth pain have been reported in association with riboflavin deficiency, but no specific deficiency syndrome has been identified.

The recommended daily intakes for riboflavin are 0.3-1.0 mg for children, 1.3 mg for adult men, 1.1 mg for adult women, 1.9 mg during pregnancy, and 2.0 mg during lactation.[4] Riboflavin is found in many foods, including meats, fish, eggs, milk, green vegetables, yeast, and enriched foods. Plasma riboflavin concentrations tend to reflect recent dietary intake. Therefore, urinary riboflavin excretion and erythrocyte glutathione reductase activity are better functional indicators of riboflavin deficiency.

Some mitochondrial beta-oxidation defects may respond to large doses of riboflavin. In addition, patients with human immunodeficiency virus infection treated with antiviral medications may develop a lactic acidosis which is reversible by riboflavin therapy.[45] Absorption of riboflavin is limited to about 25 mg per ingestion and storage is limited. Therefore, toxicity is unlikely to occur, even when taking megadoses.

Niacin

The classic syndrome of niacin deficiency, pellagra, is characterized by the "3 Ds"—diarrhea, dermatitis, and dementia. First described in Spain and Italy in the 18th century, pellagra literally means "raw skin." Goldberger's classic epidemiologic studies in the 1920s related pellagra to a deficiency of a dietary factor in maize and allowed mental hospitals in the southern United States to be emptied of many demented patients.

Niacin deficiency is now rare in developed countries, and is found mostly in some alcoholics and patients with Hartnup disease (a defect in tryptophan absorption) or prolonged isoniazid treatment.

In 1937, nicotinic acid was shown to be the dietary factor that could cure pellagra. Other bioactive forms include niacin and nicotinamide. Niacin is a precursor for nicotinamide adenine dinucleotide (NAD) and NAD phosphate (NADP), which form high-energy compounds that serve as hydrogen donors for the electron transport chain and are necessary for glycolysis, tissue respiration, and lipid metabolism.

Recommended daily intakes are 2 to 12 mg for children, 16 mg for adult men, 14 mg for adult women, 18 mg during pregnancy, and 17 mg during lactation.[4]

Tryptophan, an amino acid, can be converted into nicotinic acid in the liver and can meet most or all of the dietary niacin requirement. One niacin equivalent is equal to 1 mg of niacin or 60 mg of tryptophan. Niacin is widely distributed in plant and animal foods. Good sources include yeast, meats (especially liver), cereals, legumes, and seeds. It is theoretically possible to maintain adequate niacin status on a high protein diet of 100 g/day because tryptophan can be converted to a niacin derivative in the liver.

Direct assay of plasma niacin concentration is normally quite low and generally has not been a useful marker of nutritional status. Niacin deficiency may be better detected by measuring 24-hour urinary excretion of metabolites N-methylnicotinamide (NMN) and 2-pyridone. Less than 5.8 mmol/24 hours is indicative of deficiency and 5.8 to 17.5 mmol/24 hours is considered low.

Large doses of niacin—1.5 to 3.0 g/day—can be used to reduce serum total and low-density lipoprotein cholesterol and to raise high-density lipoprotein cholesterol.[46] Side effects of niacin therapy include flushing of the skin, hyperuricemia, hepatic and ocular abnormalities, and occasional niacin-induced myopathy.

Vitamin B6 (Pyridoxine)

In the 1930s, Paul Gyorgy separated pyridoxine from the antipellagra factor and named it vitamin B6. The related compounds pyridoxal and pyridoxamine were also shown to have similar activity. By forming a Schiff base, pyridoxal phosphate (PLP) allows the crucial transamination of many amino acids. PLP is also involved in amino acid decarboxylation, gluconeogenesis, conversion of tryptophan to niacin, synthesis of sphingolipids and neurotransmitters, steroid hormone modulation, and immune function.[47]

Overt deficiencies of vitamin B6 are probably rare. Marginal deficiencies may be more common, manifested by nonspecific stomatitis, glossitis, cheilosis, irritability, confusion, and depression. A number of genetic syndromes affecting PLP-dependent enzymes—such as homocystinuria, cystathionuria, and xanthurenic aciduria—mimic vitamin B6 deficiency. Depressed concentrations of PLP have been reported in patients with asthma, diabetes, alcoholism, heart disease, pregnancy, breast cancer, Hodgkin's disease, and sickle-cell anemia.[48] Cystathionine synthase is a PLP-dependent enzyme that produces cystathionine from serine and homocysteine. As a result, vitamin B6 deficiency can lead to elevation of plasma homocysteine, a risk factor for the development of atherosclerosis and heart disease.[49]

Pyridoxine has been used to treat patients with Down syndrome, autism, gestational diabetes, carpal tunnel syndrome, premenstrual syndrome, depression, and diabetic neuropathy with variable results.[48] Recommended daily intakes are 1.3 to 1.7 mg for adult males, 1.3 to 1.5 mg for adult females, 0.1 to 1.0 mg for children, 1.9 mg during pregnancy, and 2.0 mg during lactation. Pyridoxine and pyridoxamine are primarily found in plant foods, with pyridoxal commonly in animal foods. Meats, whole grains, vegetables, and nuts are the best source. Cooking, food processing, and storage can reduce vitamin B6 availability by 10% to 50%. A number of pyridoxine assessment tests have been used: plasma pyridoxal-5-phosphate (normal 27 to 75 nmol/L in males and 26 to 93 nmol/L in females), erythrocyte transaminase activity, urine 4-pyridoxic acid excretion (normal >3.0 mmol/day), or urine xanthurenic acid (normal <65 mmol/day) after a 2-g tryptophan load.

Vitamin B12 (Cobalamin)

A type of digestive disorder was known as pernicious anemia in the 19th century because it was invariably fatal. The 1926 Nobel Prize was awarded to Minot and Murphy for demonstrating a cure by feeding large quantities of liver to those suffering from the disorder. Ironically, the cure was probably because of iron and not the vitamins in the liver. Vitamin B12 was isolated much later as the active principle in liver, and its structure, as a corrin ring similar to hemoglobin but with a central cobalt, was finally elucidated by x-ray crystallography in 1964 by Hodgkin.

Pernicious anemia is the most common cause of vitamin B12 deficiency, accounting for over 75% of cases (see Table 3-2). Deficiency most commonly occurs in the elderly because of gastric atrophy and a lack of gastric production of intrinsic factor needed for B12 absorption in the ileum. Vegetarians, alcoholics, and patients with acquired immunodeficiency syndrome are also susceptible for B12 deficiency. Strict vegetarians may develop vitamin B12 deficiency over a period of months to years. This is partly ameliorated by a small amount of vitamin B12 produced by gut microorganisms.

Deficiency may be subclinical or may cause megaloblastic anemia, neuropathy, and demyelinization. This is possibly due to methyl group deficiency and the inability to synthesize methonine and S-Adenosyl Methionine, or to homocysteine toxicity. Both vitamin B12 and folate are required for the metabolism of homocysteine to methionine. Deficiency in these vitamins may lead to elevation in serum homocysteine concentrations, which may increase risk of atherosclerosis and heart disease.[50] Serum B12 can be measured by radioimmunoassay, but occasionally a Schilling test for absorption of radiolabeled B12 with or without intrinsic factor is necessary for determination of the exact problem.

Meat and dairy products provide the only dietary source of vitamin B12 for humans. The usual western diet contains 5 to 20 mcg of cobalamin a day, while the minimum daily requirement is much less.[51] Recommended daily intakes are 2.4 mg for adults, 0.4 to 1.8 mg for children, 2.6 mg during pregnancy, and 2.8 mg during lactation. Total body stores of vitamin B12 are 2000 to 5000 mcg, with approximately one-half of that stored in the liver: therefore, it takes years to develop vitamin B12 deficiency after absorption of dietary B12 ceases.[6]

Pernicious anemia and other forms of vitamin B12 deficiency are typically treated with 1 mg of vitamin B12 weekly for 4 weeks, and if necessary, monthly after that. An alternative therapy of high oral cobalamin 1 to 2 mg/day may utilize a second lower efficiency transport system that does not require intrinsic factor for absorption in the terminal ileum.[52] There is essentially no toxicity associated with excess vitamin B12 ingestion, as large doses often are used in placebos and megavitamin preparations.

Folate

Folate is a vitamin that is responsible for one-carbon methyl transfer in a variety of cellular reactions, including formation of purines and pyridimines, which make up DNA and RNA. Folate deficiency may result in megaloblastic anemia, as forming red cells fail to divide. As the best source of folate is in green leafy vegetables, folate nutrition may be marginal in many adolescents. Recommended daily intakes are 400 mcg for adults, 65 to 300 mcg for children, 600 mcg during pregnancy, and 500 mcg during lactation.

Recent epidemiologic evidence suggests that folate supplementation, at levels that are higher than usual dietary intake (200 to 400 mcg/day), reduce the incidence of neural tube defects (anencephaly and spina bifida) in newborns. Supplementation needs to be started early in pregnancy, before most pregnancies are apparent, so it should involve most women of childbearing age. The recent decision to supplement folate in grains and cereals in the United States will also reduce serum homocysteine levels, lowering the risk of cardiovascular disease. There is also a benefit of reduction in prostate cancer and colorectal cancer.[53]

Biotin, Pantothenate, and Other Vitamins

A number of other chemicals may also be considered essential vitamins, such as biotin (a cofactor for pyruvate carboxylase), pantothenic acid (a precursor for acetyl coenzyme A), and lipoic acid. Deficiencies are quite rare because these are widely available in foods; however, occasionally supplements are prescribed in cases of suspected mitochondrial disease. Lecithin, choline (for acetylcholine), glutamine, and carnitine (fatty acid transporter) can be synthesized to some extent in the body but might be conditionally essential in some cases. There are many other substances that may be important in health, such as carotenoids (including lycopene, lutein, and zeaxanthine) and flavinoids, but deficiency states have not been well established. However, there are many claims for substances like laetrile and pangamic acid, which have little support in the scientific literature.

Calcium

Calcium is the major component of bone, providing structural skeletal support to the human body. The approximately 4 lb of bone calcium in each person also provides a storage reservoir for the small percentage of ionized calcium that allows muscle to contract, nerves to communicate, enzymes to function, and cells to react. The body has developed several hormonal mechanisms—including vitamin D, parathyroid hormone, and calcitonin—to protect the small amount of ionized calcium in the blood from changing drastically. Tight control of blood calcium levels is needed because unduly low blood calcium might result in uncontrolled tetanic muscle contractions and seizures, while high blood calcium levels may cause kidney stones and muscle calcifications. To increase blood calcium levels, vitamin D and its metabolites increase calcium absorption from the intestinal tract, parathyroid hormone increases calcium reabsorption from the kidney, and both increase resorption of calcium from the bone. Thus, dietary calcium deficiency only rarely causes hypocalcemia (vitamin D deficiency can cause hypocalcemia), but instead may lead to progressive depletion of bone calcium, or osteoporosis.

During the early years of life, calcium is deposited in the bone as it grows, but after about the third decade, there is a steady decline in bone calcium.[54,55] This is especially marked after menopause in women, when estrogen declines, and often leads to bone loss (osteopenia) to below a threshold that predisposes women in particular to fractures (osteoporosis). Osteoporosis is not just a disease of the elderly and may occur in much younger patients, especially in athletic young women, those with anorexia nervosa, those on steroids and other medications, and in anyone on prolonged bed rest, including astronauts experiencing long periods of weightlessness.

Dietary calcium is often seen as the most limiting factor in the development of peak bone mass, and strategies to increase dietary calcium have been promoted. Other factors in the development of bone mineral include height, weight, ethnic background and inheritance, gender, activity, vitamin D deficiency, parathyroid hormone deficiency, vitamin A, vitamin K, growth hormone, calcium, phosphorus, and magnesium. Phosphorus, the other major component of bone mineral, is relatively common in the diet.

The 1997 DRIs of calcium were raised from 800 mg to 1300 mg in 9- to 18-year-olds, 1000 mg in 19- to 50-year-olds, and 1200 mg in 51- to 70-year-olds. For many years, the World Health Organization had a more modest goal of 500 mg/day but is probably raising this level.

Only a small percentage of the population consumes the RDA for calcium. The estimated average calcium intake in American women is only about 500 to 600 mg/day, and is as low as 200 mg/day in the developing world. From calcium tracer studies performed since the 1950s, intestinal calcium absorption ranges from 10% to 40% of ingested calcium, with a higher percentage absorption with lower calcium intakes. A large percentage (usually 70% to 80%) of dietary calcium is from milk and dairy products, which provides about 250 mg calcium per 8-oz glass of milk, and most studies show better absorption from dairy products than from vegetable sources. However, many people, especially non-Caucasians, develop relative lactose intolerance after childhood and are reluctant to increase their dairy food intake.

Compared to that in most American and European diets, calcium intake in the rest of the world is much less, often 200 to 300 mg/day. Most of the world does not consume as much milk and dairy products per capita as Americans and Europeans. Although osteoporosis seems to be more common among the elderly in North America and Europe, this may be because of the larger percentage of elderly among the population and/or the increased tendency to suffer falls that lead to fractures. African-Americans tend to have slightly higher bone density (about 10% higher) than do Caucasians, but the elderly in Africa and Asia seem to experience a similar decrease in bone density with aging.

Thus, attention has focused on whether supplementation or fortification of calcium, especially during adolescence, will ensure achievement of peak bone mass. Calcium supplementation up to the RDA in adolescent females has shown short-term increases in bone mineral density, but this may be because it increases mineralization in a limited amount of trabecular bone, and it remains to be seen whether this leads to long-term improvement or protection against future fractures.[56,57] Also, most studies still assume that increased bone mineral density is synonymous with reduced fracture risk, although fractures may depend on many other factors such as optimal bone architecture and lack of falls. Although the majority of scientific opinion probably favors increased dietary calcium intake in adolescence, the factors that control bone mineralization are not yet completely understood, and long-term protection against eventual bone loss and fractures remains to be demonstrated by randomized clinical trials.

Magnesium

Although dietary magnesium deficiency is uncommon, it may occur in connection with a number of gastrointestinal, endocrine, or renal disorders and may result in sudden life-threatening arrhythmias. Hypomagnesemia is sometimes a cause of hypocalcemia, probably through its effect on parathyroid hormone secretion, and correction of the magnesium deficiency will correct the hypocalcemia. Like calcium, magnesium is bound to albumin, and the ionized magnesium level is more important than the total serum magnesium; however, it is rarely available as a routine laboratory test.

Phosphorus

Like magnesium, phosphorus is fairly common in the diet, and dietary deficiency is uncommon. However, in starvation situations like protein-calorie malnutrition or anorexia nervosa, sudden refeeding of large amounts of carbohydrate calories may deplete phosphates used for ATP and lead to unexpected sudden deaths from arrhythmias, often just when the patient is thought to be recovering. Therefore, in malnourished patients who are hypometabolic, hypothermic, or hypotensive, gradual increases in calories and in phosphate, potassium, and multivitamin supplements are advised.

Iron

Iron deficiency is one of the most common vitamin or mineral deficiencies in the world, affecting over 2 billion people in the world and 9 million in the United States. Twenty percent or more of women and children may be iron deficient, especially in developing countries.[58] Adolescent women who have started menses are particularly at risk. Anemia may lead to reduced school and work performance and may affect cognitive function, as well as lead to cardiovascular and growth problems. Because iron is a key component of hemoglobin, anemia may affect the oxygen-carrying capacity of blood. Consequences of chronic iron deficiency anemia may include growth failure, reduced appetite, fatigue, weakness, increased susceptibility to infection, and poor cognitive performance.

Diagnosis is made most simply by hemoglobin level or packed red cell volume (hematocrit) and red cell morphology, or alternatively by transferrin saturation, serum ferritin, or serum iron level. Microscopic examination of a red cell smear typically shows red cells that are small (microcytic) and pale (hypochromic). Anemia, or an actual drop in hematocrit, is a late finding in iron deficiency after stores are depleted, so that more sensitive indicators of iron deficiency are often helpful, such as transferrin saturation or total iron binding capacity. Serum ferritin is a good indicator of iron stores in the bone marrow but may be falsely affected by inflammation or liver disease, as it is an acute phase reactant.

Iron absorption is affected by many factors—such as iron status, source of iron, and binding by phytates—and may range from 10% to 40% of dietary intake.[59,60] Different preparations should be checked for the amount of elemental iron contained. Only 8 gm/day elemental iron is the DRI for adult males, compared to 18 mg/day for women aged 19 to 50 years and 27 mg/day for pregnancy.

The standard treatment for iron deficiency is ferrous sulfate 300 mg three times a day until corrected by an appropriate rise in the reticulocyte count and hemoglobin, followed by a maintenance dose of 300 mg daily. Iron dextran 1 to 10 mg/day may be given intramuscularly or intravenously but care should be given to detect and treat frequent allergic reactions. Universal supplementation may not be in the best interest of all because adult males do not regularly lose blood through menses and may accumulate iron throughout the lifetime, which occasionally leads to iron overload, hemochromatosis, and liver disease.[61,62]

Zinc

Zinc is a component of many metalloenzymes including those needed for growth, pancreatic enzymes, and intestinal secretions.[63] Although it is unusual to find a documented case of clinical zinc deficiency apart from occasional cases of acrodermatitis enteropathica, there has been recent concern over the possibility of relative zinc deficiency, especially among chronically ill patients with excessive intestinal secretions. These might include patients with inflammatory bowel disease, cystic fibrosis, and anorexia nervosa or those undergoing bone marrow transplantation[64] or PN.

Zinc deficiency can lead to impaired taste (hypogeusia) and appetite and immunodeficiency, as well as affect growth. A large group of adolescents in Shiraz, Iran, was described to be of very short stature because of dietary zinc deficiency. There may also be neurologic, endocrinologic, hematologic, or rheumatologic impairment.[63] Although there are problems with interpreting serum zinc levels, they are probably more useful than are other methods of assessment, such as nail or hair analysis. Because alkaline phosphatase is a zinc metalloenzyme, low serum alkaline phosphatase levels might be indicative of zinc deficiency.

Selenium

Individuals in a group of people in Keshan, China, were found to develop cardiomyopathy because of a selenium deficiency in the soil.[65] Apparently, selenium deficiency increases susceptibility to heart damage from coxsackie virus myocarditis.[66,67] Cardiomyopathy was also reported from selenium deficiency in patients on PN.[68-70] Selenium deficiency is also associated with Kaschin-Beck disease, causing osteoarthritis or epiphyseal dysplasia. Selenium is necessary for synthesis of a number of selenoproteins, most notably glutathione peroxidase, an antioxidant. Therefore, many nutritional supplements include selenium or glutathione peroxidase.

Iodine

Iodine deficiency is surprisingly common worldwide, perhaps involving up to one-half of the world population or 3 billion people, especially in areas of Southeast Asia away from coastal areas or where iodine is not supplemented in salt. It may cause hypothyroidism, goiter (neck mass), cretinism, and impaired intelligence if severe. Iodine is bound to thyroxine and triiodothyronine as an essential mechanism in thyroid hormone metabolism. Iodine deficiency can be easily prevented with supplementation in salt, but this is often neglected in developing countries where salt production is not centralized and enforcement is difficult.

Copper

Dietary copper deficiency is quite rare, but a rare disorder of copper transport—Menkes kinky-hair syndrome—illustrates many of the cellular functions of copper, with poor growth, pallor, mental retardation, seizures, and characteristic kinky hair.[71-74] Rarely, it is associated with thin, kinky hair. There are at least 50-100 copper metalloenzymes, including lysyl oxidase, superoxide dismutase, and cytochrome c oxidase.[71,72] Intestinal copper absorption by metallothionein can be affected by other minerals such as iron and zinc.

Patients with chronic intestinal malabsorption syndromes such as celiac disease (Chapter 19) and cystic fibrosis (Chapter 25), premature newborns (Chapter 37), and those on prolonged PN have been reported to develop copper deficiency. One prominent effect is a hypochromic, microcytic anemia similar to iron deficiency.[75]

Other Minerals

There are many other trace elements that may play an essential role in human metabolism, but deficiency is very difficult to produce and may take years even in highly artificial situations, such as in long-term PN. Manganese is a constituent of numerous metalloenzymes, and a patient on long-term PN with poor growth and diffuse bone mineralization benefited from manganese supplementation.[76] Molybdenum is an enzyme cofactor and component of enzymes such as sulfite oxidase, reversed progressive mental disturbances, and coma in a patient on PN.[77] Cobalt is a component of cobalamin (vitamin B12), but dietary cobalt deficiency has been difficult to establish. Silicon, an element that is commonly found in sand and glass, may play a role in collagen and bone formation. Although silicon deficiency occurs in chicks and rats, it is not clear whether a deficiency state occurs in humans.

References

1. Nobel Lectures, Physiology or Medicine 1922-1941. Amsterdam: Elsevier; 1965.
2. Alpha Tocopherol Beta-Carotene Cancer Prevention Study Group. The effect of vitamin E and beta carotene on the incidence of lung cancer and other cancers in male smokers. *N Engl J Med.* 1994;330:1029-35.
3. Kushi LH, Folsom AR, Prineas RJ, et al. Dietary antioxidant vitamins and death from coronary heart disease in postmenopausal women. *N Engl J Med.* 1996;334:1156-1162.
4. *Institute of Medicine, Dietary Reference Intakes for Thiamin, Riboflavin, Niacin, Vitamin B6, Folate, Vitamin B12, Pantothenic Acid, Biotin, and Choline.* Washington DC: National Academy Press; 1998.
5. Institute of Medicine, Dietary Reference Intakes for Calcium, Phosphorus, Magnesium, Vitamin D, and Fluoride. Washington DC: National Academy Press; 1997.
6. *National Research Council, Recommended Dietary Allowances.* 10th ed. Washington DC: National Academy Press; 1989.
7. www.nap.edu
8. Herrera MG. Vitamin A deficiency: prevention and treatment. *International Seminars in Pediatric Gastroenterology and Nutrition.* 1995;4:3-8.
9. Fawzi WW, Herrera MG, Willett WC et al. Dietary vitamin A intake and the risk of mortality among children. *Am J Clin Nutr.* 1994;59:401-408.
10. Holick MF, ed. *Vitamin D: Molecular Biology, Physiology, and Clinical Application.* Totawa, NJ: Humana Press; 1999.
11. Holick M. Vitamin D and bone health. *J Nutr.* 1996;126:1159S-1164S.
12. Thomas MK, Lloyd-Jones DM, Thadhani RI, et al. Hypovitaminosis in medical inpatients. *N Engl J Med.* 1998;338:777-83.
13. LeBoff MS, Kohlmeier L, Hurwitz S, et al. Occult vitamin D deficiency in postmenopausal US women with acute hip fracture. *JAMA.* 1999;281:1505-1511.
14. Gordon CM, DePeter KC, Feldman HA. Prevalence of vitamin D deficiency among healthy adolescents. *Arch Pediatr Adolesc Med.* 2004;158:531-537.
15. Tangpricha Y, Pearce EN, Chen TC, Holick MF. Vitamin D deficiency among free-living healthy young adults. *Am J Med.* 2002; 112:659-662.
16. Gartner LM, Greer FR, et al. Prevention of rickets and vitamin D deficiency: new guidelines for vitamin D intake. *Pediatrics.* 2003;111:908-910.
17. Sokol RJ. Metabolism and disorders of vitamin E in infancy and childhood. *Intl Sem Pediatr Gastroenterol Nutr.* 1995;4:8-15.
18. Stephens NG, Parson A, Schofield PM, et al. Randomised controlled trial of vitamin E in patients with coronary disease: Cambridge Heart Antioxidant Study (CHAOS). *Lancet.* 1996; 374:781-6.
19. Jha P, Flather M, Lonn E, et al. The antioxidant vitamins and cardiovascular disease: a critical review of epidemiologic and clinical trial data. *Ann Intern Med.* 1995;123:*860-872.*
20. Stampfer MJ, Hennekens CH, Manson JE, et al. Vitamin E consumption and the risk of coronary heart disease in men. *N Engl J Med.* 1993;328:1450-1456.
21. Packer L. Protective role of vitamin E in biological systems. *Am J Clin Nutr.* 1991;53:1050S-1055S.
22. Suttie JW. Vitamin K and human nutrition. *J Am Diet Assoc.* 1992; 92:585-590.
23. Furie B, Furie BC. Molecular basis of vitamin K-dependent gamma carboxylation. *Blood.* 1990;75:1753-1762.
24. Lipsky JJ. Nutritional sources of vitamin K. *Mayo Clin Proc.* 1994; 69:462-466.
25. Mann KG, Nesheim ME, Church WR, et al. Surface-dependent reactions of the vitamin K dependent enzyme complexes. *Blood.* 1990:76:1-16.
26. Hirsch J. Oral anticoagulant drugs. *N Engl J Med.* 1991;324:1865-1875.
27. Carpenter KJ. *The History of Scurvy and Vitamin C.* Cambridge: Cambridge University Press; 1986.
28. Lind J. *Treatise on the Scurvy.* Edinburgh: Sandy, Murray and Cochran; 1753.
29. Hunter DJ, Manson JE, Colditz GA, et al. A prospective study of the intake of vitamins C, E, and A and the risk of breast cancer. *N Engl J Med.* 1993;329:334.
30. Gey KF, Moser UK, Jordan P, et al. Increased risk of cardiovascular disease at suboptimal plasma concentrations of essential antioxidants: an epidemiological update with special attention to carotene and vitamin C. *Am J Clin Nutr.* 1993;57:787S.
31. Gaziano JM. Antioxidants and coronary artery disease risk. *Am J Med.* 1994;97:18S.
32. Jeng KC, Yang CS, Siu WY, et al. Supplementation with vitamins C and E enhances cytokine production by peripheral blood mononuclear cells in healthy adults. *Am J Clin Nutr.* 1996;64:960.
33. Creagan ET, Moertel CG, Ofallon JR, et al. Failure of high-dose vitamin C (ascorbic acid) therapy to benefit patients with advanced cancer, a controlled trial. *N Engl J Med.* 1979;310:687.
34. Karlowski TR, Chalmers TC, Frenkel LD. Ascorbic acid for the common cold, a prophylactic and therapeutic trial. *JAMA.* 1975;231:1038.
35. Carpenter KJ. *Beriberi, White Rice and Vitamin B.* Berkeley: University of California Press; 2000.
36. Reuler JB, Girard DE, Cooney TG. Wernicke's encephalopathy. *N Engl J Med.* 1985;312:1035-1039.
37. Sechi GP, Serra A, Pirastru MI, Sotgiu S, Rosati G. Wernicke's encephalopathy in a woman on slimming diet. *Neurology.* 2002;58:1697.
38. Gropman AL, Gaillard WD, Campbell P, Charya SV. Wernicke's encephalopathy due to self starvation in a child. *Lancet.* 1998;351:1704-1705.
39. Vasconcelos MM, Silva KP, Vidal G, Silva AF, Domingues RC, Berditchevsky CR. Early diagnosis of pediatric Wernicke's encephalopathy. *Pediatric Neurology.* 1999;20:289-294.
40. Heye N, Terstegge K, Sirtl C, et al. Wernicke's encephalopathy: causes to consider. *Intensive Care Med.* 1994;20:282.
41. Hoffman RS, Goldfrank LR. The poisoned patient with altered consciousness: controversies in the use of a 'coma cocktail'. *JAMA.* 1995;274:562.
42. Lactic acidosis traced to thiamin deficiency related to nationwide shortage of multivitamins for total parenteral nutrition. *MMWR.* 1997;46:523.
43. Romanski SA, McMahon MM. Metabolic acidosis and thiamin deficiency. *Mayo Clin Proc.* 1999;74:259.
44. Sauberlich HE. *Laboratory Tests for the Assessment of Nutritional Status.* 2nd ed. Boca Raton: CRC Press; 1999.
45. Fouty B, Frerman F, Reves R. Riboflavin to treat nucleoside analogue-induced lactic acidosis. *Lancet.* 1998:32:291.
46. Brown SL, Sobel BE, Fujii S. Attenuation of the synthesis of plasminogen activator inhibitor type 1 by niacin. A potential link between lipid lowering and fibrinolysis. *Circulation.* 1995;92:767.
47. Rall LC, Meydani SN. Vitamin B6 and immune competence. *Nutr Rev.* 1993;51:217.
48. Leklem JE. Vitamin B6. In Machlin LJ, ed. *Handbook of Vitamins.* 2nd ed. New York: Marcel Dekker; 1991.
49. Rimm E, Willett WC, Hu FB, et al. Folate and vitamin B6 from diet and supplements in relation to risk of coronary heart disease among women. *JAMA.* 1998;279:359.
50. Vermeer C, Gijbers BLMG, Craciun AM, et al. Effects of vitamin K on bone mass and bone metabolism. *J Nutr.* 1996;126:1187S-91S.

51. Green R, Kinsella LJ. Current concepts in the diagnosis of cobalamin deficiency. *Neurology.* 1995;45:1435.
52. Selhub J, Jacques PF, Wilson PW, et al. Vitamin status and intake as primary determinants of homocysteinemia in an elderly population. *JAMA.* 1993;270:2693.
53. Giovanucci E, Stampfer M, Colditz G, et al. Folate, methionine, and alcohol intake and the risk of colorectal adenoma. *J Natl Cancer Inst.* 1993;87:895-904.
54. Bronner F. Calcium and osteoporosis. *Am J Clin Nutr.* 1994;60:831-836.
55. Harward MP. Nutritive therapies for osteoporosis, the role of calcium. *Med Clin N Amer.* 1993;77:889-897.
56. Johnston CC, Miller JZ, Slemenda CW, et al. Calcium supplementation and increases in bone mineral density in children. *N Engl J Med.* 1992;327:82-87.
57. Gilsanz V, Roe TF, Mora S, et al. Changes in vertebral bone density in black girls and white girls during childhood and puberty. *N Engl J Med.* 1991;325:1597-1600.
58. Cook JD, Skikne BS, Baynes RD. Iron deficiency: the global perspective. In: Herschko C, et al, eds. *Progress in Iron Research.* New York: Plenum Press; 1994: 219-228.
59. Andrews NC. Disorders of iron metabolism. *N Engl J Med.* 1999;341:1986-1995.
60. Eisenstein RS, Blemings KP. Iron regulatory protein, iron responsive elements, and iron homeostasis. *J Nutr.* 1998;128:2295-2298.
61. Letendre ED. The importance of iron in the pathogenesis of infection and neoplasia. *TIBS.* 1985;10:166-168.
62. Oppenheimer SJ. Iron and its relation to immunity and infectious disease. *J Nutr.* 2001;131:616S-635S.
63. Vallee BL, Falchuk KH. The biochemical basis of zinc physiology. *Physiol Rev.* 1993;73:79-118.
64. Papadopoulou A, Nathavitharana K, Williams MD, et al. Diagnosis and clinical associations of zinc depletion following bone marrow transplantation. *Arch Dis Child.* 1996;74:328-331.
65. Lee BJ, et al. Molecular biology of selenium and its role in human health. *Molecules Cells.* 1996:6:509-520.
66. Burk RF. Selenium and myocardial infarction. *JAMA.* 1989;262:775.
67. Gaunt C, Tracy S. Deficient diet evokes nasty heart virus. *Nature Med.* 1995;1:405-406.
68. Van Rij AM, Thomson CD, Lyons JM et al. Selenium deficiency in total parenteral nutrition. *Am J Clin Nutr.* 1986;32:2076-2085.
69. Fleming CR, McCull JT, O'Brien JF, et al. Selenium status in patients receiving home parenteral nutrition. *JPEN.* 1984;8:258-262.
70. Johnson RA, Baker SS, Fallon JT, Maynard EP, Ruskin JN, Wen Z, Ge K, Cohen HJ. An occidental case of cardiomyopathy and selenium deficiency. *N Engl J Med.* 1981;304:1210-1213.
71. Walshe JM. Copper: not too little, not too much, but just right. *J Royal Coll Phys London.* 1995;29:280-288.
72. Askwith C, Kaplan J. Iron and copper transport in yeast and its relevance to human disease. *TIBS.* 1998:23:135-138.
73. Menkes JH, Alter M, Steigleider GK, et al. A sex-linked recessive disorder with retardation of growth, peculiar hair, and focal cerebral and cerebellar degeneration. *Pediatrics.* 1962;29:764-779.
74. Danks DM , Campbell PE, Stevens BJ, et al. Menkes kinky hair syndrome: an inherited defect in copper absorption with widespread effects. *Pediatrics.* 1972;50:188-201.
75. Hirase N, Abe Y, Sadamura S, et al. Anemia and neutropenia in a case of copper deficiency: role of copper in normal hematopoiesis. *Acta Haematol.* 1992;87:195-197.
76. Norose N, Terai M, Norose K. *Manganese deficiency in a child with very short bowel syndrome receiving long-term parenteral nutrition. Trace Elem Exp Med.* 1992;5:100-101.
77. Abumrad NN, Schneider AJ, Steel D, Roger LS. Amino acid intolerance during prolonged total parenteral nutrition reversed by molybdate therapy. *Am J Clin Nutr.* 1981;34:2551-2559.

Chapter 4

Clinical Consequences of Undernutrition

Alice Buchanan, MS, RD, and
Gordon L. Jensen, MD, PhD

Introduction

Undernutrition is a common concern in the clinical setting. Patients have disease processes and injuries that elicit inflammatory responses and, as a result, impact nutritional status. They may be unable to eat for extended periods because of disease, injury, or treatment. Undernutrition results from compromised nutrient intake, impaired nutrient assimilation, or excessive nutrient losses. The clinical consequences of undernutrition syndromes are myriad and may culminate in adverse outcomes that include increased complications impacting length of hospital stay, readmission rate, and mortality.

Undernutrition Syndromes

Undernutrition can be categorized into five syndromes: wasting/marasmus, sarcopenia, cachexia, protein-energy undernutrition (PEU), and failure to thrive.[1] In order to recognize clinical consequences and to select helpful interventions and management, the medical practitioner must recognize the appropriate undernutrition syndrome. However, there is frequently overlap among undernutrition syndromes, and a given underlying condition may precipitate more than one type of syndrome. Therefore, the physician must be familiar with and be able to recognize key characteristics for each syndrome (Table 4-1).[2]

Wasting/Marasmus

Poor dietary intake or assimilation with resulting loss of body cell mass is the common feature of wasting conditions.[1] In pure wasting (clinical marasmus), there are no manifestations of acute-phase metabolic response or underlying inflammatory condition. Resting energy expenditure (REE) is reduced and visceral proteins are preserved. Increased extracellular fluid is therefore not observed.

The body's adaptive response to semistarvation is multifaceted. Without nutrient intake for approximately 48 hours, the body will shift into a fasted state. In the fasted state, energy stores of glucose (primarily muscle glycogen) have been depleted. Low levels of blood glucose signal the release of glucagons and glucosteroid hormones, which promote muscle breakdown and gluconeogenesis. The amino acids leucine and lysine cannot be used for gluconeogenesis because they form ketone bodies. These ketones can be used by the brain, heart, and skeletal muscle for fuel. The breakdown of protein for fuel is accompanied by large urinary nitrogen losses.[3] As this is not the preferred energy source, energy expenditure is decreased in an effort to conserve as much energy as possible. The REE in undernourished persons is often lower than that in a well-nourished person.[4,5] Interestingly, studies have shown that severely undernourished patients at the limit of life may experience a paradoxical increase in REE.[5] This increase is associated with high urinary nitrogen losses, low serum fatty acid concentrations, and near zero fat mass. These clinical findings are suggestive of elevated net protein oxidation.

If the fasting state persists, it will progress into the starvation state. Starvation is characterized by the body's effort to spare body protein by shifting the primary fuel source from gluconeogenesis to lipolysis. Only essential proteins are synthesized. Starvation is marked by sharp increases in serum fatty acid levels. Insulin levels are decreased. Fatty acids are oxidized by the heart, liver,

TABLE 4-1.

Differential Diagnosis of Nutritional Syndromes

Disease	*Characteristics*	*Notes*
Wasting/Marasmus	Loss of body cell mass without underlying inflammatory condition. REE reduced. Visceral proteins preserved. Extracellular fluid not increased.	Examples: marasmus, cancer, critical illness without nutrition support, chronic organ failure syndromes.
Sarcopenia	Age-related loss of muscle mass without other precipitating conditions.	Role of undernutrition in sarcopenia is unknown.
Cachexia	Loss of body cell mass with underlying inflammatory condition. Cytokine-mediated acute phase metabolic response. Elevation of REE. Decline in visceral proteins. Increased extracellular fluid.	Examples: rheumatoid arthritis, congestive heart failure, chronic obstructive pulmonary disease, critical illness with nutrition support.
Protein-Energy Undernutrition (PEU)	Clinical and laboratory evidence for reduced intake of protein and energy. Reduced visceral proteins.	Includes many patients with injury, disease, or inflammatory states who have compromised dietary intakes.
Failure to Thrive	Weight loss and decline in physical and/or cognitive functioning with signs of hopelessness and helplessness.	Applied in clinical practice to undernourished older persons in functional or cognitive decline.

Reprinted with permission from Jensen GL. Physician's Information and Education Resource. Undernutrition Syndromes. Philadelphia, PA: American College of Physicians-American Society of Internal Medicine. Available at www.pier.acponline.org/index.html. Accessed March 1, 2006.

and skeletal muscle for energy. The brain is not able to oxidize fatty acids. Glycerol becomes a precursor for gluconeogenesis to supply glucose to the brain. Survival time in starvation state depends on existing fat stores.[3] The human body is amazingly resilient and will sacrifice most everything to preserve vital organ functions (Table 4-2).

SARCOPENIA

Aging may be associated with a loss of muscle mass, called sarcopenia.[6-11] Loss of strength, reduced physical activity, and functional decline may result. It is not clear whether this condition is an inevitable part of aging or a consequence of sedentary living and/or poor nutritional status. Because the relationship between undernutrition and sarcopenia has not been established, patients with this syndrome may or may not benefit from a nutritional intervention. Skeletal muscle mass has been increased by experimental approaches that include administration of trophic factors, like growth hormone and testosterone[12-16] and resistance strength training.[17,18]

CACHEXIA

Cachexia will manifest when there is an underlying inflammatory process, injury, or condition. The syndrome is characterized by increased cytokine production that favors a catabolic state.[8] The inflammatory cytokines (tumor necrosis factor, interleukin-1, and interleukin-6) appear to play key roles in triggering the acute-phase metabolic response to inflammation. REE is elevated, amino acids are exported from muscle to liver, gluconeogenesis is increased, and there is a shift toward increased production of positive acute-phase proteins with a concomitant decline in the synthesis of albumin.[19] Increased extracellular fluid will often result in obvious edema, such that, despite erosion of body cell mass, there may not be a decline in body weight.

PROTEIN-ENERGY UNDERNUTRITION

PEU is characterized by both clinical (physical signs such as weight loss and low body mass index [BMI]) and biochemical (low albumin or other protein) signs of insufficient energy and protein intake.[20,21] Many patients with inflammatory diseases will also suffer anorexia with compromised dietary intakes. These patients' signs may be considered a subtle overlap of wasting and cachexia syndromes. It is noteworthy that in routine clinical practice, many patients with only reduced albumin or prealbumin are often designated PEU, despite that they have only manifestations of inflammatory response.

FAILURE TO THRIVE

Failure to thrive originated in the pediatric literature to describe infants who did not achieve milestones in height, weight, or behavior. This construct has since been extended to describe older persons who lose weight, exhibit decline in physical and/or cognitive functions, and demonstrate signs of hopelessness and helplessness.[22] The National Institute on Aging has described failure to

TABLE 4-2.

Key Characteristics of Energy States

Nutritional State	Fuel Source	Clinical Signs
Well nourished	Glucose, muscle glycogen	Normal REE Normal urinary nitrogen losses
Fasting (48 hours after nutrient intake)	Amino acids from muscle breakdown, gluconeogenesis	Large urinary nitrogen losses Ketosis
Sustained starvation	Lipids, lipolysis	Increased serum fatty acid levels Decreased serum insulin levels

thrive as "a syndrome of weight loss, decreased appetite and poor nutrition, and inactivity, often accompanied by dehydration, depressive symptoms, impaired immune function, and low cholesterol".[23] Because failure to thrive does not readily encompass a single identifiable clinical syndrome, some have proposed to abandon this term in favor of a group of potentially more treatable conditions: impaired physical functioning, undernutrition, depression, and cognitive impairment.[24]

Impact of Undernutrition

Life-threatening undernutrition is classified as a loss of about one-third of body weight or a BMI ≤15 kg/m^2. Death is certain when 50% of lean tissue is lost and/or when the BMI falls to 13 kg/m^2.[25,26] Much of what we know of the natural history of starvation dates from dramatic examples of malnutrition and starvation that were observed during World War II. The most well-documented examples of extreme human malnutrition and starvation during this time came from observations made by physicians confined to the Warsaw ghetto.[25,26] The entire amount of food that the residents of the Warsaw ghetto received from January to August of 1941 was less than 10% of the minimum caloric requirements necessary to sustain human life. Records indicate that during 1941, 25.3% of deaths in the Warsaw ghetto were attributed to starvation.[25,26] In 1944, Keys and colleagues[4] conducted the Minnesota experiment. They studied 32 male volunteers during a 6-month period of semi-starvation with average daily consumption of 1570 kcal, including 50 gm protein and 30 gm fat. The decline in organ system functions that resulted was systematically characterized.

Organ System Functions

Cardiovascular

The Minnesota experiment found that a 24% loss of body weight was associated with a 17% reduction in heart volume.[4] The observed changes in the cardiovascular system included a faint heart beat, significant bradycardia, hypotension, decreased oxygen consumption, low stroke volume, and decreased cardiac output. Severe starvation often results in ventricular arrhythmias and cardiac dysfunction.[27] Refractory ventricular arrhythmias unresponsive to standard interventions are often the cause of death in severe starvation. Common nonspecific electrocardiogram findings include prolonged QT interval and low voltage.[28,29] During periods of starvation heart muscle is catabolized for energy resulting in left ventricular, left atrial, and aortic dimensions that are often below normal.[30] Because the dimensions of the heart are decreased, the heart has a reduced ability to handle fluid challenge, often resulting in significant pedal and facial edema.[25] Overzealous rapid nutritional resuscitation may result in congestive failure. It should be noted that many severely undernourished patients have other underlying comorbid diseases and deficiencies that may also influence cardiovascular hemodynamics: for example, alcohol-related cardiomyopathy and thiamine deficiency.

Pulmonary

Gross changes in lung morphology are modest with undernutrition. Nonetheless, the ventilatory mechanical function and drive of the pulmonary system is decreased during starvation. This occurs primarily because of the loss of lean tissue, especially in the diaphragm and chest wall. In the Minnesota experiment, vital capacity, respiratory rate, minute ventilation, and tidal volume progressively declined with semi-starvation.[4] Doekel and colleagues[31] observed a 42% decrease in hypoxic ventilatory response among seven volunteers subjected to 10 days of semi-starvation.

Gastrointestinal

Severe undernutrition may result in impairment of gastric acid secretion and gastric emptying.[26,31,32] If enteral nutrition is lacking, then atrophy of the small intestinal mucosa may occur with flattening of the mucosa, and reduced villi may result. Disaccharide malabsorption may develop. This atrophy may also predispose the patient to increased translocation of bacteria and associated endotoxin.[33] Changes at the cellular level may be observed in a patient after 48 to 72 hours without intraluminal nutrition.[34] Severe undernutrition may also cause pancreatic acinar atrophy and fibrosis with resulting exocrine insufficiency. Pancreatic islet endocrine functions are, however, generally well preserved. Impact on hepatic functioning is dictated by the type of undernutrition syndrome. With marasmic undernutrition, the liver becomes smaller, with a decrease in fat and protein. If there is a deficit only of quality protein intake (kwashiorkor-like), then the liver may be enlarged with increased fatty infiltration.

Kidney

Renal function may be well-maintained with undernutrition, though severe starvation in an otherwise healthy individual can lead to a wide range of renal abnormalities. Glomerular filtration rate and renal plasma flow may be reduced. Urine output may be increased and urinary concentration decreased. Uncompensated metabolic acidosis can result because of a reduction in the urinary excretion of hydrogen ion without appropriate compensatory reduction in pCO_2 due to decreased ventilatory function of the lungs.[25]

Hematologic

Severe undernutrition if often characterized by a normocytic, normochromic anemia.[35] Leukopenia, thrombocytopenia, acanthocyte formation, and cellular hypoplasia of the marrow may also be seen. White cell abnormalities can include impaired neutrophil functions. Relative lymphopenia is common as noted below.

Immune

The skin is the largest body barrier organ. Periods of severe undernutrition may be associated with thin, friable skin that is prone to breakdown and with related wound infection. Mounting an immune response is energetically costly and undernutrition may impact a variety of immune functions.[36] Cell-mediated immunity may be particularly impacted during starvation as manifest by reduced total lymphocyte count and reduced number of helper T-cells.[37-42] Skin test delayed hypersensitivity response to recall antigens may be anergic.[37-39,43-45] Decreased lymphocyte response to mitogenic stimuli may also be detected. Deficits in humoral immunity have been described but are less consistently observed. For example, reduced levels of antibodies in response to influenza vaccine have been observed with undernutrition. Lastly, some severely undernourished patients have reduced levels of total serum complement as well as individual serum complement components.

Clinical Outcomes: Complications

Poor Response to Therapy

Severe undernutrition can have far-reaching impact on a patient's response to medical therapies. Limited metabolic reserve may attenuate adaptive response to injury, disease, and inflammation. Recovery from illness, injury, elective surgery, or organ or bone marrow transplant may be compromised. Patients may be unable to undertake or complete potentially life-sustaining interventions (eg, the patient with advanced laryngeal malignancy and profound starvation who is unable to complete a course of chemoradiation or surgical interventions). It can also be extremely difficult to mobilize a patient with severe erosion of body cell mass and weakness, with a consequent increase in risk for pressure wound development. Undernutrition may also be associated with altered drug metabolism and pharmacokinetics. Changes in drug absorption, protein-binding, and clearance have been described.[46,47]

Compromised Wound Healing

Jonathan Rhoads' landmark studies in undernourished animals in the 1930s first demonstrated the association between nutritional status and wound healing.[48] Protein deficiency impairs multiple facets of wound healing, including neovascularization, fibroblast proliferation, collagen synthesis, and wound remodeling.[49,50] Mechanical strength of wounds may be greatly reduced in with severe undernutrition.[49-53] Edema associated with hypoalbuminemia may further complicate wound healing. Low albumin is a risk factor for poor wound healing; however, analysis must be interpreted with caution because albumin levels are subject to perturbation by cytokine-mediated inflammatory response, and the measurement lacks sensitivity and specificity as an indicator of nutritional status. Specific micronutrient deficiencies (eg, those of vitamins C and A and zinc) have also been implicated in compromised wound healing.

Susceptibility to Infection

The broad impact of undernutrition on immune functions can impact a host of organ systems. Blunted airway defenses increase a patient's risk of contracting airborne pathogens.[54] Ventilator-associated pneumonia is a particularly serious complication that is associated with appreciable morbidity. Increased septic complications including pneumonia have been observed in severely undernourished patients undergoing elective gastrointestinal surgeries.[55] Low caloric intake is associated with nosocomial blood stream infections in medical intensive care patients.[56] Undernutrition is also a potential risk factor for infections of both pressure and surgical wounds.

Adverse Clinical Outcomes

Length of Hospital Stay

Poor response to therapy, compromised wound healing, and increased susceptibility to infection all culminate in complications that promote increased length of hospital stay and healthcare resource consumption. For example, mechanically ventilated patients who are undernourished may have compromised airway defenses and be more difficult to wean from the ventilator, which results in an increased hospital stay.[54]

Early Readmission

Undernutrition is associated with increased healthcare resource use, especially among older persons.[57,58] Studies suggest that up to 24% of all Medicare inpatient expenditures are for early non-elective readmissions.[57] Early non-elective readmission can be defined as the first subsequent urgent hospitalization occurring between 1 week and 4 months of discharge from the hospital. The strongest predictors of early hospital readmission include changes in weight and in serum albumin.[58-61] In patients with chronic obstructive pulmonary disease (COPD), weight change during hospitalization is significantly associated with unplanned early readmission. A greater weight loss and a lower initial BMI were also strong predictors of early hospital readmission.[62]

Mortality

Hypoalbuminemia has consistently been related to adverse clinical outcomes; however, much of its prognostic value likely reflects its utility as a proxy indicator for injury, disease, or inflammation.[63-65] True protein-calorie undernutrition may, nonetheless, be a contributing factor. In the community setting, hypoalbuminemia has been associated with functional limitation, sarcopenia, increased healthcare use, and mortality.[59-61] In the hospital setting, it has also been associated with increased length of hospital stay, complications, readmissions, and mortality.[59-61]

Patients with end-stage renal disease are at increased risk of cachexia because of the cytokine-mediated inflammatory nature of chronic renal disease.[66-68] Hypoalbuminemia and low total body nitrogen levels are associated with increased mortality in these patients. A 10% decrease in nitrogen level is associated with a 60% increase in death.[66] Similarly, low BMI and weight loss are risk factors for mortality in patients with other cytokine-mediated cachexia states, like COPD,[69] malignancy,[70-72] and human immunodeficiency virus.[73]

Undernourished hip-fracture patients have poor medical outcomes. Bastow et al[74] observed that patients who were objectively classified as "very thin" had significantly higher rates of in-hospital mortality (21%), compared to those of patients who were classified as "thin" (11%) or "well nourished" (5%). Longer hospital stays and increased incidence of complications among undernourished hip-fracture patients have also been observed.[75-81]

Summary

An understanding of undernutrition syndromes and their untoward effects on organ system functions is prerequisite to an appreciation of their clinical consequences. Poor response to therapy, compromised wound healing, and increased susceptibility to infections culminate in serious complications impacting length of hospital stay, readmission rate, and mortality.

References

1. Roubenoff R, Heymsfield SB, Kehayias JJ, Cannon JG, Rosenberg IH. Standardization of nomenclature of body composition in weight loss. *Am J Clin Nutr.* 1997;66:192-196.
2. Jensen GL. Physician's Information and Education Resource. Undernutrition Syndromes. Philadelphia, PA: American College of Physicians-American Society of Internal Medicine, Available at www.pier.acponline.org/index.html. Accessed May 30, 2004.
3. Groff JL, Gropper SS. Integration and regulation of metabolism and the impact of exercise and sport. In: *Advanced Nutrition and Human Metabolism.* Belmont, CA: Wadsworth/Thompson Learning; 2000:226-230.
4. Keys A, Brozel J, Henschel A, Mickelsen O, Taylor HL. *The Biology of Human Starvation.* Vols 1 and 2. Minneapolis: University of Minnesota Press; 1950.
5. Rigaud D, Hassid J, Meulemans A, Poupard AT, Boulier A. A paradoxical increase in resting energy expenditure in malnourished patients near death: the king penguin syndrome. *Am J Clin Nutr.* 2000;72:355-360.
6. Roubenoff R. The pathophysiology of wasting in the elderly. *J Nutr.* 1999;129:256S-259S.
7. Rosenberg IH. Sarcopenia: origins and clinical relevance. *J Nutr.* 1997;127:990S-991S.
8. Roubenoff R. Inflammatory and hormonal mediators of cachexia. *J Nutr.* 1997;127:1014S-1016S.
9. Lexell J. Human aging, muscle mass, and fiber type composition. *J Gerontol A Biol Sci Med Sci.* 1995;50 Spec No:11-6.
10. Evans WJ, Campbell WW. Sarcopenia and age-related changes in body composition and functional capacity. *J Nutr.* 1993;123:465-468.
11. Sarcopenia and physical performance in old age. Proceedings of a workshop. Bethesda, Maryland, July 9-10, 1996. *Muscle Nerve Suppl.* 1997;5:S1-120.
12. Papadakis MA, Grady D, Black D, et al. Growth hormone replacement in healthy older men improves body composition but not functional ability. *Ann Intern Med.* 1996;124:708-716.
13. Snyder PJ, Peachey H, Hannoush P, et al. Effect of testosterone treatment on body composition and muscle strength in men over 65 years of age. *J Clin Endocrinol Metab.* 1999;84:2647-2653.
14. Rudman D, Feller AG, Nagraj HS, et al. Effects of human growth hormone in men over 60 years old. *N Engl J Med.* 1990;323:1-6.
15. Urban RJ, Bodenburg YH, Gilkison C, et al. Testosterone administration to elderly men increases skeletal muscle strength and protein synthesis. *Am J Physiol.* 1995;269:E820-6.
16. Sih R, Morley JE, Kaiser FE, Perry HM, Patrick P, Ross C. Testosterone replacement in older hypogonadal men: a 12 month randomized controlled trial. *J Clin Endocrinol Metab.* 1997;82:1661-7.
17. Evans WJ, Cyr-Campbell D. Nutrition, exercise, and healthy aging. *J Am Diet Assoc.* 1997;97:632-638.
18. Fiatarone MA, O'Neill EF, Ryan ND, et al. Exercise training and nutritional supplementation for physical frailty in very elderly people. *N Engl J Med.* 1994;330:1769-1775.
19. Kushner I. Regulation of the acute phase response by cytokines. *Perspect Biol Med.* 1993;36:611-622.
20. Bistrian BR, Blackburn GL, Hallowell E, Heddle R. Protein status of general surgical patients. *JAMA.* 1974;230:858-860.
21. Abbasi AA, Rudman D. Observations on the prevalence of protein-calorie undernutrition in VA nursing homes. *J Am Geriatr Soc.* 1993;41:117-121.
22. Braun JV, Wykle MH, Cowling WR III. Failure to thrive in older persons: a concept derived. *Gerontologist.* 1988;28:809-812.
23. Lonergan ET. Extending life, enhancing life: a national research agenda on aging. Washington, DC: National Academy Press; 1991.
24. Sarkisian CA, Lachs MS. 'Failure to thrive' in older adults. *Ann Intern Med.* 1996;124:1072-1078.
25. Massry SG, Smogorzewski M. The hunger disease of the Warsaw Ghetto. *Am J Nephrol.* 2002;22:197-201.
26. Winick M (ed). *Hunger Disease: Studies by the Jewish Physicians in the Warsaw Ghetto.* New York: John Wiley and Sons; 1979.
27. Galetta F, Franzoni F, Prattichizzo F, Rolla M, Santoro G, Pentimone F. Heart rate variability and left ventricular diastolic function in anorexia nervosa. *J Adolesc Health.* 2003;32:416-421.
28. Isner JM, Roberts WC, Heymsfield SB, Yager J. Anorexia nervosa and sudden death. *Ann Intern Med.* 1985;102:49-52.
29. Thurston J, Marks P. Electrocardiographic abnormalities in patients with anorexia nervosa. *Br Heart J.* 1974;36:719-723.
30. Gottdiener JS, Gross HA, Henry WL, Borer JS, Ebert MH. Effects of self induced starvation on cardiac size and function in anorexia nervosa. *Circulation.* 1978;58:425-433.
31. Doekel RC, Zwillich CW, Scoggin CH, et al. Clinical semi-starvation: depression of hypoxic ventilatory response. *N Engl J Med.* 1976;295:358-361.

32. Levenson SM, Crowley LV, Seifter E. Starvation. In: Ballinger WF, Collins JA, Drucker WR, et al, eds. *Manual of Surgical Nutrition*. Philadelphia: WB Saunders; 1975, 236-264.
33. Deitch EA. The role of intestinal barrier failure and bacterial translocation in the development of systemic infection and multiple organ failure. *Arch Surg*. 1990;125:403-4.
34. Hernandez G, Velasco N, Wainstein C, et al. Gut mucosal atrophy after a short enteral fasting period in critically ill patients. *J Crit Care*. 1999;14:73-77.
35. Sheldon GF, Petersen SR. Malnutrition and cardiopulmonary function: relation to oxygen transport. *JPEN*. 1980;4:376-383.
36. Demas GE, Drazen DL, Nelson, RJ. Reductions in total body fat decrease humoral immunity. *Proc R Soc Lond B Biol Sci*. 2003;270:905-911.
37. Nova E, Samartin S, Gomez S, Morande G, Marcos A. The adaptive response of the immune system to the particular malnutrition of eating disorders. *Eur J Clin Nutr*. 2002;56(Suppl 3):S34-S37.
38. Chandra RK. Nutrition, immunity, and infection: from basic knowledge of dietary manipulation of immune responses to practical application of ameliorating suffering and improving survival. *Proc Natl Acad Sci*. 1996;93:14304-14307.
39. Edelman R. Cell mediated immune response in protein calorie malnutrition: a review. In: Suskind RM, ed. *Malnutrition and the Immune Response*. New York: Raven Press; 1977:47-75.
40. Baker CC, Hohn DC. Sepsis in trauma patients (trauma rounds-San Francisco General Hospital). *West J Med*. 1979;130:378-383.
41. Lewis RT, Klein H. Risk factors in postoperative sepsis: significance of preoperative lymphocytopenia. *J Surg Res*. 1979;26:365-371.
42. Smythe PM, Schonland M, Brereton-Stiles GG, et al. Thymolymphatic deficiency and depression of cell mediated immunity in protein calorie malnutrition. *Lancet*. 1979;2:939-944.
43. Bistrian BR, Sherman M, Blackburn GL, et al. Cellular immunity in adult marasmus. *Arch Intern Med*. 1977;137:1408-1411.
44. Law DK, Dudrick SJ, Abdou Ni. Immunocompetence of patients with protein calorie malnutrition: the effects of nutritional repletion. *Ann Intern Med*. 1973;79:545-550.
45. Law DK, Dudrick SJ, Abdou NI. The effect of protein calorie malnutrition on immune competence of the surgical patient. *Surg Gynecol Obstet*. 1974;139:257-266.
46. Parke DV, Ioannides C. The role of nutrition in toxicology. *Ann Rev Nutr*. 1981;1:207-234.
47. Roe DA. Nutrient and drug interactions. In: *Nutrition Reviews' Present Knowledge in Nutrition*. 5th ed. Washington, DC: The Nutrition Foundation, Inc; 1984:797-818.
48. Rhoads JE, Fliegelman MT, Panzer LM. The mechanism of delayed wound healing in the presence of hypoproteinemia. *JAMA*. 1942;118:21-24.
49. Levenson S, Seifter E, Van Winkle W. Nutrition. In: Hunt TK, Dunphy JE, ed. *Fundamentals of Wound Management*. New York, Appleton Century Crofts; 1979:286-363.
50. Ruberg RL. Role of nutrition in wound healing. *Surg Clin N Am*. 1984;64:705-714.
51. Thompson WD, Ravdin IS, Frank IL. Effect of hypoproteinemia on wound disruption. *Arch Surg*. 1938;36:500-508.
52. Irvin TT. Effects of malnutrition and hyperalimentation on wound healing. *Surg Gynecol Obstet*. 1978;146:33-37.
53. Ward DW, Danzi M, Lewin MR, et al. The effects of subclinical malnutrition and refeeding on the healing of experimental colonic anastomoses. *Br J Surg*. 1982;69:308-310.
54. Engelen M, Wouters E, Deutz N, Menheere P, Schols A. Factors contributing to alterations in skeletal muscle and plasma amino acid profiles in patients with chronic obstructive pulmonary disease. *Am J Clin Nutr*. 2000;72:1480-1487.
55. Perioperative total parenteral nutrition in surgical patients. The Veterans Affairs Total Parenteral Nutrition Cooperative Study Group. *N Engl J Med*. 1991;325:525-532.
56. Rubinson L, Diette GB, Song X, Brower RG, Krishnan JA. Low caloric intake is associated with nosocomial bloodstream infections in patients in the medical intensive care unit. *Crit Care Med*. 2004;32:350-357.
57. Anderson GF, Steinberg EP. Hospital readmissions in the Medicare population. *N Engl J Med*. 1984;311:1349-1353.
58. Friedmann JM, Jensen GL, Smiciklas-Wright H, McCamish MA. Predicting early nonelective hospital readmission in nutritionally compromised older adults. *Am J Clin Nutr*. 1997;65:1714-1720.
59. Sullivan DH. Risk factors for early hospital readmission in a select population of geriatric rehabilitation patients: the significance of nutritional status. *J Am Geriatr Soc*. 1992;40:792-798.
60. Sullivan DH, Walls RC, Bopp MM. Protein energy undernutrition and the risk of mortality within one year of hospital discharge: a follow up study. *J Am Geriatr Soc*. 1995;43:507-512.
61. Sullivan DH, Walls RC, Lipschitz DA. Protein energy undernutrition and the risk of mortality within 1 year of hospital discharge in a select population of geriatric rehabilitation patients. *Am J Clin Nutr*. 1991;53:599-605.
62. Pouw EM, Ten Velde GPM, Croonen B, Kester A, Schols A, Wouters E. Early non elective readmission for chronic obstructive pulmonary disease is associated with weight loss. *Clin Nutr*. 2000;19:95-99.
63. Doweiko JP, Nompleggi DJ. The role of albumin in human physiology and pathophysiology: III. Albumine and disease states. *JPEN*. 1991;15:476-483.
64. Rall C, Roubenoff R, Harris T. Albumin as a marker of nutritional and health status. In: Rosenberg IH, ed. *Nutritional Assessment of Elderly Populations: Measure and Function*. New York, NY: Raven Press; 1991.
65. Rothschild MA, Oratz M, Schreiber SS. Serum albumin. *Hepatology*. 1988;8:385-401.
66. Cooper BA, Penne EL, Bartlett LH, Pollock CA. Protein malnutrition and hypoalbuminemia as predictors of vascular events and mortality in ESRD. *Am J Kidney Dis*. 2004;43:61-66.
67. Eustace JA, Astor B, Muntner PM, Ikizler TA, Coresh J. Prevalence of acidosis and inflammation and their association with low serum albumin in chronic kidney disease. *Kidney Int*. 2004;65:1031-1040.
68. Oberg BP, McMenamin E, Lucas FL, McMonagle E, Morrow J, Ikizler TA, Himmelfarb J. Increased prevalence of oxidant stress and inflammation in patients with moderate to severe chronic kidney disease. *Kidney Int*. 2004;65:1009-1016.
69. Landbo C, Prescott E, Lange P, Jorgen V, Almdal T. Prognostic value of nutritional status in chronic obstructive pulmonary disease. *Am J Respir Crit Care Med*. 1999;160:1856-1861.
70. Haskell CM, Girman TL. *Nutrition Cancer Treatment*. 5th ed. Philadelphia, PA: WB Saunders Company; 2001.
71. Inui A. Cancer anorexia cachexia syndrome: current issues in research and management. *CA Cancer J Clin*. 2002;52:72-91.
72. Jatoi A, Loprinzi CL, Sloan JA, Klee GG, Windschiti HE. Neuropeptide Y, Leptin, and Cholecystokinin 8 in patients with advanced cancer and anorexia. *Cancer*. 2001;92:629-633.
73. Corcoran C, Grinspoon S. Treatments for wasting in patients with the acquired immunodeficiency syndrome. *N Engl J Med*. 1999;340:1740-1750.
74. Bastow MD, Rawlings J, Allison SP. Undernutrition, hypothermia, and injury in elderly women with fractured femur: an injury response to altered metabolism? *Lancet*. 1983;1(8317):143-146.
75. Stableforth PG. Supplement feeds and nitrogen and calorie balance following femoral neck fracture. *Br J Surg*. 1986;73:651-655.
76. Sullivan DH, Moriarty MS, Chernoff R, Lipschitz DA. Patterns of care: an analysis of the quality of nutritional care routinely provided to elderly hospitalized veterans. *JPEN*. 1989;13:249-254.
77. Bastow MD, Rawlings J, Allison SP. Benefits of supplementary tube feeding after fractured neck of femur: a randomized controlled trial. *Br Med J*. 1983;278:1589-1592.
78. Delmi M, Rapin CH, Bengoa JM, Delmas PD, Vasey H, Bonjour JP. Dietary supplementation in elderly patients with fractured neck of the femur. *Lancet*. 1990;335:1013-1016.
79. Gallagher J, Schermbeck J, Dixon L, Labbe-Bell M. Aggressive early management of malnutrition in hip fracture patients (abstract). *JPEN*. 1992;16:19S.

80. Foster MR, Heppenstall RB, Friedenberg ZB, Hozack WJ. A prospective assessment of nutritional status and complications in patients with fractures of the hip. *J Orthop Trauma*. 1990;4:49-57.

81. Sullivan DH, Patch GA, Walls RC, Lipschitz DA. Impact of nutritional status on morbidity and mortality in a select population of geriatric rehabilitation patients. *Am J Clin Nutr*. 1990;51:749-758.

Chapter 5

The Malabsorption Syndrome

Robert Craig, MD

Introduction

Malabsorption of nutrients can be classified by different formats; however, the most useful is in terms of the major categories "maldigestion" and "primary small intestinal absorptive defect." Maldigestion refers to improper breaking down and solubilizing the nutrients into components that can be absorbed readily across the intestinal microvilli. Bile salts are the most important solubilizers, which allow for fat digestion and proper delivery to the small intestinal mucosa. Breaking down the macromolecules into small components is accomplished by digestive enzymes secreted by the salivary glands, the stomach, the small intestine, and the pancreas; gastric acid secretion; and the grinding effect of the stomach. Therefore, maldigestion can occur from gastric, hepatobiliary, pancreatic, or small intestinal causes. Clinically, the two most common categories of maldigestion are pancreatic insufficiency and small intestinal bacterial overgrowth (SIBO). The most common primary intestinal causes for malabsorption are celiac disease in the United States and tropical sprue throughout the world. A malabsorption evaluation categorizes the defect into these three broad areas: pancreatic insufficiency, SIBO, and primary intestinal. Further evaluation characterizes the absorptive defect more specifically to allow for appropriate therapy.

Normal Absorption

The site in the human body at which a nutrient is absorbed impacts the physiology and pathophysiology of absorption. Most nutrients are primarily absorbed in the jejunum; these include water, electrolytes, water-soluble vitamins, minerals, fat-soluble vitamins, glycerol, fatty acids, cholesterol, carbohydrates, amino acids, and small peptides. Iron is preferentially absorbed in the duodenum. Bile salts and vitamin B12 are actively absorbed in the ileum. The ileum can partially take over all of the functions of the jejunum if the jejunum is lost; however, the proximal small bowel cannot reciprocate for ileal loss, as there is no active transport of bile salts and vitamin B12 in the jejunum or duodenum.

Water and sodium-chloride absorption occur by both active sodium absorptive processes across the enterocyte, with secondary solvent drag of water, and passive processes, mostly paracellularly. Minerals are absorbed both actively via carrier mechanisms and passively by mass action. Calcium absorption is controlled by vitamin D and parathormone and is actively absorbed by a carrier mechanism. Iron is preferentially absorbed in the reduced form, also by a carrier mechanism, although heme iron is the most readily absorbed. The importance of the duodenum in iron absorption is underscored by the high frequency of iron malabsorption when the duodenum is bypassed surgically. Iron is also more readily absorbed when there is normal acid secretion from the stomach, which makes dietary iron more available.

Water-soluble vitamins are also absorbed by both carrier-mediated and passive mechanisms. Fat-soluble vitamins require bile salts and mixed micelle formation for their transport to the small intestinal microvilli and absorption. Fat-soluble vitamins and cholesterol reside in the central lipid core of mixed micelles. Cholestatic syndromes make malabsorption of fat-soluble vitamins a clinical problem because of insufficient bile salt delivery to the small intestine.

Most carbohydrate absorption requires extensive digestion before the smaller components can be absorbed by the small intestine. Starch requires digestion into glucose by salivary and pancreatic amylases and amylopectins. Lactose and sucrose require mucosal digestion by the small intestinal mucosal disaccharidases, lactase and sucrase-isomaltase, respectively. Glucose is absorbed predominantly by a co-transport mechanism with sodium, which is the basis for the oral rehydration solutions used in diarrheal diseases. Fructose and galactose are also absorbed by carrier-mediated processes. A small amount of disaccharide absorption occurs by the paracellular route and is not dependent upon active transport processes. Lactulose, a disaccharide of galactose and fructose, is mostly malabsorbed, but it is absorbed to an increased extent by the paracellular route in circumstances in which the intestinal mucosa is "leaky." This physiological principle has been the basis for clinical testing of leakiness of the small intestine. D-xylose is a monosaccharide that is absorbed predominantly passively across the small intestinal enterocyte. Its incomplete absorption under normal circumstances has allowed it to be used in a good clinical tolerance test for small intestinal absorptive capacity.[1] Its absorption is also diminished in SIBO (see below, clinical testing).[2] Lactose malabsorption is perhaps the most common worldwide malabsorption disease, because of incomplete digestion of lactose into its component monosaccharides, glucose and galactose. The maldigestion is a result of an inadequate amount of the villous, brush border disaccharidase, lactase. Sucrase/isomaltase deficiency has also been described and may be a more common problem than was originally believed, being responsible for increased flatulence, diarrhea, and some irritable bowel symptoms.

Lipid absorption is a more complex process than carbohydrate absorption. Long-chain triglycerides (LCTs) require solubilization by bile salts, digestion into fatty acids and glycerol by pancreatic lipase, incorporation into mixed micelles by bile salts, traversing the unstirred water layer of the small intestine, carrier-mediated uptake into the enterocyte, repackaging into lipoproteins, and delivery into the lacteals and thence into the thoracic duct. A disturbance of bile salt solubilization secondary to decreased bile salt delivery or SIBO (see below), diminished pancreatic function with insufficient delivery of pancreatic lipase, or inadequate small intestinal capacity result in fat malabsorption and steatorrhea. Medium-chain triglycerides (MCTs) are absorbed with more alacrity than are long chain fatty acids and are delivered into the venous system and the portal vein. Cholesterol is solubilized within the mixed micelles in the lipid central component, as are fat-soluble vitamins.

Protein digestion involves the measured release of proenzymes from the pancreas, activation of the proenzymes in the small intestine by the small intestinal brush border enzyme enterokinase, and digestion of the proteins into smaller peptides. Further digestion occurs at the brush border by peptidases, resulting in amino acids, di-peptides, and tri-peptides. Specific carrier-mediated processes promote absorption into the enterocyte. Quantitatively, absorption of di-peptides may exceed or equal the absorption of individual amino acids.

The entire absorptive process is carefully regulated. Acid from the stomach stimulates duodenal secretin release, which induces a bicarbonate rich pancreatic solution delivered to the small intestine, providing the appropriate milieu for digestion. Fats and proteins stimulate duodenal release of cholecystokinin (CCK), which induces gall bladder contraction and delivery of bile salts into the duodenum. CCK also stimulates the release of pancreatic proteinases and lipases. These pro-enzymes are activated by the enterocyte enterokinase, and the activation of trypsin from trypsinogen promotes further activation of the other pro-enzymes. The presence of activated enzymes within the duodenum enlists a feedback loop, which damps pancreatic secretion. Neurogenic and motility processes are also engaged in this process.

The processes of normal absorption are discussed in greater detail in Chapter 8 of this book.

Malabsorption Syndrome

Malabsorption can be isolated to selective substances, such as lactose secondary to insufficient intestinal disaccaridase or iron in celiac disease. These specific abnormalities may be the only manifestation of malabsorption in the individual. However, discussions of malabsorption syndrome typically refer to fat malabsorption. Malabsorption syndromes usually have multiple components, including impaired carbohydrate and protein digestion and diminished mineral and vitamin absorption. Fat malabsorption results in large, bulky, malodorous stools that may have accompanying visible oil in the toilet water. The amount of diarrhea is variable, dependent upon the individual's colonic bacterial flora and its capacity to metabolized the malabsorbed fats to hydroxy-fatty acids, which can invoke a secretory diarrhea. The patient may note that he or she has lost weight, in spite of eating well and with good appetite. Increased flatulence ensues because of malabsorbed carbohydrates, which provide the fuel for colonic bacteria fermentation. The increased intestinal gas may result in gas cramping in susceptible patients, and often patients complain of unpleasant, post-prandial, abdominal bloating. Floating stools are a result of the presence of fecal gas not fat. With progression of the disease, systemic symptoms of fatigue, listlessness, and diminished well-being ensue. Physical examination might reveal little: the patient may appear pale and may have some abdominal distention and mild abdominal tenderness. Often, however, the signs and symptoms are subtle, and the practitioner must suspect the illness on the basis of little data. Frequently, a malabsorptive evaluation is embarked upon because of laboratory abnormalities.

Laboratory findings are variable. The patient may be anemic; iron deficiency anemia is, at this time, probably the most common presentation for celiac disease. Evidence of osteopenia or osteomalacia may be evident if vitamin D levels are measured or if a bone densitometry is obtained. Occasionally, liver abnormalities can be present in cystic fibrosis and celiac disease or with severe protein calorie malnutrition. The serum albumin may be low, especially in the presence of protein-losing enteropathy. Malabsorption of vitamin K would result in prolongation of the prothrombin time.

Most malabsorption syndromes are due to problems within the three categories: SIBO, pancreatic insufficiency,

TABLE 5-1.

Categories of Fat Malabsorption

Process	*Primary Absorptive Mechanism*	*Clinical Example*
Digestion	Lipolysis	Pancreatic insufficiency
Solubilization	Bile salt solubility	Small intestinal bacterial overgrowth
Absorption	Enterocyte capacity	Celiac disease

and intrinsic small intestinal disease. These categories also correspond to abnormalities in the major processes involved in absorption: solubilization, digestion, and enterocyte absorption, respectively (Table 5-1). The diagnostic evaluation proceeds along the lines of distinguishing among these three entities.

Malabsorptive Testing

A variety of tests can be used to indicate malabsorption. At times, the results of the measurements are inconclusive for malabsorption and must be accompanied by additional evaluation. Tests include small-bowel radiographs (which indicate structural defects); a 72-hour assessment of fecal fat (including Sudan staining); sugar-intolerance testing including D-xylose testing (which measures jejunal integrity and bacterial overgrowth); pancreatic testing, including endoscopic pancreatography; and the Schilling test (which assesses ileal function and bacterial overgrowth). These laboratory tests are discussed below.

Small-Bowel Radiographs

Small intestinal radiographs may show fragmentation of the barium column because of dilution, and effacement of the normal mucosal pattern of sharp valvulae conniventes can be seen in intrinsic small intestinal disease (Figure 5-1). However, these findings are nonspecific. The major value of small intestinal radiographs is to elucidate structural defects, such as Bilroth II hemigastrectomy, small intestinal diverticula, or intestinal narrowing. These structural defects would be responsible for SIBO.

Fecal Fat Assessment

The "gold standard" test for fat malabsorption is the 72-hour collection of stool for fat. Simpler tests such as Sudan stain of the stool for fat globules can be employed, but the technician must be well trained to distinguish normal from abnormal fat presence. Up to 8% of fat can be malabsorbed normally on a 100-g fat diet. Therefore, it must always be a quantitative determination. If the technician has been trained to use suitable controls to distinguish the sizes of fat globules and relate them quantitatively to the amount of fecal fat, then Sudan staining may be employed.

Another caveat in stool fat determinations is the necessity to relate the amount of fat in the stool to dietary fat. Because percentage malabsorption is the critical determination, a low fecal fat level in someone who is consuming little fat in his or her diet would have little meaning. Conversely, a slightly elevated fecal fat content would be normal in someone consuming 200 g of fat daily. Other tests that label fats and measure digestive products in the urine have come in and out of favor, and, for the most part, have not had their validity demonstrated.REF

Sugar-Tolerance Tests

Sugar tolerance tests are also used in a malabsorption evaluation. The lactose tolerance test involves the oral ingestion of lactose and measurement of serum glucose every half hour for 90 minutes. The serum glucose should rise 20 mg/dl above baseline if sufficient galactose and glucose are split from lactose. Often H2 breath testing is employed with the lactose tolerance test; however, some have questioned breath testing, as suitable controls have often not been used in establishing the validity of the results.

Another effective sugar tolerance test is the D-xylose test. D-xylose is a monosaccharide found normally in plants. It is passively absorbed across the enterocyte. In the normal subject, it is partially absorbed, partially metabolized by the liver, and partially excreted in the urine. In spite of these aspects, it is a reasonably good test of enterocyte functional mass. To conduct the test, 25 g of D-xylose is administered orally to the patient, and 5-hour urine contents and 1-hour serum concentrations of D-xylose are measured. Low levels are also found in SIBO, but are normal in patients with pancreatic insufficiency. Because levels can be abnormal in two of the major absorptive categories and normal in one, the test is useful in distinguishing the cause of malabsorption.

Pancreatic Testing

Unfortunately, no sensitive pancreatic malabsorption test currently exists that is not cumbersome. Although the duodenal drainage test with secretin and CCK stimulation is the "gold standard" for pancreatic insufficiency, it is rarely performed because of its difficulty. Tolerance tests, such as the bentiromide test, are theoretically attractive and easy to perform; however, they lack sensitivity and are abnormal only with severe pancreatic disease. One can perform a 72-hour fecal fat test before and after a therapeutic trial of pancreatic enzymes, which will give reliable information, although collection of the 72 hours of stool is unpleasant. Additionally patients may undergo endoscopic pancreatography, which delineates abnormal pancreatic ducts in patients with chronic pancreatitis.

Schilling Test

Ileal function can be tested by using a strategy dependent upon its known active absorption of vitamin B12 and bile salts. The Schilling test employs labeled vitamin B12 taken orally by the patient, followed by a 24-hour urine collection for the label. By using differential testing with and without gastric intrinsic factor and pre and post antibiotics, an abnormal test can distinguish among a gastric lesion, SIBO, and ileal disease. The test will be abnormal when there is insufficient active transport (ileal function) or when the vitamin B12 is bound or metabolized by small intestinal bacteria. The test can be used in concert with the D-xylose test, as the Schilling test is abnormal in patients with SIBO but normal in those with proximal small bowel disease, such as celiac sprue.

Another test that has come into disfavor also uses the physiology of ileal absorption. Bile salts with a nuclear label on the conjugate (glycine or taurine) are malabsorbed and spill into the colon excessively when there is diminished ileal capacity. The colonic bacteria metabolizes the conjugate, resulting in an increased amount of labeled CO_2 expelled in the breath, which can be measured. In addition, there is increased catabolism of the bile salts in the presence of SIBO. Therefore, the glycine labeled bile salt test will be abnormal in patients with SIBO or ileal dysfunction.

Malabsorption-Specific Case Studies

Pancreatic Malabsorption

Case Study

A 50-year-old female who consumes alcohol heavily complains of constipation and weight loss. On careful questioning, it is clear that her concept of constipation is the passage of one large, greasy, noisome stool daily. She does not complain of abdominal pain. Pancreatic malabsorption is suspected.

Abdominal radiographs show pancreatic calcifications. Baseline laboratory studies are normal. She submits a 72-hour fecal fat analysis that shows 30 g daily on a 100-g fat diet. A Schilling test is performed with a result of 10% (normal >7 %). A D-xylose test yields a 1-hour serum D-xylose of 40 mg/dl (normal >25 mg/dl) and a 5-hour content of 8 g (normal >4 g). She is started on an enterically coated pancreatic supplement with meals and snacks, and, as a result, her stools become normal and she regains her weight. She enters an alcohol treatment program and is currently a recovering alcoholic. A repeat 72-hour fecal fat determination is improved to 15 g daily.

Discussion

Although this patient's case is rather straightforward, it illustrates a number of important clinical points. The elevated fecal fat content confirms malabsorption. The normal Schilling test and D-xylose absorption pinpoint the diagnosis to be pancreatic malabsorption. The pancreatic calcifications further corroborate this diagnosis. It was not necessary to perform the pancreatic stimulation test with secretin/CCK stimulation or to perform an endoscopic pancreatogram.

Her improvement with pancreatic supplements confirms the diagnosis. Enterically coated pancreatic supplements are necessary, as gastric acid destroys orally administered pancreatic enzymes. An alternative strategy would be to give agents to diminish acid secretion concurrently with the pancreatic supplements.

Pancreatic insufficiency can be caused by familial, alcoholic, and idiopathic pancreatitis; hemochromatosis; cystic fibrosis; and post resection for carcinoma of the pancreas. A total pancreatectomy will clearly produce pancreatic insufficiency, although a 90% pancreatectomy with a Whipple procedure may leave the patient with enough pancreatic function to prevent pancreatic malabsorption. If weight loss ensues following pancreatic surgery, a therapeutic trial of pancreatic enzyme replacement is always reasonable. Alcoholic and idiopathic chronic pancreatitis are two relatively common causes of pancreatic insufficiency. However, biliary tract disease with acute pancreatitis rarely results in pancreatic insufficiency. The congenital disorders, cystic fibrosis and hemochromatosis, are also important causes of pancreatic malabsorption.

Intrinsic Small Intestinal Absorptive Defects

Case Study

A 30-year-old female presents with mild gaseous distention and increased flatulence. She has no weight loss or diarrhea. Her menses are normal. Her physical examination is normal. Specifically, her abdomen is soft and nontender, with no organomegaly. Bowel sounds are normal. Stool on rectal examination is negative for occult blood. Her serum multi-organ chemistry panel and urinalysis are normal. Her hemoglobin is 10 g/dl, but her white blood cell (WBC) and platelet counts are normal. Her serum ferritin is 10 mcg/dl and iron saturation is 5%.

Although it would not be unreasonable to treat her with oral iron, her gastrointestinal (GI) symptoms prompt her physician to order a serologic test for celiac sprue, the endomysial antibody, which is elevated at a titer of 1:160. A small bowel biopsy is performed confirming gluten-sensitive enteropathy (GSE) (Figures 5-1 and 5-2). A small bowel radiograph is also obtained, and it is normal. The patient is placed on a gluten-free diet, and her flatulence and iron deficiency resolve.

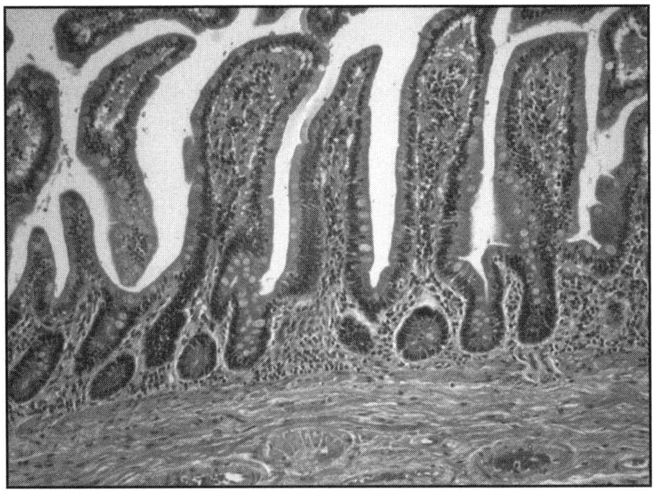

Figure 5-1. Small intestinal biopsy showing normal histology. Note that the villi lengths are greater than twice the crypt depths. The epithelial cells are columnar and the brush border is apparent. There are few intraepithelial lymphocytes. The number of lamina propria lymphocytes is normal. H and E x 150.

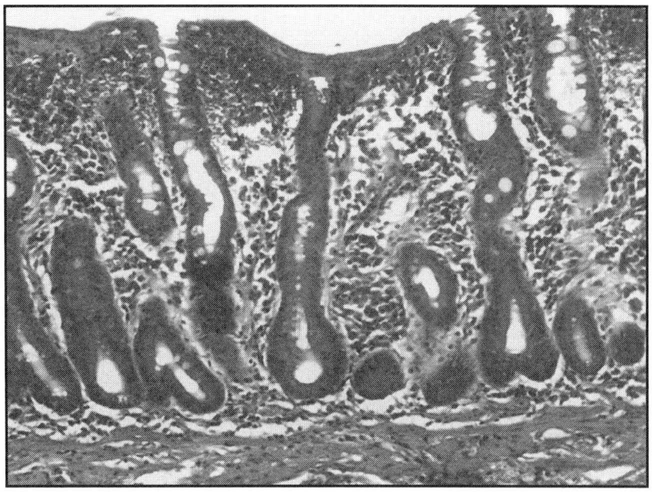

Figure 5-2. Small intestinal biopsy showing absent villi, cuboidal epithelial cells with increased intraepithelial lymphocytes, exuberant lamina propria inflammation, and deep crypts. H. and E x 150.

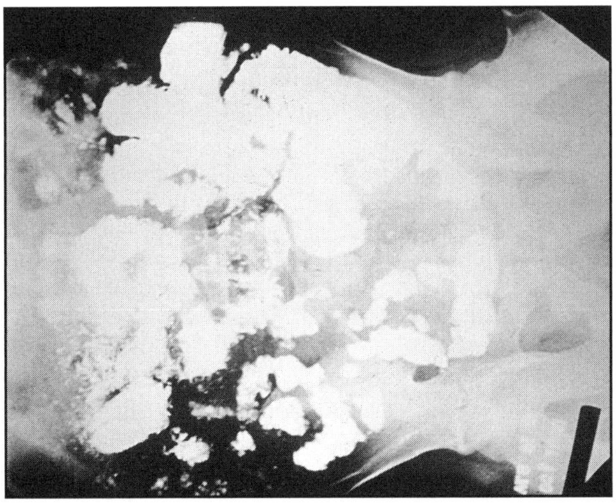

Figure 5-3. Small intestinal radiograph showing dilution of the barium column, fragmentation, and loss of the normal pattern of the valvulae conniventes.

Discussion

Most patients with GSE present relatively silently, as this patient did. Often the only manifestation is iron deficiency anemia due to iron malabsorption. GSE is a proximal small intestinal disease, affecting the duodenum more prominently than it does the jejunum, and the preferred site for iron absorption is the duodenum. Another subtle presentation for GSE is osteopenia, related to vitamin D and/or calcium malabsorption. Our patient's presentation with increased flatus is related to carbohydrate malabsorption, which is responsible for flatus in the normal and abnormal state. When the disease is more fulminant, bulky or greasy stools may be evident from steatorrhea, or frank diarrhea may be present. When the case is more severe, weight loss, anemia, and hypoalbuminemia ensue. The hypoalbuminemia is due to protein-losing enteropathy, which attends more severe disease.

The clinical evaluation of small intestinal intrinsic disease would typically show an abnormal D-xylose test, although our index patient did not require it because her endomysial antibody was abnormal. In addition, a 72-hour fecal fat collection was not required, as the diagnosis could be obtained with a small bowel biopsy. Most physicians will conduct a small bowel biopsy by panendoscopy because of the procedure's ease and reliability. Four specimens from the descending duodenum are necessary if GSE is to be excluded, and orientation is not required. Often the diagnosis is suggested by the endoscopic appearance of scalloping or blunting of the valvulae conniventes. Small intestinal radiographs are not generally required for diagnosing GSE, and they may be normal in milder disease, as in index patient. More severe disease yields dilution of the barium, effacement of the valvulae conniventes, and separation of the barium column (Figure 5-3). These findings are nonspecific and may be seen in other mucosal small intestinal diseases.

There has been considerable progress in the understanding of GSE since the seminal observation by Dicke over 50 years ago that the removal of grains containing gluten from the diet promotes resolution of symptoms and signs of celiac disease.[3] Overwhelming data support the pathogenesis of GSE to be immunologically mediated, probably autoimmune, induced by T-cell recognition of and activation by epitopes on gluten with subsequent, predominantly Th1-mediated autoreactivity against small intestinal enterocytes.[4,5] As in other autoimmune diseases, there is a susceptibility factor for GSE, expressed by the strong genetic association with HLA-DQ2 alleles.[6,7] The putative gluten peptides bind to the HLA locus, allowing for T-cell activation. This binding may be enhanced by tissue transglutaminase, which can deamidate glutamine residues on the gluten peptide to the more negatively charged glutamic acid.[8] It is also noteworthy that the target of the antibody to endomysium, which is present in most patients with GSE, is tissue transglutaminase.[9]

Table 5-2.

Intrinsic Small Intestinal Malabsorptive Diseases

Gluten-sensitive enteropathy
Tropical sprue
Giardiasis
AIDS enteropathy
Cryptosporidiosis
Mycobacterium avium complex
Ulcerating ileojejunitis
Collagenous sprue
Small intestinal T-cell lymphoma
Whipple's disease
Intestinal lymphangiectasia
Amyloidosis

Marsh has been instrumental in defining the histologic abnormalities that occur with gluten enteropathy and gluten sensitivity. He has described some patients who have lamina propia lymphocytosis (Marsh 1 lesions) and crypt hyperplasia without villous atrophy (Marsh 2 lesions) and has considered these groups sub clinical or pre-celiac disease.[10,11] Some have suggested that these lesions are not sub clinical and do indeed produce symptoms. Further, it has been suggested that some patients have symptoms secondary to gluten who have normal small bowel biopsies but have other manifestations of gluten damage, such as those with dermatitis herpetiformis.[12] Others have discussed similarities between GSE and irritable bowel syndrome: that symptoms are similar and that some patients with presumed irritable bowel have evidence of GSE serologically and histologically.[13]

GSE requires strict observation of a gluten-free diet for histologic remission to ensue. The patient's serologic markers will gradually return to normal with strict adherence to the diet, and the markers can be used to assess compliance. Not only will the patient experience resolution of his or her clinical symptoms with this dietary exclusion, but he or she will also markedly diminish risk of secondary malignancy, particularly GI lymphoma. The initial small intestinal biopsy and clinical presentation of GI lymphoma may mimic GSE; therefore, a repeat small intestinal biopsy may be required in those who do not do well with gluten restriction. Other rare complications of GSE include a severe ulcerating inflammatory process, ulcerating ileojejunitis, and collagenous sprue. The latter is a progressive small intestinal malabsorptive disorder with submucosal collagen thickening. Neither ulcerating ileojejunitis nor collagenous sprue respond well to a gluten-free diet. Corticosteroid or immunosuppressive therapy has been reported to be successful in some patients with ulcerating ileojejunitis.

Worldwide, tropical sprue is probably the most common intrinsic small intestinal malabsorptive disorder. It occurs in tropical areas, particularly in the far East. Because antibacterial therapy successfully treats patients with this disorder, it is presumably due to an overgrowth of small intestinal bacteria. However, there are distinct differences between tropical sprue and the classic SIBO syndromes. In tropical sprue, both folic-acid and vitamin-B12 absorption diminish, whereas folic-acid absorption is normal to elevated in SIBO. Further, the small intestinal biopsy of patients with tropical sprue is abnormal, showing prominent villous blunting and crypt hypertrophy, although not to the same degree as seen in GSE. On the other hand, SIBO generally does not present with significant small intestinal biopsy abnormalities. Treatment of tropical sprue with folic acid and vitamin B12 alone will bring about clinical restitution, so long as the patient is removed from the endemic area.

In the United States, GSE is by far the most common intrinsic small intestinal disease yielding malabsorption. Table 5-2 shows some other intrinsic small intestinal malabsorptive disorders, many simply curiosities because they are so rare. Acquired immunodeficiency syndrome (AIDS) enteropathy is a malabsorptive syndrome with profound D-xylose and vitamin B12 malabsorption, characterized by severe diarrhea. Small intestinal biopsies, however, show relatively mild abnormalities. Giardiasis may occur in either immunocompromised or normal hosts and can present with mild malabsorption. Other small intestinal parasites occur in patients with AIDS, including cryptosporidiosis and mycobacterium avian complex, and may produce severe diarrhea and malabsorption. Whipple's disease is a rare generalized disorder caused by a specific bacterial organism that predominantly affects the intestine, lymph nodes, and nervous system. Characteristic PAS positive macrophages may be identified in the lamina propria of patients with this disorder. Prolonged antibiotic treatment produces remission.

Small Intestinal Bacterial Overgrowth

Case Study

A 50-year-old female presents with Raynaud's syndrome, calcinosis cutis in her arms, heartburn, and weight loss. She has noted increased abdominal bloating and infrequent stool passages culminated after a few days by massive liquid bowel movements. Her physical examination shows sclerodactyly, evidence of muscle wasting, and a protuberant, tympanitic abdomen. Bowel sounds are sparse but high pitched. Her hemoglobin is 10.0 g/dl,

TABLE 5-3.

Categories and Individual Causes for Small Intestinal Bacterial Overgrowth

Category	*Disease State*
Hypochlorhydria	Pernicious anemia Aging AIDS Proton pump inhibitors
Anatomic blind loop	Billroth II partial gastrectomy or other surgical blind loop Small intestinal diverticula Intestinal obstruction or stricture
Fistulae	Gastrocolic Crohn's disease Irradiation enteritis
Small intestinal hypomotility	Scleroderma, CREST Pseudo-obstruction Diabetes mellitus

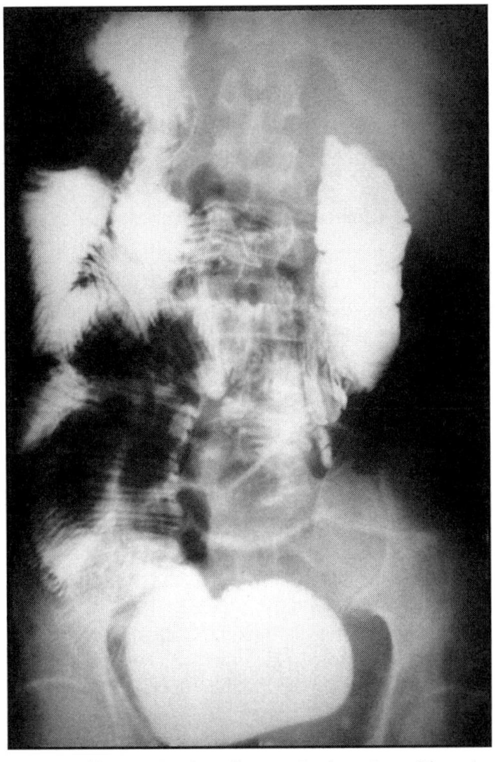

Figure 5-4. Small intestinal radiograph showing dilatation of multiple barium-filled loops of small bowel consistent with small intestinal pseudo-obstruction.

WBC count is normal, and serum albumin is 2.5 g/dl. The remaining serum chemistries on a multiorgan chemistry panel are normal. An abdominal radiograph shows multiple loops of dilated small intestine, and the barium takes greater than 24 hours to reach the cecum, yet there is no obvious obstructing point (Figure 5-4). A D-xylose absorption test shows the 5-hour D-xylose urine content to be 1.2 g (normal ≥4.0), and the 1-hour serum D-xylose concentration 7 mg/dl (normal ≥25.0), following a 25-g oral dose.

SIBO is found in many conditions and may present with malabsorption, diarrhea, and malnutrition. Whereas dietary modifications and supplements might help, the primary treatment strategy is the judicious use of antibiotics. The most effective antibiotics, shown either empirically or by clinical trials, are the quinolones, tetracycline, amoxycillin/clavulanic acid, clindamycin, and metronidazole. Some patients may fail to respond to one of these antibiotics but will respond to a second. These conditions are often chronic and require periodic or cyclical treatment. Surgical management is reserved for the select situations in which there is a clear-cut structural defect.

The SIBO syndrome is due to stasis within the small intestine, secondary to a segment of bowel out of continuity from the normal small intestinal flow or to hypomotility of the small intestine. Usually there are less than 10,000 bacteria per ml in the proximal small intestine; ileal counts may reach 103 per ml.[14,15] The most common categories and individual disease states that cause this disorder are outlined in Table 5-3. Anatomic blind loops and severe intestinal hypomotility are the usual causes of the clinical syndrome. However, most patients with diabetes mellitus and diarrhea do not have SIBO but have other causes for their diarrhea.

Usually hypochlorhydria or achlorhydria do not produce clinically important SIBO, although abnormal bacterial counts in the duodenum are common. The bacterial growth is attributed to the loss of the impeding effect of gastric acid on bacteria. Likewise, a significant proportion of patients receiving long-term protein pump inhibitors develop SIBO but do not display clinically apparent malabsorption.[16] Further, patients with AIDS can become hypochlorhydric, which results in SIBO. The elderly also frequently have increased bacterial counts in their proximal small intestine, usually related to hypochlorhydria, but do not have any apparent problem from the bacteria. Some have termed this "simple colonization of the elderly".[17] Similarly, the small intestinal contamination that sometimes accompanies pancreatic insufficiency probably does not produce clinical malabsorption by itself.[18]

The pathophysiology of the syndrome is because of the enteric bacteria binding, altering, or consuming nutritional or secreted substances in the small intestine. Carbohydrates, fats, proteins, and amino acids are metabolized; vitamin B12 is bound by or taken up by bacteria[19]; and bile salts are deconjugated.[20] The fermentation of carbohydrates leads to gas and bloating; the metabolism of nutrients leads to diminished absorption; the binding of vitamin B12 results in diminished B12 absorption; and the deconjugation of bile salts promotes passive absorption and short circuiting of unconjugated bile salts, eventuating in insufficient bile salts for proper solubilization of fats throughout the entire transit of the small intestine.

These absorptive abnormalities can be utilized in strategies for diagnosing the disease. Bacterial metabolism of carbohydrate yields abnormal D-xylose testing.[1,2] The Schilling test is abnormal because of vitamin B12 binding.[19] Fecal fat excretion is elevated because of insufficient bile salts for their appropriate absorption. Bile salt deconjugation can be seen with breath testing employing carbon labeled glycine conjugated bile salts.[20]

The "gold standard" for the diagnosis of SIGO is not well established, but the usual definition is 103 or greater bacterial colonies per ml of a sterile collection of duodenal or jejunal fluid.[21] Both aerobic and anaerobic cultures should be taken. In significant bacterial overgrowth syndromes, both aerobic and anaerobic cultures yield luxuriant growth. Bacteroides species, enterococci, anaerobic lactobacilli, and coliforms are frequently present.[21] The difficulties in obtaining small intestinal cultures have promoted the development of other tests, but none of the noninvasive tests has the equivalent sensitivity and specificity of the intestinal cultures.

General Management of Malabsorption

Identification of nutritional deficiencies and appropriate replacement are important measures in these patients. Screening tests for magnesium, calcium, iron, folic acid, vitamin B12, and occasionally other specific vitamins may be employed. Magnesium deficiency can occasionally be profound and requires parenteral therapy. It is difficult to replace magnesium orally in patients with diarrhea disorders. It is judicious to provide one multivitamin daily, which will replace most vitamin deficiencies. A prolonged prothrombin time indicates vitamin K malabsorption, which would require parenteral vitamin K administration. Cobalamin malabsorption can be corrected with monthly vitamin B12 injections and/or addition of vitamin B12 to parenteral formulations. Trace element deficiencies, such as zinc or copper deficiency, may be present and can usually be replenished orally.

A reduced lactose diet in those with lactase deficiency is often useful in reducing diarrhea. If possible, the substitution of a large part of dietary fat with MCTs is an effective intervention.[22] MCT may be consumed as the oil, but it is rather unpalatable. There are some newer commercial products that contain MCT and are more palatable and may be used. In addition, MCT oil can be used in cooking instead of LCT oils or shortenings. Other dietary modifications are idiosyncratic varying from patient to patient. Often a patient will experience more diarrhea if he or she ingests raw fruits and vegetables, caffeinated beverages, alcoholic beverages, fatty foods, or spicy foods. However, these should not be restricted in a blanket manner, as then the diet becomes unnecessarily narrowed.

Prokinetic agents have been shown to normalize intestinal motility in some patients with motor disorders and SIBO, such as those suffering from scleroderma.[23,24] Restoration of normal motor function may theoretically enhance the defense against SIBO by decreasing intestinal stasis. The commonly employed prokinetic agents include metoclopramide and erythromycin. Octreotide, a synthetic long-acting somatostatin analog, functions as a prokinetic agent in patients with scleroderma and SIBO when given at a low dose of 50 mcg.[25] It also functions as an inhibitor of GI secretion.

Conclusion

Malabsorption may be understood in terms of derangements in the normal physiology of nutrient absorption. It is classified into two categories: "maldigestion" and "primary small intestinal absorptive defect." Malabsorption syndromes fall into one of three categories: pancreatic insufficiency, SIBO, and intrinsic small intestinal diseases. The judicious use of the testing outlined in this chapter allows for the differentiation among these categories, the further refinement of the specific abnormality, and a rationale for therapy.

References

1. Craig RM, Ehrenpreis ED. D-xylose testing, a review. *J Clin Gastroent.* 1999;29:143-150.
2. King CE, Toskes PP. Small intestinal bacterial overgrowth. *Gastroenterology.* 1979;76:1035-1055.
3. Dicke WK. Coeliakie: een onderzoek naar de nadilege invloed van sommige graansoorten op de lijder an coeliakie. MD thesis. The Netherlands: University of Utrecht; 1950.
4. Lundin KEA, Scott H, Hansen T, Paulsen G, Halstensen TS, Fausa O, Thorsby E, Solid LM. Gliadin specific HLA-DQ (alpha 1*0501,beta 1*0201) restricted T-cells isolated from the small intestinal mucosa of celiac disease patients. *J Exp Med.* 1993;178:187-196.
5. Nielsen KM, Lundin KEA, Kracji P, Scott H, Sollid LM, Branatzaeg P. Gluten specific, HLA-DQ restricted T-cells from celiac mucosa produce cytokines with Th1 and Th0 profile dominated by interferon gamma. *Gut.* 1995;37:766-776.
6. Sollid MM, Markussen G, Ek J, Gjerde H, Vartdal F, Thorsby E. Evidence for a primary association of celiac disease to a particular HLA-DQ alpha/beta heterodimer. *J Exp Med.* 1989;169:345-350.
7. Sollid LM, Thorsby E. HLA susceptibility genes in celiac disease: genetic mapping and role in pathogenesis. *Gastroenterol.* 1993;105:910-922.

8. Bruce SE, Bjarnason I, Peters TJ. Human jejunal transglutaminase: demonstration of activity, enzyme kinetics and substrate specificity with special relation to gliadin and celiac disease. *Clin Sci (Colch)*. 1985;68:573-579.
9. Dieterich W, Ehnis T, Bauer M, Donner P, Volta U, Riecken EO, Schuppan D. Identification of tissue transglutaminase as the autoantigen of celiac disease. *Nat Med.* 1997;3:797-801.
10. Marsh MN. Gluten, major histocompatibility complex, and the small intestine. A molecular and immunobiological approach to the spectrum of gluten sensitivity (celiac sprue). *Gastroenterol.* 1992;102:330-354.
11. Marsh MN. The natural history of gluten sensitivity: defining, refining, and re-defining. *Q J Med.* 1995;88:9-13.
12. Marks J, Schuster S, Watson AJ. Small bowel changes in dermatitis herpetiformis. *Lancet.* 1966;2:1280-1282.
13. Sanders DS, Carter MJ, Hurlstone DP, Pierce A, Ward AM. Association of adult celiac disease with irritable bowel syndrome: a case control study in patients fulfilling Rome II criteria referred to secondary care. *Lancet.* 2001;358:1504-1508.
14. Simon GL, Gorbach SL. The human intestinal microflora. *Dig Dis.* 1986;30(Suppl 9):147S.
15. Savage DC. Gastrointestinal microflora in mammalian nutrition. *Ann Rev Nutr.* 1986;6:155.
16. Fried M, Slegrish H, Frei R, et al. Duodenal bacterial overgrowth during treatment with omeprazole in outpatients. *Gut.* 1996;35:23.
17. Salzman JR, Kowdley KV, Petrosa MC, et al. Bacterial overgrowth without clinical malabsorption in elderly hypochlorhydric subjects. *Gastroenterol.* 1994;106:615.
18. Yoshida K, Watanabe S, Takeuchi T. Antibacterial activity of human pancreatic juice. *Pancreas.* 1994;9:808.
19. Donaldson RM, Jr. Malabsorption of 60-Co-labelled cyanocobalamin in rats with intestinal diverticula. I. Evaluation of possible mechanisms. *Gastroenterol.* 1962;43:271.
20. Sherr HP, Sasaki Y, Newman A, Banwell JG, Wagner HN, Jr, Hendrix TR. Detection of bacterial deconjugation of bile salts by a convenient breath-analysis technique. *N Engl J Med.* 1971;285:656-661.
21. Bouhnik Y, Alain S, Attar A Flourie B, Raskine L, Sanson-LePors M, Rambaud JC. Bacterial populations contaminating the upper gut in patients with the small intestinal bacterial overgrowth syndrome. *Am J Gastroenterol.* 1999;94:1327-1331.
22. Ehrenpreis ED, Popovich TL, Cravero R. A practical guideline to the recognition of nutritional deficiencies. *Comprehensive Therapy.* 1997;23(3):218-222.
23. Kaye SA, Lim SG, Taylor M, et al. Small bowel bacterial overgrowth in systemic sclerosis: detection using direct and indirect methods and treatment outcome. *Br J Rheum.* 1995;34:265-269.
24. Rose S, Young MA, Reynolds JC. Gastrointestinal manifestations of scleroderma. *Gastroenterology Clin NA.* 1998;27(3):563-594.
25. Soudah HC, Hasler WL, Owyang C. Effect of octreotide on intestinal motility and bacterial overgrowth in scleroderma. *N Engl J Med.* 1991;325:1461.

Section II

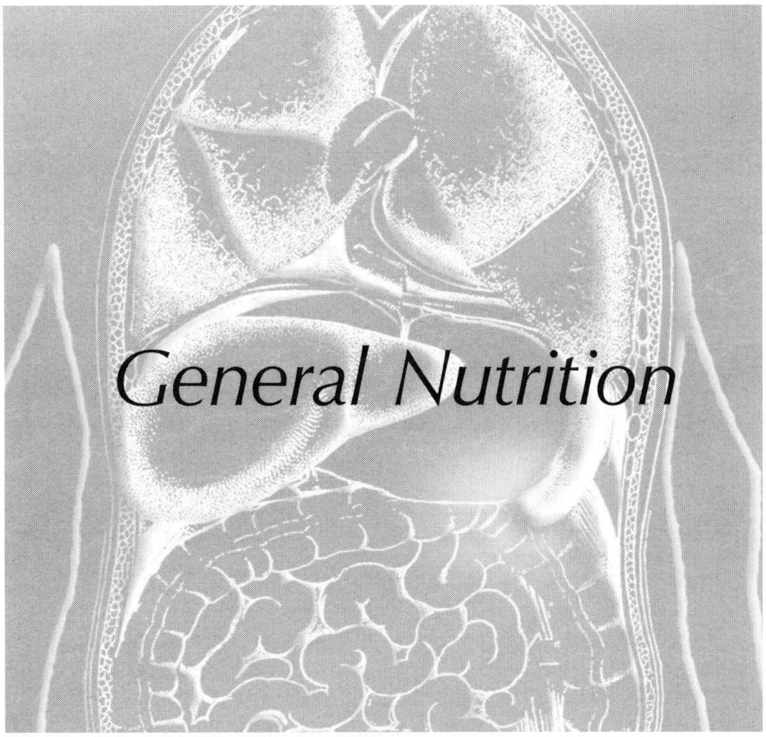

General Nutrition

Chapter 6

The Dietary Reference Intakes: What Are They and What Do They Mean?

Johanna T. Dwyer, DSc, RD

Introduction

The Dietary Reference Intakes (DRIs) refer to a set of nutrient reference values that have been developed for individuals at specific ages and life stages by the Food and Nutrition Board of the Institute of Medicine, National Academies of Sciences, and Health Canada. The DRIs are quantitative recommendations for planning and evaluating the diets of healthy people. The DRI values replace both the 1989 Recommended Dietary Allowances that were used previously in the United States[1] and prior reference data used in Canada.

Each of the DRI values has a particular role, which is discussed below and in the first volume of the new series.[2] The DRI Recommended Dietary Allowance (RDA) and Adequate Intake (AI) values are goals for nutrient intakes to meet the known nutrient requirements for vitamins, minerals/elements, water, protein, and essential fatty acids and to avoid inadequacy of almost all healthy individuals in the various age, gender, and physiological groups.

The estimated energy requirement (EER) and total energy expenditure (TEE) values of the DRIs serve as estimates of an individual's energy requirements. The estimated average requirement (EAR) is the term for vitamins, minerals, and macronutrients including protein, essential fatty acids, carbohydrate, and fiber when possible. The EAR is the value upon which the RDA is based; it is used more for research than for clinical purposes. Nevertheless, all three of these values (RDA, AI, and EAR) are defined by specific functional criteria of nutrient adequacy. The upper tolerable level or the tolerable upper intake level (UL) is defined by a specific endpoint of an adverse effect when one is available. It assures that potential risk of excess is avoided. Whenever possible, functional end points are used for the criteria of adequacy for these UL values as well.

Finally, acceptable macronutrient distribution ranges (AMDR) are also provided. These are recommendations for intakes of carbohydrate, total fat, n-6 and n-3 polyunsaturated fatty acids, and protein. These ranges are not given the same weight in the report as are other DRI values because firm end points do not exist; however, they may also be useful for certain purposes.

These, therefore, are the DRIs. A common set of measures is now available that can be referred to in assessing and planning dietary intakes. Although it is beyond the scope of this chapter, the new values, which are accompanied by new statistical procedures for assessing and planning intakes, now permit better estimation of dietary intakes.

Importance of Dietary Reference Intakes in Gastroenterology

The DRIs provide an update on the validity and reliability of existing dietary standards. They present a new paradigm for assessing dietary adequacy and excess and for planning adequate, balanced intakes that are thought to minimize chronic degenerative disease risks. This new model is needed because older nutrient standards were often based on criteria that were not functional in nature or related to chronic degenerative disease endpoints. Various applications of the DRIs are presented elsewhere.[3]

The DRI reviews for the various nutrients are the most extensive evidence base yet assembled on requirements of nutrients and other substances in the diet for achieving different functional outcomes. As such, they are a useful starting point for investigations of medical issues involving nutrients. The data used to develop DRIs come from observational and experimental studies in humans.[2] The amount of data varies greatly, and, in some age and gender groups, it is quite limited.

Categories of Dietary Reference Intake Reference Values

There are many DRI reference values. This chapter focuses on those of interest in clinical medicine. A full discussion of the DRI values of interest to researchers, planners, and policy makers and their uses is provided in the various Institute of Medicine publications.

Dietary Reference Intake Reference Heights and Weights

The reference heights and weights used in the DRI are representative of weights in the United States and Canada as obtained from national survey and other data.[2] Reference heights and weights are usually provided in the DRI tables because more specificity than that given in gender and age breakouts is sometimes needed. Also reference heights and weights are needed when nutrient requirements are reported on a body weight basis. When values are lacking for certain age or gender groups, weight is often used as the means for extrapolating the data to children or others for whom direct data do not exist.

Dietary Reference Intake Values by Age, Gender, and Life Stage

Nutrient requirements differ by age and gender, as well as physiological conditions, such as pregnancy or lactation. The DRI tables include values for categories that are based on usual differences in needs by these groupings, and the appropriate values should be used in assessing or planning diets for patients. Divisions in infancy include age 0 to 6 and 7 to 12 months; toddlers ages 1 to 3 years; early childhood 4 to 8 years; puberty/adolescence ages 9 to 13 (females) and 14 to 18 (males) years; young adulthood and middle age 19 to 30 and 31 to 50 years; adulthood and older adult ages 51 to 70 and over 70 years; and pregnancy and lactation.[2,3] All of the values are given for healthy people. Modifications for illness are discussed below.

Dietary Reference Intake Definitions and How the Values Are Derived

Recommended Dietary Allowances

The RDA is the average daily dietary intake level sufficing to meet nutrient requirements of most healthy persons. This is calculated by taking the values two standard deviations above the EAR (discussed below), assuming a normal distribution of nutrient requirements.

The RDA and AI for vitamins and for mineral elements are presented in a number of volumes of the DRI reports.[2,4-9] The more intakes fall below the RDA, the greater the risk of inadequacy. RDAs have also been set for carbohydrate, protein, and amino acids.[8,9] This is the first time that an RDA for carbohydrate has been established. The basis for its essentiality is that the brain is a carbohydrate-dependent organ and there is a requirement for carbohydrate based on the average amount of glucose used by the brain.

The proteins serve many functions in the body. The RDA for protein is based on nitrogen balance data. The amino acids, the dietary components of protein, consist of both indispensable and dispensable amino acids. Nine amino acids are considered indispensable; these must be provided in the diet.

The RDA is the target individuals should aim for in planning their diets. The RDA is not useful in assessing the diets of either individuals or groups because it is too generous; by definition the RDA exceeds actual requirements of all but 2% to 3% of the population. Therefore, patients whose intakes of a nutrient are below the RDA may still be getting enough of that nutrient to be above their requirement levels, and dietary change is not necessary.

Adequate Intake

The data on nutrient requirements for some functional criteria of health significance may not always be available, and under such circumstances an RDA cannot be set. However, there is often enough information that permits scientists to make quantitative recommendations about intake levels of nutrients that are likely to be healthful, and then an AI is set. The AI is an appropriate goal or target for the nutrient intake of individuals. However, it is not a requirement and should not be interpreted as such. Instead it is usually the average or median intake of a group of healthy people, all of whom are assumed, by definition, to be meeting their nutrient needs. Although falling below the AI does not necessarily signify deficiency, no positive benefit derives either.

An AI has been set for a number of vitamins and minerals including total fiber, n-6 (linoleic) and n-3 (alpha linoleic acid) polyunsaturated fatty acids, but not for total fat. Because saturated fatty acids, monounsaturated fatty acids, and cholesterol are synthesized by the body and have no known beneficial role in preventing chronic diseases or other functions that are known, they are not required in the diet, and no AI, EAR, or RDA have been set. Linoleic acid is an essential fatty acid. Other polyunsaturated fatty acids of the n-3 family are also important in a variety of functions and interact in metabolism with the n-6 series.

This 2004 edition is the first time a recommendation has been made for fiber, and AI are based on levels observed to protect against coronary artery disease.[8,9] For the first time, the DRI committee distinguished between dietary fiber that consists of nondigestible carbohydrates and lignin that are intrinsic and intact in plants, and functional fiber consisting of isolated, non-digestible carbohydrates that have beneficial physiological effects in humans.

Total fiber is the sum of both of these. There is no UL for fiber or its constituents.

New values and AI have recently been provided by the DRI committee for electrolytes, sulfur, and water.[7] No RDA was set for the electrolytes because dose-response data needed to set an EAR was limited. However, AI for potassium, sodium, and chloride have been established. At present dietary intakes of potassium by most persons in the United States are below the AI, with a mean intake only about two thirds or less of the AI.[7] The AI level is thought to be one that lowers blood pressure, blunts the adverse effects of sodium chloride on blood pressure, reduces risk of kidney stones, and reduces bone loss. However, the beneficial effects of the potassium in this respect seem to be mainly from forms found naturally in foods such as fruits and vegetables that are associated with bicarbonate precursors rather than forms associated with other ions than chloride.[7]

The AI and UL for sodium were established using blood pressure as the criterion. Very active individuals who have high sodium sweat losses may need more. Chronic consumption of sodium intakes above the UL may place individuals at risk of adverse effects. It is likely that some individuals are chronically consuming more sodium than they should for health. Data presented in the volume on electrolytes shows that between 95% and 99% of all adults in the United States consume dietary sodium at levels greater than the AI, and 75% or more of the adults in recent population based surveys have sodium intakes that exceed the UL, even when the amount of sodium added to foods during meals is excluded.[7]

The AI for chloride is set to be in the same molar ratio as that of sodium because virtually all of the chloride in the diet comes from sodium-containing foods. Although data were insufficient to set an AI for sulfate, current recommended intakes for the sulfur amino acids should suffice. Data were insufficient to set an UL for sulfate.

An AI now exists for water.[7] Water is perhaps the most essential nutrient, and yet it is often forgotten. Total water intake includes drinking water, water in beverages, and water (moisture) in food based on criteria of hydration status using serum or plasma osmolarity as the marker. The AI for total water intake prevents deleterious acute effects of dehydration, including metabolic and functional abnormalities. Because physical activity and environmental conditions have substantial influences on water needs, these need to be taken into account in individual cases. In health, homeostatic responses compensate for under or over hydration and permit adjustments to be made. (Note that the AI is not equivalent to the RDA.) Data presented in that volume also shows that the median intake of the American population is equal to or exceeds the AI[7]; therefore, the prevalence of inadequacy is likely to be low, especially because the AI is set as a median intake of a healthy group, as it is for water.

Estimated Energy Requirement

The EER is the average dietary energy intake that is predicted to maintain energy balance in a healthy adult of a defined age, gender, weight, height, and level of physical activity.[8,9] In children and pregnant and lactating women, the EER includes the needs associated with the deposition of tissues or the secretion of milk at rates consistent with good health. The EER is presented with four different likely levels of energy expenditure so that TEE can be calculated.

Estimated Average Requirement

The EAR is the median amount of a nutrient that meets the requirement for a specific criterion of adequacy for half of the healthy individuals in a specific age, gender, and life-stage group. These EAR values are available in the various DRI volumes; however, they are not discussed further in this chapter because they are not useful for estimating nutrient adequacy or planning diets for individuals and therefore are rarely used clinically.

Acceptable Macronutrient Distribution Ranges

The acceptable macronutrient distribution ranges (AMDRs) are provided in the DRI report as ranges for individuals.[8,9] The AMDR is associated with reduced risk of chronic disease and presents a range of intake for a particular energy source with the AI of essential nutrients. The AMDR is expressed as a percentage of total energy intakes because it is not independent of other energy sources in the diet or of the total energy need of the individual. Each need must be expressed in relationship to the others; therefore, each AMDR has an upper and lower boundary. These boundaries are set because the lowest or highest value for other energy-providing nutrients has an expected impact on an individual's health: consuming outside these ranges potentially increases an individual's risk of chronic degenerative diseases, which affect long-term health, and of insufficient intakes of essential nutrients. For example, when fat intakes are high, many individuals gain weight and saturated fatty acids are likely to be high, and when fat intakes are low and carbohydrate intakes are high, there is some evidence that plasma HDL cholesterol decreases. The notion underlying the AMDR is that individuals can consume moderate levels without risk of adverse health effects, while increased risks may occur with the consumption of diets that are either too low or too high in these macronutrients. Most of the evidence is based on clinical end point and associations with risk of various conditions; many other factors may also be involved in determining the development of chronic disease. Therefore, these values are somewhat more tentative than the other DRI values.

Tolerable Upper Level of Intake

Getting too much of a nutrient can disturb bodily functions and cause acute progressive or permanent disability, just as getting too little can cause health problems (see Chapter 3). For the first time, in the current DRIs, a safe UL has been calculated.[10] The UL is the highest level of chronic daily nutrient intake that poses no risk of adverse health effects to a majority of the population. This margin was chosen to assure that even sensitive persons would not experience adverse effects within this UL. Below this level, the individual should be able to tolerate the nutrient amount from the biological standpoint. Just as the EAR and RDA are set using a particular functional criterion, so too are the adverse effects chosen to be those most likely to harm health, assuming sufficient data are available.

For many nutrients, data on adverse effects of very large amounts of nutrients are not yet available, even though many individuals consume rather large amounts. Therefore, for many nutrients, it is not yet possible to establish an UL. The absence of an UL does not mean that the risk of adverse effects is not present; there is no established benefit for consuming nutrient levels above the RDA or AI, and there is possible danger in consuming amounts above the UL. For most nutrients, exceeding the UL is difficult when consuming ordinary foods. However, concentrated nutrient supplements that exceed suggested amounts or are over-consumed can cause a greater potential risk of excess.

Using the Dietary Reference Intakes in Assessing and Planning for Individuals: Clinical Medicine

Assessment

An entire volume of the DRI series is devoted to the uses of the DRI in assessment.[11] For individuals, the EER is used to examine the probability that usual energy intakes are inadequate. The RDA is used as the intake of micronutrients, protein, fatty acids, and carbohydrate, which are consumed on a usual basis at or above which there is a low probability of inadequacy. The AI is the usual intake at or above which there is a low probability of inadequacy. The UL is the usual intake above which the individual is placed at risk of adverse effects from excessive nutrient intakes.

Planning

For planning individual intakes, the goal is the RDA or the AI.[12] The UL is also useful as a guide to limit intakes.[10,12] Chronic intakes of higher amounts may increase the individual's potential risk of adverse effects and should therefore be avoided. The AMDR may also be helpful in planning ranges of macronutrients for healthful diets. The DRI report on macronutrients also includes the AMDR, which provides recommendations for intakes of macronutrients such as carbohydrate, fat, protein, and fiber so that intakes of macronutrients are within their respective acceptable ranges.[8,9]

Nutrient-Based Food Guidance Systems

In some instances, in clinical medicine, rather than focusing specifically on nutrients, it suffices to use nutrient-based food guidance systems. The DRIs and similar values were used as the basis of food based dietary guidance including national food guides, such as the US Department of Agriculture's Food Guide Pyramid and the Dietary Guidelines for Americans.[13-15] Guides like the Pyramid recommend that users select the appropriate amount of food for their age, gender, physiological status, body size, and physical activity level from a range of servings from several different food groups. The food groups designated are those available in the US and are chosen to be rich sources of certain protective nutrients, such as protein, vitamins, and minerals.[15] The Dietary Guidelines for Americans in the year 2000 included the Pyramid as a way of achieving variety. The 2005 Dietary Guidelines do not do so quite as explicitly. However, the same themes remain present in the Dietary Guidelines Committee's deliberations.

Both the Pyramid and the Dietary Guideline were recently revised to reflect the 2005 updates of the Pyramid and the Dietary Guidelines. DRI standards for nutrients are used in planning individual diets when the new food guides are used. Changes are minimal from guidance issued in 2000 but with increased emphasis on weight control, physical activity, and moderation in dietary intakes.

Using the Dietary Reference Intakes for Assessment and Planning for Groups

Clinically, the major uses of the DRI are applications for individuals. For groups, different DRIs are used; details are provided in the publications of the DRI on assessment and planning[11,12] and other resources.[16]

Planning Energy Intakes for Individuals

The estimation of energy intake and assessment and planning to meet energy needs is also dealt with in the DRIs.[8,9] Additional terms are employed that focus specifically on energy. There are a variety of issues to address when calculating energy intakes for individuals.

First, energy-intake reports by patients are unreliable. Dietary planning and assessment often rely on self-reported intake. There is abundant evidence that such energy intakes are underreported, and thus their accuracy is poor. When there is a means for measuring intakes (eg, by observing foods selected or inputs and outputs in institutional settings) data may be stronger. In general, however, proxies for energy intake must be used.

Second, estimates of energy intake are unreliable. Therefore, the best way to assess and plan energy intakes of individuals is to assess the person's body weight. When individuals consume intakes above their energy needs, weight gain occurs, and when intakes are below energy needs, weight loss (and eventually loss of fat tissue and lean body mass) occurs. Thus, unless these changes are obscured by alterations in body water or other body composition compartments, they reflect changes in energy intake to some degree.

Third, there is no RDA for an individual's energy intake, although there is an RDA or AI for most other nutrients. Rather, the appropriate value is the minimal energy requirement to achieve energy balance. The reason for this lies in the RDAs definition. The RDA and AI are beyond most individuals' requirements, because they exceed the requirements of 97% of all individuals. For energy, because there is no way to rid the body of excess, an RDA set using that definition would result in weight gain in most individuals, and therefore there is no RDA set.

Finally, usual energy intakes of individuals are almost never available, and reported energy intakes are so error ridden that they cannot be used. Therefore, an individual's usual energy intake is almost never known and must be estimated. This necessitates the calculation of the EER and application of estimated physical activity levels (PAL) to obtain an individual's estimated TEE. The EER tables used for planning energy needs consist of equations that reflect TEE as estimated from doubly labeled water data and associated with an individual's gender, age, height, weight, and PAL. The equations predict TEE from these characteristics, included as a coefficient by which the value is multiplied by in the equation. By definition, the EER provides the intake that is required to maintain an individual's current weight and PAL. The variability that is reflected in the standard deviation is considerable, because energy needs vary from one person to another. Thus, the requirement is actually a range of possible values. The equations were developed for normal weight and overweight individuals, but the equations for normal weight individuals are the ones that are recommended for use. The EER at four levels of energy expenditure are presented to permit calculation of the TEE. The latest edition of the DRI also provides recommendations for PALs that decrease risk of chronic disease.

Calculating Energy Intakes for Healthy Individuals

The goal of planning energy intake is to obtain a low risk of inadequate energy intake with a low risk of excess. However, the approach to planning for energy needs is different than it is for other nutrients. One difference is that no efficient physiological mechanism exists for ridding the body of excess consumed energy. Also, reports of energy intakes are inaccurate and usually grossly underestimated; so, if planning intakes were based on reported intakes, weight loss would result. The best estimate of energy needs is obtained indirectly as discussed above.

To plan energy intake, the healthcare provider must calculate an initial estimate of TEE using the equation for individual with appropriate characteristics. In health, energy intakes are likely to be very close to energy outputs, and body weight will be maintained within a relatively normal range. In healthy people who are weight stable, at a healthy weight to begin with, and performing the minimal amount of total activity recommended, their recommended energy intake is their usual total energy intake or TEE. That is, their TEE is their energy requirement. Among the overweight who are maintaining their elevated weight but not gaining or losing, their TEE is also their recommended energy intake for maintaining their weight.

After calculating the individual's estimated TEE, the clinician must refine the estimate by monitoring the patient's body weight and adjusting accordingly. By definition because of the variability of these estimates and the fact that equations are based on group data, the TEE will underestimate true energy expenditure 50% of the time and overestimate it 50% of the time. If the values were not adjusted, this would lead to changes in body weight that might be undesirable.

Usually all that is necessary for planning diets for weight loss is to induce the overweight individual in energy balance to regularly consume an energy intake that is 500 cal/day less than his or her usual actual TEE, and this will result in the loss of 1 lb/week, on average. Under certain circumstances, such as for patients in institutions, an energy intake level may need to be specified as well, and the EER and TEE tables may be useful for doing this. Also, although it is rarely necessary to do so, the EER and TEE can also be used to estimate initial energy intakes to lose weight that are needed by individuals who are very heavy and who must lose weight; using a standard 1200- or 1500-calorie-reducing diet would cause very rapid weight loss among them. The initial TEE is calculated, and then 500 cal/day is subtracted to develop the prescription for intake that should result in loss of about 1 lb/week.

Calculating Energy Intakes for Individuals With Illness

The goal of planning energy intakes for the ill is to obtain a low risk of inadequate energy intake with a low risk of excess. For individuals with some health problems, they are in a state of energy imbalance, their weights are increasing or decreasing, and their appetites cannot be counted on to meet bodily needs. For other patients, it is impossible to assess weight changes because of shifts in body water or other compartments of weight obscure them. It is sometimes possible to obtain estimates of resting energy expenditure directly among hospitalized or institutionalized patients, but this is an expensive procedure and rarely done. An alternative for estimating energy intakes in illness is to start with the EER and TEE equations, modifying PAL to conform to what is usually very sedentary levels. This is a target level toward which intakes should be aimed initially. After monitoring, further adjustments up or down may be needed.

Planning Intakes of Vitamins, Minerals, Essential Fatty Acids, Carbohydrate, Protein, Water, and Electrolytes for Healthy Individuals

The new Food Guide Pyramid and the Dietary Guidelines are helpful for providing guidance on foods that meet nutrient needs within their energy requirements of individuals.[17,18] These guides usually suffice for healthy people. The goal in planning nutrient intakes of vitamins, minerals, and protein for individuals is to ensure that the risk of inadequacy is low by meeting the RDA or AI. At the same time, it is important to also assure that there is a low probability of excess. This means that intakes should remain below the UL. Intakes at or above the RDA or AI are almost certainly above the individual's requirements.

There is little likelihood of benefit and no adverse effects to the individual of consuming an intake above his or her requirement, provided that the intake remains below the UL. The RDA, the AI, and the UL are the appropriate DRIs to use for dietary planning for healthy individuals. RDA/AI intake recommendations should be appropriate for the individual's gender, age, PAL, and physiological state (eg, pregnancy, lactation). These values already account for factors such as normal individual variability, individual adjustment factors (such as age, nutrient status, genetic variation, and body size) and, in most cases, can be used without alteration or addition of safety factors. In actuality, some food guidance system that ensures that these values are met is usually used, such as the Food Guide Pyramid, various food exchange lists, or dietary instructions calculated by a dietician. Detailed calculations of nutrients provided are usually carried out only for research purposes or for constructing therapeutic menus for medical nutrition therapy, such as those provided in therapeutic diet manuals in hospitals.

Adjustments for Those Who Are Ill

The DRIs are based on requirements for healthy individuals and assume normal gastrointestinal function. However, when absorption, metabolism, or excretion of a nutrient is altered by a specific illness or disease process, the DRIs can also be used as the basis for developing therapeutic diets. If the patient is ill and physiological or health factors that alter nutrient needs are present, the DRI values as given will not apply and must be modified. To plan a diet for a patient who is ill, the provider must begin by assessing the problem(s) that exists and how it may affect nutrient needs. Because some individuals who are ill (particularly with gastroenterological problems) have conditions that affect the absorption, storage, metabolism, or excretion of one or more nutrients, the DRI for the affected nutrients must be appropriately modified. For most diseases and conditions, needs for only a few nutrients are altered. Other nutrient needs remain similar to those of healthy people and do not change.

Next, the clinician must set therapeutic goals, including goals for nutrient intakes that are appropriate for the individual's health status and nutrient needs. Unless a specific deviation in a nutrient is known, the individual's nutrient needs are assumed to be those of healthy people and an unadjusted RDA or AI is a reasonable goal. Therefore in most cases, as is the case with healthy people, the age/gender specific recommendation applies. For example, a uremic patient in end-stage renal disease might require a very low protein diet: to decrease blood urea nitrogen and other biochemical indices of uremia, for symptomatic relief, and for altered sodium and phosphorus needs. However, the RDA and AI would be used for other nutrients.

Finally, the therapeutic goals must be converted into a diet and eating pattern that the individual can acquire, afford, and eat. The services of a registered dietitian are helpful. No matter how carefully the diet is formulated, if the patient refuses to eat it, it will do the patient no good. Therapeutic dietary planning relies on specialized food guidance and menu-planning systems specific to the various disease states that affect nutrient needs.

An example of the need for adjustments in recommendations would include patients with malabsorption of a fat-soluble vitamin owing to disease or trauma. It is unlikely in the absence of a genetic defect or an inborn error of metabolism that needs would ever be less than the EAR, but they might greatly exceed the RDA because of high absorptive losses. Under such circumstances, recommendations must be adjusted upward.

Recommended Dietary Allowance/Adequate Intake Suitable for Obese as Well as Normal Weight Persons

The RDA and AI allowances for nutrients include typical variation for body size and energy output in specific groups that may be associated with skeletal mass, lean body mass, body water, or other factors. In general, larger people have greater requirements because of larger body nutrient pools or functional compartments; however, at present, information on most nutrients is inadequate to set precise recommendations in relation to an individual's body size or energy expenditure. Therefore, the values in the tables should be used and weight monitored with intakes adjusted accordingly.

Nutrition Requirements for Hospitalized Patients

Parenterally fed patients require special forms of nutrients, and needs must be adjusted. Bioavailability factors are not applicable and absorptive losses do not occur with nutrients administered by vein. Thus, the DRIs cannot be used directly to plan parenteral intakes.

"House" diets fed to patients in hospitals or other institutional situations who are at low nutritional risk and do not require specific therapeutic diets are often required by regulation or convention to meet the RDA or some other nutrient standard. For such individuals, the RDA or AI is the appropriate goal, with any special modifications that need to be made for other reasons, such as texture, etc.

Hospital diet manuals and related materials should be updated to reflect the latest DRI values. For those who are ill and require medical nutritional therapy for various conditions, diet manuals provide therapeutic diet plans which may be linked to menus served in the hospital that are appropriate for the disease in question. For nutrients that are affected by the illness, values may have been adjusted for therapeutic reasons. For other nutrients that are not affected by the illness, the RDA is used.

Conclusions

The DRIs provide the gastroenterologist with quantitative estimates of nutrient needs. The evidence on which these are based are a series of authoritative volumes that now cover all nutrients known to be required by human beings. These authoritative DRI volumes provide a sound science base for human nutritional requirements and methods for assessment and planning nutrient intakes that can be used for many years to come. Nutrition guidance materials based on them provide useful tools for advising patients about healthy diet[17,18] and especially tailored tools based on the DRI are appropriate for therapeutic purposes.

References

1. Committee on Dietary Allowances, Food and Nutrition Board. *Recommended Dietary Allowances*. 10th rev ed. Washington, DC: National Academy Press; 1989.
2. Institute of Medicine. *Dietary Reference Intakes for Calcium, Phosphorus, Magnesium, Vitamin D, and Fluoride*. Washington, DC: National Academy Press; 1997.
3. Devaney BL, Barr SI. DRI, EAR, RDA, AI, UL: Making sense of this alphabet soup. *Nutrition Today*. 2003;37:225-232.
4. Institute of Medicine. *Dietary Reference Intakes for Thiamin, Riboflavin, Niacin, Vitamin B6, Folate, Vitamin B12, Pantothenic Acid, Biotin, and Choline*. Washington, DC: National Academy Press; 1998.
5. Institute of Medicine. *Dietary Reference Intakes for Vitamin A, Vitamin K, Arsenic, Boron, Chromium, Copper, Iodine, Iron, Manganese, Molybdenum, Nickel, Silicon, Vanadium, and Zinc*. Washington, DC: National Academy Press; 2001.
6. Institute of Medicine. *Dietary Reference Intakes for Vitamin C, Vitamin E, Selenium and Carotenoids*. Washington, DC: National Academy Press; 2002.
7. Institute of Medicine. *Dietary Reference Intakes for Water, Potassium, Sodium, Chloride and Sulfate*. Washington, DC: National Academy Press; 2004.
8. Institute of Medicine. *Dietary Reference Intakes for Energy, Carbohydrate, Fiber, Fat, Fatty Acids, Cholesterol, Protein, and Amino Acids, Part 1: Summary and Chapters 1 to 9*. Washington, DC: National Academy Press; 2002.
9. Institute of Medicine. *Dietary Reference Intakes for Energy, Carbohydrate, Fiber, Fat, Fatty Acids, Cholesterol, Protein, and Amino Acids, Part 2: Chapters 10 to 14 and Appendices*. Washington, DC: National Academy Press; 2002.
10. Institute of Medicine. *Dietary Reference Intakes: A Risk Assessment Model for Establishing Upper Intake Levels for Nutrients*. Washington, DC: National Academy Press; 1999.
11. Institute of Medicine. *Dietary Reference Intakes: Applications in Dietary Assessment*. Washington, DC: National Academy Press; 2000.
12. Subcommittee on Interpretation and Uses of Dietary Reference Intake, and the Standing Committee on the Scientific Evaluation of Dietary Reference Intakes. *Dietary Reference Intakes: Applications in Dietary Planning*. Washington, DC: National Academy Press; 2003.
13. US Department of Agriculture. *The Food Guide Pyramid*. Home and Garden Bulletin No. 252. Washington, DC: US Government Printing Office; 1992.
14. US Department of Agriculture and US Department of Health Human Services. *Nutrition and Your Health: Dietary Guideline for Americans*. 5th ed. Home and Garden Bulletin No. 232. Washington, DC: US Government Printing Office; 2000.
15. Welsh SO, Davis C, Shaw A. *USDA's Food Guide: Background and Development*. Miscellaneous Publication No. 1514. Hyattsville, MD: US Department of Agriculture; 1993.
16. Dwyer J. Dietary Reference Intakes (DRI's): concepts and implementation. In: Johnson LR, ed. *Encyclopedia of Gastroenterology*. New York: Elsevier; 2004: 613-623.
17. US Department of Health and Human Services and US Department of Agriculture. *Dietary Guidelines for Americans*. HHS Publication Number HHS/ODPHP 2005-01-DGAA. Washington, DC; 2005.
18. MyPyramid.gov. (2005).

Chapter 7

Dietary Treatment of Gastrointestinal Diseases

Carol Porter, PhD, RD, FADA

Introduction

Medical Nutrition Therapy includes diet modification, nutrient supplementation, nutrition support, and nutrition counseling as modes of therapy for disease. This chapter will focus on dietary modifications that are used to treat hospitalized or ambulatory patients with diseases of the mouth, esophagus, stomach, intestine, liver, and pancreas. Pathophysiology and other forms of treatment will be covered in other chapters.

Treatment of disease with diet has been reported since ancient times. Hippocrates considered diet to be important in maintaining harmony in body fluids of the organism.[1] An English textbook from the 1800s described diet modification for diseases of the gastrointestinal (GI) tract. "In disease...the stomach requires rest as much as the brain and the limbs and it is rested by having its work done for it, [by using]...gruels, soups, jellies, blanc manges, syrups, extracts."[2] If foods were pre-digested, these authors wrote, the GI tract would be allowed to rest. Products such as pepsin or pancreatic ferments (peptonising powders) were used to predigest foods containing protein. Milk, eggs, and cereals were cooked to prevent indigestion. Specific foods were restricted or recommended for those with dyspepsia, constipation, diarrhea, or liver disease. Some of these recommendations continue to this day, whether or not they are supported by scientific evidence.

This chapter will review current scientific evidence to support dietary modification for GI disease. If current practice is to modify diet based on empiric evidence, this will be noted. More detailed information about diet modification can be found in the Manual of Clinical Dietetics and the Pediatric Manual of Clinical Dietetics from the American Dietetic Association.[3]

Modifications in Consistency

Clear Liquid Diet

A clear liquid diet consists of foods that are liquid at body temperature and generally look clear. Examples are clear or strained juices, broth, gelatin, and popsicles. This diet leaves little residue in the bowel and causes minimal stimulation of the GI tract. It is used prior to surgery or some endoscopic procedures and may be used when foods are being reintroduced following surgery.

Clear liquid diets do not meet nutrient needs as defined by the Dietary Reference Intakes (DRI)[4] for any nutrient (discussed in Chapter 6), with the possible exception of water. A clear liquid diet should not be used for longer than 5 days in an adult (3 days for a child) with good nutritional status or 3 days in an adult (1 day in child) with poor nutritional status. If oral intake is restricted to clear liquids for a longer period, nutrient-fortified clear liquid supplements (Enlive! [Ross Products Division of Abbott Laboratories]; Resource Fruit Beverage [Novartis Medical Health Inc]; NuBasics Juice Drink [Nestle Nutrition]), or other forms of nutrition support should be considered.

Liquids versus NPO Prior to Surgery

In the past, patients received nothing by mouth after midnight prior to surgery. However, practice guidelines for healthy adults and children undergoing elective procedures have been revised[5] and recommend that light meals (toast and clear liquids), milk, or formula can be given up to 6 hours before surgery, breast milk up to 4 hours before surgery, and clear liquids up to 2 hours before surgery. These guidelines do not apply to patients who have conditions that may affect the disposition of gastric content or gastric emptying, such as gastroesophageal reflux disease (GERD) or diabetes mellitus.[6]

Clear-Liquid Diet Following Surgery

Traditionally, postoperative feeding of clear liquids was started when there were clinical signs of intestinal motility. It has become more common to offer oral fluids within the first 6-8 hours following surgery, irrespective of presence of bowel sounds. Bohm and coworkers[7] studied tolerance to early feeding in patients who had small or large bowel resections. Patients progressed from clear fluids on day 1 through a mechanically altered diet to a regular diet by day 4 following surgery. The authors reported a low incidence of nausea, vomiting, or other feeding problems that would retard progression or lead to nutrition support. Gocmen and coworkers[8] studied feeding tolerance in women after Caesarean section. One group received low residue feedings 6 hours after surgery. The second group was fed only after bowel sounds were heard. Postoperative ileus was similar in the two groups. Initiation of oral intake and hospital stay were significantly shorter in the early-feeding group. Lee and coworkers[9] reviewed the outcome of early feeding in children following surgery for hypertropic phyloric stenosis. Those fed 8 hours of surgery experienced more vomiting than did those who were fed 13 to 20 hours following surgery. There was no difference between the groups in time to establish full feeding and post-operative stay in the hospital.

The early introduction of clear fluids needs to be individualized, based on type of surgery. However, when patients enter surgery in a malnourished state and it is expected that they will be unable to meet their nutrient needs by oral intake soon after surgery, early jejunostomy feedings with an elemental or peptide-based formula should be considered.[10]

Soft, Low-Residue Diet

The term "soft diet" is often confused with a diet that is mechanically altered, sometimes referred to as a "mechanical soft" diet. The soft, low-residue diet contains whole foods that are only lightly seasoned and low in fiber. Most raw foods, whole grains, legumes, seeds, nuts, gas-forming foods, and foods that are highly seasoned, have strong flavors or odors, or are fried are avoided. Depending upon the food choices, this diet will meet the DRI. The soft, low-residue diet is often used postoperatively and when a patient cannot tolerate regular food. The use of this diet is based on clinical experience. Therefore, it should be individualized for patient preference.

Mechanically Altered Diets

The most common uses of mechanically altered diets are following oral or esophageal surgery, for patients with few or no teeth, or for patients with oral-pharyngeal or esophageal dysphagia. The consistency of these diets can range from liquid to pureed to chopped (sometimes referred to as mechanical soft) diets. Depending upon the food choices and total food intake, all of these diets can meet the DRI.

Liquid Diet Following Oral Surgery

Following oral surgery, a patient may have difficulty consuming enough volume to meet his or her nutrient and energy needs. Foods of a consistency that can be taken through a large straw (no more dense than a creamed soup) may be used. For the first 2 weeks following surgery, sucking on a straw may put too much pressure on sutures. During this period, a large syringe is used for "eating."

Milk or milk-based beverages, soy milk, thinned custards, sherbet or thinned milkshakes, mashed potatoes or blended rice or pasta thinned with milk or broth, and cooked refined cereals (Wheatena [Homestat Farm Ltd]; Kraft Foods, Cream of Wheat and Cream of Rice [Kraft Foods]) thinned with milk are mainstays of the diet. Strained and blended soups, blended meats, poultry, or beans thinned with broth, thinned cheese sauces, and egg products are also used. Non-fibrous fruits and vegetables that do not contain seeds can be blended with fruit or vegetable juices.

Dietary protein intake can be enhanced with the addition of dry milk powder, Instant Breakfast (Nestle Carnation), yogurt, or pasteurized eggs. Using whole milk or adding ice cream, cream, thinned gravy, honey or sugar, maple syrup, butter, or margarine can increase calories. The diet can also be adjusted to decrease saturated fat and cholesterol, but obtaining enough protein and energy may be more important temporarily. Commercial liquid dietary supplements such as Ensure (Ross Products Division of Abbott Laboratories) or Boost and Resource (Novartis Medical Health Inc) can also be used.

Diet Following Esophageal Surgery

Patients who have undergone esophageal surgery most often tolerate tender and moist meats, casseroles, cooked cereals, and soft fruits and well-cooked vegetables that do not contain seeds or skins and are not highly fibrous. These people may have lost significant amounts of weight prior to the surgery. Emphasis should be placed on small, frequent meals that are energy and nutrient dense.

Diets for Dysphagia

Patients with oral-pharyngeal or esophageal dysphagia are at nutritional risk, particularly for weight loss and dehydration.[11] In most hospitals, the registered dietitian works closely with the physician and the speech-language pathologist or occupational therapist to determine which food consistency will result in adequate intake without choking, aspiration, or the feeling that food is "sticking" in the esophagus. Assessments of food intake ("calorie count") should be done prior to patients' discharge to assure that they can meet their nutrient needs. If not, they may require enteral nutrition support to meet some or all of their nutrient needs.

Diets are highly individualized and depend upon the etiology of the dysphagia and upon results of the clinical evaluation of swallowing problems.[12] Generally, patients who have problems with the oral preparation or transit or the pharyngeal transit phase of swallowing will need foods that are soft to semi-solid in texture: ie, moist foods that form a cohesive bolus in the mouth. Often thin liquids

TABLE 7-1.

National Dysphagia Diets

Foods	*Description*
Dysphagia Pureed Diet	Blended or pureed foods that are homogenous, cohesive, and a smooth pudding-like consistency (smooth soufflés, mashed potatoes with gravy, puddings).
Dysphagia Mechanically Altered	Foods that are moist, soft-textured and are easily formed into a bolus in the mouth. Foods such as tender ground or finely diced meats, soft tender-cooked vegetables, scrambled or soft-cooked eggs, ripe or canned fruit, slightly moistened dry untextured cereal.
Dysphagia Advanced	The "dysphagia advanced diet" contains foods that are close to a regular texture except that hard, sticky or crunchy foods are avoided.
Liquids	Spoon-thick (consistency of gelatin) Honey-thick (consistency of buttermilk) Nectar-thick

are restricted. Patients with esophageal obstructions that affect esophageal transit may need pureed or soft moist foods and thin liquids. Patients with dysphagia may benefit from eating slowly, in a relaxed atmosphere, and sitting upright. A multi-disciplinary task force has standardized terminology for dysphagia diets (Table 7-1).[13,14]

Foods and fluids can be thickened using gelatin or commercial thickeners that thicken the food without binding free water [Resource Thicken Up (Novartis Medical Health, Inc); Thick and Easy (Hormel HealthLabs); Thick-It (Precision Foods)]. Pureed vegetables, fruits, and baby rice cereal can also be used. Texture-modified commercial foods and drinks have been developed for people with dysphagia. These include thickened juices, milk, coffee, water, and preformed pureed foods that resemble the original product in both appearance and flavor (Hormel Healthlabs, Novartis Medical Health Inc, Milani/Precision Foods Products).

Diet for Gastroesophageal Reflux Disease and Peptic Ulcer Disease

Diet therapy for GERD should be considered only as an adjunct to pharmacologic therapy. The most common dietary recommendations are to restrict alcohol, coffee, chocolate, peppermint, citrus, and fatty foods and to refrain from eating large meals or meals close to bedtime. Recommendations also include eating in an upright position and losing weight if the patient is obese.[15] Data supporting the effects of these restrictions on gastric-acid secretion, lower esophageal pressure, or reduction in esophagitis are conflicting.[16,17] However, eating in an upright position and avoiding large, high fat and highly concentrated meals or excessive alcohol within 3 hours of bedtime are most likely sound recommendations and ones that most patients can follow. Weight reduction should be encouraged for any obese patient.

Patients should be advised that there is little evidence to support diet therapy for PUD, with the exception of moderate, though conflicting, evidence that alcohol and regular and decaffeinated coffee may increase gastric acid secretions.[18-21] In most cases, patients should be encouraged to eat a wide variety of healthful foods and only avoid foods and beverages that cause intolerance for them.

Stomach acid is important in the initial phases of digestion of some nutrients, especially protein-bound vitamin B12, iron, and calcium. Although there are no studies known that document altered nutritional status in patients treated with medications that reduce production or secretion of stomach acid, a multivitamin and mineral supplement should be encouraged. Dietary supplements should not contain more than 100% of the Daily Value (DV)• for any nutrient.

Diet Following Gastrectomy

Residual stomach volume following partial or total gastrectomy is an important factor in determining intolerance to foods. Generally, reintroduction of food following gastric surgery begins with water and progresses to clear liquids. We have also found that these patients can tolerate plain foods containing carbohydrate, such as soda crackers, white bread, bagels, baguettes, Cream of Wheat or oatmeal, and white rice with these clear liquids.[22]

DIET FOR DUMPING SYNDROME

Patients who have had gastric surgery that affects their ability to control the rate of release of food from the stom-

Table 7-2.

Diet For Dumping Syndrome

- Meals should be small and frequent.
- Liquids and solid food consumption should be separated by > ½ hour.
- Liquids can include decaffeinated coffee, soup, unsweetened fruit juice, milk, soy milk, sugar-free carbonated beverages and water. Liquids should not contain concentrated sugars, caffeine, or theobromine (eg, breakfast drinks, milkshakes, sodas, regular coffee, tea).
- Diets should be high in protein and moderate in fat content.
- Complex carbohydrates (eg, starches in breads, potatoes, rice, pasta) are better tolerated than simple carbohydrates (eg, sugar, candy, honey, jelly, jam, syrup, molasses).
- Foods should be consumed in a relaxed atmosphere and eaten slowly.
- Some people have an intolerance to very hot or very cold foods.
- When foods such as sweets, fluids, raw fruits and vegetables, coffee, cola, tea are reintroduced, small amounts should be consumed and the response noted (bloating , diarrhea, sweating or dizziness). If these symptoms occur, the food should be omitted and reintroduced at a later time.

ach may experience "dumping syndrome." Management of "dumping" with diet is described in Table 7-2.

Diet for Gastric Bypass or Gastric Stapling for Obesity

Following gastric bypass or stapling (Chapter 50), there is an intentional reduction in the stomach's capacity to hold food. The pouch size is typically <45 mL, with the ability to expand to >120 mL in the first year following resection. Patients who have had gastric-bypass surgery may experience "dumping" symptoms and should follow recommendations described in Table 7-2, with the exception of limiting energy intake and increasing protein intake. Because food intake is restricted, nutrient intake does not meet the DRI. Reduced food intake, changes in food selections, and decreases in stomach acid can contribute to micronutrient deficiencies. Folic acid, iron, and calcium are most often compromised. Vitamin B12 status can be affected if there is decreased intrinsic factor. A prenatal vitamin and mineral supplement is usually recommended because it has higher concentrations of folic acid, calcium, and iron than does a standard vitamin and mineral supplement.

Diet for Hypolactasia (Lactose Intolerance)

Incidence of hypolactasia varies from <15% in people of northwest European descent to >60% in Asians, African Americans, Native Americans, Latinos.[23] However, people with lactase deficiency have varying levels of intolerance to lactose and may be able to consume lactose in small amounts or along with solid foods, complex carbohydrates, or soluble fiber that can delay gastric emptying.[24-28] Often, however, fresh milk is not a part of cultural food patterns of groups that have the highest incidence of hypolactasia. Milk can be replaced with soy drinks that are fortified with calcium and vitamin D or with lactase hydrolyzed milk, such as Lactaid (McNeil Nutritionals) and Dairy Ease (Land-O'-Lakes). (Although fortified rice-milk may contain similar amounts of calcium and vitamin D, it is a poor source of protein.) Other milk products such as yogurt, sour cream, cheeses, cream cheese, and butter contain less than half the lactose of fresh or evaporated milk (Table 7-3).[29,30] In the United States, lactose may also be used in processed foods and medications; the person who is intolerant to lactose should read labels carefully.

When dairy products or fortified dairy substitutes, such as soy drinks, are restricted in the diet, the calcium and vitamin D intake may not meet the DRI. People who do not consume products containing concentrated sources of calcium and vitamin D will most likely need to take a dietary supplement to meet their nutrient needs.

Gluten-Restricted Diet for Celiac Disease

The only treatment for celiac disease (Chapter 19) is a gluten-restricted diet. Gluten is a storage protein found in cereal grains that serves as a nitrogen source for germinating seeds.[31] Development of gluten during production of breads gives them their structure. The prolamin fraction of gluten contains the offending agent: gliadin (wheat), secalin (barley), and hordein (rye). Oats contain a similar protein (avenin), but wheat, rye, and barley have a closer genetic link. Whether oats need to be restricted in people with celiac disease is controversial.[32]

The sequence of amino acids in a peptide fraction of prolamin produces an inflammatory response in those who are genetically predisposed to the disease. This leads to morphologically altered mucosal architecture and malabsorption.[33-35] Untreated patients may also have lactose intolerance, which usually resolves when a gluten-restricted diet is followed.

TABLE 7-3.

Calcium and Vitamin D Content of Milk Products or Milk Substitutes

Product	Lactose (grams)	Calcium (milligrams) DRI: ranges from 1000 to 1300 mg depending upon age	Vitamin D, (micrograms) (International Units) DRI: ranges from 5 to 10 ug (200 to 400 IU) depending upon age
Sweetened condensed milk (1/2 cup or 125 mL)	15	432	0
Evaporated milk (1/2 cup or 125 mL)	12	320	2.4 (96)
Milk, whole, 2%, 1%, fat-free (1 cup or 250 mL)	11	300	2.5 (100)
Buttermilk (1 cup or 250 mL)	10	285	0
Ice Cream (1/2 cup or 125 mL)	6	40-60	0
Half-and-half cream (1/2 cup or 125 mL)	5	130-160	0
Yogurt, low fat (1 cup or 250 mL)	4	270	2.7 (106) (if fortified)
Sour cream (1/2 cup or 125 mL)	4	112	0
Cottage cheese, creamed (1/2 cup or 125 mL)	3	100	0
Whipping cream (1/2 cup or 125 mL)	3	80	0
Sherbet, orange (1/2 cup or 125 mL)	2	0	0
American cheese (1 oz or 30 g)	2	124	0
Other cheese, Swiss, cheddar, parmesan (1 oz or 30 g)	1	200 – 300	0
Cream cheese (1 oz or 30 g)	1	0	0
Butter (1 tsp or 5 g)	Trace	1	0
Lactaid Milk (McNeil Nutr) (1 cup or 250 mL)	<1	300	2.5 (100)
Soy-based ice cream (Tofutti [Tofutti Brands, Inc]);	0	0	0
Soy Dream (Imagine Foods) Soy-based yogurt (O'Soy, [Stoneyfield Farms]) 4 oz	0	100	0
Fortified soy milk-substitute (Silk-White Wave [Dean Foods]; 8th Continent [The Solae Company]) (1 cup or 250 mL)	0	300	2.5 – 3 (100 – 120) if fortified
Rice Dream, Enriched (Imagine Foods), (1 cup) Unlike cow's milk or soy milk-substitutes, rice beverages are a poor source of protein (1 gram protein/cup vs. 7 to 10 g protein/cup in cow's milk or soy milk-substitute).	0	300	2.5 (100)

In the United States, wheat, rye, barley, and usually oats are eliminated from the diet. The most difficult part of following this diet is that these grains are used in the production of stabilizers, thickeners, and preservatives in many foods and in some medications. The patient must learn to read labels, check with manufacturers about incidental ingredients not included on labels, or talk with their pharmacist about medications containing gluten.

Patients often find this diet difficult to follow and may also have trouble identifying gluten-free foods.[36] Some grocery companies in the United States (eg, Trader Joes, Whole Foods Market) have lists of gluten-free products available in their stores. Some European countries require that food labels contain information about gluten. In the United States, The Food Allergen Labeling and Consumer Protection Act of 2004 (Public Law 108-282, August 2, 2004) will require the Secretary of Health and Human Services to issue a final rule to define and permit the use of the term "gluten free" on food labels no later than August 2008.[37] A patient with celiac disease should be referred to a registered dietitian who has knowledge about its dietary treatment. In-depth counseling, follow-up, and referral to other sources of information and support groups are important for good compliance to this diet.

A comprehensive list of foods to avoid and foods allowed is beyond the scope of this chapter. However, general foods that need to be avoided are wheat, rye, barley, and possibly oats.

The soft and hard wheat (genus: triticum) grown in the United States today are hybrids of earlier versions of wheat cultivated over the last 10,000 years (kamut, spelt, einkorn, emmer). These soft and hard wheats contain higher concentrations of gluten than earlier forms of wheat.[38] Some older forms of wheat, such as spelt, are still grown and may be found in health food stores. Although they may be tolerated by those with a wheat allergy, they should be avoided by patients who have celiac disease.

Patients should be advised to avoid foods that contain the following wheat flours or products containing wheat: Abyssinian hard, all-purpose flour; bleached flour; bulgur, cake or pastry flour; couscous; durum wheat; einkorn wheat; farina; fu (dried wheat gluten); graham flour; granary flour; high-gluten flour kamut wheat; matzo; self-rising flour; semolina; spelt; sprouted wheat; triticale (mixture of wheat and barley); triticum; wheat bran; wheat germ; wheat grass; wheat nuts; and cereals and pastas made from wheat. In the United States and Canada, patients should avoid wheat starch. In Europe, wheat starch that meets standards of quality set by the Codus Alimentarius is considered safe for patients.[39]

Buckwheat comes from a fruit. Kasha is roasted buckwheat. Buckwheat does not contain gluten and is tolerated by those with celiac disease. However, the lack of gluten results in bread products with little structure. For this reason, recipes may include both buckwheat and gluten-containing grains, such as wheat flour.

Barley is the earliest domesticated grain. Its use as the primary cereal grain was supplanted when wheat was cultivated. Today, pearled barley (barley that has the hull and bran removed) is still used as a cereal.[40] However, most barley in the United States is now used as livestock feed, to produce beer and whiskey, and for malt used to flavor cereals. Patients with celiac disease should be advised to avoid barley, pearl barley, barley grass, barley malt, malt extract, malt syrup, malt flavoring, malt vinegar, beer, lager, ale, stout, and cereals that are flavored with malt, barley groats, and sprouted barley.

Rye appears to have developed as a cultivated crop from weeds in wheat and barley fields. Rye bread almost always contains wheat flour to give it structure.[41]

Oats also developed from weeds.[42] A hulled oat is called an oat groat. A wide variety of products are made from oats: rolled oats, oat flour, and oat bran. Studies using biopsy and serologic tests have shown no adverse effects when oats were used over a 5-year period in adults who had established diagnoses of celiac disease and were in remission.[43,44] It is unknown if oats are safe for children with celiac disease. Oats in some northern European countries are thought to be free of gluten. In the United States, oats may be contaminated with other grains in the field, storage, or processing. A reasonable recommendation is that adults should avoid oats until they are in remission, and then they should consume only a moderate amount of oats that are thought to be free of wheat contamination: eg, McCann's Irish Oats (McCann's Products, Odlum Group, Ireland).[45,46] Children and adolescents with celiac disease should avoid oats until there is evidence of safety in this age group.

Other cereal or plant products that can be used by patients with celiac disease are millet, rice flour or starch, wild rice, buckwheat, corn flour or starch, quinoa, flax, potato flour or starch, ragi, sesame, sunflower, sorghum, soy, teff, wheat starch (if meets Codex Alimentarius quality), and tapioca.

Many products can be made from grains that contain gluten, such as artificial colors, bullion cubes, citric acid (outside of the US), some ground spices, hydrolyzed plant or vegetable protein, modified food starch, monosodium glutamate, mustard powder, and soy sauce. In the United States, mono- and diglycerides used in food products can contain a wheat carrier. Caramel may or may not contain gluten, depending upon the grain used to produce it. Dextrin comes from starch that has been incompletely hydrolyzed and can be made from wheat.[47]

In addition to learning about foods and food labeling, patients should be advised to watch for sources of gluten contamination. For example, grains sold in bulk may be cross-contaminated when scoops are used in several bins. Wheat bread crumbs can contaminate butter, jams, or the toaster. Contamination is thought to be one reason why some patients with celiac disease are not responsive to the gluten-restricted diet.[48]

There are many national organizations that provide support to people with celiac disease: the American Celiac Society, the Celiac Disease Foundation, the Celiac Sprue Association, and Friends of Celiac Disease Research, Inc., Gluten Intolerance Group of North America, and Raising Our Celiac Kids (ROCK). There are also many websites and a listserv that provide information and support to people with celiac disease.

People with celiac disease may have experienced malabsorption prior to treatment. In addition, there has been one report indicating that vitamin status may be altered in patients with celiac disease, particularly vitamins that are normally added to processed grains (eg, folic acid).[49] Patients should be advised to make healthy food choices. In addition, it is probably wise to recommend a vitamin and mineral supplement that does not contain gluten (Centrum [Wyeth Consumer Healthcare], Theragran [Bristol-Myers Squibb Co.], Freeda Vitamins [Freeda Pharmacy, New York], and other brands). If milk intake is restricted, a gluten-free calcium supplement, eg, Caltrate (Wyeth Consumer Healthcare), should be recommended. If the multivitamin does not contain adequate vitamin D, a calcium and vitamin-D supplement should be taken. Non-prescription dietary supplements should not contain more than 100% DV for any nutrient.

Diet for Inflammatory Bowel Disease (Crohn's Disease and Ulcerative Colitis)

Inflammatory bowel disease (IBD) refers to both Crohn's disease (CD) and ulcerative colitis (UC). CD is a chronic inflammatory condition that involves patches of the GI tract in the ileum, colon, or both. The inflammation can involve all layers of the intestinal tract. Complications can include bowel strictures caused by intestinal stenosis and bacterial overgrowth of the small intestine following strictures, fistulas, or surgery. Primary treatment focuses on control of the inflammation using medications. Resection of the affected bowel may be necessary, but disease can reoccur in other areas of the intestine.

UC is an inflammation and ulceration of the colon. The disease may involve only the rectum or occur throughout the entire colon. Unlike CD, the inflammation involves only the mucosal layer and is continuous rather than patchy. Treatment focuses on control of inflammation using medications. Some patients may require surgery.

The goal of nutrition therapy is to address nutritional deficiencies that may be caused by poor dietary intake, malabsorption, and secretion of nutrients (such as protein) into the intestine or by nutrient deficits caused by medical and surgical treatment. During acute inflammatory stages of the diseases, diet modification may help relieve symptoms. Fat malabsorption, strictures, and ostomies may require further dietary modification.

Role of Foods or Dietary Patterns in Etiology of Inflammatory Bowel Disease

Although it has been suggested that length of breast feeding and consumption of refined carbohydrates, fiber, and fat play a role in etiology of IBD, there are no clear data that these or any other foods or dietary patterns cause IBD.[50]

Treatment of Inflammatory Bowel Disease With Diet

There is no specific diet for IBD. Patients in remission stages of UC and CD (except with stenosis) should be encouraged to eat a variety of healthful foods, including dietary fiber, and only avoid those things that cause individual intolerances.[51,52] However, because undernutrition is common in patients with IBD, practitioners should know what foods are being avoided and address nutrient deficiencies that result from avoidance of these foods. For example, patients with CD may experience intolerance to lactose-containing foods and should be encouraged to consume fermented milk products, lactase-treated milk, or fortified soy products to obtain an adequate protein, calcium, and vitamin D intake (see Table 7-3).

During acute inflammatory phases of IBD, patients may find relief from diarrhea and abdominal pain if they follow a soft, low-residue diet (discussed earlier in this chapter). Patients with bowel stenosis should limit fiber in their diet. Foods that contain the highest amount of total fiber are raw fruits (except ripe banana), dried fruits, raw vegetables, vegetables with tough skins (corn, peas), cooked lentils and other dried peas and beans, whole grain breads and cereals, and nuts and seeds (Table 7-4).[53]

Inflammation, bacterial overgrowth, or resection of the ileum in CD may affect absorption of fat and fat-soluble vitamins. A moderate restriction in total fat and supplementation with water-miscible vitamins A, D, E, and K may be used. Patients should be advised to restrict full-fat milk products, foods that are fried or produced with excess fat (eg, doughnuts, chips, high-fat desserts), excess butter, margarines, salad dressings or oils, and high fat meats. The diet should not be so restrictive that energy and nutrient intake are limited. Medium-chain triglycerides (MCT), a fraction of coconut oil containing fatty acids that are 8-10 carbons long, may also be used. MCT was originally developed as a dietary supplement by Mead Johnson & Company but can now be purchased as an oil from a number of different companies that sell foods and dietary supplements. It should be introduced slowly (<20-30 g/day and no more than 3-4 teaspoons at one time). The oil has little flavor and can be incorporated into salad dressing, added to non-fat milk or juice, or used in cooking in place of other oils. However, its smoke point is low and this decreases its usefulness in frying.

An additional complication of ileal disease and fat malabsorption is an increased incidence of oxalate stones in the kidney. With fat malabsorption, the unabsorbed dietary long-chain fatty acids will bind calcium to form soaps. Not only does this decrease calcium absorption, but it also affects the disposition of oxalate from the diet. Normally, some of the dietary calcium would be bound to oxalate, decreasing its absorption. When fatty acids are binding calcium, the displaced oxalate binds to sodium. In this form, it is more soluble and better absorbed in the colon. Patients with ileal dysfunction may need to restrict oxalate in their diets.[54] Foods that contain oxalate are draft beer, chocolate and cocoa, carob, soy milk, instant tea and coffee, nuts including soy nuts and nut butters, berries, Concord grapes, red currants, citrus peels, rhubarb, tofu, baked beans, wax beans, legumes, beet root and top, okra, celery, dark-green leafy vegetables, eggplant, leeks, summer squash, and potatoes including sweet potatoes.[55-57]

Protein energy undernutrition, growth failure, osteopenia/osteoporosis, anemia (blood loss, B12, folic acid), and clinical or sub-clinical micronutrient deficiencies (of iron, zinc, magnesium, B vitamins, vitamin C) are common in patients with IBD, especially CD.[58] Antioxidant need may increase in the inflammatory phases of CD and UC. There

TABLE 7-4.

Dietary Fiber in Foods

Food Groups and Examples of Foods	*Dietary Fiber (approximate g/serving)*
Fresh Fruits 1 medium apple, peach or pear, 3 medium apricots, 1 cup grapes – all with skin 1 medium orange, 1/2 – 1 cup berries	1.5 to 4.0 grams
Dried fruits 2/3 cup raisins, 10 dried plums	5 to 6 grams
Vegetables 1/2 cup broccoli or Brussels sprouts, 1 cup cabbage, 1 cup carrots, 1 cup cauliflower, 1/2 cup corn, 1 cup green beans, 3/4 cup green peas	3 grams
Beans and lentils 1/2 cup, cooked	5 to 8 grams
Whole grain breads 1 slice	2 grams
Brown Rice 1/2 cup	2 grams
Cooked whole grain cereals 1/2 cup	3 to 6 grams
All-Bran cereal 1/3 cup	10 grams
Wheat bran 1/3 cup	11 grams
Wheat germ 1/4 cup	4 grams
Nuts and seeds 1 oz almonds, chestnuts, corn nuts, macadamia nuts, mixed nuts, peanuts, pecans, walnuts	2 to 3 grams

may also be drug-nutrient interactions. Sulfasalazine, which affects folic-acid absorption, can exacerbate an already tenuous folic-acid status resulting from inadequate intake of fresh fruits, vegetables, and fortified cereals. High doses of prednisolone (not budesonide)[59] stimulate gluconeogenic pathways and increase requirements for dietary protein.

During acute phases of IBD, especially in patients with CD, food intake alone may not meet nutrient and energy needs. Nutritional supplementation or nutrition support may be required (Chapter 19). Most evidence indicates that use of corticosteroids is more effective than is nutritional support in decreasing inflammation and inducing remission.[60-63] However, if food intake is inadequate, if patients are resistant to corticosteroids, and when corticosteroids affect growth, nutrition support should be used. It is common practice to use nocturnal enteral feeding with children and adolescents who have CD and high potential for growth failure. Enteral support is preferred over parenteral support unless there are contraindications for its use (eg, small bowel obstruction, short bowel). Evidence published to date indicates that polymeric formulas are as efficacious as elemental or peptide-based formulas. Data to support the efficacy of glutamine, omega-3 and monounsaturated fatty acids, and prebiotics in decreasing the inflammatory response or inducing remission have been discordant.[64-69] However, a recent randomized, controlled trial reported that oral supplements containing omega-3 fatty acids, antioxidants, and fermentable soluble fiber significantly reduced inflammation and corticosteroid requirements in patients with UC.[70]

Diet for Ileostomy and Colostomy

Following the placement of an ileostomy or colostomy the patient progresses from liquids to a soft, low-residue diet that contains soluble fiber (eg, oatmeal, applesauce, banana, rice). Fried foods, foods containing insoluble fiber (eg, bran, high fiber cereals, legumes), or foods containing nuts and seeds are eliminated for ileostomies. Colostomy patients usually can consume a regular diet.

Within 6 to 8 weeks following the ostomy placement, a patient may be able to add other foods as tolerated. Patients should be encouraged to eat what they can tolerate. However, the foods patients have most difficulty with are those that produce gas or odors, are incompletely digested, or have the potential to block the stoma (eg, carbonated drinks, strong cheeses, cooked dried peas and beans, vegetables in the cabbage family, corn, coconut, nuts, seeds, fruits and vegetables with tough skins, highly spiced foods, garlic). Patients should also be encouraged to chew foods well. They should also have a good fluid and electrolyte intake, particularly those patients with total colectomies. Patients with ileostomies are more likely to experience bile salt deficiency and problems with fat absorption. A low fat intake and use of MCT products may be used.

Diet for Short Bowel Syndrome

Short bowel syndrome is a malabsorptive disorder resulting from resection of ≥ 2/3 of the small intestine. It is characterized by diarrhea, malabsorption, and electrolyte and fluid losses that can compromise nutritional status. Extensive resection may require nutrition support, which is described in other chapters. The area of the bowel affected, bowel adaptation, and presence or absence of the ileum and colon will dictate response to diet.

Patients who have a colon should consume several meals each day that are low in fat and high in protein (as discussed earlier). Medium chain triglycerides (MCT) may be useful. Complex carbohydrates, but not simple sugars, should be consumed. Oxalate may need to be restricted and a good fluid intake should be encouraged. Those patients without an intact colon can usually tolerate more fat.[71,72] (This subject is discussed in detail in Chapter 29.)

Diet to Control Diarrhea

Diarrhea is characterized by an increase in the frequency and liquidity of stools. It can result from a variety of diseases or conditions (eg, celiac disease, IBD, ostomies, following radiation of the pelvis, short bowel syndrome) and is categorized by its origin as either osmotic with malabsorption and steatorrhea, secretory from a change in electrolyte transport, or inflammatory, resulting from enterocyte damage.

Treatment includes fluid replacement to offset excess losses and modification of the diet to minimize residue (discussed earlier), prolong intestinal transit time, and reduce stool frequency. Residue is defined as material that is left in the intestinal lumen following digestion (eg, undigested food, endogenous secretions). Soluble fiber found in fruits such as applesauce, bananas, and canned fruits, refined breads, and cereal products may also help to control the diarrhea.

Diet for Constipation and Diverticulosis

Dietary fiber is important for GI health. Consumption of dietary fiber, particularly cellulose, oligofructose, bran, and psyllium promotes laxation and fecal weight. Prospective, case control and intervention trials have shown protective effects of dietary fiber, particularly cellulose and unprocessed bran, for diverticular disease. However, the mechanism for this protective effect is unknown. There is conflicting evidence about the role of dietary fiber in prevention of colon cancer. The most recent DRI recommends 19 to 38 g/day, depending on the individual's age.[73]

When patients need to increase fiber in their diets, recommendations should emphasize the use of high fiber foods rather than fiber supplements. Not only do high fiber foods contain phytonutrients, thought to be protective against chronic disease, but many high fiber foods (eg, fruits and vegetables) also contain water. (Table 7-4 provides approximate content of dietary fiber in common foods.) Adults and children can meet the DRI recommendations for fiber by following the USDA food guide, "MyPyramid" (http://www.mypyramid.gov) that recommends 5 to 7 servings of fruits and vegetables and 3 to 5 servings of whole grain cereals per day.

Fluid intake is also important in treatment of constipation. The most recent DRI[74] recommends a total water intake for adults of ~3 to 4 L/day from both food and beverages. Beverage intake should be approximately 2 to 3 L/day (~9 to 13 cups/d) and can be supplied by any drink (eg, water, milk, coffee, juice). Recommendations for total water intake for children range from ~1 to 3 L and beverage consumption from 0.6-2.6 L/d (~3 to 11 cups), depending upon age. Although fluid recommendations for older people are no different than those for younger adults, the older person may need encouragement to consume fluid because of decreasing sense of thirst with age.

Diet for Liver Disease—Sodium- and Protein-Restricted Diets

Undernutrition is common in advanced chronic liver disease.[75] Although this is particularly true in patients who have had a long history of excessive alcohol consumption, it may also be true when patients are placed on unnecessarily restrictive diets. There is evidence that dietary restriction of sodium can help with the management of ascites. There is weak evidence that dietary restriction of protein or alterations in the amino-acid composition of the diet is helpful in treating chronic liver disease or hepatic encephalopathy.

Ascites and Sodium Intake

Dietary treatment of ascites involves creating a negative sodium balance using a sodium-restricted diet. Response to a sodium restriction is greatest in patients with recent-onset ascites and normal renal function.[76]

Recommendations for sodium restrictions in many textbooks are so low that the diet is difficult to follow without using expensive low-sodium foods. In addition, the restriction often compromises overall food intake. The average sodium intake in the American population is more than three times higher than recently recommended by the Institute of Medicine. Approximately 75% of dietary sodium is added during food processing and 20% comes from salting food during cooking or at the table.[77] Because most Americans have a relatively high sodium intake, a milder sodium restriction of ~ 2000 to 3000 mg/day (87 to 130 mmol or mEq) will be a contrast to their usual sodium intake and will be easier to follow.

A diet that contains ~2000 to 3000 mg of sodium eliminates foods and beverages that have high concentrations of sodium [eg, meats that are cured with salt such as bacon, salt pork, chipped beef, corned beef, ham, hot dogs, sausages, ham, luncheon meats, salted fish, cheese spreads and sauces, snack foods containing salt, instant hot cereals, canned or dehydrated soups, olives, flavored vinegars and high sodium salad dressings, pickled or salted vegetables such as sauerkraut, salt (regular, sea salt, kosher salt) or sodium-containing flavorings such as garlic salt, meat tenderizers, monosodium glutamate, soy sauce, teriyaki sauce]. Foods that are highly processed, such as those found in most fast-food restaurants usually contain excessive amounts of sodium.

Patients can also be taught how to read labels and determine the sodium content of foods. They should choose products that contain <10% DV for sodium. In the United States, the sodium content of a serving of food is expressed as a percentage of the DV (2400 mg/day), so products that contain <240 mg of sodium per serving would be acceptable. Food labels may also contain claims about sodium content: "low-sodium" (≤140 mg sodium/serving), very low sodium (≤35 mg sodium per serving), and sodium-free (<5 mg sodium per serving).

Protein Restrictions and use of Branched Chain Amino Acid Formulas in Chronic Liver Disease and Hepatic Encephalopathy

Neither European nor American parenteral and enteral nutrition societies support the use of protein restrictions in chronic liver failure.[78,79] However, some textbooks and journal articles continue to promote these restrictions and many clinicians follow them.[80] The unfortunate result of a dietary protein restriction is that patients will use their own endogenous stores to meet nitrogen needs. Often a patient's nutritional status is already compromised by long-term disease, poor appetite, and inadequate food intake. A protein restriction will only exacerbate this poor nutritional status.

The DRI for protein has been determined for healthy people.[81] It is 1.52 g/kg/day for term infants, 0.85 to 1.10 g/kg/day for children, and 0.80 g/kg/day for adults. People with chronic liver disease may have higher protein requirements. The following recommendations have been made for children and adults: 1.5 to 3.0 g/kg/day for infants and children[82] and ≥1.0 g protein/kg/day for adults.[83] Patients with cirrhosis are better able to achieve nitrogen balance with frequent feedings, including an evening meal.[84 85]

Hepatic encephalopathy is usually treated with medications and either no or only slight modifications in protein intake. Protein intake for children should be near the DRI, but no less than 1.0 g protein/kg/day. Adults should receive protein intakes of ~1.0 g/kg/day and no less than 0.6 g/kg/day (total of 40 g/day of protein).

Formulas supplemented with branched-chain amino acids (BCAA) have been proposed as beneficial for patients with hepatic encephalopathy. Not only are these unappetizing products, a recent Cochrane review[86] found that evidence was inadequate to support their use. Both European and American nutrition societies recommend use of BCAA formulas only in the few patients with liver disease who are intolerant to standard protein intake (ie, unable to tolerate 1.0 g protein/kg/day without encephalopathy).[87,88]

Diet for Acute and Chronic Pancreatitis

Most patients with mild acute pancreatitis will be able to return to a normal oral intake within 7 days. In patients with severe acute pancreatitis, nutrition intervention may be warranted. Evidence supports enteral feeding with a polymeric formula via jejunostomy feeding tube.[89-92] Extreme cases of acute pancreatitis may warrant complete gut rest and support with total parenteral nutrition. A small number of patients have acute pancreatitis caused by hypertriglyceridemia. These patients will require medical treatment that includes a significant restriction in dietary fat.

Patients with chronic pancreatitis may have an increased incidence of diabetes. They may also be undernourished because of decreased intake related to chronic pain or to malabsorption. One of the main goals in the management of chronic pancreatitis is to control pain. The cause of pain is incompletely understood but thought to be related, in part, to intraductal pressure caused by strictures or calculi.[93] Cholecystokinin (CCK) stimulates pancreatic enzyme secretion. Although dietary protein and fat stimulate CCK, dietary fat appears to have the greatest effect on interdigestive and postprandial output of enzymes by the pancreas.[94] Therefore, a moderate restriction in dietary fat and an alcohol restriction are most often recommended. There is some evidence that enteral formulas with MCT and hydrolyzed peptides [Peptamen (Nestle Nutrition) and Pro-Peptide (Hormel Healthlabs)] are useful in blunting CCK release.[95]

Concluding Comments

This chapter has reviewed the evidence for dietary modification in the treatment of gastrointestinal diseases or conditions. When practitioners prescribe these diets, they should understand the strength of evidence to support their use. These diets should also be used with moderation, particularly when they do not provide all nutrients. They may exacerbate existing nutrition problems caused by decreased food intake, dysphagia, maldigestion and malabsorption, altered metabolism, and increased secretory losses of nutrients. In addition, other forms of medical and surgical treatment can affect nutritional status of these patients.

Acknowledgments

The author would like to thank Andrea Aiello RD, CSP (UCSF Children's Hospital, pediatric gastroenterology) and Viveca Ross, RD, CNSD (UCSF Medical Center, adult gastroenterology) for their helpful contributions to the preparation of this chapter.

Footnotes

- The term Daily Value (DV) is used by FDA for food and dietary supplement labeling. Because only one value for each nutrient can be used in labeling, the value chosen is the highest nutrient value for nonpregnant, nonlactating adults from the 1968 Recommended Dietary Allowances (earlier name for the DRI). DV for energy, protein, fat, fiber, sodium, and cholesterol are based on the US Dietary Guidelines.
- In an attempt to avoid skin cancer, avoidance of the sun or use of sunscreen restricts conversion of skin cholesterol to vitamin D. Therefore, fortified food products are important in meeting an individual's vitamin D needs.
- Distilled whiskeys are usually well tolerated by those with celiac disease.
- Most other vinegars in the United States are made from products (eg, corn, apples, grapes, rice) that are well tolerated by those with celiac disease.
- The most recent DRI recommends that Americans decrease their sodium intake to 1500 mg/day and obtain a good potassium intake. This committee also noted that this level of sodium intake will be difficult to achieve considering the present intake and food supply. (See DRI73 for sodium.)

References

1. Bujalkova M, Straka S, Jureckova A. Hippocrates' humoral pathology in nowaday's reflections. *Bratisl Lek Listy.* 2001;102 (10):489-492.
2. *The Art of Feeding the Invalid by a Medical Practitioner and A Lady Professor of Cookery.* London: The Scientific Press, Ltd. (circa 1800s).
3. Hornick B, ed. *Manual of Clinical Dietetics.* 6th ed. Chicago, IL: American Dietetic Association; 2000.
4. Nevin-Folino NL, ed. *Pediatric Manual of Clinical Dietetics.* 2nd ed. Chicago, IL: American Dietetic Association; 2003.
5. Practice guidelines for preoperative fasting and the use of pharmacologic agents to reduce the risk of pulmonary aspiration: application to healthy patients undergoing elective procedures: a report by the American Society of Anesthesiologist Task Force on Preoperative Fasting. *Anesthesiology.* 1999;90(3):896-905.
6. Winslow EH, Crenshaw JT, Warner MA. Best practices shouldn't be optional: prolonged fasts aren't more effective – or even safer. *Amer J Nurs.* 2002;102(6):59-60.
7. Bohm B, Haase O, Heine G, Junghans T. Muller JM. Tolerance of early oral feeding after operations of the lower gastrointestinal tract. *Chirug.* 2000;71(8):955-962.
8. Gocmen A, Gocmen M, Saraoglu M. Early post-operative feeding after caesarean delivery. *J Int Med Res.* 2002;30(5):506-511.
9. Lee AC, Munro FD, MacKinlay GA. An audit of post-pyloromyotomy feeding regimens. *Eur J Pediatr Surg.* 2001;11(1):12-14.
10. Moore EE, Jones TN. Benefits of immediate jejunostomy feeding after major abdominal trauma – a prospective, randomized study. *J Trauma.* 1986;26(10):874-880.
11. Food Trial Collaboration. Poor nutritional status on admission predicts poor outcomes after stroke. *Stroke.* 2003;34:1450-1456.
12. AGA Technical review on management of oropharyngeal dysphagia. *Gastroenterology.* 1999;116(2):455-478.
13. The National Dysphagia Diet Task Force. *The National Dysphagia Diet: Standardization for Optimal Care.* Chicago IL: American Dietetic Association; 2002.
14. McCallum SL. The national dysphagia diet: implementation at a regional rehabilitation center and hospital system. *J Amer Diet Assoc.* 2003;103(3):381-384.
15. DeVault KR, Castell DO. Updated guidelines for the diagnosis and treatment of gastroesophageal reflux disease. The Practice Parameters Committee of the Am Coll Gastroenterol. *Am J Gastroenterol.* 1999;94(6):1434-1442.
16. Meining A, Classen M. The role of diet and lifestyle measures in the pathogenesis and treatment of gastroesophageal reflux disease. *Am J Gastroenterol.* 2000;95(10):2692-2697.
17. Katz PO. Optimizing medical therapy for gastroesophageal reflux disease: state of the art. *Rev Gastroenterol Disord.* 2003;3(2):59-69.
18 Boekema JC, Samsom M, van Berge Henegouwen GP, Smout AJ. Coffee and gastrointestinal function. A Review. *Scand J Gastroenterol* (Suppl). 1999;230:35-39.
19 Chari S, Teyssen S, Singer MV. Alcohol and gastric acid secretion in humans. *Gut.* 1993;34(6):843-847.
20. Stermer E. Alcohol consumption and the gastrointestinal tract. *Isr Med Assoc J.* 2002;4(3):200-202.
21 Van Deventer G, Kamemoto E, Kuznicki JT, Heckert DC, Schulte MC. Lower esophagel sphincter pressure, acid secretion, and blood gastrin after coffee consumption. *Dig Dis Sci.* 1992;37(4):558-569.
22. UCSF Medical Center Post Gastrointestinal Surgery Diet, 2004 (developed by Viveca Ross, RD, CNSD).
23. Sahi T. Genetics and epidemiology of adult-type hypolactasia. *Scand J Gastroenterol.* (Suppl). 1994;202:7-20.
24. McBean LD, Miller GD. Allaying fears and fallacies about lactose intolerance. *J Am Diet Assoc.* 1998;98(6):671-676.
25. Hertzler SR, Huynh BC, Savaiano DA. How much lactose is low lactose? *J Am Diet Assoc.* 1996;96(3):243-246.
26. Vesa TH, Korpela RA, Sahi T. Tolerance to small amounts of lactose in lactose maldigesters. *Am J Clin Nutr.* 1996;64(2):197-201.
27. Solomons NW, Guerrero AM, Torum B. Dietary manipulation of postprandial colonic lactose fermentation: I. Effect of solid food in a meal. *Am J Clin Nutr.* 1985;41(2):199-208.
28. Martini MC, Savaiano DA. Reduced intolerance symptoms from lactose consumed during a meal. *Am J Clin Nutr.* 1988;47(1):57-60.
29. Hornick B, ed. *Manual of Clinical Dietetics.* 6th ed. Chicago, IL: American Dietetic Association; 2000.
30. Pennington JAT. *Bowes and Church's Food Values of Portions Commonly Used.* Philadelphia: JB Lippincott; 1994.
31. Vader LW, Stepniak DT, Bunnik EM, Kooy YMC, deHaan W, Drijfhout JW, Van Veelen PA, Koning F. Characterization of cereal toxicity for celiac disease patients based on protein homology in grains. *Gastroenterology.* 2003;125(4):1105-1113.
32. Hill ID, Bhatnagar S, Cameron DJ, DeRosa S, Maki M, Russell GJ, Troncone R. Celiac disease: working group report of the First World Congress of Pediatric Gastroenterology, Hepatology, and Nutrition. *J Pediatr Gastroenterol Nutr.* 2002;35:S78-S88.
33. Murray JA. The widening spectrum of celiac disease. *Am J Clin Nutr.* 1999;69(3):354-365.
34. Williamson D, Marsh MN. Celiac disease. *Mol Biotechnol.* 2002; 22(3):293-299.
35. Vader LW, Stepniak DT, Bunnik EM, Kooy YMC, deHaan W, Drijfhout JW, Van Veelen PA, Koning F. Characterization of cereal toxicity for celiac disease patients based on protein homology in grains. *Gastroenterology.* 2003;125(4):1105-1113.
36 Cranney A, Zarkadas M, Graham ID, Switzer C. The Canadian celiac health survey – the Ottawa chapter pilot. *BMC Gastroenterology.* 2003;3:8.

37. Food Allergen Labeling and Consumer Protection Act of 2004 (Title II of Public Law 108-282), US Food and Drug Administration, Center for Food Safety and Applied Nutrition. http://www.cfsan.fda.gov/~dms/alrgact.html (Accessed July 19, 2005).
38. Seigler DS. Plants and their uses, Department of Plant Biology, University of Illinois, Urbana, 2003. http://www.life.uiuc.edu/plantbio/263/CERGRAIN.html (Accessed June, 2004).
39. Peraaho M, Kaukinen K, Paasikivi K, Sievanen H, Lohiniemi S, Maki M, Collin P. Wheat-starch-based gluten-free products in the treatment of newly detected celiac disease: prospective and randomized study. *Aliment Pharmacol Ther.* 2003;17(4):587-594.
40. Seigler DS. Plants and their uses, Department of Plant Biology, University of Illinois, Urbana, 2003. http://www.life.uiuc.edu/plantbio/263/CERGRAIN.html (Accessed June, 2004).
41. Seigler DS. Plants and their uses, Department of Plant Biology, University of Illinois, Urbana, 2003. http://www.life.uiuc.edu/plantbio/263/CERGRAIN.html (Accessed June, 2004).
42. Seigler DS. Plants and their uses, Department of Plant Biology, University of Illinois, Urbana, 2003. http://www.life.uiuc.edu/plantbio/263/CERGRAIN.html (Accessed June, 2004).
43. Janatuinen EK, Pikkarainen PH,Kemppainen TA, Kosma VM, Jarvinen RM, Uusitupa MI, Julkunen RJ. A comparison of diets with and without oats in adults with celiac disease. *N Engl Med J.* 1995;333(16):1033-1037.
44. Janatuinen EK, Kemppainen TA, Julkunen RJ, Kosma VM, Maki M, Heikkinen M, Uusitupa MI. No harm from five year ingestion of oats in coeliac disease. *Gut.* 2002;50(3):332-335.
45. Farrell RJ, Kelly CP. Celiac sprue. *N Engl J Med.* 2002;346(3):180-188.
46. Thompson T. Oats and the gluten-free diet. *J Amer Diet Assoc.* 2003;103(3):376-379.
47. Managing Celiac Disease. UCSF Medical Center educational material, 2002 (developed by Ashleigh Sellman, RD).
48. Abdulkarim AS, Burgart LJ, See J, Murray JA. Etiology of nonresponsive celiac disease: results of a systematic approach. *Am J Gastroenterol.* 2002;97(8):2016-2021.
49. Hallert C, Grant C, Grehn S, Granno C, Hulten S, Midhagen G, Strom M, Svensson H, Valdimarsson T. Evidence of poor vitamin status in coeliac patients on a gluten-free diet for 10 years. *Aliment Pharmacol Ther.* 2002;16(7):1333-1339.
50. Cashman KD, Shanahan F. Is nutrition an aetiological factor for inflammatory bowel disease? *Eur J Gastroenterol Hepatol.* 2003;15(6):607-613.
51. Campos FG, Waitzberg DL, Teixeira MG, Mucerino DR, Habr-Gama A, Kiss DR. Inflammatory bowel diseases. Principles of nutrition therapy. *Rev Hosp Clin Fac Med Sao Paulo.* 2002;57(4):187-198.
52. Levenstein S, Prantera C, Luzi C, D'Ubaldi A. Low residue or normal diet in Crohn's disease: a prospective controlled study in Italian patients. *Gut.* 1985;26(10):989-993.
53. Goh J, O'Morain CA. Review article: nutrition and adult inflammatory bowel disease. *Aliment Pharmacol Ther.* 2003;17(3):307-320.
54. Worcester EM, Stones from bowel disease. *Endocrinol Metab Clin North Am.* 2002;31(4):979-999.
55. Johnson MD. Management of short bowel syndrome – a review. *Support Lind.* 2000;22(6):11-25.
56. Holmes RP, Kennedy M. Estimation of the oxalate content of foods and daily oxalate content of foods and daily oxalate intake. *Kidney Int.* 2000;57:1662-1667.
57. Manual of Clinical Dietetics (6th edition) & Pediatric Manual of Clinical Dietetics (2nd edition). American Dietetic Association.
58. Gassull MA, Cabre E. Nutrition in inflammatory bowel disease. *Curr Opin Clin Nutr Metab Care.* 2001;4(6):561-569.
59. Al-Jaouni R, Schneider SM, Piche T, Rampal P, Hebuterne X. Effect of steroids on energy expenditure and substrate oxidation in women with Crohn's disease. *Am J Gastroenterol.* 2002;97(11):2843-2849.
60. O'Morain C, Segal AW, Levin AJ. Elemental diet as primary treatment of acute Crohn's disease: a controlled trial. *Br Med J.* 1984;288(6434):1859-1862.
61. Wright N, Scott BB, Wright N. Dietary treatment of active Crohn's disease. *Brit Med J.* 1997;314(7079):454-456.
62. Bernstein CN, Shanahan F. Critical appraisal of enteral nutrition as primary therapy in adults with Crohn's disease. *Am J Gastroenterol.* 1996;91(10):2075-2079.
63. Griffiths AM, Ohlsson A, Sherman PM, Sutherland LR. Meta-analysis of enteral nutrition as a primary treatment of active Crohn's disease. *Gastroenterology.* 1995;108(4):1056-1067.
64. Cabre E, Gassull MA. Nutritional and metabolic issues in inflammatory bowel disease. *Curr Opin Clin Nutr Metab Care.* 2003;6(5):569-576.
65. Gassull MA, Frenandez-Banares F, Cabre E, et al. European Group on Enteral Nutrition in Crohn's Disease. Fat composition may be a clue to explain the primary therapeutic effect of enteral nutrition in Crohn's disease: results of a double blind randomized multicentre European trial. *Gut.* 2002;51(2):164-168.
66. Bamba T, Shimoyama T. Sasaki M, et al. Dietary fat attenuates the benefits of an elemental diet in active Crohn's disease: a randomized, controlled trial. *Eur J Gastroenterol Hepatol.* 2003;15(2):151-157.
67. Ziegler TR, Evans ME, Fernandez-Estivariz C, Jones D. Trophic and cytoprotective nutrition for intestinal adaptation, mucosal repair, and barrier function. *Ann Rev Nutr.* 2003;23:229-261.
68. Gorard DA. Enteral nutrition in Crohn's disease: fat in the formula. *Eur J Gastronenterol Hepatol.* 2003;15(2):115-118.
69. Teitelbaum JE, Allan W. Review: the role of omega 3 fatty acids in intestinal inflammation. *J Nutr Biochem.* 2001;12(1):21-32.
70. Seidner DL, Lashner BA, Brzezinski A, et al. An oral supplement enriched with fish oil, soluble fiber, and antioxidants for cotricosteroid sparing in ulcerative colitis: a randomized, controlled trial. *Clin Gastro Hepat.* 2005;3:358-369.
71. Willmore DW. Indications for specific therapy in the rehabilitation of patients with the short-bowel syndrome. *Best Practice & Research Clinical Gastroenterology.* 2003;17(6):895-906.
72 Johnson MD. Management of short bowel syndrome – a review. *Support Line.* 2000;22(6):11-13.
73. *Dietary Reference Intakes. Energy, carbohydrate, fiber, fat, fatty acids, cholesterol, protein, and amino acids.* Washington, DC: National Academy Press, 2003.
74. *Dietary Reference Intakes for Water, Potassium, Sodium, Chloride, Sulfate.* Washington, DC: National Academy Press, 2004.
75 Stickel F, Hoehn B, Schuppan D, Seitz HK. Review article: nutrition therapy in alcoholic liver disease. *Aliment Pharmacol Ther.* 2003;15;18(4):357-373.
76 Podolsky DK, Isselbacher KJ. Alcohol-related liver disease and cirrhosis. In: *Harrison's Principles of Internal Medicine.* 13th ed. New York: McGraw-Hill, Inc.; 1994.
77. Saltos E, Bowman S. Dietary guidance on sodium: should we take it with a grain of salt? *Family Economics and Nutrition Review.* 1998;11(4):49-51.
78 Plauth M, Merli M, Kondrup J, Weimann A, Ferenci P, Muller MJ. ESPEN guidelines for nutrition in liver disease and transplantation. *Clin Nutr.* 1997;16:43.
79. A.S.P.E.N. Board of Directors and the Clinical Guidelines Task Force. Specific guidelines for disease–adult. *JPEN.* 2002;26(1)(suppl):67SA-69SA.
80 Soulsby CT, Morgan MY. Dietary management of hepatic encephalopathy in cirrhotic patients: survey of current practice in United Kingdom. *Br Med J.* 1999;318(7195):1391.
81. *Dietary Reference Intakes. Energy, carbohydrate, fiber, fat, fatty acids, cholesterol, protein, and amino acids.* Washington, DC: National Academy Press, 2003.
82. Novy MA, Schwarz KB. Nutritional considerations and management of the child with liver disease. *Nutrition.* 1997;13(3):177-184.
83. Gabuzda GJ, Shear L. Metabolism of dietary protein in hepatic cirrhosis. Nutritional and clinical considerations. *Am J Clin Nutr.* 1970;23(4):479-487.

84. Swart GR Zillikens MC, van Vuure JK,van den Berg JW. Effect of a late evening meal on nitrogen balance in patients with cirrhosis of the liver. *Br Med J.* 1989;299(6709):1202-1203.
85. A.S.P.E.N. Board of Directors and the Clinical Guidelines Task Force. Specific guidelines for disease–adult. *JPEN.* 2002;26(1)(suppl):67SA-69SA.
86. Als-Nielsen B, Koretz RL, Kjaergard LL, Gluud C. Branced-chain amino acids for hepatic encephalopathy. *Cochrane Database Syst Rev.* 2003;(2):CD001939.
87. A.S.P.E.N. Board of Directors and the Clinical Guidelines Task Force. Specific guidelines for disease–adult. *JPEN.* 2002;26(1)(suppl):67SA-69SA.
88. Plauth M, Merli M, Kondrup J, Weimann A, Ferenci P, Muller MJ. ESPEN guidelines for nutrition in liver disease and transplantation. *Clin Nutr.* 1997;16:43.
89. Dejong CH, Greve JW, Soeters PB. Nutrition in patients with acute pancreatitis. *Curr Opin Crit Care.* 2001;7(4):251-256.
90. Abou-Assi S, O'Keefe SJ. Nutrition in acute pancreatitis. *J Clin Gastroenterol.* 2001;32(3):203-209.
91. Mitchell RM, Byrne MF, Baillie J. Pancreatitis. *Lancet.* 2003;361(9367):1447-1455.
92. Avgerinos C, Delis S, Rizos S, Dervenis C. Nutritional support in acute pancreatitis. *Dig Dis.* 2003;21(3):214-219.
93. Pitchumoni CS. Chronic pancreatitis: pathogenesis and management of pain. *J Clin Gastroenterol.* 1998;27(2):101-107.
94. Boivin M, Lanspa SJ, Zinsmeister AR, Go VL, DiMagno EP. Are diets associated with different rates of human interdigestive and postprandial pancreatic enzyme secretion? *Gastroenterology.* 1990;99(6):1763-1771.
95. Shea JC, Bishop MD, Parker EM, Freedman SD. An enteral therapy containing medium-chain triglycerides and hydrolyzed peptides reduces postprandial pain associated with chronic pancreatitis. *Pancreatology.* 2003;3(1):36-40.

Chapter 8

Macronutrient Digestion, Absorption, and Metabolism

Brian M. Chung, PhD, and
Kelly A. Tappenden, PhD, RD

Introduction

The absorptive epithelium of the gastrointestinal (GI) tract serves the dual purpose of providing a barrier that impedes the free passage of ingested toxins and pathogens to the systemic circulation, while digesting and subsequently absorbing ingested nutrients required for the continuation of life. The primary site of macronutrient absorption is the small intestine. The morphology of the small intestine is characterized by a series of folds serving to progressively increase absorptive area over that of a smooth tube. Plica muscularis, which are button-like projections of the epithelium into the lumen of the intestine, are lined with finger-like projections of the epithelial monolayer called villi. The luminal or apical plasma membrane of absorptive enterocytes is arranged in an array of finger-like projections termed collectively as the brush-border or microvilli. While plica muscularis magnify the surface area of the small intestine by a factor of 10, villi magnify surface area by a factor of 30 and the brush-border array magnifies absorptive area by a factor of 300.[1,2]

Given the diversity of the human diet, the ability for a single layer of specialized epithelial cells to function as a semi-permeable membrane with specificity over a surface area roughly 600 square meters is nothing short of monumental.[1,2] The transport of dietary macronutrients across the epithelium of the GI tract relies on the coordinated activities of specialized digestive enzymes, the products of which are then transported into the specialized absorptive cells lining the intestinal tract via transport proteins. The digestion of macronutrients into their basic units—monosaccharides, amino acids and peptides, and fatty acids, cholesterol esters and phospholipids—permits the absorptive enterocytes of the intestinal tract to express a limited array of specialized transporter proteins that mediate the transfer of these products from the lumen of the intestine into the enterocyte and eventually throughout the body.

Carbohydrate Digestion, Absorption and Metabolism

Dietary Carbohydrates

Mankind's quest for sugar or sweets has been proposed as a driving force for our diversification.[3] Our fascination with readily available sugar has its roots in honey, and while an officer of Alexander the Great reported sugar cane 300 years B.C., the domestication of sugar production dates back at least 5,000 years.[4] The current world sugar production totals over 150 billion kilograms of sugar per annum, amounting to nearly 70 grams per person daily.[4] While nutritionists laud the trend of developed societies to incorporate increasing amounts of processed simple sugars into their daily dietary routine, plant-derived starches still provide the majority of carbohydrates. The average dietary intake of carbohydrates is roughly 200 to 300 grams, accounting for around 50% total caloric energy intake.[5] It is somewhat fitting that our knowledge of carbohydrate absorption has come so far given the role of glucose as the primary metabolic energy source for the body.

Dietary Carbohydrate Digestion

Initial carbohydrate digestion begins with salivary α-amylase digestion. However, the enzymatic function of salivary amylase is rapidly degraded as the bolus is delivered to the low pH environment of the stomach.

TABLE 8-1.

Enzymatic Digestion of Dietary Carbohydrates

Enzyme	*Target*	*Product*
a-amylase	a(1,4)-glycosidic linkages	Di- and trisaccharides, a-limit dextrins
Sucrase-isomaltase	Sucrose, maltose& a-limit dextrins	Glucose, fructose
Lactase-phlorizin	Lactose	Glucose, galactose
Maltase-glucoamylase	a(1,4)-linked glucose polymers	Glucose

This table outlines the various enzymes expressed in the intestinal tract that are involved in the sequential digestion of dietary carbohydrates into monomeric sugars, their solutes, and their digestion products.

Upon entrance into the duodenum, the various contents of the chyme stimulate the secretion of pancreatic digestive enzymes. Pancreatic α-amylase proceeds to digest starches to shorter chain lengths and disaccharides. Final digestion of dietary carbohydrates occurs at the brush border with membrane-bound disaccharidases that cleave specific bonds to release the monomeric sugars glucose, galactose and fructose (Table 8-1). Disaccharidase enzymes can be classified as either α-glucosidases (sucrase-isomaltase, maltase-glucoamylase and trehalase), or β-glucosidase (lactase). The location of these disaccharidase enzymes creates a microclimate of high monomeric sugar intimately concentrated at the level of the brush border. Disaccharidase activities are highest in the proximal jejunum, and throughout the small intestine, brush-border disaccharidase activity is highest at the villus tip.[6] Lactase activity is highest at birth and during infancy and decreases in adulthood, as witnessed by the increased incidence of lactose intolerance in adults.[7]

Carbohydrates are digested and subsequently transported as monomeric hexoses across the brush-border membrane and into the cytosol via specialized transport proteins. Intact or partially digested oligosaccharide chains are not readily transported across the intestinal epithelium. Consequently, the importance of complete digestion of dietary carbohydrate is vital for the assimilation of dietary carbohydrates. In order to determine a treatment for a defect in carbohydrate assimilation, one must first determine if the defect is primarily the result of insufficient absorptive surface area, defective enzymatic digestion and/or defective monosaccharide transporter activity.

INTESTINAL MONOSACCHARIDE ABSORPTION

The salient protein involved in glucose and galactose transport across the brush border has been well characterized by Wright and associates as the sodium glucose/galactose-linked cotransporter 1 (SGLT1), also called SLC5A1.[8,9] SGLT1 is a secondary active transporter that harnesses the inward driving force of sodium created by the sodium potassium ATPase enzyme (Na+,K+-ATPase) on the basolateral membrane, to transfer glucose from the lumen to the cytosol. SGLT1 transports its solutes with a stoichiometric ratio of 2 sodium molecules: 1 glucose/galactose molecule, at a relatively high affinity, low volume for glucose.[10] The transport of fructose is mediated primarily through a high affinity, low volume facilitative transporter GLUT5, the product of gene SLC2A5 that mediates the transport of fructose down a concentration gradient.[11]

Classic absorptive physiology holds that, once these monomeric hexoses enter the cytoplasm of the absorptive enterocyte, they are then transported down their concentration gradient through the low-affinity, high-volume facilitative hexose transporter GLUT2 (SLC2A2). GLUT2 is a multi-solute facilitative transporter that transports both glucose and fructose across the basolateral membrane and into the intracellular space where the nutrients diffuse into the portal circulation. Also important is the fact that this process is normally carried out by enterocytes occupying the upper one-third of the villus. To this end, it should also be noted that SGLT1 has been described as a water carrier, transporting almost 300 water molecules per glucose monomer per cycle, an activity that might be vital for the absorption of water.[12,13] The net movement of water in complement to nutrient absorption has been utilized for treatment of dehydration and infectious diarrhea, as witnessed through the use of Oral Rehydration Solution as advocated by the World Health Organization (WHO).[14]

While the plasticity of the described hexose transport system is capable of effective glucose uptake from the lumen when glucose concentrations are between 40 to 80 mM, a number of additional hexose transport pathways have also been described which have been implicated to occur in exceptional circumstances.[15-17] The initial deposition of glucose and other nutrients into the intracellular space beneath the tight junction complex can create a microclimate reaching 600 to 1000 mOsm, which creates an enormous osmotic gradient across the epithelium.[15] Complementing the creation of an intense osmotic gradient in the intracellular space is the data indicating that the entrance of glucose has been shown to stimulate a contraction of the actin-myosin fibers in the terminal web cytoskeletal array, which supports the brush-border and tight junction complex, resulting in a reduction of the enterocyte circumference.[18] These two mechanisms have been used to describe a model of solvent drag, in which the osmotic gradient across the tight junction complex as well as the contraction of the terminal web lead to increased pore size between adjacent enterocytes and subsequent flow of nutrients down the osmotic gradient to dilute the intracellular space. This model would provide an enormous absorptive capacity, albeit with somewhat reduced specificity.

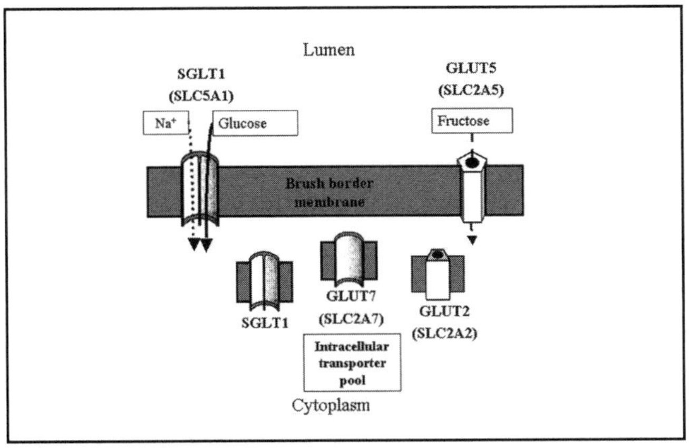

Figure 8-1A. Glucose and fructose are initially transported across the brush-border membrane via SGLT1, GLUT5. Additional transport capacity is retained within the enterocyte in the form of intracellular hexose transporters (SGLT1, GLUT7 and GLUT2).

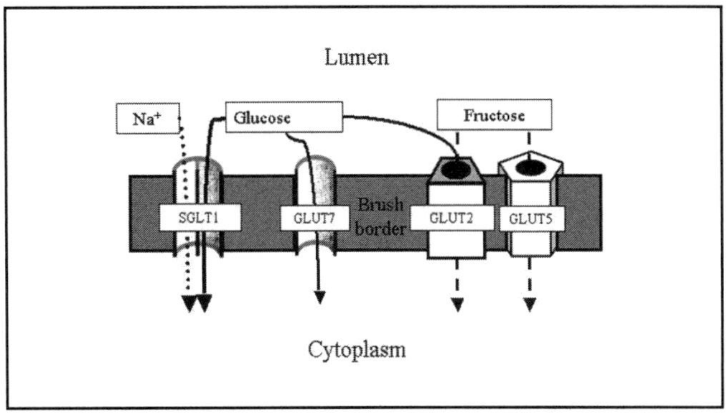

Figure 8-1B. Should the normal brush-border hexose transport mechanism (SGLT1 and GLUT5) become overwhelmed, SGLT1, GLUT2 and GLUT7 from a sub-apical intracellular store can be inserted into the brush border to increase epithelial hexose absorptive capacity by increasing the number of hexose transport proteins.

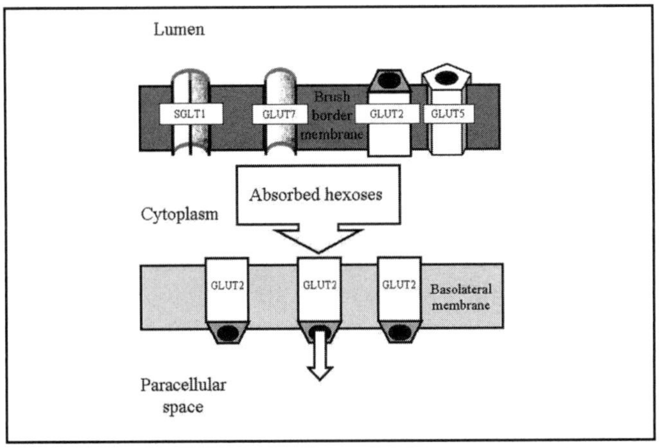

Figure 8-1C. Hexoses transported across the brush border and into the cytoplasm of the absorptive enterocyte are then transported across the basolateral membrane and into the paracellular space via the facilitative hexose transporter GLUT2.

An additional monosaccharide transport pathway stems from the interesting findings that GLUT2, the classic facilitative glucose transporter initially believed to be sequestered to the basolateral membrane, as well as a novel facilitative glucose-specific transporter GLUT7 (SLC2A7), can both be inserted into the brush border in response to high glucose loads in the lumen of the small intestine.[11,16,19] This model requires glucose to initially be transported by SGLT1, whose activity triggers protein kinase C (PKC) and mitogen-activating protein kinase (MAP-K), the end effect of which is the rapid insertion of GLUT2 into the brush border.[16] The rapid insertion of facilitative glucose (GLUT2 and GLUT7) and fructose (GLUT2) transport proteins in the apical brush border would then provide a pair of high-volume facilitative hexose transporters capable of handling the microclimate of high monosaccharide concentrated by brush-border dissacharidases.[16,19,20] Figure 8-1A-C illustrates the various carrier-mediated pathways which dietary monosaccharides can be transported across the absorptive enterocyte. Figure 8-2 illustrates the difference between specific carrier-mediated monosaccharide transport that occurs via absorptive enterocytes lining the upper villus region, as well as paracellular solvent drag between adjacent enterocytes.

Patients diagnosed with the rare genetic disorder known as Fanconi-Bickel disease demonstrate a defect in GLUT2 function. Accordingly, these patients present no classic basolateral hexose transport pathway. However, despite this defect, these patients can be managed with correct dietary manipulation. To this end, this condition has been studied and data indicates an alternative hexose delivery pathway wherein luminal glucose is transported into the cytoplasm via SGLT1. Subsequently, glucose is phosphorylated and transferred into the endoplasmic reticulum whereupon membrane-trafficking delivers glucose-containing vesicles to the basolateral membrane and hence delivered into the basolateral space.[20-23]

The crucial step in intestinal hexose transport remains sodium-coupled glucose transport through SGLT1. Following transport across the brush-border membrane, numerous signaling pathways, microclimate changes, and metabolic enzymes can act to regulate the rate of glucose hexose transport as well as the transfer of the absorbed hexoses into the basolateral space.[24-28]

Regulation of Monosaccharide Transport

Numerous studies have demonstrated an innate capacity for increased transport capacity in response to numerous stimuli.[17] Glucose itself has been shown to elicit rapid increases in active glucose transport mediated via SGLT1, as have other clinically relevant conditions such as prior exercise, forskolin treatment (and possibly other conditions that cause prolonged elevations in cyclic AMP), surgical anesthetics, heat shock injury, epinephrine, and various hormones such as epidermal growth factor and glucagon-like peptide-2 over a longer time.[27,29-40] In addition to expression patterns changing in accordance to circadian rhythm, changes in dietary intake of carbohydrates, leading to alterations in the luminal hexose load, have been

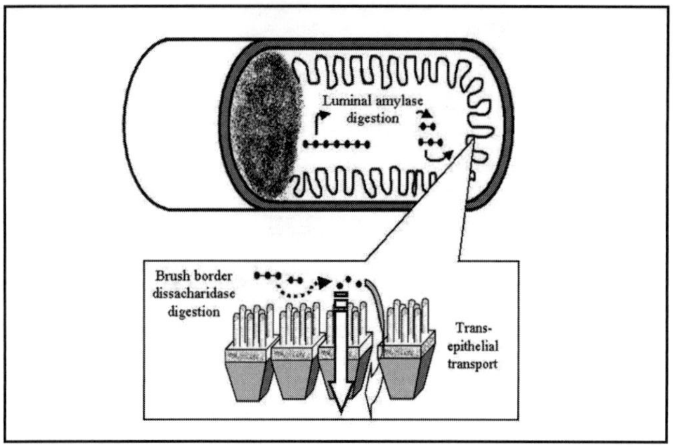

Figure 8-2. Luminal hexoses, the product of luminal a-amylase and brush-border dissacharidase digestion are initially absorbed by carrier-mediated mechanisms utilizing specific transport proteins. The deposition of hexoses into the paracellular space between each enterocyte can create an osmotic force that can draw water and solutes (such as hexoses) across the tight junctions between each enterocyte.

shown to alter the expression of SGLT1.[41,42] In a similar manner, resection of a significant length of small intestine, reducing the total absorptive surface area of the remaining gut, stimulates the remnant intestine to mount a number of adaptive responses including increased absorptive surface area through increased villus and brush-border height and corresponding alterations nutrient transport capacity.[31, 43-45] Conversely, removal of enteral nutrition and provision of nutrients by parenteral route has been shown to induce atrophy of the intestinal tract. The corresponding reduction in absorptive surface with total parenteral nutrition induced intestinal atrophy area also influences transporter expression, and subsequent carbohydrate absorptive capacity.[38,44,46-48] Natural age progression and inhibition of the metabolic enzyme ornithine decarboxylase[49] have been linked to a decrease in intestinal glucose transport indicative of decreased expression of the hexose transporters.[50,51] Specific interactions with the hexose transporters have been demonstrated by altering the outer hemileaflet fluidity of the brush-border membrane[52] and through possible interaction with immunosuppressives.[53,54]

While the overall increase or decrease in transporter expression can have profound effects on substrate transport, the involvement of this regulatory mechanism in the context of the small intestine must also be rendered in the context of the unique absorptive morphology of this organ. Indeed, some studies have found that, in addition to specifically increasing the amount of SGLT1 in the brush border and thus rapidly increasing active glucose transport capacity, these mechanisms increase brush-border height as well as recruit enterocytes further down the villus by utilizing actin polymerization and a possible chaperone protein known as RSC1A1.[29,30,39,55] Therefore, the rapid increase in active glucose transport capacity also involves increasing absorptive surface area by the dual recruitment of additional membrane into the brush border and additional enterocytes into the absorptive population.[29,30] Another interesting mechanism arises when one examines the effect of altering the location of SGLT1 expression along the villus axis. In a system where no alteration in the overall amount of SGLT1 is seen, reducing expression at the villus tip and biasing expression to the base of the villus equates to decreased active glucose transport capacity, while the normalization of this expression pattern (increasing towards the villus tip) restores transport capacity to normal.[43,44,56] Hence, while absorptive surface area and capacity appear to be intimately associated, morphological location of these transporters can also have a profound effect on transport capacity.

Assimilation of Resistant Starch and Dietary Fiber

While the discussion to this point has focused on readily digested and transported carbohydrate, one must not forsake dietary fiber as an important dietary carbohydrate. The term dietary fiber has been used to describe species of plant starches for which humans do not express adequate digestive enzymes to digest. Subsequently, a portion of plant-based carbohydrate actually escapes enzymatic digestion in the upper intestinal tract. Instead, some forms of dietary fiber, termed fermentable fiber, undergo fermentation in the large intestine by resident microflora. In addition, despite the excess capacity for digestion and absorption in the small intestine, with the majority of absorbable carbohydrates being absorbed in the jejunum, a minor amount of digestible carbohydrates escapes digestion and passes into the large intestine; these resistant starches also serve as a fermentable carbohydrate source for the resident microflora.[57] Nonfiber carbohydrates that have been processed under high heat can be chemically altered to prevent enzymatic digestion in the small intestine, thereby passing into the large intestine where they undergo fermentation.[58] As well, endogenous carbohydrates in the form of glycoproteins, such as mucins, enter the large intestine and can also be fermented.[58]

The fermentation of resistant starches in the large intestine leads to the production of short-chain fatty acids (SCFA), with the major forms acetate (60% to 75%)—propionate (15% to 25%) and butyrate (10% to 15%)—produced in fairly consistent ratios across a wide range of species.[59] In an elegant example of symbiosis, these fermentation products, butyrate in particular, serve as the primary metabolic energy source for the epithelial cells of the large intestine and can also be readily utilized by the epithelium of the small intestine. Differing amounts of fermentable fiber along the length of the intestine allow concentrations of SCFA to also change as one samples along the gut.[57]

To enter the colonocyte for metabolism or transfer to the portal blood, SCFA must first cross the apical membrane of these cells. The lumen of the colon is generally neutral (pH 7.0), and at this proton concentration, butyrate and the other SCFA species dissociate to anionic form and cannot readily pass across the apical membrane of the colonocyte. However, the presence of sodium proton exchange (mediated by NHE3) in the apical membrane of colonocytes and small intestinal enterocytes acts to acidify the microclimate overlaying these cells that might aid in the diffusion of SCFA across the apical membrane.[60-63] Despite the acidic microclimate overlying the apical membrane, evidence for the transport of SCFA across the apical

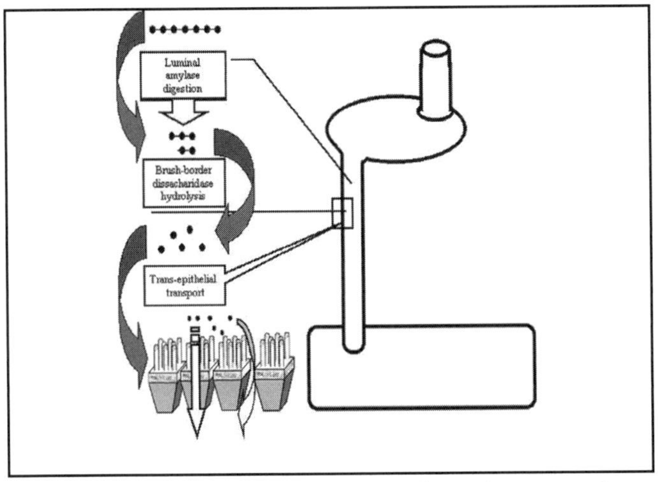

Figure 8-3A. As carbohydrates progress down the intestinal tract, they are sequentially digested and absorbed as monomeric glucose and fructose in the small intestine.

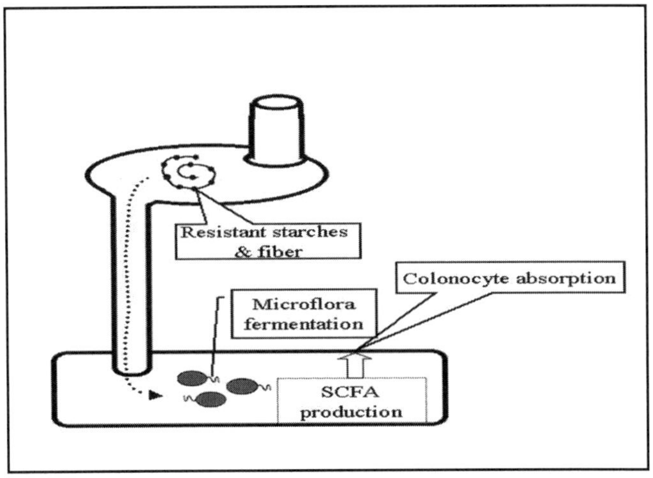

Figure 8-3B. Resistant starches and fermentable fiber in the large intestine undergo bacterial fermentation releasing short chain fatty acids (SCFA) that are then absorbed by the colonic epithelium.

plasma membrane is more indicative of the presence of a carrier-mediated process. Consequently, numerous anion transporters have been implicated in the absorption of SCFA in the large intestine, and these processes also have been demonstrated in the distal small intestine.

Analysis of SCFA transport in the intestinal tract is difficult because the epithelial cells of the intestine quickly metabolize SCFA, particularly butyrate. Despite these complications, much progress has been made in the analysis of carriers that mediate the transport of SCFA. Recently, a sodium-dependent SCFA co-transporter, termed sodium-coupled monocarboxylate transporter (SMCT), also called SLC5A8, has been cloned and identified in the colon.64 The membrane location of SMCT is yet unknown, but this transporter does transport SCFA in a sodium-dependent manner with a stoichiometric ratio of 4:1.[64] In the distal ileum, and throughout the colon, an anion-monocarboxylate exchanger known as MCT1, also known as SLC16A1, has been implicated as an important mediator of SCFA uptake from the lumen.[60,65-67] MCT1 mediates the exchange of bicarbonate with SCFA, with the interesting fact that exchange activity is increased when the microclimate overlying the apical membrane is slightly acidic.[66,68,69] Despite the preference for an acidic external environment, there does not appear to be reliance between NHE and MCT activities.[68] Studies have also indicated the presence of a chloride/SCFA exchange mechanism in both surface and crypt epithelial cells of the colon that is perceived to play a minor but nonetheless important role in SCFA transport when compared to MCT1.[60,70,71]

Once across the apical plasma membrane, SCFA are either rapidly metabolized, or, in a manner similar to hexoses, can be transported out of the epithelial cells and into the circulation. Because cytoplasmic pH is neutral, SCFA transported into the epithelial cells undergo dissociation to, or remain in, anionic form. Consequently, the transfer of SCFA across the basolateral membrane is likely carrier mediated. There is evidence for bicarbonate/butyrate exchange on the basolateral membrane that is functionally distinct from MCT1 located on the apical membrane.[69,72] This exchanger is believed to function to extrude SCFA (butyrate in particular) from the epithelial cell to the portal circulation, rather than transport monocarboxylates like ketone bodies into these cells during fasting.[65,69]

As with hexose transporters, studies have shown that SCFA transport can be regulated by diet, although through a more complicated mechanism. The requirement for microfloral fermentation to produce SCFA allows dietary alterations that alter the microfloral constituent of the gut (pre- and probiotics) to have profound effects on the amount of SCFA produced. Alterations in luminal butyrate production have been shown to directly influence MCT1 expression in the colon,[73] as have long-term inhibition of PKC activity.[67] Ileal inflammation has been linked to decreased butyrate uptake; however, the mechanism governing this response does not appear to involve altering MCT1 expression.[71]

The assimilation of carbohydrate energy by the human body is vital for normal function as glucose is the primary metabolic fuel for almost all cell types in the body. Therefore, it is appropriate that the intestinal tract has developed efficient mechanisms through which to absorb carbohydrate energy in the form of hexoses. This marvelous efficiency can been witnessed in both effectiveness and plasticity of the small intestine to digest dietary carbohydrates and rapidly absorb the monomeric hexoses through a number of different pathways and with the capacity to transport and utilize the products of resistant carbohydrate fermentation as a primary metabolic energy source. Figure 8-3A,B illustrates the pattern of carbohydrate assimilation along the length of the intestinal tract, with regard to digestible carbohydrates, as well as resistant starches and fermentable fiber.

Intestinal Carbohydrate Metabolism

Although often obscured by reports emphasizing glutamine as the enterocyte-preferred nutrient, short-term cultures of isolated enterocyte have demonstrated that glucose is also an important oxidative fuel.[74-77] When assessing oxidative fuel use of the portal drained viscera, glucose accounts for 29% of CO_2 produced, a level that is secondary to both glutamine and glutamate. Further, glutamine can suppress glucose oxidation in culture enterocytes, whereas glucose has little impact on glutamine oxidation.[75,76] These data have lead to speculation that glutamine and glutamate are preferentially channeled towards mitochondrial oxidation, while most of the glucose is utilized for other metabolic or biosynthetic purposes relating to mucin glycoproteins and lipids.

Reports from Burrin and colleagues indicate that the route of glucose administration impacts glucose oxidation rate.[78] These studies, conducted in neonatal piglets, confirm that significant quantities of glucose are indeed oxidized by the GI tract. However, they further indicate a preferential oxidation of arterial rather than dietary glucose. The enterocytes preference to oxidize glucose obtained from systemic circulation, rather than that provided from the intestinal lumen, indicates that the intestine has a preferred mandate to pass glucose onto the liver for metabolic judgment regarding whole body nutrient partitioning and glycemic control. These results also indicate that the relationship between nutrient transport and oxidative processes in the enterocyte are not simply related by virtue of concentration gradients. Future work must focus on molecular chaperones that may distinguish brush-border versus basolaterally-derived glucose as it relates to enterocyte oxidation. Finally, the enterocytes preference to oxidize systemically provided glucose has implications for patients receiving total parenteral nutrition. The role of intestinal metabolism in critically ill patients receiving parenteral nutrition warrants attention, as intensive metabolic control remains an issue of priority.[79]

SCFA are readily metabolized by colonocytes.[80-86] Uptake and metabolism of SCFA is rapid and complete as $^{14}CO_2$ appears in the breath 10 to 15 minutes after administration, and 50% of $^{1\text{-}14}C$-labelled acetic and propionic acids and 63% of butyric acid appear as $^{14}CO_2$ in the breath within 6 hours.[87] Butyrate, specifically, appears to be the fuel of choice for colonocytes,[77,81,88,89] and its presence suppresses glucose oxidation by about 50%.[90] It has been estimated by colonic luminal perfusion studies that the human colon has the ability to absorb up to 540 kcal/day in the form of SCFAs.[91] However, in addition to providing energy, SCFA production may influence GI function beyond the colon and systemic administration of SCFA enhance both small intestinal structure and nutrient transport, as discussed earlier.[44,92,93]

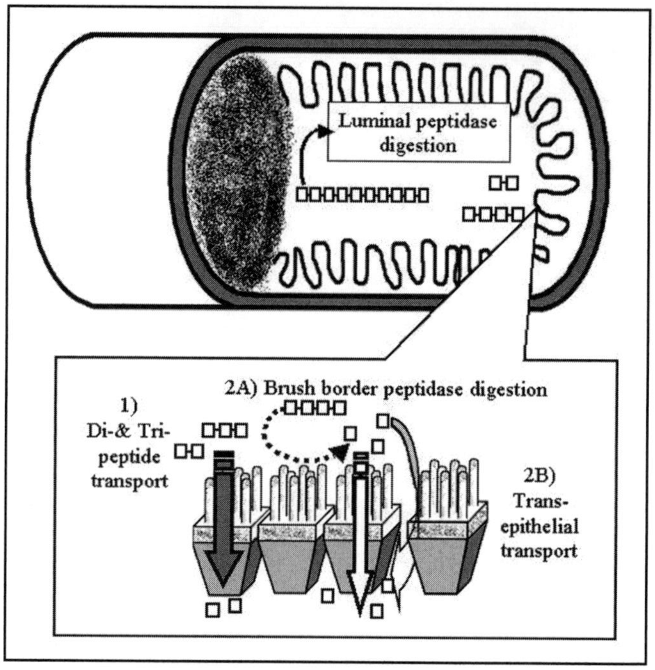

Figure 8-4. Digestion of luminal proteins and epithelial transport. Luminal protease and peptidase activity digests proteins into large peptides (upper panel). Di and tri-peptides are transported across the apical brush-border membrane via specific carrier-mediated transport (PEPT1 and HPT1) (Lower panel, 1). Large peptides are subsequently digested by brush-border peptidases into di- and tri-peptides and free amino acids (Lower panel, 2A). Di- and tri-peptides (Lower panel 1A), along with free amino acids (Lower panel 2B) can be transported across the epithelium via specific carrier-mediated transport. Note that small amounts of intact proteins and large peptides can also be absorbed from the lumen by pinocytotic endocytosis.

Protein Digestion, Absorption, and Metabolism

Dietary Protein

The human body utilizes 20 amino acids, 9 of which are considered essential because they cannot be made endogenously. Physiological amino acids are those in the L-isomeric configuration, as D-stereoisomers are generally bacterial-derived.[94] The average daily intake of protein is roughly 70 to 100 g/day. This amount of protein is coupled to 50 to 60 g/day—excreted into the lumen of the intestinal tract in the form of digestive enzymes, carrier proteins, antibodies and cellular debris—which places a large digestive and absorptive load on the intestinal tract.[95] The intestinal tract absorbs proteins and their products through a complex series of mechanisms, some of which are just recently being elucidated. The intestinal tract has the ability to absorb proteins intact, as the peptide products of digestion in the lumen by luminal and brush-border peptidases and as amino-acid monomers. It is important to remember the concept of solvent drag and how a portion of the protein assimilation might also occur by non-carrier–mediated passage across the tight junction complex in response to the increased osmotic load and terminal web contraction. Figure 8-4 illustrates the mechanisms by which protein absorption takes place across the absorptive epithelium of the small intestine.

Dietary Protein Digestion

The absorption of intact proteins has been described as a mechanism through which infants acquire maternal immunity factors as well as α-lactalbumin in breastmilk.[94] This process occurs in newborn neonates in part because of the delayed development of acid production in the stomach and proteolytic activity in pancreatic secretions and brush-border peptidases.[94] In a process termed "closure," this transport pathway gradually declines immediately following parturition. Despite the gradual decline in intact protein absorption across the GI tract, there continues to be a small portion of intact protein absorption by the epithelium into adulthood. This process is implicated in the antigenic sampling of the dietary load by microfold or M-cells overlying Peyer's patches throughout the small intestine. M-cells constantly sample the contents of the lumen through pinocytosis. These M-cells rapidly deliver their sampled contents via basolateral exocytosis to underlying immunocompetent cells comprising the lymphoid mass. M-cells appear particularly competent at absorbing antigens that have been bound by secretory IgA.[94] This process is important in the development and maintenance of oral immunity. Absorptive enterocytes are also capable of pinocytosis of intact proteins from the lumen. Interestingly, the protein uptake rate is similar between M-cells and enterocytes, and the ability for M-cells to deliver intact proteins for immunological antigen sampling is a result of the reduced cytoplasmic protease activity in the M-cells.[94]

Intact protein absorption plays a minor role in nutrient absorption, therefore most protein energy is assimilated following significant degradation. The initial stage of protein degradation occurs in the acid environment of the stomach, where low pH initiates protein hydrolysis. Gastric pepsin acts to cleave proteins into large peptides. Enzymatic secretions from the pancreas comprise the next stage of luminal protein digestion. Trypsin, chymotrypsin, elastase, and carboxypeptidase comprise the major proteases and peptidases that digest proteins and large peptides in the lumen of the small intestine. The luminal digestion of proteins results in 3 to 6 amino-acid peptides and free amino acids.[2] Subsequent brush-border peptidase digestion of the remnant peptide chains releases free amino acids; however, a significant portion of 2 to 3 amino-acid peptides can be absorbed across the brush border. Brush-border peptidases include enterokinase, which activates trypsin secreted by the pancreas, as well as aminopeptidase and dipeptidase. These brush-border enzymes digest peptides into di- and tripeptides and monomeric amino acids.[2] There is evidence that peptide transport comprises the significant mechanism for protein assimilation in the proximal small intestine, and that amino-acid transporters comprise the significant transport mechanisms from the jejunum and especially into the ileum.[2,95] The gradient of preferential peptide versus amino-acid transport along the length of the small intestine is likely related to the gradual digestion of the chyme. The gradual digestion of protein results in increasing amounts of monomeric amino acids as the chyme proceeds down the intestinal tract. In association with the transport function of villus tip enterocytes, brush-border peptidase activity is highest in the villus tip region and demonstrates a decreasing activity gradient along the length of the small intestine.[6]

Intestinal Peptide Absorption

The absorption of 2 to 3 amino-acid peptides is mediated through the proton-driven peptide transporter PEPT1 (SLC15A1) and another peptide transporter HPT-1. PEPT1 is particularly fascinating given that peptides can be transported regardless of their net charge or size. Recent studies have derived recognition requirements under which PEPT1 operates.[96] PEPT1 cotransports hydrogen with peptides across the brush border in a 1:1 stoichiometric ratio, and the hydrogen is recycled out of the enterocyte by NHE3. Once in the cytoplasm of enterocytes, peptides can either be rapidly digested to monomeric amino acids by cytoplasmic proteases or transported across the basolateral membrane through a peptide transporter distinct from PEPT1 and whose identity has not yet been established.[96] The capacity to transport the intact peptides is particularly important for patients of Hartnup disease, with which patients cannot absorb the particular amino-acid histidine, tryptophan, and phenylalanine, and also for patients suffering cystinuria type 1, where cytosine transport is defective. These genetic conditions are both due to genetic defects in two different amino-acid transporters;[96] however, these patients can assimilate these amino acids if they are delivered in di- and tripeptide form.[97]

Another interesting role for PEPT1 is in the absorption of oral drugs and prodrugs.[96,98-101] Certain oral angiotensin-converting enzyme inhibitors and antibiotics can be transported across the intestinal epithelium via a PEPT1-mediated process. In the case of prodrugs, subsequent proteolytic digestion in the cytoplasm of the enterocyte activates the compound before its release into the circulation. This mechanism has been employed to improve the bioavailability of L-DOPA (L-3,4-dihydroxyphenylalanine) for patients suffering from Parkinson's disease.[101]

Normal expression of PEPT1 also follows a distinct circadian rhythm, with maximal daily expression observed during peak feeding times.[102] In accordance with its role in luminal peptide absorption, PEPT1 has been localized to the apical membrane of villus enterocytes in the small intestine, with very little expression in crypt cells or the colon; this expression follows an increasing expression pattern as one proceeds towards the villus tip.[102-104] Despite this, PEPT1 expression in the colon is stimulated in patients with inflammatory bowel disease. This latter response is interesting because PEPT1 can also transport the bacterial toxin formyl-Met-Leu-Phe (fMLP), which acts as a chemoattractant for neutrophil recruitment.[95,105,106] Expression of PEPT1 can be regulated by particular amino acids and peptides that act on specific response elements

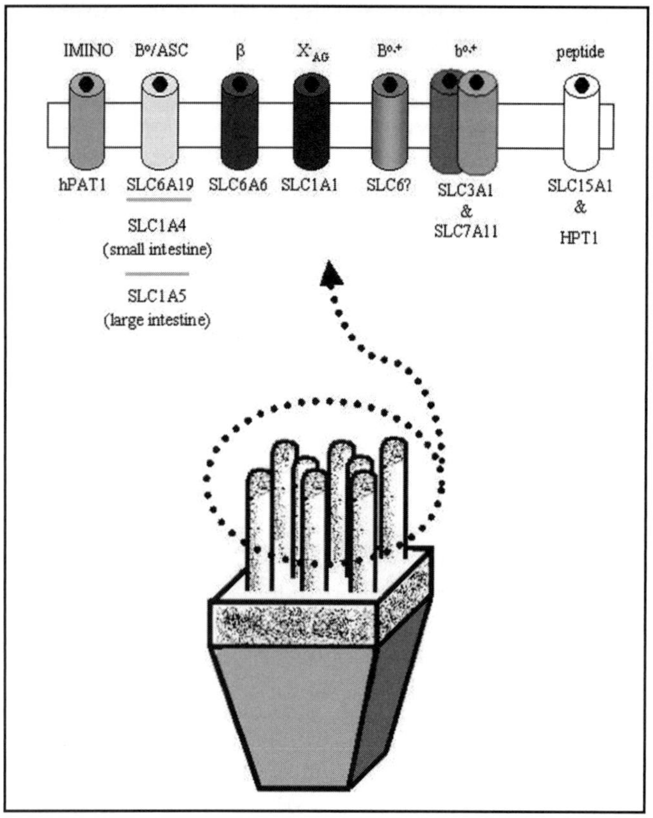

Figure 8-5. Brush-border peptide and amino-acid transport proteins. Brush-border transport of di- and tri-peptides along with amino-acid transport proteins mediate the specific uptake of the products of luminal and brush-border protein digestion. Amino-acid transporters are grouped by their various system identifications.

within the PEPT1 gene promoter, which implies dietary manipulation of PEPT1 expression.[107] Other regulatory mechanisms that have been shown to stimulate PEPT1 expression include insulin, short-term fasting, growth hormone, epidermal growth factor, chemically induced diabetes mellitus, decreased intracellular cAMP levels, and decreased intracellular calcium.[108-111] Conversely, cholera infection and PKC stimulation, increased intracellular calcium levels and thyroid hormone (3,5,3′-L-triiodothyronine) have been shown to decrease PEPT1 expression activity.[95,96,112]

While the role of PEPT1 in luminal peptide transport has been studied in depth, there are also reports of another peptide transporter in the apical membrane of enterocytes. This alternative peptide transporter traces its genetic lineage to the cadherins family of membrane proteins and has been labeled HPT-1.[98,113,114] Little is known about the function of HPT-1 other than different substrate affinity from PEPT1, as well as subtle distinctions in cellular localization of HPT-1 versus PEPT1.[114]

Intestinal Amino-Acid Absorption

The absorption of monomeric amino acids represents a complex interaction of numerous transport proteins, not all of which have been identified. The 20 amino acids present in a normal diet can be grouped into large or small neutral, anionic, or cationic, as well as acidic or basic. The current model of intestinal amino-acid transport involves transport proteins that discriminate, based on those aforementioned groups. Thus, many of the currently described amino-acid transporters are capable of transporting numerous amino acids. However, despite this, the identification of the array of amino-acid transporters expressed throughout the gut is a continual process.

Classically, amino-acid transporters have been grouped into systems, based on solute. To transport amino acids across the brush border, the carrier systems were identified as $B^{o/ASC}$ for sodium-dependent neutral amino acids including alanine, serine, and cystine; $B^{o,+}$ for sodium-dependent neutral and dibasic amino acids; X-$_{AG}$ for sodium- and potassium-dependent anionic amino acids; the IMINO or PAT system for proline and glycine; and system $b^{o,+}$ for sodium-independent neutral and dibasic amino acids (not to be confused with $B^{o,+}$ which is sodium-dependent).[115] A unique system for the brush border has been described for the transport of taurine, termed β, and identified as SLC6A6.[116] Until recently, the proteins comprising these systems were cryptic, and the systems had been identified based on substrate requirements and kinetics. Identification of the amino-acid transporters is somewhat complicated because of their wide solute specificities, and new findings indicate the probability of other unidentified transporters. Figure 8-5 illustrates the brush-border amino-acid transport systems and their respective proteins.

The proteins that represent a number of these aforementioned amino-acid transport systems have been identified through different methods. System B^o is currently represented by the proteins ASCT1 (SLC1A4) in the small intestine and ASCT2 (SLC1A5) in the large intestine, as well as the protein B^oAT (SLC6A19),[97,111,117-121] all of which transport neutral amino acids. Expression of System B^o can be manipulated by hypoxia and jejunal resection, which decrease transporter expression, whereas chronic metabolic acidosis has been shown to increase transporter expression.[111,122,123] System B^o has been implicated in Hartnup disease, where a genetic defect in SLC6A19 (B^oAT) leads to defective neutral amino-acid uptake from the lumen, as well as excessive loss in the kidneys.[97,118] System $B^{o,+}$ has been identified as a 680 amino-acid protein member of the SLC6 family that transports not only neutral amino acids, but dipolar and basic amino acids as well (hence the superscript).[124-126]

System X-$_{AG}$ has been identified as EAAC1 (SLC1A1), which cotransports three sodium molecules with a single anionic amino acid, coupled to a single potassium molecule transported out.[119,124,127,128] This transport system was originally identified through its specific uptake of the acidic amino acids aspartate and glutamate, and System X-$_{AG}$ represents a high affinity transporter for these substrates that appears to operate in conjunction with System B.[124]

The IMINO or PAT system was identified as a proton-coupled proline- and glycine-transport system that can also mediate the uptake of alanine and γ-aminobutyrate (GABA).[124,129] Expression of the protein hPAT1, the proposed IMINO-system transporter, has been shown to occur in the small and large intestines and is believed to function in conjunction with NHE3, which creates the inward proton gradient that drives hPAT1 activity.[129]

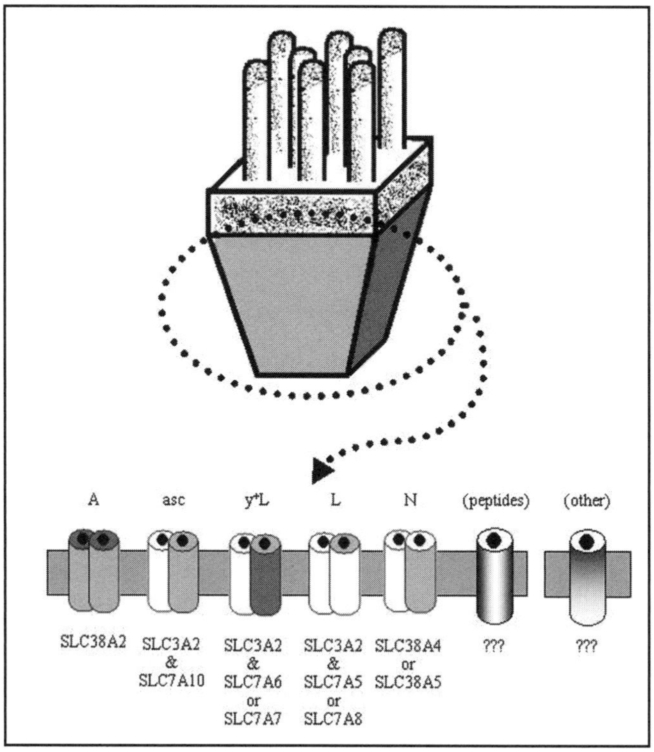

Figure 8-6. Basolateral peptide and amino-acid transport proteins. Once absorbed across the apical brush-border membrane, peptides are rapidly digested by cytoplasmic peptidases, however some peptides can be transported intact across the basolateral membrane by an uncharacterized transport protein. Currently, the basolateral amino-acid transport systems are identified by specific amino-acid exchangers that act in conjunction with an uncharacterized amino-acid uniport proteins to mediate the net transport of amino acids from the cytoplasm to the intracellular space.

System $b^{o,+}$ is represented by an interesting transport mechanism comprised of a heterodimer of the glycoprotein rBAT (SLC3A1) and $b^{o,+AT}$ (SLC7A11).[115,121,130,131] This transport unit acts as an obligatory exchanger that is not dependent on sodium.[132] System $b^{o,+}$ mediates the uptake of cationic amino acids in exchange for neutral amino acids with 1:1 stoichiometry.[133,134] System $b^{o,+}$ has been localized to the villus tip enterocytes throughout the small intestine, with the highest expression levels in the ileum and no expression in crypt epithelial cells.[115] Because this system acts as an exchanger, it cannot, by itself, mediate a net flux of amino acids and therefore combines with the activity of System B^o to broaden the solute range of the brush-border amino transport.[130] According to this model, the solutes that are excreted by System $b^{o,+}$ are then recycled back into the enterocyte via System B^o. System $b^{o,+}$ is particularly relevant for patients suffering from Cystinuria Type 1, where a genetic defect in rBAT (SLC3A1) expression results in defective cystine, arginine, and lysine absorption from the lumen, as well as excessive loss in the kidneys.[115,132] In addition to relying on System B^o to mediate a net absorption of amino acids from the lumen to the cytoplasm, System $b^{o,+}$ also relies on the coordinated activity of basolateral amino-acid transporters in order to result in net vectoral transport of amino acids from the lumen to the circulation.

Upon entry to the cytoplasm of the absorptive enterocyte, almost all peptides and proteins are digested into amino acids by cytoplasmic proteases, whose activity is suspected to be in excess of brush-border peptidase activity.[95] As with carbohydrate absorption, the basolateral amino-acid transporters represent distinctly different proteins than do those present on the apical brush-border membrane. Three sodium-dependent amino-acid transport systems have been labeled: System A for alanine, glutamine, and dipolar amino-acid transport; System N for glutamine transport; and System y^+L for dibasic amino acids.[115] In addition, two sodium-independent amino-acid transport systems have been identified: System asc for sodium-independent small neutral amino acids and System L for sodium-independent large neutral amino acids.[115,124] Figure 8-6 illustrates this model system by identifying the aforementioned basolateral amino-acid transport systems with their respective proteins.

System A is represented by ATA2 or SAT2 (SLC38A2), and transports neutral amino acids, such as alanine.[135-137] SLC38A2 appears to mediate enterocyte uptake of amino acids from the circulation rather than being involved directly with the vectoral transport of amino acids from the lumen to the circulation. Expression of SLC38A2 can be influenced by amino-acid starvation and elevated cAMP levels, both of which lead to increased expression of this protein in numerous other tissues as well.[136,138] System N is likely represented by SNAT2 or SN2 (SLC38A5), which transports neutral amino acids in a sodium-dependent manner, and couples this activity to hydrogen excretion.[137,139]

The remaining amino-acid transporters that have been identified include Systems asc (not to be confused with ASC on the brush border), y^+L, and L. These transporters are similar to System $b^{o,+}$ on the brush-border membrane in that they are comprised to heterodimers consisting of a glycoprotein (4F2hc, called SLC3A2) and a unique catalytic unit that identifies each transporter system. As such, these transporters also function as obligate exchangers, thus requiring concerted activity with other amino-acid transporters (some of which have yet to be identified) to mediate net amino-acid transport into the circulation.[115,130] System asc is represented by a heterodimer of 4F2hc (SLC3A2) and Asc-1 [also called ascAT-1 (SLC7A10)], exchanging glutamate for alanine, serine, or cystine.[115,130,140] Expression of System asc is quite low throughout the intestinal tract.

System y^+L,—represented by two heterodimers consisting of 4F2hc (SLC3A2) associated with either y^+LAT1 (SLC7A6) or y^+LAT2 (SLC7A7),—mediates the sodium-dependent export of dibasic amino or cationic acids for the influx of neutral amino acids.[132,141] 4F2hc (SLC3A2) coupled y^+LAT1 (SLC7A5) heterodimers have been localized to villus tip enterocytes in both the jejunum and ileum, with no expression in crypt epithelium.[115] System y^+L has been shown to be the cause for lysinuric protein intolerance, an autosomal recessive disorder caused by defective cationic amino-acid absorption from the lumen and excessive renal excretion. The genetic defect has been traced to a defect in y^+LAT2 (SLC7A7) expression.[142]

In the intestinal tract, System L is represented by a heterodimer of 4F2hc (SLC3A2) associated with LAT2 (SLC7A8) and is responsible for high-affinity, low-capacity, sodium-independent neutral amino-acid exchange.[143] System-L heterodimers have been localized to the basolateral membrane of parietal cells lining the stomach, as well as throughout the small intestine, on the basolateral membrane of villus tip enterocytes.[115]

As explained earlier, the basolateral amino-acid exchangers cannot mediate net amino-acid transport into the circulation alone and instead serve to augment the solute range of other transport systems. In this exchanger augmentation transporter system, System L has been described to complement System y+L in conjunction with a yet unidentified amino-acid uniport with limited specificity.[121,143,144] This unknown uniport serves to recycle the amino acids that System L transports into the enterocyte back out to the circulation.[143,145]

This seemingly overly complicated intestinal protein assimilation model has some relevance when one factors in the metabolic fate of amino acids in the intestinal epithelium. Recalling the importance of glucose as a metabolic fuel source for the body, enterocytes of the small intestine have apparently developed to favor the utilization of amino-acid–derived energy, especially glutamine and glutamate. By preferentially utilizing amino-acid–derived metabolic energy, the net vectoral transport of glucose and fructose is favored over net metabolism of this vital energy source.[146,147]

Enterocyte Amino-Acid Metabolism

Upon entering the enterocyte, amino acids can be utilized for three major metabolic purposes: 1) incorporation into synthesized protein; 2) conversion via transamination into other amino acids, metabolic substrates and biosynthetic intermediates; and 3) complete oxidation to CO_2. In situ studies have estimated that at least 50% of the dietary glutamate and glutamine taken up by the gut is completely oxidized to CO_2.[148] These results have been confirmed in piglets, wherein 95% of enteral glutamate is oxidized to CO_2.[78] Similarly, studies in premature infants and adult humans indicate that approximately 50% to 95% of the dietary glutamine and glutamate is extracted by splanchnic tissues, and most of this is oxidized to CO_2.[149-151] It is important to note that the role of glutamine and glutamate in the GI tract extend beyond their distinction as enterocyte specific fuels. These amino acids function as important precursors of nucleic acids, nucleotides, amino sugars, amino acids, and glutathione.[152-157]

The GI tract has a disproportionate impact on whole-body protein metabolism, because of its enormous requirements for protein synthesis. The tissues drained by the portal vein, which are largely comprised of the GI tract, contribute 3% to 6% of body weight but account for 20% to 35% of whole-body protein turnover and energy expenditure.[78,158-160] These high rates of protein metabolism are related to the high rates of epithelial turnover and protein secretion within the small intestine.[161-163] In contrast to the enterocyte preference for systemically derived glucose for oxidation, studies in piglets with isotopically labeled substrates have shown that, when it comes to amino acids, those arising from the lumen are the preferred oxidative choice.[78] The rationale for this difference is largely unstudied but may relate to specific nutrient transporters on the brush-border versus luminal poles of the enterocyte, the protein-synthesis requirements of the metabolically active enterocyte. The observation that, during total parenteral nutrition, atrophy occurs primarily in the proximal region of the small intestine where the oxidative requirements are greatest supports the concept that the small intestine has elevated requirements for these amino acids and therefore greedily oxidizes them without the opportunity for first-pass metabolism.[164,165]

Lipid Digestion, Absorption, and Metabolism

Dietary Lipids

The essentiality of specific fatty acids in the human diet was not described until 1963, when a large formula trial revealed that infants receiving <0.1% of their energy as the polyunsaturated linoleic acid (18:2 n-6) developed dry thickened skin and had unsatisfactory growth. Notably, these problems were reversed with the addition of linoleic acid to these infants' diets.[166] Knowledge regarding essential fatty acids was further advanced by studies of children receiving total parenteral nutrition wherein reversible deficiencies of both linoleic acid[167] and its essential omega-3 counterpart, α-linolenic acid,[168] were observed. Indeed, the scabby feet and biochemical profile associated with linoleic-acid deficiency returned to normal upon rubbing the skin with sunflower oil, a rich source of linoleic acid.[169]

Research advances over the past 30 years have shifted our focus from essentiality to that of optimal fatty-acid composition of the diet. Infant formulas now contain docosahexaenoic acid (22:6n-3) and arachidonic acid (22:4n-6) for enhanced neurological, retinal, membrane, and immunity development.[170,171] Americans adults are encouraged to limit consumption of the cholesterol-raising saturated and trans fatty acids while staying wary of the energy density associated with all fatty acids, regardless of the inclusion or position of double bonds.[173]

The predominant form of lipid in the human diet is triglycerides, with modest amounts of sterols, phospholipids, and free fatty acids (Table 8-2). Compared to dietary carbohydrate or protein digestion, dietary lipid digestion is complicated by the aqueous nature of the digestive milieu. As a result, dietary lipids undergo a complex process wherein they "shift" from aqueous to non-aqueous environment in directions opposite to that of their carbohydrate and protein counterparts. As such, several distinguishing processes in the basic digestion and absorption of dietary lipids include their emulsification, hydrolysis, micellization, and uptake by the enterocyte.

Dietary Triglyceride Digestion

Dietary triglycerides are digested by lipase enzymes produced in the mouth, stomach, and pancreas to yield diglycerides (2,3-diacylglycerols), monoglycerides (2-monoacylglycerols), and free fatty acids.[174,175] Lingual lipase, secreted from acinar cells of the serous von Ebner's glands of the tongue,[176] is frequently viewed as an auxiliary enzyme for digestion of dietary triglycerides in

TABLE 8-2.

Dietary Lipid Sources and Relevance

Lipid Structure	*Structure*	*Lipid in Typical Western Diet*	*Biological Importance*	*Dietary Sources*
Fatty acids	Hydrocarbon (from 4-24 C) terminating with carboxylic acid group. Saturated, Monounsaturated, polyunsaturated Cis, trans n-3, n-6	Negligible as free fatty acid (found in triglycerides) Oleate (C18:1) and palmitate (C16:0) are major FA present in dietary TGs	Essential fatty acids Major energy source	Both plant and animal tissues
Triglycerides	Glycerol plus three fatty acids	95% (~150 g/d)	Storage form of fat	Both plant and animal tissues
Sterols and Steroids	Four-ring core structure cholesterol fatty acid esters	5% (~300-600 mg/d) Mainly cholesterol	Cell membrane (particularly nervous tissue) bile acids steroid sex hormones adrenocortical hormones vitamin D	Plant and animal tissues Cholesterol only present in animal tissues– meat, egg yolk, dairy products
Phospholipids	Lipids plus phosphate and fatty acid(s) glycerophosphatides sphingophosphatides	Mainly phosphatidylcholine (lecithin) 2-8 g/d	Cell membranes Organelle membranes (due to their highly polar nature) Chylomicron surface (stabilize lipid particles in aqueous medium) Intracellular signaling Component of NS (myelin and medullary sheaths) red blood cell antigens	Plant and animal tissues

adults. However, a recent report indicates that the lipolysis envoked in the oral cavity may allow for orosensory detection of triglycerides and thereby assist in the humans' evolutionary quest to find nutritive lipids in food.[177] Conversely, in preterm infants, lingual lipase activity is closely coupled to the digestion of approximately 50% of ingested dietary triglycerides prior to exiting the stomach—a phenomenon enhanced by both sucking[178] and a high fat diet.[179] The heightened contribution of lingual lipase to triglyceride digestion in the infant may reflect adaptations to the increased proportion of lipids contributing to the suckling infants' diet, compensation for the developmental deficiency in gastric and/or pancreatic lipase activity[178] and/or developmental shifts caused at birth, when nutrient provision shifts from the parenteral to enteral route. Consistent with a compensatory upregulation during triglyceride malabsorption, lingual lipase is also noted to be of particular importance in patients with cystic fibrosis and exocrine pancreatic insufficiency who exhibit varying degrees of steatorrhea because of the lack of pancreatic lipase activity.[180]

In adults, approximately 25% of dietary triglyceride digestion is completed by human gastric lipase,[175] an acid-stable lipolytic enzyme synthesized primarily by the chief cells of the fundic mucosa[174,181] and secreted into the gastric lumen.[182] Although the digestive capacity of the stomach is often still disregarded, the first observation that gastric lipase was the 'ferment' responsible for fat hydrolysis was described by Volhard in 1901[183] and confirmed by Hull and Keaton in 1917.[184]

The vast majority of triglyceride digestion is initiated and completed in the small intestine where emulsification of these lipid molecules is essential for successful digestion. Emulsification is initiated by lipolysis products of dietary lipid and the shearing produced during the passage of chyme through the pyloric sphincter; however, the emulsion is stabilized by interfacing with bile in the duodenum. With the alkalizing action of bicarbonate contained within pancreatic secretions, the pH of the chyme is raised to 6 to 7, at which the optimal activity of the acid lipase—gastric lipase—is exceeded but continues to work in concert with the newly secreted human pancreatic lipase.[175] However, even with well-emulsified lipid molecules, lipases face a challenge similar to that of other proteins involved in lipid metabolism and intracellular signaling mechanisms. Specifically, these water-soluble enzymes are charged with catalyzing reactions involving water and the water-insoluble target that is present as part of a large emulsified particle.[185] Further impairing the action of human pancreatic lipase is the presence of phospholipids, protein, and bile salts (the types of surface constituents which, presumably, dominate the particle surface: ie, phospholipids, proteins, and bile salts are all known to inhibit lipolysis in model systems).[186,187] The mystery underlying the efficiency of human pancreatic lipase despite the antagonistic environment of the small intestinal lumen was solved by the discovery of colipase. Colipase is secreted from the pancreas as procolipase and activated by trypsin. By binding to lipase in a 1:1 ratio,[188] colipase provides an anchor within the two-dimensional phase by binding to the triglyceride/aqueous interface and allowing lipase to bind to the lipid/aqueous interface. In this regard, colipase overcomes the inhibition provided by both structure and composition of the emulsified micelle.[189] The importance of colipase in facilitating human pancreatic lipase absorption is supported by the reported manifestation of severe steatorrhea in two young Assyrian brothers with a confirmed genetic deficiency of colipase.[190] Further details regarding proteins regulating triglyceride digestion are developing with the recent description of a lipase gene family and two proteins—pancreatic lipase-related proteins 1 and 2—that share significant homology to human pancreatic lipase.[191]

Dietary Phospholipid and Cholesterol Ester Digestion

The small intestinal lumen also serves as the venue to digestion of both phospholipids and cholesterol esters. Found within the mixed micelle, phosphatidylcholine (lecithin)—the predominant phospholipid—is hydrolyzed by phospholipase A2, which is secreted from the pancreas as prophospholipase A2 and then activated by trypsin. The resulting products are lysolecithin (lecithin without the C-2 fatty acid) and a fatty acid. Recent advances in this area describe multiple classes of phospholipase A2 isozymes with various functions relating to phospholipids digestion and metabolism, host defense, and signal transduction.[192,193]

Ten percent to 15% of cholesterol present in the diet is found as a cholesterol ester and must therefore be liberated of the associated fatty acid prior to being absorbed as free cholesterol by the intestinal epithelium. Cholesterol esterase is secreted by the pancreas as an active enzyme that is stimulated upon interaction with bile salts within the mixed micelles. This bile salt stimulation also causes self-aggregation of the enzyme into polymeric forms, which protect the enzyme from proteolytic inactivation. Cholesterol esterase exhibits activity across many lipid molecules and is, therefore, also referred to as carboxyl ester hydrolase and nonspecific esterase. Beyond cholesterol esters, cholesterol esterase can also hydrolyze triglycerides, phosphoglycerides, esters of fat-soluble vitamins, and monoacylglycerols.[194]

Intraluminal Formation of Mixed Micelles

The formation of mixed micelles during intestinal lipid digestion is very important to the absorption of these lipid substances across the brush-border membrane.[195,196] At a diameter of ~5 nm, the mixed micelle structure allows these monomeric lipid particles to access the intramicrovillus spaces (50 to 100 nm) of brush-border membrane. In addition, the polar bile salts that serve as the foundation for the mixed micelle provide the water-solubility necessary for the digested lipid particles to penetrate the unstirred water layer bathing small intestinal epithelium. The unstirred water layer is reported to be the rate limiting uptake of long-chain fatty acids (LCFA) but not of SCFA or medium-chain fatty acids (MCFA), whose limiting step occurs at the brush-border membrane.[197] The microclimate in the unstirred water layer is slightly acidic because of actions of the sodium-hydrogen exchanger at the brush-border membrane. This slightly acidic environment (pH 5 to 6) destabilizes the mixed micelle by decreasing the fatty acid solubility and encourages liberation of the fatty acids at the mucosal surface where they can cross the brush-border membrane.

Intestinal Fatty Acid Absorption

The cellular mechanism(s) whereby fatty acids traverse the brush-border membrane has been a topic of much interest in recent years. The two mechanisms that have been proposed are passive diffusion or carrier-mediated uptake. Traditionally, the absorption of lipids was thought to be passive based on the concept that lipids are soluble in the bilipid membrane and diffuse down a concentration gradient into the cell. The inwardly directed concentration gradient is maintained in the fed state by the high concentration of fatty acids within the intestinal lumen and the rapid scavenging of free fatty acids for triglyceride reformation once inside the enterocyte.

Shaking the dogma that fatty acid absorption occurs via passive diffusion, recent evidence has revealed that enterocyte lipid uptake involves energy-dependant carrier-mediated processes.[194] Uptake studies with brush-border membrane vesicles indicate that oleic and arachidonic acid absorption are saturable, which suggests an active transport process. Putative fatty acid transport proteins that have been identified include plasma membrane fatty acid binding protein,[198,199] megalin,[200,201] CD35,[202,203] caveolin,[204] and a family of fatty acid transporters.[202,205] Further in vivo studies determining the relative impact of these fatty acid transport proteins in fatty acid absorption are needed to determine the relative importance of lipid absorption via passive diffusion and/or carrier-mediated mechanisms. Current theories indicate that both mechanisms contribute to lipid absorption. At low fatty acid concentrations, carrier-mediated mechanisms take precedence with little passive diffusion occurring. However, when free fatty acid concentration in the intestinal lumen is high, absorption of fatty acids via passive diffusion becomes the predominant route.[206]

Intestinal Sterol Absorption

As with fatty acids, the absorption of sterols have often thought to occur via simple passive diffusion down a concentration gradient.[207] However, the observations that cholesterol, but not beta-sitosterol (a related plant sterol), is well absorbed by the small intestine raised the argument that cholesterol absorption across the brush-border membrane was an active process.[208] Convincing support for this concept is the genetic defect of beta-sitosterolemia, where the intestine fails to discriminate between cholesterol and beta-sitosterol. The gene mutations are now known to affect adjacent genes encoding for members of the ATP-binding cassette (ABC) transporters, ABCG5 and ABCG8.[209,210] Studies in the ABCG5/8 knockout mouse have revealed that ABCG5/8 are critical for preventing bulk intestinal absorption of plant sterols but also facilitate biliary secretion of cholesterol and neutral sterols.[211] Other intestinal cholesterol transporters that have been identified include pancreatic cholesterol esterase,[212] scavenger receptor class B, type I,[213] and ABCA1.[214] However, evidence that these proteins contribute significantly to overall intestinal cholesterol absorption is lacking.[215-218]

Intestinal Phospholipid Absorption

Phosphatidylcholine is absorbed as lysolecithin by the epithelium that lines the proximal intestine. The presence of dietary phosphatidylcholine in the intestinal lumen increases triglyceride[219] and lycopene[220] absorption via influence on the rate of chylomicron formation and the partitioning of fatty acids between lymphatic and dietary phosphatidylcholine portal transport.[221-224] Phosphatidylcholine also impacts the production of intestinal mucus, which is a hydrophobic, phosphatidylcholine-enriched barrier against antigens and toxins within the intestinal lumen. Interestingly, recently work indicates that the phosphatidylcholine contributing to this barrier is secreted by the intestinal epithelium, which indicates that mechanisms for both phosphatidylcholine absorption and secretion occur within the enterocyte.[225]

Enterocyte Lipid Metabolism

Once inside the enterocyte, fatty acids bind to specific fatty acid binding proteins (FABP), named I-FABP and L-FABP for the intestine and liver, respectively, where they were first isolated. These FABPs have greater affinity for unsaturated versus saturated fatty acids and very little for SCFA or MCFA.[226] Nuclear magnetic resonance imaging indicates that I-FABP is involved in intracellular transport of fatty acids, whereas the L-FABP is involved in the intracellular transport of monoglycerides and lysophosphatidylcholine across the cytoplasm to the endoplasmic reticulum for triglyceride resynthesis.[227]

Triglyceride resynthesis occurs at the cytosolic surface of the endoplasmic reticulum via two pathways. The major route is the monoglyceride pathway, wherein a monoglyceride is re-esterified with a free LCFA after it has been activated to form acyl-coenzyme A. Microsomal acyl-coenzyme A-ligase is necessary to synthesize coenzyme A from the fatty acid before esterification. A diglyceride and then triglyceride is sequentially formed. There is controversy over whether the same enzyme synthesizes both diglycerides and triglycerides; however, in animals with knockout acyl-coenzyme A:diglyceride acyl transferase (the enzyme credited with catalyzing the diglyceride to triglyceride reaction), triglyceride resynthesis is not impaired.[228,229] Interestingly, this reaction favors LCFA absorbed from the lumen. Upon entrance into the enterocyte, fatty acids with 12 or more fatty acids are activated to coenzyme A by the enzyme acyl coenzyme A synthestase. Phosphatidylcholine and cholesterol esters are resynthesized using the same pathway. In a second pathway, triglycerides can be formed by glycerol 3-phosphate, which is produced from the phosphorylation of free glycerol or from reduction of dihydroxyacetone phosphate, an intermediate in the pathway of glycolysis. The importance of this secondary pathway depends on the sufficiency of 2-monoacylglycerol; therefore, this pathway only becomes significant during fasting states.

MCFA (those with 12 or less carbon atoms) pass into portal circulation and onto liver without esterification. For this reason, use of MCFA (8 to 12 carbon length) are clinically valuable for individuals who lack necessary bile salts for emulsification and micellular formation required for LCFA transport or for those with abetalipoproteinemia where there is an inability to transport triglycerides from the epithelium into lymphatic circulation. MCFA supplements available for clinical use are normally provided in the form of oil or a dietary beverage containing other macronutrients and micronutrients.

Absorbed dietary cholesterol joins endogenous cholesterol (ie, cholesterol derived from bile, lipoproteins, and de novo cholesterol synthesis) in a free cholesterol pool within the enterocyte. Cholesterol is transported as esterified cholesterol through the lymphatic system. Cholesterol esterase and acyl-coenzyme A:cholesterol acyltransferase (ACAT) are the enzymes responsible for cholesterol esterification. ACAT is stimulated by a high-cholesterol diet and thought to be more important in mucosal cholesterol esterification than in cholesterol esterase.[230] ACATs' role in cholesterol esterification is supported by resistance to diet-induced hypercholesterolemia due to defective cholesterol esterification and absorption in the small intestine in ACAT-2 knockout mice.[231]

Inside the enterocyte, lysophosphatidylcholine can be reacylated to form phosphatidylcholine. Alternatively, lysophophatidylcholine can be hydrolyzed to form glycerol 3-phosphorylcholine wherein the liberated fatty acid can be used to triglyceride synthesis.

Enterocyte Lipoprotein Synthesis

Resynthesized lipids and fat-soluble vitamins collect in the enterocyte endoplasmic reticulum as large fat particles. While in the endoplasmic reticulum, a layer of protein is added to enable these lipids to enter the aqueous environment of circulation. The particles pinch off as lipid vesicles and fuse with the Golgi apparatus where carbohydrate is attached to the protein coat—the final step in chylomicron formation. Chylomicrons, a specific class of lipoprotein, are exocytosed into lymphatic circulation. Chylomicrons range from 750 to 6000 nm in diameter. The chylomicron core is comprised of triglycerides, whereas cholesterol ester and phospholipids form more than 80% of the surface coat. Also contained within the surface is the essential apolipoprotein, ApoA. ApoA, synthesized in the small intestine and found in bile, is important for all lipoproteins, including chylomicrons, very low-density lipoproteins (VLDL), and high-density lipoproteins (HDL).[232] ApoB is essential for synthesis and secretion of chylomicrons, however does not appear to be a rate-limiting step.[233,234] During fasting, VLDL containing apo B-48 are the major triglyceride-rich lipoprotein emerging from the epithelium. However, with feeding, chylomicrons are secreted from the enterocyte with a fatty acid pattern similar to that of the consumed dietary triglycerides.[197]

Abetalipoproteinemia is a rare genetic disorder resulting in complete failure of the liver and intestine to make triglyceride-rich lipoproteins.[235] Although originally thought to be to the result of a lack of apoB synthesis, this protein is produced in small amounts, and a mutation in the microsomal triglyceride transfer protein gene has been reported.[234,236] Anderson's disease (also known as chylomicron retention disorder) is a small intestinal disorder wherein synthesis or secretion of chylomicrons is impaired. No defect has been found in the genes known to carry apoprotein and microsomal triglyceride transfer protein,[237] which indicates an unknown factor central to chylomicron secretion.

Lipids are transported in the blood as components of various lipoprotein particles—such as VLDL, low-density lipoproteins (LDL), and HDL—for distribution among various tissues of the body. Key metabolic processes include lipids as a rich source of energy; as a precursor of bioactive substances such as prostaglandins, thromoxanes, and leukotrienes; and as key components of cell membranes and adipose tissue. Ultimately, the metabolic perspective on lipid molecules relates these compounds to their macronutrient counterparts (carbohydrate and protein) wherein regulation of nutrient metabolism choreographs intermediary metabolites so efficiently (ie, macronutrient to acetyl CoA) that the original macronutrient class (carbohydrate, protein, or lipids) crossing the brush-border member is indistinguishable.

References

1. Hardin JA, Gall DG. The regulation of brush border surface area. *Ann N Y Acad Sci*. 1992;664:380-387.
2. DeSesso JM, Jacobson CF. Anatomical and physiological parameters affecting gastrointestinal absorption in humans and rats. *Food Chem Toxicol*. 2001;39(3):209-228.
3. Hladik CM, Pasquet P, Simmen B. New perspectives on taste and primate evolution: the dichotomy in gustatory coding for perception of beneficent versus noxious substances as supported by correlations among human thresholds. *Am J Phys Anthropol*. 2002;117(4):342-348.
4. Cox TM. The genetic consequences of our sweet tooth. *Nat Rev Genet*. 2002;3(6):481-487.
5. Rumessen JJ. Fructose and related food carbohydrates. Sources, intake, absorption, and clinical implications. *Scand J Gastroenterol*. 1992;27(10):819-828.
6. Fan MZ, Stoll B, Jiang R, Burrin DG. Enterocyte digestive enzyme activity along the crypt-villus and longitudinal axes in the neonatal pig small intestine. *J Anim Sci*. 2001;79(2):371-381.
7. Gupta SK, Chong SK, Fitzgerald JF. Disaccharidase activities in children: normal values and comparison based on symptoms and histologic changes. *J Pediatr Gastroenterol Nutr*. 1999;28(3):246-251.
8. Lam JT, Martin MG, Turk E, et al. Missense mutations in SGLT1 cause glucose-galactose malabsorption by trafficking defects. *Biochim Biophys Acta*. 1999;1453(2):297-303.
9. Hediger MA, Coady MJ, Ikeda TS, Wright EM. Expression cloning and cDNA sequencing of the Na+/glucose co-transporter. *Nature*. 1987;330(6146):379-381.
10. Wright EM, Loo DD, Panayotova-Heiermann M, et al. 'Active' sugar transport in eukaryotes. *J Exp Biol*. 1994;196:197-212.
11. Li Q, Manolescu A, Ritzel M, et al. Cloning and functional characterization of the human GLUT7 isoform SLC2A7 from the small intestine. *Am J Physiol Gastrointest Liver Physiol*. 2004;287(1):G236-242.
12. Zeuthen T, Meinild AK, Loo DD, Wright EM, Klaerke DA. Isotonic transport by the Na+-glucose cotransporter SGLT1 from humans and rabbit. *J Physiol*. 2001;531:631-644.
13. Wright EM, Turk E. The sodium/glucose cotransport family SLC5. *Pflugers Arch*. 2004;447(5):510-518.
14. Gagnon MP, Bissonnette P, Deslandes LM, Wallendorff B, Lapointe JY. Glucose accumulation can account for the initial water flux triggered by Na+/glucose cotransport. *Biophys J*. 2004;86(1):125-133.
15. Pappenheimer JR. On the coupling of membrane digestion with intestinal absorption of sugars and amino acids. *Am J Physiol*. 1993;265(3):G409-417.

16. Kellett GL. The facilitated component of intestinal glucose absorption. *J Physiol.* 2001;531:585-595.
17. Steyermark AC, Lam MM, Diamond J. Quantitative evolutionary design of nutrient processing: glucose. *Proc Natl Acad Sci U S A.* 2002;99(13):8754-8759.
18. Keller TC, III, Conzelman KA, Chasan R, Mooseker MS. Role of myosin in terminal web contraction in isolated intestinal epithelial brush borders. *J Cell Biol.* 1985;100(5):1647-1655.
19. Pappenheimer JR. Role of pre-epithelial "unstirred" layers in absorption of nutrients from the human jejunum. *J Membr Biol.* 2001;179(3):185-204.
20. Gouyon F, Caillaud L, Carriere V, et al. Simple-sugar meals target GLUT2 at enterocyte apical membranes to improve sugar absorption: a study in GLUT2-null mice. *J Physiol.* 2003;552(Pt 3):823-832.
21. Stumpel F, Burcelin R, Jungermann K, Thorens B. Normal kinetics of intestinal glucose absorption in the absence of GLUT2: evidence for a transport pathway requiring glucose phosphorylation and transfer into the endoplasmic reticulum. *Proc Natl Acad Sci U S A.* 2001;98(20):11330-11335.
22. Sakamoto O, Ogawa E, Ohura T, et al. Mutation analysis of the GLUT2 gene in patients with Fanconi-Bickel syndrome. *Pediatr Res.* 2000;48(5):586-589.
23. Santer R, Hillebrand G, Steinmann B, Schaub J. Intestinal glucose transport: evidence for a membrane traffic-based pathway in humans. *Gastroenterology.* 2003;124(1):34-39.
24. Lane JS, Whang EE, Rigberg DA, et al. Paracellular glucose transport plays a minor role in the unanesthetized dog. *Am J Physiol.* 999;276(3 Pt 1):G789-794.
25. Pappenheimer JR, Michel CC. Role of villus microcirculation in intestinal absorption of glucose: coupling of epithelial with endothelial transport. *J Physiol.* 2003;553(2):561-574.
26. Millar GA, Hardin JA, Johnson LR, Gall DG. The role of PI 3-kinase in EGF-stimulated jejunal glucose transport. *Can J Physiol Pharmacol.* 2002;80(1):77-84.
27. Pencek RR, Koyama Y, Lacy DB, et al. Prior exercise enhances passive absorption of intraduodenal glucose. *J Appl Physiol.* 2003;95(3):1132-1138.
28. Hines OJ, Whang EE, Bilchik AJ, et al. Role of Na+-glucose cotransport in jejunal meal-induced absorption. *Dig Dis Sci.* 2000;45(1):1-6.
29. Chung BM, Wallace LE, Hardin JA, Gall DG. The effect of epidermal growth factor on the distribution of SGLT-1 in rabbit jejunum. *Can J Physiol Pharmacol.* 2002;80(9):872-878.
30. Chung BM, Wong JK, Hardin JA, Gall DG. Role of actin in EGF-induced alterations in enterocyte SGLT1 expression. *Am J Physiol.* 1999;276(2 Pt 1):G463-469.
31. Hardin JA, Wong JK, Cheeseman CI, Gall DG. Effect of luminal epidermal growth factor on enterocyte glucose and proline transport. *Am J Physiol.* 1996;271(3):G509-515.
32. Opleta-Madsen K, Hardin J, Gall DG. Epidermal growth factor upregulates intestinal electrolyte and nutrient transport. *Am J Physiol.* 1991;260(6):G807-814.
33. Ishikawa Y, Eguchi T, Ishida H. Mechanism of beta-adrenergic agonist-induced transmural transport of glucose in rat small intestine. Regulation of phosphorylation of SGLT1 controls the function. *Biochim Biophys Acta.* 1997;1357(3):306-318.
34. Mabjeesh SJ, Guy D, Sklan D. Na+/glucose co-transporter abundance and activity in the small intestine of lambs: enhancement by abomasal infusion of casein. *Br J Nutr.* 2003;89(5):573-580.
35. Pencek RR, Koyama Y, Lacy DB, et al. Transporter-mediated absorption is the primary route of entry and is required for passive absorption of intestinal glucose into the blood of conscious dogs. *J Nutr.* 2002;132(7):1929-1934.
36. Mahraoui L, Takeda J, Mesonero J, et al. Regulation of expression of the human fructose transporter (GLUT5) by cyclic AMP. *Biochem J.* 1994;301 (Pt 1):169-175.
37. Ikari A, Nakano M, Kawano K, Suketa Y. Up-regulation of sodium-dependent glucose transporter by interaction with heat shock protein 70. *J Biol Chem.* 2002;277(36):33338-33343.
38. Martin GR, Wallace LE, Sigalet DL. Glucagon-like peptide-2 induces intestinal adaptation in parenterally fed rats with short bowel syndrome. *Am J Physiol Gastrointest Liver Physiol.* 2004;286(6): G964-972.
39. Kipp H, Khoursandi S, Scharlau D, Kinne RK. More than apical: Distribution of SGLT1 in Caco-2 cells. *Am J Physiol Cell Physiol.* 2003;285(4):C737-749.
40. Hardin J, Kroeker K, Chung B, Gall DG. Effect of proinflammatory interleukins on jejunal nutrient transport. *Gut.* 2000;47(2):184-191.
41. Pan X, Terada T, Okuda M, Inui K. The diurnal rhythm of the intestinal transporters SGLT1 and PEPT1 is regulated by the feeding conditions in rats. *J Nutr.* 2004;134(9):2211-2215.
42. Tavakkolizadeh A, Berger UV, Shen KR, et al. Diurnal rhythmicity in intestinal SGLT-1 function, V(max), and mRNA expression topography. *Am J Physiol Gastrointest Liver Physiol.* 2001;280(2): G209-215.
43. Chung BM, Wallace LE, Winkfein RK, O'Loughlin EV, Hardin JA, Gall DG. The effect of massive small bowel resection and oral epidermal growth factor therapy on SGLT-1 distribution in rabbit distal remnant. *Pediatr Res.* 2004;55(1):19-26.
44. Bartholome AL, Albin DM, Baker DH, Holst JJ, Tappenden KA. Supplementation of total parenteral nutrition with butyrate acutely increases structural aspects of intestinal adaptation after an 80% jejunoileal resection in neonatal piglets. *JPEN J Parenter Enteral Nutr.* 2004;28(4):210-222; discussion 222-213.
45. Ray EC, Avissar NE, Sax HC. Methods used to study intestinal nutrient transport: past and present. *J Surg Res.* 2002;108(1):180-190.
46. Burrin DG, Stoll B, Chang X, et al. Parenteral nutrition results in impaired lactose digestion and hexose absorption when enteral feeding is initiated in infant pigs. *Am J Clin Nutr.* 2003;78(3):461-470.
47. Tappenden KA, McBurney MI. Systemic short-chain fatty acids rapidly alter gastrointestinal structure, function, and expression of early response genes. *Dig Dis Sci.* 1998;43(7):1526-1536.
48. Kotler DP, Levine GM, Shiau YF. Effects of luminal nutrition and metabolic status on in vivo glucose absorption. *Am J Physiol.* 1981;240(6):G432-436.
49. Johnson LR, Brockway PD, Madsen K, Hardin JA, Gall DG. Polyamines alter intestinal glucose transport. *Am J Physiol.* 1995;268(3):G416-423.
50. Drozdowski L, Woudstra T, Wild G, Clandindin MT, Thomson AB. The age-associated decline in the intestinal uptake of glucose is not accompanied by changes in the mRNA or protein abundance of SGLT1. *Mech Ageing Dev.* 2003;124:1035-1045.
51. Esposito G, Faelli A, Tosco M, Orsenigo MN, Battistessa R. Age-related changes in rat intestinal transport of D-glucose, sodium, and water. *Am J Physiol.* 1985;249(3):G328-334.
52. Jourd'heuil D, Meddings JB. Oxidative and drug-induced alterations in brush border membrane hemileaflet fluidity, functional consequences for glucose transport. *Biochim Biophys Acta.* 2001;1510:342-353.
53. Gabe SM, Bjarnason I, Tolou-Ghamari Z, et al. The effect of tacrolimus (FK506) on intestinal barrier function and cellular energy production in humans. *Gastroenterology.* 1998;115(1):67-74.
54. Stockmann M, Engelmann BE, Langrehr JM, Neuhaus P. Influence of immunosuppressive drugs on intestinal epithelial transport function. *Transplant Proc.* 2002;34(5):1449-1450.
55. Veyhl M, Wagner CA, Gorboulev V, Schmitt BM, Lang F, Koepsell H. Downregulation of the Na(+)- D-glucose cotransporter SGLT1 by protein RS1 (RSC1A1) is dependent on dynamin and protein kinase C. *J Membr Biol.* 2003;196(1):71-81.
56. Hardin JA, Chung B, O'Loughlin E V, Gall DG. The effect of epidermal growth factor on brush border surface area and function in the distal remnant following resection in the rabbit. *Gut.* 1999;44(1):26-32.
57. Topping DL, Clifton PM. Short-chain fatty acids and human colonic function: roles of resistant starch and nonstarch polysaccharides. *Physiol Rev.* 2001;81(3):1031-1064.

58. Stevens CE, Hume ID. Contributions of microbes in vertebrate gastrointestinal tract to production and conservation of nutrients. *Physiol Rev.* 1998;78(2):393-427.
59. Bugaut M. Occurrence, absorption and metabolism of short chain fatty acids in the digestive tract of mammals. *Comp Biochem Physiol B.* 1987;86(3):439-472.
60. Charney AN, Micic L, Egnor RW. Nonionic diffusion of short-chain fatty acids across rat colon. *Am J Physiol.* 1998;274(3):G518-524.
61. Harig JM, Ng EK, Dudeja PK, Brasitus TA, Ramaswamy K. Transport of n-butyrate into human colonic luminal membrane vesicles. *Am J Physiol.* 1996;271(3):G415-422.
62. Harig JM, Soergel KH, Barry JA, Ramaswamy K. Transport of propionate by human ileal brush-border membrane vesicles. *Am J Physiol.* 1991;260(5):G776-782.
63. Ritzhaupt A, Wood IS, Ellis A, Hosie KB, Shirazi-Beechey SP. Identification and characterization of a monocarboxylate transporter (MCT1) in pig and human colon: its potential to transport L-lactate as well as butyrate. *J Physiol.* 1998;513:719-732.
64. Miyauchi S, Gopal E, Fei YJ, Ganapathy V. Functional identification of SLC5A8, a tumor suppressor down-regulated in colon cancer, as a Na(+)-coupled transporter for short-chain fatty acids. *J Biol Chem.* 2004;279(14):13293-13296.
65. Halestrap AP, Meredith D. The SLC16 gene family-from monocarboxylate transporters (MCTs) to aromatic amino acid transporters and beyond. *Pflugers Arch.* 2004;447(5):619-628.
66. Becker HM, Broer S, Deitmer JW. Facilitated lactate transport by MCT1 when coexpressed with the sodium bicarbonate cotransporter (NBC) in Xenopus oocytes. *Biophys J.* 2004;86(1):235-247.
67. Alrefai WA, Tyagi S, Gill R, et al. Regulation of butyrate uptake in Caco-2 cells by phorbol 12-myristate 13-acetate. *Am J Physiol Gastrointest Liver Physiol.* 2004;286(2):G197-203.
68. Schroder O, Opritz J, Stein J. Substrate and inhibitor specificity of butyrate uptake in apical membrane vesicles of the rat distal colon. *Digestion.* 2000;62(2-3):152-158.
69. Tyagi S, Venugopalakrishnan J, Ramaswamy K, Dudeja PK. Mechanism of n-butyrate uptake in the human proximal colonic basolateral membranes. *Am J Physiol Gastrointest Liver Physiol.* 2002;282(4):G676-682.
70. Rajendran VM, Binder HJ. Characterization and molecular localization of anion transporters in colonic epithelial cells. *Ann N Y Acad Sci.* 2000;915:15-29.
71. Manokas T, Fromkes JJ, Sundaram U. Effect of chronic inflammation on ileal short-chain fatty acid/bicarbonate exchange. *Am J Physiol Gastrointest Liver Physiol.* 2000;278(4):G585-590.
72. Sellin JH. SCFAs: The enigma of weak electrolyte transport in the colon. *News Physiol Sci.* 1999;14:58-64.
73. Cuff MA, Lambert DW, Shirazi-Beechey SP. Substrate-induced regulation of the human colonic monocarboxylate transporter, MCT1. *J Physiol.* 2002;539(2):361-371.
74. Darcy-Vrillon B, Posho L, Morel MT, et al. Glucose, galactose, and glutamine metabolism in pig isolated enterocytes during development. *Pediatr Res.* 1994;36(2):175-181.
75. Kight CE, Fleming SE. Oxidation of glucose carbon entering the TCA cycle is reduced by glutamine in small intestine epithelial cells. *Am J Physiol.* 1995;268(6):G879-888.
76. Wu G, Knabe DA, Yan W, Flynn NE. Glutamine and glucose metabolism in enterocytes of the neonatal pig. *Am J Physiol.* 1995;268(2):R334-342.
77. Marsman KE, McBurney MI. Dietary fiber increases oxidative metabolism in colonocytes but not in distal small intestinal enterocytes isolated from rats. *J Nutr.* 1995;125(2):273-282.
78. Stoll B, Burrin DG, Henry J, Yu H, Jahoor F, Reeds PJ. Substrate oxidation by the portal drained viscera of fed piglets. *Am J Physiol.* 1999;277(1):E168-175.
79. van den Berghe G, Wouters P, Weekers F, et al. Intensive insulin therapy in the critically ill patients. *N Engl J Med.* 2001;345(19):1359-1367.
80. Cummings JH. Short chain fatty acids in the human colon. *Gut.* 1981;22(9):763-779.
81. Roediger WE. Utilization of nutrients by isolated epithelial cells of the rat colon. *Gastroenterology.* 1982;83(2):424-429.
82. Engelhardt WV, Rechkemmer G. Absorption of inorganic ions in short-chain fatty acids in the colon of mammals. In: Gilles-Baillien M, Gilles R, eds. *Intestinal Transport. Fundamental and Comparative Aspects.* Berlin: Springer-Verlag; 1983:26-45.
83. McNeil NI. The contribution of the large intestine to energy supplies in man. *Am J Clin Nutr.* 1984;39(2):338-342.
84. Marty J, Vernay M. Absorption and metabolism of the volatile fatty acids in the hind-gut of the rabbit. *Br J Nutr.* 1984;51(2):265-277.
85. Awad AB, Ferger SL, Fink CS. Effect of dietary fat on the lipid composition and utilization of short-chain fatty acids by rat colonocytes. *Lipids.* 1990;25(6):316-320.
86. Topping DL, Illman RJ, Clarke JM, Trimble RP, Jackson KA, Marsono Y. Dietary fat and fiber alter large bowel and portal venous volatile fatty acids and plasma cholesterol but not biliary steroids in pigs. *J Nutr.* 1993;123(1):133-143.
87. Hoverstad T, Bohmer T, Fausa O. Absorption of short-chain fatty acids from the human colon measured by the 14CO2 breath test. *Scand J Gastroenterol.* 1982;17(3):373-378.
88. Desmoulin F, Canioni P, Cozzone PJ. Glutamate-glutamine metabolism in the perfused rat liver. 13C-NMR study using (2-13C)-enriched acetate. *FEBS Lett.* 1985;185(1):29-32.
89. Ardawi MS, Newsholme EA. Fuel utilization in colonocytes of the rat. *Biochem J.* 1985;231(3):713-719.
90. Roediger WE. Role of anaerobic bacteria in the metabolic welfare of the colonic mucosa in man. *Gut.* 1980;21(9):793-798.
91. Ruppin H, Bar-Meir S, Soergel KH, Wood CM, Schmitt MG, Jr. Absorption of short-chain fatty acids by the colon. *Gastroenterology.* 1980;78(6):1500-1507.
92. Tappenden KA, Thomson AB, Wild GE, McBurney MI. Short-chain fatty acid-supplemented total parenteral nutrition enhances functional adaptation to intestinal resection in rats. *Gastroenterology.* 1997;112(3):792-802.
93. Tappenden KA, Drozdowski LA, Thomson AB, McBurney MI. Short-chain fatty acid-supplemented total parenteral nutrition alters intestinal structure, glucose transporter 2 (GLUT2) mRNA and protein, and proglucagon mRNA abundance in normal rats. *Am J Clin Nutr.* 1998;68(1):118-125.
94. Gardner MLG. Absorption of intact proteins and peptides. In: Johnson LR, ed. *Physiology of the Gastrointestinal Tract.* New York: Raven Press; 1994.
95. Daniel H. Molecular and integrative physiology of intestinal peptide transport. *Ann Rev Physiol.* 2004;66:361-384.
96. Daniel H, Kottra G. The proton oligopeptide cotransporter family SLC15 in physiology and pharmacology. *Pflugers Arch.* 2004;447(5):610-618.
97. Kleta R, Romeo E, Ristic Z, et al. Mutations in SLC6A19, encoding B0AT1, cause Hartnup disorder. *Nat Genet.* 2004;36(9):999-1002.
98. Ganapathy ME, Brandsch M, Prasad PD, Ganapathy V, Leibach FH. Differential recognition of beta -lactam antibiotics by intestinal and renal peptide transporters, PEPT 1 and PEPT 2. *J Biol Chem.* 1995;270(43):25672-25677.
99. Zhu T, Chen XZ, Steel A, Hediger MA, Smith DE. Differential recognition of ACE inhibitors in Xenopus laevis oocytes expressing rat PEPT1 and PEPT2. *Pharm Res.* 2000;17(5):526-532.
100. Shu C, Shen H, Hopfer U, Smith DE. Mechanism of intestinal absorption and renal reabsorption of an orally active ace inhibitor: uptake and transport of fosinopril in cell cultures. *Drug Metab Dispos.* 2001;29(10):1307-1315.
101. Tamai I, Nakanishi T, Nakahara H, et al. Improvement of L-dopa absorption by dipeptidyl derivation, utilizing peptide transporter PepT1. *J Pharm Sci.* 1998;87(12):1542-1546.
102. Pan X, Terada T, Irie M, Saito H, Inui K. Diurnal rhythm of H+-peptide cotransporter in rat small intestine. *Am J Physiol Gastrointest Liver Physiol.* 2002;283(1):G57-64.
103. Groneberg DA, Doring F, Eynott PR, Fischer A, Daniel H. Intestinal peptide transport: ex vivo uptake studies and localization of peptide carrier PEPT1. *Am J Physiol Gastrointest Liver Physiol.* Sep 2001;281(3):G697-704.

104. Hussain I, Kellett L, Affleck J, Shepherd J, Boyd R. Expression and cellular distribution during development of the peptide transporter (PepT1) in the small intestinal epithelium of the rat. *Cell Tissue Res.* 2002;307(1):139-142.
105. Buyse M, Charrier L, Sitaraman S, Gewirtz A, Merlin D. Interferon-gamma increases hPepT1-mediated uptake of di-tripeptides including the bacterial tripeptide fMLP in polarized intestinal epithelia. *Am J Pathol.* 2003;163(5):1969-1977.
106. Buyse M, Tsocas A, Walker F, Merlin D, Bado A. PepT1-mediated fMLP transport induces intestinal inflammation in vivo. *Am J Physiol Cell Physiol.* 2002;283(6):C1795-1800.
107. Shiraga T, Miyamoto K, Tanaka H, et al. Cellular and molecular mechanisms of dietary regulation on rat intestinal H+/Peptide transporter PepT1. *Gastroenterology.* 1999;116(2):354-362.
108. Wenzel U, Kuntz S, Diestel S, Daniel H. PEPT1-mediated cefixime uptake into human intestinal epithelial cells is increased by Ca2+ channel blockers. *Antimicrob Agents Chemother.* 2002;46(5):1375-1380.
109. Gangopadhyay A, Thamotharan M, Adibi SA. Regulation of oligopeptide transporter (Pept-1) in experimental diabetes. *Am J Physiol Gastrointest Liver Physiol.* 2002;283(1):G133-138.
110. Thamotharan M, Bawani SZ, Zhou X, Adibi SA. Functional and molecular expression of intestinal oligopeptide transporter (Pept-1) after a brief fast. *Metabolism.* 1999;48(6):681-684.
111. Avissar NE, Ziegler TR, Wang HT, et al. Growth factors regulation of rabbit sodium-dependent neutral amino acid transporter ATB0 and oligopeptide transporter 1 mRNAs expression after enteretomy. *JPEN J Parenter Enteral Nutr.* 2001;25(2):65-72.
112. Ashida K, Katsura T, Motohashi H, Saito H, Inui K. Thyroid hormone regulates the activity and expression of the peptide transporter PEPT1 in Caco-2 cells. *Am J Physiol Gastrointest Liver Physiol.* 2002;282(4):G617-623.
113. Dantzig AH, Hoskins JA, Tabas LB, et al. Association of intestinal peptide transport with a protein related to the cadherin superfamily. *Science.* 1994;264(5157):430-433.
114. Behrens I, Kamm W, Dantzig AH, Kissel T. Variation of peptide transporter (PepT1 and HPT1) expression in Caco-2 cells as a function of cell origin. *J Pharm Sci.* 2004;93(7):1743-1754.
115. Dave MH, Schulz N, Zecevic M, Wagner CA, Verrey F. Expression of heteromeric amino acid transporters along the murine intestine. *J Physiol.* 2004;558:597-610.
116. Vinnakota S, Qian X, Egal H, Sarthy V, Sarkar HK. Molecular characterization and in situ localization of a mouse retinal taurine transporter. *J Neurochem.* 1997;69(6):2238-2250.
117. Avissar NE, Ryan CK, Ganapathy V, Sax HC. Na(+)-dependent neutral amino acid transporter ATB(0) is a rabbit epithelial cell brush-border protein. *Am J Physiol Cell Physiol.* 2001;281(3):C963-971.
118. Kekuda R, Torres-Zamorano V, Fei YJ, et al. Molecular and functional characterization of intestinal Na(+)-dependent neutral amino acid transporter B0. *Am J Physiol.* 1997;272(6):G1463-1472.
119. Kanai Y, Hediger MA. The glutamate/neutral amino acid transporter family SLC1: molecular, physiological and pharmacological aspects. *Pflugers Arch.* 2004;447(5):469-479.
120. Munck BG, Munck LK. Effects of pH changes on systems ASC and B in rabbit ileum. *Am J Physiol.* 1999;276(1 Pt 1):G173-184.
121. Verrey F, Meier C, Rossier G, Kuhn LC. Glycoprotein-associated amino acid exchangers: broadening the range of transport specificity. *Pflugers Arch.* 2000;440(4):503-512.
122. Wasa M, Wang HS, Shimizu Y, Okada A. Amino acid transport is down-regulated in ischemic human intestinal epithelial cells. *Biochim Biophys Acta.* 2004;1670(1):49-55.
123. Pan M, Meng Q, Choudry HA, Karinch AM, Lin C, Souba WW. Stimulation of intestinal glutamine absorption in chronic metabolic acidosis. *Surgery.* 2004;136(2):127-134.
124. Ganapathy V, Brandsch M, Leibach FH. Intestinal transport of amino acids and peptides. In: Johnson LR, ed. *Physiology of the Gastrointestinal Tract.* New York: Raven Press; 1994.
125. Munck BG. Transport of imino acids and non-alpha-amino acids across the brush-border membrane of the rabbit ileum. *J Membr Biol.* 1985;83(1-2):15-24.
126. Hu M, Borchardt RT. Transport of a large neutral amino acid in a human intestinal epithelial cell line (Caco-2): uptake and efflux of phenylalanine. *Biochim Biophys Acta.* 1992;1135(3):233-244.
127. Kanai Y, Hediger MA. Primary structure and functional characterization of a high-affinity glutamate transporter. *Nature.* 1992;360(6403):467-471.
128. Shigeri Y, Seal RP, Shimamoto K. Molecular pharmacology of glutamate transporters, EAATs and VGLUTs. *Brain Res Brain Res Rev.* 2004;45(3):250-265.
129. Chen Z, Fei YJ, Anderson CM, et al. Structure, function and immunolocalization of a proton-coupled amino acid transporter (hPAT1) in the human intestinal cell line Caco-2. *J Physiol.* 2003;546:349-361.
130. Wagner CA, Lang F, Broer S. Function and structure of heterodimeric amino acid transporters. *Am J Physiol Cell Physiol.* 2001;281(4):C1077-1093.
131. Palacin M, Kanai Y. The ancillary proteins of HATs: SLC3 family of amino acid transporters. *Pflugers Arch.* 2004;447(5):490-494.
132. Chillaron J, Estevez R, Mora C, et al. Obligatory amino acid exchange via systems bo,+-like and y+L-like. A tertiary active transport mechanism for renal reabsorption of cystine and dibasic amino acids. *J Biol Chem.* 1996;271(30):17761-17770.
133. Pfeiffer R, Loffing J, Rossier G, et al. Luminal heterodimeric amino acid transporter defective in cystinuria. *Mol Biol Cell.* 1999;10(12):4135-4147.
134. Fernandez E, Carrascal M, Rousaud F, et al. rBAT-b(0,+)AT heterodimer is the main apical reabsorption system for cystine in the kidney. *Am J Physiol Renal Physiol.* 2002;283(3):F540-548.
135. Bain PJ, LeBlanc-Chaffin R, Chen H, Palii SS, Leach KM, Kilberg MS. The mechanism for transcriptional activation of the human ATA2 transporter gene by amino acid deprivation is different than that for asparagine synthetase. *J Nutr.* 2002;132(10):3023-3029.
136. Hatanaka T, Huang W, Martindale RG, Ganapathy V. Differential influence of cAMP on the expression of the three subtypes (ATA1, ATA2, and ATA3) of the amino acid transport system A. *FEBS Lett.* 2001;505(2):317-320.
137. Varoqui H, Erickson JD. Selective up-regulation of system a transporter mRNA in diabetic liver. *Biochem Biophys Res Commun.* 2002;290(3):903-908.
138. Palii SS, Chen H, Kilberg MS. Transcriptional control of the human sodium-coupled neutral amino acid transporter system A gene by amino acid availability is mediated by an intronic element. *J Biol Chem.* 2004;279(5):3463-3471.
139. Gu S, Roderick HL, Camacho P, Jiang JX. Characterization of an N-system amino acid transporter expressed in retina and its involvement in glutamine transport. *J Biol Chem.* 2001;276(26):24137-24144.
140. Verrey F, Closs EI, Wagner CA, Palacin M, Endou H, Kanai Y. CATs and HATs: the SLC7 family of amino acid transporters. *Pflugers Arch.* 2003.
141. Torrents D, Mykkanen J, Pineda M, et al. Identification of SLC7A7, encoding y+LAT-1, as the lysinuric protein intolerance gene. *Nat Genet.* 1999;21(3):293-296.
142. Borsani G, Bassi MT, Sperandeo MP, et al. SLC7A7, encoding a putative permease-related protein, is mutated in patients with lysinuric protein intolerance. *Nat Genet.* 1999;21(3):297-301.
143. Meier C, Ristic Z, Klauser S, Verrey F. Activation of system L heterodimeric amino acid exchangers by intracellular substrates. *Embo J.* 2002;21(4):580-589.
144. Lash LH, Jones DP. Characteristics of cysteine uptake in intestinal basolateral membrane vesicles. *Am J Physiol.* 1984;247(4):G394-401.
145. Rossier G, Meier C, Bauch C, et al. LAT2, a new basolateral 4F2hc/CD98-associated amino acid transporter of kidney and intestine. *J Biol Chem.* 1999;274(49):34948-34954.

146. Souba WW, Smith RJ, Wilmore DW. Glutamine metabolism by the intestinal tract. *JPEN J Parenter Enteral Nutr.* 1985;9(5):608-617.
147. Windmueller HG, Spaeth AE. Uptake and metabolism of plasma glutamine by the small intestine. *J Biol Chem.* 1974;249(16):5070-5079.
148. Windmueller HG, Spaeth AE. Respiratory fuels and nitrogen metabolism in vivo in small intestine of fed rats. Quantitative importance of glutamine, glutamate, and aspartate. *J Biol Chem.* 1980;255(1):107-112.
149. Haisch M, Fukagawa NK, Matthews DE. Oxidation of glutamine by the splanchnic bed in humans. *Am J Physiol Endocrinol Metab.* 2000;278(4):E593-602.
150. Darmaun D, Roig JC, Auestad N, Sager BK, Neu J. Glutamine metabolism in very low birth weight infants. *Pediatr Res.* 1997;41(3):391-396.
151. Battezzati A, Brillon DJ, Matthews DE. Oxidation of glutamic acid by the splanchnic bed in humans. *Am J Physiol.* 1995;269(2):E269-276.
152. Gate JJ, Parker DS, Lobley GE. The metabolic fate of the amido-N group of glutamine in the tissues of the gastrointestinal tract in 24 h-fasted sheep. *Br J Nutr.* 1999;81(4):297-306.
153. Smith RJ. Glutamine metabolism and its physiologic importance. *JPEN J Parenter Enteral Nutr.* 1990;14(4 Suppl):40S-44S.
154. Souba WW. Interorgan ammonia metabolism in health and disease: a surgeon's view. *JPEN J Parenter Enteral Nutr.* 1987;11(6):569-579.
155. Souba WW, Klimberg VS, Plumley DA, et al. The role of glutamine in maintaining a healthy gut and supporting the metabolic response to injury and infection. *J Surg Res.* 1990;48(4):383-391.
156. Rouse K, Nwokedi E, Woodliff JE, Epstein J, Klimberg VS. Glutamine enhances selectivity of chemotherapy through changes in glutathione metabolism. *Ann Surg.* 1995;221(4):420-426.
157. Klimberg VS, McClellan JL, Organ CH, Jr. Honorary lectureship. Glutamine, cancer, and its therapy. *Am J Surg.* 1996;172(5):418-424.
158. Burrin DG, Ferrell CL, Eisemann JH, Britton RA, Nienaber JA. Effect of level of nutrition on splanchnic blood flow and oxygen consumption in sheep. *Br J Nutr.* 1989;62(1):23-34.
159. Yen JT, Nienaber JA, Hill DA, Pond WG. Oxygen consumption by portal vein-drained organs and by whole animal in conscious growing swine. *Proc Soc Exp Biol Med.* 1989;190(4):393-398.
160. Nieto R, Lobley GE. Integration of protein metabolism within the whole body and between organs. In: Lobley GE, White A, MacRae JC, eds. *Proceedings of the 8th International Symposium on Protein Metabolsim and Nutrition.* EAAP Publication No. 96; 1999:69-99.
161. Attaix D, Arnal M. Protein synthesis and growth in the gastrointestinal tract of the young preruminant lamb. *Br J Nutr.* 1987;58(1):159-169.
162. Burrin DG, Fiorotto ML, Hadsell DL. Transgenic hypersecretion of des(1-3) human insulin-like growth factor I in mouse milk has limited effects on the gastrointestinal tract in suckling pups. *J Nutr.* 1999;129(1):51-56.
163. Attaix D, Aurousseau E, Rosolowska-Huszcz D, Bayle G, Arnal M. In vivo longitudinal variations in protein synthesis in developing ovine intestines. *Am J Physiol.* 1992;263(6):R1318-1323.
164. Goldstein RM, Hebiguchi T, Luk GD, et al. The effects of total parenteral nutrition on gastrointestinal growth and development. *J Pediatr Surg.* 1985;20(6):785-791.
165. Morgan W, 3rd, Yardley J, Luk G, Niemiec P, Dudgeon D. Total parenteral nutrition and intestinal development: a neonatal model. *J Pediatr Surg.* 1987;22(6):541-545.
166. Hansen AE, Wiese HF, Boelsche AN, Haggard ME, Adam JD, Davis H. Role of linoleic acid in infant nutrition. *Pediatrics.* 1963;312:171-192.
167. Paulsrud JR, Pensler L, Whitten CF, Stewart S, Holman RT. Essential fatty acid deficiency in infants induced by fat-free intravenous feeding. *Am J Clin Nutr.* 1972;25(9):897-904.
168. Holman RT, Johnson SB, Hatch TF. A case of human linolenic acid deficiency involving neurological abnormalities. *Am J Clin Nutr.* 1982;35(3):617-623.
169. Friedman Z, Shochat SJ, Maisels MJ, Marks KH, Lamberth EL, Jr. Correction of essential fatty acid deficiency in newborn infants by cutaneous application of sunflower-seed oil. *Pediatrics.* 1976;58(5):650-654.
170. Field CJ, Clandinin MT, Van Aerde JE. Polyunsaturated fatty acids and T-cell function: implications for the neonate. *Lipids.* 2001;36(9):1025-1032.
171. Neuringer M. Infant vision and retinal function in studies of dietary long-chain polyunsaturated fatty acids: methods, results, and implications. *Am J Clin Nutr.* 2000;71(1 Suppl):256S-267S.
172. Grundy SM, Abate N, Chandalia M. Diet composition and the metabolic syndrome: what is the optimal fat intake? *Am J Med.* 2002;113 (Suppl 9B):25S-29S.
173. Human Nutrition Information Service and Health and Human Services. *Dietary Guidelines for Americans, 2005.* 6th ed. Washington DC: Agriculture Dept; 2005.
174. Moreau H, Laugier R, Gargouri Y, Ferrato F, Verger R. Human preduodenal lipase is entirely of gastric fundic origin. *Gastroenterology.* 1988;95(5):1221-1226.
175. Carriere F, Barrowman JA, Verger R, Laugier R. Secretion and contribution to lipolysis of gastric and pancreatic lipases during a test meal in humans. *Gastroenterology.* 1993;105(3):876-888.
176. Hamosh M, Scow RO. Lingual lipase. *Symp Oral Sens Percept.* 1973(4):311-322.
177. Kawai T, Fushiki T. Importance of lipolysis in oral cavity for orosensory detection of fat. *Am J Physiol Regul Integr Comp Physiol.* 2003;285(2):R447-454.
178. Smith LJ, Kaminsky S, D'Souza SW. Neonatal fat digestion and lingual lipase. *Acta Paediatr Scand.* 1986;75(6):913-918.
179. Harries JT. Fat absorption in the newborn. *Acta Paediatr Scand Suppl.* 1982;299:17-23.
180. Abrams CK, Hamosh M, Hubbard VS, Dutta SK, Hamosh P. Lingual lipase in cystic fibrosis. Quantitation of enzyme activity in the upper small intestine of patients with exocrine pancreatic insufficiency. *J Clin Invest.* 1984;73(2):374-382.
181. Moreau H, Bernadac A, Gargouri Y, Benkouka F, Laugier R, Verger R. Immunocytolocalization of human gastric lipase in chief cells of the fundic mucosa. *Histochemistry.* 1989;91(5):419-423.
182. Hamosh M. Lingual and gastric lipases. *Nutrition.* 1990;6(6):421-428.
183. Volhard F. Uber das fettspaltende Ferment des Magens. *Z. Klind. Med.* 1901;42:414-429.
184. Hull M, Keaton RW. The existence of a gastric lipase. *J Biol Chem.* 1917;32:127-140.
185. Entressangles B, Desnuelle P. Action of pancreatic lipase on aggregated glyceride molecules in an isotropic system. *Biochim Biophys Acta.* 1968;159(2):285-295.
186. Borgstrom B, Erlanson-Albertsson C. Pancreatic colipase. In: Borgstrom B, Brockman HL, eds. *Lipases.* Amsterdam: Elsevier Science Publishers; 1984:151-183.
187. Verger R. Pancreatic lipases. In: Borgstrom B, Brockman HL, eds. *Lipases.* Amsterdam: Elsevier Science Publishers; 1984:83-150.
188. Chapus C, Rovery M, Sarda L, Verger R. Minireview on pancreatic lipase and colipase. *Biochimie.* 1988;70(9):1223-1234.
189. Brockman HL. Kinetic behavior of the pancreatic lipase-colipase-lipid system. *Biochimie.* 2000;82(11):987-995.
190. Hildebrand H, Borgstrom B, Bekassy A, Erlanson-Albertsson C, Helin I. Isolated co-lipase deficiency in two brothers. *Gut.* 1982;23(3):243-246.
191. Lowe ME. Properties and function of pancreatic lipase related protein 2. *Biochimie.* 2000;82(11):997-1004.
192. Murakami M, Nakatani Y, Atsumi G, Inoue K, Kudo I. Regulatory functions of phospholipase A2. *Crit Rev Immunol.* 1997;17:225-283.

193. Valentin E, Lambeau G. What can venom phospholipases A(2) tell us about the functional diversity of mammalian secreted phospholipases A(2)? *Biochimie*. 2000;82:815-831.
194. Phan CT, Tso P. Intestinal lipid absorption and transport. *Front Biosci*. 2001;6:D299-319.
195. Hofmann AF, Borgstrom B. Physico-chemical state of lipids in intestinal content during their digestion and absorption. *Fed Proc*. 1962;21:43-50.
196. Hofmann AF, Borgstrom B. Hydrolysis of long-chain monoglycerides in micellar solution by pancreatic lipase. *Biochim Biophys Acta*. 1963;70:317-331.
197. Thomson AB, Schoeller C, Keelan M, Smith L, Clandinin MT. Lipid absorption: passing through the unstirred layers, brush-border membrane, and beyond. *Can J Physiol Pharmacol*. 1993;71(8):531-555.
198. Stremmel W, Lotz G, Strohmeyer G, Berk PD. Identification, isolation, and partial characterization of a fatty acid binding protein from rat jejunal microvillous membranes. *J Clin Invest*. 1985;75(3):1068-1076.
199. Stremmel W, Strohmeyer G, Borchard F, Kochwa S, Berk PD. Isolation and partial characterization of a fatty acid binding protein in rat liver plasma membranes. *Proc Natl Acad Sci U S A*. 1985;82(1):4-8.
200. Lundgren S, Carling T, Hjalm G, et al. Tissue distribution of human gp330/megalin, a putative Ca(2+)-sensing protein. *J Histochem Cytochem*. 1997;45(3):383-392.
201. Moestrup SK, Cui S, Vorum H, et al. Evidence that epithelial glycoprotein 330/megalin mediates uptake of polybasic drugs. *J Clin Invest*. 1995;96(3):1404-1413.
202. Abumrad N, Coburn C, Ibrahimi A. Membrane proteins implicated in long-chain fatty acid uptake by mammalian cells: CD36, FATP and FABPm. *Biochim Biophys Acta*. 1999;1441(1):4-13.
203. Abumrad NA, Sfeir Z, Connelly MA, Coburn C. Lipid transporters: membrane transport systems for cholesterol and fatty acids. *Curr Opin Clin Nutr Metab Care*. 2000;3(4):255-262.
204. Murata M, Peranen J, Schreiner R, Wieland F, Kurzchalia TV, Simons K. VIP21/caveolin is a cholesterol-binding protein. *Proc Natl Acad Sci U S A*. 1995;92(22):10339-10343.
205. Stahl A, Hirsch DJ, Gimeno RE, et al. Identification of the major intestinal fatty acid transport protein. *Mol Cell*. 1999;4(3):299-308.
206. Frohnert BI, Bernlohr DA. Regulation of fatty acid transporters in mammalian cells. *Prog Lipid Res*. 2000;39(1):83-107.
207. Stenge EF, Dietschy JM. Cholesterol absorption and metabolism by the intestinal epithelium. In: Danielsson H, Sjovall J, eds. *Sterols and Bile Acids*. New York: Elsevier Science Publishers; 1985:121-149.
208. Turley SD, Dietschy JM. Sterol absorption by the small intestine. *Curr Opin Lipidol*. 2003;14(3):233-240.
209. Berge KE, Tian H, Graf GA, et al. Accumulation of dietary cholesterol in sitosterolemia caused by mutations in adjacent ABC transporters. *Science*. 2000;290(5497):1771-1775.
210. Lee MH, Lu K, Hazard S, et al. Identification of a gene, ABCG5, important in the regulation of dietary cholesterol absorption. *Nat Genet*. 2001;27(1):79-83.
211. Yu L, Li-Hawkins J, Hammer RE, et al. Overexpression of ABCG5 and ABCG8 promotes biliary cholesterol secretion and reduces fractional absorption of dietary cholesterol. *J Clin Invest*. 2002;110(5):671-680.
212. Lopez-Candales A, Bosner MS, Spilburg CA, Lange LG. Cholesterol transport function of pancreatic cholesterol esterase: directed sterol uptake and esterification in enterocytes. *Biochemistry*. 1993;32(45):12085-12089.
213. Hauser H, Dyer JH, Nandy A, et al. Identification of a receptor mediating absorption of dietary cholesterol in the intestine. *Biochemistry*. 1998;37(51):17843-17850.
214. Repa JJ, Dietschy JM, Turley SD. Inhibition of cholesterol absorption by SCH 58053 in the mouse is not mediated via changes in the expression of mRNA for ABCA1, ABCG5, or ABCG8 in the enterocyte. *J Lipid Res*. 2002;43(11):1864-1874.
215. Howles PN, Carter CP, Hui DY. Dietary free and esterified cholesterol absorption in cholesterol esterase (bile salt-stimulated lipase) gene-targeted mice. *J Biol Chem*. 1996;271(12):7196-7202.
216. Weng W, Li L, van Bennekum AM, et al. Intestinal absorption of dietary cholesteryl ester is decreased but retinyl ester absorption is normal in carboxyl ester lipase knockout mice. *Biochemistry*. 1999;38(13):4143-4149.
217. Mardones P, Quinones V, Amigo L, et al. Hepatic cholesterol and bile acid metabolism and intestinal cholesterol absorption in scavenger receptor class B type I-deficient mice. *J Lipid Res*. 2001;42(2):170-180.
218. Drobnik W, Lindenthal B, Lieser B, et al. ATP-binding cassette transporter A1 (ABCA1) affects total body sterol metabolism. *Gastroenterology*. 2001;120(5):1203-1211.
219. Nishimukai M, Hara H, Aoyama Y. Enteral administration of soybean lecithin enhanced lymphatic absorption of triacylglycerol in rats. *Br J Nutr*. 2003;90(3):565-571.
220. Nishimukai M, Hara H. Enteral administration of soybean phosphatidylcholine enhances the lymphatic absorption of lycopene, but reduces that of alpha-tocopherol in rats. *J Nutr*. 2004;134(8):1862-1866.
221. Tso P, Kendrick H, Balint JA, Simmonds WJ. Role of biliary phosphatidylcholine in the absorption and transport of dietary triolein in the rat. *Gastroenterology*. 1981;80(1):60-65.
222. Mansbach CM, 2nd, Dowell RF. Portal transport of long acyl chain lipids: effect of phosphatidylcholine and low infusion rates. *Am J Physiol*. 1993;264(6 Pt 1):G1082-1089.
223. Parlier RD, Frase S, Mansbach CM, 2nd. Intraenterocyte distribution of absorbed lipid and effects of phosphatidylcholine. *Am J Physiol*. 1989;256(2 Pt 1):G349-355.
224. Mansbach CM, 2nd, Arnold A, Cox MA. Factors influencing triacylglycerol delivery into mesenteric lymph. *Am J Physiol*. 1985;249(5):G642-648.
225. Ehehalt R, Jochims C, Lehmann WD, et al. Evidence of luminal phosphatidylcholine secretion in rat ileum. *Biochim Biophys Acta*. 2004;1682(1-3):63-71.
226. Tso P. Intestinal lipid absorption. In: Johnson L, ed. *Physiology of the Gastrointestinal Tract*. New York: Raven Press; 1994:1873.
227. Storch J, Thumser AE. The fatty acid transport function of fatty acid-binding proteins. *Biochim Biophys Acta*. 2000;1486(1):28-44.
228. Smith SJ, Cases S, Jensen DR, et al. Obesity resistance and multiple mechanisms of triglyceride synthesis in mice lacking Dgat. *Nat Genet*. 2000;25(1):87-90.
229. Oelkers P, Tinkelenberg A, Erdeniz N, Cromley D, Billheimer JT, Sturley SL. A lecithin cholesterol acyltransferase-like gene mediates diacylglycerol esterification in yeast. *J Biol Chem*. 2000;275(21):15609-15612.
230. Field FJ, Cooper AD, Erickson SK. Regulation of rabbit intestinal acyl coenzyme A-cholesterol acyltransferase in vivo and in vitro. *Gastroenterology*. 1982;83(4):873-880.
231. Buhman KK, Accad M, Novak S, et al. Resistance to diet-induced hypercholesterolemia and gallstone formation in ACAT2-deficient mice. Nat Med. Dec 2000;6(12):1341-1347.
232. Go MF, Schonfeld G, Pfleger B, Cole TG, Sussman NL, Alpers DH. Regulation of intestinal and hepatic apoprotein synthesis after chronic fat and cholesterol feeding. *J Clin Invest*. 1988;81(5):1615-1620.
233. Davidson NO, Magun AM, Brasitus TA, Glickman RM. Intestinal apolipoprotein A-I and B-48 metabolism: effects of sustained alterations in dietary triglyceride and mucosal cholesterol flux. *J Lipid Res*. 1987;28(4):388-402.
234. Hayashi H, Fujimoto K, Cardelli JA, Nutting DF, Bergstedt S, Tso P. Fat feeding increases size, but not number, of chylomicrons produced by small intestine. *Am J Physiol*. 1990;259(5):G709-719.
235. Ohashi K, Ishibashi S, Osuga J, et al. Novel mutations in the microsomal triglyceride transfer protein gene causing abetalipoproteinemia. *J Lipid Res*. 2000;41(8):1199-1204.

236. Bouma ME, Beucler I, Aggerbeck LP, Infante R, Schmitz J. Hypobetalipoproteinemia with accumulation of an apoprotein B-like protein in intestinal cells. Immunoenzymatic and biochemical characterization of seven cases of Anderson's disease. *J Clin Invest.* 1986;78(2):398-410.

237. Dannoura AH, Berriot-Varoqueaux N, Amati P, et al. Anderson's disease: exclusion of apolipoprotein and intracellular lipid transport genes. *Arterioscler Thromb Vasc Biol.* 1999;19(10):2494-2508.

Chapter 9

FOOD ALLERGIES

Stephan C. Bischoff, MD
and Sheila E. Crowe, MD

Introduction

Food proteins, although indispensable for life, can become harmful when recognized by the immune system as foreign antigens. In this case, food proteins trigger an abnormal immune response and subsequently an inflammatory reaction, which can be detrimental to the host depending on the extent and the duration of inflammation. Food proteins that induce such damaging immune responses are referred to as food allergens, and the reactions are called allergic (from greek "allos" = different from, "ergos" = work) reactions.

Allergic reactions to food frequently occur in early childhood and disappear spontaneously within the first 4 to 6 years of life. Sometimes, these reactions are replaced by inhalant allergies to plant pollens, mites, or animal epithelia. Relatively few children retain their food allergies until adulthood. Some adults, however, develop food allergies without experiencing food allergy in childhood. The prevalence of food allergy decreases from 4% to 8% in children to 1% to 4% in adults.[1-5]

At least 20% of the population in developed nations reports adverse reactions to food (ARF).[6] ARF are caused by a variety of mechanisms, with only about a third of the reactions in children and 10% of those in adults due to actual food allergy in which there is an abnormal immunological reaction to food. Most ARF are non-immunologic in origin, and lactose intolerance is globally the most common type of adverse reaction to food. The symptoms of allergy range from minor symptoms to life-threatening shock reactions.[7] Of the patients suffering from true food allergy, roughly one-third complain predominantly of gastrointestinal (GI) symptoms (nausea, vomiting, cramps, bloating, diarrhea), with the others also reporting skin symptoms (urticaria, atopic dermatitis), respiratory complaints (rhinitis, asthma), or less well-defined systemic complaints, which may not be related to food allergy (migraine headaches, fatigue, edema, arthritis). Although dermatologic, respiratory, and systemic manifestations of food allergy are well recognized, those reactions manifesting primarily in the digestive tract can be difficult to diagnose and treat. This reflects the various ways food can cause GI symptoms, the relatively poorly understood pathophysiological mechanisms, and the limited diagnostic methods available to objectively identify affected subjects, which are, in turn, a consequence of the difficulty accessing the GI tract to establish mechanisms of disease and develop methods to diagnose and treat food allergy.[8,9]

Along with allergic reactions in general, allergic reactions to food are increasing in prevalence. However, except for peanut allergy,[10,11] clear data confirming this increase in food allergies are lacking. Recent epidemiologic studies suggest that the greater level of hygiene in urbanized populations in industrialized countries might play a central role in mediating this increase in allergic diseases.[12-14] Food allergies and other types of adverse reactions to foods manifest primarily with GI symptoms in up to 50%,[15,16] and therefore, many afflicted patients consult specialists in gastroenterology who are, as a group, often less aware of how to approach such cases. Often, such patients become classified as being "psychosomatic" or "functional" or having irritable bowel syndrome (IBS) without defining the real problem. It has been recognized for some time now that IBS is often associated with ARF and in some instances, food allergy might be a mechanism for symptoms in a subgroup of afflicted patients.[17-19]

Dealing with food allergy becomes an even more important issue now that food allergy has become the most common cause of life-threatening anaphylaxis in industrialized countries.[20] Unquestionably, confirmed food allergy is treated successfully by avoidance of food allergens, the mainstay of treatment of food allergy, but supportive medical treatment with epinephrine, antihistamines, and corticosteroids can also be beneficial for severe reactions. In spite of an evolving understanding of the field, further investigation into the underlying mechanisms is needed in order to optimize the prevention, diagnosis, and treatment of food allergies.

Cellular and Molecular Mechanisms of Food Allergy

The best-characterized, abnormal immunologic reaction to food is immediate IgE-mediated hypersensitivity to food, also termed a Type-I reaction according to the classification of Coombs and Gell. The IgE-mediated type-I reaction is involved in the pathogenesis of many cases of asthma, rhinitis, urticaria, and atopic eczema as well as GI adverse reactions to food. Delayed reactions following immediate IgE-mediated hypersensitivity occur in selected individuals and are characterized by an enhanced cell infiltration of the tissue with inflammatory cells and subsequent tissue damage. These and other cell-mediated immune reactions to food antigens may operate in the GI tract and beyond. Such mechanisms are thought to play a role in milk and soy protein enteropathies and in celiac disease (Chapter 19).[14,21,22] Immunologic reactions to foods can also involve mixed IgE- and non-IgE-mediated and other mechanisms than classical immediate or delayed type-I hypersensitivity. In particular, type-IV hypersensitivity reactions against food proteins have been suggested based on findings such as the presence of food antigen-specific T cells with either T helper or cytotoxic phenotype.[23]

Allergic inflammation of the gut requires a sufficient load of triggering allergen into the gut lumen and a hyper-responsive mucosal immune system. Enhanced antigen exposure may result from genetically determined alterations of key molecules comprising the GI barrier, immaturity, acquired disturbances of the GI defense system such as enteric infection, or a combination thereof. Nonspecific inflammation induced by bacteria, viruses, or toxins can predispose to a loss of tolerance and subsequent development of immunological hypersensitivity. Naïve lymphocytes of the gut-associated lymphoid tissue (GALT) get primed for cytokine-producing Th2 effector cells required for IgE-producing plasma cells. Indeed, allergen-specific T cells can be isolated from blood, skin, and mucosal sites in patients with food allergy, and, characteristically, they express a Th2 cell phenotype releasing interleukin- (IL-) 4, IL-5, and IL-13(23). Such cytokines play a central role in the induction and maintenance of allergic responses by regulating IgE synthesis (IL-4, IL-13) and chemoattraction of inflammatory cells, such as mast cells (IL-4) and eosinophils (IL-5) (24-26).

Any delayed development of the protective IgA system of GALT in the postnatal phase or an enhanced switch to IgE-producing Bε cells is associated with an increased risk of developing allergic disease. The major inducer of IgA synthesis, apart from external triggers, is TGF-ß derived from Th3 cells, whereas the switch to IgE synthesis is dependent on CD40L, IL-4, and IL-13 derived from Th2 cells and inflammatory cells such as mast cells or basophils.[21] In contrast, Th1 cytokines such as IFN-γ inhibit the action of Th2 cells, and thereby, controlled Th1-driven immune responses are required to limit the default Th2 GI response and to prevent overproduction of IgE.[25] Such mechanisms further argue for the hygiene hypothesis, which proposes that an overly "clean" environment with reduced microbial challenge is a risk factor for atopy, defined as an enhanced Th2 milieu and subsequent IgE-mediated allergy.

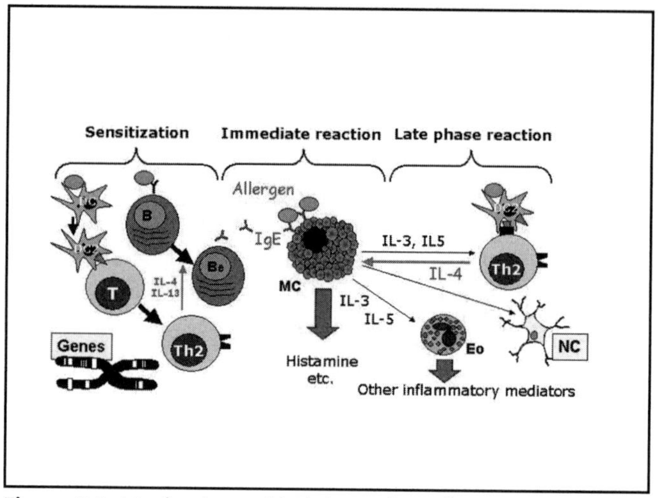

Figure 9-1. Mechanisms of IgE-dependent allergic reactions.

Clinical studies strongly suggest that IgE is also produced locally in the GI mucosa,[27] providing an explanation for the fact that serum IgE measurements and skin tests do not correlate well with mucosal allergic responses in the intestine.[8] In atopic individuals, elevated IgE levels are closely correlated with IL-13, a gene subject to polymorphisms that are linked to atopy.[28] The IgE-mediated allergic immune response can be divided into three phases: the sensitization phase, the effector phase consisting of an acute and a facultative late phase reaction, and a chronic phase that may be the result of repetitive late phase reactions (Figure 9-1).

The sensitization phase is dependent on the uptake and processing of the antigen by antigen-presenting cells such as dendritic cells, macrophages, or B cells, and the subsequent presentation of antigenic peptides to naive CD4+ T cells. Under the influence of particular cytokines, such as IL-4 and IL-13, the naive Th0 cells are transformed to Th2-type lymphocytes required for B cell switch to plasma cells producing larger amounts of specific IgE directed against particular food antigens. Once mast cells and basophils expressing the high-affinity IgE receptor have bound sufficient specific IgE, recurrent antigen exposure may induce an effector phase by cross-linking of surface IgE molecules. This "acute phase" causes activation of mast cells and basophils with release of histamine, leukotrienes, and other mediators known to be responsible for a number of effects in the GI tract. Acute reactions occurring within seconds to minutes may be followed by a "late-phase reaction" starting within 2 to 24 hours after allergen challenge and characterized by a cellular infiltration of the tissue with granulocytes (basophils, eosinophils) and lymphocytes (mainly Th2 cells).[29] These phases have been studied less extensively in the GI tract, but there is some evidence that suggests that they occur in a fashion similar to those of other organs.[8,30]

The chronic phase of allergic disease, thought to be a result of repetitive late-phase reactions, is not necessarily Th2 dominated because Th1-type lymphocytes are also found as described for chronic airways disease or Crohn's disease. The pathology typically consists of a mixture of Th2- and Th1-type cytokines and cells, accompanied by arteriolar dilatation, increased vascular permeability, enhanced stimulation of sensory nerves, and impaired GI function. The ongoing inflammation induces a permanent upregulation of adhesion molecules and the release of chemokines, which causes persistent infiltration of all types of granulocytes, macrophages, and lymphocytes, and finally, structural changes such as fibrosis and organ dysfunction.

Inflammatory mediators produced by mast cells and eosinophils are responsible for the clinical symptoms and the organ dysfunction that occurs during allergic reactions. Elevated levels of histamine and its metabolite, methylhistamine, tryptase, eosinophil cationic protein (ECP), eosinophil-derived neurotoxin (EDN), IL-5, and tumor necrosis factor (TNF)-α have been measured in serum, urine, gut lavage fluid, and stool from patients with food allergy.[31-34] Further evidence of activation of mast cells and eosinophils are histological studies that show degranulation, cytokine production by these cell types, and enhanced levels of proinflammatory mediators after allergen provocation tests.[30]

Mast cells, eosinophils, and basophils are now recognized not only as effector cells of allergic inflammation, but also as immunoregulatory cells contributing to the maintenance of GI homeostasis and also involved in defense mechanisms (eg, against bacteria and parasites).[35,36] In recent years, it has become evident that the ENS also regulates key cells involved in allergic inflammation such as lymphocytes, mast cells, and eosinophils. The morphologic and functional associations between immune cells and nerves were first recognized for mast cells in the skin, lung, intestine, and lymphoid and synovial tissues of animals and humans. The extent to which eosinophils are in such close proximity to nerves in different tissues has been studied less extensively. Of particular interest is the finding that GALT is innervated and, in turn, that the ENS is also modulated by mediators derived from immune and inflammatory cells. Such enteric neuroimmune interactions provide a potential mechanism for the reported psychological or functional aspects to allergic responses.[37]

In conclusion, the development of food allergy depends on the presence of several risk factors, such as immature mucosal immune system; early introduction of solid food; impaired GI barrier; IgA or TGF-β deficiency; GI infections or inadequate challenge of the intestinal immune system with commensal flora; genetically determined bias towards a Th2 environment, polymorphisms of Th2 cytokine, or IgE receptor genes; and altered enteric nervous system.[38]

Biochemistry of Food Allergens

The structural and biochemical properties of the triggering antigen influence the type of immune response; however, the specific requirements for allergenicity are still unclear.[39] This is an important issue given the advent of genetically modified foods that raise the question of how to predict or test allergenicity.[40] In general, soluble proteins are more tolerogenic than are particulate or globular antigens.[21] Other biochemical characteristics of food allergens affect their absorption and their stability. For example, the peanut protein Ara h1 was recently shown to resist to degradation because of the formation of stable homo-trimers.[41] Dose of antigen is of relevance for the subsequent immunological response with activation of regulatory T cells (Th3) by low doses of antigen, whereas high doses induce anergy or apoptosis.[21]

The development of specific food allergies depends on exposure to specific foods and, thus, the cultural habits of eating various kinds of food. As a result, peanut allergy is common in North America, while sesame allergy is more common in the Middle East.[42] The relative importance of specific food allergens also depends on the age of afflicted individuals: allergies to cow's milk, eggs, and wheat are more common in infants and children, while seafood allergies are more common in adults. Of particular interest is the cross-reactivity amongst foods belonging to the same botanical group of foods and between foods and other types of allergens such as pollens, mites, or latex.[43,44] Understanding the potential for cross-reactivity directs the history for specific foods and other substances inducing allergic symptoms, enhances the accuracy of dietary elimination advice, and allows new insights into the molecular structures of typical allergens.

Major allergen epitopes have been identified and characterized on a molecular level over the past decade. Such major epitopes are found in allergens belonging to the same group or even in different types of allergens such as pollens and foods, thereby explaining on a molecular basis the well-known phenomenon of cross-reactivity between allergens. The first major proteins found were Bet v1 and Bet v2 (profilin), which were found in birch pollen and a number of food allergens such as fruits and celery.[45] Most of the specific IgE in allergic patients is to birch pollen and foods and is directed against Bet v1, which emphasizes the importance of this epitope as a major B-cell epitope and cross-linking agent of mast cells in sensitized individuals. More than 1000 epitopes, of which 50 to 100 are major epitopes, have since been cloned and sequenced (for details on recombinant allergen epitopes see http://www.allergome.org).[46]

Recombinant food antigens offer a number of new possibilities both for the diagnosis and treatment of food allergy, including their use in skin testing and in vitro laboratory tests (such as measurement of specific IgE or mediator release assays) and as replacement for allergen extracts, which are known to contain low amounts of allergen of limited stability and unknown immunologic activity.[47] In addition, recombinant allergens can be modified so they will be recognized by T cells but not by B cells, and thus they offer the potential for safe and effective desensitization in patients with food allergy.[48] As an example, the cloned peanut allergen Ara h3 can be modified to a hypoallergenic molecule that binds less efficiently to IgE but retains the ability to stimulate T-cell activation in peripheral blood mononuclear cells from Ara h3 allergic donors.[49]

In recent studies, allergens have been shown to act not only as T-cell antigens or IgE-crosslinking agents but also as modulators of inflammation. For example, allergens release bioactive molecules such as eicosanoids, which are known to act as proinflammatory and immunomodulatory molecules. The amounts released seem to be sufficient to modulate cell functions; however, the regulation of such "biomediators" and their clinical impact remain to be elucidated in allergic reactions.

Clinical Classification of Food Allergy

Food allergy typically affects three major targets (Table 9-1), either alone or in combination: the skin, the respiratory tract, and the GI tract. Occasionally, food allergy presents as migraine, diffuse arthritis, generalized edema, hypotension, and fatigue; however, such symptoms are usually associated with nonimmune reactions to food. The most important manifestation of food allergy is systemic anaphylaxis, and it is now recognized that food allergy is the major cause of anaphylactic reactions in developed nations including the United States, Australia, and Europe.[50-52] The prevalence of peanut allergy (0.5% to 7% of adults in the United States and Great Britain)[53] and its potentially fatal consequences has had significant impact on society, including schools[54] and the airline industry.[55] Minute amounts of antigen such as that imparted by a kiss can induce fatal anaphylaxis.[56,57]

Food-associated exercise-induced anaphylaxis is a rare type of anaphylaxis in which the food only elicits an anaphylactic reaction when the subject exercises within several hours of ingesting that food. A recent study suggests that exercise-induced activation of tissue transglutaminase in the intestinal mucosa—which can lead to cross-linking of omega-5 gliadin derived peptides forming larger allergen complexes that are capable of eliciting an anaphylactic response—may be the mechanism of wheat-dependent exercise-induced anaphylaxis because of the major allergen omega-5 gliadin.[58] Acetylsalicylates and other non-steroidal anti-inflammatory drugs can also augment type-I allergic symptoms when combined with food and exercise in individuals with food-dependent exercise-induced anaphylaxis.[59,60]

Nongastrointestinal Manifestations

A variety of dermatologic diseases (see Table 9-1) result from immunologic reactions to foods, including atopic dermatitis associated with increased gut permeability and, to some extent, urticaria that occurs often in association with food-dependent exercise-induced anaphylaxis.[61,62] Dermatitis herpetiformis is well recognized to occur in association with gluten-sensitive enteropathy, and the skin lesions can be effectively treated by a gluten-free diet alone. Respiratory manifestations of food allergy (see Table 9-1) include airway hyperresponsiveness, asthma, rhinitis, and possibly serous otitis media.[63] While asthma is commonly thought to be caused by inhalant allergens, a recent study indicates that food allergy was a major risk for life-threatening asthma in children.[64]

Gastrointestinal Manifestations

Typical manifestations of GI food allergy in infants and young children are food (dietary) protein-induced proctitis or proctocolitis and food protein-induced enteropathy.[65] More recently, eosinophilic esophagitis and allergic constipation have been described.[66,67] In older children and adults, the most common manifestation of food allergy is the oral allergy syndrome.[68] Typically, the GI symptoms of food allergic reactions (nausea, vomiting, abdominal pain, and diarrhea) occur in conjunction with allergic manifestations in other target organs. The foods primarily responsible for this type of GI food allergy include cow's milk, eggs, peanuts, seafood, and fish, depending on the local eating habits. Other forms of GI immunologically mediated adverse reactions to food include eosinophilic gastroenteropathies and celiac disease.[69,70]

The oral allergy syndrome (OAS) is triggered by plant proteins that cross-react with certain inhalant antigens, particularly birch, ragweed, and mugwort. Pruritis, tingling, and/or swelling of the tongue, lips, palate, or oropharynx, and occasionally to bronchospasm or more systemic reactions, occurring a few minutes after ingestion of the allergen, result from exposure to the cross-reacting foods. The diagnosis can be confirmed by skin-prick tests or measurement of specific IgE, as these reactions are almost all mediated by IgE.

Latex-Food Allergy Syndrome

Latex-food allergy syndrome, also known as the latex-fruit syndrome, is a specific form of food allergy that is increasing in prevalence throughout the world, with a frequency of associated-food allergy that varies from ~20% to 60%.[71] Globally, banana, avocado, chestnut, and kiwi are the most common causes of food-induced symptoms associated with latex allergy. In latex-sensitive individuals, exposure to these foods can result in the same symptoms—eg, pruritis, eczema, oral-facial swelling, asthma, GI complaints, and anaphylaxis—as are caused by exposure to latex.

Food Protein Enteropathy and Food Protein Enterocolitis/Proctitis

Food protein enteropathy is a disease of infants characterized by protracted diarrhea and vomiting. The associated malabsorption and protein-losing enteropathy may lead to edema, abdominal distension, and anemia. Other causes—such as infectious and metabolic disorders, lymphangiectasia, celiac disease, and other conditions—should be considered in the differential diagnosis. The underlying mechanisms involve immune complex mechanisms and/or abnormal T-cell immune responses, most

TABLE 9-1.

Manifestations of Adverse Reactions to Food

GI Manifestations	*Extraintestinal Manifestations*
Immediate GI hypersensitivity (primarily IgE mediated)	Skin
Oral allergy syndrome (OAS)	Urticaria and angioedema
Allergic gastritis	Atopic eczema
Allergic entrocolitis	Dermatitis herpetiformis
Eosinophilic gastroenteropathies (~50% IgE mediated)	Respiratory tract
Eosinophilic esophagitis	Rhinitis
Eosinophilic gastritis	Asthma
Eosinophilic enterocolitis	Alveolitis
Eosinophilic proctitis	
	Miscellaneous
Dietary protein enterocolitis and proctitis	Migraine headache
Chronic constipation	Chronic fatigue syndrome
Dietary protein enteropathy	Psychiatric and behavioral problems
Celiac disease	Hyperkinetic syndrome
Other mechanisms of adverse food reactions	Cardiovascular system
GERD	Vasculitis
Non-ulcer dyspepsia (NUD)	Systemic anaphlyaxis
Inflammatory bowel disease	
IBS	

commonly to cow's milk and soy but also to a wide variety of other foods.[72] Induction of specific IgE does not typically occur in this condition. Endoscopy with characteristic biopsy findings (increased intraepithelial lymphocytes and eosinophils and villous injury similar to that seen in celiac disease) and responses to elimination diets and rechallenges form the basis for diagnosis.

Celiac disease may occur in up to 1% of the population, making this form of food allergy much more common in adults than previously appreciated.[73] Ingestion of gliadin found in wheat, hordelein in rye, and secalin on barley induces an enteropathy in genetically susceptible individuals. Removal of the offending grain peptides from the diet restores normal small-bowel function and appearance, with improvement in symptoms that can range from diarrhea, weight loss, and failure to thrive to the more common, but less often recognized, complaints of fatigue, dyspepsia, neurological dysfunction, and musculoskeletal problems. Elimination of the offending food substance (gluten), as with other immune-mediated ARF, is the primary method of management in celiac disease. However, unlike most other food protein-induced enteropathies, gluten must be eliminated from the diet on a life-long basis in celiac disease.

Eosinophilic Esophagitis and Gastroesophageal Reflux Disease (GERD)

Studies on cow's milk elimination in infants suggest that about one-third of reflux disease is attributable to cow's milk allergy.[74] In infants and children, symptoms of esophagitis may not improve following standard treatment for acid reflux. Their esophageal mucosa reveals a dense infiltration with eosinophils, giving rise to the label of eosinophilic esophagitis. This condition differs from esophageal inflammation due to gastroesophageal acid reflux in that treatment strategies such as food elimination (if food allergy can be confirmed as causative) or corticosteroids (if the triggering agent[s] are unclear) are beneficial rather than measures to inhibit acid reflux. Symptoms include vomiting, pain, and dysphagia, and some affected individuals present with food impactions and strictures. Allergy, particularly food allergy, is an associated finding in most patients, and many have concomitant asthma or other chronic respiratory disease. Recent studies suggest that this disease entity is not restricted to infants and children but can affect adults to an unknown degree.[67]

Eosinophilic Gastroenterocolitis

Eosinophilic gastroenteritis is a heterogeneous and uncommon disorder characterized by eosinophilic inflammation of the GI tissues. The varied manifestations of this condition reflect the location and depth of infiltration, the latter also being the basis for the classification into mucosal, muscular, and serosal forms of eosinophilic gastroenteritis. In nearly 50% of cases, abdominal pain, vomiting, and diarrhea occur together, and peripheral eosinophilia is seen in up to two-thirds of patients with eosinophilic gastroenteritis. Eosinophilic gastroenteritis is often associated with food allergies and concomitant atopic diseases, or a family history of allergies is elicited in 50% to 70% of cases. Parasitic infections, inflamma-

Table 9-2.

Food Intolerances (Nonimmune ARF)

- Food toxicity (bacteria or bacterial toxins)
- Nonspecific mast cell activation (Pseudoallergic reactions by strawberries, chocolate, tomatoes, and other foods. Also, additives such as salicylates, benzoates, and tartrazine
- Histamine intolerance triggered by fish, cheese, red wine etc. in diamineoxidase-deficient individuals
- Other intolerances to biogene amines (tyramine, serotonin etc.)
- Lactose intolerance (constitutive or acquired)
- Psychological food intolerance
- Physiological food intolerance, eg, starches found in legumes serve as substrate for gas production by colonic flora, and favoring histamine synthesis by fermentation

tory bowel disease, connective tissue diseases, some malignancies, and adverse effects of drugs should also be considered in the differential diagnosis of eosinophilic gastroenteritis. The gold standard for diagnosis, usually demonstrated on endoscopic biopsies, is prominent tissue eosinophilia with a mild mastocytosis.[69,75]

Nonimmune Adverse Reactions to Food

The majority of ARF are not immunologic in origin; however, given how commonly they occur, these should be considered in any discussion of ARF (Table 9-2). Microbial contamination of food causing primarily GI manifestations due to preformed toxins (eg, *Staphylococcal enterotoxin*) or replication of enteric pathogens (*Campylobacter, Salmonella, Shigella, Escherichia coli*) is classified as food toxicity or food poisoning. These reactions can be distinguished from other ARF as they have characteristic presentations, including a short duration and rare recurrence. Post-infectious IBS may ensue from a self-limited infection, however. Recurrent infectious GI illnesses should prompt an evaluation for immunodeficiencies, such as IgA deficiency, which occurs at a frequency of approximately 1 in 500-600 and is the most common form of inherited immunodeficiency.

Pseudoallergic and Pharmacologic Reactions

Anaphylactoid or pseudoallergic reactions to food result from foods that mimic the effects of mast-cell degranulation but do not involve IgE antibodies.[76] Pharmacological reactions to food or food additives represent a relatively common type of ARF although most of these reactions cause symptoms outside of the GI tract. Frequently, food additives such as sulfites, tartrazine, and monosodium glutamate are the causative agents. These have all been associated with asthma, and glutamate can also cause a characteristic syndrome consisting of a burning or warm sensation, chest tightness, headache, and gastric discomfort shortly after its ingestion. As with immune-mediated ARF, patients exhibiting such reactions should be instructed to avoid the offending food substance if identifiable. Biogenic amines such as histamine, serotonin, or tyramine can cause symptoms similar to those of immune-mediated food allergy including headaches, hypotension, skin erythema, and GI symptoms. The pathophysiology of histamine intolerance includes an increased sensitivity towards rather small amounts of histamine in food because of an impaired inactivation of histamine as a consequence of decreased diamineoxidase activity, the major histamine-degrading enzyme in the gut, or its co-enzymes (vitamin B6 and probably C). Measurement of plasma histamine and diaminooxidase levels, as well as challenge tests, are useful for confirmation of the diagnosis.

Lactose Intolerance

This disorder is the most common adverse reaction to a specific food worldwide, with most cases due to declining levels of intestinal lactase activity in later childhood and adult life (metabolic food intolerance), although rare congenital deficiencies can occur. Symptoms of lactase insufficiency are usually dose-related and include bloating, flatulence, and diarrhea. Secondary lactase deficiency can result from viral gastroenteritis, radiation enteritis, Crohn's disease, and celiac sprue. It is worth clarifying that individuals with lactose intolerance do not suffer severe and potential life-threatening complications of ingesting lactose and are able to consume naturally low lactose diary products including most cheeses and yogurts. In contrast, patients with cow's-milk allergy may suffer anaphylactic or asthmatic reactions to dairy products and, therefore, must avoid all foods containing the allergenic cow's-milk protein, usually casein or B-lactoglobulin.

Psychological Intolerance

Reactions to food may be psychological.[37,77] This is a difficult type of ARF to diagnose because the mechanisms giving rise to such reactions are poorly understood. Some studies suggest individuals reporting ARF without confirmation by food challenge had a higher rates of psychiatric disorders than did those with ARF confirmed by food challenge,[37] while other studies suggest there is no increase of psychological disturbance in those who perceive they have ARF than in other populations.[78] An individual who experienced a severe food-poisoning reaction may avoid the culprit food for fear of further reactions. There is also some evidence that hypersensitivity reactions to food may be triggered through central neural mechanisms so that eventually, just the thought of ingesting the food can trigger allergic symptoms in the absence of antigen.[79]

Physiological Food Intolerance

Perhaps the most common form of ARF results from physiological reactions to food components or additives. For example, it is well known that starches found in legumes serve as substrate for gas production by colonic flora. Many other foods are associated with "gas" including cabbage, bran fiber, and other vegetables and grains. Other foods and food additives affect the lower esophageal sphincter, while foods high in fat delay gastric emptying, all with the potential to cause symptoms of heartburn and dyspepsia. Physiological reactions to foods are often noted by patients with functional bowel disease, many of whom exhibit heightened endocrine, motor, and sensory responses to normal digestive events. It is important to determine whether specific food intolerances exist in this group of patients because elimination of the offending food(s) can provide some benefit. A survey of patients in a gastroenterology clinic in the UK revealed that those with functional diagnoses were most likely to report adverse reactions to foods and drugs, with foods reported to worsen GI symptoms.[80] There are some studies suggesting that patients with IBS may benefit from a specific elimination diet including a recent controlled study in which elimination of foods to which IgG antibodies were detected in serum provided a clinically and statistically significant improvement.[19]

Diagnosis and Treatment

The American Gastroenterological Association has published guidelines for the evaluation of food allergies, stressing the role of a careful history correlating symptoms with specific foods.[73] Open food challenges, although helpful as a first approach, are subject to bias and should be corroborated by another more objective method before the food is permanently eliminated from the patient's diet.

Skin-prick testing provides a readily available and relatively inexpensive means to assess a panel of food allergens in both children and adults. The major limitation of skin testing is its poor positive predictive value, but a negative test in the absence of antihistamine usage strongly suggests that immediate hypersensitivity is an unlikely mechanism for the patient's food-induced complaints. The value of the classical skin-prick test is further limited because of the poor standardization and stability of many food-allergen extracts, a problem that might be overcome by use of recombinant food allergens. Alternatively, skin tests can be improved with use of native food instead of extracts by performing the prick-to-prick test (first the food is pricked, then the skin) or the recently established epicutaneous test, which also tests delayed reactions to food.[81]

Measurement of specific IgE can be used as an alternative to skin testing. The advantages of specific IgE compared to skin-prick testing are the higher specificity and the higher reliability because of its independence from the examiner. Moreover, this test has advantages in patients with skin involvement, such as atopic dermatitis, in which prick tests are not recommended. A possible explanation of the discrepancy between skin tests or radioallergosorbent test and a patient's history may be that hypersensitivity reactions of the gut are mediated by local IgE that is not necessarily reflected by serum levels.[8,27] In addition, IgE-independent mechanisms may be responsible and can be assessed including measurement of serum IgG antibodies to specific foods[19] and eosinophil-derived mediators such as ECP and EPX in serum and stool.[33] However, these methods are not well standardized and, given the current limitations of all laboratory means to confirm GI food allergy, the diagnosis is based largely on diagnosis by exclusion.

In unclear cases, a double-blinded placebo-control food challenge in which food antigens are administered by nasogastric tube or gelatin capsules should be performed, if possible. This technique is considered the gold standard for diagnosing food allergy;[82,83] however, this procedure has several limitations with regard to food allergy manifestating in the GI tract. The read-out is not well standardized and validated, which makes the test less objective. Secondly, the test does not confirm food allergy but food intolerance and therefore only confirms a patient's history without allowing clues on the mechanism of the adverse reaction.

A number of investigators have performed the GI equivalent of skin testing by injecting the GI mucosa with a panel of antigens and observing for a wheal-and-flare response by endoscopy. This technique was reported as early as the 1930s, with subsequent series describing gastric, duodenal, and, most recently, colonic mucosal allergen challenge.[30,84] Although such methods represent an advance in the field of food hypersensitivity, their incorporation into routine clinical practice has been limited. In contrast, endoscopy and mucosal biopsy techniques remain the major diagnostic method to evaluate other GI immune-mediated reactions to food including celiac disease, food protein gastroenteropathies, and eosinophilic gastroenteritis.

Management of Food Allergy

Key in the management of food allergy is the avoidance of the offending allergen (Table 9-3). This is especially important in cases of food allergies like peanut allergy where trace amounts of allergen can cause significant reactions.[11] Unfortunately, it is often difficult to comply with a restrictive diet, particularly if multiple and/or common foods are eliminated. If an elimination diet cannot be performed properly, or because the responsible foods cannot be identified, antiallergic medication is required. In more severe cases, a therapy with steroids might be inevitable. Topical or alternate steroids (eg, budesonide) may be helpful in GI food allergy but have not been studied yet.

Given the difficulties preventing accidental exposure to food antigens, patients with a history of an anaphylactic reaction should be instructed to carry an epinephrine-containing syringe for emergency administration. Patients with food allergies should learn to read and understand labels for hidden food allergens and to recognize the potential for foods to cross-react with other antigens. A useful website to refer patients and their families to is www.foodallergy.org.[85] To date, there is no clear evidence that

Table 9-3.

Strategies for Dietary Counseling for Food Allergies

Elimination of Food Allergens

- Instruction about allowed food, partially restricted and totally forbidden food (Principle: eliminate the least possible, just as much as required!)
- Instruction about hidden allergens, cross-reacting allergens
- Propose alternatives for basic foods (eg, milk, wheat, eggs)

Avoidance of Malnutrition

- Formal dietary consultation
- Use of appropriate nutritional supplements

Preparation of Food

- Preferentially eat cooked food instead of raw food (eg, fruits and vegetables are often tolerated if cooked but not if raw; however, some foods such as milk, egg, fish and nuts are heat-stable!)
- Eat at home, not out

Individual Consideration of Quality of Life

- Personal motivation
- Age
- Eating habits
- Family and work environment

Avoidance of Food Additives

- Avoidance of fast food and precooked food
- Avoidance of mixed food
- Avoidance of unknown or foreign food depending on source of food and local reputation

oral desensitization, injection immunotherapy, prophylactic medication, or similar techniques are beneficial in the prevention or modulation of food allergy. Hypoallergenic diets have been recommended during pregnancy and with breast-feeding for atopic mothers to reduce the incidence of food allergy in their offspring. Foods with a higher allergenic potential should be introduced later into the diets of infants at high risk for developing food allergy to decrease the possibility of developing such an allergy.[86,87] Formulas with reduced antigenicity include those in which milk proteins are partially hydrolyzed by heat or enzymes as well as more extensively hydrolyzed preparations.

Future Possibilities

Recently, studies have been published indicating that probiotics—such as the *Lactobacillus GG* strain—are capable of preventing allergy in newborns from families with a high risk for allergy development. For example, the prevalence of food-induced atopic dermatitis was reduced by 50% in a cohort study including high-risk families when mother and newborns were treated for 12 months (6 months before delivery and 6 months after) with *Lactobacillus GG*.[88]

New therapeutic approaches include tolerogenic peptides, recombinant epitopes, anti-IgE, and DNA vaccination as well neutralizing antibodies or receptor antagonists of Th2 cytokines like IL-4.[89,90] Methods to genetically or chemically modify the antigenic structures of foods to reduce their allergic potential are also being developed. For example, it is known that single amino-acid substitutions in the IgE binding site of a peanut allergen can lead to the loss of binding to these epitopes.[91] Antibodies specific for the portion of the IgE molecule that binds to receptors on mast cells and basophils have been used in animal models and in clinical trials with asthmatic subjects with benefit[92] and have the potential for use in food allergy. The latter therapy has been successfully used for treatment of patients with peanut allergy.[93]

Whereas classical immunotherapy and oral immunotherapy are still entertained for treatment of food allergy, new approaches aiming to direct the antigen more precisely to the gut are under development. For example, DNA vaccination to induce host-cell expression of antigenic protein offers promise as a therapy for food allergy as well as evidenced by a recent study in a mouse model of peanut allergy. Mice vaccinated orally with DNA coding for a major peanut allergen, Ara h2, complexed with a polysaccharide delivery vehicle, were shown to express the food protein in their GI tract and exhibit less immunologic and clinical reactivity to subsequent challenge with antigen when compared to control mice.[94] Another way of tolerance induction was achieved by treatment of ovalbumin T cellreceptor transgenic mice with the probiotic *lactobacillus casei* inducing IL-12 and thereby inhibiting IgE and IgG1 responses.[95]

Conclusion

Adverse reactions to food are common in the general population and often underestimated, particularly in adults, of whom 1% to 4% have symptoms due to food allergy. Food allergies are mediated by IgE-dependent and IgE-independent mechanisms involving mast cells, eosinophils, and other immune cells. Despite continued progress in understanding the underlying mechanisms, many questions remain unanswered. New understanding such as the role of innate defense systems and the gut microflora have opened exiting new therapeutic strategies, such as the use of probiotic bacteria for treatment and prevention of food allergy. The developments in the field of recombinant allergens and their modulation by genetic engineering will improve both diagnostic methods and therapeutic options, such as hyposensitization and induction of tolerance.

In the sensitization phase, exposure to a food antigen may result in the production of specific IgE antibodies to that food depending on antigen properties, host genetics, the type of antigen presenting cells involved (eg, dendritic cells), and the interaction with T cell subsets. Specific IgE antibodies then bind to circulating basophils and tissue mast cells. The immediate hypersensitivity reaction results from subsequent exposure to the food antigen that leads to cross-linking bound specific IgE and activation of mast cells with release of the contents of their granules including various metabolites and cytokines. In addition, release of cytokines such as IL-3 and IL-5 recruit other cell populations including eosinophils and other mast cell products such as nerve growth factor, affect nerve cells in the gut. Together, such events may lead to a so-called late phase reaction associated with allergy.

Abbreviations: B=B lymphocytes; DC=dendritic cells; Eo=eosinophil; IgE=immunoglobulin E; IL=interleukin; MC=mast cell; NC=nerve cell; T lymphocytes Th2=T helper lymphocytes type 2.

References

1. Nowak-Wegrzyn A, Conover-Walker MK, Wood RA. Food-allergic reactions in schools and preschools. *Arch Pediatr Adolesc Med.* 2001;155(7):790-795.
2. Schafer T, Bohler E, Ruhdorfer S, et al. Epidemiology of food allergy/food intolerance in adults: associations with other manifestations of atopy. *Allergy.* 2001; 56(12):1172-1179.
3. Kanny G, Moneret-Vautrin DA, Flabbee J, Beaudouin E, Morisset M, Thevenin F. Population study of food allergy in France. *J Allergy Clin Immunol.* 2001;108(1):133-140.
4. Sampson HA. Update on food allergy. *J Allergy Clin Immunol.* 2004; 113(5):805-819.
5. Zuberbier T, Edenharter G, Worm M, et al. Prevalence of adverse reactions to food in Germany—a population study. *Allergy.* 2004;59(3):338-345.
6. Young E, Stoneham MD, Petruckevitch A, Barton J, Rona R. A population study of food intolerance. *Lancet.* 1994; 343(8906):1127-1130.
7. Sampson HA, Mendelson L, Rosen JP. Fatal and near-fatal anaphylactic reactions to food in children and adolescents. *N Engl J Med.* 1992; 327:380-384.
8. Bischoff SC, Mayer JH, Manns MP. Allergy and the gut. *Int Arch Allergy Immunol.* 2000;121(4):270-283.
9. Crowe SE. Gastrointestinal food allergies: do they exist? *Curr Gastroenterol Rep.* 2001;3(4):351-357.
10. Grundy J, Matthews S, Bateman B, Dean T, Arshad SH. Rising prevalence of allergy to peanut in children: Data from 2 sequential cohorts. *J Allergy Clin Immunol.* 2002;110(5):784-789.
11. Burks W. Peanut allergy: a growing phenomenon. *J Clin Invest.* 2003;111(7):950-952.
12. Helm RM, Burks AW. Mechanisms of food allergy. *Curr Opin Immunol.* 2000;12(6):647-653.
13. Bjorksten B. The epidemiology of food allergy. *Curr Opin Allergy Clin Immunol.* 2001;1(3):225-227.
14. Kalliomaki M, Isolauri E. Role of intestinal flora in the development of allergy. *Curr Opin Allergy Clin Immunol.* 2003;3(1):15-20.
15. Sicherer SH. Clinical aspects of gastrointestinal food allergy in childhood. *Pediatrics.* 2003;111(6 Pt 3):1609-1616.
16. Crespo JF, Rodriguez J. Food allergy in adulthood. *Allergy.* 2003;58(2):98-113.
17. Iacono G, Cavataio F, Montalto G, et al. Intolerance of cow's milk and chronic constipation in children. *N Engl J Med.* 1998;339(16):1100-1104.
18. Read NW. Food and hypersensitivity in functional dyspepsia. *Gut.* 2002;51(Suppl 1):i50-i53.
19. Atkinson W, Sheldon TA, Shaath N, Whorwell PJ. Food elimination based on IgG antibodies in irritable bowel syndrome: a randomised controlled trial. *Gut.* 2004;53(10):1459-1464.
20. Sicherer SH, Sampson HA, Bock SA, Munoz-Furlong A. Underrepresentation of the risk and incidence of anaphylaxis to foods. *Arch Intern Med.* 2001;161(16):2046-2047.
21. Brandtzaeg PE. Current understanding of gastrointestinal immunoregulation and its relation to food allergy. *Ann N Y Acad Sci.* 2002;964:13-45.
22. Shah U, Walker WA. Pathophysiology of intestinal food allergy. *Adv Pediatr.* 2002;49:299-316.
23. Eigenmann PA, Frossard CP. The T lymphocyte in food-allergy disorders. *Curr Opin Allergy Clin Immunol.* 2003;3(3):199-203.
24. Bischoff SC, Sellge G, Lorentz A, Sebald W, Raab R, Manns MP. IL-4 enhances proliferation and mediator release in mature human mast cells. *Proc Natl Acad Sci USA.* 1999;96(14):8080-8085.
25. De Vries JE, Carballido JM, Aversa G. Receptors and cytokines involved in allergic TH2 cell responses. *J Allergy Clin Immunol.* 1999;103(5 Pt 2):S492-S496.
26. Hogan SP, Foster PS, Rothenberg ME. Experimental analysis of eosinophil-associated gastrointestinal diseases. *Curr Opin Allergy Clin Immunol.* 2002;2(3):239-248.
27. Schwab D, Raithel M, Klein P, et al. Immunoglobulin E and eosinophilic cationic protein in segmental lavage fluid of the small and large bowel identify patients with food allergy. *Am J Gastroenterol.* 2001;96(2):508-514.
28. Vercelli D. Genetics of IL-13 and functional relevance of IL-13 variants. *Curr Opin Allergy Clin Immunol.* 2002;2(5):389-393.
29. Macfarlane AJ, Kon OM, Smith SJ, et al. Basophils, eosinophils, and mast cells in atopic and nonatopic asthma and in late-phase allergic reactions in the lung and skin. *J Allergy Clin Immunol.* 2000;105:99-107.
30. Bischoff SC, Mayer J, Wedemeyer J, et al. Colonoscopic allergen provocation (COLAP): a new diagnostic approach for gastrointestinal food allergy. *Gut.* 1997;40:745-753.

31. Bengtsson U, Knutson TW, Knutson L, Dannaeus A, Hallgren R, Ahlstedt S. Eosinophil cationic protein and histamine after intestinal challenge in patients with cow's milk intolerance. *J Allergy Clin Immunol.* 1997; 100(2):216-221.
32. Bischoff SC, Grabowsky J, Manns MP. Quantification of inflammatory mediators in stool samples of patients with inflammatory bowel disorders and controls. *Dig Dis Sci.* 1997;42(2):394-403.
33. Majamaa H, Laine S, Miettinen A. Eosinophil protein X and eosinophil cationic protein as indicators of intestinal inflammation in infants with atopic eczema and food allergy. *Clin Exp Allergy.* 1999;29(11):1502-1506.
34. Santos J, Bayarri C, Saperas E, et al. Characterisation of immune mediator release during the immediate response to segmental mucosal challenge in the jejunum of patients with food allergy. *Gut.* 1999;45(4):553-558.
35. Rothenberg ME. Gastrointestinal eosinophils. *Allergy.* 2001;56 (Suppl 67):21-22.
36. Wedemeyer J, Tsai M, Galli SJ. Roles of mast cells and basophils in innate and acquired immunity. *Curr Opin Immunol.* 2000;12(6):624-631.
37. Kelsay K. Psychological aspects of food allergy. *Curr Allergy Asthma Rep.* 2003;3(1):41-46.
38. Bischoff SC, Crowe SE. Gastrintestinal food allergy: new insights into pathophysiology and clinical perspectives. *Gastroenterology.* 2005;128(4):1089-113. Review.
39. Lehrer SB, Ayuso R, Reese G. Current understanding of food allergens. *Ann NY Acad Sci.* 2002;964:69-85.
40. Helm RM. Food biotechnology: is this good or bad? Implications to allergic diseases. *Ann Allergy Asthma Immunol.* 2003;90(6 Suppl 3):90-98.
41. Maleki SJ, Kopper RA, Shin DS, et al. Structure of the major peanut allergen Ara h 1 may protect IgE-binding epitopes from degradation. *J Immunol.* 2000;164(11):5844-5849.
42. Dalal I, Binson I, Reifen R, et al. Food allergy is a matter of geography after all: sesame as a major cause of severe IgE-mediated food allergic reactions among infants and young children in Israel. *Allergy.* 2002;57(4):362-365.
43. Rodriguez J, Crespo JF. Clinical features of cross-reactivity of food allergy caused by fruits. *Curr Opin Allergy Clin Immunol.* 2002;2(3):233-238.
44. Vieths S, Scheurer S, Ballmer-Weber B. Current understanding of cross-reactivity of food allergens and pollen. *Ann NY Acad Sci.* 2002;964:47-68.
45. Valenta R, Duchene M, Ebner C, et al. Profilins constitute a novel family of functional plant pan-allergens. *J Exp Med.* 1992;175(2):377-385.
46. http://www.allergome.org. Accessed June 29, 2005.
47. Bohle B, Vieths S. Improving diagnostic tests for food allergy with recombinant allergens. *Methods.* 2004;32(3):292-299.
48. Valenta R. The future of antigen-specific immunotherapy of allergy. *Nat Rev Immunol.* 2002;2(6):446-453.
49. Rabjohn P, West CM, Connaughton C, et al. Modification of peanut allergen Ara h 3: effects on IgE binding and T cell stimulation. *Int Arch Allergy Immunol.* 2002;128(1):15-23.
50. Bock SA, Munoz-Furlong A, Sampson HA. Fatalities due to anaphylactic reactions to foods. *J Allergy Clin Immunol.* 2001;107(1):191-193.
51. Tejedor A, Sastre DJ, Sanchez-Hernandez JJ, Perez FC, de L. Idiopathic anaphylaxis: a descriptive study of 81 patients in Spain. *Ann Allergy Asthma Immunol.* 2002;88(3):313-318.
52. Clark S, Bock SA, Gaeta TJ, Brenner BE, Cydulka RK, Camargo CA. Multicenter study of emergency department visits for food allergies. *J Allergy Clin Immunol.* 2004;113(2):347-352.
53. Sicherer SH, Munoz-Furlong A, Sampson HA. Prevalence of peanut and tree nut allergy in the United States determined by means of a random digit dial telephone survey: a 5-year follow-up study. *J Allergy Clin Immunol.* 2003;112(6):1203-1207.
54. Plicka M. Mr. Peanut goes to court: accommodating an individuals peanut allergy in schools and day care centers under the Americans with Disabilities Act. *J Law Health.* 1999;14(1):87-106.
55. James JM. Airline snack foods: tension in the peanut gallery. *J Allergy Clin Immunol.* 1999;104(1):25-27.
56. Hallett R, Haapanen LA, Teuber SS. Food allergies and kissing. *N Engl J Med.* 2002;346(23):1833-1834.
57. Steensma DP. The kiss of death: a severe allergic reaction to a shellfish induced by a good-night kiss. *Mayo Clin Proc.* 2003;78(2):221-222.
58. Palosuo K, Varjonen E, Nurkkala J, et al. Transglutaminase-mediated cross-linking of a peptic fraction of omega-5 gliadin enhances IgE reactivity in wheat-dependent, exercise-induced anaphylaxis. *J Allergy Clin Immunol.* 2003;111(6):1386-1392.
59. Aihara M, Miyazawa M, Osuna H, et al. Food-dependent exercise-induced anaphylaxis: influence of concurrent aspirin administration on skin testing and provocation. *Br J Dermatol.* 2002;146(3):466-472.
60. Shirai T, Matsui T, Uto T, Chida K, Nakamura H. Nonsteroidal anti-inflammatory drugs enhance allergic reactions in a patient with wheat-induced anaphylaxis. *Allergy.* 2003;58(10):1071.
61. Leung DY, Bieber T. Atopic dermatitis. *Lancet.* 2003;361(9352):151-160.
62. Chong SU, Worm M, Zuberbier T. Role of adverse reactions to food in urticaria and exercise-induced anaphylaxis. *Int Arch Allergy Immunol.* 2002;129(1):19-26.
63. James JM. Food allergy and the respiratory tract. *Curr Allergy Rep.* 2001;1(1):54-60.
64. Roberts G, Patel N, Levi-schaffer F, Habibi P, Lack G. Food allergy as a risk factor for life-threatening asthma in childhood: a case-controlled study. *J Allergy Clin Immunol.* 2003;112(1):168-174.
65. Vanderhoof JA, Young RJ. Allergic disorders of the gastrointestinal tract. *Curr Opin Clin Nutr Metab Care.* 2001;4(6):553-556.
66. Daher S, Tahan S, Sole D, et al. Cow's milk protein intolerance and chronic constipation in children. *Pediatr Allergy Immunol.* 2001;12(6):339-342.
67. Croese J, Fairley SK, Masson JW, et al. Clinical and endoscopic features of eosinophilic esophagitis in adults. *Gastrointest Endosc.* 2003;58(4):516-522.
68. Blanco C. Latex-fruit syndrome. *Curr Allergy Asthma Rep.* 2003;3(1):47-53.
69. Rothenberg ME. Eosinophilic gastrointestinal disorders (EGID). *J Allergy Clin Immunol.* 2004;113(1):11-28.
70. Fasano A, Catassi C. Current approaches to diagnosis and treatment of celiac disease: an evolving spectrum. *Gastroenterology.* 2001;120(3):636-651.
71. Condemi JJ. Allergic reactions to natural rubber latex at home, to rubber products, and to cross-reacting foods. *J Allergy Clin Immunol.* 2002;110(2 Suppl):S107-S110.
72. Nowak-Wegrzyn A, Sampson HA, Wood RA, Sicherer SH. Food protein-induced enterocolitis syndrome caused by solid food proteins. *Pediatrics.* 2003;111(4 Pt 1):829-835.
73. American Gastroenterological Association position statement: Guidelines for the evaluation of food allergies. *Gastroenterology.* 2001; 120:1023-1025.
74. Hill DJ, Heine RG, Cameron DJ, et al. Role of food protein intolerance in infants with persistent distress attributed to reflux esophagitis. *J Pediatr.* 2000;136(5):641-647.
75. Khan S, Orenstein SR. Eosinophilic gastroenteritis: epidemiology, diagnosis and management. *Paediatr Drugs.* 2002;4(9):563-570.
76. Zuberbier T, Pfrommer C, Specht K, et al. Aromatic components of food as novel eliciting factors of pseudoallergic reactions in chronic urticaria. *J Allergy Clin Immunol.* 2002;109(2):343-348.

77. Kelso JM, Connaughton C, Helm RM, Burks W. Psychosomatic peanut allergy. *J Allergy Clin Immunol.* 2003;111(3):650-651.
78. Knibb RC, Armstrong A, Booth DA, Platts RG, Booth IW, MacDonald A. Psychological characteristics of people with perceived food intolerance in a community sample. *J Psychosom Res.* 1999;47(6):545-554.
79. Barrett JE, King MG, Pang G. Conditioning rhinitis in allergic humans. *Ann NY Acad Sci.* 2000;917:853-859.
80. Bhat K, Harper A, Gorard DA. Perceived food and drug allergies in functional and organic gastrointestinal disorders. *Aliment Pharmacol Ther.* 2002;16(5):969-973.
81. Niggemann B. The role of the atopy patch test (APT) in diagnosis of food allergy in infants and children with atopic dermatitis. *Pediatr Allergy Immunol.* 2001;12(Suppl 14):37-40.
82. Sampson HA. Food allergy. Part 2: diagnosis and management. *J Allergy Clin Immunol.* 1999; 103:981-989.
83. Sicherer SH. Food allergy: when and how to perform oral food challenges. *Pediatr Allergy Immunol.* 1999;10(4):226-234.
84. Crowe SE, Perdue MH. Gastrointestinal food hypersensitivity: Basic mechanisms of pathophysiology. *Gastroenterology.* 1992;103:1075-1095.
85. www.foodallergy.org. Accessed June 29, 2005.
86. Fiocchi A, Martelli A, De Chiara A, Moro G, Warm A, Terracciano L. Primary dietary prevention of food allergy. *Ann Allergy Asthma Immunol.* 2003;91(1):3-12.
87. Zeiger RS. Food allergen avoidance in the prevention of food allergy in infants and children. *Pediatrics.* 2003;111:1662-1671.
88. Kalliomaki M, Salminen S, Poussa T, Arvilommi H, Isolauri E. Probiotics and prevention of atopic disease: 4-year follow-up of a randomised placebo-controlled trial. *Lancet.* 2003;361(9372):1869-1871.
89. Nguyen MD, Cinman N, Yen J, Horner AA. DNA-based vaccination for the treatment of food allergy. *Allergy.* 2001; 56 Suppl 67:127-130.
90. Nowak-Wegrzyn A. Future approaches to food allergy. *Pediatrics.* 2003;111:1672-1680.
91. Burks AW, King N, Bannon GA. Modification of a major peanut allergen leads to loss of IgE binding. *Int Arch Allergy Immunol.* 1999;118:313-314.
92. MacGlashan DW, Jr., Bochner BS, Adelman DC, et al. Down-regulation of Fc(epsilon)RI expression on human basophils during in vivo treatment of atopic patients with anti-IgE antibody. *J Immunol.* 1997;158(3):1438-1445.
93. Leung DY, Sampson HA, Yunginger JW, et al. Effect of anti-IgE therapy in patients with peanut allergy. *N Engl J Med.* 2003;348(11):986-993.
94. Roy K, Mao HQ, Huang SK, Leong KW. Oral gene delivery with chitosan—DNA nanoparticles generates immunologic protection in a murine model of peanut allergy. *Nat Med.* 1999;5:387-391.
95. Shida K, Takahashi R, Iwadate E, et al. Lactobacillus casei strain Shirota suppresses serum immunoglobulin E and immunoglobulin G1 responses and systemic anaphylaxis in a food allergy model. *Clin Exp Allergy.* 2002;32(4):563-570.

Chapter 10

Dietary Supplements: Herbs and Vitamins

Timothy O. Lipman, MD

Introduction

The gastroenterologist should know about dietary supplements, because his or her patient will probably be taking a supplement[1] or because, in some instances, a supplement may be part of the therapeutic armamentarium. Estimates of supplement usage rates and costs vary; however, it is estimated 50% or more of the Western population is taking some form of supplement at a total cost of billions of dollars. Over 50% of supplement takers do not report this use to their physician.[2] Only a handful of available dietary supplements have undergone rigorous scientific evaluation. According to the Dietary Supplement Health and Education Act (DSHEA) of 1994, a dietary supplement is a product "intended to supplement the diet to enhance health," and includes vitamins, minerals, amino acids, herbs, and other botanicals.[3] Further, a dietary supplement is "not represented as a conventional food or a sole item of a meal or the diet." Some products that are isolated components of food—eg, wheat bran, oat bran, flax seed—might be taken as supplements to "enhance health" but are not really considered supplements, at least not for the present overview. A medical food, as defined by the Food and Drug Administration (FDA) is a food that is prescribed by a physician when a patient has special nutrient needs and the patient is under the physician's ongoing care. The label must clearly state that the product is intended to manage a specific medical disorder or condition.[4] Probiotics and supplements, such as fish oil, fall under the rubric of a medical food. Nutraceuticals, although not officially defined, have enjoyed recent popularity and may be considered a manufactured, chemically defined formula enriched with certain nutrients thought to endow specific biologic and/or pharmacological benefits. Functional foods are real or whole foods—tree nuts, soy, olive oil, fish, etc—that are thought to have definite health benefits: eg, cholesterol reduction, anti-neoplastic, cardioprotective.

This chapter addresses two forms of supplements—herbals and vitamins. An herbal product is one form of what has been termed complementary and alternative medicine (CAM). CAM therapies involve a variety of heterogeneous modalities, including, but not necessarily limited to, acupuncture, traditional Chinese and Ayurvedic (Indian) medicine, homeopathy, chiropractic, manipulative osteopathy, therapeutic touch, remote intercessional prayer, faith healing, detoxification, and reflexology. An encompassing and accurate definition of CAM has been difficult. "Interventions neither taught widely in medical schools nor generally available in US hospitals",[5] is one definition, albeit somewhat unsatisfactory, as 1) many forms of CAM are increasingly taught in medical schools, 2) the National Institutes of Health has a division devoted to CAM, and 3) CAM therapies are increasingly integrated into western healthcare facilities.[6] Others talk of "traditional," meaning ancient, therapies as opposed to more contemporary, recent Western therapy.[7] Another definition speaks of CAM therapies as those which deviate from the conventional—alternative when they are used instead of and complementary when they are applied as an adjunct to standard management.[8]

An "herbal" may be defined as a substance derived from any plant source—roots, bark, leaves, seeds, flowers, and/or fruits. A vitamin may be defined as a chemically defined organic substance that is contained in small quantities in food with specifically defined metabolic functions and is essential in trace amounts for normal metabolism. Herbal products, on the other hand, may consist of a number of constituents, none of which is defined down to the biochemical level.

Individuals consume herbal and vitamin supplements for multiple reasons, including: 1) perceptions that "natural" products are healthier than manufactured drugs; 2) dissatisfaction with "conventional" medicine, with feelings that doctors do not listen to the patient and do not respect cultural traditions; 3) thoughts that doctors focus on curing disease rather than treating the "whole patient;" 4) wishes to maintain "control" over own health; 5) recommendations from family, friends, sales person, TV infomercials, and/or "a nutritionist;" 6) perceived dietary insufficiency from either inadequate intake or an inadequate food supply; 7) special circumstances of pregnancy, inadequate sunlight, or aging; 8) prevention of classical nutrition deficiency syndromes; 9) prevention of chronic diseases, including cardiac, dementia, and cancer; 10) prevention of aging; and 11) enhanced performance.[9,10] Many view these therapies as a continuation of collective wisdom and ancient healing arts, which have been proven through passage from generation to generation.

Regulation, Quality, and Efficacy

Herbal therapy is classified under the rubric of CAM because all herbals are unregulated and have not undergone the rigorous testing for safety and efficacy required of pharmaceutical products. Herbals are usually obtained as capsules, tablets, elixirs, and teas but also may be obtained as "free-standing" mixtures of bulk dried herbs, as is typical in traditional Chinese medicine. Vitamins, usually in pill or liquid form, are classified as nutritional supplements but are more accepted in Western medicine because of a long tradition of documentation of vitamin deficiency states and their correction with vitamin replacement. Nonetheless, much contemporary use of vitamins and minerals may not be based upon as rigorous evidence as is required of other pharmaceutical products.

Consequent to the DSHEA of 1994, herbal products are not considered drugs and are unregulated by the US federal government.[9] A product is considered safe with the burden upon the federal government (FDA) to prove otherwise. Nor is there any requirement to prove efficacy, as long as there are no claims for diagnosis, treatment, cure, and/or prevention of any disease. A product is allowed to claim utility in maintaining "normal health" as long as it carries a specific disclaimer that the product has not been evaluated by the FDA. Few herbals have been scientifically tested, and advocates frequently deny the need for such testing. Herbal promoters suggest that if a product helps even some, it should be made available, even if the product helps no more than a placebo.[11] Anecdotal reports are considered sufficient to establish efficacy. The distinction between disease claims (allowable for drugs) and health claims (allowable for herbals) is often arbitrary and unclear, as proof of efficacy for an herbal is usually by treatment of a disease. Information on true efficacy, optimum dosing, side effects and toxicity, and interactions with other herbs or traditional pharmaceuticals is, on the whole, lacking. There is, in short, in the United States, neither regulation with requirements for safety and efficacy before introduction nor organized surveillance post-marketing.[12] Dietary supplements are held to a much lower standard than are traditional pharmaceuticals. Surveys have revealed that most consumers do not realize that these products are scientifically unproven and unregulated.

Quality control and standardization in the US is voluntary on the part of the manufacturer. Quality control should ensure that the content of a specific herbal is the same from lot to lot as well as manufacturer to manufacturer. Standardization is difficult because the products are often complex mixtures in which the responsible agent for the putative therapeutic benefit is unknown. Because herbals derive from plant sources, batch-to-batch preparations may not have consistent pharmacologic properties. Bioassay techniques, which could be used, depend upon biologic models, which often are not available for the health claims of herbals.[13] Food and drugs must adhere to "good manufacturing practices" and are regulated by the FDA; it is not so with herbals, as defined by the DSHEA. When analyzed for content, herbal preparations have been found to have none, or significantly less, of the substance that is stated on the label[14-16] or are contaminated with a variety of adulterants, including other botanicals, microorganisms, microbial toxins, pesticides, fumigation agents, toxic metals, and drugs.[17] Many countries in the European Union have more substantive oversight.

Herbals

Botanicals as pharmaceuticals have a distinguished history. Plants with medicinal properties have been found in a Neanderthal tomb dating back 60,000 years, and herbal evidence has been found in a 5000-year-old Alpine "ice man." Ancient records of botanical use can be found in China, Egypt, Mesopotamia, and classical Greece.[8,13] Classic botanical products, with extraction and biochemical purification, have entered western medicine—purple foxglove treated dropsy (digitalis); opium poppy treated pain, cough, and diarrhea (morphine); cinchona-bark and willow-bark treated fever (quinine and aspirin); reserpine (formally used for hypertension) was isolated from *Rauwolfia serpentina*; the chemotherapeutic agent taxol was derived from the bark of the Pacific *yew*. Therapeutic success was founded on empiricism, and the exact component(s) of the botanical that resulted in therapeutic efficacy was/were unknown. At the same time, many other botanicals had no evidence for efficacy and some were toxic. It is estimated that 80% or more of the worldwide population use botanicals as medicines.[18] More recently, pharmaceutical companies have systematically searched botanical preparations for potential drugs. The difference between a drug originally derived from an herb and an herb is that the former is chemically defined and rigorously tested for safety and efficacy. Despite similarities between drugs and herbals, there is no guarantee in the United States that an herbal will have a predictable response or that what is on the label is in the preparation.

TABLE 10-1.

Herbal Hepatotoxicity

Some Herbs Reported Causing Liver Injury	Types of Liver Injury Resulting from Herbs
Anthranoid rich herbals	Hepatitis
Protoberberine alkaloid rich herbals	Fibrosis/cirrhosis
Celandine	Cholestasis
Chaparal leaf or stem	Fulminant hepatic failure
Chinese Herbals	Steatosis
Jin Bu Huan	Carcinoma
"eternal life"	Veno-occlusive disease
Com	
Coumarin rich herbals	
Germander species	
Herbal tealmpila root	
Kava rhizome	
Kombucha	
LipoKinetix*	
Mahuang	
Mistletoe	
Pennyroyal oil	
Podophylltoxin rich herbals	
Prostata**	
Sassafras	
Skullcap	
Toxic pyrrolizidine alkaloids	
Vallerian	

* Multicomponent commercial product (Syntras, Cape Girardeau, MO) containing yohimbine, usiniate, norephedrine, and caffeine.
** Multicomponent product used in Europe for "urinary flow" containing Saw Palmetto, ginseng, and other ingredients.

Adapted from De Smet PAGM. *N Eng J Med.* 2002;347:2046; Langmead L, Rampton DS. *Aliment Pharmacol Ther.* 2001;15:1239; Ernst E. *Am J Med.* 1998;104:170; Stedman C. *Semin Liver Dis.* 2002;22:195.

SAFETY

Therapy reviews usually discuss efficacy before safety. Although most herbals are taken by healthy individuals without serious illness, and most herbals are probably harmless, safety issues are of such paramount concern that it is rational to discuss them first.

Safety concerns are several, aside from the issues discussed above. There is always the concern that use of herbals without demonstrated efficacy may compromise, delay, or replace a proven effective therapy. Additionally, there may be health risks consequent to herbals, including direct adverse risks of cardiotoxicity, neurotoxicity, renal toxicity, and carcinogenesis. For the gastroenterologist, the greatest concern, and where the clinician may see patients, is with hepatotoxicity (Table 10-1) or, less frequently, with drug interactions with the gastrointestinal (GI) pharmaceutical armamentarium (Table 10-2).

The epidemiology of adverse effects and toxicity is difficult to establish because of the lack of effective reporting and monitoring. As is especially illustrated by the reported hepatotoxicity resulting from Chinese herbals, "tests of time" and thousands of years of tradition do not ensure safety. Toxic effects may only recently have been recognized, even though the herbal has been used for centuries. Further compounding the problem are complexities of terminology: Chinese and Indian herbs may have differing transliterations, and many names may identify a single product—the English common name(s), the scientific name, the pharmaceutical name, the species, and the brand name.[19] Since quality controls are lacking, adverse and toxic affects may be due to a variety of bioactive compounds in any given preparation, contamination with known toxins, or adulterants inadvertently or purposefully added.

Because the liver is the major metabolic site for chemical biotransformation, it is considered to be at unique risk for toxic injury.[20] A variety of mechanisms appear to be involved, including direct dose-dependent hepatotoxicity, immune and allergic mechanisms, exacerbation of herb-drug interactions, and development of veno-occlusive disease.

Liver injury in various forms is usually reported as isolated cases or case series. Germander—a preparation used for its purported choleretic and antiseptic properties and contained in pills, liqueurs, teas, and tonics—has been

TABLE 10-2.
Potential Herb – Drug Interactions

Herbal	Conventional Drug	Interaction
Echinacea	Anabolic steroids Ketoconazole Methotrexate	Hepatoxicity
Ferfew Garlic Ginseng	Warfarin	Increased bleeding
Ginko Ginger Devils claw	Iron	Decreased absorption
St. John's wort	Cyclosporine Midazolam Tacrolimus	Reduced blood levels and decreased area under the curve (transplant rejection with cyclosporine effect)
Tamarind	Aspirin	Increased bleeding
Chilli/capsaicin (peptic ulcer)	ACE inhibitors	Increased ACE inhibitor induced cough
Shosaiko-to (hepatitis)	Prednisolone Interferon	Reduced bioavailabilityInterstitial pneumonitis
Liquorice (peptic ulcer)	Prednisolone	Enhanced aldosterone effects

Adapted from De Smet PAGM. *N Eng J Med.* 2002;347:2046; Langmead L, Rampton DS. *Aliment Pharmacol Ther.* 2001;15:1239; Ernst E. *Am J Med.* 1998;104:170; Stedman C. *Semin Liver Dis.* 2002;22:195.

associated with acute liver failure, including one fatality.[21,22] Chaparral, either alone or in a combination tea with other botanicals—valerian root and skull cap—has been associated with acute hepatitis and sometimes fulminant hepatic failure.[19,23] A Chinese herb, Jin Bu Huan, which has been used for over 1000 years as a sedative and analgesic, has been associated with cases of acute hepatitis.[24] Another Chinese herb, Syo-saiko-to (xiao-chai-hu-tang), used for the common cold in China and hepatitis in Japan, also has been associated with hepatitis and cholestasis.[25]

Greater celandine, in extract form and widely used in Europe for gallstone disease and dyspepsia, has been associated with development of mild to severe hepatitis.[26] Illustrative of the difficulty in ferreting out the true cause of a hepatoxic effect is the fact that, for example, the European commercial greater celandine product is an extract containing multiple different ingredients, including more than 20 alkaloids with known biologic activity. Hepatotoxicity may occur from supplements that contain both herbal and non-herbal components. Seven patients were reported to develop acute hepatitis, one with fulminant hepatic failure associated with a "dietary supplement" LipoKinetix (Syndtrax, Cape Girardeau, MO), a combination product sold for weight loss containing both herbals (yohimbine and usinate) and nonherbals.[27] A combination product, "Prostata"—used in Europe for "urinary flow" and containing Saw Palmetto, ginseng, and other ingredients—was associated with development of jaundice, presumably secondary to the estrogenic and antiandrogenic activity of the Saw Palmetto.[28] A variety of Chinese herbal products, in combination and some with unknown ingredients, have been associated with hepatitis and fulminant hepatic failure.[29-31]

GI symptoms of dyspepsia, abdominal pain, nausea, and/or diarrhea may be seen with a number of herbals, including ginkgo, hawthorn extracts, St. John's wort, and Saw palmetto. Peptic ulcers and esophagitis were found in patients taking "Chinese Black Balls," a preparation of over 20 herbs sold for "liver and kidney ailments" and found to be contaminated with mefanamic acid, a non-steroidal anti-inflammatory agent.[32] Chronic diarrhea and colitis have been reported as toxic manifestations of herbals.[19]

Given known underreporting, the true incidence of adverse effects is unknown. The clinician needs to be aware that any unexplained perturbation of the GI tract or evidence of hepatobiliary injury might be due to herbal ingestion. Suspected GI and hepatic toxicity from herbals should be reported to MedWatch, the FDA adverse drug reporting mechanism (www.fda.gov/medwatch or telephone: 1-800-FDA-1088).

HERBAL USE FOR THE GI TRACT

Randomized controlled trials (RCT) of a small fraction of the thousands of botanicals available do exist. Although a RCT is the only way to truly demonstrate a therapeutic benefit, the herbal industry is not required to conduct such trials. Most herbal therapy in GI disease is directed towards functional symptoms—irritable bowel syndrome (IBS) and dyspeptic symptoms,—or usually self-limited illness involving diarrhea, nausea or vomiting.

A systematic review found placebo-controlled trials of herbal therapy in a broad range of GI conditions: constipation (celandin, aloe vera); nausea and vomiting, including postoperative (ginger); IBS (compound Ayurvedic preparation with Aegle marmelos correa and Bacopa monniere as well as Padma 179, a Tibetan compound); peptic ulcer disease (curcuma and mastic gum); and inflammatory bowel disease (IBD) (Jian P Ling).[8] Many of these herbal interventions demonstrated a significantly better treatment response than did placebo. Other analyses below are more circumspect.

Irritable Bowel Syndrome

A German RCT assessed a multi-herb product.[33] In this study, there were four study groups: 1) the commercial product, containing nine herbs (bitter candytuft, chamomile flower, peppermint leaves, caraway fruit, licorice root, lemon balm leaves, celandine herbs, angelica root, and milk thistle fruit); 2) a "research" herbal preparation, containing the first six herbs in the commercial product (listed above); 3) a monoextract of bitter candytuft; and 4) a placebo. Using a careful definition of IBS, both of the multi-herb preparations were significantly better in improving total abdominal pain scores and IBS symptom score as compared to the mono-extract or placebo at 4 weeks. Outcomes over a longer term are unknown. Interestingly, as is true for "herbals," the commercially available product in the United States is labeled as a "dietary supplement to support the digestive system."

A RCT compared 1) a "standardized" Chinese herbal formulation, 2) an "individualized" Chinese herbal formulation (formulated to specific patients by a Chinese herbal practitioner), and 3) a placebo in subjects with well-defined IBS.[34] Compared to the placebo, both of the Chinese herbal medicine groups had significantly improved in IBS scores and global improvement score as rated by both patients and gastroenterologists. Although there was no difference in efficacy between the standard and individualized Chinese herbals, on follow-up 14 weeks after completion of the study, only the individualized treatment group maintained improvement.

Peppermint oil is a smooth muscle relaxant and is often used for symptoms of IBS. A systematic review evaluating peppermint for this syndrome found evidence that peppermint oil improved symptoms over placebo but concluded that methodologic problems with the analyzed studies prohibited firm conclusions.[35] Two subsequently published short-term (2 to 4 weeks) RCTs also found benefit from peppermint oil over placebo in adults[36] and children.[37]

"Padma Lax" is a Tibetan-based proprietary product, containing 13 different herbal constituents, used in Switzerland and said to "promote regularity, soothe and stimulate digestion, and help maintain proper digestive function." A low-quality RCT (small sample size, high drop-out rate) found "Padma Lax" to be a safe and effective treatment for constipation-predominant IBS.[38]

Dyspepsia

A RCT demonstrated that the 9-herb German commercial product STW 5 and the 6-herb "research product" STW 5-II were equivalent to cisapride for the treatment over 4 weeks of "dysmotility-type" functional dyspepsia.[39] A blinded RCT comparing the same 6-herb preparation to placebo in a block scheme lasting up to 12 weeks found that the herbal preparation improved functional dyspeptic symptoms significantly better than did placebo.[40] A systematic review, limited to RCTs, evaluated the evidence for use of herbals in non-ulcer dyspepsia.[41] Seventeen RCTs were identified: four of various montherapies (greater celandine, tumeric, banana, *Emblica officinalis*) and the remainder of various combinations. Nine of the 13 combination trials involved peppermint and caraway as ingredients. A wide range of other constituents were involved. Overall, in these trials, the various herbal treatments appeared to relieve non-ulcer dyspeptic symptoms without toxicity. Despite this apparent therapeutic benefit, caution in interpretation has been suggested.[42] Most of the trials involved relatively small numbers of participants and were of short duration. Methodologic quality scores were overall low. The exact symptoms of dyspepsia were not consistent across studies, with probable inclusion of individuals with reflux and IBS, and the definition of non-ulcer dyspepsia was often not clear. Finally, there is the major issue of publication bias—would a "no effect" study be published?

Artichoke is a historical medicinal plant promoted for a variety of conditions, including cholesterol lowering, improvement in digestion, liver protection with promotion of bile flow, and suppression of free radicals. A 6-week RCT comparing artichoke leaf extract with placebo in subjects with functional dyspepsia found that the verum arm significantly alleviated symptoms and improved disease-specific digestive quality of life.[43]

Diarrhea

Most CAM therapy of diarrhea involves probiotics, a topic beyond the scope of this chapter. Chamomile extract combined with pectin was found better than placebo in the treatment of acute pediatric diarrhea.[44] Carob bean juice (a traditional Anatolia/Turkish diarrheal remedy) in combination with standard World Health Organization oral rehydration solution (ORS) may improve responses in acute pediatric diarrhea as compared to ORS alone.[45]

Nausea and Vomiting

Ginger has been used since antiquity in both Chinese and Indian traditional medicine, with one of its indications being the treatment of nausea and vomiting. Evidence for use of ginger from animal experiments, experimental induction of nausea in humans, and non-randomized human studies support its potential efficacy. A systematic review focusing on RCTs found evidence that ginger might be useful for nausea and vomiting associated with postoperative states, seasickness, morning sickness, and chemotherapy-induced nausea but concluded that more rigorous evidence is still needed.[46]

Inflammatory Bowel Disease

Most alternative therapies for IBD have consisted of fish oil or probiotics, again beyond the purview of this chapter. Wheat grass juice is touted to have a variety of health benefits. In a small, short-term RCT, wheat grass juice was found to significantly improve overall disease activity and severity of rectal bleeding in distal ulcerative colitis.[47] A small RCT testing aloe vera gel in active ulcerative colitis found significant improvement in secondary outcome measures of clinical response and histological disease activity, suggesting reasonableness for further studies.[48]

Liver Disease

Of 1500 plant species introduced into the health food market, some 800 are touted as hepatoprotective.[49] Probably the most well known and most commonly used traditional herb for the liver is milk thistle, or Silybum. Its active components are collectively known as silymarin. Milk thistle extracts are hepatoprotective against toxic insults in animal models. Uncontrolled studies have suggested use in acute hepatic failure from Amonita phalloides mushroom poisoning. A systematic review identified RCTs of milk thistle in alcoholic liver disease, viral hepatitis, drug-induced liver disease, and mixed etiologies.[50] Although treatment durations lasted from 1 week to 4 years, no definite benefit from milk thistle could be established.

S-adenosyl-L-methionine (SAMe) is involved with methlyation reactions and has major antioxidant functions, including hepatic protection against alcohol and its metabolite acetaldehyde.[51] Because SAMe may be depleted in liver disease, replacement may attenuate liver injury, which has been demonstrated in animal models. SAMe has been studied in Europe for cholestatic and alcoholic liver disease.

A systematic review identified eight RCTs investigating the use of SAMe in alcoholic liver disease, but only one trial had a large sample size and reported adequately on mortality and liver transplantation.[52] The systematic review could not demonstrate any clinical benefit from SAMe use in alcoholic liver disease. There was no evidence, however, for toxicity in the trials studied.

Chinese herbs have been used for thousands of years to treat chronic liver disease. Worldwide, and especially in Asia, hepatitis B chronic infection and asymptomatic carriage are major health problems, with increased risks of death from cirrhosis and hepatocellular carcinoma.

A systematic review assessed the efficacy and safety of Chinese medicinal herbs for treatment of asymptomatic hepatitis B virus carriers.[53] Only three randomized or quasirandomized trials of poor methodologic quality lasting for more than 3 months involving 307 patients could be found. An herbal compound, "Jianpi Wenshen recipe," had significant effects on clearing hepatitis B surface and e antigens as well as seroconversion from hepatitis e positive to hepatitis e antibody positive. Two other herbals, Phyllanthus amarus and Astragalus membranaceus, showed no significant antiviral effects compared to placebo. Eight RCTs of less than 3 months duration demonstrated no antiviral benefit. No data was available on long-term clinical outcomes or quality of life.

A meta-analysis identified 27 RCTs in the Chinese literature, assessing the effectiveness of Chinese herbal medicine for hepatitis B viral clearance when used alone or in combination with interferon alfa, and found significant rates of viral clearance.[54] Because of poor methodologic qualities in the studies, the authors could not reach firm conclusions but suggested that further research was warranted.

A systematic review assessed traditional Chinese medicinal herbs for treatment of chronic hepatitis B infection.[55] Nine randomized trials were identified, involving over 900 patients, but study methodology was considered adequate in only one trial. Ten different herbs were tested in these nine trials. Three—Fuzheng Jiedu Tang (herbal compound), Polyporus umbellatus polysaccharide, and Phyllanthus amarus—demonstrated a variety of anti-viral effects. No other significant benefits were found.

Phyllanthus is an herb grown in India and elsewhere and has been used for thousands of years in Ayurvedic medicine for a variety of maladies, including jaundice. Phyllanthus' phytochemical properties have been elucidated, and it has been shown to block DNA polymerase in vitro. A variety of Phyllanthus species have been used for anti-hepatitis B therapy. A systematic review identified 22 RCTs involving genus Phyllanthus' use in chronic hepatitis B infection.[56] Based upon studies of poor methodologic quality, there was a suggestion that Phyllanthus may have positive antiviral and liver biochemical effects. A more recent double-blind, placebo-controlled, clinical trial could find no anti-viral or biochemical benefit from a Phyllanthus species after 6 months of therapy.[57]

Hepatitis C is often treated with herbal therapy. A systematic review identified 10 randomized trials involving over 500 patients, mostly with chronic hepatitis C, in which 12 different herbals were compared to placebo, interferon, or other herbs.[58] Methodologic quality was found to be adequate in four trials. With one short-term exception, in the trials comparing herbs with placebo, the herbal therapy did not demonstrate improved viral or biochemical markers. Bing Gan Tang combined with interferon-alpha cleared hepatitis C virus RNA and normalized alanine transferase better than did interferon-alpha alone. Yi Zhu as well as Yi Er Gan Tang were the only remaining herbs that demonstrated any biochemical improvements. Adverse events consequent to herbal therapy were reported in six trials and included palpitations, diarrhea, abdominal pain, and thrombocytopenia.

"Liv.52" is a combination product containing seven herbals, touted for its protective benefits in the liver. A RCT testing its efficacy in alcoholic liver disease found no clinical or biochemical benefit after 6 months of use.[59]

A recent review discussed the potential antifibrotic effects of botanicals in chronic liver disease, discussing some of the herbals mentioned above.[60]

Reasons for Herbal Efficacy

Why might herbals be effective in GI and liver disease?[8] One must always consider a placebo effect, which can occur at a rate of 40% or more, especially when dealing with functional syndromes. If blinding is inadequate, study subjects know or can guess which treatment they receive, biasing the results. Herbal remedies contain a myriad of potentially biologically active compounds, including mono- and polysaccharides, amino acids, a variety of enzymes, antioxidants, and minerals. Thus, while it is scientifically invalid to extrapolate in vivo effects merely from the presence of potential biologically active compounds, the fact remains that these compounds may have physiologic roles. Finally, a range of evidence suggests that individual chemicals from a variety of plants may have various pharmacologic actions, including antibacterial, antiviral, antifibrotic, antioxidant, anticytokine, antispasmodic, cytotoxic, immunomodulatory, and neuromodulatory.

TABLE 10-3.

Patient Advice For Herbal Use

- Make sure the following information is on the label
  - Name and address of manufacturer
  - Botanical name of the herb with plant part used
  - Batch or lot number and expiration date
- Use standardized extracts whenever possible
- Avoid using a large variety of herbals
- If immunocompromized, use caution because of potential microbial contamination
- Let your clinician know what you are taking
- Do not exceed recommended doses
- Use with extreme caution during pregnancy or lactation
- Web site: www.Consumerlab.com or others for quality checks on products
- Report adverse effects to your clinician and FDA MedWatch program (1-800-332-1088 or www.fda.gov/medwatch

Adapted from Grundling K, Rand V. Dietary supplements: review and update. Presented at the American College of Physicians, Annual Meeting, Atlanta, GA; 2001.

HERBAL CONCLUSIONS

Rather than speaking of CAM, it has been suggested that there is therapy that has been adequately tested and that which has not, medicine that works and medicine that may or may not work.[6] If a treatment has been adequately tested, it no longer matters whether or not it was once considered alternative, complementary, or a supplement. What is necessary is evidence, not anecdote, speculation, and testimonial. The clinician needs to be vigilant in assessing evidence for efficacy. Care need be taken to avoid "leap of faith" conclusions, going from in vitro results to in vivo conclusions, from animal experiments to human conclusions, or from epidemiologic and observational associations as well as anecdote to causation.[9]

Almost 20% of Canadians with IBD take an herbal supplement,[61] and almost two-thirds of these say they would continue even if scientific evidence were to show no benefit from that particular form of CAM therapy.[62] Clinicians need to be able to explain to patients that "natural" does not necessarily mean better; if some is good for health, more is not necessarily better; and that there are important differences between herbs and drugs. Table 10-3 lists advice that the clinician might provide patients who wish to continue herbal supplements.

Vitamins

The vitamin business is the other major player in the multimillion dollar dietary supplement industry. Near the herbals in any supermarket, pharmacy, or health store are the vitamins. Aggressive claims are often made for the health benefits of these products.

Vitamins are a collection of organic compounds essential for normal metabolism. Vitamins cannot be synthesized by humans and must be ingested in the diet. The fat-soluble vitamins—A, D, E, and K—are stored. Water-soluble vitamins—thiamine (B1), riboflavin (B2), niacin (B3), pantothenic acid (B5), pyridoxine (B6), folic acid, cyanocobalamin (B12), biotin, and vitamin C—are not stored and need ongoing replenishment. Many of these vitamins are pertinent to GI practice, and discussion will be limited to these.

Historically, vitamin deficiency syndromes are well described. Gross vitamin deficiency syndromes are uncommon in western societies and when seen, are confined to specific populations, eg, the elderly, alcoholics, or inborn errors of metabolism. This is in stark contrast to developing world countries where classic deficiency syndromes remain frequent and manifest.

Recommended Daily Allowances (RDA) for vitamins are considered to be the amount needed to prevent deficiency syndromes in a population, with an error towards overestimating needs. Daily allowances for known essential micronutrients have been established scientifically and updated since the 1940s. The scientific basis for these recommendations include: 1) observations of food intake by the healthy; 2) balance studies; 3) biomarker studies designed to establish normal tissue sufficiency; 4) studies of induced deficiency; and 5) assessment of "normal" whole blood, serum, or plasma concentrations in healthy defined populations; 6) allowance for the 5% of the population that requires more than daily requirements yet prevention of micronutrient toxicity.[9] RDA are discussed in detail in Chapter 6.

Much contemporary vitamin advocacy stems from postulated occult vitamin deficiency secondary to high caloric, unbalanced western diets. These purported deficiency syndromes lack the presenting features of historical classic deficiency syndromes. Others suggest that the RDAs for deficiency are insufficient to prevent chronic disease and aging. Consequently, many may ingest vitamins in physiologic or pharmacologic doses with the hope of preventing aging and/or chronic disease.

MULTIVITAMINS

It has been estimated that 25% of US adults take a daily vitamin, and probably most supplemental vitamin intake is in the form of a multivitamin. The personal cost of such supplementation is relatively inexpensive—$15 to $30 per year. There is no standard multivitamin, nor are there formal standards for categorizing multivitamins. There is no oral "MVI." "M.V.I.-12" and "M.V.I. Pediatric" (AAIPharma Inc., Wilmington, NC) are registered trademark products, intended for intravenous use. "MVI" was the first intravenous multivitamin preparation that was able to achieve water solubilization of fat-soluble vitamins. The specific manufacturer of this brand-name intravenous product has changed over the years.

A classification of oral multivitamins includes:

1. B complex, and B complex with C
2. Hexavitamins (6 vitamins, both fat and water soluble)
3. Decavitamins (10 vitamins, both fat and water soluble)
4. Multivitamins (all "essential" vitamins)
5. Multivitamins with minerals (addition of various minerals)
6. Therapeutic multivitamins, usually with minerals (most vitamins in quantities greater than RDA, based upon the belief that more is better).

Within the above schema are also "pediatric," "geriatric," "stress," and "antioxidant" formulations, among others.

It should also be remembered that supplemental vitamins represent only a small fraction of the micronutrients found in food, many of which may have important physiologic functions for health. Far more carotenoids are ingested in the normal diet than are found in a multivitamin.[63] Virtually hundreds to perhaps thousands of bioflavenoids, phytochemicals, and other "nonessential" antioxidants may have physiologic functions.[64] A varied diet, especially rich in fruits and vegetables may be far more important for overall health than is the intake of one or more individual known micronutrients.

Few studies have reported the effects of multivitamins as opposed to their specific components. Nonetheless, there are theoretical reasons why a multivitamin in some form may be beneficial. If diet is inadequate or inappropriate, a multivitamin is a means to obtain known essential micronutrients. If chronic disease can be prevented by individual vitamins, a single pill would be an easy intervention. If patients with chronic GI and/or liver disease need specific vitamin supplementation, a multivitamin might be an easy means to achieve adequate intake. As will be discussed below, studies suggest that several individual vitamins and/or calcium may reduce GI cancer risk.

Malnutrition impairs immune function. Vitamin supplementation may improve immune status and response to infection, especially in developing countries.[65] Most studies in the West have looked only at the effect of multivitamins on upper respiratory infections, demonstrating benefit, no benefit, or harm.[66-69] One study suggested reduced GI infections in type 2 diabetics taking a multivitamin.[66] The relationship of these findings to GI practice is unknown.

Because multivitamins are inexpensive, convenient, and relatively safe, intake of daily multivitamin may be reasonable in GI practice, particularly in 1) the elderly who may malabsorb vitamin B12 and may be vitamin D deficient secondary to malabsorption, inadequate sunlight, and dietary inadequacy; 2) in vegans with inadequate B12 intake; and 3) persons who substitute alcohol for a varied diet, resulting in many micronutrient deficiencies. Multivitamins users should be cautious not to exceed the recommended daily allowance with other supplements. The increased fracture risk seen with high normal vitamin A intake is of particular concern. Large-scale RCTs are needed before any definitive recommendations can be made for global multivitamin supplementation.[70]

Specific vitamins are discussed below, and Table 10-4 lists vitamin effects of interest to the gastroenterologist. (Vitamin deficiencies are discussed in detail in Chapter 3.)

Vitamin A

Vitamin A is a fat-soluble vitamin, obtained from animal sources and in fortified foods. Beta-carotene, or provitamin A, is derived from fruits and vegetables. Beta-carotene is only one of 600 carotenoids found in nature, 40 carotenoids consumed in a varied diet, and 20 carotenoids identified in human sera and tissues.[63] Beta-carotene happens to be the carotenoid most studied and the only carotenoid usually found in supplements, but many others presumably have important biologic effects.[71]

Vitamin A helps regulate cell differentiation; higher intake potentially could reduce cancer risk. Data with respect to vitamin A, carotenoids, and GI cancer risk is, at best, discordant. The Physicians' Health Study found no link between beta-carotene supplementation and incidence of malignant neoplasms, including lung, colorectal, pancreas, stomach, and prostate.[72] Although the alpha-tocopherol beta-carotene (ATBC) trial found an increased risk of lung cancer among male smokers who received beta-carotene supplementation,[73] there was no association between beta-carotene supplementation and gastric cancer incidence.[74] The Polyp Prevention Study did not find any association between beta carotene and incidence of colorectal adenomas.[75]

Chronic overdose of vitamin A may present with ataxia, alopecia, hyperlipidemia, hepatotoxicity, bone pain, hypercalcemia, and bone fractures. The gastroenterologist should not forget or ignore the chronic liver disease seen in chronic hypervitaminosis A, manifested by hepatomegaly, portal hypertension, ascites, and histologic abnormalities of increased numbers and size of stellate cells, fibrosis, or cirrhosis.[76,77]

Vitamin A excess may result in bone fracture. Recent evidence documents increased risk of osteoporotic fractures at high normal intakes.[78,79] The gastroenterologist should be aware of this increased fracture risk in individuals with GI risk factors for osteoporosis—Crohn's disease, celiac disease, cholestatic liver disease, etc.

Vitamin D and Calcium

Vitamin D, or calciferol, is a fat-soluble vitamin involved in calcium homeostasis and bone metabolism. Sources of vitamin D include production in the skin by photoisomerization of provitamin D to D3, intestinal absorption, and fortification of the diet, particularly milk products. Vitamin D uptake requires full fat absorptive mechanisms, including

TABLE 10-4.

Vitamin Supplementation In Gastrointestinal Disease

Vitamin Recommendation	*Gastrointestinal Disease*	*Supporting Evidence*
B12	-Gastric disease (post-gastrectomy, gastritis, acchlorydia)	Strong
	-Chronic pancreatitis	Moderate
	-Intestinal disease (Crohn's, celiac sprue, ileal resection)	Strong
	-Pernicious anemia	Strong
Vitamin D/calcium* *calcium citrate	-Chronic steroids (Crohn's, ulcerative colitis, primary biliary cirrhosis, primary sclerosing cholangitis)	Strong
	-Malabsorption (celiac sprue, pancreatic insufficiency, small bowel resection)	Strong
	-Colorectal adenoma recurrence prevention	Weak
Folic acid	-Medications (methotrexate, asulfasalazsine),	Strong
	-Colon cancer prevention	Weak
Thiamine	Intravenous artificial feeding (TPN)	Strong
Antioxidants	-Colorectal adenoma prevention	Weak
	-Gastric cancer prevention	Weak
	-Esophageal cancer prevention	Weak

Adapted from Sharma N, Trope B, Lipman TO. Vitamin supplementation. What the gastroenterologist needs to know. *J Clin Gastroenterol.* 2004;38(10):844-54.

transport into enterocytes, packaging into chylomicrons, and transport to the liver via the portal circulation. In the liver, vitamin D is hydroxylated to form 25-hydroxy-vitamin-D. The proximal tubules of the kidney perform further hydroxylatation to produce 1,25-dihydroxy-vitamin-D, the physiologically active form of vitamin D. (Vitamin D is closely linked to calcium homeostasis. Although calcium is a mineral, not a vitamin, it is so closely tied to vitamin D metabolism and function that it is included in this discussion.)

Cross-sectional studies in IBD have shown that a substantial percentage of these patients may have low bone mineral density.[80,81] Likely causes include malnutrition, malabsorption, bowel resection, and corticosteroid use.[82] Additionally, an increased inflammatory state with disease activity and cytokine production is an independent risk factor for osteoporosis. It is not clear whether osteopenia risk in ulcerative colitis is similar to that observed with Crohn's disease.[82] Males and females are at similar risk for osteoporosis. The relationship between vitamin D and calcium intake and bone mineral density in premenopausal women with IBD is unclear.[83] The frequent onset of Crohn's disease and celiac sprue during adolescence or young adulthood predisposes these patients to osteoporosis at an earlier age.[82] (Crohn's disease and celiac sprue are discussed in Chapters 18 and 19, respectively.)

Calcium supplementation may prevent recurrent colorectal adenomas, presumably by an inhibition of carcinogenic effects of bile acids via calcium binding in the bowel lumen.[84,85] Other studies have not been able to confirm these findings.[86-88] Supplements are usually necessary also for persons on chronic glucocorticoid therapy and those with an increased risk of osteoporosis or proven osteoporosis: ie, 400-800 IU of vitamin D and 1000-1500 mg/day. For IBD, several unique factors suggest that calcium citrate is the preferred supplement rather than calcium carbonate, including better absorption, correction of metabolic acidosis from persistent diarrhea, and decreased urolithiasis. In addition, higher dose supplements may be required in patients with Crohn's disease.[89] Noncompliant patients may benefit from high dose intermittent vitamin D therapy, without calcium supplementation.[90]

VITAMIN E (TOCOPHEROL)

Vitamin E is a fat-soluble antioxidant that works as a free radical scavenger to protect polysaturated fatty acids, major structural components of cell membranes, from peroxidation. Eight naturally occurring compounds exist, including alpha, beta, delta, and gamma tocopherol.

There is conflicting data regarding antioxidant supplementation and the incidence of colorectal adenomas. Greenberg et al found no evidence that supplemental beta-carotene, vitamin C, and vitamin E given over a 4-year period decreased the incidence of recurrent colorectal adenomas.[76] These findings contrast with other studies, which suggest an inverse association between vitamin E intake and colon cancer.[74,91,92]

The ATBC Cancer Prevention Study found no association between daily alpha-tocopherol intake and gastric cancer after 6 years.[75] On the other hand, the Chinese Nutrition Intervention Trial found a 16% reduction in gastric cancer incidence among persons who consumed a combination of beta carotene, vitamin E, and selenium.[93] However, this population may have had underlying vitamin insufficiency.

Some consider vitamin E supplementation of up to 1000 IU per day to be safe.[94] However, safety in pharmacologic doses has not been studied rigorously and caution must be urged.[95,96] The ATBC study found increased mortality because of hemorrhagic strokes with vitamin E supplementation.[74] An antioxidant cocktail (vitamins E and C, beta-carotene, and selenium) attenuated the beneficial effects of a statin and niacin in individuals with known coronary artery disease and low high-density lipoprotein levels.[97]

Vitamin K

Vitamin K, or "koagulationsvitamin," is a fat-soluble vitamin. Vitamin K1 is found in green, leafy vegetables and absorbed by the distal small intestine, while vitamin K2 is synthesized by gut microflora. Vitamin K is essential for activity of clotting factors but is also an important cofactor in bone mineralization.[98]

Very high doses of vitamins E and A may antagonize vitamin K.[27] Clinicians managing patients on intravenous artificial feeding (total parenteral nutrition support) need to be cognizant of the vitamin K content of the intravenous multivitamin preparation being used, as some do and some do not contain vitamin K.

Thiamine

Vitamin B1 (thiamine) is a water-soluble precursor of thiamine pyrophosphate, a co-enzyme in oxidative decarboxylation of alpha-ketoacids to aldehydes. Thiamine is found in a wide variety of animal and vegetable products but is abundant in only a few. It is critical in glucose and energy metabolism. It is required for pyruvate entry into the Kreb's cycle; without thiamine, pyruvate accumulates and is converted into lactate.[99]

Folate and Folic Acid

Folate, found in green, leafy vegetables, fruits, and legumes, is necessary for DNA synthesis in conjunction with vitamin B12. Folic acid is the synthetic form and is 50% more bioavailable than folate.

Folate sufficiency at conception prevents neural tube defects and other fetal abnormalities.[100,101] Because of inadequate intake among young women, the FDA mandated the fortification of cereal grain products with folic acid.[102,103] Decreased folate levels lead to aberrant DNA synthesis and potential carcinogenesis. Higher dietary folate may be associated with a reduction in the risk of colorectal adenomas and colon cancer, breast cancer, as well as esophageal, pancreatic, and stomach cancer.[104-106] Patients with ulcerative colitis receiving folate supplementation have a 62% lower incidence of colorectal dysplasia and cancer.[106,107]

Although toxicity is unusual, pharmacologic intake of folic acid may increase carcinogenesis, especially in individuals with a history of colorectal adenomas.[108]

Vitamin B12 (Cobalamin)

Vitamin B12 is required for DNA synthesis in cells undergoing rapid turnover. Sources for vitamin B12 include meat and dairy products. B12 absorption is a complex process. Release of food-bound B12 requires an acid environment, and any decrease of gastric acid may result in failure of the release of B12 bound to food. After cobalamin is released from food binding, it binds to R proteins found in the stomach. Pancreatic enzymes are necessary to break the B12-R protein bonds.[109]

The recommended dietary allowance for cobalamin is 2 ug per day for adults, which can be achieved with the usual western diet.[110] The elderly may require higher intake via supplements; one RCT suggests greater than 50 ug/day for the elderly.[111] Supplements contain crystalline B12, which is not bound to food and thus does not need acid or pancreatic enzyme cleavage. Patients who have undergone gastric or ileal resection have been treated routinely with intramuscular B12. High-dose oral crystalline B12 (1000-2000 ug daily) may sometimes be used effectively in these patients,[101] and a gel for intranasal administration is now available.

Vitamin C

Vitamin C, or ascorbic acid, is a water-soluble antioxidant vitamin with numerous biological actions, including collagen synthesis, fatty acid transport, norepinephrine synthesis, and prostaglandin metabolism.

A low intake of vitamin C has been associated with gastric cancer in several studies; however, the effects of vitamin C supplementation specifically have not been studied.[101] The Polyp Prevention Study Group found no benefit in polyp formation with 4 years of supplemental vitamin C.[76] These results contrast with a study in which vitamin C supplementation decreased the number of rectal polyps in patients with familial polyposis.[112] Numerous RCTs also have not shown any effect of vitamin C on the common cold.[106] While vitamin C plus E impairs eradication of *Helicobacter pylori (H pylori*) infection,[41] high-dose vitamin C supplementation may protect against *H pylori* and progression of gastric mucosal atrophy.[107]

Vitamin C toxicity can result in diarrhea, abdominal bloating, false negative stool guaiac results, and fatal cardiac arrythmias in patients with iron overload, secondary to oxidative injury.[113,114]

Vitamin Conclusions

Vitamins are necessary for survival. Observational studies suggest additional benefit from vitamin supplementation in acute and chronic illness. Consequent to or in spite of these findings, there has been a great increase in vitamin consumption over the last several years. Unfortunately, randomized trials do not necessarily correlate with observational findings, and few definitive recommendations can be made. Inconsistencies between observational studies and the majority of randomized trials may reflect the frequent overestimate of benefit occurring with observational studies. Problems with many available RCTs include small sample sizes, differing dosages of vitamins, short duration of vitamin consumption and follow-up, and exclusion of other vitamins, which may be necessary cofactors in prevention of disease. Vitamin supplements are appropriate for recognized deficiencies, but it is by no means clear that they are useful for prevention of many chronic diseases. Vitamins should not be a substitute for a healthy lifestyle and diet.

References

1. Kaufman DW, Kelly JP, Rosenberg L, Anderson TE, Mitchell AA. Recent patterns of medication use in the ambulatory adult population of the United States: the Stone survey. *JAMA*. 2002: 287:337-344.
2. Hensrud DD, Engle DD, Scheitel SM. Unerreporting the use of dietary supplemens and nonprescription medications among patients undergoing a periodic health examination. *May Clin Proc*. 1999;74:443-447.
3. Halsted CH. Dietary supplements and The American Journal of Clinical Nutrition. *Am J Clin Nutr*. 2000;71:399-400.
4. Medical Foods. www.fda.gov
5. Koretz RL. Is Alternative Medicine Alternative Science? *J Lab Clin Med*. 2002;139:329-333.
6. Angell M, Kassirer JP. Alternative medicine—the risks of untested and unregulated remedies. *N Engl J Med*. 1998;339:838-841.
7. Strader DB, Zimmerman JH. Complementary and alternative medicine in Hepatitis C. In Liang TJ, Hoffnagle JH (eds.). *Hepatitis C*. Philadelphia PA: Academic Press; 2000: 427-451.
8. Langmead L, Rampton DS. Review article: herbal treatment in gastrointestinal and liver disease—benefits and dangers. *Aliment Pharmacol Ther*. 2001;15:1239-1252.
9. Buchman AL. Personal and government regulation of nutritional supplements; What we want and what we should expect. *J Lab Clin Med*. 2002;139:339-342.
10. Sardesai VM. Herbal medicines: Poisons or potions? *J Lab Clin Med*. 2002;139:343-348.
11. Specter M. Miracle in a bottle. *The New Yorker*. February 24, 2004:64-75.
12. Lewis JD, Strom BL. Balancing safety of dietary supplements with the free market. *Ann Intern Med*. 2002;136:616-618.
13. Goldman P. Herbal medicines today and the roots of modern pharmacology. *Ann Intern Med*. 2001;135:594-600.
14. Liberti LE, DerMarderosian AD. Evaluation of commercial ginseng products. *J Pharm Sci*. 1978;67:1487-1489.
15. Herbal roulette. *Consumer Reports*. November 1995:698.
16. Cui J, Garle M, Eneroth P, Bjorkhem I. What do commercial ginseng preparations contain? *Lancet*. 1994;344:134.
17. De Smet PAGM. Drug therapy: Herbal remedies. *N Eng J Med*. 2002;347:2046-2056.
18. Atherdon D. Towards the safer use of traditional remedies. *BMJ*. 1994;308:673-674.
19. Ernst E. Harmless herbs? A review of the recent literature. *Am J Med*. 1998;104:170-178.
20. Stedman C. Herbal hepatotoxicity. *Semin Liver Dis*. 2002;22:195-206.
21. Larrey D, Vial T, Pauwels A, Castot A, Biour M, David M, Michel H. Hepatitis after germander administration. *Ann Intern Med*. 1992;117:129-132.
22. Mostefa-Kara N, Pauwels A, Pines E, Biour M, Levy VG. Fatal hepatitis after germander gea. *Lancet*. 1992;340:674.
23. Gordon DW, Rosenthal G, Hart J, Sirota R, Baker AL. Chaparral ingestion: thebroadening spectrum of liver injury caused by herbal medications. *JAMA*. 1995;273:489-490.
24. Woolf GM, Petrovic LM, Rojter SE, Wainwright S, Villamil FG, Katkov WN, Michieletti P, Wanless IR, Stermitz FR, Beck JJ, et al. Acute hepatitis associated with Chinese herbal product Jin Bu Huan. *Ann Intern Med*. 1994;121:729-735.
25. Itoh S, Marutani K, Nishijima T, Matsuo S, Itabashi M. Liver injuries induced by herbal medicine, syo-saiko-to (xiao-chai-hu-tang). *Dig Dis Sci*. 1995;40:1845-8.
26. Benninger J, Schneider HT, Schuppan D, Kirchner T, Hahn EG. Acute hepatitis induced by greater celandine (Chelidonium majus). *Gastroenterology*. 1999;117:1234-1237.
27. Favreau JT, Ryu ML, Braunstein G, et al. Severe hepatotoxicity associated with the dietary supplement LipoKinetix. *Ann Intern Med*. 2002;136:590-595.
28. Hamed S, Rojiter S, Vierling J. Protracted cholestatic hepatitis after the use of Prostata. *Ann Intern Med*. 1997;127:169-170.
29. Graham-Brown R. Toxicity of Chinese herbal remedies. *Lancet*. 1992;340:673-4.
30. Vautier G, Spiller RC. Safety of complementary medicines should be monitored. *BMJ*. 1995;311:633.
31. Chan TY, Chan JC, Tomlinson B, Critchley JA. Chinese herbal medicines revisited: a Hong Kong perspective. *Lancet*. 1993;342:1532-4.
32. Gertner E, Marshall PS, Filandrinos D, Potek AS, Smith TM. Complications resulting from the use of Chinese herbal medications containing undeclared prescription drug. *Arthritis Rheum*. 1995;38:614-617.
33. Madisch A, Holtmann G, Plein K, Hotz J. Treatment of irritable bowel syndrome with herbal preparations: results of a double-blind, randomized, placebo-controlled, multi-centre trial. *Aliment Pharmacol Ther*. 2004:19:271-279.
34. Bensoussan A, Talley NJ, Hing M, Menzies R, Guo A, Meng N. Treatment of irritable bowel syndrome with Chinese herbal medicine: A randomized controlled trial. *JAMA*. 1998;280:1585-1589.
35. Pittler MH, Ernst E. Peppermint oil for irritable bowel syndrome: a criticial review and meta-analysis. *Am J Gastroenterol*. 1998;93:1131-1135.
36. Liu JH, Chen GH, Yeh HZ, Huang CK, Poon SK. Enteric coated peppermint oil capsules in the tratment of irritable bowel syndrome: A prospective randomized trial. *J Gastroenterol*. 1997;32:765-768.
37. Kline RM, Kline JJ, DiPalma J, Barbero GJ. Enteric-coated, pH-dependent peppermint oil capsules for the treatment of irritable bowel syndrome in children. *J Pediatr*. 2001;138:125-128.
38. Sallon S, Ben-Arye E, Davidson R, et al. A novel treatment for constipation-predominant irritable bowel syndrome using Padma Lax, a Tibetan herbal formula. *Digestion*. 2002;65:161-171.
39. Rosch W, Vinson B, Sassin I. A randomized clinical trial comparing the efficacy of a herbal preparation STW 5 with the prokinetic drug cisapride in patients with dysmotility type of functional dyspepsia. *Z Gastroenterol*. 2002;40:401-408.
40. Madisch A, Holtman G, mayr G, Vinson B, Hotz J. Treatment of functional dyspepsia with a herbal preparation: a double-blind, randomized, placebo-controlled, multicenter trial. *Digestion*. 2004;69:45-52.
41. Thompson Coon J, Ernst E. Systematic review: herbal medicinal products for non-ulcer dyspepsia. *Aliment Pharmacol Ther*. 2002;16:1689-1699.
42. Locke III GR. Review: Herbal medicinal products seem to be effective and safe in non-ulcer dyspepsia. *ACP Journal Club*. September/October 2003:43.
43. Holtmann G, Adam B, Haag S, et al. Efficacy of artichoke leaf extract in the treatment of patients with functional dyspepsia: a six-week placebo-controlled, double-blind, multicentre trial. *Aliment Pharmacol Ther*. 2003;18:1099-1105.
44. De la Motte S, Bose-O'Reilly S, Heinisch M, et al. [Double-blind comparison of an apple pectin-chamomile extract preparation with placebo in children with diarrhea.] *Arzneimittelforschung*. 1997;11:1247-1249. [Article in German, English abstract]
45. Aksit S, Caglayan S, Cukan R, et al. Carob bean juice: a powerful adjunct to oral rehydration solution treatment in diarrhoea. *Paediatr Perinat Epidemiol*. 1998;12:176-181.

46. Ernst E, Pittler MH. Efficacy of ginger for nausea and vomiting: a systematic review of randomized clinical trials. *Br J Anesth.* 2000;84:367-371.
47. Ben-Ayre E, Goldin E, Wengrower D, et al. Wheat grass juice in the treatment of active distal ulcerative colitis: a randomized double-blind placebo-controlled trial. *Scand J Gastroenterol.* 2002;37:444-449.
48. Langmead L, Feakins RM, Goldthorpe S, et al. Randomized, double-blind, placebo-controlled trial of oral aloe vera gel for active ulcerative colitis. *Aliment Pharmacol Ther.* 2004;19:719-747.
49. Liang TJ. Complementary and alternative medicine: The roots of healing. *Gastrroenterology.* 1999;117:1041.
50. Mulrow C, Lawrence V, Jacobs B, et al. Milk thistle: effects on liver disease and cirrhosis and clinical adverse effects. Evidence Report/Technology Assessment No. 21. AHRQ Publication No. 01-E025. Rockville MD: Agency for Healthcare Research and Quality; October 2000.
51. Lieber CS. S-adenosyl-L-methionine: its role in the treatment of liver disorders. *Am J Clin Nutr.* 2002;76:1183S-1187S.
52. Rambaldi A, Gluud C. S-adenosyl-L-methionine for alcoholic liver diseases (Cochrane Review). In: The Cochrane Library, Issue 1, 2004. Chichester, UK: John Wiley & Sons, Ltd.
53. Liu JP, McIntosh H, Lin H. Chinese medicinal herbs for asymptomatic carriers of hepatitis B virus infection (Cochrane Review). In: The Cochrane Library, Issue 1, 2004. Chichester, UK: John Wiley & Sons, Ltd.
54. McCulloch M, Broffman M, Gao J, et al. Chinese herbal medicine and interferon in the treatment of chronic hepatitis B: A meta-analysis of randomized, controlled trials. *Am J Public Health.* 2002;92:1619-1627.
55. Liu JP, McIntosh H, Lin H. Chinese medicinal herbs for chronic hepatitis B (Cochrane Review). In: The Cochrane Library, Issue 1, 2004. Chichester, UK: John Wiley & Sons, Ltd.
56. Liu J, Lin H, McIntosh H. Genus Phyllanthus for chronic hepatitis B virus infection: A systematic review. *J Viral Hepat.* 2001;8:358-366.
57. Chan HL, Sung JJ, Fong WF, et al. Double-blinded placebo-controlled study of Phyllanthus urinaris for the treatment of chronic hepatitis B. *Aliment Pharmacol Ther.* 2003;18:339-345.
58. Liu JP, Manheimer E, Tsutani K, et al. Medicinal herbs for hepatitis C virus infection (Cochrane Review). In: The Cochrane Library, Issue 1, 2004. Chichester, UK: John Wiley & Sons, Ltd.
59. De Silva HA, Saparamadu PA, Thabrew MI, et al. Liv.52 in alcoholic liver disease: a prospective, controlled trial. *J Ethnopharmacol.* 2003;84:47-50.
60. Stikel F, Brinkhaus B, Krähmer N, et al. Antifibrotic properties of botanicals in chronic liver disease. *Hepato-Gastroenterology.* 2002;49:1102-1108.
61. Hilsden RJ, Verhoef MJ, Best A, et al. Complementary and alternative medicine use by Canadian patients with inflammatory bowel disease: Results from a national survey. *Am J Gastroenterol.* 2003;98:1563-1568.
62. Vanderheyden LC, Verhoef MJ, Hilsden RJ. Perceived role of scientific evidence in the decision to continue use of complementary therapies by Canadians with inflammatory bowel disease. *Gastroenterology.* 2004;126:A606.
63. Cooper DA, Eldridge AL, Peters JC. Dietary carotenoids and lung cancer: A review. *Nutr Rev.* 1999;57:133-145.
64. Decker EA. The role of phenolics, conjugated linoleic acid, carnosine, and pyrroloquinoline quineone as nonessential dietary antioxidants. *Nutrition Reviews.* 1995;53:49-58.
65. Fawzi W, Stampfer MJ. A role for multivitamins in infection? *Ann Intern Med.* 2003;138:430-431.
66. Barringer TA, Kirk JK, Santaniello AC, et al. Effect of a Multivitamin and mineral supplementation on infection and quality of life. A randomized, double-blind, placebo-controlled trial. *Ann Intern Med.* 2003;138:365-371.
67. Chandra RK. Effect of vitamin and trace element supplementation on immune responses and infection in elderly subjects. *Lancet.* 1992;340:1124-1127.
68. Chavance M, Herbeth B, Lemoine A et al. Does multivitamin supplementation prevent infections in healthy elderly subjects? A controlled trial. *Int J Vitam Nutr Res.* 1993;63:11-6.
69. Graat JM, Schouten ME, Kok F. Effect of daily vitamin E and multivitamin-mineral supplementation on acute respiratory tract infections in elderly persons. *JAMA.* 2002;288:715-721.
70. Christen WG, Gaziano JM, Hennekens CH. Design of Physicians' Health Study II—A randomized trial of beta-carotene, vitamins E and C, and multivitamins, in prevention of cancer, cardiovascular disease, and eye disease, and review of results of completed trials. *Ann Epidemiol.* 2000;10:125-134.
71. Giovannucci E. Tomatoes, tomato-based products, lycopene, and cancer: Review of the epidemiologic literature. *J Natl Cancer Inst.* 1999;91:917-933.
72. Hennekens CH, Buring JE, Manson JE, et al. lack of effect of long-term supplementation with beta carotene on the incidence of malignant neoplasms and cardiovascular disease. *N Engl J Med.* 1996;334:1145-1149.
73. The Alpha-Topherol, Beta-Carotene Cancer Prevention Study Group. The effect of vitamin E and beta-carotene on the incidence of lung cancer and other cancers in male smokers. *N Engl J Med.* 1994;330:1029-1035.
74. Malila N, Taylor PR, Virtanen MJ et al. Effects of alpha-tocopherol and beta-carotene supplementation on gastric cancer incidence in male smokers (ATBC Study, Finland). *Cancer Causes Control.* 2002;13(7):617-23.
75. Greenberg ER, Baron JA, Tosteson TD et al. A clinical trial of antioxidants to prevent colorectal adenoma. Polyp Prevention Study Group. *N Engl J Med.* 1994;331:441-147.
76. Leo MA, Lieber CS. Hypervitaminosis A: A liver lover's lament. *Hepatology.* 1998;8:412-417.
77. Fallon MB, Boyer JL. Hepatic toxicity of vitamin A and synthetic retinoids. *J Gastroenterol Hepatol.* 1990;5:334-342.
78. Michaelsson K, Kithell H, Vessby B, et al. Serum retinol levels and the risk of fracture. *N Engl J Med.* 2003;348:287-294.
79. Feskanich D, Singh V, Willett WC, et al. Vitamin A Intake and hip fractures among postmenopausal women. *JAMA.* 2002;287:47-54.
80. Compston, JE, Judd D, Crawley EO, et al. Osteoporosis in patients with inflammatory bowel disease. *Gut.* 1987;28:410-415.
81. Pigot F, Roux C, Chaussade S, et al. Low bone mineral density in patients with inflammatory bowel disease. *Dig Dis Sci.* 1992;37:1396-1403.
82. Jahnsen J, Falch JA, Aadland E, et al. Bone mineral density is reduced in patients with Crohn's disease but not in patients with ulcerative colitis: A population based study. *Cut.* 1997; 40:313-319.
83. Bernstein CN, Bector S, Leslie WD. Lack of relationship of calcium and vitamin D intake to bone mineral density in premenopausal women with inflammatory bowel disease. *Am J Gastroenterol.* 2003;98:2468-2473.
84. Baron JA, Beach M, Mandel JS, et al. Calcium supplements for the prevention of colorectal adenomas. *N Engl J Med.* 1999;340:101-107.
85. Shaukat A, Scouras N, Schunermann H. Role of supplemental calcium in the recurrence of colorectal adenomas: A meta-analysis of randomized controlled trials. *Gastroenterology.* 2004;126:A397-A398.
86. Grau MV, Baron JA, Sandler RS, et al. Vitamin D, Calcium supplementation, and colorectal adenomas: Results of a randomized trial. *J Natl Cancer Inst.* 2003;95:1765-1771.
87. Graham S, Marshall J, Haughey B, et al. Dietary epidemiology of cancer of the colon in western New York. *Am J Epidemiol.* 1988;128:490-503.
88. Boutron MC, Faivre J, Marteau AP, et al. Calcium, phosphorus, vitamin D, dairy products and colorectal carcinogenesis: a French case-control study. *Br J Cancer.* 1996;74:141-151.
89. Rosen HN, Robinson A. Metabolic bone disease in inflammatory bowel disease. In: Rose BD, ed. *UpToDate.* Wellesley MA: UpToDate; 2004.

90. Trivedi DP, Doll R, Khaw KT. Effect of four monthly oral vitamin D3 (cholecalciferol) supplementation on fractures and mortality in men and women living in the community: randomized double blind controlled trial. *BMJ*. 2003;326:469-474.
91. Bostick RM, Potter JD, McKenzie DR, et al. Reduced risk of colon cancer with high intake of vitamin E: the Iowa Women's Health Study. *Cancer Res*. 1993;53:4230-4237.
92. Wu K, Willett WC, Chan JM, et al. A prospective study on supplemental vitamin E intake and the risk of colon cancer in women and men. *Cancer Epidemiol Biomarkers Prev*. 2002;11:1298-1304.
93. Blot WJ, Li J-Y, Taylor PR, et al. Nutrition intervention trials in Linxian, China: Supplementation with specific vitamin/mineral combinations, cancer incidence, and disease-specific mortality in the general population. *J Natl Cancer Inst*. 1993;85:1483-1492.
94. Willett WC, Stampfer MJ. What vitamins should I be taking, doctor? *N Engl J Med*. 2001;345:1819-1824.
95. Schwartz JL The dual roles of nutrients as antioxidants and prooxidants: Their effects on tumor cell growth. *J Nutr*. 1996;126:1221S-1227S.
96. Christen S, Woodall AA, Shigenaga MK, et al. γ-Tocopherol traps mutagenic electrophiles such as No_x and complements α-tocopherol: Physiological implications. *Proc Natl Acad Sci*. 1997;94:3217-3222.
97. Brown BG, Zhao X-Q, Chait A, et al. Simvastatin and niacin, antioxidant vitamins, or the combination for the prevention of coronary disease. *New Eng J Med*. 2001;345:1583-1592.
98. Compston, J E. Boning up on vitamin K. *Gut*. 2001;48:448.
99. Bender DA. Optimum nutrition: thiamin, biotin and pantothenate. *Proc Nutr Soc*. 1999;58:427-433.
100. Glade MJ. Workshop on Folate, B12, and Choline. Sponsored by the Panel on Folate and other B vitamins of the Standing Committee on the Scientific Evaluation of Dietary Reference Intakes, Food and Nutrition Board, Institute of Medicine, Washington, D.C., March 3-4, 1997 Nutrition 1999; 15:92-96.
101. MRC Vitamin Study Research Group. Prevention of neural tube defects: results of the Medical Research Council Vitamin Study. *Lancet*. 1991;338:131-137.
102. Oakley GP Jr. Eat right and take a multivitamin. *N Engl J Med*. 1998;338:1060-1061.
103. Jacques PF, Selhub J, Bostom AG, et al. The effect of folic acid fortification on plasma folate and total homocysteine concentrations. *N Engl J Med*. 1999;340(19):1449-1454.
104. Giovannucci E, Stampfer MJ, Colditz GA, et al. Multivitamin use, folate, and colon cancer in women in the Nurses' Health Study. *Ann Intern Med*. 1998;129:517-524.
105. Giovannucci E, Rimm EB, Ascherio A, et al. Alcohol, low-methionine-low-folate diets, and risk of colon cancer in men. *J Natl Cancer Inst*. 1995;87:265-273.
106. Pazirandeh S, Lo CW, Burns DL. Overview of water-soluble vitamins-II. In: Rose BD, ed. *UpToDate*. Wellesley MA: UpToDate; 2003.
107. Sasazuki S, Sasaki S, Tsubono Y, et al. The effect of 5-year vitamin C supplementation on serum pepsinogen level and Helicobacter pylori infection. *Cancer Sci*. 2003;94:378-382.
108. Kim Y. Role of folate in colon cancer development and progression. Internation research conference on food, nutrition, and cancer. *J Nutr*. 2003;133:3731S-3739S.
109. Schrier SL. Etiology and clinical manifestations of vitamin B12 and folic acid deficiency. In: Rose BD, ed. *UpToDate*. Wellesley MA: UpToDate; 2004.
110. Green R. Kinsella LJ. Editorial: Current concepts in the diagnosis of cobalamin deficiency. *Neurology*. 1995;45:1435-1440.
111. Seal EC, Metz J, Flicker L, et al. A randomized, double-blind, placebo-controlled study of oral vitamin B12 supplementation in older patients with suboptimal or borderline serum B12 concentrations. *J Am Geriatr Soc*. 2002;50:146-151.
112. Bussey HJ, DeCosse JJ, Deschner EE, et al. A randomized trial of ascorbic acid in polyposis coli. *Cancer*. 1982;50:1434-1439.
113. Jaffe RM, Kasten B, Young DS, et al. False-negative stool occult blood tests caused by ingestion of ascorbic acid (vitamin C). *Ann Intern Med*. 1975;83:824-826.
114. McLaren CJ, Bett JH, Nye JA, et al. Congestive cardiomyopathy and haemochromatosis—rapid progression possibly accelerated by excessive ingestion of ascorbic acid. *Aust N Z Med*. 1982;12:187-188.

Chapter 11

Prebiotics, Probiotics, and Dietary Fiber

Martin H. Floch, MS, MD, MACG

Introduction

The intestinal microflora is essential in maintaining health. Intestinal microecology consists of a complex of the microflora, gastrointestinal (GI) secretions, foods, and the products of the gut wall. Understanding the roles of: 1) prebiotics, 2) probiotics, and 3) dietary fiber in this GI physiology is essential to understand the role of intestinal microecology in health and disease. All three affect the intestinal microflora and its effect on the host. The definition and role of each are described in this chapter.

Prebiotics

Definition

"Prebiotics are non-digested food ingredients that beneficially affect the host by selectively stimulating the growth or activity of one or a limited number of bacteria in the colon that can improve the host's health."[1] This concept was introduced only in 1995,[1] but there has been much animal and human research and publication on the subject so that the principle is now widely accepted.[2-4]

Prebiotics are food substances that are not absorbed in the small intestine. Hence, they reach the large intestine. A study performed on patients with conventional ileostomy in which either inulin, oligofructose, or sucrose were added to a controlled diet during three experimental periods of 3 days each revealed that inulin and oligofructose had no affect on cholesterol absorption or excretion of cholesterol, bile acids, fat, calcium, magnesium, zinc, and iron.[5] From this and other studies, it can be concluded that nonabsorbable prebiotics have little affect on mineral and lipid metabolism in the small bowel. Furthermore, careful studies evaluating calcium bioavailability also reveal that prebiotics have little affect on the absorption of calcium in the small bowel.[6] The effect of prebiotics occurs in the large intestine.[2-4]

Prebiotic Substances Used and Available

Prebiotic substances are carbohydrates that are not digested by human enzymes. There are a wide range of prebiotic carbohydrates that can stimulate beneficial bacteria growth. Some of these carbohydrates may be digested by enzymes specific to bacterial species and, hence, account for the wide range of species of organisms available in the colon.[7-10] Table 11-1 lists the prebiotic substances, and Table 11-2 lists the commercial products available.

A synthetic lactose derivative, Lactulose, is well known for its treatment of both constipation and hepatic encephalopathy.[11,12]

Prebiotics stimulate bacterial growth. The same bacteria in turn stimulate fermentation and production of short-chain fatty acids (SCFA).[8] Oligofructose and inulin stimulate Bifidobacterial growth and metabolism in humans.[9] Fructooligosaccharide (FOS) promotes the growth of both *Bifidobacteria* and *Lactobacilli*. Prebiotics lower the colonic pH of feces, and appear to discourage the growth of pathogenic clostridia. In addition, they produce a lower glycemic index, are water soluble, and have a very low viscosity. Since FOS is usually pleas-

TABLE 11-1.
Prebiotic Substances

Disaccharides
Lactulose
Oligosaccharide
Fructooligosaccharide (FOS)
Glactooligosaccaride
Soybean oligosaccharide
Other Main Digestible Oligosaccharides:
 Xylooligosaccharide, Isomaltooligosaccharide, Lactulosesucrose, Palatinose
 Polycondensats
Inulin
Resistant Starch

TABLE 11-2.
Prebiotic Substances[3,8]

Prebiotic	Country
Fructooligosaccharide	Orafti, Belgium
Isomaltooligosaccharide	Showa Sangyo, Japan
Oligomate	Yakult, Japan
Palatinose	Sudzucker, Germany
Pyrodextrin	Matsutani, Japan
Raftiline	Orafti, Belgium
Soybean oligosaccharide	Calpis, Japan
Xylooligosaccharide	Sutory, Japan
Fructooligosaccharides	Ross Laboratories, Columbus, OH (US)
Guar	Novartis Nutrition, Minneapolis, MN (US)
Lactulose (Duphalac)	Solvay, Marietta, GA (US)
(Kristalose)	Bartek (US)

antly sweet tasting, it can be used to add texture to foods. It occurs naturally in artichokes, onions, garlic, chicory, wheat and some cereals. A major effect of feeding FOS is to increase the production of SCFA.[3] It is also known that prebiotic feeding can stimulate *Bifidobacteria* to produce B vitamins.[10]

EFFECT ON INTESTINAL FLORA

The goal of administering a prebiotic is to stimulate the growth and metabolism of organisms that are saccharolytic. Most prebiotics stimulate the growth of Lactobacilli and Bifidobacteria at the greatest rates, but bacteria of the generium of *Bacteroides, Bifidobacterium, Neubacterium, Lactobacillus*, and *Clostridia* all ferment prebiotics.

In vitro and in vivo studies show that oligofructose and inulin will stimulate the growth of *Bifidobacteria*, whereas they inhibit the growth of *Escherichia coli* (*E. coli*) and *Clostridium prefringens*.[3]

In a randomized, double-blind, and placebo-controlled experiment, lactulose and lactitol were shown to significantly increase *Bifidobacteria, Lactobacilli, and Streptococci*, whereas populations of *Bacteroides, Clostridia, Chloroforms*, and *Neubacteria* were decreased.[11] In studies using lactulose in the treatment of hepatic encephalopathy, there was also a clear shift in bacteria populations. Exact mechanisms of lactulose benefit in hepatic encephalopathy are unknown, yet the shift in bacteria populations clearly indicates that a prebiotic changes the metabolism of the intestinal ecology.[12]

It is also clear that FOS stimulates *Bifidobacteria* metabolism and growth. This is highly suspected from the fact that oligosaccharides are in breast milk and result in primarily a beneficial flora in infants.[2] Furthermore, in human volunteer studies, administration of oligofructose while on controlled diets in a dose of 15 grams a day for 2 weeks clearly demonstrated a significant increase in stool *Bifidobacteria*.[9]

The lactooligosaccharides have also been shown to be bifidogenetic.[13] When eight human volunteers were each fed 10 g/day for 21 days, they had significant increases in fecal *Bifidobacteria*.[14] Soybean has also been shown to increase the *Bifidobacteria* flora but less consistently.[14] Inulin similarly increases the *Bifidobacteria*.[9,15] It is also known that inulin is fermented more slowly and, hence, its greatest effect appears to be in the left rather than the right side of the bowel.

Clinical Utilization

Prebiotics have been shown to be helpful in treating constipation. Kleesen and associates fed constipated subjects inulin. They found that *Bifidobacteria* increased log counts from 7.9 to 9.2 per gram of feces with a concomitant decrease in *enterobacteria* and *enterococci*.[15] This change in the flora was associated with higher production of SCFA. Stools became soft and more frequent with only mild discomfort during defecation.

Many patients with irritable bowel syndrome (IBS) seek alternative methods of therapy. FOS was tested to determine how it would affect the symptoms of IBS patients because there was concern it may increase symptoms.[16] In a multi-center, prospective, randomized, double-blind, placebo-controlled trial at 24 sites, a 2-week single-dose plan phase and a 12-week double-blind comparative phase were done feeding 20 g of FOS as compared to a placebo. The authors found some symptoms did indeed increase in patients with IBS at the onset, but when 20 g of FOS were fed over a 12-week period, there was no worsening of symptoms.[16] In another study—a double-crossover trial—using oligofructose, the authors found no significant change in any of the clinical parameters that they studied—even in patients with prominent diarrhea or prominent constipation IBS.[17] At the present state of our knowledge, there is no evidence that prebiotics are harmful or helpful in IBS.

Prebiotics have been shown to be effective in treating inflammatory bowel disease (IBD) in several clinical trials.[18] Kuisma and associates randomly administered germinated barley foodstuff (TBF) to 18 patients in a pilot study and found it increased luminal butyrate production and stimulated growth of probiotic bacteria.[18] Although they examined a small group of patients, they found that, in a 4-week period, there was a significant decrease in the clinical activity index and found no side effects. Barley was also used in a simple open-labeled protocol for 24 weeks.[18,19] Once again, investigators found a decrease in clinical activity of the ulcerative colitis. Although the participant numbers were small and the results marginal in these studies, the findings indicate that there may be a place for prebiotic therapy in IBD.

These trials in IBS and IBD indicate that the symbiotic relationship between prebiotics and probiotics needs further study and elaboration in all intestinal disease.

In humans, there is controversy as to whether prebiotics are helpful in controlling lipid cardiovascular risk factors. FOS has been shown to reduce serum cholesterol in diabetic patients.[20] Similarly, inulin has been shown to reduce serum lipids in women with high cholesterol levels.[21] Furthermore, the symbiotic effect of feeding the probiotic with a drink that contains fermented oats significantly lowered concentrations of LDL cholesterol and fibrinogen,[22] and a similar effect could be demonstrated on several cardiovascular disease risk factors in smokers.[23] However, these are limited human experiments and much more data is necessary to prove whether a prebiotic substance alone or a symbiotic relationship between prebiotic substances and probiotics can be effective in regulating lipid metabolism. The concept is appealing because dietary fiber appeared to have such a beneficial effect; however, much more research is needed to substantiate these scattered results.

There is no question that probiotics are important in maintaining a normal immune response and in maintaining or helping in the treatment of infections. The enhancement of probiotic activity as an added effect by prebiotics is an important theoretical concept, but experimental study is needed to establish this effect and to determine if there is clinical usefulness.[8]

Probiotics

Definition

Probiotics were defined in 1989 as "microbial supplements that benefit the host animal by improving its intestinal microbial balance."[24] Probiotics are live microbial organisms obtained from humans and used in supplements. Metchnikoff is credited for promulgating the concept of the importance of the intestinal microbial balance in maintaining health.[25] In his thesis, published in 1907, he proposed that substances produced by putrefying active intestinal bacteria were absorbed and helped cause aging. He also proposed that saccrolytic organisms such as *lactobacilli* would improve microbial balance and help prolong life. It wasn't until 1926 that Kipeloff began to promulgate the importance of *Lactobacillus acidophilus,* and later Rettger et al suggested its therapeutic applications.[26,27] In 1955, the relationship of pathogenic bacteria to infectious bacteria was demonstrated in animals,[28] and in 1965, Lilly and Stillwell demonstrated the growth-promoting factors produced by probiotic microorganisms.[29]

Organisms Used as Probiotics

The most common strains employed are from the species *Lactobacilli* or *Bifidobacteria*. However, there are many other species of organisms, including some yeast organisms from the species *Saccharomyces*, that are also used. These organisms are administered commonly in yogurt or in capsules. The yogurts contain live organisms, and the capsules contain freeze-dried organisms.

A review of the literature from 1980 to the present reveals that there are more than 100 published reports of probiotic organisms used in humans.[30] The most common organism employed in single or multiple products

TABLE 11-3.

Most Common Probiotic Microorganisms Used In Supplements

Lactobacillus Species	*Bifidobacterium Species*
L. acidophilus	*B. adolescentis*
L. amylovorus	*B. animalis*
L. casei	*B. lectis*
L. crispatus	*B. bifidum*
L. gasseri	*B. breve*
L. johnsonii	*B. infantis*
L. paracasei	*B. longum*
L. plantarum	
L. reuteri	
L. rhamnosus	
Non-Lactic Acid Bacteria & Yeasts	*Other Lactic Acid Bacteria*
Bacillus cereus var. toyoi	*Enterococcus faecium*
Escherichia coli strain nissle	*Leuconstoc mesenteroides*
Propoinibacterium fredenreichii	*Streptococcus thermophilus*
Saccharomyces cerevisiae	
Saccharomyces boulardii	

is *Lactobacillus acidophilus*. Such an organism has been described in detail—*Lactobacilus acidophilus* (L. acidophilus) NCFN—and is used as available in many food supplements.[31] Its status has been established as an A-1 strain by both hemolytic and genotypic techniques. It survives transit through the GI tract and adheres to CACO-2 and lupus-secreting H29 cell culture systems. Table 11-3 lists the most common organisms used of the *Lactobacillus* species, *Bifidobacteria* species, nonlactic acid bacteria and other bacteria.[32]

Although there are more than 100 studies now published, some have been more specific of their effects and importance in demonstrating the importance of probiotic organisms. Table 11-4 lists examples of such studies in which single organisms were employed.[32-46]

The use of multiple microorganisms in one probiotic supplement has gained popularity in more recent studies, particularly of use in IBD.[47,48] Where some investigators have used two or four organisms, which are commonly available in many products, the widely accepted published data in IBD has employed eight organisms to demonstrate the benefit.[48]

PHYSIOLOGIC EFFECTS RESULTING IN BENEFIT TO HOST

General

The intestinal tract represents an important ecosystem within the human body. The ecosystem has four major components: the wall of the gut, secretions from the gut, ingested food and nutrients that enter the gut, and the microflora.[8] Normal indigenous intestinal microflora have a symbiotic relationship with the host. In that relationship, the flora has certain definite effects. The normal flora (from which probiotic organisms are taken): 1) protect the host by producing antibacterial substances and creating barrier protection; 2) stimulate natural immune processes; 3) is directly responsible for maintaining the enterohepatic circulation of bile acids; and 4) performs a metabolic function in that the flora helps ferment and digest carbohydrates to produce SCFA that are essential for health. It is assumed and proven in some experiments that, when the normal flora is deficient in certain bacteria, the administration of probiotic organisms will assist with one or more of these functions.

Immune Process

A large part of normal immunophysiologic regulation of the gut depends on the indigenous flora.[49] Specific immunomodulary properties of probiotic bacteria can be characterized.[50] The microflora stimulate the activity of the lymphoid system and immunoglobulin response.[50] It is becoming increasingly clear that human response is a result of reactivity to DNA from probiotic bacteria.[51] It is also becoming evident that the same effect can be induced by injection of probiotic bacterial content. By injecting *Lactobacillus salivarius* into the interleukin 10 knockout model of colitis, suppression of anti-inflammatory effects can be shown. The probiotic effect is associated with decreased production of inflammatory cytokines and maintaining the production of anti-TGFß.[52]

The fact that alpha-tissue necrosis factor (alpha-TNF) antibody has proven to be effective in the treatment of Crohn's disease is of interest and is important for understanding its relationship to probiotic organisms.[53] Tissues obtained from surgical specimens at surgery and then cultured showed that numerous probiotic organisms can reduce the production of alpha-TNF. From these experiments, it was clear that the organisms interact with immunocompetent cells and effect alpha-TNF physiology.[54]

Table 11-4.

Studies Demonstrating Probiotic Importance Using Single Organism

Study or Studies	Probiotic	Clinical Relevance
Bernet et al.[33]	*Lactobacillus acidophilus* LC1	Adherence to human intestinal cells, balancing of intestinal microflora, and immune enhancing
Lidbeck et al.[34] Salminen et al.[35]	*L. acidophilus* NCF01748	Treatment of constipation, decreased food and enzymes, and prevention of radiotherapy-related diarrhea
Kaila et al.[36,37] Majamaa et al.[38] Gorbach[39]	*L. rhamnosus* GG	Treatment and prevention of rotavirus diarrhea, treatment of relapsing C. difficile colitis, prevention of acute diarrhea, prevention of antibiotic-associated diarrhea, antagonistic against carcinogenic bacteria
Marteau et al.[40]	*Bifidobacterium bifidum*	Treatment of rotavirus and viral diarrhea and balancing intestinal microflora
Shornikova et al.[41] Wolf et al.[42]	*L. reuteri*	Colonization of the intestinal tract, shortening of rotavirus diarrhea
Surawicz et al.[43]	*Saccharomyces boulardi*	Prevention and treatment of C. difficile colitis and antibiotic-associated diarrhea
Rembacken et al.[44]	*Escherichia coli strain Nissle*	Used to maintain remission in IBD
Nobaek et al.[45]	*L. plantarum*	Decreased IBS symptoms
Hilton et al.[46]	*L. acidophilus*	Prevention of recurrent candidal vaginitis

Probiotic organisms have been demonstrated to have immunoregulating function associated with the gut lymphoid tissue. IGA-producing cells appear to be effective through components of their cell, which can be demonstrated by oral feeding and parenteral mechanisms. There is also no question that the intestinal microflora can stimulate phagocytosis. However, there are still many questions that remain concerning the role of individual organisms in the live ecosystem.[52-54]

Barrier Protection

Permeability caused by bacteria can be abolished in vitro when intestinal mucosa is pretreated with probiotic organisms.[55] Probiotic organisms also produce substances that may attack invasive organisms or pathogens. Defenses and antibiotic-like substances are produced by various probiotic species.

In summary, probiotics function and protect the host by resisting upper GI tract secretions, adhering to intestinal cells, colonizing the human intestinal tract, producing antimicrobial substances, and enhancing immunologic modulation and act as a barrier protection in the intestine.[10]

Importance of Fermentation

Non-starch polysaccharides and carbohydrates not absorbed in the small intestine are fermented by intestinal bacteria. Probiotics are particularly effective in this fermentation, and they produce SCFA.[8] SCFA produced are butyric, acetic, and propionic acids.[2,3] Butyric acid is the main nutrient for colonocytes. The epithelial cells choose to metabolize it at a greater rate than they do glucose. The role of acetic is that it is absorbed and used for production of cholesterol. The role of propionic remains somewhat uncertain but is suspected to be lipid controlling through some feedback mechanism. In a randomized, double-blind, controlled study of 36 healthy volunteers, investigators found that those participants who received a probiotic plus the prebiotic had significant decrease in blood pressure, leptin, cardiovascular risk factors, and monocyte adhesive properties.[23] The authors theorized that effects were because of increased production of SCFA. The production of SCFA is essential in maintaining body homeostasis and is protective in many metabolic processes.[56,57]

Clinical Utilization

Infections

Because probiotics stimulate immunomodulation and enhance phagocytosis, it is logical to use them in treating infections. Most accept that they have been effective in treating rotavirus infection.[37,38] As this is a common infection in children, it was not surprising to see that a meta-analysis in which the entrance criteria included healthy children less than 5 years of age in 18 eligible studies clearly suggested that coadministration of probiotics with standard rehydration therapy reduced the duration of acute infection by 1 day. This data stood up when the authors reanalyzed the material and limited it to hospitalized children, double-blinded trials, and studies evaluating Lactobacillus.[58]

Clostridia difficile (C. difficile) can cause significant post-antibiotic diarrhea and *pseudomembranous colitis,* which may result in severe life-threatening disease. It is usually effectively treated with antibiotics, but at times C. difficile becomes resistant to treatment, and, because it is a spore-forming organism, reinfections are common.[39] In certain individuals, control of the reinfection becomes a very significant clinical problem. For that reason, Surawicz et al employed a probiotic, *Saccharomyces boulardii,* to successfully reduce the incidence of recurrent infection.[43] In a prospective, double-blinded, controlled study of 180 patients, investigators found that the probiotic reduced the incidence of reinfection from 22% to 9%. Gorbach and colleagues have also shown that *Lactobacillus GG* is effective in reducing the relapses of C. difficile.[39] Hence, probiotic therapy has been effective in assisting the treatment of recurrent C. difficile diarrhea.

The effectiveness of probiotics in preventing travelers' diarrhea is controversial, and no studies have justified their use.[32]

There is some evidence that indicates that probiotic agents can be effective in the treatment of genito-urinary infections in women. One study compared a controlled group of 11 women, who received a placebo, to 11 women who were treated with yogurt-containing probiotic. Those on the placebo had 36 infections during the trial period, whereas the women who ate the yogurt had only four infections.[46] There are other non-controlled studies that have demonstrated the effectiveness of probiotics in genito-urinary tract infections. However, Reid has analyzed the literature and notes that *Lactobacilli* are the major constituents of the normal vaginal flora of premenopausal women.[59,60] The normal strains are important for their adhesive abilities and production of anti-microbial substances that prevent infection. However, efforts to use Lactobacilli and other probiotics have definitely revealed mixed results. Several strains of Lactobacilli with the ability to inhibit overgrowth by pathogens have been isolated, and it is suspected that therapy treatment would be strain specific. Of note in the initial studies is that treatment has been effective by direct vaginal insert of the probiotic, as well as by the oral administration of the probiotic.[46] This indicates that the oral probiotic affects the immune regulatory mechanisms that control the vaginal infection.

Inflammatory Bowel Disease

Studies on the microflora in Crohn's disease reveal that bacteria are more invasive and that there are increased number of bacteria that survive in the mucus layer.[61-65] These facts support that probiotics would be helpful in overcoming the growth of other organisms in the mucus layer as well as block their entry through the epithelium. Other studies have also revealed that there is a great biodiversity of the flora in patients with Crohn's disease and in ulcerative colitis.[64,65]

Ulcerative Colitis

There are three controlled studies on the use of E. coli Nissle strain in the treatment of ulcerative colitis.[44,66,67] Kruis and colleagues reported an initial study that did not have statistical significance; however, when they continued their work, a second report was found to be clinically significant. They compared the use of E. coli to the maintenance dose of mesalamine (2400 mg/day) and found that the probiotic was as effective in maintaining remission as was the E. coli. In a very small random-controlled study, Ishikawa et al used 100 cc/day of bifidobacteria fermented milk for 1 year and found a definite change in flora with 3 of 11 probiotic and 9 of 10 controls experiencing an exacerbation.[68]

Venturi et al used VSL#3 (eight organisms) in an uncontrolled study of 20 ulcerative colitis patients evaluated for 1 year and found definite changes in the flora with 15 of the 20 remaining in remission.[69] A preliminary study using VSL#3 for the arthralgia associated with IBD revealed improvement of symptoms.[70]

Unfortunately, to date research only reports controlled studies with one probiotic and uncontrolled studies with VSL#3. Certainly, more work is needed to establish its effectiveness in ulcerative colitis.

Crohn's Disease

There are four studies in the literature on the use of probiotics in Crohn's disease. Two are with the use of *Saccharomyces boulardii*[71,72] and one with VSL#3.[73] Both of the *Saccharomyces* studies indicate benefit. One showed improvement of the activity index scores and the other was helpful in maintaining remission. They used a dose of 3-4 x 1011 organisms per day.[71,72] A fourth study in the literature on Crohn's disease employed 12 billion organisms per day of *Lactobacillus GG* and showed no effect of either improving the activity index or endoscopic findings.[74] The study with VSL#3 was one in which the probiotic supplement contains 300 billion organisms (now produced at 450 billion per capsule) containing eight organisms: *Lactobacillus casei, Lactobacillus plantarum, L. acidophilus, Lactobacillus dulbreueckii,* subspecies *Bulgaris, Bifidobacterium longtum, Bifidobacterium breve, Bifidobacterium infantis, and Streptococcus salivarius.* They studied 40 patients in a randomized, controlled fashion versus mesalamine and found that only 20% of the subjects had endoscopic relapse on VSL#3 and 40% with relapse on mesalamine. Therefore, it appears that probiotics do have a positive effect in three of the four studies and that the variation may be because of the type of probiotic that is used.

Pouchitis

Pouchitis is inflammation that occurs in a pouch made of ileum to increase the reservoir for feces after total colectomy and attaching the ileum to the anus.

There has been a great deal of effort in evaluating the use of VSL#3 in the treatment and prevention of pouchitis. The studies were double-blinded and placebo-controlled and showed that probiotic therapy maintains remission after antibiotic therapy and is effective in preventing the onset of pouchitis.[75,76] The first reports studied patients who were receiving antibiotic therapy before the maintenance was attempted. In those studies, the relapse rate on the probiotic was 10% to 15%, and the relapse rate on placebo was 94% to 100%.[47,48] In those patients who were employed in a preventative program, only 10% developed pouchitis on the probiotic, whereas 40% developed it on a placebo.[75] In a long-term reuse study, 36 patients were randomized (20 received VSL and 16 received placebo), all of which experienced at least two attacks of pouchitis in the year before the study. Remission was maintained by 85% of subjects on probiotic and by only one patient (6%) on the placebo. The last study was an international study employing patients in two countries, and the data appears to reveal that this eight-organism probiotic is effective in treating and preventing pouchitis.

It also has been demonstrated that there are changes in the mucosal bacteria that result in a switch from internal to surface antigen/antibody reactivity of a predominantly IGG1 type, which leads to greater opsonisation of a respiratory burst in lymphocytes, which provides a mechanism for maintaining the inflammatory state in ulcerative colitis.[61] Recent reviews on the subject have also concluded that probiotics can be effective in IBD, but the type of organism and the dose used are to be considered in each type of IBD.[77]

Irritable Bowel Syndrome

Recent literature includes reports of five controlled studies on the use of probiotics. Three studies demonstrated some benefit,[45,78,79] one showed a trend to improve patients' diarrhea,[80] and one reported no benefits.[81] The first study that demonstrated a benefit reported that patients experienced decreased abdominal pain and symptoms with the use of *Lactobacillus plantarum* (*L. plantarum*).[45] However, another study using the same organism but in lower doses showed no effect.[81] A double-blind study reported that *L. plantarum* appeared to provide significant benefit over placebo in that abdominal pain was markedly reduced.[78] In other studies with *Lactobacillus GG*, there were little symptom changes in most patients but those with diarrhea did seem to normalize bowel movement.[80] In the study utilizing VSL#3 (eight organisms in a 450 billion dose per day), 25 patients were randomized to either the probiotic or placebo twice daily for 8 weeks; after a 2 week run-in, patients experienced significant decreases in abdominal bloating.[79] All these patients had diarrhea, but sophisticated transit studies revealed no difference between the placebo and the experimental group.[79] In a large, anecdotal, uncontrolled evaluation of patients, a significant improvement was recorded.[82] All of the data reveals a controversial picture as to whether probiotics are helpful in IBS, with some proponents and some who feel there is no significant help.

Miscellaneous Claims

Numerous claims have been made for the effectiveness of probiotics. Tannock[83] reports that these claims include increased resistance to infectious diseases, decreased duration of diarrhea, reduced blood pressure, reduced serum cholesterol concentration, reduced allergy, stimulation of phagocytosis by peripheral blood leukocytes, modulation of cytosine gene expression, adjuvant effect, regression of tumors, and reduced carcinogen or co-carcinogen production. Unfortunately, the literature does not substantiate most of these claims. The acceptance of these claims is confounded by use of numerous organisms in the studies and a lack of proven viability of the preparations. The huge number of variables makes interpretation difficult, and consequently the claims cannot be accepted without more controlled studies. Review of the literature does substantiate use in infections and IBD, but more controlled data collection is necessary to prove the reliability of the other claims.

Dietary Fiber

Definition

Dietary fiber is nonstarch polysaccharide in plant food that is poorly digested by human enzymes. There is still some controversy in defining dietary fiber, but this author chooses this simple definition. The history of its importance in human health and disease began with the work of surgeon Cleave.[84] In his theories and writings, he attributed most of the degenerative diseases of our western society to increased simple sugar intake. He pointed out that a marked increase in the intake of sugar was associated with the processing of food so that westernized people ate more sugar and more starch.[84] He began to promulgate these theories in the second half of the 20th century. In 1975, the noted epidemiologists Dennis Burkett and Hugh Trowell began to publish their observations on the importance of a refined carbohydrate as a possible cause of disease associated with the deficiency of dietary fiber intake.[85,86] These theories began to reach the scientific community of the western world, and by late in the 20th century, they were accepted.[87-89]

Classification: Chemical and Physical Properties

The fiber component of plant foods is extremely complex chemically. Its analysis has been a problem for food scientists. At the onset of interest in dietary fiber, the estimates of the food content were made by crude fiber analysis. This consisted mostly of cellulose and lignin. However, this underestimated fiber content of food. Further study of fiber physiology elucidated that both soluble and insoluble components were necessary to determine the total fiber content and the crude fiber methods did not measure soluble fiber. Food scientists then created appropriate techniques to measure both of these components. Early chemists working in the field—Asp, Englyst, Southgate, and Theander—gradually developed techniques that were able to define the total fiber, nonstarch polysaccharides, and soluble and insoluble components.[90] The final determination that there is both an insoluble and soluble component and their relationship to bacterial fermentation and the effects on the GI tract function was instrumental in understanding the role of fiber in health and disease.

The methods of Englyst demonstrated that, after extraction of substances, the dietary fiber could be broken down into soluble and insoluble as well as cellulose components. It is in these forms that the physiologic properties

TABLE 11-5.

Dietary Fiber Components of Foods[88]

Classical Nomenclature	*Solubility Characteristics*	*Classes of Polysaccharide*
		Plant Cell Wall Components
Pectic substances	Water Soluble	Galacturonans Arabinogalactans ß-glucans Arabinoxylans
Hemicelluloses	Insoluble in water	Arabinoxylans Galactomannans
	Soluble in alkali	Xyloglucans
a-cellulose	Insoluble in alkali	Cellulose (glucan)
Lignin	Insoluble in 12 M H_2SO_4	Lignin (Klason) Noncarbohydrate
		Nonstructural Components
Gums	Water Soluble or	Galactomannans Arabinogalactans
Mucilages	Dispersible	Wide range of branched and substituted galactans

are best understood. Insoluble components are primarily in the plant cell walls and are cellulose, noncellulose polysaccharides, lignin, waxes, proteins, and ash. The soluble components are primarily hemicelluloses, and today we include gums and mucilages in that category. The components are listed in Table 11-5. Our present understanding clearly indicates that there is very poor fermentation by the intestinal microflora of the insoluble component, whereas the soluble components are readily fermented.[89,90]

Dietary fiber produces very special effects in the intestinal ecology because of its physical properties.[91] Each property is important.

1. The particle size will vary with processing and can affect the physical properties.
2. Polysaccharides may be hydrophilic and, hence, have a water-holding capacity. Cellulose is very limited in its swelling property, whereas other polysaccharides will swell greatly; therefore, the food's ability to hold water will depend on the type of polysaccharide content. The water-holding capacity of insoluble fibers is important in maintaining a larger and softer stool. Insoluble fibers that are poorly fermented by bacteria and that hold onto water will best serve this purpose, as the insoluble fibers are not fermented.
3. Ion binding appears to be an important function of certain fibers. These tend to hold onto ions; yet, when they are fermented, the ions become completely free. Polysaccharides containing neuronic acid and lignin components of the fiber have an acidophilic function that reacts with ions. Zinc, iron, and calcium are readily bound and readily freed in the intestinal ecology. Bile acids may also be bound and free. This is a very dynamic process: it brings certain ions to where they are best absorbed or removes them if they are harmful.
4. Fermentation occurs because of a wide range of the intestinal microflora. When the diet contains more soluble fiber that enhances the growth of bacteria, the result is a larger stool, which is made up of bacterial mass.

From a practical point of view, it is important to note that wheat bran is 90% insoluble, oat bran is 50% insoluble and 50% soluble, and psyllium is 90% soluble. Fruits are a major contributor to our intake of soluble fiber.

Nonstarch polysaccharides, cellulose, hemicellulose, pectins, beta-glucans, fructans, gums, mucilages, and oligopolysaccharides are a few of the many carbohydrates in food. The other polysaccharides are starch, amylose, amylopectin, and modified food starches. Other carbohydrates are monosaccharide, disaccharides, and oligosaccharides; the latter (oligosaccharides) are poorly digested by human enzymes and are digested in the fermentation process.[90,91]

MECHANISMS RESULTING IN BENEFIT

Effect on Gastrointestinal Function

Almost all the plants that humans consume contain a mixture of carbohydrates. The nonstarch polysaccharides have specific effects, as opposed to the starch component. They tend to increase satiety and slow gastric emptying; they may have an inhibitory effect on pancreatic enzyme activity and may slow the rate of absorption, particularly if they are free of simple carbohydrates; and they increase stool bulk either by their hydrophilic action or by enhancing bacterial growth as a nutrient in fermentation. In addition, the fermentation process produces SCFA. (Those benefits are described under fermentation, which is discussed above.) Fibers may vary in their ability to slow mouth-to-fecal transit time. It is a complicated interface. For example, guar gum can delay hydrogen-to-breath time, whereas bran and other gums can have lesser effect, and pectin and cellulose have no effect.[91]

From a metabolic point of view, the glycemic index and glycemic load have a great effect on glucose blood levels and insulin metabolism. Jenkins first emphasized the importance of the glycemic index, and it is now firmly established that foods vary in this chemical index; however, controversy still exists as to its importance.[92] Most researchers agree that the glycemic index is a measure of overall glycemic response and insulin demand.[93] The glycemic index varies with the dietary fiber content; in general, refined grain products and potatoes have a high glycemic index, whereas legumes and unprocessed grains have a moderate glycemic index, and nonstarch fruit and vegetables have a low glycemic index.[94]

There is no question that there is physiologic benefit in the ability of pectin and gums to lower serum cholesterol and modify blood lipids in humans.[95,96] Although controversy still exists on which water-soluble dietary fibers have the greatest benefit, most nutrition experts accept the frequently demonstrated lipid-lowering effect of soluble fiber. This has repeatedly been demonstrated for soluble fibers.[97-100]

Fermentation and Short-Chain Fatty Acids

The matrix that exists in the colon, with its huge bacterial population of aerobes and anaerobes, ferments soluble fibers at a rate 10 times greater than that of insoluble fibers. SCFA are produced and are pivotal for the health of the colon and for control of cholesterol metabolism. The most abundant SCFA are acidic, propionic, and butyric.[101-103] In the right colon, they are at a molecular ratio of 57 for acetate, 22 for propionate, and 21 for butyrate. The ratios remain relatively the same in the left colon. However, when measured in the portal vein, the acetic rises to 71, the propionate stays at 21, and the butyrate falls to 8. The peripheral blood acitic has a molecular ratio of 91 to 5 to 4. More SCFA are produced than are excreted; the difference is presumably because of the amount absorbed.[102] SCFA are rapidly absorbed from the colon lumen in a concentration dependent upon and associated with the appearance of bicarbonate in the lumen and with the absorption of water and sodium.[101,102] Total SCFA titers appear to be negligible in the jejunum, higher in the ileum, and more than 10 times higher in the cecum.[101] Butyrate is the preferred energy source for colonocytes. Using isolated surface epithelial cells, it was shown that 70% to more than 80% of the energy needs for colonic mucosa were obtained from butyrate. Butyrate is more important in the distal as compared to the proximal colon.[104,105] In addition, acetate and propionate appear to have some controlling mechanisms on the development and maintenance of cholesterol.[106]

Intake, Contents in Foods, and Therapeutic Recommendations

The amount of dietary fiber that is ingested varies greatly from society to society and from individual to individual. The landmark studies of Burkett, Trowell, and Walker revealed that in underdeveloped countries as much as 60 to 80 g of dietary fiber were ingested daily.[85,86,89] This was as a result of the high cereal and grain intake in Asia and Africa. In western societies, studies clearly indicate that as little as 5 to 10 g of dietary fiber are eaten daily.[107] In westernized societies, the great variation is certainly due to lifestyle and availability of foods, as well as the advent of processed foods.[84] The classic busy executive of western society who is too hurried to eat breakfast, rushes through lunch, and then eats a large, protein fat dinner is a victim of low dietary fiber, as compared to the native of Africa who eats only maize for his or her meal. However, as the importance of dietary fiber is gaining worldwide interest, more balanced diets appear to be developing on a worldwide basis. Table 11-6 lists the common foods available and their total fiber, soluble fiber, and insoluble fiber content. (For more detailed information, the reader is referred to the appropriate references.[88,108,109])

On a practical basis, depending on the individual, his or her lifestyle, and the society, the dietary fiber intake varies with the foods available and consequently eaten. Therapeutic recommendation for intake is currently between 20 to 35 g/day of dietary fiber, but that depends on the consumer's size and caloric intake. Someone who requires 1,000 kcal/day will certainly eat less fiber than will someone who requires 2,000. Most fruits and vegetables will average approximately 3 to 5 g per portion, cereals and grains 5 to 10 g per portion, and wheat breads 2 to 5 g per portion. Therefore, an individual can train him- or herself to eat from 6 to 8 food choices of dietary fiber per day to maintain the recommended intake.

On another note, some individuals may require more soluble fiber and others more insoluble fiber. Bloating may be caused by one type of fiber and not the other. Therefore, ideal intake requires individual experimentation. Some subjects can metabolize legumes with ease, for example, whereas others cannot. Hyperlipidemia patients should have more soluble fiber intake; the recommendation is oats and psyllium for that individual rather than wheat. All of these variations must be considered on an individual basis, but the generalities are certainly acceptable for the healthy individual practicing preventative medicine.

Clinical Utilization

Prevention of Coronary Heart Disease and Lipid Control

The classic Zutphen Study on 10-year mortality and dietary fiber intake was started in 1960 and published 1982.[110] In that study in the Netherlands, 871 middle-aged men were enrolled and interviewed using a careful cross-check dietary history method. During the 10 years of follow-up, 107 men died from all causes. Of those, 37 had coronary heart disease, and 44 had cancer. The dietary fiber intake was divided into quintiles, and the mortality from coronary heart disease was four times higher in men from the quintile receiving the lowest amount than in those from the highest quintile. Rates from cancer and all other causes were approximately three times higher in the lowest quintile. An earlier study in Great Britain clearly indicated the importance of high dietary fiber in the pre-

TABLE 11-6.

Soluble, Insoluble, and Total Dietary Fiber Contents of Common Foods[88,108,109]

	Size of Serving	Soluble Fiber Content per Serving (g)	Insoluble Fiber Content per Serving (g)	Total Fiber Content per Serving (g)
Vegetables				
(cooked, unless otherwise noted)				
Asparagus	¾ cup	.8	2.3	3.1
Bean Sprouts, raw	½ cup	.3	1.3	1.6
Beans				
Green	½ cup	.5	1.6	2.1
Kidney	½ cup	2.5	3.3	5.8
Lima	½ cup	1.1	3.2	4.4
Pinto	½ cup	2.0	3.3	5.3
White	½ cup	1.4	3.6	5.0
Broccoli	½ cup	.9	1.1	2.0
Brussel Sprouts	½ cup	1.6	2.3	3.9
Cabbage	½ cup	.9	1.1	2.0
Carrots	1-7 in.	1.1	1.2	2.3
Cauliflower	½ cup	.4	.6	1.0
Celery, raw	½ cup	.4	.9	1.3
Corn, kernels	½ cup	1.7	2.2	3.9
Eggplant	½ cup	.8	1.2	2.0
Kale	½ cup	1.4	1.4	2.8
Lettuce, raw	½ cup	.1	.2	.3
Okra	½ cup	1.0	3.1	4.1
Onions, raw	½ cup	.8	1.8	2.6
Peas	½ cup	.4	2.8	3.2
Potatoes				
Sweet, baked	½ large	.7	1.0	1.7
White, baked	½ medium	1.0	1.0	1.9
Radishes, raw	5 medium	.1	.5	.6
Squash				
Acorn	½ cup	.5	3.8	4.3
Zucchini	½ cup	1.3	1.4	2.7
Tomato, raw	1 medium	.2	.6	.8
Turnip	½ cup	.8	.9	1.7
Zucchini	½ cup	.5	.7	1.2
Fruits (raw)				
Apple, with skin	1	.8	2.0	2.8
Apricots	2	.7	.8	1.5
Avocado	1/8 fresh	.5	.7	1.2
Banana	½ medium	.3	.7	1.0
Blackberries	½ cup	.7	3.9	4.5
Cherries	10	.3	.9	1.2
Figs	1 ½	1.1	1.2	2.3
Grapefruit	½ medium	.6	1.1	1.7
Grapes	12	.1	.4	.5
Mango	1 medium	1.9	2.2	4.1
Melon, cantaloupe	1 cup	.3	.8	1.1
Orange	1 small	.3	.9	1.2
Peach	1 medium	.6	1.0	1.6
Pear	½ medium	.5	2.0	2.5
Pineapple	½ cup	.3	.9	1.2
Plums	3 small	.7	1.1	1.8
Raspberries	¾ cup	.4	6.4	6.8
Strawberries	¾ cup	.7	1.3	2.0

continued

TABLE 11-6, CONTINUED.

	Size of Serving	Soluble Fiber Content per Serving (g)	Insoluble Fiber Content per Serving (g)	Total Fiber Content per Serving (g)
Grain Products				
Bread				
Bagel, plain	½	.3	.4	.7
French	1 slice	.3	.7	1.0
Rye	1 slice	.3	.6	.9
White enriched	1 slice	.3	.3	.5
Whole wheat	1 slice	.3	1.4	1.2
Cereal				
All-Bran (100%)	1/3 cup	1.7	7.0	8.6
Corn Flakes	1 cup	.2	.3	.4
Shredded Wheat	1 biscuit	.4	2.4	2.8
Fiber One	½ cup	.8	11.1	11.9
Raisin Bran	¾ cup	.9	4.4	5.3
Oatmeal (oats)	1/3 cup	1.4	1.3	2.7
Crackers				
Graham	2 squares	.5	2.3	2.8
Saltine	6 crackers	.3	.4	.7
Rice				
Brown	½ cup	.2	2.2	2.4
White	½ cup.	.01	.09	.1
Spaghetti	½ cup	.3	.5	.8
Nuts				
Almonds	1 tbsp.	.1	1.0	1.1
Cashews	1 cup	.5	7.3	7.8
Pistachio	1 cup	3.4	10.4	13.8
Peanuts, roasted	10	.2	.4	.6
	1 cup	4.8	7.9	12.7

All-Bran, Shredded Wheat, Fiber One, and Raisin Bran are all registered trademarks.

vention of heart disease and as a factor in coronary heart disease.[111]

A pooled analysis of cohort studies published in 2004 reveals results consistent with the earlier studies.[112] The authors analyzed the original data from 10 perspective studies in the United States and Europe over a 6- to 10-year follow-up of 5,249 coronary cases and 2,011 coronary deaths among 91,058 men and 245,186 women; the data were adjusted for participants' body mass index, demographics, and lifestyle factors. The authors reported a 14% decrease in risk of low coronary events, and a 27% decrease in coronary artery death. They concluded that consumption of dietary fiber from cereals and fruits is inversely associated with the risk of coronary heart disease.

In a careful study measuring the intima-media thickness (IMT) of common carotid arteries using ultrasonography, it was found that there was clearly an inverse association between IMT progression and the intake of visgus fiber and pectin. The authors of this study concluded that the intake of visgus fiber, especially pectin, appears to protect against IMT progression.[113]

Similarly to coronary artery disease and arteriosclerosis, fruits and vegetable intake appears to correlate with a decreased incidence of stroke in men.[114]

The mechanism by which dietary fiber impairs the progression of arteriosclerosis and stroke appears to be in lipid control. Pectin, guar gum, and cereals containing a high percentage of soluble fiber clearly have a positive protective effect on the lipid profile.[115-117] However, some controversy exists on the use of whole grain substances. The Iowa Women's Health Study reveals the clear inverse association between whole grain intake and the risk of ischemic heart disease.[118] The authors of that study pointed out that whole grain foods contain many vital chemicals and antioxidants that may be helpful, in addition to the dietary fiber. It should also be pointed out that grains vary in their soluble fiber content and, hence, the grains containing more soluble fiber would clearly be more helpful than are those containing less. In addition, selective dietary fiber foods such as nuts have also demonstrated that there is an inverse association between their consumption and total coronary heart disease death rates.[119]

From all of this information, the composite opinion of epidemiologists and molecular biologists is that the higher intake of dietary fiber is beneficial in the prevention and probably in treatment of atherosclerotic diseases.

Diabetes Mellitus

A careful assessment and meta-analysis of the evidence of carbohydrate and fiber intake in diabetic individuals recommends that they should be encouraged to achieve and maintain a desirable body weight and the diet should provide 55% carbohydrate, 12% to 15% protein, and less than 30% fat, with monosaturated fat 12% to 15%.[120] In addition, the diet should provide 25 to 50 g/day of dietary fiber or 15 to 25 g per 1,000-kcal intake. In addition, the glycemic index information should be incorporated into all food exchange education. The glycemic index is discussed above, and studies clearly indicate that it is an important factor in both young and old.[92,121] The data clearly reveals that the dietary effect is due to dietary fiber, but there are many subtle physiologic events that are related to specific foods. An example of this is the role of fruit and fruit juice in satiety and glucose and insulin metabolism.[122] The fiber content can be demonstrated to be effective since whole fruits have a positive effect, whereas the juice of the fruit does not. (Nutrition as it relates to diabetes is discussed in detail in Chapter 16.)

Constipation and Bowel Movement Regulation

As mentioned above, it is well accepted that dietary fiber, through its water-holding capacity and its ability to increase the colonic microflora, will successfully treat constipation of dietary origin. The effects are clearly described for all dietary fiber foods, but there is a definite variation with the type of food and the degree of soluble or insoluble content.[88,89,91,123] A careful study combining wheat bran with resistant starch has also shown that the combination is more beneficial—it can have more effect on transit time and stool size, as well as output of important SCFA.[124] Therefore, it is important that the physician and nutritionist recognize that there is individual variation and that the diet recommendations will have to vary from individual to individual. Starting with a high-soluble fiber supplemented diet maybe beneficial, but an individual may have to have a high bran intake.[124] Remembering simple facts—such as wheat bran is 90% insoluble, oat bran is 50% insoluble, and psyllium seed is 90% soluble—are important to designing the correct plan for individual patients. In addition, transit time may increase or decrease and bulk may increase or decrease with various fibers.

Diverticular Disease

Epidemiologic and anatomic studies reveal that diverticular formation in the colon is primarily a disease of industrialized and westernized population.[89,125,126] The association is made with the decreased dietary fiber intake of westernized societies so that it is well accepted that diverticular formation is related to the long-term decrease in dietary fiber. This association is made also with the understanding that physiologic phenomena, such as increased colonic force of contraction and decreased colon fiber, are important in the development of the diverticular.[126,127] Sixty percent of humans living in westernized countries over the age of 60 years will develop diverticular, and 5% of those will develop some complications.[128-130]

A lifespan study in rats offered strong support for the theory that diverticular disease is due to fiber deficiency. Studying 1,800 rats in nine diet groups demonstrated significant relationships between fiber intake, fecal output, and transit time and the development of true acquired diverticular both in single and multiple occurrences.[131]

There have been few recent trials, but older studies using unprocessed bran to treat patients with symptomatic diverticular disease showed benefit.[132-135] There have been some conflicting studies[136] and not enough in the literature to perform a clear meta-analysis.

Given the high incidence of diverticular formation and diverticulitis with all of its complications of abscess and perforation, it behooves clinicians to recommend a high fiber intake. The use of fiber once diverticular have developed has not yet been established as a preventative of diverticulitis. In addition, once diverticulitis has developed, the patient's fiber intake should decrease in the acute phase, and, once the acute attack and symptoms are relieved, the patient should return to a regular or recommended high fiber diet intake.[127]

Irritable Bowel Syndrome

The literature is controversial on the use of bran in the treatment of IBS.[137] Although there was great enthusiasm on the possibility of bran helping patients with IBS, particularly those with constipation,[136] more detailed studies such as the one performed on 100 consecutive outpatients fulfilling the ROME criteria, revealed that actually 55% were made worse, whereas only 10% found it helpful.[138] IBS is a very complex syndrome, with some patients having diarrhea, some having constipation, and some having abdominal pain. Therefore, the treatment with diet will require individual association and breakdown of groups before there can be any clear picture as to which patients are helped. Nevertheless, if there is an irritable bowel patient with a dietary constipation, the treatment of that patient as described under constipation will be helpful.

Colon Neoplasia

Early epidemiologic evidence[85,86,139,140] clearly indicated an association of low dietary fiber intake with colorectal polyp and cancer formation. The epidemiologic studies of Burkett and Trowell seemed overwhelming, but prospective questionnaire studies[139] and prospective case controlled studies showed varied support.[140] A careful analysis of the literature completed a decade later that included more recent prospective studies supports the theory but questioned the importance of dietary fiber because of the muddled relationship of high-fat, low fat-fiber overlap.[140] Prospective studies employing a variety of questionnaires, including 1-day and 3-day diet histories and food choice analyses, revealed no standard effect by fruit, vegetables, and cereal fibers but selective effects as emphasized by the Australian polyp study, which showed that large polyps were decreased but small polyps were not.[140,141]

Interventional studies in which high fiber diets were used as chemo-preventive agents are lacking. One convincing follow-up study performed by DeCosse, in which patients with familial adnomenous polyposis were placed on fiber supplements, revealed a decrease in the number of polyps formed in patients on supplemental fiber.[143] The study was convincing but is not yet reproduced, and other interventional studies have revealed conflicting results.[141]

The American Gastroenterology Association issued a position statement as follows:

> "Currently available evidence from epidemiological, animal and interventional studies does not unequivocally support the protective role of fiber in its development of colorectal cancer. However, when the whole body of evidence from these studies is analyzed critically, the overall conclusion supports an inverse association between dietary fiber intake and colorectal cancer risk."[141]

The recommendations include decreasing consumption of fat and red meat, avoiding obesity, consuming minimal to moderate amounts of alcohol, quitting smoking, engaging in daily physical activity, and increasing total fiber intake to greater than 30 to 35 g/day for the standard North American diet. These recommendations will potentially prevent colorectal cancer and will provide other health benefits.[141]

Inflammatory Bowel Disease

SCFA are an important product of bacterial fermentation, as discussed above. The connection between SCFA and colitis was first established by Harig et al with the treatment of four patients with diversion colitis.[144] These were patients whose distal colon was taken out of the normal fecal stream for surgical reasons. When the distal separated bowel was treated with SCFA, remission of the colitis occurred. Histologic, endoscopic, and metabolic similarities between diversion colitis and ulcerative colitis are suggestive of a nutritional SCFA deficiency.[105]

Experimental inhibition of fatty acid oxidation in the colonic mucosa results in acute colitis similar to acute ulcerative colitis.[145] Decreased fecal concentrations of SCFA have also been demonstrated in patients with ulcerative colitis.[146] There is also evidence that suggest that the ulcerative colitis mucosa is unable to metabolize SCFA in some form of a metabolic block.[146] Therefore, the experimental evidence indicates that treatment with SCFA would be helpful in ulcerative colitis. Butyric acid has been shown to be the main fuel for colonocytes; therefore, the treatment with butyric acid enemas has been tried in ulcerative colitis. Initial treatment in small studies reveal very encouraging results in that bathing the colon with butyric acid in molecular concentrations of 40 to 80 resulted in significant improvement in both children and adults.[147-152] However, a carefully controlled study with 103 patients from several institutions using topical SCFA twice daily revealed conflicting results.[153] Some seemed to improve with early treatment and others did not. In addition, there appeared to be a subset of patients with distal ulcerative colitis of short episodes that seemed to gain the most improvement. The consensus opinion from the data was that this treatment could not be recommended consistently.[153]

Although the use of SCFA is controversial, its importance in the treatment of diversion colitis and the observations that it is important in colonocyte metabolism indicate that dietary fiber and substances that stimulate the normal growth of the intestinal microflora are extremely important for the health of the colonocytes. If not used as the treatment, it should be considered in the recovery and maintenance of normal colonocytes growth. Therefore, it follows that dietary fiber is important in normal colonocytes function and health.

Conclusion

Dietary fiber is probably the best prebiotic. In tying prebiotics, probiotics, and dietary fiber together, it is important to emphasize that intestinal microecology is dependent on a matrix within the colon. An important part of that matrix is food to maintain a healthy bacterial flora. The key food appears to be dietary fiber. When disease occurs, prebiotics and probiotics may be helpful.

References

1. Gibson GR, Roberfroid MB. Dietary modulation of the human colonic microbiotia: introducing the concept of prebiotics. *J Nutr.* 1995;125:1401-1412.
2. Crittenden RG. Prebiotics. In: Tannock GW, ed. *Probiotics: A Critical Review.* Wymondham, UK: Horizon Scientific Press; 1999:141-156.
3. Cummings JH, Macfarlane GT, Englyst HN. Prebiotic digestion and fermentation. *Am J Clin Nutr.* 2001;73(Suppl):415S-420S.
4. Rastall RA, Gibson GR. Prebiotic oligosaccharides: evaluation of biological activities and potential future developments. In: Tannock GW, ed. *Probiotics and Prebiotics: Where Are We Going?* Wymondham, England: Caister Academic Press; 2002:107-148.
5. Ellegard L, Andersson H, Bosaeus I. Inulin and oligofructose do not influence the absorption of cholesterol, or the excretion of cholesterol, Ca, Mg, Zn, Fe, or bile acids but increases energy excretion in ileostomy subject. *Eur J Clin Nutr.* 1997:51(1)1-5.
6. Cashman K. Prebiotics and calcium bioavailability. In: Tannock GW, ed. *Probiotics and Prebiotics: Where Are We Going?* Wymondham, England: Caister Academic Press; 2002:149-174
7. Roberfroid MB, Van Loo JAE, Gibson GR. The bifidogenic nature of inulin and its hydrolysis products. *J Nutr.* 1998;128:11-19.
8. Floch MH, Hong-Curtiss J. Probiotics, irritable bowel syndrome, and inflammatory bowel disease. *Curr Treat Op in Gastro.* 2003;6:283-288.
9. Gibson GR, Beatty ER, Wang X. Cummings JH. Selective stimulations of bifidobacteria in the human colon by oligofructose and inulin. *Gastroenterology.* 1995;108:975-982.
10. Macfarlane GT, Cummings JH. Probiotics and prebiotics: can regulating the activities of intestinal bacteria benefit health? *BMJ.* 1999;318:999-1003.
11. Ballongue J, Schumann C, Quignon P. Effects of lactulose and lactitol on colonic microflora and enzymatic activity. *Scand J Gastroenterol.* 1997;32(Suppl):222:41-44.
12. Elkington SG, Floch MH, Conn HO. Lactulose in the treatment of chronic portal-systemic encephalopathy. *N Engl J Med.* 1969;281:408-411.
13. Benno Y, Endo K, Shiragami N, et al. Effects of raffinose intake on human fecal microflora. *Bifidobacteria Microflora.* 1987;6:59-63.
14. Hara T, Ikeda N, Hatsumi K, et al. Effects of small amount ingestion of soybean oligosaccharides on bowel habits and fecal flora of volunteers. *Jap J Nutr.* 1997;55:79-84 (In Japanese).
15. Klessen B, Sykura B, Zunfit HJ. Effects of inulin and lactose on fecal microflora, microbial activity, and bowel habit in elderly constipated persons. *Am J Clin Nutr.* 1997;65:1397-1402.
16. Olesen M, Gudmand-Hoyer E. Efficacy, safety, and tolerability of fructooligosaccharides in the treatment of irritable bowel syndrome. *Am J Clin Nutr.* 2000;72(6):1570-5.

17. Hunter JO, Tuffnell Q, Lee AJ. Controlled trial of oligofructose in the management of irritable bowel syndrome. *J Nutr.* 1999;129(7 Suppl):1451S-3S.
18. Kanauchi O, Mitsuyama K, Araki Y, Andoh A. Modification of intestinal flora in the treatment of inflammatory bowel disease. *Curr Pharm Design.* 2003;9:333-346.
19. Kanauchi O, Mitsuyama K, Homma T, et al. Treatment of ulcerative colitis patients by long-term administration of germinated barley foodstuff: multi-center open trial. *Intern J Molec Med.* 2003;12(5):701-4.
20. Yamashita K, Kawai K, Itakura M. Effects of fructooligosaccharides on blood glucose and serum lipids in diabetic subjects. *Nutr Res.* 1984;4:961-966.
21. Davidson MH, Maki KC, Synecki C, et al. Effects of dietary inulin on serum lipids in men and women with hypercholesterolemia. *Nutr Res.* 1998;18:503-517.
22. Bukowska H. Pieczul-Mroz J, Jastrzebska M, et al. Decrease in fibrinogen and LDL-cholesterol levels upon supplementation of diet with Lactobacillus plantarum in subjects with moderately elevated cholesterol. *Atherosclerosis.* 1997;137:437-8.
23. Naruszewicz M, Johansson M-L, Zapolska-Downar D, et al. Effect of Lactobacillus plantarum 299v on cardiovascular disease risk factors in smokers. *Am J Clin Nutr.* 2002;76:1249-55.
24. Fuller R. Probiotics in man and animals. *J Appl Bacteriol.* 1989;66:365-378.
25. Metchnikoff E. *The Prolongation of Life: Optimistic Studies.* London: Butterworth-Heinemann; 1907.
26. Kipeloff N. *Lactobacillus Acidophilus.* Baltimore: Williams & Wilkins; 1926.
27. Rettger LF, Levy MN, Weinstein L, et al. *Lactobacillus Acidophilus and Its Therapeutic Application.* London: Yale University Press; 1935.
28. Freter R. The fatal enteric cholera infection in the guinea pig achieved by inhibition of normal enteric flora. *J Infect Dis.* 1955;97:57-64.
29. Lilly DM, Stillwell RH. Probiotics: growth promoting factors produced by micro-organisms. *Science.* 1965;147:747-748.
30. Montrose D, Floch MH. Probiotics used in human studies. *J Clin Gastroenterol.* 2005;39:469.
31. Sanders ME, Klaenhammer TR. The scientific basis of Lactobacillus acidophilus NCFM functionality as a probiotic. *J Dairy Sci.* 2001;84:319-331.
32. Floch MH, Hong-Curtiss J. Probiotics and functional foods in gastrointestinal disorders. *Curr Gastro Rep.* 2001;3:343-350.
33. Bernet MF, Brassart D, Nesser JR, et al. Lactobacillus acidophilus LA-1 binds to cultured human intestinal cell-lines and inhibits cell attachment and cell invasion by enterovirulent bacteria. *Gut.* 1994;35:483-489.
34. Lidbeck A, Overnick E, Rafter J, et al. Effect of Lactobacillus acidophilus supplements on mutagen excretion in feces and urine in humans. *Microb Ecol Health Dis.* 1992;5:59-67.
35. Salminen S, Deighton MA, Gorbach SL. Lactic acid bacteria in health and disease. In: von Wright SS, ed. *Lactic Acid Bacteria.* New York: Marcel Dekker; 1993:199-225.
36. Kaila M, Isolauri E, Soppi E, et al. Enhancement of the circulatory antibody screening cell response in human diarrhea by a human Lactobacillus strain. *Pediatr Res.* 1992;32:141-144.
37. Kaila M, Isolauri E, Saxelin M, et al. Viable versus inactivated Lactobacillus GG in acute rotavirus diarrhea. *Arch Dis Child.* 1995;72:51-53.
38. Majamaa H, Isolauri E, Saxelin M, Vesikari T. Lactic acid bacteria in the treatment of acute rotavirus gastroenteritis. *J Pediatr Gastroenterol Nutr.* 1995;14:107-111.
39. Gorbach SL. Probiotics and gastrointestinal health. *Am J Gastroenterol.* 2000;95(suppl):S2-S4.
40. Marteau P. Flourie B, Pochart P, et al. Effect of chronic ingestion of a fermented dairy product containing Lactobacillus acidophilus and Bifidobacterium bifidum on metabolic activities of the colonic flora in humans. *Am J Clin Nutr.* 1990;52:685-688.
41. Shornikova A-V, Casas I, Isolauri E, et al. Lactobacillus reuteri as a therapeutic agent in acute diarrhea in young children. *J Pediatr Gastroenterol Nutr.* 1997;24:399-404.
42. Wolf BW, Garleb DG, Casas I. Safety and tolerance of Lactobacillus reuteri in healthy adult male subjects. *Microb Ecol Health Dis.* 1995;8:41-50.
43. Surawicz CM, Elmer GW, Speelman P, et al. Prevention of antibiotic associated diarrhea by Saccharomyces boulardi: a prospective study. *Gastroenterology.* 1989;96:981-988.
44. Rembacken BJ, Snelling AM, Hawkey PM, et al. Non-pathogenic Escherichia coli versus mesalazine for the treatment of ulcerative colitis: a randomised trial. *Lancet.* 1999;354:635-9.
45. Nobaek S, Johansson M-L, Molin G, Ahrne S, et al. Alteration of intestinal microflora is associated with reduction in abdominal bloating and pain in patients with irritable bowel syndrome. *Am J Gastroenterol.* 2000;95:1231-1238.
46. Hilton E, Isenberg HD Alperstein P, et al. Ingestion of yogurt containing Lactobacillus acidophilus as prophylaxis for candidal vaginitis. *Ann Intern Med.* 1992;116:353-357.
47. Gionchetti P, Rizzello F, Venturi A, et al. Oral bacteriotherapy as maintenance treatment in patients with chronic pouchitis: a double-blind, placebo-controlled trial. *Gastroenterology.* 2000;119:305-309.
48. Mimura T, Rizzello F, Schreiber S, et al. Once daily high dose probiotic therapy maintains remission and improves quality of life in patients with recurrent or refractory pouchitis: a randomised, placebo-controlled, double-blind trial. *Gastroenterology.* 2002;122: A81.
49. McCracken UJ, Gasrins HR. probiotic and the immune system. In: Tannock GW, ed. *Probiotics: A Critical Review.* Norfolk, England: Horizon Scientific Press; 1999: 85-111.
50. Isolauri E, Sütas Y, Kankaapää P, et al. Probiotics: effects on immunity. *Am J Clin Nutr.* 2001;73(Suppl):444S-450S.
51. Jijon H, Backer J, Diaz H, et al. DNA from probiotic bacteria modulates murine and human epithelial and immune function. *Gastroenterology.* 2004;126:1358-1373.
52. Sheil B, McCarthy J, O'Mahony L, et al. Is the mucosal route of administration essential for probiotic function? Subcutaneous administration is associated with attenuation of murine colitis and arthritis. *Gut.* 2004;53:694-700.
53. Rutgeerts P, D'Haens G, Targan S, et al. Efficacy and safety of retreatment with anti-tumor necrosis factor antibody (infliximab) to maintain remission in Crohn's disease. *Gastroenterology.* 1999;117:761-769.
54. Borruel N, Carol M, Casellas F, et al. Increased mucosal tumour necrosis factor z production in Crohn's disease can be downregulated ex vivo by probiotic bacteria. *Gut.* 2002;51:659-664.
55. Mangell P, Nejdfors P, Wang M, et al. Lactobacillus plantarum 299v inhibits Escherichia coli-induced intestinal permeability. *Dig Dis Sci.* 2002;47:511-516.
56. Duggan C, Gannon J, Walker WA. Protective nutrients and functional foods for the gastrointestinal tract. *Am J Clin Nutr.* 2002;75:789-808.
57. Hasler CM. Functional foods: benefits, concerns and challenges—a position paper from the American Council on Science and Health. *Am Soc Nutr Sci.* 2002;3772-3781.
58. Huang JS, Bousvaros A, Lee JW, et al. Efficacy of probiotic use in acute diarrhea in children. A meta-analysis. *Dig Dis Sci.* 2002; 47:2625-2634.
59. Reid G. Probiotic agents to protect the urogenital tract against infection. *Am J Clin Nutr.* 2001;73(Suppl):437S-443S.
60. McLean NW, Rosenstein IJ. Characterization and selection of a Lactobacillus species to re-colonise the vagina of women with recurrent bacterial vaginosis. *J Med Microbiol.* 2000;49:543-552.
61. Furrie E, Macfarlane S, Cummings JH, Macfarlane GT. Systemic antibodies towards mucosal bacterial in ulcerative colitis and Crohn's disease differentially activate the innate immune response. *Gut.* 2004;53:91-98.

62. Schultsz C, Van Den Berg FM, Kate FW, et al. The intestinal mucus layer from patients with inflammatory bowel disease harbors high numbers of bacteria compared with controls. *Gastroenterology.* 1999;117:1089-1097.
63. Kleessen B, Koresen AJ, Buhr JH, Blaut M. Mucosal and invading bacteria in patients with inflammatory bowel disease compared with controls. *Scand J Gastroenterol.* 2002;37:1034-1041.
64. Seksik P, Rigottier-Gois L, Gramet G, et al. Alterations of the dominant feacal bacterial groups in patients with Crohn's disease of the colon. *Gut.* 2003;52:237-242.
65. Swidsinski A, Ladhoff A, Pernthaler A, et al. Mucosal flora in inflammatory bowel disease. *Gastroenterology.* 2002;122:44-54.
66. Kruis W, Schutz E, Fric P, et al. Double-blind comparison of an oral Escherichia coli preparation and mesalazine in maintaining remission of ulcerative colitis. *Aliment Pharmacol Ther.* 1997;11:853-858.
67. Kruis W, Kalk EK, Stolte M, et al. Maintenance of remission in ulcerative colitis is equally effective with Escherichia coli Nissle 1917 and with standard mesalamine. *Gastroenterology.* 2001;120: A127.
68. Ishikawa H, Akedo I, Umesaki Y, et al. Randomized controlled trial of the effect of bifidobacteria-fermented milk on ulcerative colitis. *J Amer Coll Nutr.* 2003;22:56-63.
69. Venturi A, Gionchetti P, Rizzello F, et al. Impact on the composition of the fecal flora by a new probiotic preparation: preliminary data on maintenance treatment of patients with ulcerative colitis. *Aliment Pharm and Ther.* 1999;13:1103-1108.
70. Karimi O, Pena AS, vanBodegraven AA. Probiotics (VSL#3) in arthralgia. Preliminary results of an ongoing open trial in patients with ulcerative colitis and Crohn's disease. *Gastroenterology.* 2004;126:A-627.
71. Plein K, Hotz J. Therapeutic effects of Saccharomyces boulardii on mild residual symptoms in a stable phase of Crohn's disease with special respect to chronic diarrhea-a pilot study. *Z Gastroenterol.* 1993;31:129-134.
72. Guslandi M, Messi G, Sorghi M, Testoni PA. Saccharomyces boulardii in maintenance treatment of Crohn's disease. *Dig Dis Sci.* 2000;45:1462-1464.
73. Campieri M, Rizzello F, Venturi A, et al. Combination of antibiotic and probiotic treatment is efficacious in prophylaxis of post-operative recurrent of Crohn's disease: a randomised controlled study versus mesalazine. *Gastroenterology.* 2000;118:A781.
74. Pantera C, Scribano ML, Falasco G, et al. Ineffectiveness of probiotics in preventing recurrence after curative resection for Crohn's disease. A randomized controlled trial with Lactobacillus GG. *Gut.* 2002;51:405-409.
75. Gionchetti P, Rizzello E, Ventoni A, et al. Prophylaxis of pouchitis onset with probiotic therapy: a double-blind placebo controlled trial. *Gastroenterology.* 2000;118:1214.
76. Mimura T, Rizzello F, Helwig U, et al. Once daily high dose probiotic therapy (VSL#3) for maintaining remission in recurrent or refractory pouchitis. *Gut.* 2004;53:108-114.
77. Hart AL, Stagg A, Kamm MA. Use of probiotics in the treatment of inflammatory bowel disease. *J Clin Gastroenterol.* 2003;36:111-119.
78. Niedzielin K, Kordecki H, Birkenfeld B. A controlled, double-blind, randomized study on the efficacy of Lactobacillus plantarum 299V in patients with irritable bowel syndrome. *Eur J Gastroenterol Hepatol.* 2001;13:1143-7.
79. Kim HJ, Camilleri M, McKinzie S, et al. A randomized controlled trial of a probiotic, VSL#3, on gut transit and symptoms in diarrhea-predominant irritable bowel syndrome. *Alim Pharm Ther.* 2003;17:895-904.
80. O'Sullivan MA, O'Morain CA. Bacterial supplementation in the irritable bowel syndrome. A randomised double-blind placebo-controlled crossover study. *Dig Liver Dis.* 2000;32:294-301.
81. Sen S, Mullan MM, Parker TJ, et al. Effect of Lactobacillus plantarum 299v on colonic fermentation and symptoms of irritable bowel syndrome. *Dig Dis Sci.* 2002;47:2615-20.
82. Faber SM. Irritable bowel syndrome and reinoculation with probiotics. *Am J Gastroenterol.* 2002;97:A211.
83. Tannock GW. *Probiotics: A Critical Review.* Wymondham, UK: Horizon Scientific Press; 1999.
84. Cleave TL. *The Saccharine Disease.* New Canaan, CT: Keats Publishing, Inc.; 1975.
85. Burkett DP, Trowell HC. *Refined Carbohydrate Foods and Disease: Some Implications of Dietary Fiber.* London: Academic Press, 1975.
86. Burkett DP, Walker ARP, Painter NS. Dietary fiber and disease *JAMA.* 1974;229:1068-1074.
87. Vahouny GV, Kritzhevsky D. *Dietary Fiber.* New York: Plenum Press; 1986.
88. Spiller GA. *Dietary Fiber in Human Nutrition.* 2nd ed. Boca Raton, FL: CRC Press, Inc.; 1993.
89. Trowell H, Burkett D, Heaton K. *Dietary Fibre, Fibre-Depleted Foods and Disease.* London: Academic Press; 1985.
90. Asp, N-GL. Classification and methodology of food carbohydrates as related to nutritional effects. *Am J Clin Nutr.* 1995;61(Suppl):930S-7S.
91. Cummings JH, Englyst HN. Gastrointestinal effects of food carbohydrate. *Am J Clin Nutr.* 1995;61(Suppl)938S-45S.
92. Jenkins DJ, Wolever TM, Taylor RH, et al. Glycemic index of foods: a physiological basis for carbohydrate exchange. *Am J Clin Nutr.* 1981;34:362-6.
93. Ludwig DS, Eckel RH. The glycemic index at 20 y. *Am J Clin Nutr.* 2002;76(Suppl);264S-5S.
94. Foster-Powell K, Holt SHA, Brand-Miller JC. International table of glycemic index and glycemic load values: 2002. *Am J Clin Nutr.* 2002;76:5-56.
95. Baig MM, Cerda JJ. Pectin: its interaction with serum lipoproteins. *Am J Clin Nutr.* 1981;34:50-53.
96. Ross AHM, Eastwood MA, Anderson JR, et al. A study of the effects of dietary gum arabic in humans. *Am J Clin Nutr.* 1983;37:368-375.
97. Jensen CD, Spiller GA, Gates JE, et al. The effect of acacia gum and a water-soluble dietary fiber mixture on blood lipids in humans. *J Am Coll Nutr.* 1993;12:147-154.
98. Anderson JW, Story L, Sieling B, et al. Hypocholesterolemic effects of oat-bran or bean intake for hypercholesterolemic men. *Am J Clin Nutr.* 1984;40:1146-1155.
99. Demark-Wahnefried W, Bowering J, Cohen PS. Reduced serum cholesterol with dietary change using fat-modified and oat bran supplemented diets. *J Am Diet Assoc.* 1990;90:223-229.
100. Swain JF, Rouse IL, Curley CB, Sacks FM. Comparison of the effects of oat bran and low-fiber wheat on serum lipoprotein levels and blood pressure. *N Engl J Med.* 1990;322:147-152.
101. Cummings JH, Pomare EW, Branch WJ, et al. Short chain fatty acids in human large intestine, portal, hepatic and venous blood. *Gut.* 1987;28:1221-1227.
102. Hoverstad T. Studies of short-chain fatty acid absorption in man. *Scand J Gastroenterol.* 1986;21:257-260.
103. McNeil NI, Cummings JH, James WPT, et al. Short chain fatty acid absorption by the human large intestine. *Gut.* 1978;19:819-822.
104. Roediger WEW. Role of anaerobic bacteria in the metabolic welfare of the colonic mucosa in man. *Gut.* 1980;21:793-798.
105. Rabassa AA, Rogers AI. The role of short-chain fatty acid metabolism in colonic disorders. *Am J Gastroenterol.* 1992;87:419-423.
106. Wolever TMS, Schrade KB, Vogt JA, et al. Do colonic short-chain fatty acids contribute to the long-term adaptation of blood lipids in subjects with type 2 diabetes consuming a high-fiber diet? *Am J Clin Nutr.* 2002;75:1023-30.
107. Dorfman SH, Ali M, Floch MH. Low fiber content of Connecticut diets. *Am J Clin Nutr.* 1976;29:87.
108. Anderson JW. *Plant Fiber in Foods.* Lexington KY: HCF Diabetes Research Foundation Inc.; 1986: 10-30.
109. Pennington JAT, Douglass JS. *Bowes & Church's Food Values of Portions Commonly Used.* Philadelphia: Lippincott Williams & Wilkins; 2005.

110. Kromhout D, Bosschieter EB, Coulander, CdeL. Dietary fibre and 10-year mortality from coronary heart disease, cancer, and all causes. Lancet 1982;518-521.
111. Morris JN, Marr JW, Clayton DG. Diet and heart: a postscript. *Br Med J.* 1977;ii:1307-14.
112. Pereira MA, O'Reilly E, Augustsson K, et al. Dietary fiber and risk of coronary heart disease. *Arch Intern Med.* 2004;164:370-376.
113. Wu H, Dwyer KM, Fan Z, et al Dietary fiber and progression of atherosclerosis: the Los Angeles Atherosclerosis Study. *Am J Clin Nutr.* 2003;78:1085-91.
114. Gillman MW, Cupples LA, Gagnon D, et al. Protective effect of fruits and vegetables on development of stroke in men. *JAMA.* 1995;273:1113-7.
115. Jenkins DJA, Newton AC, Leeds AR, Cummings JH. Effect of pectin, guar gum, and wheat fibre on serum cholesterol. *Lancet.* 1975;1:116-117.
116. Olsen BH, Anderson SM, Becker MP, et al. Psyllium-enriched cereals lower blood total cholesterol and LDL cholesterol, but not HDL cholesterol, in hypercholesterolemic adults: results for a meta-analysis. *J Nutr.* 1997;127:1973-1980.
117. Anderson JW, Floore TL, Geil PB, et al. Hypocholesterolemic effects of different hydrophilic fibers. *Arch Intern Med.* 1991;151:1597-602.
118. Jacobs Jr DR, Meyer KA, Kushi LH, Folsom AR. Whole-grain intake may reduce the risk of ischemic heart disease death in postmenopausal women: the Iowa Women's Health Study. *Am J Clin Nutr.* 1998;68:248-57.
119. Albert CM, Gaziano JM, Willett WC, Manson JE. Nut consumption and decreased risk of sudden cardiac death in the physicians' health study. *Arch Intern Med.* 2002;162:1382-6.
120. Anderson JW, Randles KM, Kendall CWC, Jenkins DJA. Carbohydrate and fiber recommendations for individuals with diabetes: a quantitative assessment and meta-analysis of the evidence. *J Am Coll Nutr.* 2004;23:5-17.
121. Brand-Miller JC, Thomas M, Swan V, et al. Physiological validation of the concept of glycemic load in lean young adults. *J Nutr.* 2003;133:2728-2732.
122. Bolton RP, Heaton KW, Burroughs LF. The role of dietary fiber in satiety, glucose, and insulin: studies with fruit and fruit juice. *Am J Clin Nutr.* 1981;34:211-217.
123. Cummings JH, Southgate DAT, Branch W, et al. Colonic response to dietary fibre from carrot, cabbage, apple, bran and guar gum. *Lancet.* 1978;1:5-9.
124. Muir JG, Yeow EGW, Keogh J, et al. Combining wheat bran with resistant starch has more beneficial effects on fecal indexes than does wheat bran alone. *Am J Clin Nutr.* 2004;79:1020-8.
125. Almy TP, Howell DA. Diverticular disease of the colon. *N Engl J Med.* 1980;302:324-330.
126. Painter NS, Trowell H. Burkett DP, et al. Diverticular disease of the colon. In: *Dietary Fibre, Fibre-Depleted Foods and Disease.* London: Academic Press, 1985:145-160.
127. Floch MH, Bina I. The natural history of diverticulitis: fact and theory. *J Clin Gastroenterol.* 2004;38(suppl):S2-S7.
128. Pohlman T. Diverticulitis. *Gastroenterol Clin.* 1988;17:357-385.
129. Hughes LE. Postmortem survey of diverticular disease of the colon. *Gut.* 1969;10:336-351.
130. Garcia G. Diverticulitis. In: Blaser MT, Smith DD, Ravdin JI, et al, eds. *Infections of the Gastrointestinal Tract.* 2nd ed. Philadelphia: Lippincott Williams & Wilkins; 2002:306-316.
131. Fisher N, Berry CS, Fearn T, et al. Cereal dietary fiber consumption and diverticular disease: a lifespan study in rats. *Am J Clin Nutr.* 1985;42:788-804.
132. Patiner NS, Almeida AZ, Colebourn KW. Unprocessed bran in treatment of diverticular disease of colon. *Br Med J.* 1972;2:137-140.
133. Findlay JM, Smith AN, Mitchell WD, et al. Effects of unprocessed bran on colon function in normal subjects and in diverticular disease. *Lancet.* 1974;1:146-149.
134. Taylor, I, Duthie HL. Bran tablets and diverticular disease. *Br Med J.* 1976;1:988-990.
135. Brodribb AJM. Treatment of symptomatic diverticular disease with high-fibre diet. *Lancet.* 1977;2:664-666.
136. North WRS, Cox AG. Are fibre supplements really necessary in diverticular disease of the colon? a controlled clinical trial. *Br Med J.* 1981;282:1353-1356.
137. Painter NS. Bran and the irritable bowel syndrome. *Lancet.* 1976;i:540.
138. Francis CY, Whorwell PJ. Bran and irritable bowel syndrome: time for reappraisal. *Lancet.* 1994;344:39-40.
139. Thun MJ, Calle EE, Namboodiri MM, et al. Risk factors for fatal colon cancer in a large prospective study. *J Natl Cancer Inst.* 1992;84:1491.
140. Howe GR, Benito E, Castelleto R, et al. Dietary intake of fiber and decreased risk of cancers of the colon and rectum: evidence from the combined analysis of 13 case-control studies. *J Natl Cancer Inst.* 1992;84:1887.
141. Kim YI. AGA technical review: impact of dietary fiber on colon cancer occurrence. *Gastroenterology.* 2000;118:1235.
142. MacLennan R, Macrae F, Bain C, et al. Randomized trial of intake of fat, fiber, and beta carotene to prevent colorectal adenomas. *J Natl Cancer Inst.* 1995;87:1760.
143. DeCosse JJ, Miller HH, Lesser ML. Effect of wheat fiber and vitamin C and E on rectal polyps in patients with familial adenomatous polyps. *J Natl Cancer Inst.* 1989;81:1290-1297.
144. Harig JM, Soergel KH, Komorowski RA, Wood CM. Treatment of diversion colitis with short-chain fatty acid irrigation. *N Engl J Med.* 1989;320:23-27.
145. Roediger WEW, Nance S. Metabolic induction of experimental ulcerative colitis by inhibition of fatty acid oxidation. *Br J Exp Path.* 1986;67:773-782.
146. Roediger WEW. The colonic epithelium in ulcerative colitis: an energy-deficiency disease? *Lancet.* 1980;2:712-715.
147. Scheppach W, Sommer H, Kirchner T, et al. Effect of butyrate enemas on the colonic mucosa in distal ulcerative colitis. *Gastroenterology.* 1992;103:51-56.
148. Scheppach W, German-Austrian SCFA Study Group. Treatment of distal ulcerative colitis with short-chain fatty acid enemas: a placebo-controlled trial. *Dig Dis Sci.* 1996;41:2254-2259.
149. Breuer RI, Buto SK, Christ ML, et al. Rectal irrigation with short-chain fatty acids for distal ulcerative colitis: preliminary report. *Dig Dis Sci.* 1991;36:185-187.
150. Patz J, Jacobsohn WZ, Gottschalk-Sabag S, et al. Treatment of refractory distal ulcerative colitis with short chain fatty acid enemas. *Am J Gastroenterol.* 1996;91:731-734.
151. Steinhart AH, Brzezinski A, Baker JP. Treatment of refractory ulcerative proctosigmoiditis with butyrate enemas. *Am J Gastroenterol.* 1994;89:179-183.
152. Treem WR, Ashsan N. Shoup M. Hyams JS. Fecal short-chain fatty acids in children with inflammatory bowel disease. *J Pediatr Gastroenterol Nutr.* 1994;18:159-164.
153. Breuer RI, Soergel KH, Lashner BA, et al. Short chain fatty acid rectal irrigation for left-sided ulcerative colitis: a randomized, placebo controlled trial. *Gut.* 1997;40:485-491.

Chapter 12

Food and Water Safety: Potential for Bioterrorist Attack

Cynthia Sears, MD

Introduction

Food and water safety, as well as investigations of food- and water-borne diseases, have received increased attention by public health authorities in the United States over the last 10 years. Food safety and reduction of food-borne illnesses are specific goals within Healthy People 2010, the United States public health blueprint for the decade 2000 to 2010.[1] The Centers for Disease Control and Prevention (CDC) define a food-borne disease outbreak as two or more cases of a similar illness resulting from ingestion of a common food. The only exception to this definition is a single case of botulism.[2]

Food- and water-borne disease outbreaks have been a key source of information on food- and water-borne diseases in the United States. However, data from outbreaks are not typically reflective of the epidemiology and impact of endemic (community-acquired) food- and water-borne diseases.[3] The CDC estimates that 76 million cases of endemic food-borne disease occur in the United States annually. These cases are estimated to result in 325,000 hospitalizations and 5,000 deaths, with an annual economic loss estimated to be between $1.2 to $37 billion.[4-6]

The CDC also reports periodically on water-borne disease outbreaks. The most recent data from 2001-2002 reported 96 outbreaks involving 3556 persons with 61 hospitalizations and 15 deaths.[7,8] The goal of this chapter will be to outline, for the clinician, the major sources of food- and water-borne disease. The clinical syndromes resulting from food or water contamination will be described. Lastly, reports available in which food has been deliberately contaminated will be discussed along with the pathogens projected as potential bioterrorism concerns for dissemination by food or water.

Epidemiology of Food-Borne Illnesses in the United States

In response to inadequate information on endemic food-borne disease, FoodNet, an emerging infectious diseases food-borne diseases active surveillance network, was developed by the CDC in 1996, in collaboration with the Food and Drug Administration (FDA), the United States Department of Agriculture (USDA), and nine State Public Health Departments.[9] Over time, this surveillance network expanded to encompass 13% of the United States population (or 37.4 million persons) and 10 diseases. The 10 diseases (or the causing bacteria) are *Campylobacter jejuni* (*C. jejuni*), *Salmonella spp., Shigella spp*, Shiga toxin-producing *Escherichia coli* (STEC—0157 and non-0157), the hemolytic uremic syndrome (HUS), *Vibrio spp., Listeria monocytogenes (L. monocytogenes)*, *Yersinia enterocolitica (Y. enterocolitica)*, *Cryptosporidium*, and *Cyclospora*.[3,10] This surveillance network is based in microbiology laboratories where stools, primarily from ill persons, are received as ordered by physicians. Subsequently, illnesses caused by the FoodNet pathogens are defined as likely food-borne disease prompting phone calls to the patient from whom additional epidemiological information is accrued.

FoodNet data estimates that the prevalence of acute endemic diarrhea in the United States is 11%, resulting in 375 million episodes of diarrhea annually or approximately 1.4 episodes per person per year.[6,11] Approximately 200 million of these episodes last longer than a single day and significantly impair daily activities. Approximately 10% to 20% of all affected patients see physicians; approximately 2% are cultured (or 10% to 20% of those seeing physicians),[9] and approximately

TABLE 12-1.

FoodNet Results (2003)

Organism	Total Cases
Salmonella spp.	6,017 cases
Campylobacter jejuni	5,215 cases
*Shigella spp.**	3,021 cases
Escherichia coli O157†	443 cases
Total	15,600 cases‡

Adapted from CDC.[8,15]

* Of *Shigella spp.* cases, 85% are *Shigella sonnei* cases, 13% are *Shigella flexneri* cases.

† The 2003 FoodNet final report, issued in late 2004,[9] includes non-O157 STEC infections and cases of the hemolytic uremic syndrome. (In the final 2002 report, there were 717 cases of STEC [O157, non-O157] infection and hemolytic uremic syndrome reported.)

‡ Laboratory-confirmed cases.

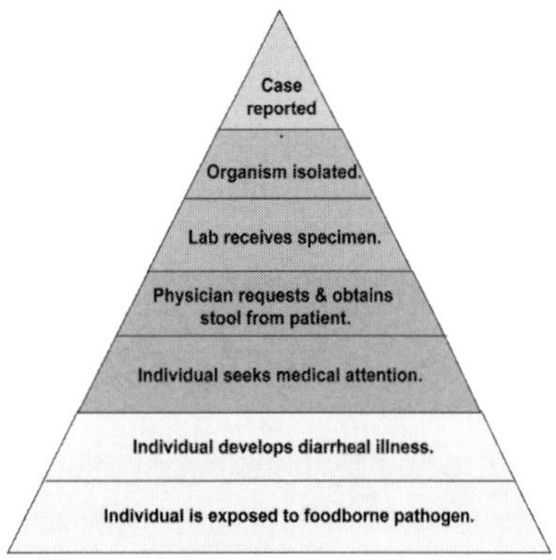

Figure 12-1. FoodNet Burden-of-Illness Pyramid. Reproduced with permission from Allos BM.[3]

0.5% are hospitalized. Of note, 79% of physicians will order a stool culture if the diarrhea is bloody (as versus 40% if nonbloody diarrhea is reported)[12]; and, in one study, 100% of patients with bloody diarrhea complied with providing a sample, whereas only 20% with nonbloody diarrhea provided stool samples for analysis.[13]

Table 12-1 summarizes FoodNet results for 2003.[14] In 2002, isolation of *Salmonella spp.* exceeded that of *C. jejuni* for first time.[15] *Shigella spp.*, of which the majority are *Shigella sonnei* in the United States, is the third most common enteric bacterial pathogen, with STEC isolation being fourth in the United States. However, there is marked variation in the rates at which different enteric pathogens are isolated among the different FoodNet sites. For example, rates of STEC 0157 infection can vary as much as five- to 10-fold among different sites.[16]

Reporting Food-Borne Disease: The Process

Figure 12-1 illustrates how FoodNet data is only "the tip of the iceberg" in reflecting the burden of illness caused by food-borne disease in the United States.[10] This burden-of-illness pyramid indicates the various steps in the detection of food-borne disease. Initially, the individual must be exposed to a food-borne pathogen. A subset of individuals exposed to a food-borne pathogen will develop disease and a smaller group will seek medical attention. The physician must request and obtain a stool for culture. The laboratory must receive the specimen and isolate the organism to generate a single report of food-borne disease. Using available epidemiological information and estimates of the likelihood of completing each of these steps, the CDC then estimates the total disease burden of a food-borne pathogen. For example, for each case of *Salmonella* identified in the laboratory, 38.6 cases are predicted to occur in the community. Thus, the reported *Salmonella* cases are only 2.6% of the estimated total annual burden of food-borne salmonellosis in the United States (estimate 1.4 million nontyphoidal *Salmonella* infections).[13]

FoodNet

FoodNet[9] data represents the most current estimates of food-borne disease available in the United States. However, there are several limitations to FoodNet data.[10] First, these data are limited to diagnosed illnesses, and most food-borne disease is not diagnosed. Second, there are variations in how laboratory testing for pathogens is performed and which pathogens are tested for in individual laboratories. This has been particularly notable for STEC infections in the United States.[16] Thus, the available laboratory-based FoodNet data from site-to-site is variable. Third, the isolation of a particular pathogen in the laboratory does not, in all instances, indicate that the reported illness was specifically food-borne (see *Link Between Food Source and Specific Pathogens* on the following page). Fourth, these data are limited to a minority of the US population and, when these populations have been further analyzed, there is some probable bias in the distribution of minorities in these data. For example, overall, Hispanics are underrepresented.[10] Fifth, the data analysis is delayed such that the most current data are not immediately available. Lastly, because of the absence of available rapid diagnostic tests, one important exclusion from the FoodNet data set is norovirus infection (formerly known as Norwalk virus and Norwalk-like viruses). This

TABLE 12-2.

Foods of Concern for Transmission of Food-Borne Diseases

	Potential Organisms*
Eggs, poultry	*Campylobacter jejuni, Salmonella spp.*
Hamburger	STEC, *Salmonella spp.*
Raw seafood	Noroviruses, *Vibrio spp.*, Hepatitis A
Ready-to-eat foods†	*Listeria monocytogenes*
Unpasteurized foods‡	STEC, *Salmonella spp., Listeria monocytogenes, Yersinia enterocolitica, Brucella spp.*
Alfalfa sprouts	STEC, *Salmonella spp.*
Pork	*Yersinia enterocolitica, Taenia solium*
Produce	*Salmonella spp.*, STEC, Hepatitis A, *Cryptosporidium, Cyclospora*

* Common or most likely organisms are listed; however, this list is not exhaustive.
† Lunchmeat, deli, and hot dogs are common, potentially contaminated "ready-to-eat" foods.
‡ For example, milk, apple cider, cheese.

exclusion is important because it is estimated that nearly two-thirds of cases of food-borne disease in the United States are due to norovirus infections.[4,17]

Link Between Food Source and Specific Pathogens

The potential for food contamination exists in each step in the food chain. The most common source of contamination is fecal contamination of food, predominantly from food animals (eg, livestock, poultry) or, less frequently, from a food handler. Further adding to the risk of food-borne disease is the fact that many of the pathogens commonly associated with food-borne disease have low infectious inoculums. Table 12-2 summarizes foods of particular concern that should be discussed with select patient populations including parents of young children, immunocompromised patients, the elderly, and pregnant women. Important foods to discuss include poultry and eggs, hamburger, seafood, unpasteurized products (eg, milk, cheese, apple cider), alfalfa sprouts, lunch meat/deli, and "ready-to-eat" foods.

Poultry is not infrequently contaminated with either *C. jejuni* or *Salmonella spp.*[18,19] It is estimated that as much as 60% to 80% of poultry is contaminated with *C. jejuni.* Recent studies evaluating ground chicken, beef, turkey, and pork from grocery stores identified a rate of contamination of at least 20% with *Salmonella spp.*[20] Of particular concern, the isolated organisms exhibited high levels of antibiotic resistance, with 84% being resistant to at least one antibiotic and 53% being resistant to at least three antibiotics.[20] Similarly, when isolation of *Enterococcus faecium* is used as a marker for bacterial contamination of food, contamination has been identified in 17% to 87% of chicken samples (n=407) in four states.[21] Both the albumen and yolk of eggs can commonly be contaminated with *Salmonella spp.* Typically, each egg has less than 100 organisms and only about 1 in 10,000 eggs are currently estimated to be infected. However, because of batching of eggs for cooking, eggs remain a significant source for salmonellosis in the United States.[22]

Hamburger is a food of concern. Each pound of hamburger is estimated to represent 100 cows. Evaluation of hamburger for bacterial contamination indicates that approximately 25% will be positive by culture for STEC with up to 60% potentially contaminated when hamburger is evaluated for STEC organisms by molecular techniques.[23] Although hamburger is the most common source of STEC infection,[24] multiple other foods as well as water have been documented to be contaminated and result in human disease. These include lettuce and salads, alfalfa sprouts, and apple cider (unpasteurized) as well as recreational and municipal water.[7,8,25,26]

Ingestion of contaminated seafood is estimated to account for 10% to 19% of food-borne disease in the United States.[27,28] The leading source of food-borne disease due to seafood is raw or undercooked shellfish, especially oysters. As filter feeders, shellfish are able to concentrate both viruses and bacteria in their tissue. Of diagnosed illnesses linked to the ingestion of seafood, viral gastroenteritis, often caused by noroviruses, is most common, accounting for about 50% of diagnosed illnesses.[28] Hepatitis A is another viral illness potentially transmitted by contaminated shellfish. In contrast, bacterial illnesses account for about 9% of diagnosed foodborne diseases linked to ingestion of seafood.[28] While numerous bacterial species have been associated with illnesses transmitted by seafood ingestion, *Vibrio* (V.) species are most common including *V. parahemolyticus, V. vulnificus, V. cholerae,* and non-01 *V. cholerae* strains. Parasitic diseases linked to seafood (eg, anisakiasis; liver, lung and intestinal fluke diseases; and infection with *Diphyllobothrium latum*) are documented infrequently in the United States but are common in other regions, particularly Japan, China, and southeast Asia.[27]

Seafood is also the source of scombroid fish poisoning due to finned fish, such as tuna, blue fish, mahi-mahi, marlin, and salmon. Scombroid fish poisoning occurs when the meat of the fish is contaminated with bacteria and the fish is not kept cold after harvest. Under these conditions,

TABLE 12-3.

Frequency of Acquisition of Pathogens From Food

Pathogen	% of Illnesses Food-Borne
*Salmonella spp.**	nearly all
Shigella spp.	20%
Campylobacter jejuni	nearly all
STEC	nearly all
Yersinia enterocolitica	90%
*Listeria monocytogenes**	nearly all
Cryptosporidium	10%
Giardia lamblia	10%
Cyclospora	90%
Noroviruses	40%

*Together, *Salmonella spp.* and *Listeria monocytogenes* account for approximately 60% to 80% of deaths due to food-borne disease.

Adapted from Mead PS, Slutsker L, Dietz V, et al. Food-related illness and death in the United States. *Emerg Infect Dis*. 1999;5(5):607-625.

the bacteria metabolize the amino acid histidine in the fish flesh to histamine. Histamine is a heat-stable molecule that upon ingestion (even if the fish is cooked) rapidly triggers symptoms such as flushing, shortness of breath, pruritis, urticaria, and gastrointestinal (GI) distress.[29] Fish contaminated with histamine is often described as having a "peppery" taste. Additional forms of seafood poisoning that occur relatively infrequently are shellfish poisoning or ciguatera associated with toxic dinoflagellate ingestion.[30] In these contaminations, toxic dinoflagellates (single-cell microalgae) multiply, creating (in some cases) a red tide or algal bloom and produce toxins that are filtered and concentrated in fish or shellfish. Shellfish poisoning associated with red tides may present with several syndromes including paralytic, neurotoxic, diarrheal, and amnestic poisoning. Ciguatera is associated with ingestion of large reef fish—such as barracuda, grouper, and amberjack—and presents with self-limited GI symptoms as well as neurological signs. In particular, unusual sensory disorders, including a sensation of loose teeth and hot-cold reversal, can persist for days and sometimes as long as 6 months.[31]

L. monocytogenes infection has been linked, in particular, to contaminated soft cheeses, lunch meat, deli, hot dogs, and other ready-to-eat foods.[32,33] This is of keen concern in pregnant women and immunocompromised hosts where systemic infection, meningitis, or brain abscesses may result. *L. monocytogenes* is an organism capable of growing at refrigerator temperatures such that contamination can increase with the duration of storage of these foods in the refrigerator. Consistent with this, direct links between specific *L. monocytogenes* strains isolated from individual refrigerators and cases of *L. monocytogenes* disease have been reported.[33]

Other foods of concern include any unpasteurized foods including milk and apple cider. Alfalfa sprouts have been a source of both STEC and *Salmonella spp.* infections because the seeds can be intrinsically infected with organisms that multiply exponentially upon germination.[26] Illnesses following consumption of chitterlings (raw pork intestines) are often linked to infection with *Y. enterocolitica*. In general, undercooked pork products are a major reservoir of *Y. enterocolitica*, although infection has also been linked to contaminated milk and other sources.[34] Similar to *L. monocytogenes, Y. enterocolitica* can proliferate at refrigerated temperatures. Imported fruits and vegetables have increasingly been recognized to be a source of food-borne disease. Examples are the *Cyclospora* outbreaks due to contaminated raspberries in the late 1990s[35] and snow peas in 2004,[36] both imported from Guatemala, and an outbreak of Hepatitis A infection associated with importation of green onions from Mexico.[37]

Table 12-3 lists the likelihood that a particular pathogen is acquired by ingestion of contaminated food.[4] Of note, nearly all *Salmonella spp., C. jejuni*, STEC, *L. monocytogenes*, and *Y. enterocolitica* infections are thought to be food-borne illnesses. In contrast, only 20% of *Shigella spp.* infections are linked to contaminated food, with the majority of *Shigella spp.* illnesses thought to be secondary to person-to-person transmission of infection. Although only a minority of *Cryptosporidium* and *Giardia lamblia* (*G. lamblia*) infections are linked to food, these organisms are clearly associated with water-borne transmission (see *Water-Borne Disease*).[7,8] Estimates for the occurrence of *Cyclospora* and noroviruses as food-linked illnesses are uncertain, at present, because most investigations to date have focused primarily on epidemics of these infections. However, one recent study suggests that norovirus is also a likely common cause of community gastroenteritis accounting potentially for 10% to 20% of endemic food- and water-borne disease.[17]

Syndromic Analysis of Food-Borne Disease

Table 12-4 lists common syndromic presentations of food-borne disease and the pathogens likely to cause

TABLE 12-4.

Clinical Presentation of Common Food-Borne Diseases

Timing	Agent	Clinical Presentation
<6 h	*Staphylococcus aureus*	emesis > diarrhea
	Bacillus cereus	emesis > diarrhea
6 to 24 h	*Clostridium perfringens*	noninflammatory diarrhea
	Bacillus cereus	noninflammatory diarrhea
24 to 72 h	Noroviruses	emesis > diarrhea
	Salmonella spp.	inflammatory diarrhea
	Campylobacter jejuni	inflammatory diarrhea
	Shigella spp.	inflammatory diarrhea
	STEC	bloody diarrhea
3 to 30 days	*Listeria monocytogenes*	fever, systemic illness
	Hepatitis A	hepatitis
	*Clostridium botulinum**	paralysis

*Incubation period can vary from hours to weeks depending on the amount of botulinum toxin ingested.

TABLE 12-5.

Syndromic Analysis: Foodborne Outbreaks of Unknown Etiology (1982-1989)

	% Outbreaks*
Noroviruses	48%
Vomiting toxin	22%
Salmonella-like	12%
Diarrhea toxin	5%
STEC	1%
Unclassified	12%

*N = 337 known and 712 unknown outbreaks.

Adapted from Hall JA, Goulding JS, Bean NH, Tauxe RV, Hedberg CW. Epidemiologic profiling: evaluating foodborne outbreaks for which no pathogen was isolated by routine laboratory testing: United States, 1982-9. *Epidemiol Infect.* 2001;127(3):381-387.

these syndromes.[29] Using a syndromic analysis of food-borne outbreaks of unknown etiology involving 300 diagnosed and 712 outbreaks of unknown etiology analyzed between 1982 and 1989, the CDC was able to classify 88% of outbreaks into one of the common patterns shown in Table 12-5.[38] In this analysis, only 12% of food-borne outbreaks were of unknown etiology.

Illnesses associated with notable vomiting fall into two major categories: namely, norovirus infection and bacterial toxin-mediated emetic disease. Specific criteria were published in 1982 for the diagnosis of norovirus infection.[38] These criteria included an estimated incubation period of 1 to 2 days, duration of illness of 12 to 60 hours, with more than 50% of individuals affected experiencing vomiting. Overall, it is estimated that 70% to 90% of individuals with norovirus infection will experience both vomiting and diarrhea. In addition, 30% to 50% of individuals with norovirus infection will experience a fever. These criteria assist in distinguishing norovirus infections from those due to *Staphylococcus aureus (S. aureus)* or *Bacillus cereus (B. cereus)* toxin-induced emetic disease.

Most illnesses resulting in predominant emesis rather than diarrhea with a rapid onset (on average approximately 6 hours) after ingestion of the implicated food are due to contamination of food by toxin-producing strains of *S. aureus* or *B. cereus*.[29] *S. aureus* food contamination generally occurs during food preparation when food is contaminated with *S. aureus* strains colonizing the food handler. Although many foods may support the growth of *S. aureus*, foods classically associated with these intoxications include potato salad and other salads. *B. cereus* infections are specifically associated with rice that is contaminated with the spores of *B. cereus*.

These illnesses are not caused by infection with the organisms but rather represent an intoxication with preformed protein toxins produced in food contaminated by these bacteria and then kept at an inappropriately warm temperature. Under these conditions, *S. aureus* rapidly multiply and produce one of its enterotoxins and, similarly, the spores of *B. cereus* germinate releasing organisms that also produce a toxin. The heat-stable toxins produced by these organisms are super-antigens that induce cytokines

TABLE 12-6.

Waterborne Disease Outbreaks

Drinking Water (ground water, nearly all GI disease)

Escherichia coli O157, *Salmonella spp.*, *Campylobacter jejuni*
Giardia lamblia, *Cryptosporidium*
Noroviruses
Unidentified (23%-44%)

Recreational Water (2/3 involving chlorinated water, ~50% GI disease)

*Cryptosporidium**
STEC†
Shigella spp.
Noroviruses
Unidentified (17%-24%)

*Leading pathogen in treated (eg, chlorinated) recreational water.
†STEC and noroviruses leading pathogens in fresh (eg, lake) recreational water.

Adapted from Centers for Disease Control and Prevention: Surveillance for Waterborne-Disease Outbreaks Associated with Recreational Water--United States, 2001-2002. *MMWR*. 2004;53:1-22; Hall JA, Goulding JS, Bean NH, Tauxe RV, Hedberg CW. Epidemiologic profiling: evaluating foodborne outbreaks for which no pathogen was isolated by routine laboratory testing: United States, 1982-9. *Epidemiol Infect*. 2001;127(3):381-387.

and an abrupt onset of nausea and vomiting. Because the toxins are heat-stable, they are resistant to denaturation by heating of food. A minority of patients will experience fever with these illnesses. The duration of these illnesses is relatively short, typically less than 24 hours, which, like fever, assists in distinguishing them from norovirus infections. There is little or no immunity to the toxins that produce these clinical syndromes; thus, it is possible for an individual to repeatedly experience these illnesses.

In contrast to these illnesses, noninflammatory diarrheal illnesses have an onset of approximately 6 to 24 hours after ingestion of contaminated food.[29] Common etiologic food-borne agents for this type of syndrome are *Clostridium perfringens* and *B. cereus*. In these illnesses, the individual ingests the organism that multiplies in the upper small intestine, producing heat-labile enterotoxins that stimulate intestinal secretion, which produce watery non-inflammatory diarrhea, typically without fever. These illnesses contrast to illnesses produced by ingestion of the common enteric pathogens, *Salmonella spp., C. jejuni, Shigella spp.* and STEC. These infections have a somewhat longer incubation period of 24 to 72 hours and commonly produce diarrhea that is not infrequently associated with one or more signs of inflammation. Inflammation may be manifested by fever, abdominal pain, occult or gross blood in the stool, or fecal leukocytes or lactoferrin detected by laboratory examination of the stool.[39] However, all of the pathogens that can induce inflammatory diarrhea may also present clinically with milder manifestations.[40] These latter illnesses are clinically indistinguishable from illnesses due to pathogens causing noninflammatory diarrhea.

Lastly, certain food-borne illnesses have potentially protracted incubation periods of a few days to up to a month. These include *L. monocytogenes* (see *Link Between Food Source and Specific Pathogens*), Hepatitis A infection, and botulism.

Water-Borne Disease

Water-borne disease outbreaks can be broken into those attributable to drinking water and those attributable to recreational water (Table 12-6).[7,8,41] The majority of drinking water-related outbreaks are associated with GI disease. Common pathogens include STEC, *Salmonella spp., C. jejuni, G. lamblia, Cryptosporidium*, and noroviruses. Large-scale drinking water contamination in the United States has been recognized relatively infrequently. However, the Milwaukee outbreak of *Cryptosporidium* infection in 1992 caused by contaminated municipal water in the city of Milwaukee resulted in an estimated 400,000 cases of *Cryptosporidium* infection.[42] The severity of this outbreak illustrated the seriousness of the public health threat when central water resources become contaminated. There remains concern that contaminated tap water in the United States is a source of endemic GI illnesses and is estimated to be linked to 14% to 40% of GI illnesses.[43] This concern is augmented by observations that water turbidity fluctuations and increased rain are associated with increased diarrheal disease rates in communities, increased visits to emergency rooms, and hospital admissions.[44] The CDC is presently seeking to better define the role of tap water in endemic water-borne disease through a blinded controlled study to evaluate the impact of treating home drinking water with ultraviolet light and filtration through one micrometer filters to prevent drinking water-linked illnesses (pilot water evaluation trial [WET]).[45]

Approximately two-thirds of water-borne disease outbreaks linked to recreational water are associated with chlorinated water (eg, swimming pools).[7,41] These outbreaks result in GI disease approximately 50% of the time, with the remainder of illnesses being predominantly skin infections (eg, *Pseudomonas aeruginosa* folliculitis). The leading pathogen identified in outbreaks linked to treated water is *Cryptosporidium. Cryptosporidium* is often causal in chlorinated water outbreaks because the oocyst form of this parasite is very hardy and some *Cryptosporidium* strains have a very low infectious inoculum, in which as few 10 oocysts are estimated to be able to cause infection in an immunocompetent host.[46] The leading pathogens linked to fresh recreational water resources (such as swimming in lakes) are STEC and norovirus infections. For example, a recent norovirus outbreak was associated with children playing in a recreational water fountain.[47]

Selected Infectious Pathogens Associated With Food- or Water-Borne Disease

Noroviruses

Overall, noroviruses are thought to account for greater than 90% of outbreaks of nonbacterial gastroenteritis worldwide, with most of these caused by contaminated food and water.[17,48] The most common presentation of norovirus is epidemic disease, but noroviruses may also account for as much as 10% to 20% of community-associated gastroenteritis.[17] Interestingly, susceptibility to norovirus infection is, in part, genetically determined by an individual's expression of blood group antigens. Individuals who are secretor status negative and/or blood group B antigen positive are resistant or relatively resistant to infection and disease.[48] Noroviruses have been associated with multiple modes of transmission. These include food and water, person-to-person spread, aerosolization, and transmission by fomites. Only 10-100 viral particles are necessary to transmit infection and the virus is resistant to heat, chlorine, and freezing. This makes norovirus a very efficient pathogen in food-borne illnesses. For example, a single food handler was identified as contaminating 76 L of icing that resulted in 3000 illnesses in a single town.[49] Similarly, numerous outbreaks of norovirus infection on cruise ships have been reported. These outbreaks have been, in some instances, recalcitrant to infection control measures with repeat outbreaks occurring on single ships because of the hardiness of the virus and the multiple potential modes of transmission.[17]

Nontyphoidal Salmonella spp.

Nontyphoidal *Salmonella spp.* are a leading cause of food-borne illnesses and infect approximately 1% of the US population per year. There are 2400 serotypes of nontyphoidal *Salmonella spp.* It is estimated that only 5% of cases of food-borne *Salmonella* illness are related to outbreaks with 95% of illnesses occurring sporadically in the United States. The five leading *Salmonella* serotypes associated with food-borne illness are: 1) *Salmonella* (S.) *typhimurium* (20%), which is linked to multiple vehicles including ground beef and pork, chicken, and others; 2) *S. enteritidis* (14%), which is linked most often to contaminated chicken and eggs; 3) *S. newport* (12%), recently linked to ingestion of contaminated beef; 4) *S. heidelberg* (6%), also linked to contaminated eggs; and 5) *S. javiana* (6%), which is associated with contact with reptiles.[14] Nontyphoidal *Salmonella* infections are associated with fever, diarrhea, and vomiting. Bloody diarrhea occurs in 45% to 65% of *S. enteritidis* and *S. typhimurium* infections. In a recent report, the median duration of illness is 7 days, with a range of 1 to 76 days.[13]

Campylobacter jejuni

Similar to *Salmonella spp., C. jejuni* affects approximately 1% of the US population per year. The strongest risk factor for acquisition of *C. jejuni* infection is ingestion of contaminated chicken and eggs. However, recent data indicate that this is not the only source of *C. jejuni* infection, with other sources including nonpoultry meat, raw seafood, untreated water, unpasteurized milk, and contact with pet puppies or animal stool on farms.[19] The clinical presentation of *C. jejuni* disease is similar to that described above for salmonellosis. An important (but infrequent) sequela of *C. jejuni* infection is the Guillain-Barré syndrome (GBS).[50] GBS is thought to be an autoimmune disease caused by antibodies induced by the organism that cross react with peripheral nerve gangliosides leading to weakness and ascending paralysis. Approximately 20% to 40% of patients with GBS have evidence of prior evidence of *C. jejuni* infection and *C. jejuni* is now the leading recognized cause of GBS. However, GBS occurs in only a small number of *C. jejuni* infections (estimated to be 1 per 1000 cases of intestinal *C. jejuni* infection).

Shiga Toxin-Producing Escherichia coli

The most severe intestinal manifestation of STEC infection is the development of bloody diarrhea, although many individuals will develop only watery diarrhea or even may be asymptomatic upon infection.[40,51] STEC infection can be complicated by the development of thrombotic microangiopathy (hemolysis and thromobocytopenia) or the HUS (hemolytic anemia, thrombocytopenia, renal failure). The clinical course of some patients who develop HUS is further complicated by neurologic disease. The infectious inoculum for many STEC strains is thought to be very small, even a few organisms, as infection resulting in fatal disease has been reported in young children with a single bite of contaminated food. Young children (less than 15 years of age) and those older than 60 years are more prone to severe disease and the development of systemic complications of the infection. Although STEC infection remains most strongly linked to undercooked hamburger ingestion, other foods—including unpasteurized apple cider, alfalfa sprouts, and salads—that had been contaminated with infected fecal matter have transmitted infection.[24-26] Similarly, transmission by contaminated water has been reported.[7,8] The low infectious inoculum also facilitates person-to-person spread of infection as well as transmission occurring at farm petting zoos (likely fecal-oral transmission).

Most recently, environmental spread of *E. coli* 0157 has been reported as an outbreak source.[52] A county fair outbreak of *E. coli* 0157 infection was reported that had no association with water, hamburger, or contact with cows. The only apparent risk factor was visiting a particular building at the county fair. Importantly, environmental samples were culture positive at 6 (44% of environmental samples positive) and 42 (30% of environmental samples positive) weeks after livestock excreting *E. coli* 0157 were housed in this building. Cultures of wooden rafters were positive, indicating the ability of the organism to be airborne, possibly on dust particles, and leaving widespread contamination of surfaces within this building.

Listeria monocytogenes

L. monocytogenes has only recently been appreciated to cause food-borne disease in immunocompetent as well as immunocompromised patients.[53] The majority of *L. monocytogenes* infections represent food-borne illnesses.[4] Immunocompetent hosts who ingest food contaminated with *L. monocytogenes* develop brief fever, as high as 39°C, followed by self-limited watery diarrhea (typically less than 2 to 3 days).[53] *L. monocytogenes,* in contrast to many of the other pathogens discussed, is a high inoculum disease. Foods associated with the development of *L. monocytogenes* disease are commonly contaminated with 10^8 to 10^9 organisms per gram of food. A survey of refrigerators of patients with diagnosed *L. monocytogenes* infection revealed that 11% of food in the refrigerators was culture positive for *L. monocytogenes,* with commonly contaminated foods including soft cheeses, cooked poultry, cabbage, hot dogs, and other ready-to-eat foods.[32,33] *Listeria,* however, does not grow well in all foods. For example, it does not grow well on lettuce or roast beef, whereas the organism will proliferate well in soft cheeses. Surveys have revealed that 2% to 10% of the population are colonized when stools are cultured for *L. monocytogenes.* Systemic illness with *L. monocytogenes* typically affects women who are pregnant, individuals at the extremes of age or those that are immunocompromised. In contrast to the less than 1% mortality rate associated with other food-borne disease pathogens, *L. monocytogenes* has a mortality rate of approximately 20%.[4]

Bovine Spongiform Encephalopathy

Bovine spongiform encephalopathy (BSE), or "mad cow disease," is a new prion disease that was identified in the United Kingdom in 1986.[54-56] Prion diseases are thought to be caused by self-replicating, misfolded forms of a normal cellular protein. The abnormal protein is termed PrP^{Sc} or PrP^{res} for "prion protein 'scrapie'" or "prion protein 'resistant' to proteinase K." The BSE epidemic in the United Kingdom and Europe is believed to have been initiated by "ruminant recycling" in which sheep and/or cow meat and bone meal was fed to cows. Subsequent spread of the BSE infectious agent from cows to humans occurred with emergence in 1996 of a new form of Creutzfeldt-Jakob disease (vCJD for variant CJD). Approximately 150 cases of vCJD have been reported in Europe, predominantly in the United Kingdom. At present, case numbers appear to be declining. Specific criteria for diagnosis of vCJD have been published.[55]

In December 2003, the first blood transfusion-linked case of vCJD and the first case of disease in a cow in the United States were reported.[54,57] An additional North American BSE case has been reported from Canada. No human vCJD case linked to transmission of the BSE agent from a beef product produced in the United States has been identified. The risk of acquisition of vCJD by ingestion of beef produced in the United States for the individual consumer is unknown but thought to be extremely small given that testing for BSE has detected 1 positive cow in 40,000 cattle tested to date.[54] In Great Britain, approximately 4 million BSE-infected cows were consumed and only approximately 150 human cases of vCJD have been documented. Only one human genotype is known to be susceptible to the BSE prion. These individuals are homozygous for methionine at codon 129 of the prion protein.[55] This form of the normal cellular prion protein (PrP^{c}) is thought to be susceptible to induction of misfolding if associated with PrP^{Sc}.

The pathogenesis of BSE infection remains unclear. However, the abnormal PrP^{sc} is ingested, resulting in what now appears to be a systemic dissemination of the prion protein with tonsils, spleen, and muscle identified as containing abnormal prion proteins in humans.[58] The exact mode of spread of the abnormal prion protein to the brain is unclear; however, it is at this site that the significant clinical pathology occurs, resulting in degenerative neurologic disease.

The BSE agent is resistant, for example, to heat (350°C), radiation, and formalin. Currently, sheep, pig, and chicken products are considered free of any risk of transmitting prions and, similarly, European beef and beef products (including milk and daily products) are no longer thought to carry any risk. Beef gelatin and cow derivatives are also utilized in other foodstuffs such as jellybeans and, again, are thought to be of low risk. The testing of 200,000 cattle in the United States proposed by the USDA will further define if BSE is a public health threat in the United States.[54]

Hepatitis A

In general, Hepatitis A has been an infrequently transmitted food-borne disease. However, in 2003, green onions imported from Mexico, contaminated with hepatitis A, led to approximately 1000 cases of hepatitis A disease and three deaths in four states (Tennessee, North Carolina, Georgia, and Pennsylvania).[59,60] Fresh produce now exceeds raw shell fish as a source for hepatitis A food-borne outbreaks.[37] However, it is important to note that the leading mode of spread of hepatitis A remains person-to-person, with the principal reservoir for this infection being children.

Prevention of Food-Borne Disease

One key aspect to preventing food-borne disease involves changing the behavior of the consumer. Consumers need education on the proper handling and preparation of food as well as food selection. Table 12-7 shows results

TABLE 12-7.

Food Practices of American Adults

Ingestion of	*% Surveyed Population*
Raw milk	1.5%
Raw shellfish	1.9%
Runny eggs	19%
Pink hamburger	30%*
Wash hands or cutting board	93%
Willing to buy irradiated meat	50%

*Ingested by 35% of men, 38% of individuals with a college education, 49% of individuals with annual income >$100,000 and 10% of African-Americans.

Adapted from Shiferaw B, Yang S, Cieslak P, et al. Prevalence of high-risk food consumption and food-handling practices among adults: a multistate survey, 1996 to 1997. The Foodnet Working Group. *J Food Prot.* 2000;63(11):1538-1543; Frenzen PD, DeBess EE, Hechemy KE, et al. Consumer acceptance of irradiated meat and poultry in the United States. *J Food Prot.* 2001;64(12):2020-2026.

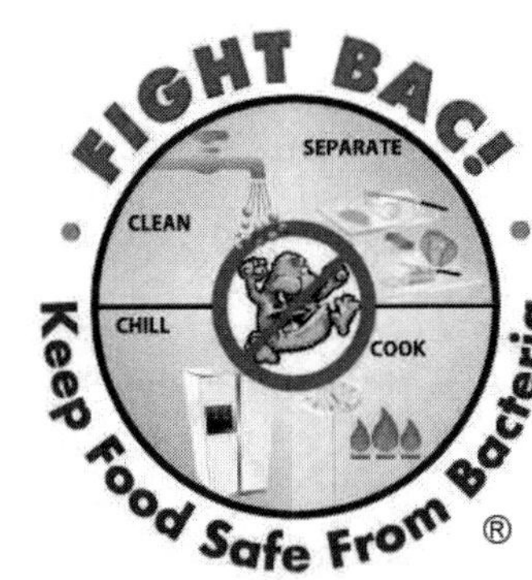

Figure 12-2. Partnership for Food Safety Education: Fight BAC! Reproduced with permission of the Partnership for Food Safety Education. http://www.fightbac.org

assessing consumer errors in food selection and preparation.[61,62] The data further suggest that these errors may, in part, vary by gender, race, and socioeconomic status. The most common food preparation errors include: 1) cross contamination of foods in the kitchen such as can occur with STEC, *Salmonella spp*, and *C. jejuni*; 2) time-temperature abuse such as keeping foods at warm temperatures that permit organism multiplication (ie, as occurs in *S. aureus* and *B. cereus* food poisoning); and 3) ingestion of uncooked and unpasteurized foods resulting in food-borne disease. Cooking of foods to 160 to 165°F is necessary to kill STEC and *L. monocytogenes* and to 180°F to decontaminate poultry. Microwave ovens, because of their inherent uneven heating, are inadequate for consistently killing organisms that cause food-borne disease. Several resources are available to obtain information on food safety including the Centers for Disease Control website,[63] nonprofit websites such as the Partnership for Food Safety Education,[64] and the USDA Hotline (1-888-674-6854). The emblem of the Partnership for Food Safety Education (Figure 12-2) emphasizes key steps to prevent bacterial contamination of food.

Studies have indicated that widespread kitchen contamination occurs when handling of poultry occurs.[65,66] In addition, *Salmonella spp*, possibly because of its greater hardiness than *C. jejuni*, are detectable on surfaces in the kitchen longer than *C. jejuni*. How to adequately decontaminate the kitchen is a matter of debate. Mechanical removal of bacteria with adequate soap and hot water is probably key. The use of antibacterial soaps and diluted bleach may be helpful. Adequate rinsing is considered essential.[65,66] One potential culprit in the kitchen is the dishrag, which may remain persistently contaminated with organisms. Use of disposable dishrags is advised when working with contaminated foods. Utilization of antibacterial soaps in the kitchen is controversial because of concern that their use will promote cross-resistance to other antibacterial agents as well as antibiotics because genes conferring resistance to antibacterial agents and antibiotics can be carried on plasmids.[67] However, at present, there is no firm data indicating that use of antibacterials for kitchen cleaning actually promotes increased resistance of indigenous human flora of family members in the home.

In addition to personal measures to reduce the occurrence of food-borne disease and to improve food safety, institution of regulatory standards have been important to progress on the control of food-borne diseases.[37] One available, but underutilized, approach to control of food contamination is food irradiation.[68-70] This approach has been endorsed as safe by numerous American and international organizations and is presently approved for numerous foods in the United States including red meat, poultry, pork, fruits and vegetables, spices, eggs, and others. In addition, use of irradiated hamburgers (directed at reducing the possibility of STEC disease) for school lunch programs in the United States has been approved. Both the CDC and the World Health Organization consider food irradiation to be an important technology to protect the public against food-borne diseases. It is estimated that irradiation of only 50% of meat and poultry in the United States would eliminate nearly a million illnesses and approximately 350 deaths due to food-borne pathogens.[70]

Table 12-8.

Potential Biological Agents for Public Health Preparedness in Food Safety

Category A*
- *Bacillus anthracis* (anthrax)
- *Clostridiium botulinum* neurotoxins (botulism)
- *Francisella tularensis* (tularemia)

Category B
- *Coxiella burnetti* (Q-fever)
- *Brucella spp.* (brucellosis)
- Ricin from *Ricinus communis* (ricin intoxication)
- Epsilon toxin of *Clostridium perfringens*
- *Staphylococcal enterotoxin* B
- Food and waterborne agents†

Category C
- Nipah virus

* Category A includes many well-recognized biowarfare agents. Category B agents have potential for large-scale dissemination and could be used to contaminate food or water sources. Category C agents are considered emerging pathogens with future potential for mass dissemination.
† Examples include *Salmonella spp, Shigella dysenteriae, Escherichia coli* O157:H7, *Vibrio cholerae,* and *Cryptosporidium.*

Adapted from Centers for Disease Control and Prevention: Biological and chemical terrorism: strategic plan for preparedness and response recommendations of the CDC strategic planning workgroup. *MMWR.* 2000:49:1-14.

To address shellfish contamination, monitoring of fecal coliforms is mandated in shellfish harvest areas and only shellfish from beds with less than 230 *E. coli*/100 g seafood may be delivered for direct human consumption.[27] Higher-level contamination requires depuration or heat treatment prior to the shellfish being relayed for human consumption. Depuration is an approach where filter-feeding shellfish are placed in clean water for varying periods of time to flush out infectious pathogens. Depuration will significantly decrease bacterial counts in shellfish but is ineffective in reducing, for example, shellfish norovirus contamination. Thus, it is estimated that the risk of acquiring an enteric virus by ingesting raw shellfish from an approved harvesting site in the United States is still 1%.[27]

In 1997, the USDA also instituted Hazard Analysis and Assessment of Critical Point Control (HAACP). This program challenges industry to identify the points in food processing where contamination occurs and to institute changes to prevent future contamination from occurring. In 2002, the FDA instituted the Public Health Security and Bioterrorism Preparedness Response Act.[37] This statue necessitates several steps to promote food safety, including that domestic and foreign food suppliers must register with the FDA; the FDA must be notified of all imported food; detailed records of food movement and sources must be kept; and procedures are defined for detaining food if credible threats occur. These regulations are in the process of being implemented.

Bioterrorism and the US Food Supply

The US food supply is vulnerable to bioterrorist attack. Table 12-8 summarizes agents of potential concern for widespread contamination of the food supply.[71] The outcome of intentional contamination of food will depend on several factors including where in the food chain the food product is contaminated and what agent is used to contaminate food.[72] The US food supply is increasingly characterized by centralized production with wide distribution of products. Deliberate contamination of a commercial food product at its source could lead to widely dispersed illnesses. These illnesses could present as an increase in sporadic cases that are difficult to detect or as an explosive epidemic, depending on the contaminating agent. Alternatively, contamination of food at a distribution point may result in a more geographically constrained outbreak of disease. Preparedness for detection of a bioterrorist attack on the food supply requires a strong public health infrastructure for disease surveillance; diagnostic methods that are sensitive, specific, and available; and the capacity for response that includes the personnel, procedures, and facilities to rapidly investigate and instigate measures to control outbreaks and to treat affected individuals.[72]

Initial detection of a potential bioterrorist attack involving food is likely to be by astute clinicians and/or laboratory workers who then alert public health authorities or through national surveillance mechanisms such as PulseNet, the Public Health Laboratory Information System or FoodNet.[72] PulseNet is a network of public health and regulatory laboratories that utilize molecular subtyping to evaluate food-borne pathogens isolated from clinical specimens or food products. Detection of an increased number of new strains with identical molecular patterns would suggest a common source outbreak. Similarly, the Public Health Laboratory Information System and/or FoodNet can assist in detecting an increase in specific food-borne pathogens suggesting a new outbreak.

The potential public health implications of intentional contamination of food can be estimated, in part, by considering the impact of prior outbreaks of food-borne or water-borne disease. For example, in 1994, transport of pasteurized liquid ice cream in tanker trucks previously contaminated with unpasteurized liquid eggs resulted in an estimated 224,000 illnesses due to *Salmonella enteriditis* distributed throughout the United States.[73] In 1997, traceback of an outbreak of *E. coli* O157:H7 disease resulted in the recall of 25 million pounds of ground beef.[74] As discussed earlier, contamination of the Milwaukee water supply with *Cryptosporidium* resulted in an estimated 400,000 illnesses and subsequent excess deaths within the HIV-infected community due to the acquisition of intractable GI and biliary tract disease.[42,75] As became obvious during the mailing of *Bacillus anthracis (B. anthracis)* spores in 2001, even limited dissemination of a biological agent resulting in few illnesses can induce public fear and strain the public health system.[72,76] Further security concerns about providing "a roadmap for terrorists" have limited open discussions about the vulnerabilities of the US food supply.[77]

Deliberate contamination of food with biological agents has been reported in only a few instances to date. In the 1960s, several outbreaks of typhoid fever and dysentery in Japan were traced to food contaminated by a research bacteriologist.[78] In 1970, a postgraduate student deliberately contaminated food consumed by his roommates with the ova of *Ascaris suum*, a large roundworm of pigs. Severe disease with massive pulmonary infiltrates, asthma, and eosinophilia resulted.[79] In 1984, salad bars in multiple restaurants in The Dalles, Oregon, were deliberately contaminated with *S. typhimurium* by members of a religious cult as trial runs for an attack planned to disrupt an upcoming political election. Although the ensuing outbreak of salmonellosis was not initially appreciated to be intentional contamination of food, public health authorities closed all salad bars, effectively aborting the later attack. In this outbreak in a community of 10,500 persons, 751 individuals developed Salmonella gastroenteritis, of whom 6% were hospitalized; no fatalities were reported.[80] In 1996, a stock culture of *Shigella dysenteriae* type 2, a rare pathogen in the United States, was taken from a medical center laboratory and used to contaminate pastries, resulting in a cluster of 12 cases of infection. The circumstances suggested deliberate contamination by a worker linked to the laboratory and resulted in the introduction of enhanced security measures in the workplace.[78] These limited events further illustrate the complex challenge of insuring the safety of the food supply and the potential profound impact on public health that can result from deliberate contamination of food with biological agents.

The biological agents of greatest concern for food contamination are Category A agents (considered the highest priority agents for US security) that may be easily disseminated, are anticipated to cause high morbidity and mortality, and require a specific public health response.[71] *Clostridium botulinum (C. botulinum)* neurotoxins and *B. anthracis* are the Category A agents (see Table 12-8) of greatest concern to the food supply.[2,76,81,82] *Botulinum* toxin is the most lethal substance known, with an estimated LD50 of 0.001 µg/kg. Ingestion of this toxin results in afebrile descending flaccid paralysis with multiple cranial nerve palsies but a clear sensorium. Timing of disease onset depends on the amount of toxin absorption and varies from a few hours to more than a week. Death results from respiratory arrest if the intoxication is not recognized and treated promptly. As 95% of individuals with botulism require admission and 60% require mechanical ventilation, widespread food contamination could tax available antitoxin supplies and medical resources.[72] Because *C. botulinum* toxin is heat-labile, transmission is always by foods that are not heated or not heated thoroughly prior to eating. Water-borne botulism has not been reported likely because the toxin is also labile to standard water treatments, including chlorination and aeration.[2,81] Importantly, a single case of botulism is considered a public health emergency. In contrast to botulism, GI anthrax has not been reported in the United States but does occur abroad.[76,83] Symptoms appear 2 to 5 days after ingestion of food (meat of infected animals in naturally occurring disease) contaminated with the endospores of *B. anthracis*. Fever, diffuse abdominal pain, rebound tenderness, bloody diarrhea, and systemic toxicity are potential presenting features of GI anthrax; ascites may develop a few days after onset of the illness and even mediastinal widening (considered pathognomonic of inhalational anthrax) has been reported in GI anthrax. GI anthrax results in mesenteric lymphadenitis as well as mucosal ulceration and massive edema with the potential for intestinal perforation. Both blood and peritoneal fluid may reveal large gram-positive bacilli on Gram stain. Even with aggressive intravenous antibiotic therapy, the prognosis is poor. Remotely, deliberate contamination of food or water with a high inoculum of *Francisella tularensis*, the agent of tularemia, is also projected to result in systemic disease.[83]

Category B biological agents (second highest priority agents for US security) include several classic food-borne pathogens as well as rarer pathogens with the potential for inducing illness by the ingestion of intentionally contaminated food.[71] In contrast to Category A agents, Category B agents are anticipated to cause only moderate morbidity and low mortality if appropriately diagnosed and treated. *Coxiella burnetti (C. burnetti)*, the agent of Q fever, is most often transmitted from infected animals to humans through aerosolization of the organism. If used as a bioweapon, transmission by aerosolization, food, or water contamination or by mail has been anticipated.[34] However, the infectious inoculum to produce clinical disease by the oral route is projected to be very high and there is nothing known about contamination of food or water with massive doses of *C. burnetti*. *Brucella spp.* are also considered potential bioweapon agents and are zoonotic pathogens that may be transmitted to humans by aerosolization of infected animal secretions, skin or mucous membrane inoculation, or ingestion of, most often, unpasteurized dairy products, particularly if derived from goats.[82-84] The long incubation period of the disease and low mortality are suspected to limit the utility of *Brucella spp.* as a bioattack agent. Ricin toxin poisoning is anticipated to present similarly to STEC because the mechanism of action of ricin and Shiga toxin are quite similar, if not identical.[85] The epsilon toxin secreted by *Clostridium perfringens* types B and D is a lethal toxin that acts via formation of pores in cell membranes.[86] Consistent with observations in animals, deliberate contamination of food with the organism and/or toxin is projected to induce enterocolitis in humans, whereas aerosolization of epsilon toxin is expected to produce acute pulmonary edema.[85] *Staphylococcal enterotoxin* B (SEB), a heat-stable protein secreted by *S. aureus*, is one of the exotoxins associated with *S. aureus* food poisoning (see *Syndromic Analysis of Food-borne Disease*).[82,85] SEB is relatively stable in aerosols and it is proposed that this toxin could be used as a bioweapon by aerosolization or potentially to contaminate food or water, resulting in incapacitating pulmonary and/or GI illnesses. Inhalation of only 30 ng/person is estimated to result in incapacitating illness.[82] Known food- or water-borne pathogens projected as potential bioweapon agents are bacteria causing inflammatory or bloody diarrhea (*Salmonella spp., Shigella spp.,* and *E. coli* O157:H7); *Vibrio cholerae* because it induces profuse watery, potentially rapidly life-threatening, diarrhea; and *Cryptosporidium* because of its hardy nature and known ability to cause widespread disease by water contamination.[83] Details of the clinical presentations of Category B agents are available from multiple sources including several recent reviews.[82,83,85]

Category C agents (or third highest priority agents for US security) are emerging pathogens that may potentially be engineered for mass dissemination.[71] Of these, only Nipah virus has been reported as potentially transmitted by ingestion of contaminated food or drink. Transmission from pigs to humans in Indonesia and potentially by infected bats to humans in rural Bangladesh have been reported.[87,88] Nipah virus infection results in severe, and often fatal, encephalitis.

Conclusion

While at least 200 microbial pathogens or toxins may cause food- or water-borne disease, most food- or water-borne disease is caused by common pathogens.[3,4] Familiarity with the foods likely to transmit food-borne pathogens and the clinical disease patterns by which food- or water-borne disease may present assists the clinician in focusing on the most likely pathogens and directs diagnostic testing and institution of therapy. Most food- or water-borne disease remains undiagnosed, and, for some illnesses, readily available diagnostic testing is not available. Most often, therapy is directed at maintaining hydration because of GI loss of fluids caused by vomiting and diarrhea.[39,89]

Physicians also play a key role in educating patients to assist in prevention of food-borne disease. It is critical that the clinician be aware of the potential for food- or water-borne agents to be used as bioweapons and the potential manifestations of diseases transmitted by deliberate contamination of food or water. Clinicians should not hesitate to report to public health authorities unusual illnesses or unexpected disease epidemiology and must be knowledgeable about how to contact their local public health authorities immediately if concerns arise.

References

1. Office of Disease Prevention and Health Promotion, U.S. Department of Health and Human Services [DHHS Web site]. Available at: http://www.healthypeople.gov. Accessed June 28, 2005.
2. Shapiro RL, Hatheway C, Becher J, Swerdlow DL. Botulism surveillance and emergency response. A public health strategy for a global challenge. *JAMA*. 1997;278(5):433-435.
3. Allos BM, Moore MR, Griffin PM, Tauxe RV. Surveillance for sporadic foodborne disease in the 21st century: the FoodNet perspective. *Clin Infect Dis*. 2004;38(Suppl)3:S115-S120.
4. Mead PS, Slutsker L, Dietz V, et al. Food-related illness and death in the United States. *Emerg Infect Dis*. 1999;5(5):607-625.
5. Sandler RS, Everhart JE, Donowitz M, et al. The burden of selected digestive diseases in the United States. *Gastroenterology*. 2002;122(5):1500-1511.
6. Herikstad H, Yang S, Van Gilder TJ, et al. A population-based estimate of the burden of diarrhoeal illness in the United States: FoodNet, 1996-7. *Epidemiol Infect*. 2002;129(1):9-17.
7. Centers for Disease Control and Prevention: Surveillance for Waterborne-Disease Outbreaks Associated with Recreational Water--United States, 2001-2002. *MMWR*. 2004;53:1-22.
8. Centers for Disease Control and Prevention: Surveillance for Waterborne-Disease Outbreaks Associated with Drinking Water--United States, 2001-2002. *MMWR*. 2004;53:23-45.
9. Department of Health and Human Services, Centers for Disease Control and Prevention Web site. Available at: http://www.cdc.gov/foodnet. Accessed June 28, 2005.
10. Hardnett FP, Hoekstra RM, Kennedy M, Charles L, Angulo FJ. Epidemiologic issues in study design and data analysis related to FoodNet activities. *Clin Infect Dis*. 2004;38(Suppl)3:S121-S126.
11. Imhoff B, Morse D, Shiferaw B, et al. Burden of self-reported acute diarrheal illness in FoodNet surveillance areas, 1998-1999. *Clin Infect Dis*. 2004;38(Suppl)3:S219-S226.
12. Hennessy TW, Marcus R, Deneen V, et al. Survey of physician diagnostic practices for patients with acute diarrhea: clinical and public health implications. *Clin Infect Dis*. 2004;38(Suppl)3:S203-S211.
13. Voetsch AC, Van Gilder TJ, Angulo FJ, et al. FoodNet estimate of the burden of illness caused by nontyphoidal Salmonella infections in the United States. *Clin Infect Dis*. 2004;38(Suppl)3:S127-S134.
14. Centers for Disease Control and Prevention: Preliminary FoodNet Data on the Incidence of Infection with Pathogens Transmitted Commonly through Food--Selected Sites, United States, 2003. *MMWR*. 2004;53:338-343.
15. Centers for Disease Control and Prevention: Preliminary FoodNet Data on the Incidence of Foodborne Illnesses--Selected Sites, United States, 2002. *MMWR*. 2003;52:340-343.
16. Bender JB, Smith KE, McNees AA, et al. Factors affecting surveillance data on Escherichia coli O157 infections collected from FoodNet sites, 1996-1999. *Clin Infect Dis*. 2004;38(Suppl)3:S157-S164.
17. Bresee JS, Widdowson MA, Monroe SS, Glass RI. Foodborne viral gastroenteritis: challenges and opportunities. *Clin Infect Dis*. 2002;35(6):748-753.
18. Kimura AC, Reddy V, Marcus R, et al. Chicken consumption is a newly identified risk factor for sporadic Salmonella enterica serotype Enteritidis infections in the United States: a case-control study in FoodNet sites. *Clin Infect Dis*. 2004;38(Suppl)3:S244-S252.
19. Friedman CR, Hoekstra RM, Samuel M, et al. Risk factors for sporadic Campylobacter infection in the United States: A case-control study in FoodNet sites. *Clin Infect Dis*. 2004;38(Suppl)3:S285-S296.
20. White DG, Zhao S, Sudler R, et al. The isolation of antibiotic-resistant salmonella from retail ground meats. *N Engl J Med*. 2001;345(16):1147-1154.
21. McDonald LC, Rossiter S, Mackinson C, et al. Quinupristin-dalfopristin-resistant Enterococcus faecium on chicken and in human stool specimens. *N Engl J Med*. 2001;345(16):1155-1160.
22. Blaser MJ, Newman LS. A review of human salmonellosis: I. Infective dose. *Rev Infect Dis*. 1982;4(6):1096-1106.

23. Acheson DW. How does Escherichia coli O157:H7 testing in meat compare with what we are seeing clinically? *J Food Prot.* 2000;63(6):819-821.
24. Kassenborg HD, Hedberg CW, Hoekstra M, et al. Farm visits and undercooked hamburgers as major risk factors for sporadic Escherichia coli O157:H7 infection: data from a case-control study in 5 FoodNet sites. *Clin Infect Dis.* 2004;38(Suppl)3:S271-S278.
25. Ackers ML, Mahon BE, Leahy E, et al. An outbreak of Escherichia coli O157:H7 infections associated with leaf lettuce consumption. *J Infect Dis.* 1998;177(6):1588-1593.
26. Taormina PJ, Beuchat LR, Slutsker L. Infections associated with eating seed sprouts: an international concern. *Emerg Infect Dis.* 1999; 5(5):626-634.
27. Butt AA, Aldridge KE, Sanders CV. Infections related to the ingestion of seafood. Part II: parasitic infections and food safety. *Lancet. Infect Dis.* 2004;4(5):294-300.
28. Butt AA, Aldridge KE, Sanders CV. Infections related to the ingestion of seafood Part I: Viral and bacterial infections. *Lancet Infect Dis.* 2004;4(4):201-212.
29. Bishai WR, Sears CL. Food poisoning syndromes. *Gastroenterol Clin N Am.* 1993;22(3):579-608.
30. Morris JG, Jr. Pfiesteria, "the cell from hell," and other toxic algal nightmares. *Clin Infect Dis.* 1999;28(6):1191-1196.
31. Centers for Disease Control and Prevention: Ciguatera Fish Poisoning--Texas, 1997. *JAMA.* 1998;280:1394-1395.
32. Gombas DE, Chen Y, Clavero RS, Scott VN. Survey of Listeria monocytogenes in ready-to-eat foods. *J Food Prot.* 2003; 66(4):559-569.
33. Pinner RW, Schuchat A, Swaminathan B, et al. Role of foods in sporadic listeriosis. II. Microbiologic and epidemiologic investigation. The Listeria Study Group. *JAMA.* 1992;267(15):2046-2050.
34. Madariaga MG, Rezai K, Trenholme GM, Weinstein RA. Q fever: a biological weapon in your backyard. *Lancet Infect Dis.* 2003;3(11):709-721.
35. Herwaldt BL. Cyclospora cayetanensis: a review, focusing on the outbreaks of cyclosporiasis in the 1990s. *Clin Infect Dis.* 2000;31(4):1040-1057.
36. Centers of Disease Control and Prevention: Outbreak of Cyclosporiasis Associated with Snow Peas--Pennsylvania, 2004. *MMWR.* 2004;53:876-878.
37. Acheson DW, Fiore AE. Preventing foodborne disease--what clinicians can do. *N Engl J Med.* 2004;350(5):437-440.
38. Hall JA, Goulding JS, Bean NH, Tauxe RV, Hedberg CW. Epidemiologic profiling: evaluating foodborne outbreaks for which no pathogen was isolated by routine laboratory testing: United States, 1982-9. *Epidemiol Infect.* 2001;127(3):381-387.
39. Guerrant RL, Van Gilder T, Steiner TS, et al. Practice guidelines for the management of infectious diarrhea. *Clin Infect Dis.* 2001;32(3):331-351.
40. Slutsker L, Ries AA, Greene KD, Wells JG, Hutwagner L, Griffin PM. Escherichia coli O157:H7 diarrhea in the United States: clinical and epidemiologic features. *Ann Intern Med.* 1997;126(7):505-513.
41. Centers for Disease Control and Prevention: Surveillance for Waterborne-Disease Outbreaks--United States, 1999-2000. *MMWR.* 2002;51[SS-8]:1-48.
42. MacKenzie WR, Hoxie NJ, Proctor ME, et al. A massive outbreak in Milwaukee of cryptosporidium infection transmitted through the public water supply. *N Engl J Med.* 1994;331(3):161-167.
43. Payment P, Richardson L, Siemiatycki J, Dewar R, Edwardes M, Franco E. A randomized trial to evaluate the risk of gastrointestinal disease due to consumption of drinking water meeting current microbiological standards. *Am J Public Health.* 1991;81(6):703-708.
44. Gaffield SJ, Goo RL, Richards LA, Jackson RJ. Public health effects of inadequately managed stormwater runoff. *Am J Public Health.* 2003;93(9):1527-1533.
45. Colford JM, Jr., Rees JR, Wade TJ, et al. Participant blinding and gastrointestinal illness in a randomized, controlled trial of an in-home drinking water intervention. *Emerg Infect Dis.* 2002;8(1):29-36.
46. Okhuysen PC, Chappell CL, Crabb JH, Sterling CR, DuPont HL. Virulence of three distinct Cryptosporidium parvum isolates for healthy adults. *J Infect Dis.* 1999;180(4):1275-1281.
47. Hoebe CJ, Vennema H, Roda Husman AM, van Duynhoven YT. Norovirus outbreak among primary schoolchildren who had played in a recreational water fountain. *J Infect Dis.* 2004;189(4):699-705.
48. Lindesmith L, Moe C, Marionneau S, et al. Human susceptibility and resistance to Norwalk virus infection. *Nat Med.* 2003;9(5):548-553.
49. Kuritsky JN, Osterholm MT, Greenberg HB, et al. Norwalk gastroenteritis: a community outbreak associated with bakery product consumption. *Ann Intern Med.* 1984;100(4):519-521.
50. Rees JH, Soudain SE, Gregson NA, Hughes RA. Campylobacter jejuni infection and Guillain-Barre syndrome. *N Engl J Med.* 1995;333(21):1374-1379.
51. Thorpe CM. Shiga toxin-producing Escherichia coli infection. *Clin Infect Dis.* 2004;38(9):1298-1303.
52. Varma JK, Greene KD, Reller ME, et al. An outbreak of Escherichia coli O157 infection following exposure to a contaminated building. *JAMA.* 2003;290(20):2709-2712.
53. Dalton CB, Austin CC, Sobel J, et al. An outbreak of gastroenteritis and fever due to Listeria monocytogenes in milk. *N Engl J Med.* 1997;336(2):100-105.
54. Chesebro B. Biomedicine. A fresh look at BSE. *Science.* 2004;305(5692):1918-1921.
55. Beisel CE, Morens DM. Variant Creutzfeldt-Jakob disease and the acquired and transmissible spongiform encephalopathies. *Clin Infect Dis.* 2004;38(5):697-704.
56. Donnelly CA. Bovine spongiform encephalopathy in the United States—an epidemiologist's view. *N Engl J Med.* 2004;350(6):539-542.
57. Llewelyn CA, Hewitt PE, Knight RS, et al. Possible transmission of variant Creutzfeldt-Jakob disease by blood transfusion. *Lancet.* 2004;363(9407):417-421.
58. Glatzel M, Abela E, Maissen M, Aguzzi A. Extraneural pathologic prion protein in sporadic Creutzfeldt-Jakob disease. *N Engl J Med.* 2003;349(19):1812-1820.
59. Centers for Disease Control and Prevention. Hepatitis: an outbreak associated with green onions at a restaurant, Monaca, Pennsylvania, 2003. *MMWR.* 2003;52:1155-1157.
60. Fiore AE. Hepatitis A Transmitted by food. *Clin Infect Dis.* 2004;38:705-715.
61. Shiferaw B, Yang S, Cieslak P, et al. Prevalence of high-risk food consumption and food-handling practices among adults: a multistate survey, 1996 to 1997. The Foodnet Working Group. *J Food Prot.* 2000;63(11):1538-1543.
62. Frenzen PD, DeBess EE, Hechemy KE, et al. Consumer acceptance of irradiated meat and poultry in the United States. *J Food Prot.* 2001;64(12):2020-2026.
63. National Center for Infections Diseases, Centers for Disease Control and Prevention Web site. Available at: http://www.cdc.gov/ncidod/diseases/food/safety.htm. Accessed July 1, 2005.
64. Partnership for Food Safety Education Web site. Available at: http://www.fightbac.org. Accessed June 28, 2005.
65. Cogan TA, Bloomfield SF, Humphrey TJ. The effectiveness of hygiene procedures for prevention of cross-contamination from chicken carcases in the domestic kitchen. *Lett Appl Microbiol.* 1999;29(5):354-358.
66. Bloomfield SF. Home hygiene: a risk approach. *Int J Hyg Environ Health.* 2003;206(1):1-8.
67. Dixon B. Biocides in the kitchen. *ASM News.* 2004;70:4-5.
68. Tauxe RV. Food safety and irradiation: protecting the public from foodborne infections. *Emerg Infect Dis.* 2001;7(3 Suppl):516-521.
69. Thayer DW. Irradiation of food—helping to ensure food safety. *N Engl J Med.* 2004;350(18):1811-1812.
70. Osterholm MT, Norgan AP. The role of irradiation in food safety. *N Engl J Med.* 2004;350(18):1898-1901.

71. Centers for Disease Control and Prevention: Biological and chemical terrorism: strategic plan for preparedness and response--recommendations of the CDC strategic planning workgroup. *MMWR*. 2000:49:1-14.
72. Sobel J, Khan AS, Swerdlow DL. Threat of a biological terrorist attack on the US food supply: the CDC perspective. *Lancet*. 2002;359(9309):874-880.
73. Hennessy TW, Hedberg CW, Slutsker L, et al. A national outbreak of Salmonella enteritidis infections from ice cream. The Investigation Team. *N Engl J Med*. 1996;334(20):1281-1286.
74. Centers for Disease Control and Prevention: Escherichia coli O157:H7 infections associated with eating a nationally distributed commercial brand of frozen ground beef patties and hamburgers: Colorado, 1997. *MMWR*. 1997;46:777-778.
75. Vakil NB, Schwartz SM, Buggy BP, et al. Biliary cryptosporidiosis in HIV-infected people after the waterborne outbreak of cryptosporidiosis in Milwaukee. *N Engl J Med*. 1996;334(1):19-23.
76. Dixon TC, Meselson M, Guillemin J, Hanna PC. Anthrax. *N Engl J Med*. 1999;341(11):815-826.
77. Mervis J, Stokstad E. Bioterrorism. NAS censors report on agriculture threats. *Science*. 2002;297(5589):1973-1975.
78. Kolavic SA, Kimura A, Simons SL, Slutsker L, Barth S, Haley CE. An outbreak of Shigella dysenteriae type 2 among laboratory workers due to intentional food contamination. *JAMA*. 1997;278(5):396-398.
79. Phills JA, Harrold AJ, Whiteman GV, Perelmutter L. Pulmonary infiltrates, asthma and eosinophilia due to Ascaris suum infestation in man. *N Engl J Med*. 1972;286(18):965-970.
80. Torok TJ, Tauxe RV, Wise RP, Livengood JR, Sokolow R, Mauvais S et al. A large community outbreak of salmonellosis caused by intentional contamination of restaurant salad bars. *JAMA*. 1997;278(5):389-395.
81. Arnon SS, Schechter R, Inglesby TV, et al. Botulinum toxin as a biological weapon: medical and public health management. *JAMA*. 2001;285(8):1059-1070.
82. Franz DR, Jahrling PB, Friedlander AM, et al. Clinical recognition and management of patients exposed to biological warfare agents. *JAMA*. 1997;278(5):399-411.
83. Greenfield RA, Drevets DA, Machado LJ, Voskuhl GW, Cornea P, Bronze MS. Bacterial pathogens as biological weapons and agents of bioterrorism. *Am J Med Sci*. 2002;323(6):299-315.
84. Centers for Disease Control and Prevention: Suspected brucellosis case prompts investigation of possible bioterrorism-related activity--New Hampshire and Massachusetts, 1999. *MMWR*. 2004;49:509-512.
85. Greenfield RA, Brown BR, Hutchins JB, et al. Microbiological, biological, and chemical weapons of warfare and terrorism. *Am J Med Sci*. 2002;323(6):326-340.
86. Fernandez Miyakawa ME, Uzal FA. The early effects of Clostridium perfringens type D epsilon toxin in ligated intestinal loops of goats and sheep. *Vet Res Commun*. 2003;27(3):231-241.
87. Hsu VP, Hossain MJ, Parashar UD, et al. Nipah virus encephalitis reemergence, Bangladesh. *Emerg Infect Dis*. 2004;10[12].
88. Goh KJ, Tan CT, Chew NK, et al. Clinical features of Nipah virus encephalitis among pig farmers in Malaysia. *N Engl J Med*. 2000;342(17):1229-1235.
89. Thielman NM, Guerrant RL. Clinical practice. Acute infectious diarrhea. *N Engl J Med*. 2004;350(1):38-47.

Chapter 13

Metabolic Bone Disease in Gastrointestinal Illness

Asim S. Khokhar, MD, and
Douglas L. Seidner, MD, FACG

Introduction

Metabolic bone disease (MBD) is an important but often unrecognized complication of gastrointestinal (GI) illness. Maldigestion, malabsorption, inflammation, and abnormal metabolism as a result of the underlying disease and the medications used to treat them all contribute to the development of, most often, osteoporosis and other forms of MBD. An understanding of how these issues lead to the development of MBD should assist in the prevention and treatment of these conditions. A concerted effort should be made in patients with GI disease to diagnose and treat MBD and, in those patients whose bone density is normal or mildly decreased, to provide vitamin and mineral supplements to limit bone mineral loss. This chapter reviews the normal physiologic processes that surround bone metabolism and the development of osteoporosis and osteomalacia. The specific pathophysiologic causes of MBD in patients with celiac disease, postgastrectomy, pancreatic insufficiency, short gut, and advanced liver disease will then be discussed followed by treatment strategies for each of these conditions.

Normal Bone Anatomy and Physiology

Bone is a rigid structure that, in addition to providing structural support for locomotion and protection for the body's vital organs, acts as a reservoir for minerals and a site for hematopoiesis. There are two types of bone: cortical (also called compact bone) and trabecular (also called cancellous, spongy or medullary bone).[1] Cortical bone constitutes 80% of the total bone mass, and includes the outer layer (cortex) of all bones and the interior of the shafts of the long bones. It provides strength for weight bearing and has a low turnover rate of resorption and synthesis. Trabecular bone makes up the remaining bone mass and is present in the interior of the bones, especially the vertebral bodies. It is composed of thin spicules of bone that are lined with osteoblasts and osteoclasts. Trabecular bone has a relatively high turnover rate compared with cortical bone.

Bone is composed of an organic matrix, bone salts, and cells. The organic matrix, which is also called osteoid, provides tensile strength to the bone and is composed of collagen fibers, extracellular fluid, and proteoglycans. The predominant bone salts are calcium and phosphate: they provide compressional strength to the bone and are combined as hydroxyapatite crystals. Lastly, the bone cells—osteoblasts, osteoclasts, and osteocytes—take part in the bone turnover.

The osteoblasts secrete a number of proteins that make up the osteoid. Osteoid acts as a nidus for the precipitation of the hydroxyapatite crystals. Osteocalcin, a protein secreted by osteoblasts after induction by 1,25-dihydroxyvitamin D [1,25(OH)2D], binds calcium and hydroxyapatite. Osteonectin, another protein secreted by osteoblasts, is also involved in bone mineralization. This process is counterbalanced by extracellular glycoproteins that inhibit mineralization. These proteins must be inhibited to promote mineralization.

The coordinated interplay of parathyroid hormone (PTH), vitamin D, calcium, and phosphate has a central role in bone metabolism.[2] An imbalance in any of these compounds or minerals can lead to MBD. Other hormones, such as testosterone and estradiol, are also

TABLE 13-1.

Causes of Osteoporosis

Primary (Involutional)
Type 1, due to low estrogen in post-menopausal population
Type 2 (senile involutional), progressive bone loss after age 35
Secondary
Malabsorption
Hypogonadism
Hyperthyroidism
Hyperparathyroidism
Insulin dependent diabetes
Hypercortisolism
Growth hormone deficiency
Hypothalamic amenorrhea
Hepatobiliary disorders
Multiple myeloma
Decreased mobility
Drug induced, eg, corticosteroids, alcohol, tobacco, heparin, thyroxine, loop diuretics, anticonvulsants

important for maintaining normal bone mass, and their deficiency can lead to a decrease in the ratio of bone formation to bone resorption, which results in decreased bone mineral density.

In response to the biomechanical forces of daily living and to repair the resultant microfractures, bone is constantly undergoing a coordinated process of resorption and bone formation known as remodeling.[1] Vitamin D and PTH stimulate the osteoblasts to secrete factors such as macrophage colony stimulating factor, which cause proliferation of osteoclast precursors that go on to become mature osteoclasts. The osteoclasts secrete acid and proteases that cause resorption of bone in a localized area and create a defect known as a pit. Osteoclasts then move away from the pit and osteoblasts take their place to build new bone matrix and promote its mineralization. Osteoblast and stromal cells secrete two newly described proteins. Osteoprotegrin ligand or nuclear factor kappa-beta (RANK) ligand (a member of the tumor necrosis factor [TNF] family) stimulates the differentiation of pre-osteoclast to osteoclasts and also stimulates the activity of mature osteoclasts by binding to the receptor for activation of RANK on the osteoclast. The other protein, osteoprotegrin, protects the bone from osteoclastic activity by binding to RANK ligand. MBD can occur if there is an imbalance in the closely regulated process of bone remodeling.

Metabolic Bone Disease

The two most common types of MBD are osteoporosis, which is a quantitative defect in which there is decreased bone density, and osteomalacia, which is a qualitative defect where there is defective mineralization of bone. Osteoporosis occurs predominantly in postmenopausal females and elderly adults. Osteomalacia can be seen with severe malabsorption, renal disease, and other metabolic disorders.

OSTEOPOROSIS

The World Health Organization (WHO) defines osteoporosis as "a systemic skeletal disease characterized by low bone mass and micro architectural deterioration of bone tissue, with a consequent increase in bone fragility and susceptibility to fracture." Bone mineral density is most easily measured by dual energy x-ray absorptiometry (DEXA) scan. (DEXA is discussed in detail in Chapter 2.) A T-score between -1 and -2.5 is termed osteopenia, while a T-score less than -2.5 is called osteoporosis. An imbalance in bone remodeling—when the net amount of bone resorption is more than bone formation (negative remodeling balance)—will lead to bone loss.

The development of osteoporosis has been categorized as either the result of low or high bone turnover. Low turnover osteoporosis occurs when there is reduced synthesis accompanied by normal resorption, whereas high turnover osteoporosis occurs when there is enhanced resorption along with increased synthesis that is insufficient to compensate for the degree of resorption. In both situations, there is a net loss of bone.

The prevalence of osteoporosis in United States is 13% to 18% in women above 50 years of age and 3% to 6% in men of the same age.[3] Primary (involutional) osteoporosis accounts for nearly 80% of the patients with osteoporosis and is further subdivided into types 1 and 2. Type 1 is secondary to low estrogen in post-menopausal population and is a high turnover type, whereas type 2 (senile involutional) is a progressive bone loss after the age of 35 years in both men and women and is a low turnover type. A variety of GI and endocrinologic diseases, toxins, and drugs cause secondary osteoporosis. The causes of osteoporosis are listed in Table 13-1.

Osteomalacia

Osteomalacia is characterized by diffuse, dull aching skeletal pain worsened by physical activity.[1] The term itself means soft bones. It is caused by defective mineralization of newly formed osteoid, usually because of vitamin D deficiency. Other etiologies of osteomalacia include renal tubular acidosis; hypophosphatemia; hypophosphatasia (low alkaline phosphate), which is a rare disorder resulting in abnormal bone mineralization; and inhibitors of mineralization such as anticonvulsants, fluoride, etidronate, and aluminum toxicity. In children, the defect in mineralization occurs at the epiphysis, where bone growth takes place, thus resulting in deformities characteristic of rickets. Osteomalacia is now relatively uncommon because of dietary supplementation of vitamin D, thus making osteoporosis the predominant MBD.

Evaluation of Metabolic Bone Disease

A thorough history, physical exam, laboratory assessment, and diagnostic testing are required for the evaluation of MBD.[1] Osteoporosis is generally asymptomatic, while osteomalacia can present with diffuse skeletal pain and proximal muscle weakness. Bone fractures with minimal or no trauma can be a feature of both conditions. A complete dietary and medication history should be taken, especially inquiring about glucocorticoids, diuretics, and adequacy of vitamin and mineral intake. Physical exam may show kyphosis, which is suggestive of past compression fractures of vertebral bodies. Moreover, signs of the underlying diseases may be present in secondary osteoporosis.

Laboratory studies should include a complete blood count, comprehensive metabolic panel, and thyroid-stimulating hormone to exclude liver, kidney, and thyroid diseases and the presence of metabolic acidosis and low concentrations of calcium and phosphate. If there is a strong suspicion of MBD or the bone mineral density is found to be abnormal, an intact parathyroid hormone (iPTH) and 25-hydroxyvitamin D [25(OH)D] should be checked. A high iPTH and low calcium would suggest inadequate calcium intake or absorption, while a high iPTH with high calcium would point towards primary hyperparathyroidism. A high iPTH with a low 25(OH)D could indicate the presence of secondary malabsorption with osteomalacia. Serum magnesium should be assessed if there is significant malabsorption or if diuretics are used that cause increase losses of urinary magnesium. Aluminum toxicity may cause osteomalacia and can be associated with an elevated 1,25(OH)2D, blood aluminum concentration, or abnormal deferoxamine test.

Bone resorption leads to breakdown of collagen into peptides, which can be measured in the urine and blood as markers of bone turnover.[1] Because osteoporosis can be present at any bone turnover rate and the values of these markers overlap between normal and osteoporotic patients, they are not very useful in the diagnosis of osteoporosis. These markers can be used to monitor the effectiveness of medications that decrease the rate of bone resorption in patients with high bone turnover. Some of the available markers, which are byproducts of collagen breakdown and can be measured in serum and urine, include N-telopeptides (NTX), carboxy-terminal cross-links (CTX), and deoxypyridinoline cross-links (DPD).

Bone density measurement is a very important modality in the diagnosis and management of osteoporosis. The most commonly used diagnostic test for bone mineral density is a DEXA scan.[4] On a DEXA scan, bone mineral density is considered normal when it is within one standard deviation of the young adult mean of the same gender and race. This measurement is also called a T-score. In children, a Z-score is used to determine the bone mineral density; this compares patient populations of the same age and gender with normal measurements. A T-score between -1 and -2.5 SD is a modest reduction of bone mineral density and has been termed osteopenia, and a value below -2.5 is osteoporosis. The value of -2.5 is also used as an arbitrary fracture threshold, even though the relationship between bone mineral density and fracture risk is continuous. The advantages of DEXA are its low cost, low levels of radiation exposure (<3 mrem), time efficiency (<10 minutes), and excellent reproducibility (standard error of 1% to 2%).[3] The disadvantage of DEXA scan is that ideally follow-up scans should be conducted on the same machine to avoid variation in results and that it cannot differentiate between osteoporosis and osteomalacia; this can only be done reliably by a bone biopsy. Other less commonly used diagnostic procedures are ultrasonography, single-photon absorptiometry (SPA), dual-photon absorptiometry, quantitative computed tomography (QCT), and radiographic absorptiometry.

Several expert groups have published recommendations for bone mineral density measurement in the general population, the details of which are beyond the scope of this text. Most of these recommendations are based on studies done on postmenopausal white women. Readers may refer to the recommendations by the National Osteoporosis Foundation,[5] United States Preventive Services Task Force,[6] the American Academy of Family Physicians,[7] and the Health Care Finance Administration (HCFA).[8]

Gastrointestinal Disorders Associated With Metabolic Bone Disease

The predominant type of MBD in most GI illnesses is osteoporosis, while osteomalacia can be found on occasion. Table 13-2 lists the GI diseases that will be discussed and is organized by the primary pathogenic process that leads to MBD. This section will also review the effect that certain medications, used to treat these diseases, has on bone metabolism. A few unusual forms of MBD associated with GI illness will also be discussed. These include avascular necrosis, hypertrophic osteoarthropathy, and hepatitis C-associated osteosclerosis (conditions seen most often in adults) and hepatobiliary rickets, which is seen in children.

Table 13-2.

Common Gastrointestinal Disorders Associated With Metabolic Bone Disease

Malabsorption and Maldigestion	Chronic Liver Disease
Celiac disease	Cholestatic diseases
Postgastrectomy	Primary biliary cirrhosis
Short bowel syndrome	Primary sclerosing cholangitiso
Pancreatic insufficiency	Hepatocellular diseases
Cystic Fibrosis	
Inflammatory Bowel Disease	*MBD Secondary to Therapy for GI Illnesses*
Crohn's disease	Post liver transplant
Ulcerative colitis	Medications (eg, corticosteroids, cholestyramine)
	TPN

Celiac Disease

Celiac sprue and the nutrition needs of those suffering from the disease are presented in detail in Chapter 19.

Although there is a lack of population-based data on the prevalence of osteoporosis in patients with celiac disease, several studies have shown lower bone mineral density in patients with untreated celiac disease compared to that in healthy controls.[9-11] A case control study comparing the fracture rates in 165 patients with celiac disease to those in 165 control patients found a significantly higher incidence of fractures in the celiac patients (25% versus 8%).[12] On the other hand, Thomason, West and Logan et al[13] performed a population-based survey for the presence of fractures in 244 patients with celiac and 161 controls and showed no overall risk of increased fractures in celiac patients.

The main pathophysiologic mechanism responsible for celiac-induced osteoporosis is calcium malabsorption. Celiac disease results in villous atrophy, which mainly affects the proximal small bowel, the region of the GI tract with the greatest capacity to absorb calcium.[14] In addition to malabsorption, the amount of calcium available for absorption is also decreased. Patients with celiac disease initially may have lactose intolerance, leading to reduced intake of dairy products, and thus consume a diet with an insufficient amount of calcium. Moreover, there is decreased bioavailability of calcium because it readily binds to unabsorbed fatty acids.[15]

Reduced calcium intake and impaired calcium absorption trigger a sequence of events that leads to a reduction in bone mass.[16] Hypocalcemia causes secondary hypersecretion of PTH-enhanced 1,25(OH)2D synthesis, and decreased 25(OH)D. The defective enterocytes do not respond to 1,25(OH)2D, which leads to a further reduction in calcium absorption. A higher level of 1,25(OH)2D upregulates vitamin D 24-hydroxylase activity and causes more rapid metabolism of vitamin D stores. The vitamin D dependent transporter protein, calbindin-D9K, may also be reduced in celiac disease, further diminishing vitamin D levels. The high levels of PTH also cause an increase in calcium and phosphorus release from bone, an increase in the renal clearance of phosphorus, a lower calcium: phosphate product, and a decrease in bone mineralization.[17] PTH is inversely correlated with bone mineral density, with higher levels of PTH associated with lower bone mineral density.[18]

There are several other factors that can contribute to the development of osteoporosis in celiac disease. Systemic inflammation plays an important role in causing low bone mineral density by the increased production of cytokines that leads to the activation of osteoclasts.[14,19] Elevated levels of interleukin (IL) -6, which has been associated with untreated celiac disease, is associated with low bone mineral density.[18] Insulin-like growth factor (IGF)-1, which has anabolic effects on bone, is reduced in celiac disease in patients with malnutrition or zinc deficiency. Zinc malabsorption can be exacerbated by calcium supplementation because they are both absorbed across the intestinal mucosa by the same transport protein. Another factor contributing to osteoporosis in men with celiac disease is an impaired conversion of testosterone to dihydrotestosterone. This problem is compounded by the presence of androgen resistance, which also occurs in celiac disease.[20,21] These processes appear to develop independently of malabsorption associated with celiac disease.

Postgastrectomy Syndrome

MBD was a common complication in patients with peptic ulcer disease following gastric resection. In one study, the prevalence of osteopenia or vertebral fractures was found to be as high as 55% in postgastrectomy patients.[22] Fortunately, surgery is rarely done for peptic ulcer disease because medical therapies, including treatment of *Helicobacter pylori* and with proton pump inhibitors, have become most effective in preventing complications of the underlying disease.

Calcium malabsorption is the major cause of postgastrectomy–associated MBD. Following antrectomy or sub-total gastrectomy, creation of a gastrojejunostomy (Billroth II anastomosis) leads to calcium malabsorption as a result of the anatomic bypass of the primary site of intestinal calcium absorption. When a gastroduodenostomy (Billroth I anastomosis) is created, malabsorption occurs because of the rapid transit of the meal through the upper digestive tract, which functionally bypasses the proximal duodenum.[23] Serum calcium levels are usually normal in postgastrectomy patients; however, this may be at the expense of the calcium stores in the bones. Malabsorption of vitamin D secondary to intestinal hurry may also occur but it has not been found to be of great clinical consequence. Most studies looking at vitamin D absorption in post-gastrectomy states have found normal absorption or mild malabsorption.[18] Decreased levels of vitamin D found in some studies has been attributed to reduced oral intake.

The role of gastrin in the development of MBD is not very clear, because bone disease has been recognized in patients with partial gastrectomy (hypergastrinemia) and total gastrectomy (hypogastrinemia). Gastrocalcin, a hormone elaborated in the fundic region of the stomach, appears to enhance the uptake of calcium by the bone in the presence of gastrin.[24] The precise role of this hormone is unknown. A lack of gastric acid does not appear to play a major role in the development of MBD in post-gastrectomy patients because chronic, high-dose administration of H2 antagonists does not appear to significantly affect bone mineral density.[25]

Calcitonin, which has osteoclast-inhibiting effects, has been shown to be reduced following antrectomy with Billroth I or II anastomoses.[26] This suggests that low concentrations of calcitonin may play a role in bone resorption in these patients. Reduced protein intake may also have a role in mediating postgastrectomy MBD because proteins help in the formation of collagen matrix of the bone.[23]

Short Bowel Syndrome

There is very little evidence available in literature regarding the incidence of MBD in patients with short bowel syndrome. Obviously, these patients are at risk for the development of both osteoporosis and osteomalacia as consequences of extensive intestinal resection. Calcium and vitamin D are poorly absorbed as a result of diminished intestinal surface area and losses of these nutrients are increased in the presence of steatorrhea. A diminution of the bile salt pool may also contribute to this process. The intestinal tract itself may play a role in the regulation of renal handling of calcium excretion. A study comparing rodents undergoing extensive intestinal resection to controls undergoing intestinal diversion showed that animals undergoing resection lost significantly more calcium in their urine.[27] Patients with short bowel syndrome are also prone to develop metabolic acidosis because a large amount of bicarbonate is lost in the stool. This metabolic abnormality contributes to the development of MBD because phosphate salts provide buffering capacity and are leached from the bone when tissue stores are depleted.

Pancreatic Insufficiency

There is limited data on the incidence of MBD and long-term effect of this problem in adults with chronic pancreatitis (discussed in Chapter 21). In one study that examined the metabolic effect of pancreatic insufficiency in adults predominantly with alcohol-induced chronic pancreatitis, osteopenia was noted in 69% of patients with meal-stimulated intraduodenal lipase <10% of lowest normal range and steatorrhea and 56% of patients with chronic pancreatitis who had adequate lipase secretion.[28] The mean values for calcium, alkaline phosphorus, and PTH were found to be in the normal range, while the mean concentrations of 25(OH)D and 1,25(OH)2D metabolites were low in both groups of patients. These patients also had other risk factors for the development of MBD including alcohol exposure, tobacco use, and hypogonadism.

Cystic Fibrosis

Children and young adults with cystic fibrosis have decreased bone mineralization, which in one study was found to be on average 19% less than in age and gender-matched controls.[29] Another study found lower bone mineral density accompanied by a higher fracture rate.[30] In addition to lower bone mineral density, other less common skeletal manifestations of cystic fibrosis are hypertrophic osteoarthropathy and a painful arthropathy.[31,32] The former presents with joint deformity while the latter is manifested as swollen painful joints accompanied by a rash. These less common conditions have been reported in up to 5% of cystic fibrosis patients. The causes of MBD patients with cystic fibrosis have pancreatic insufficiency and abnormalities of bile salt metabolism. (Nutrition needs of patients with cystic fibrosis are discussed in Chapter 25.)

Inflammatory Bowel Disease

Osteoporosis is a common occurrence in inflammatory bowel disease (IBD), with up to 30% of patients with Crohn's disease or ulcerative colitis having low bone mineral density.[33,34] The overall risk of fractures in IBD is 40% greater than that of the general population and the overall incidence is approximately 1 per 100 patient years, but advanced age is a major factor determining the incidence of fractures.[35] Some studies have shown osteopenia to be more common in Crohn's disease than ulcerative colitis,[36-38] while others have failed to show any difference between the two.[34,39-41]

Predisposing factors that contribute to the development of osteoporosis in the general population—such as sedentary lifestyle, low body mass index, hypogonadism, low dietary intake of calcium and vitamin D, and smoking—are also important in patients with IBD. Additional risk factors predisposing these patients to develop MBD include the inflammatory cytokines IL-1, IL-6, and TNF-α. TNF-α inhibits expression of a critical transcription factor required for osteoblast differentiation and induces osteoclast differentiation, thus promoting bone resorption. It also increases the life span of mature osteoclasts and protects them against apoptosis; inhibits bone collagen synthesis; and antagonizes the vitamin D by activation of a nuclear inhibitor; and, with IL-1, TNF-α sensitizes osteoblasts to apoptosis. TNF-α also stimulates osteoblasts to secrete IL-6, which in turn increases osteoclast activation. On the other hand, some cytokines, such as IL-12 and IL-18, have protective effects on bone mineral density by inhibiting osteoclast activation. TGF-β has both positive and negative effects on osteoclast activation. The clinical significance of these cytokines in preventing MBD is not very clear.

Another factor contributing to MBD is vitamin D deficiency, which is common in IBD, with one study showing 65% of patients with Crohn's disease having low vitamin D stores.[42] The low vitamin D levels are either because of poor vitamin D absorption secondary to diseased bowel or resection of small bowel segments. Along with vitamin D, avoidance of dairy intake in Crohn's disease patients also predisposes them to calcium deficiency.

Glucocorticoids are another important cause of MBD in IBD. The mechanism whereby glucocorticoids cause MBD is discussed later in this chapter.

Chronic Liver Disease

MBD in patients with chronic liver disease has been termed hepatic osteodystrophy. Although the liver has an essential role in the vitamin D absorption and metabolism, the primary disorder is osteoporosis and not osteomalacia.[43] As stated earlier, the latter is now uncommon because of better dietary management and vitamin D supplementation.[44] The prevalence of MBD in chronic liver disease ranges from 5% to 50%, depending on the underlying disease and type of study used to assess the frequency of this complication.[43] Uncontrolled cross-sectional studies appear to overestimate the prevalence of MBD, while controlled cross-sectional and longitudinal studies appear to provide more accurate estimates. Differences in study results also reflect the heterogeneity of patients with chronic liver disease, exposure to corticosteroids, and the gender of patients with certain forms of liver disease. For example, osteoporosis occurs in a moderately large number of patients with primary biliary cirrhosis (PBC) because it affects middle-aged women who are already prone to MBD.[43] Some studies suggest that patients with cholestatic disorders, such as PBC and primary sclerosing cholangitis (PSC), have a lower bone mineral density than do those with noncholestatic disorders; however, the differences do not appear to be as great as once thought. While PBC has been more extensively studied as a cause of osteoporosis, PSC seems to have a similar predisposition to osteoporosis.[45]

The pathophysiology of MBD in chronic liver disease is multifactorial, with a number of mechanisms described. Nutritional deficiencies are common in chronic liver disease.[43] Toxins—including unconjugated bilirubin, copper, and bile salts—that are retained because of cholestasis, prevent the osteoblasts from functioning properly and results in decreased bone formation.[44,46,47] The hypothesis that decreased bile salt flow leads to decreased vitamin D absorption has been discounted because of the observation that most patients with PBC and osteoporosis have normal levels of vitamin D.[48]

Hypogonadism is another factor contributing to bone loss in chronic liver disease.[43] Hypogonadism in males results in lower levels of testosterone and estrogens, as testosterone is converted to estrogen, and thus contributes to osteoporosis. Other factors include lower levels of IGF-1 in advanced chronic liver disease.[46] Its significance in osteoporosis is highlighted by an animal study showing improvement in bone density with IGF-1 therapy.[49] Similarly, osteoprotegrin is produced by the liver, and its lower levels will also predispose patients to osteoporosis. Renal tubular acidosis and malabsorption of vitamin K in liver disease may also contribute to development of osteoporosis.[46]

Liver Transplant

Rapid bone loss occurs following the first 3 to 6 months after orthotopic liver transplant and then stabilizes. This is associated with an increased risk of fractures, with 35% of patients having fractures in the first year following transplant. Improved bone density is then seen 6 months after transplant and is attributed to the tapering doses of corticosteroids and immunosuppressants used during transplant and because the underlying liver condition causing the pretransplant bone loss has resolved.[50] Over the subsequent 5 years, there is also a reduction in fracture rate.[51]

There are a numbers of pretransplant and posttransplant factors contributing to MBD in orthotopic liver transplant patients. The most important pretransplant factor is the presence of osteopenia at baseline.[46] As discussed earlier, cholestatic diseases may have a higher incidence of MBD. These patients also have an increased risk of osteonecrosis after transplant.[50] In hemochromatosis, hypogonadism and low testosterone levels contribute to the development of MBD. In alcoholic liver disease, hypogonadism, poor nutrition, sedentary life style, and direct toxic effects of alcohol are factors that contribute to the development of low bone density.[46,50] Prolonged use of loop diuretics may also contribute to MBD by causing an increase in urinary calcium loss. Liver transplantation by itself can also cause bone loss, as demonstrated in an animal study that suggested that denervation after liver transplant causes impaired functioning of osteoblasts via a process involving altered local signaling through the autonomic nervous system in bone tissue.[52] Patients may also develop secondary hyperparathyroidism after transplant, which can also contribute to bone loss.[53]

Medications That Affect Bone Metabolism

A number of medications have adverse side effects on bone metabolism, including corticosteroids, heparin, warfarin, cholestyramine, immunosuppressants, loop diuretics, and parenteral nutrition (PN). Most of these medications lead to bone loss through a variety of mechanisms. On the other hand, thiazide diuretics can minimize bone loss. These medications are important adjuncts to the management of GI disease; therefore, it is imperative for gastroenterologists to recognize the role that these medications play in MBD. A few of these medications will be discussed here.

Glucocorticoid-induced osteoporosis is multifactorial. It inhibits bone formation, increases bone resorption, decreases intestinal absorption of calcium, and increases renal excretion of calcium. Glucocorticoids alter bone metabolism, favoring bone loss by increasing the production of osteoprotegrin ligand while decreasing the produc-

TABLE 13-3.

Parenteral Nutrition Preparation to Minimize Metabolic Bone Disease

Calcium gluconate	Initial dose 15 mEq, adjust to blood and urine levels
Magnesium sulfate	Initial dose 15 mEq, adjust to blood and urine levels
Phosphate	Calcium to phosphate ratio 1:2, adjust to blood level
Sodium	Meet daily losses, adjust to blood level
Acetate	Adjust to normalized serum bicarbonate
Vitamin D	200 IU (in parenteral multiple vitamins)
Amino acids	Reduce to maintenance dose (1 gm/kg/d) once weight and visceral protein level replete

tion of osteoprotegrin.[54] In one study, the incidence of osteopenia in patients with IBD on glucocorticoids was found to be twice as high as those not treated by glucocorticoids.[55] Both glucocorticoids and IBD have an inhibitory effect on the pituitary-gonadal axis. The resulting hypogonadism may be an important factor in predisposing patients to MBD.

Immunosuppressants such as cyclosporine and tacrolimus are an important category of medications in the post-liver transplant period. They are used to prevent rejection and are steroid-sparing drugs. Because immunosuppressants are given alongside corticosteroids, it may be difficult to separate out their effects from those of steroids on bone density. Because of the importance of limiting the severity of glucocorticoid-induced MBD, Park, Hay and Lee et al[56] conducted a study comparing bone mineral density in two groups of posttransplant patients. One group of patients received conventional cyclosporine with corticosteroids while the other received tacrolimus with low dose corticosteroids. No significant difference was found in the bone mineral density between both groups. This suggests that either tacrolimus has a stronger effect on bone density negating the presumed beneficial effect of using a low dose of corticosteroids, or that the associated renal dysfunction seen with tacrolimus use contributes to the loss of bone density. Closer investigation of the metabolic effects of these medications needs to be undertaken.

Loop diuretics increase urinary calcium by impairing reabsorption in the loop of Henle. Prolonged use can cause a negative calcium balance and promote osteoporosis. Thiazide diuretics, on the other hand, increase calcium reabsorption and decrease calcium excretion. In cross-sectional studies and clinical trials, thiazides have shown a beneficial effect on bone mineral density,[57,58] while some observational studies have also shown decreased fracture risk with thiazides.[59] The evidence is not sufficient to recommend use of thiazides for prevention or treatment of osteoporosis, but they can be used in the place of loop diuretics in osteoporotic patients, if needed.

PN has been known to have a negative impact on bone metabolism (Chapter 38). Contamination of PN solutions with aluminum through the use of protein hydrolysate as a source of nitrogen was a cause of MBD in the past but is now uncommon (Chapter 36). The primary cause of MBD in patients on PN is the patient's underlying disease that leads to the use of PN. Having said this, PN solutions have been shown to increase the urinary excretion of calcium, especially when this therapy is first initiated. The cause for the development of hypercalciuria has been attributed to an increase in the glomerular filtration rate that is believed to be caused by an increase in renal blood flow.[60] Over time, homeostatic mechanisms develop, which leads to conservation of calcium through a slight increase in PTH secretion. While these changes have been demonstrated in a primate model, clinical observations support these events in humans.[61] In addition, there are numerous factors that promote hypercalciuria during PN administration. They include rapid infusion of the solution; high versus modest doses of amino acids; dextrose, calcium, and sodium infusion; and inadequate dosing of phosphorous. While some of these factors cannot be avoided, measures can be taken to minimize hypercalciuria and thus the development of MBD in patients receiving PN.[62] Some of these measures are outlined in Table 13-3.

Metabolic Bone Disease Other than Osteoporosis and Osteomalacia in Gastrointestinal Illnesses

Avascular necrosis—also called osteonecrosis, aseptic necrosis, ischemic necrosis, and osteochondritis dissecans—is caused by compromise of the bone vasculature, which results in the death of bone segments.[63] Etiologies relating to GI illnesses include corticosteroid use, post-transplantation (most likely secondary to steroids), and alcohol intake. Most common presentation is pain, and site of involvement is femoral head, although other joints may be involved. Alkaline phosphatase, frog-leg and lateral x-rays, and bone scans are needed for diagnosis; however, plain radiographs may not show joint involvement for months after the disease has started. Magnetic resonance imaging is better for diagnosis but may lead to overdiagnosis and unnecessary treatment. Prevention strategies include avoidance of the etiological factors and minimizing corticosteroid use, which may be possible by using steroid-sparing medications in the posttransplant setting. Treatment modalities include core decompression, osteotectomy, and joint replacement.

Rickets secondary to hepatobiliary diseases or hepatobiliary rickets has skeletal manifestations similar to those of nutritional rickets.[64] Hepatobiliary conditions impair vitamin D absorption from the GI tract, and, in addition, there is insufficient 25-hydroxylation of vitamin D2 by the hepatocytes, although a small study from 1979 involving 3 pediatric patients showed that the cause of low vitamin D was only malabsorption of vitamin D and not impairment of hepatic metabolism.[65]

Hepatitis-C–associated osteosclerosis is a rare disease that is characterized by a marked increase in bone mass during adult life. Common presentation during active disease is forearm and leg pain. With the exception of the cranium, all bones are involved and there is periosteal, endosteal, and trabecular bone thickening. The underlying etiology is alteration in IGF-1 and IGF-II or their binding proteins (IGFBPs); these have potent anabolic effects on bone by stimulation of osteoblasts.[66] Bone turnover is high, with bone mineral density as high as two to three times of age-matched controls. There is spontaneous remission, and, if not, then bisphosphonates or calcitonin may be tried.

Hypertrophic osteoarthropathy (HOA) is a syndrome characterized by abnormal proliferation of skin and osseous tissues in the distal extremities. Secondary HOA is due to some underlying disease process and is seen in about 5% of cystic fibrosis patients.[31] It is also seen in patients with IBD, where it is accompanied by sacroiliitis, spondylitis, arthropathy, and juxta articular osteoporosis.

Recommendations for Prevention and Treatment of Metabolic Bone Disease in Gastrointestinal Illness

General Recommendations

Behavioral modifications are very important for the prevention and treatment of MBD. Regular exercise and the avoidance of smoking and alcohol intake should be recommended in all patients with osteoporosis. If the lumbar spine density is diminished, a referral to physical therapy is warranted. Vitamin D deficiency should be diagnosed and treated.[20] Vitamin D should be supplemented (400 to 800 IU/day) in patients with less than 400 IU/day dietary intake of vitamin D. In patients with low 25(OH)D levels, repeat levels in 1 month and adjust the dose to keep the level in the upper half of normal (normal range 10 to 50 ng/ml). Gonadal steroid deficiency should be treated if present. Ensure adequate dietary intake of calcium (1500 mg/day).[20] Patients on chronic steroids should receive calcium and vitamin D supplementation. Glucocorticoid use should be minimized if possible. Patients who require steroids for more than 3 months should be considered for bisphosphonate therapy. One study prefers calcium citrate over calcium carbonate because of better absorption and bioavailability.[67] If the patient has secondary hyperparathyroidism, it should be treated with calcium and vitamin D.[20] When prescribing estrogen to post-menopausal women, the benefits should be weighed against the cardiovascular and breast cancer risks. If osteoporosis has developed, pharmacologic therapy should be used.

Bone Mineral Density Measurement in Gastrointestinal Illness

Bone mineral density measurement should be considered in patients with GI disease under the following circumstances: in patients who have used corticosteroids for more than 3 months or have had repeated use; in patients with fragility fractures (fractures with minimal or no trauma); in postmenopausal females or males >50 years; and in those individuals who have hypogonadism.[18] In adults with a new diagnosis of celiac disease, consider DEXA at diagnosis and at 1 year after initiation of a gluten-free diet.[18] Bone mineral density should also be measured in patients with cirrhosis and PBC and all patients being evaluated for liver transplantation. Follow-up DEXA scans should be done at 2 to 3 years for patients with a normal initial DEXA and at 1 year for patients with initial high-dose corticosteroid therapy. For patients on long-term corticosteroids, DEXA scans should be repeated yearly until bone mineral density stabilizes.

Treatment Recommendations Based on DEXA Results

Patients with a T score higher than -1 only require basic measures to prevent osteopenia. This includes adequate calcium and vitamin D intake, regular weight bearing exercises, smoking cessation, avoidance of excess alcohol intake, minimization of corticosteroid use, and correction of hypogonadism. When the T score ranges from -1 to -2.5, osteopenia is present and all of the basic preventive measures noted above should be applied. Referral to a physician with a special interest in MBD might be considered at this time. Repeat DEXA should be done in 2 years to assess for further loss in bone density. If prolonged or repeated corticosteroid therapy is required for the management of the underlying disease in patients with osteopenia, then one should consider prescribing a bisphophonate and repeating the DEXA in 1 year. Patients with osteoporosis, defined as a T score below -2.5, and those with vertebral compression and fragility fractures, regardless of T score results, should be counseled on all of the basic preventive measures noted above and should be screened for other causes of low bone density. Testing should include a complete blood count: serum calcium, alkaline phosphate, creatinine, vitamin D, protein electrophoresis, and (in males) testosterone. Bisphosphonate or recombinant human PTH should be prescribed or referral to a bone specialist should be considered.

Pharmacologic Therapy for Metabolic Bone Disease

Several different medications are currently used for the treatment of osteoporosis. These are listed in Table 13-4. The first class of drugs is the antiresorptive medications, which includes estrogen, selective estrogen receptor modulators, bisphosphonates, and calcitonin. Their basic mechanism of action is inhibition of osteoclastic bone

TABLE 13-4.

Pharmacologic Therapy for Osteoporosis

- Calcium/Vitamin D
- Selective estrogen receptor modulators (Evista)
- Bisphosphonates (Alendronate, Risedronate)
- Estrogen: only selective use
- Calcitonin
- Recombinant human PTH 1-34 (Forteo, Teriparatide of rDNA origin)
- Isoflavones
- Calcitriol: only selective use
- Thiazide diuretics
- Androgens: in male hypogonadism

resorption. The second class of drugs works at the level of bone formation. The only currently effective drug in this category is teriparatide (Forteo, Ely Lilly, Indianapolis IN).[68] Teriparatide is manufactured from recombinant human DNA from amino acids 1-34 of the native peptide. It has been approved for use in postmenopausal women with osteoporosis and men with senile osteoporosis or osteoporosis from hypogonadism. PTH can increase both osteoblast and osteoclast function. When PTH is chronically elevated, as in primary hyperparathyroidism, it causes bone resorption. Intermittent administration of PTH augments osteoblast function more than osteoclasts, which leads to an increase in bone density. Teriparatide works on the latter principle and is given as a daily injection. It has a peak serum level in 30 minutes and declines to undetectable levels in 3 hours. Off-label uses of teriparatide include that for patients who have failed antiresorptive therapy or who are considered high risk for fractures. Because of a risk of development of osteosarcoma seen in animal studies, the use of teriparatide should be avoided in children, teenagers, young adults, and patients with open epiphysis, Paget's disease, prior radiation, unexplained elevation of alkaline phosphatase, bone metastasis, skeletal malignancies, preexisting hypercalcemia, or MBD other than osteoporosis.

Recommendations below are disease specific.

Malabsorption Due to Any Cause

Patients with malabsorption may need higher doses of calcium and vitamin D. Calcium requirements can be as high as 2 to 3 g/day. Blood calcium levels are maintained at the expense of the bones even in low calcium states by the release of calcium from bones. Therefore the adequacy of calcium dosing is not always reflected in the serum. A 24-hour urine sample can be checked to see if the amount of calcium excreted is in the normal range. Urinary values fall below the normal range of 100 to 300 mg/day when oral dosing is not adequate. In severe malabsorption, oral vitamin D at 50,000 IU 2 to 3 times a week may be needed. If this does not work, 1,25(OH)2D at a dose of 0.5 mcg/day may be required. On rare occasions, parenteral vitamin D is needed when these other measures fail. Vitamin D metabolites should be monitored as outlined previously to avoid excessive dosing and toxicity. Hypomagnesemia can also accompany malabsorption. Low serum levels of magnesium interfere with PTH secretion and its effect on the kidneys. It can be difficult to replete low magnesium because many of the available supplements are composed of salts that dissociated poorly in the GI tract and exacerbate diarrhea. Magnesium lactate dihydrate, gluconate, and chloride salts dissociated well at a neutral pH, and, as in the case of calcium, a 24-hour urine magnesium determination may be needed to assess for adequate dosing. One must keep in mind that treatment of the underlying disease can improve intestinal absorption and result in a decrease in the requirement for these nutrients.

(Additional discussion of general nutrient deficiency is discussed in Chapter 3, and Chapter 5 provides a general discussion of the diagnosis and treatment of malabsorption.)

Celiac Disease

Bone mineral density is commonly decreased in patients with untreated celiac disease and, following treatment with a gluten-free diet, bone mineral density almost always increases and may even reach normal values. In one study the fractional absorption of calcium returned to normal after 1 year of treatment with a gluten-free diet, but bone mineral density was not affected. Conversely, a 5-year prospective study of celiac disease patients consuming a gluten-free diet showed an increase in bone mineral density with the most increase in the first year.[19] Other studies have shown this range of improvement, from modest to clinically significant.[69,70] One study found an overall improvement in bone mineral density after 1 year of treatment, but mucosal recovery had occurred in only 57% of patients. These findings suggest that a gluten-free diet can improve bone mineral density even when villous atrophy persists,[14,71] whereas another study found a more direct correlation between villous atrophy and bone mineral density.[72] Adults with treated celiac disease who were diagnosed as children and who started and adhered to a gluten-free diet have a higher bone mineral density than do those diagnosed as adults.[18] These studies underscore the importance that adherence to a gluten-free diet has on the prevention of MBD.

Secondary hyperparathyroidism develops in patients with untreated celiac disease. Some experts recommend supplementation of calcium and vitamin D to prevent this,[14,20] but it has not been supported by controlled studies.[14,70] Most studies demonstrate that treatment with a gluten-free diet is adequate for prevention.

Even if asymptomatic, celiac disease should be diagnosed early and treated with a strict gluten-free diet to optimize the patient's bone health and thus to prevent fractures.[18] Screening of family members of celiac disease patients should be done because earlier diagnosis is important and low bone mineral density is not fully reversible in late diagnosis and treatment of celiac disease. In adults with a new diagnosis of celiac, consider DEXA at diagnosis and at 1 year after initiation of a gluten-free diet. DEXA scan is not needed in newly diagnosed uncomplicated pediatric celiac patients. For osteoporotic women, males >55 years, and those with fragility fractures, measure bone mineral density at menopause or when first seen and offer treatment if osteoporotic.[20] Serum 25(OH)D, calcium, and PTH should be measured in patients with newly diagnosed celiac disease.[18]

Postgastrectomy

There is no clear evidence that calcium and vitamin D supplementation is beneficial in preventing MBD in postgastrectomy patients.[14] Some authors have recommended increased calcium intake but other studies have not shown any advantage.[14]

Severe hypocalcemia after intravenous pamidronate has been reported in a patient with subclinical osteomalacia because of vitamin D deficiency (as a result of gastric bypass surgery).[73] Patients should be screened for vitamin D deficiency prior to receiving intravenous bisphosphonate therapy.

Cystic Fibrosis

Routine supplementation of 400-800 IU of vitamin D may not be enough to maintain a normal bone mineral density in cystic fibrosis. Therefore, serum 25(OH)D levels should be measured as part of the management of cystic fibrosis patients.[30]

Inflammatory Bowel Disease

In ulcerative colitis, usual doses of vitamin D (400 IU/day) and calcium (1000 to 1500 mg/day) should be sufficient, but patients with extensive Crohn's disease of the small bowel have a higher requirement, and serum levels of calcium, phosphate, vitamin D, and PTH should be measured to guide therapy. The extra citrate or even carbonate given with calcium supplements also acts as a bicarbonate precursor and has other advantages in IBD as well, such as decreasing urolithiasis. Citrate decreases urolithiasis directly as an inhibitor of stone formation and indirectly by correcting metabolic acidosis caused by persistent diarrhea. The correction of metabolic acidosis also decreases uric acid stone formation.

Once patients are receiving adequate calcium/vitamin D/gonadal steroids, they should have their bone mineral density checked every 2 years. If they continue to lose bone mineral density, antiresorptive therapy should be considered. Postmenopausal women with IBD may benefit from estrogen therapy by improvement in bone mineral density but the side effect profile of estrogens suggests bisphosphonate therapy instead. Low-impact exercise improves bone mineral density[74] and thus potentially reduces fracture rate in Crohn's disease patients.

Chronic Liver Disease

In general, there should be a focus on prevention of osteoporosis.[44] At diagnosis of PBC, plasma 25(OH)D, calcium, and phosphate should be measured. If normal, repeat the measurements every 2 to 3 years. Patients with severe symptomatic bone disease refractory to medical management should be referred for liver transplantation. One of the first clinical manifestations of cholestatic liver disease can be osteoporosis; therefore, antimitochondrial antibody should be checked in osteoporotic patients with elevated alkaline phosphatase and gamma glutamyl transpeptidase.[46] If estrogen must be administered to a patient with liver disease, the patient should receive transdermal estrogen, which is less hepatotoxic.

Liver Transplant

Pretransplant evaluation for MBD should include a history and physical exam focusing on the risk factors for osteoporosis and thoraco-lumbar spine X-rays, especially if loss of height or severe back pain is reported.[46] Serum calcium, phosphate, 25(OH)D level, and free testosterone level (in males) should be checked. Therapy should include education of patients regarding behavioral/lifestyle modification (smoking cessation and weight bearing exercises) and correction of vitamin D deficiency, keeping serum 25(OH)D level in the range of 25 to 30 ng/ml. For levels <15 ng/ml, vitamin D supplementation of 50,000 IU PO/wk for 8 weeks should be given. For maintenance, vitamin D supplementation (400 to 800 IU PO/day), and calcium supplementation (1000 to 1200 mg of elemental calcium), should be given.

Pharmacological therapy with estrogen, oral or intravenous bisphosphonates, and calcitonin has been shown to have conflicting results in different small trials. These therapeutic modalities have shown encouraging results and have been approved by FDA in other settings with osteoporosis; therefore, they should be considered for patients with liver transplant as well.[46] Teriparatide can also be used, but these therapies should be coordinated by a bone specialist. Hormone therapy may be used for female hypogonadism and early menopause (before age 45 years). Testosterone should be used to treat hypogonadism in men.

Conclusion

Patients with GI illnesses that result in maldigestion, malabsorption, and chronic inflammation or who use drugs known to adversely affect bone mineral density should be evaluated for secondary MBD. Over the past decade, our ability to assess and treat osteoporosis has markedly improved because DEXA scan is now widely available, and medications—such as selective estrogen receptor modulators, bisphosphonates and PTH—have been developed and approved for use. All patients who are at risk for developing MBD should be advised to discontinue tobacco use and limit alcohol intake and those with malabsorption may require oral supplements of calcium, vitamin D, and magnesium. The need to avoid the development of this potentially debilitating complication of GI disease cannot be overstated.

References

1. Raisz LG, Kream BE, Lorenzo JA. Metabolic Bone Disease. In: Larsen PR, Kronenberg HM, Melmed S, Polonsky KS, eds. *Williams Textbook of Endocrinology,* 10th ed. Philadelphia, PA: Elsevier; 2003: 1373-1410.
2. Barrett EJ, Barrett, P. The parathyroid glands and vitamin D. In: Boron WF, Boulpaep EL, eds. *Medical Physiology.* Philadelphia, PA: Saunders; 2003:1086-1102.
3. Looker AC, Orwoll ES, Johnston CC Jr, et al. Prevalence of low femoral bone density in older US adults from NHANES III. *J Bone Miner Res.* 1997;12:1761-1768
4. Richmond B. DXA scanning to diagnose osteoporosis: do you know what the results mean? *Cleveland Clinic Journal of Medicine.* 2003;70:353-360.
5. National Osteoporosis Foundation. Guidelines for osteoporosis screening. Available at http://www.nof.org/_vti_bin/shtml.dll/physguide/index.htm . Accessed June 14, 2004.
6. U.S. Preventive Services Task Force. *Guide to Clinical Preventive Services,* 3rd ed. Available at http://www.ahrq.gov/clinic/uspstfix.htm. Accessed June 14, 2004.
7. American Academy of Family Physicians. *Age charts for periodic health examination.* Kansas City, MO: American Academy of Family Physicians; 1994.
8. DHHS. Medicare program: Medicare coverage of and payment for bone mass measurements. Federal Register. Washington DC, US Government Printing Office 1998;63(121):34320-34328.
9. Kemppainen T, Kroger H, Janatuinen E, et al. Osteoporosis in adult patients with celiac disease. *Bone.* 1999;24:249-255.
10. Mustalahti K, Collin P, Sievanen H, Salmi J, Maki M. Osteopenia in patients with clinically silent disease warrants screening. *Lancet.* 1999;354:744-745.
11. Gonzalez D, Mazure R, Mautalen C, Vasquez H, Bai J. Body composition and bone mineral density in untreated and treated patients with celiac disease. *Bone.* 1995;16:231-234.
12. Vasquez H, Mazure R, Gonzalez D, et al. Risk of fractures in celiac disease patients: a cross-sectional, case-control study. *Am J Gastroenterol.* 2000;95:183-189.
13. Thomason K, West J, Logan RFA, Coupland C, Holmes GKT. Fracture experience of patients with celiac disease: a population based survey. *Gut.* 2003;52:518-522.
14. Tirpitz C, Reinshagen M. Management of osteoporosis in patients with gastrointestinal diseases. *European Journal of Gastroenterology & Hepatology.* 2003;15:869-876.
15. Walters JRF. The role of the intestine in bone homeostasis. *European Journal of Gastroenterology & Hepatology.* 2003;15:845-849.
16. Bernstein CN, Leslie WD. The pathophysiology of bone disease in gastrointestinal disease. *European Journal of Gastroenterology & Hepatology.* 2003;15:857-864.
17. Fickling WE, McFarlane XA, Bhalla AK, Robertson DAF. The Clinical impact of MBD in celiac disease. *Postgrad Med J.* 2001;77:33-36.
18. Bernstein CN, Leslie WD, Leboff MS. AGA technical review on osteoporosis in gastrointestinal diseases. *Gastroenterology.* 2003;124:795-841.
19. Kemppainen T, Kroger H, Janatuinen E, et al. Bone recovery after a gluten free diet: a 5-year follow-up study. *Bone.* 1999;25:355-360.
20. Scott EM, Gaywood I, Scott BB. Guidelines for osteoporosis in celiac disease and inflammatory bowel disease. British Society of Gastroenterology. *Gut.* 2000;46(suppl 1):1-8.
21. Farthing MJ, Rees LJ, Edwards CR, Dawson AM. Male gonadal function in celiac disease: 2. Sex hormones. *Gut.* 1983;24:127-135.
22. Zittel TT, Zeeb B, Maier GW, et al. High prevalence of bone disorders after gastrectomy. *Am J Surg.* 1997;174:431-438.
23. Tovey FI, Hall ML, Ell PJ, Hobsley M. A review of post gastrectomy bone disease. *J Gastroenterol Hepatol.* 1992;7:639-45.
24. Hakanson R, Persson P, Axelson J, Johnell O, Sundler F. Evidence that gastrin enhances 45Ca uptake into bone through release of a gastric hormone. *Regul Pept.* 1990; 28:107-118.
25. Adachi Y, Shiota E, Matsumata T, Iso Y, Yoh R, Kitano S. Bone mineral density in patients taking H2 receptor antagonist. *Calcified Tissue International.* 1998;62:283-285.
26. Filipponi P, Gregorio F, Cristallini S, et al. Partial gastrectomy and mineral metabolism: effects on gastrin-calcitonin release. *Bone Miner.* 1990;11:199-208.
27. Chu RC, Barkowski SM, Buhac J. Small bowel resection associated urinary calcium loss in rats on long term TPN. *Journal of Parenteral and Enteral Nutrition.* 1990;14:64-67.
28. Haaber AB, Rosenfalck AM, Hansen B, Hilsted J, Larsen S. Bone mineral metabolism, bone mineral density, and body composition in patients with chronic pancreatitis and pancreatic exocrine insufficiency. *International Journal of Pancreatology.* 2000; 27:21-27.
29. Henderson RC, Madsen CD. Bone mineral content and body composition in children and young adults with cystic fibrosis. *Pediatr Pulmonol.* 1999;27:80-84.
30. Donovan DS Jr, Papadopoulos A, Staron RB, et al. Bone mass and vitamin D deficiency in adults with advanced cystic fibrosis lung disease. *Am J Respir Crit Care Med.* 1998;157:1892-1900.
31. Lipnick RN, Glass RB. Bone changes associated with cystic fibrosis. *Skeletal Radiol.* 1992;2:115-116.
32. Merkel PA. Rheumatic disease and cystic fibrosis. *Arthritis Rheum.* 1999;42:1563-1571.
33. Compston JE, Judd D, Crawley EO, et al. Osteoporosis in patients with inflammatory bowel disease. *Gut.* 1987;28:410-415.
34. Pigot F, Roux C, Chaussade S, et al. Low bone mineral density in patients with inflammatory bowel disease. *Dig Dis Sci.* 1992;37:1396-403.
35. Bernstein CN, Blanchard JF, Leslie W, Wajda A, Yu BN. The incidence of fracture among patients with inflammatory bowel disease: a population-based cohort study. *Ann Int Med.* 2000;133:795-799.
36. Jahnsen J, Falch JA, Aadland E, Mowinckel P. Bone mineral density is reduced in patients with Crohn's disease but not in patients with ulcerative colitis: a population based study. *Gut.* 1997;40:313-319.
37. Ghosh S, Cowen S, Hannan WJ, Ferguson A. Low bone mineral density in Crohn's disease, but not in ulcerative colitis at diagnosis. *Gastroenterology.* 1994;107:1031-1039.
38. Gokhale R, Favus MJ, Karrison T, Sutton MM, Rich B, Kirschner BS. Bone mineral density assessment in children with inflammatory bowel disease. *Gastroenterology.* 1998;114:902-911.
39. Abitbol V, Roux C, Chaussade S, et al. Metabolic bone assessment in patients with inflammatory bowel disease. *Gastroenterology.* 1995;108:417-422.
40. Bjarnason I, Macpherson A, Mackintosh C, Buxton-Thomas M, Forgacs I, Moniz C. Reduced bone density in patients with inflammatory bowel disease. *Gut.* 1997;40:228-233.
41. Bernstein CN, Seeger LL, Sayre JW, Anton PA, Artinian L, Shanahan F. Decreased bone density in inflammatory bowel disease is related to corticosteroid use and not disease diagnosis. *J Bone Miner Res.* 1995;10:250-256.
42. Driscoll RH, Meredith SC, Sitrin M, Rosenberg IH. Vitamin D deficiency and bone disease in patients with Crohn's disease. *Gastroenterology.* 1982;83:1252-1258.
43. American Gastroenterological Association medical position statement: osteoporosis in hepatic disorders. *Gastroenterology.* 2003;125:937-940.

44. Flamm S, Kaplan MM. MBD in primary biliary cirrhosis. Up-to-date version 11.3. Available by subscription at http://www.uptodate.com. Accessed February 20, 2004.
45. Hay JE, Lindor KD, Wiesner RH, Dickson ER, Krom RA, LaRusso NF. The metabolic bone disease of primary sclerosing cholangitis. *Hepatology.* 1991;14:257-261.
46. Leslie WD, Bernstein CN, Leboff MS. AGA technical review on osteoporosis in gastrointestinal diseases. *Gastroenterology.* 2003;125:941-966.
47. Janes CH, Dickson ER, Okazaki R, Bonde S, McDonagh AF, Riggs BL. Role of hyperbilirubinemia in the impairment of osteoblast proliferation associated with cholestatic jaundice. *J Clin Invest.* 1995;95:2581-2586.
48. Kaplan MM, Goldberg MJ, Matloff DS, Neer RM, Goodman DB. Effect of 25-hydroxy vitamin D3 on vitamin D metabolites in primary biliary cirrhosis. *Gastroenterology.* 1981;81:681-685.
49. Cemborain A, Castilla-Cortazar I, Garcia M, et al. Osteopenia in rats with liver cirrhosis: beneficial effects of IGF-1 treatment. *J Hepatol.* 1998;28:122-131.
50. Reich D, Rothstein K, Manzarbeitia C, Munoz S. Common medical diseases after liver transplantation. *Seminars in Gastrointestinal Disease.* 1998;9:110-125.
51. Porayko MK, Wiesner RH, Hay JE, et al. Bone disease in liver transplant recipients: incidence, timing, and risk factors. *Transplantation Proceedings.* 1991;23:1462-1465.
52. Kissler H J, Erben R G, Hennig R, et al. Regional bone loss after orthotopic liver transplantation in inbred rats: the role of hepatic denervation. *Calcif Tissue Int.* 2002;71:193-202.
53. Arnold J C, Hauser D, Ziegler R, et al. Bone Disease after Liver Transplantation. *Transplantation Proceedings.* 1992;24:2709-2710.
54. Canalis E, Giustina A. Glucocorticoid-induced osteoporosis: summary of a workshop. *Journal of Clinical Endocrinology & Metabolism.* 2001;86:5681-5685.
55. Abitbol V, Roux C, Chaussade S, et al. Metabolic bone assessment in patients with inflammatory bowel disease. *Gastroenterology.* 1995;108:417-422.
56. Park KM, Hay JE, Lee SG, et al. Bone loss after orthotopic liver transplantation: FK 506 versus cyclosporine. *Transplantation Proceedings.* 1996;28:1738-1740.
57. Cauley JA, Cummings SR, Seeley DG, et al. Effects of thiazide diuretic therapy on bone mass, fractures and falls. *Ann Intern Med.* 1993;118:666-673.
58. Orwoll ES, Bauer DC, Vogt TM, Fox KM. Axial bone mass in older women. *Ann Intern Med.* 1996;124:187-196.
59. Jones G, Nguyen T, Sambrook PN, Eisman JA. Thiazide diuretics and fractures: can meta-analysis help? *J Bone Miner Res.* 1995;10:106-111.
60. Lipkin EW. A longitudinal study of calcium regulation in a non-human primate model of parenteral nutrition. *Am J Clin Nutr.* 1998;67:246-254.
61. Lipkin EW, Ott SM, Chesnut CH 3rd, Chait A. Mineral loss in the parenteral nutrition patient. *Am J Clin Nutr.* 1988;47:5155-5123.
62. Seidner DL. Parenteral nutrition associated MBD. *Journal of Parenteral and Enteral Nutrition.* 2002;26:S37-S42.
63. Mankin HJ. Nontraumatic necrosis of bone (osteonecrosis). *NEJM.* 1992;326:1473-1479.
64. Holda ME, Ryan JR. Hepatobiliary rickets. *Journal of Pediatric Orthopedics.* 1982;2:285-287.
65. Kooh SW, Jones G, Reilly BJ, Fraser D. Pathogenesis of rickets in chronic hepatobiliary disease in children. *Journal of Pediatrics.* 1978;94:870-874.
66. Khosla S, Hassoun AA, Baker BK, et al. Insulin like growth factor system abnormalities in hepatitis C associated osteosclerosis. Potential insights into increasing bone mass in adults. *J Clin Invest.* 1998;101:2165-2173.
67. Heller HJ, Greer LG, Haynes SD, Poindexter JR, Pak CY. Pharmacokinetic and pharmacodynamic comparison of two calcium supplements in postmenopausal women. *J Clin Pharmacol.* 2000;40:1237-1244.
68. Deal C, Gideon J. Recombinant human PTH 1-34 (Forteo): An anabolic drug for osteoporosis. *Cleveland Clinic Journal of Medicine.* 2003;70:585-594.
69. McFarlane XA, Bhalla AK, Robertson DA. Effect of a gluten free diet on osteopenia in adults with newly diagnosed celiac disease. *Gut.* 1996;39:180-184
70. Mautalen C, Gonzalez D, Mazure R. Effect of treatment on bone mass, mineral metabolism, and body composition in untreated celiac disease patients. *Am J Gastroenterol.* 1997;92:313-318.
71. Sategna-Guidetti C, Grosso SB, Grosso S, et al. The effects of 1-year gluten withdrawal on bone mass, bone metabolism and nutritional status in newly diagnosed adult celiac disease patients. *Aliment Pharmacol Ther.* 2000;14:35-43.
72. Valdimarsson T, Toss G, Ross I, Lofman O, Strom M. Bone mineral density in celiac disease. *Scand J Gastroenterol.* 1994;29:457-461.
73. Rosen CJ, Brown S. Severe hypocalcemia after intravenous bisphosphonate therapy in occult vitamin D deficiency. *N Engl J Med.* 2003; 348:1503-1504.
74. Robinson RJ, Krzywicki T, Almond L, et al. Effect of a low-impact exercise program on bone mineral density in Crohn's disease: a randomized controlled trial. *Gastroenterology.* 1998;115:36-41.

Chapter 14

Nutrition in the Elderly

Lisa M. Neff, MD, and Joel B. Mason, MD

Introduction

In the early years of the 20th century, the life expectancy of a newborn American infant was just 49 years. However, as a result of improved nutrition, sanitation, and medical care in the last century, humans now survive nearly 80 years on average.[1] In 1900, only 4% of the American population lived to 65 years of age.[2] By the year 2000, this number increased to over 12%.[3] It has been estimated that by the year 2030, 71 million or nearly 1 in 5 will reach the age of 65 years, and 19.5 million will live to see their 80th birthdays.[3] Figure 14-1 demonstrates the dramatic demographic shifts in the United States in the years since the 1900 census.[4] Similar trends are apparent in most industrialized nations, including Canada and most European nations. This graying of the population has wide-ranging implications for almost every aspect of healthcare, including nutrition.

Many factors influence nutritional status, including nutrient intake, biosynthesis of nutrients (such as vitamin D), nutrient absorption by the gastrointestinal (GI) tract, and the subsequent metabolism of nutrients. Aging affects these determinants in a variety of ways, and it may thereby alter nutrient requirements and place older individuals at risk of malnutrition.

Malnutrition in the Elderly

Estimates of the prevalence of malnutrition in elderly populations vary widely, depending on the population studied and the method used to determine nutritional status. Nevertheless, it has been estimated that 3% to 11% of community-dwelling elderly individuals are undernourished, and 17% to 65% of nursing home residents and 15% to 40% of hospitalized elderly patients are malnourished.[5-9] As is true in the younger segment of the American population, obesity is an increasing problem in the elderly population, affecting over 30% of all individuals over the age of 60.[10] Although this chapter will focus on the determinants, consequences, and management of undernutrition, it behooves the physician to diligently attend to the issue of overnutrition, overweight, and obesity in the elderly. A brief discussion of this matter appears later in this chapter. More thorough coverage of the topic can be found in Chapters 47 through 53 of this book.

Consequences of Malnutrition in the Elderly

In rehabilitation hospitals and nursing homes, poor nutritional status has been associated with increased morbidity and mortality.[11,12] In the hospital setting, malnutrition has been linked to an increased risk of nosocomial infections and other complications, increased length of stay, increased healthcare expenditures, and increased risk of morbidity and mortality.[13-19] Improving the nutritional status of undernourished elderly nursing home residents has been shown to reduce the risk of morbidity and mortality.[11,20] In the acute care setting, addressing the nutritional needs of malnourished hospitalized patients has similarly been shown to reduce morbidity and sometimes mortality.[21,22]

Clinical outcomes are typically observed to be improved with nutritional support only in those individuals who are moderately to severely malnourished (often defined as those who have unintentionally lost 10% of their usual body weight or more). This underscores the importance of stratifying inpatients by nutritional status, as it is those who are substantially malnourished who should be targeted for aggressive nutritional support. "Aggressive nutritional support" here refers to the use of whatever means are necessary and practical to meet the nutritional needs of a patient, including both enteral and parenteral modalities. Scores of small trials have attempted to deal with the question of the potential benefits of aggressive nutritional support, so this is therefore a topic that is perhaps best addressed by well-performed meta-analyses; such analyses have repeatedly confirmed the benefits of nutrition support in the acute care setting among those who are malnourished.[21,22]

Studies demonstrating the benefits of nutritional support in hospitalized patients have not been conducted in an exclusively elder population; however, elderly individuals comprise a large proportion of patient populations of most of the large studies on this matter, thereby establishing that aging adults benefit from such nutritional support as well. Therefore, it is essential to understand the factors that contribute to the development of malnutrition in the elderly and to be able to identify those patients who are at risk of malnutrition so that appropriate interventions can be made.

Nutrient Intake in Elderly Individuals

Over 80% of older Americans are free from disability, and less than 10% live in nursing homes and assisted-living facilities.[23] However, aging is associated with an increased prevalence of illness, chronic disability, functional impairment, and financial hardship, all of which can impact an individual's ability to procure and prepare nutritious foods. Medications with anorectic effects, social isolation, mood disorders, abnormal taste perceptions, impaired thirst mechanisms, and disorders of chewing and swallowing can all lead to decreased food intake. Nutrient intake can also be affected by adherence to special diets, which may reduce the palatability, variety, and nutritional quality of ingested foods. Examples of such diets include low-fat, low-cholesterol diet plans, lactose-free diets, and sodium- or fluid-restricted diets. Older individuals who avoid dairy products, for instance, often have inadequate intakes of calcium and vitamin D.

Data from the Third National Health and Nutrition Examination Survey (NHANES III) suggest that many elderly individuals have inadequate intakes of calcium and zinc.[24] Other studies of community-dwelling elderly individuals indicate that many also have insufficient intakes of folate, vitamin B6, vitamin E, and magnesium.[25,26] In one study conducted in rural Iowa, more than 60% of community-dwelling elderly individuals did not meet the current national recommendations for intake of folate, vitamins D and E, calcium, and magnesium.[27] Failure to meet the Recommended Daily Allowance (RDA) of a nutrient (Chapter 6) does not necessarily mean a deficiency will develop, although studies document particularly high rates of insufficiency of vitamins D, B6, and B12 in free-living

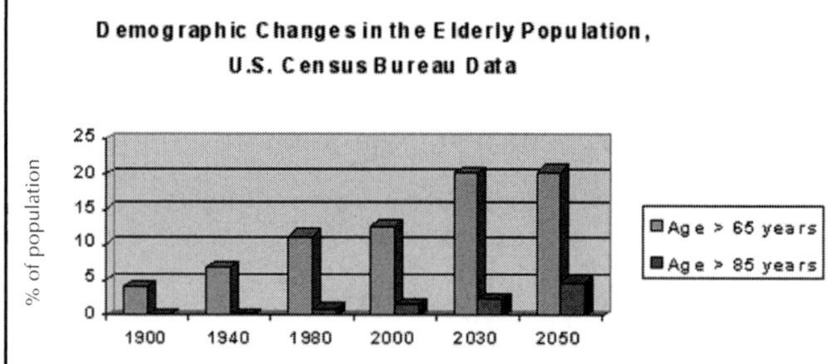

Figure 14-1. Demographic changes in the elderly population.

elderly individuals, underscoring the health consequences of low intake.[28-30]

Biosynthesis of Nutrients in Aging: Vitamin D

Hypovitaminosis D, or low serum 25-hydroxyvitamin D (25[OH]D), is very common in elderly individuals, and its prevalence increases with age.[31] As discussed above, insufficient intake of vitamin-D–rich foods, such as fatty fish or fortified milk, can contribute to this problem (Chapter 3). The mean dietary intake of vitamin D in men and women over the age of 70 years is approximately 200 IU daily, far less than the 600 IU/day currently recommended for adequate intake (AI) in elderly individuals.[32] Decreased biosynthesis of vitamin D also plays a role in the development of hypovitaminosis D in the elderly. With exposure to ultraviolet rays of wavelengths between 290 and 315 nm, 7-dehydrocholesterol undergoes photo isomerization, primarily in the epidermis, forming previtamin D3. Older adults often have reduced exposure to sunlight than younger individuals, either voluntarily because of health concerns or involuntarily because of decreased mobility, and this can limit the amount of vitamin D synthesized in the skin. In addition, as compared to the skin of younger individuals, aging skin has a reduced capacity to synthesize vitamin D in response to sunlight exposure, largely a result of the greater than 50% decline in epidermal stores of 7-dehydrocholesterol in aging.[33]

Seasonal variations in ultraviolet light exposure have been shown to affect serum 25(OH)D levels, usually on the order of 25 to 50 nmol/L (10-20 ng/mL).[34] In the United States, serum 25(OH)D levels typically peak in the late summer (August or September) and decline during the winter, reaching a nadir in February or March.[28,35] These seasonal fluctuations in 25(OH)D levels have been associated with seasonal changes in serum parathyroid hormone concentration, bone mineral density, and urine concentrations of the bone resorption marker, N-telopeptide.[35,36]

In addition to seasonal effects, geographic variations in sunlight exposure and food fortification also produce significant regional differences in the mean serum 25(OH)D concentration and the prevalence of hypovitaminosis D. For example, in Canada, where milk is fortified with vitamin D, 20% of free-living adults have serum 25(OH)D concentrations less than 40 nmol/L (16 ng/mL) during the winter.[37] In Europe, on the other hand, where milk is not fortified with vitamin D, hypovitaminosis D can be found in 36% to 86% of the elderly population in the winter months.[38,39] There remains much debate regarding the optimal serum concentration of 25(OH)D, but studies suggest that levels below 60 to 75 nmol/L (24 to 30 ng/mL) are associated with an increased prevalence of secondary hyperparathyroidism, increased markers of bone turnover, and increased risk of hip fracture.[40-44] The optimization of bone mass in the elderly often dictates a target level of serum vitamin D that is above the range reported as normal by many clinical laboratories (22.5 to 62.5 nmol/L or 9 to 25 ng/mL). There is little concern for vitamin D toxicity because the therapeutic window of vitamin D is large and daily vitamin D intakes of up to 2000 IU/day are considered entirely safe. In fact, some researchers maintain that vitamin D intakes of up to 10,000 IU/day are unlikely to cause adverse effects.[45]

Gastrointestinal Function and Nutrient Absorption in Elderly Individuals

GI physiology is largely preserved in aging humans, although a minor and largely subclinical decline in function can be demonstrated. For example, there is a higher prevalence of esophageal dysmotility in the elderly population than in younger groups.[46] In addition, gastric emptying time has been found to be prolonged in older individuals as compared to younger adults.[47,48] However, these changes have not been shown to result in alterations in total GI transit time and do not appear to be associated with any clinically meaningful impairments in nutrient absorption.

In the 1970s and earlier, a number of studies reported an increased prevalence of malabsorption in elderly individuals, suggesting that pancreatic exocrine function is compromised in aging.[49,50] However, subsequent studies revealed that pancreatic function is largely preserved in aging and that fat malabsorption does not occur under normal dietary conditions.[51-53] Therefore, fat malabsorption should not be considered to be a consequence of normal aging.

Atrophic Gastritis

On the other hand, some pathologic changes that commonly accompany aging, such as atrophic gastritis, can lead to significant nutritional sequelae in the elderly. The prevalence of *Helicobacter-pylori*–associated atrophic gastritis (type B atrophic gastritis) increases with age, and the disorder affects between 9% and 31% of elderly Americans, with prevalence rates varying by geographic region.[54,55] Atrophic gastritis leads to a reduction in the secretion of gastric acid and intrinsic factor and an increase in the density of bacterial populations in the upper small intestine, although generally not to the levels necessary to produce the classical hallmarks of small bowel bacterial overgrowth. Gastric acid releases protein-bound vitamin B12 from food and increases the solubility of certain forms of iron (non-heme iron and ferric iron) and calcium (calcium carbonate) in the diet. Furthermore, it is thought that bacteria may bind free vitamin B12 in the intestinal lumen, reducing the amount available for absorption.[56] Therefore, hypochlorhydria and achlorhydria can lead to a reduction in the amount of absorbable vitamin B12, iron, and calcium in the GI tract of affected individuals, putting them at risk for deficiency. It has been shown that atrophic gastritis can result in significant reductions in serum vitamin B12 levels and can lead to increased serum concentrations of methylmalonic acid (MMA) and homocysteine, two intermediary metabolites that accumulate in the face of a cellular deficiency of vitamin B12.[55,57] In fact, in a study by Krasinki and colleagues, vitamin B12 deficiency was found in 8% of patients with mild to moderate atrophic gastritis and in 53% of patients with severe atrophic gastritis.[55]

The prevalence of atrophic gastritis increases with age; therefore, elderly individuals are at high risk for the development of vitamin B12 deficiency. In the Framingham cohort, for example, over 11% of elderly individuals were found to have biochemical evidence of vitamin B12 deficiency, as compared to less than 6% of younger subjects.[30] Neurodegenerative syndromes, which are ameliorated by vitamin B12 therapy, can arise in elder individuals whose plasma B12 concentrations are in the low normal range (200 to 400 pg/mL) and whose serum MMA concentrations are substantially elevated.[58] Therefore, this so-called "subclinical vitamin B12 deficiency" cannot be perceived as only a biochemical curiosity. Any elder who has a neurodegenerative syndrome of unknown etiology and whose plasma B12 concentration is between 150 and 400 ng/mL should have a serum MMA check; trivial elevations are common because of confounding factors such as renal insufficiency, but a substantial increase strongly suggests the presence of a cellular deficiency of B12. A B12 level less than 150 ng/mL should be assumed to be a B12 deficiency and in most instances does not require an MMA level.

In addition to its effect on gastric acid production, atrophic gastritis can also lead to a modest reduction in the secretion of intrinsic factor. However, this does not seem to hinder vitamin B12 absorption significantly, except in the most severe cases of gastric atrophy.[59] Indeed, pernicious anemia (end stage type A atrophic gastritis) is much less common than is type B atrophic gastritis, occurring in just 2% to 3% of elderly individuals.[55,60] On a practical level, it is important to recognize that the malabsorption of vitamin B12 that occurs with atrophic gastritis pertains only to protein-bound vitamin B12 in food and not to the crystalline form of the vitamin.[56] Therefore, supplementation with crystalline vitamin B12 effectively treats vitamin B12 deficiency in patients with atrophic gastritis.

Iatrogenic hypochlorhydria and achlorhydria such as that seen after gastric surgery, vagotomy, or prolonged treatment with histamine blockers or proton pump inhibitors results in impaired absorption of vitamin B12 as well.[61-64] Whether the magnitude of the drug-induced malabsorption of B12 (due to chronic use of histamine blockers or proton pump inhibitors) is sufficient to produce a clinically significant B12 deficiency remains a matter of debate. Nevertheless, healthcare providers are advised to check vitamin B12 status yearly in those elders who are on long-term treatment with proton-pump inhibitors.

There is also ample evidence that reductions in gastric acidity are associated with reductions in the fractional absorption of dietary non-heme iron.[65] However, it is unclear whether impaired gastric acid secretion results in clinically important changes in iron status. Early work in the field suggested that patients with hypochlorhydria or achlorhydria have a higher risk of iron deficiency and iron-deficiency anemia than do normal individuals.[66] However, more recent reports suggest that clinically significant changes in iron status are not more prevalent in patients with atrophic gastritis or medication-induced hypochlorhydria.[55,67] Furthermore, surveys of elderly individuals generally suggest that iron overload is a more prevalent disorder than is iron deficiency. In the Framingham Heart Study cohort, for example, less than 3% of free-living elder adults had iron deficiency, whereas 12% had evidence of elevated iron stores.[68]

In view of the frequent inadequacy of select micronutrients among the elderly—vitamins D, B6, and B12 in particular—a daily multivitamin is not unreasonable, even for healthy elders. In general, these authors do not recommend a multivitamin that contains iron because iron supplementation is unnecessary in most cases, as described above. It is debatable whether vitamin supplementation should become standard treatment for all elderly individuals. The authors prefer to individualize the decision because potential drawbacks do exist; for example, elders with chronic kidney disease appear to be vulnerable to vitamin A toxicity due to chronic intake of vitamin A supplements, even at relatively low doses.[69,70]

Calcium Absorption in Aging

Data from the 1994 Continuing Survey of the Food Intake of Individuals (CSFII) and NHANES III suggest that, on average, elderly Americans consume around 500 to 700 mg of calcium daily.[71,72] This is far less than the recommended daily intake of 1200 to 1500 mg, so calcium supplements are often indicated. Gastric acidity is known to affect the absorption of certain calcium salts (calcium carbonate) but not others (calcium citrate), so the type of calcium supplement chosen may be of significance for individuals with achlorhydria. In the fasting state, normal control subjects absorb between 20% and 25% of ingested calcium carbonate or citrate. The fractional absorption of calcium carbonate in patients with achlorhydria, however, is reduced to only 5% in the fasting state, whereas absorption of calcium citrate is not impaired.[73] When calcium carbonate is taken with meals, there is no significant difference in absorption between patients with achlorhydria and normal subjects. Therefore, for optimal absorption of supplemental calcium, patients with achlorhydria should either select calcium citrate or take calcium carbonate with meals.

As illustrated in Figure 14-2, the fractional absorption of calcium appears to decline in a linear fashion with advancing age, from a peak of around 25% to 30% in young adults to only 15% to 20% in adults in their ninth decade of life.[74] The fractional absorption of calcium is particularly low in elder individuals with low calcium intakes.[74]

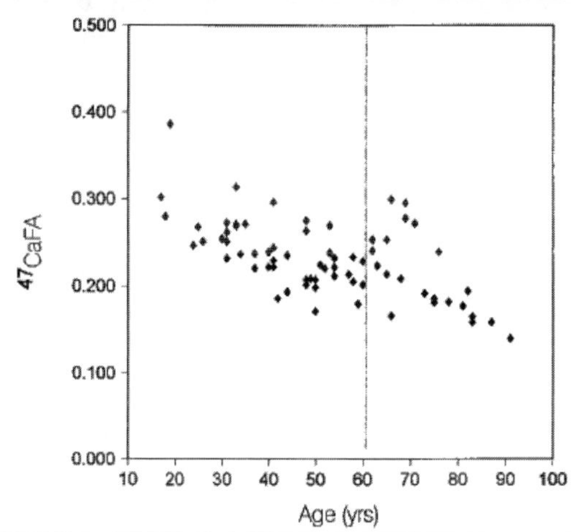

Figure 14-2. Intestinal calcium absorption as a function of age in 70 normal men. Reprinted with permission from Springer, LLC. Agnusdei D, Civitelli R, Camporeale A, et al. Age related decline of bone mass. *Calcif Tissue Int*. 1998;63(3):197-201.

The etiology of this phenomenon is not clear, but some studies suggest that it may be due to a relative intestinal resistance to 1.25-dihydroxyvitamin D (1.25[OH]$_2$D) in aging individuals.[75,76] Calcium absorption can also be decreased as a result of impaired conversion of 25(OH)D to 1,25(OH)$_2$D in chronic kidney disease, which is more common in the elderly than in the young. Other factors can also reduce the fractional absorption of calcium in young and old subjects, such as dietary fiber intake, the presence of certain vitamin D receptor polymorphisms and cigarette smoking.[77-79]

Changes in Body Composition With Aging

Sarcopenia

To understand the effect of aging on an individual's macronutrient requirements, it is important to be aware of the changes in body composition that occur over an individual's lifetime. Aging is associated with a reduction in lean body mass and is often accompanied by a concomitant increase in fat mass, as is demonstrated in Figure 14-3, which compares the magnetic resonance image of the thigh of a young patient (B) and that of an elderly patient (A). This loss of muscle mass in aging has been called sarcopenia, a term originally suggested by Irwin Rosenberg in the late 1980s.[80] The loss of appendicular skeletal muscle occurs at a rate of 0.6 to 1.6 kg/decade and is largely a result of changes in the lower extremities.[81,82] It is important to note that sarcopenia can occur in the absence of any significant change in body weight because of the relative increase in fat mass.[82]

Sarcopenia has been associated with a variety of metabolic changes, including a decline in resting energy expenditure (REE) and insulin sensitivity.[83] Although it continues to be a matter of debate as to whether sarcopenia is a physiologic accompaniment of aging or a pathologic

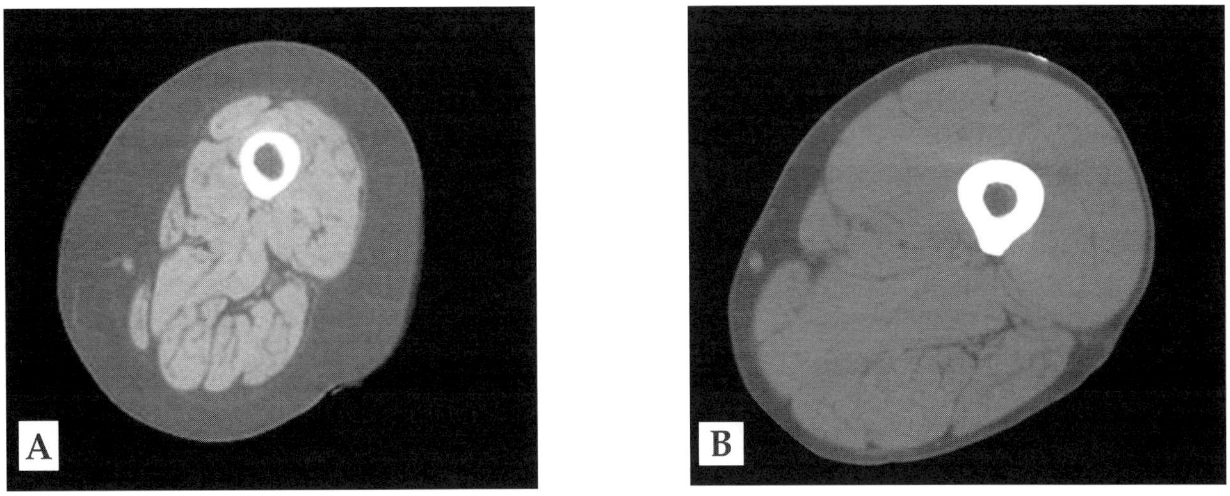

Figure 14-3. Cross-sectional MRI of the mid-thigh of a sedentary 67-year-old (A) and an active 23-year-old individual (B). Note the relative decrease in muscle mass and increase in fat mass in the older individual. Images courtesy of Miriam Nelson, PhD.

process, sarcopenia is clearly associated with diminished muscle strength and an increased risk of physical disability, falls, and mortality, particularly when the lower extremities are affected.[84-86]

Sarcopenia appears to be a multifactorial disorder. Contributing factors probably include decreased circulating levels of sex hormones, growth hormone, and insulin-like growth factor 1 and increased cytokine production with aging. Neuromuscular changes may also play a role. Physical inactivity, malnutrition, and smoking increase the risk of sarcopenia.[83]

The estimated prevalence of sarcopenia varies widely depending upon the criteria used to diagnose it. For example, one recent study defined sarcopenia as lean body mass two or more standard deviations below the gender-specific mean for young adults. Using this cutoff point, the prevalence of sarcopenia was estimated to be 4% to 16% in relatively healthy, ambulatory adults over the age of 70 years.[85] In another recent study, sarcopenia was defined as a skeletal muscle index (muscle mass/body mass x 100) either one to two standard deviations below the gender-specific mean for young adults (class I sarcopenia) or more than two standard deviations below the mean (class II sarcopenia). In this study, 72% of women and 50% of men over the age of 80 years were found to have either class I or class II sarcopenia.[87]

In recent years, a number of therapeutic modalities have been studied in patients with age-related losses of muscle mass and strength. These potential therapies include exercise, nutritional interventions, and hormone replacement. Of these approaches, exercise seems to be the most promising. In a well-designed randomized, controlled trial, Fiatarone and colleagues showed that 10 weeks of progressive resistance training may reduce age-related muscle loss, increase appendicular muscle mass and strength, and produce significant improvements in mobility and functional status.[88] A number of other studies confirm that muscle mass, strength, and functional status improve with resistance training, and some trials have suggested that cardiorespiratory fitness may also be improved.[89-92] Other recent trials show that resistance training is associated with many additional health benefits, including remarkable improvements in glycemic control in older individuals with type 2 diabetes mellitus; significant reductions in bone loss in postmenopausal women; and improvements in mood, quality-of-life scores, and sleep quality in depressed elderly individuals.[93-96]

Unfortunately, not all studies have been able to document improvements in muscle mass, strength, and functional status with exercise, and some researchers have even suggested that the risk of musculoskeletal injury may outweigh the potential benefits of resistance training in the frail elderly.[97] The preponderance of evidence, however, suggests that supervised resistance training is a safe and effective therapy for reducing the age-related loss of muscle mass and strength in older individuals, even in debilitated individuals in their eighth, ninth, and tenth decades of life. Thirty minutes of strength training, thrice weekly, has generally been sufficient to produce these beneficial results.

To date, nutritional therapy has not been shown to be as successful as exercise interventions in the treatment of sarcopenia. In the 10-week study by Fiatarone and colleagues, for example, a liquid protein, calorie, and multivitamin supplement did not improve muscle strength or reduce frailty in elderly individuals.[88] Another recent study suggested that a liquid nutritional supplement resulted in small gains in body weight without significant improvements in overall body composition or functional status.[98] However, it is clear that malnutrition, particularly protein-calorie malnutrition, results in significant losses of lean body mass, decreased muscle strength, and impaired functional status. Studies also show that even short-term consumption of low-protein diets can result in significant losses of muscle mass and function in healthy elderly individuals.[99,100] Therefore, older individuals should be counseled to consume a diet adequate in both calories and protein to avoid malnutrition-induced loss of muscle mass, which will further aggravate the problem of sarcopenia. In elderly patients who cannot consume adequate protein or calories on their own, nutritional supplements should be considered.

Targets for hormonal interventions in sarcopenia include testosterone, dehydroepiandrosterone (DHEA), estrogen, and growth hormone, as aging and sarcopenia have been associated with decreases in levels of these hormones in a sizeable minority of individuals so afflicted. A number of preliminary studies have uncovered some of the potential benefits and risks of hormone therapy in aging. For example, in elderly men with declining serum testosterone levels, testosterone supplementation appears to increase muscle mass, improve bone density, and decrease visceral adiposity; however, it also causes erythrocytosis in up to 25% of patients and can result in small but significant increases in serum levels of prostate specific antigen.[101] In very small, relatively short-term studies, the administration of DHEA to older women has been associated with small improvements in appendicular muscle and fat mass and significant decreases in both fasting glucose and fasting insulin level, without any clinically-significant side effects.[102] Estrogen replacement therapy, on the other hand, does not seem to reduce the risk of sarcopenia in postmenopausal women, although it clearly improves bone density.[103] Growth hormone therapy appears to lead to increases in muscle mass and decreases in fat mass in healthy older individuals, but it can also increase the risk of hyperglycemia, peripheral edema, arthralgias, and carpal tunnel syndrome.[104] In general, the long-term benefits and risks of supplemental hormone treatments have not been adequately documented to justify their use in the management of sarcopenia at this time, particularly in light of recent unexpected findings concerning the risks of long-term estrogen and progestin therapy in postmenopausal women.[105]

OBESITY IN THE ELDERLY

Like sarcopenia, obesity is common in elderly populations. In fact, recent data from NHANES suggest that nearly 32% of men and 35% of women over the age of 60 are obese, defined as a body mass index (BMI) of 30 or more.[10] The prevalence of obesity increases significantly from the third to the eighth decades of life and then declines slightly. However, even with this downward trend, nearly 10% of men and 20% of women over the age of 80 years are obese.[10]

Many of the factors that contribute to the development of obesity in the elderly are the same as those seen in younger individuals. These factors include the consumption of large portions of energy-dense foods, sedentary lifestyles, and genetic influences. In addition, age-related changes in energy metabolism may also play a role in the development of overweight and obesity in older individuals. These metabolic changes will be discussed at greater length below.

Obesity has been associated with an increased risk of many diseases, including diabetes, hypertension, hyperlipidemia, heart disease, sleep apnea, arthritis, and certain types of cancer. In elderly individuals, obesity is also associated with an increased risk of functional limitations.[106] In young and middle-aged adults, obesity is associated with a significantly increased risk of mortality. In elderly individuals, however, the association between increasing BMI and mortality is controversial.[107]

Treatment options for obesity include lifestyle modifications, pharmacologic therapy, and bariatric surgery. In younger obese adults, all of these therapies have been shown to produce some degree of weight loss and improvement in many comorbid conditions, including hyperlipidemia, hypertension, diabetes, sleep apnea, and arthritis. Unfortunately, current evidence regarding treatment of obesity in elderly populations is sparse. In fact, most obesity trials specifically exclude individuals over the age of 70 years. However, one study of lifestyle changes in elderly hypertensive individuals suggested that relatively small changes in weight are associated with improvements in blood pressure.[108] In another study, laparoscopic gastric banding resulted in dramatic weight loss and improved sleep apnea, diabetes, hypertension, and arthritis in morbidly obese elderly subjects.[109] However, these studies were both very small, and further investigation should be conducted before specific obesity treatments can be widely recommended to elderly individuals.

Changes in Energy Metabolism With Aging

Aging is associated with a significant reduction in energy expenditure, usually on the order of 10% to 25%.[110-112] Total energy expenditure is comprised of REE, the energy cost of digesting and absorbing nutrients (the thermic effect of food), and energy expended during physical activity. Most studies suggest that the age-related decline in total energy expenditure is primarily related to a reduction in REE. This, in turn, is widely thought to be simply the result of age-related changes in body composition, including the loss of lean mass (sarcopenia) and increase in fat mass, which is less metabolically active than lean tissue.[113,114] However, some studies suggest that the diminished REE in older individuals results not only from losses of metabolically active lean mass but also from a relative decline in metabolic activity of aging lean tissue.[111,115]

For practical purposes, it can be assumed that most elderly individuals require fewer calories than do their younger counterparts if total body weight, physical activity, and health status are matched. A number of equations have been used to estimate basal (asleep) or resting (awake) energy requirements in older individuals, including the familiar Harris-Benedict equations and the Schofield equations, which have been adopted by the World Health Organization (WHO).[116-118] Although the Harris-Benedict equations are widely used in clinical practice, they have been shown to be inaccurate in malnourished elderly individuals.[119,120] The Schofield/WHO equations are generally thought to be superior to the Harris-Benedict equations for use in elderly populations. One advantage of the Schofield/WHO equations is that modified equations have been created for which no assessment of height is required, with only a very small reduction in predictive power. These modified equations are particularly useful for wheelchair-bound, bedridden, or kyphotic patients, in whom accurate measurement of height may be very difficult. However, studies suggest that the Schofield/WHO equations may slightly underestimate the caloric requirements of elderly individuals, and experts have recommended that better predictive equations be developed.[121] In response, Lührmann et al recently proposed a promising new equation to estimate

TABLE 14-1.

Predictive Equations for Basal Energy Expenditure and Resting Energy Expenditure

*Equations**	*Men†*	*Women†*
Harris-Benedict equations[116]	BEE = 66.5 + 13.7W + 5H - 6.8A	BEE = 655 + 9.6W + 1.7H - 4.7A
World Health Organization equations for individuals over 60 years old[118]	REE = 8.8W + 1128H - 1071 ‡REE = 13.5W + 487	REE = 9.2W + 637H - 302 ‡REE = 10.5W + 596
Lührmann equation[122]	REE = 3169 + 50W - 15.3A + 746	REE = 3169 + 50W - 15.3A

* in kcal/day[116,118] or kJ/day[122] (kJ = kcal X 4.184)
† W = weight in kg; H = height in cm[116] or m[118]; and A = age in y.
‡ Generally, ≤10% loss in accuracy is obtained by using the alternative WHO equations, which lack a height factor.

REE in elderly individuals.[122] However, further research is needed to validate this equation in various ethnic groups and in elderly individuals over the age of 85 years. The Harris-Benedict, Schofield/WHO, and Lührmann equations are shown in Table 14-1.

Once basal energy expenditure (BEE) or REE is calculated using one of the available predictive equations, total energy expenditure can be estimated by multiplying the result by an activity factor and a stress factor. In general, most individuals have a total energy expenditure that is roughly 1.2 (sedentary individuals) to 1.8 (extremely active individuals) times higher than BEE.

When a more precise estimate of an individual's caloric requirements is required, indirect calorimetry should be considered. With this method, direct measurements of oxygen consumption and carbon dioxide production are used to calculate REE. Indirect calorimetry is likely to be particularly useful in critically ill patients, in whom the predictive equations are often inaccurate. It should also be considered for malnourished patients who fail to gain weight despite the institution of nutritional therapy.

Protein Requirements in Elderly Individuals

The current Recommended Daily Allowance (RDA) for protein is 0.8 g of protein per kilogram of body weight per day for all adults, regardless of age.[123] However, several studies suggest that this amount may not be sufficient for the elder adult and that intakes of at least 0.9 g/kg/day may be necessary to prevent the development of a negative nitrogen balance and the loss of muscle mass in the elderly.[99,124-126] As a result, some have suggested that the RDA for protein should be increased to 0.9 to 1.1 g/kg/day for elderly individuals.[127] However, controversy still exists, and the RDA remains at 0.8 g/kg/day for all healthy adults. It is important to note that the optimal protein intake for an individual patient may vary, depending upon the presence of certain disease states. For example, individuals with chronic kidney disease, acute renal failure (not on hemodialysis), or protein-sensitive hepatic encephalopathy may benefit from protein intakes as low as 0.6 g/kg/day, as higher intakes carry certain disadvantages in these conditions. It is worth emphasizing, however, that the vast majority of cases of mild hepatic encephalopathy are easily corrected with lactulose, thereby enabling patients to achieve protein intakes more closely matched to their actual needs. On the other hand, some conditions dictate higher protein intakes of 1.2 to 2 g/kg/day. Acute illnesses with a significant systemic inflammatory response, chronic steroid treatment, and hemodialysis and peritoneal dialysis are examples.

Micronutrient Requirements in Aging

According to current national guidelines regarding micronutrient requirements, healthy elderly individuals need more calcium, vitamin D, and vitamin B6 and less chromium than do healthy younger adults.[71,128-130] In addition, healthy postmenopausal women require less iron than do younger women because menstrual blood loss has ceased. As discussed above, elderly individuals with hypochlorhydria are likely to need more dietary vitamin B12 than do those with normal gastric acidity. The daily requirements for most other micronutrients (including thiamine, folate, riboflavin, magnesium, zinc, and vitamins C, E, and K) do not appear to change with aging.

However, elderly individuals may require less vitamin A than do younger individuals because of changes in vitamin A metabolism with aging. These changes include decreased clearance of postprandial retinol esters and increasing fasting plasma retinol concentrations with advancing age.[131] In the United States, vitamin A deficiency appears to be rare in elderly individuals. In the Baltimore Longitudinal Study of Aging, for example, less than 0.5% of elderly subjects had low or marginal plasma retinol concentrations, despite the fact that 20% had vitamin A intakes below the RDA.[132] In addition, older individuals with chronic kidney disease have occasionally developed signs of chronic vitamin A toxicity with modest levels of supplementation.[69,70] Nevertheless, the current RDA for vitamin A is the same for young and elder adults. At usual ranges of dietary vitamin A intake, however, vitamin A deficiency and toxicity are both uncommon in elderly individuals.

Nutrition Assessment

It is important to identify those elderly who are at risk of malnutrition so that nutrition interventions can be made. Formal nutrition assessment typically relies on a combination of history, physical exam, anthropometrics, and biochemical markers to diagnose overt malnutrition and to identify patients at risk for the development of malnutrition. Nutrition assessment is discussed in detail in Chapter 1.

A thorough nutrition history should address dietary habits, food preferences and dislikes, food allergies, recent weight changes, dental health, medical history, ability to perform activities of daily living, and the use of medications, dietary supplements, and alcohol. In addition, clinicians should ask about the many psychological and social factors that can affect nutrient intake, such as depression, social isolation, and financial pressures. In general, a reported or documented involuntary weight loss of 10% of body weight or more over 6 months is indicative of a high risk of malnutrition.[133]

Physical exam findings that may suggest a compromised nutrition status include a BMI of less than 18.5, body weight less than 90% of ideal weight, reduced handgrip strength, reduced scapular skin-fold thickness, mid-arm circumference less than 22 cm, and the presence of decubitus ulcers. Many other physical findings can be seen in individuals with specific vitamin and mineral deficiencies, as described in Chapter 3.

Biochemical findings that are common in patients with protein-calorie malnutrition include low albumin and prealbumin, a decreased lymphocyte count, and low cholesterol. In some elderly patients—such as those with weight loss, monotonous diets, GI disorders, or symptoms or signs of nutritional deficiency—additional laboratory tests may be indicated. These may include iron studies, a complete blood count, and serum measures of vitamin B12, folate, homocysteine, methylmalonic acid, and 25(OH)D.

Using history, anthropometrics, physical exam, and biochemical tests, dietitians, physicians, and other specially-trained practitioners can accurately identify elderly individuals who are likely to benefit from specific nutrition interventions. However, the comprehensive nutrition assessment requires trained personnel, may involve the use of special equipment (such as a handgrip dynamometer or calipers), and can be costly and time-consuming, limiting its utility in larger groups. Therefore, a variety of screening tools have been developed to help busy clinicians quickly identify those patients who are malnourished or at risk for malnutrition.

Mini Nutritional Assessment

One such tool is the Mini Nutritional Assessment (MNA), developed by scientists at Nestle for use with elderly subjects. As shown in Figure 14-4, the MNA is administered in two stages, the first of which is a six-item screening questionnaire that addresses food intake, weight loss, mobility, psychological stressors, cognitive factors, and body mass index. Patients who score less than 12 out of a possible 14 points on the first stage may be at nutritional risk, and the second stage of the MNA should then be completed. The second stage includes questions about independence, medication use, presence of decubitus ulcers, frequency of meals, protein intake, fruit and vegetable consumption, and fluid intake. Mid-arm and calf circumferences are also measured in the second stage of the MNA. Individuals with total scores that are less than 17 points are considered to have protein energy malnutrition, whereas individuals with at least 24 points have adequate nutrition. Those with scores between 17 and 24 are thought to be at increased risk for the development of malnutrition. The MNA has been validated in elderly patients and appears to correlate well with traditional anthropometric and biochemical indices of nutrition status.[134] Low MNA scores have been associated with a longer hospital length of stay and an increased risk of mortality.[135,136]

Subjective Global Assessment

Subjective Global Assessment (SGA) is a nutrition screening tool designed in the 1980s and initially intended for use with surgical inpatients.[137] The components of SGA include a brief nutrition history and a focused physical exam. The SGA tool has been shown to be reliable, even in the hands of first-year medical and surgical residents.[138] SGA has since been validated for use in elderly individuals and in patients with a variety of medical conditions, including cancer and chronic kidney disease.[136,139-141] Elderly individuals both who are classified by SGA as having moderate to severe protein-energy malnutrition have been found to have a higher risk of mortality than those classified as well-nourished.[136] Chapter 1 includes an extensive evaluation of the SGA and its validity, and Table 1-2 presents the features of the SGA.

Nutrition Screening Initiative

The Nutrition Screening Initiative (NSI) is a multi-agency project founded in 1990 by the American Academy of Family Physicians, the American Dietetic Association, and the National Council on the Aging, Inc.[142] A major aim of the NSI is the promotion of nutrition screening, education, and treatment, particularly in the elderly population. The NSI screening tools include a brief nutritional checklist that can be completed by the elderly patient or caregiver; a Level I screen for use by paramedical or medical professionals; and a comprehensive Level II screen for use by physicians, nutritionists, or other trained medical personnel. The Level II screen, which is shown in Figure 14-5, includes a brief dietary history, an assessment of functional and economic status, an evaluation of mental status and risk of depression, anthropometric and laboratory data, and physical exam findings.

Nutrition Support in the Elderly

After malnourished or at-risk patients have been identified, a wide variety of interventions can be made. These

NESTLÉ NUTRITION SERVICES

Nestlé

Mini Nutritional Assessment MNA®

Last name: First name: Sex: Date:

Age: Weight, kg: Height, cm: I.D. Number:

Complete the screen by filling in the boxes with the appropriate numbers.
Add the numbers for the screen. If score is 11 or less, continue with the assessment to gain a Malnutrition Indicator Score.

Screening

A Has food intake declined over the past 3 months due to loss of appetite, digestive problems, chewing or swallowing difficulties?
- 0 = severe loss of appetite
- 1 = moderate loss of appetite
- 2 = no loss of appetite ☐

B Weight loss during last months
- 0 = weight loss greater than 3 kg (6.6 lbs)
- 1 = does not know
- 2 = weight loss between 1 and 3 kg (2.2 and 6.6 lbs)
- 3 = no weight loss ☐

C Mobility
- 0 = bed or chair bound
- 1 = able to get out of bed/chair but does not go out
- 2 = goes out ☐

D Has suffered psychological stress or acute disease in the past 3 months
- 0 = yes 2 = no ☐

E Neuropsychological problems
- 0 = severe dementia or depression
- 1 = mild dementia
- 2 = no psychological problems ☐

F Body Mass Index (BMI) (weight in kg) / (height in m)^2
- 0 = BMI less than 19
- 1 = BMI 19 to less than 21
- 2 = BMI 21 to less than 23
- 3 = BMI 23 or greater ☐

Screening score (subtotal max. 14 points) ☐ ☐

12 points or greater Normal – not at risk – no need to complete assessment

11 points or below Possible malnutrition – continue assessment

Assessment

G Lives independently (not in a nursing home or hospital)
- 0 = no 1 = yes ☐

H Takes more than 3 prescription drugs per day
- 0 = yes 1 = no ☐

I Pressure sores or skin ulcers
- 0 = yes 1 = no ☐

J How many full meals does the patient eat daily?
- 0 = 1 meal
- 1 = 2 meals
- 2 = 3 meals ☐

K Selected consumption markers for protein intake
- At least one serving of dairy products (milk, cheese, yogurt) per day? yes ☐ no ☐
- Two or more serving of legumes or eggs per week? yes ☐ no ☐
- Meat, fish or poultry every day yes ☐ no ☐

0.0 = if 0 or 1 yes
0.5 = if 2 yes
1.0 = if 3 yes ☐.☐

L Consumes two or more servings of fruits or vegetables per day?
- 0 = no 1 = yes ☐

M How much fluid (water, juice, coffee, tea, milk...) is consumed per day?
- 0.0 = less than 3 cups
- 0.5 = 3 to 5 cups
- 1.0 = more than 5 cups ☐.☐

N Mode of feeding
- 0 = unable to eat without assistance
- 1 = self-fed with some difficulty
- 2 = self-fed without any problem ☐

O Self view of nutritional status
- 0 = view self as being malnourished
- 1 = is uncertain of nutritional state
- 2 = views self as having no nutritional problem ☐

P In comparison with other people of the same age, how do they consider their health status?
- 0.0 = not as good
- 0.5 = does not know
- 1.0 = as good
- 2.0 = better ☐.☐

Q Mid-arm circumference (MAC) in cm
- 0.0 = MAC less than 21
- 0.5 = MAC 21 to 22
- 1.0 = MAC 22 or greater ☐.☐

R Calf circumference (CC) in cm
- 0 = CC less than 31 1 = CC 31 or greater ☐

Assessment (max. 16 points) ☐ ☐.☐

Screening score ☐ ☐

Total Assessment (max. 30 points) ☐ ☐.☐

Malnutrition Indicator Score

17 to 23.5 points at risk of malnutrition ☐

Less than 17 points malnourished ☐

Ref.: Guigoz Y, Vellas B and Garry PJ. 1994. Mini Nutritional Assessment: A practical assessment tool for grading the nutritional state of elderly patients. *Facts and Research in Gerontology.* Supplement #2:15-59.

Rubenstein LZ, Harker J, Guigoz Y and Vellas B. Comprehensive Geriatric Assessment (CGA) and the MNA: An Overview of CGA, Nutritional Assessment, and Development of a Shortened Version of the MNA. In: "Mini Nutritional Assessment (MNA): Research and Practice in the Elderly". Vellas B, Garry PJ and Guigoz Y, editors. Nestlé Nutrition Workshop Series. Clinical & Performance Programme, vol. 1. Karger, Bâle, in press.

08.98 USA

Figure 14-4. Mini nutritional assessment. Reprinted with permission from Nestlé Nutrition Services.

Level II Screen

Complete the following screen by interviewing the patient directly and/or by referring to the patient chart. If you do not routinely perform all of the described tests or ask all of the listed questions, please consider including them but do not be concerned if the entire screen is not completed. Please try to conduct a minimal screen on as many older patients as possible, and please try to collect serial measurements, which are extremely valuable in monitoring nutritional status. Please refer to the manual for additional information.

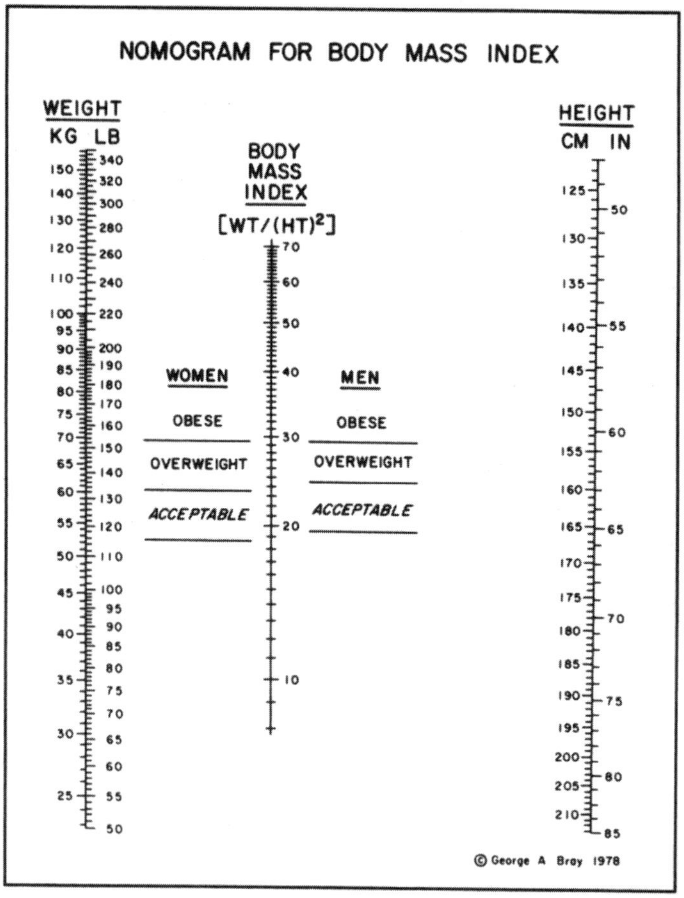

Anthropometrics

Measure height to the nearest inch and weight to the nearest pound. Record the values below and mark them on the Body Mass Index (BMI) scale to the right. Then use a straight edge (paper, ruler) to connect the two points and circle the spot where this straight line crosses the center line (body mass index). Record the number below; healthy older adults should have a BMI between 24 and 27; check the appropriate box to flag an abnormally high or low value.

Height (in):________________
Weight (lbs):________________
Body Mass Index (weight/height^2):________________

Please place a check by any statement regarding BMI and recent weight loss that is true for the patient.

- ❑ Body mass index <24
- ❑ Body mass index >27
- ❑ Has lost or gained 10 pounds (or more) of body weight in the past 6 months

Record the measurement of mid-arm circumference to the nearest 0.1 centimeter and of triceps skinfold to the nearest 2 millimeters.

Mid-Arm Circumference (cm):____________
Triceps Skinfold (mm):____________
Mid-Arm Muscle Circumference (cm):________

Refer to the table and check any abnormal values:

- ❑ Mid-arm muscle circumference <10th percentile
- ❑ Triceps skinfold <10th percentile
- ❑ Triceps skinfold >95th percentile

Note: mid-arm circumference (cm) - {0.314 x triceps skinfold (mm)}= mid-arm *muscle* circumference (cm)

For the remaining sections, please place a check by any statements that are true for the patient.

Laboratory Data

- ❑ Serum albumin below 3.5 g/dl
- ❑ Serum cholesterol below 160 mg/dl
- ❑ Serum cholesterol above 240 mg/dl

Drug Use

- ❑ Three or more prescription drugs, OTC medications, and/or vitamin/mineral supplements daily

LEVEL II SCREEN **Name:** **Date:**

Figure 14-5. Level II screen (page 1). Reprinted with permission from The Nutrition Screening Initiative, Washington, DC.

Clinical Features

Presence of (check each that apply):

- ❑ Problems with mouth, teeth, or gums
- ❑ Difficulty chewing
- ❑ Difficulty swallowing
- ❑ Angular stomatitis
- ❑ Glossitis
- ❑ History of bone pain
- ❑ History of bone fractures
- ❑ Skin changes (dry, loose, nonspecific lesions, edema)

Percentile	Men 55-65 y	Men 65-75 y	Women 55-65 y	Women 65-75 y
Arm circumference (cm)				
10th	27.3	26.3	25.7	25.2
50th	31.7	30.7	30.3	29.9
95th	36.9	35.5	38.5	37.3
Arm muscle circumference (cm)				
10th	24.5	23.5	19.6	19.5
50th	27.8	26.8	22.5	22.5
95th	32.0	30.6	28.0	27.9
Triceps skinfold (mm)				
10th	6	6	16	14
50th	11	11	25	24
95th	22	22	38	36

From: Frisancho AR. New norms of upper limb fat and muscle areas for assessment of nutritional status. Am J Clin Nutr 1981; 34:2540-2545. © 1981 American Society for Clinical Nutrition.

Eating Habits

- ❑ Does not have enough food to eat each day
- ❑ Usually eats alone
- ❑ Does not eat anything on one or more days each month
- ❑ Has poor appetite
- ❑ Is on a special diet
- ❑ Eats vegetables two or fewer times daily
- ❑ Eats milk or milk products once or not at all daily
- ❑ Eats fruit or drinks fruit juice once or not at all daily
- ❑ Eats breads, cereals, pasta, rice, or other grains five or fewer times daily
- ❑ Has more than one alcoholic drink per day (if woman); more than two drinks per day (if man)

Living Environment

- ❑ Lives on an income of less than $6000 per year (per individual in the household)
- ❑ Lives alone
- ❑ Is housebound
- ❑ Is concerned about home security
- ❑ Lives in a home with inadequate heating or cooling
- ❑ Does not have a stove and/or refrigerator
- ❑ Is unable or prefers not to spend money on food (<$25-30 per person spent on food each week)

Functional Status

Usually or always needs assistance with (check each that apply):

- ❑ Bathing
- ❑ Dressing
- ❑ Grooming
- ❑ Toileting
- ❑ Eating
- ❑ Walking or moving about
- ❑ Traveling (outside the home)
- ❑ Preparing food
- ❑ Shopping for food or other necessities

Mental/Cognitive Status

- ❑ Clinical evidence of impairment, e.g. Folstein<26
- ❑ Clinical evidence of depressive illness, e.g. Beck Depression Inventory>15, Geriatric Depression Scale>5

Patients in whom you have identified one or more major indicator (see pg 2) of poor nutritional status require immediate medical attention; if minor indicators are found, ensure that they are known to a health professional or to the patient's own physician. Patients who display risk factors (see pg 2) of poor nutritional status should be referred to the appropriate health care or social service professional (dietitian, nurse, dentist, case manager, etc.).

These materials developed by the Nutrition Screening Initiative.

A6173

Figure 14-5. Level II screen (page 2). Reprinted with permission from The Nutrition Screening Initiative, Washington, DC.

can include encouragement or assistance from caregivers during mealtimes, proper dental care, discontinuation of anorectic medications, treatment of depression, and referral to food provision programs, such as Meals-on-Wheels. Treatment of documented micronutrient deficiencies should be initiated. If macronutrient intake is poor and nutrition support is indicated, clinicians can prescribe liquid nutrition supplements, enteral formulas delivered through feeding tubes (EN), or parenteral nutrition (PN).

Treatment of Specific Micronutrient Deficiencies

Administration of daily multivitamin and calcium supplements is likely to improve the nutritional status and reduce the incidence of overt micronutrient deficiencies in elderly patients with marginal nutrient intakes.[143] However, in individuals with documented micronutrient deficiencies, short-term administration of at least three to five times the usual daily requirement is usually indicated. For example, individuals with hypovitaminosis D typically require 50,000 IU of ergocalciferol (over 80 times the RDA) on a weekly basis for a month or more to replenish their body stores of vitamin D. In patients with vitamin B12 deficiency, therapeutic options include oral, enteral, or intranasal administration and intramuscular injection of cyanocobalamin. Unlike the vitamin B12 found in food, which must first be cleaved from food proteins by gastric acid and pepsin before it can be absorbed, crystalline vitamin B12 (ie, the pharmacologic form found in vitamins) is readily absorbed even in the absence of gastric acid and pepsin, and therefore, individuals with atrophic gastritis readily respond to oral vitamin B12 therapy. It is also worth remembering that after initial parenteral repletion of vitamin B12, the vast majority of patients with pernicious anemia can be adequately treated with high doses of oral vitamin B12, such as 1 mg daily.[144] Semi-annual checks of plasma concentrations of vitamin B12 and MMA can be used thereafter to confirm the efficacy of this approach.

Oral Nutrition Supplements

Liquid nutrition supplements can be used to increase nutrient intake in malnourished elderly individuals. Although few large randomized controlled trials have been done, existing evidence indicates that oral liquid nutritional supplements can lead to weight gain, improved functional status, and decreased mortality in malnourished elderly patients.[145] One recent study suggested that energy intake may be higher when liquid nutrition supplements are administered between rather than with meals.[146]

Enteral Nutrition

Short-term nutrition support can be provided through nasogastric or nasoenteric (post-pyloric) feeding tubes. If EN is required for longer than 1 month, however, a permanent gastrostomy is usually recommended, largely because gastrostomy tubes are generally more comfortable and better tolerated by patients than are nasogastric or nasoenteric tubes.[147] In addition, gastrostomy tubes typically do not become displaced as often as do nasogastric tubes, so patients' enteral feeds are not interrupted. For this reason, patients fed via gastrostomy tubes may receive more of their prescribed enteral formula and gain more weight than do patients fed via nasogastric tubes.[148]

Gastrostomy is usually chosen over jejunostomy because of the relative ease of both initial placement and subsequent replacement if the tube becomes dislodged. In addition, the side effect profile of gastrostomy is largely thought to be better than jejunostomy, which has been associated with small bowel necrosis in a very small number of cases. It has been suggested that jejunostomy feeding tubes may be associated with a lower risk of aspiration pneumonia than gastrostomy tubes, but most studies refute this assertion.[149-151] Therefore, jejunostomy tubes are usually reserved for patients who have significant upper GI tract disease.

Another distinct advantage of nasogastric or gastrostomy tubes is that enteral formulas can be administered as bolus, continuous, or cycled (eg, overnight) feeds. Because the small intestine is much less distensible than is the stomach, however, bolus feeds should not be given through nasoenteric or jejunal feeding tubes. The choice of enteral formula depends on a variety of factors, including tube site, the patient's specific nutritional needs, and presence of certain disease states. A thorough discussion of commonly-used enteral formulas and their indications can be found in Chapter 42.

Complications of tube feeding (discussed in Chapter 38) include wound infection, bleeding, aspiration pneumonia, nausea, vomiting, diarrhea, hyperglycemia, electrolyte imbalance, refeeding syndrome, tube blockage, peristomal leakage, and the "buried bumper" syndrome. In patients undergoing percutaneous endoscopic gastrostomy (PEG) placement, minor complications occur in 13% to 32%, with tube blockage and wound infections being the most common events.[152,153] Major complications occur in 3% to 13% of patients, and the procedure-related mortality rate is 0.6% to 4%.[152-154]

Feeding tubes are often placed to prevent aspiration pneumonitis and pneumonia in high-risk patients, such as those with neurologic dysphagia. Paradoxically, aspiration is a known complication of EN. It is difficult to perform a meta-analysis and to reach a consensus about the risk of aspiration in tube-fed patients because the entity is defined differently from study to study. However, there is little evidence to support the hypothesis that tube feeding lowers the risk of aspiration.[155] It is sometimes assumed that postpyloric or intraduodenal feeding is associated with a lower risk of aspiration than is intragastric feeding. Studies suggest that postpyloric or intraduodenal feeding carries the same risk of clinically-significant aspiration as intragastric feeding.[156,157] Aspiration risk is clearly highest in tube-fed, bedridden elderly patients who have altered levels of consciousness. On the other hand, the risk of clinically-significant aspiration appears to be very low in elderly patients who have a normal sensorium, whether they are ambulatory or bed-bound.[158]

Minimizing Complications of Tube Feeding

With proper management, the risk of tube-feeding complications in the elderly can be minimized. For example, administration of broad-spectrum antibiotics during routine PEG placement reduces the occurrence of peristomal infections in a safe and cost-effective manner.[159-162] The risk of aspiration can be reduced by proper positioning of the patient, with the head of the bed up at a 30° to 45° angle. GI side effects can usually be minimized by avoiding excessive infusion rates and selecting appropriate enteral formulas. Metabolic complications such as electrolyte imbalance and dehydration can often be avoided by careful attention to formula selection and provision of adequate free water. In elderly adults with significant malnutrition, EN should be initiated gradually to limit the risk of refeeding syndrome, and blood levels of potassium, phosphorus, and magnesium should initially be monitored in these individuals on a regular basis.

Parenteral Nutrition

There is limited data about the use of PN specifically in elderly individuals, but in the right clinical situation, it should not be withheld on account of advanced age. The use of PN in older patients should be reserved for those in whom the GI tract is nonfunctional, just as it is in younger patients. Complications of PN in older patients include those seen in younger patients. In addition, older individuals may be at higher risk of PN-related hyperglycemia than are younger patients.[163] As a result of declining renal or cardiac function with aging, fluid overload may also occur. As in younger patients, complications can be minimized by adhering to standard sterile techniques; obtaining periodic measurements of electrolytes, glucose, and liver function; and assessing fluid status on a regular basis.

Ethics of Nutrition Support

There is no question that nutrition support can improve outcome and quality of life in older patients with acute illnesses. However, in some patients with severe dementia, chronic debilitating diseases, or terminal illnesses, the benefits of nutrition support are not always so clear. In fact, a review of the literature by Finucane and colleagues revealed that in patients with advanced dementia, there is little or no evidence that tube feeding reduces the risk of aspiration, prevents the occurrence of decubitus ulcers or infection, improves functional status, or prolongs life.[164] There is also little evidence that nutrition support improves quality of life in elderly patients with chronic incapacitating illnesses like dementia. In one small study of long-term tube feeding, objective measures of quality of life deteriorated in 46% and improved in only 29% of patients with dementia or other debilitating disease.[165] Perhaps the most revealing aspect of this study was the finding that 73% of family members caring for patients with dementia or chronic debilitating illnesses would not want to have a feeding tube placed if they themselves were in a similar situation. This finding mirrors the results of another recent study, which revealed that physicians often prescribe EN and other life-sustaining therapies more often than their patients would want them to. In fact, only 22% to 28% of elderly patients surveyed would want a feeding tube placed if they developed a severe irreversible mental or physical illness or metastatic cancer.[166]

As is the case with other life-sustaining therapies, the decision to accept or decline nutrition support is best made by a competent, informed patient. In an ideal world, all patients would have advanced directives concerning the use of nutrition support in the event of a severely debilitating or dementing illness. Too often, though, the wishes of the patient are unknown and family members are left to make the difficult decision for them. In these cases, the pros and cons of nutrition support should be carefully considered and discussed with the patient's loved ones before a decision is made to initiate treatment.

Chapter 46 discusses the medical, legal, and ethical aspects of nutritional support.

Conclusion

There is still much to be learned about the interaction between nutrition and aging. It is known that aging is associated with a variety of changes in GI function, body composition, energy metabolism, and macro- and micronutrient requirements, each of which can influence nutritional status. Malnutrition is associated with an increased risk of morbidity and mortality, and nutrition support can improve clinical outcome in selected elderly populations. Therefore, clinicians who are involved in the care of elderly individuals should be able to identify individuals at risk of malnutrition and should be familiar with available treatment options, including lifestyle counseling, micronutrient supplementation, and EN and PN support.

References

1. NCHS. Life expectancy by age, race, and sex, 1900-2000. *National Vital Statistics Reports*. 2002;51(3):29-32.
2. Hobbs F, Stoops N. Demographic trends in the 20th century: Census 2000 special reports, Series CENSR-4. Washington, DC: US Government Printing Office; November 2002.
3. Goulding M, Rogers M, Smith S. Public health and aging: trends in aging--United States and worldwide. *MMWR*. 2003;52(06):101-106.
4. Hobbs F, Damon B. Current Population Reports, Special Studies, P23-190, 65+ in the United States. Washington, DC: US Bureau of the Census; April 1996.
5. Manson A, Shea S. Malnutrition in elderly ambulatory medical patients. *Am J Public Health*. 1991;81(9):1195-1197.
6. Wilson M-M, Vaswani S, Liu D, Morley J, Miller D. Prevalence and causes of undernutrition in medical outpatients. *Am J Med*. 1998;104(1):56-63.
7. Morley J, Silver AJ. Nutritional issues in nursing home care. *Ann Intern Med*. 1995;123(11):850-859.
8. Azad N, Murphy J, Amos S, Toppan J. Nutrition survey in an elderly population following admission to a tertiary care hospital. *CMAJ*. 1999;161(5):511-515.
9. McWhirter J, Pennington C. Incidence and recognition of malnutrition in hospital. *BMJ*. 1994;308(6934):945-948.
10. Flegal K, Carroll M, Ogden C, Johnson C. Prevalence and trends in obesity among US adults, 1999-2000. *JAMA*. 2002;288(14):1723-1727.
11. Keller H. Weight gain impacts morbidity and mortality in institutionalized older persons. *J Am Geriatr Soc*. 1995;43(2):165-169.

12. Phillips P. Grip strength, mental performance and nutritional status as indicators of mortality risk among female geriatric patients. *Age Ageing.* 1986;15:53-56.
13. Gorse G, Messner R, Stephens N. Association of malnutrition with nosocomial infection. *Infect Control Hosp Epidemiol.* 1989;10(5):194-203.
14. Sullivan DH, Bopp M, Roberson PK. Protein-energy undernutrition and life-threatening complications among the hospitalized elderly. *J Gen Intern Med.* 2002;17:923-932.
15. Sullivan DH, Patch GA, Walls RC, Lipschitz DA. Impact of nutritional status on morbidity and mortality in a select population of geriatric rehabilitation patients. *Am J Clin Nutr.* 1990;51:749-758.
16. Reilly J, Hull S, Albert N, Waller A, Bringardener S. Economic impact of malnutrition: a model system for hospitalized patients. *JPEN J Parenter Enteral Nutr.* 1988;12(4):371-376.
17. Correia M, Waitzberg D. The impact of malnutrition on morbidity, mortality, length of hospital stay and costs evaluated through a multivariate model analysis. *Clin Nutr.* 2003;22(3):235-239.
18. Middleton M, Nazarenko G, Nivison-Smith I, Smerdely P. Prevalence of malnutrition and 12-month incidence of mortality in two Sydney teaching hospitals. *Intern Med J.* 2001;31(8):455-461.
19. Covinsky K, Martin G, Beyth R, Justice A, Sehgal A, Landefeld C. The relationship between clinical assessments of nutritional status and adverse outcomes in older hospitalized medical patients. *J Am Geriatr Soc.* 1999;47(5):532-538.
20. Gil Gregorio P, Ramirez Diaz S, Ribera Casado J. Demention and nutrition. Intervention study in institutionalized patients with Alzheimer disease. *J Nutr Health Aging.* 2003;7(5):304-308.
21. Detsky A, Baker J, O'Rourke K, Goel V. Perioperative parenteral nutrition: a meta-analysis. *Ann Intern Med.* 1987;107:195-203.
22. Heyland D, MacDonald S, Keefe L, Drover J. Total parenteral nutrition in the critically ill patient: a meta-analysis. *JAMA.* 1998;280(23):2013-2019.
23. Manton KG, Gu X. Changes in the prevalence of chronic disability in the United States black and nonblack population above age 65 from 1982 to 1999. *Proc Natl Acad Sci USA.* 2001;98(11):6354-6359.
24. Ervin RB, Kennedy-Stephenson J. Mineral intakes of elderly supplement and non-supplement users in the Third National Health and Nutrition Examination Survey. *J Nutr.* 2002;132:3422-3427.
25. Koehler K, Baumgartner R, Garry PJ, Allen R, Stabler SP, Rimm E. Association of folate intake and serum homocysteine in elderly persons according to vitamin supplementation and alcohol use. *Am J Clin Nutr.* 2001;73(3):628-637.
26. Weimer J. Factors affecting nutrient intake of the elderly. Agricultural Economic Report No. 769. Washington, DC: US Department of Agriculture; 1998.
27. Marshall T, Stumbo P, Warren J, Xie X-J. Inadequate nutrient intakes are common and are associated with low diet variety in rural, community-dwelling elderly. *J Nutr.* 2001;131:2192-2196.
28. Omdahl JL, Garry PJ, Hunsaker LA, Hunt WC, Goodwin JS. Nutritional status in a healthy elderly population: vitamin D. *Am J Clin Nutr.* 1982;36:1225-1233.
29. Chen L, Fan-Chiang W. Biochemical evaluation of riboflavin and vitamin B6 status of institutionalized and non-institutionalized elderly in Central Kentucky. *Int J Vitam Nutr Res.* 1981;51(3):232-238.
30. Lindenbaum J, Rosenberg I, Wilson P, Stabler S, Allen R. Prevalence of cobalamin deficiency in the Framingham elderly population. *Am J Clin Nutr.* 1994;60(1):2-11.
31. Baker M, Peacock M, Nordin B. The decline in vitamin D status with age. *Age Ageing.* 1980;9(4):249-252.
32. Bialostosky K, Wright J, Kennedy-Stephenson J, McDowell M, Johnson C. Dietary intake of macronutrients, micronutrients and other dietary constituents: United States, 1988-94. National Center for Health Statistics. Vital Health Stat. 2002;11(245).
33. MacLaughlin J, Holick MF. Aging decreases the capacity of human skin to produce vitamin D3. *J Clin Invest.* 1985;76:1536-1538.
34. Parfitt AM, Gallagher J, Heaney R, Johnston C, Neer R, Whedon GD. Vitamin D and bone health in the elderly. *Am J Clin Nutr.* 1982;36:1014-1031.
35. Rapuri PB, Kinyamu HK, Gallagher JC, Haynatzka V. Seasonal changes in calcitropic hormones, bone markers, and bone mineral density in elderly women. *J Clin Endo Metab.* 2002;87(5):2024-2032.
36. Rosen C, Morrison A, Zhou H, et al. Elderly women in northern New England exhibit seasonal changes in bone mineral density and calciotropic hormones. *Bone Miner.* 1994;25(2):83-92.
37. Rucker D, Allan J, Fick G, Hanley D. Vitamin D insufficiency in a population of healthy western Canadians. *CMAJ.* 2002;166:1517–1524.
38. van der Wielen R, Lowik M, van den Berg H, et al. Serum vitamin D concentrations among elderly people in Europe. *Lancet.* 1995;346(8969):207-210.
39. Freaney R, McBrinn Y, McKenna M. Secondary hyperparathyroidism in elderly people: combined effect of renal insufficiency and vitamin D deficiency. *Am J Clin Nutr.* 1993;58(2):187-191.
40. Souberville J, Cormier C, Kindermans C, et al. Vitamin D status and redefining serum parathyroid hormone reference range in the elderly. *J Clin Endocrinol Metab.* 2001;86:3086-3090.
41. Gomez-Alonso C, Naves-Diaz M, Fernandez-Martin J, Diaz-Lopez J, Fernandez-Coto M, Cannata-Andia J. Vitamin D status and secondary hyperparathyroidism: the importance of 25-hydroxyvitamin D cut-off levels. *Kidney Int.* 2003;85:S44-48.
42. Jesudason D, Need A, Horowitz M, O'Loughlin P, Morris H, Nordin B. Relationship between serum 25-hydroxyvitamin D and bone resorption markers in vitamin D insufficiency. *Bone.* 2002;31(5):626-630.
43. Lips P, van Ginkel F, Jongen M, Rubertus F, van der Vijgh W, Netelenbos J. Determinants of vitamin D status in patients with hip fracture and in elderly control subjects. *Am J Clin Nutr.* 1987;46(6):1005-1010.
44. LeBoff MS, Kohlmeier L, Hurwitz S, Franklin J, Wright J, Glowacki J. Occult vitamin D deficiency in postmenopausal US women with acute hip fracture. *JAMA.* 1999;281(16):1505-1511.
45. Vieth R. Vitamin D supplementation, 25-hydroxyvitamin D concentrations, and safety. *Am J Clin Nutr.* 1999;69(5):842-856.
46. Ferriolli E, Oliveira R, Matsuda N, Braga F, Dantas R. Aging, esophageal motility, and gastroesophageal reflux. *J Am Geriatr Soc.* 1998;46(12):1534-1537.
47. Clarkston W, Pantano M, Morley J, Horowitz M, Littlefield J, Burton F. Evidence for the anorexia of aging: gastrointestinal transit and hunger in healthy elderly vs. young adults. *Am J Physiol.* 1997;272:R243-248.
48. Brogna A, Ferrara R, Bucceri A, Lanteri E, Catalano F. Influence of aging on gastrointestinal transit time: an ultrasonographic and radiologic study. *Invest Radiol.* 1999;34(5):357-359.
49. Webster S, Wilkinson E, Gowland E. A comparison of fat absorption in young and old subjects. *Age Ageing.* 1977;6(2):113-117.
50. Werner I, Hambraeus L. The digestive capacity of elderly people. In: Carlson, ed. *Nutrition in Old Age.* Uppsala, Sweden: Almquist and Wicksell; 1972:55-60.
51. Gullo L, Priori P, Daniele C, Ventrucci M, Gasbarrini G, Labo G. Exocrine pancreatic function in the elderly. *Gerontology.* 1983;29(6):407-411.
52. Gullo L, Ventrucci M, Naldoni P, Pezzilli R. Aging and exocrine pancreatic function. *J Am Geriatr Soc.* 1986;34:790-792.
53. Arora S, Kassarjian Z, Krasinski S, Croffey B, Kaplan M, Russell RM. Effect of age on tests of intestinal and hepatic function in healthy humans. *Gastroenterology.* 1989;96:1560-1565.
54. Hurwitz A, Brady D, Schaal SE, Samloff IM, Dedon J, Ruhl C. Gastric acidity in older adults. *JAMA.* 1997;278(8):659-662.
55. Krasinki S, Russell RM, Samloff IM, et al. Fundic atrophic gastritis in an elderly population. Effect on hemoglobin and several serum nutritional indicators. *J Am Geriatr Soc.* 1986;34(11):800-806.
56. Suter PM, Golner BB, Goldin BR, Morrow FD, Russell RM. Reversal of protein-bound vitamin B12 malabsorption with antibiotics in atrophic gastritis. *Gastroenterology.* 1991;101:1039-1045.
57. Santarelli L, Gabrielli M, Cremonini F, et al. Atrophic gastritis as a cause of hyperhomocysteinaemia. *Aliment Pharmacol Ther.* 2004;19(1):107-111.

58. Lindenbaum J, Healton E, Savage D, et al. Neuropsychiatric disorders caused by cobalamin deficiency in the absence of anemia or macrocytosis. *N Engl J Med.* 1988;318(26):1720-1728.
59. Russell RM. Changes in gastrointestinal function attributed to aging. *Am J Clin Nutr.* 1992;55:1203S-1207S.
60. Carmel R. Prevalence of undiagnosed pernicious anemia in the elderly. *Arch Int Med.* 1996;156(10):1097-1100.
61. Sumner AE, Chin MM, Abrahm JL, et al. Elevated methylmalonic acid and total homocysteine levels show high prevalence of vitamin B12 deficiency after gastric surgery. *Ann Intern Med.* 1996;124(5):469-476.
62. Steinberg W, King C, Toskes P. Malabsorption of protein-bound cobalamin but not unbound cobalamin during cimetidine administration. *Dig Dis Sci.* 1980;25(3):188-191.
63. Marcuard SP, Albernaz L, Khazanie PG. Omeprazole therapy causes malabsorption of cyanocobalamin (vitamin B12). *Ann Intern Med.* 1994;120(3):211-215.
64. Schenk B, Kuipers E, Klinkenberg-Knol E, et al. Atrophic gastritis during long-term omeprazole therapy affects serum vitamin B12 levels. *Aliment Pharmacol Ther.* 1999;13(10):1343-1346.
65. Skikne BS, Lynch S, Cook J. Role of gastric acid in food iron absorption. *Gastroenterology.* 1981;81:1068-1071.
66. Jacobs A, Rhodes J, Peters K, Campbell H, Eakins J. Gastric acidity and iron absorption. *Brit J Haematol.* 1966;12:728-736.
67. Koop H, Bachem MG. Serum iron, ferritin and vitamin B12 during prolonged omeprazole therapy. *J Clin Gastroenterol.* 1992;14(4):288-292.
68. Fleming DJ, Jacques PF, Tucker KL, et al. Iron status of the free-living, elderly Framingham Heart Study cohort: an iron-replete population with a high prevalence of elevated iron stores. *Am J Clin Nutr.* 2001;73(3):638-646.
69. Gleghorn E, Eisenberg L, Hack S, Parton P, Merritt R. Observations of vitamin A toxicity in three patients with renal failure receiving parenteral alimentation. *Am J Clin Nutr.* 1986;44(1):107-112.
70. Farrington K, Miller P, Varghese Z, Baillod R, Moorhead J. Vitamin A toxicity and hypercalcemia in chronic renal failure. *Br Med J Clin Research Ed.* 1981;282(6281):1999-2002.
71. DRI. Dietary reference intakes for calcium, phosphorus, magnesium, vitamin D and fluoride. Washington, DC: National Academies Press; 1997.
72. Alaimo K, McDowell M, Briefel R, et al. Dietary intake of vitamins, minerals, and fiber of persons ages 2 months and over in the United States: Third National Health and Nutrition Examination Survey, Phase I, 1988-91. Hyattsville, MD: National Center for Health Statistics; 1994: 258.
73. Recker R. Calcium absorption and achlorhydria. *N Engl J Med.* 1985;313:70-73.
74. Agnusdei D, Civitelli R, Camporeale A, et al. Age-related deline of bone mass and intestinal calcium absorption in normal males. *Calcif Tissue Int.* 1998;63(3):197-201.
75. Eastell R, Yergey A, NE V, Cedel S, Kumar R, Riggs B. Interrelationship among vitamin D metabolism, true calcium absorption, parathyroid function, and age in women: evidence of an age-related intestinal resistance to 1,25-dihydroxyvitamin D action. *J Bone Miner Res.* 1991;6(2):125-132.
76. Pattanaungkul S, Riggs B, Yergey A, Vieira N, O'Fallon W, Khosla S. Relationship of intestinal calcium absorption to 1,25-dihydroxyvitamin D [1,25(OH)2D] levels in young versus elderly women: evidence for age-related intestinal resistance to 1,25(OH)2D action. *J Clin Endo Metab.* 2000;85(11):4023-4027.
77. Wolf R, Cauley J, Baker C, et al. Factors associated with calcium absorption efficiency in pre- and perimenopausal women. *Am J Clin Nutr.* 2000;72(2):466-471.
78. Dawson-Hughes B, Harris S, Finneran S. Calcium absorption on high and low calcium intakes in relation to vitamin D receptor genotype. *J Clin Endo Metab.* 1995;80(12):3657-3661.
79. Krall E, Dawson-Hughes B. Smoking increases bone loss and decreases intestinal calcium absorption. *J Bone Miner Res.* 1999;14(2):215-220.
80. Rosenberg IH. Summary comments: epidemiological and methodological problems in determining nutritional status of older persons. *Am J Clin Nutr.* 1989;50:1231-1233.
81. Starling R, Ades P, Poehlman E. Physical activity, protein intake, and appendicular skeletal muscle mass in older men. *Am J Clin Nutr.* 1999;70:91-96.
82. Gallagher D, Ruts E, Visser M, et al. Weight stability masks sarcopenia in elderly men and women. *Am J Physiol Endocrinol Metab.* 2000;279(2):E366-375.
83. Greenlund L, Nair K. Sarcopenia--consequences, mechanisms, and potential therapies. *Mech Ageing Dev.* 2003;124:287-299.
84. Baumgartner R, Koehler K, Gallagher D, et al. Epidemiology of sarcopenia among the elderly in New Mexico. *Am J Epidemiol.* 1998;147(8):755-763.
85. Castillo E, Goodman-Gruen D, Kritz-Silverstein D, Morton D, Wingard D, Barrett-Connor E. Sarcopenia in elderly men and women. The Rancho Bernardo Study. *Am J Prev Med.* 2003;25(3):226-231.
86. Roubenoff R, Parise H, Payette H, et al. Cytokines, insulin-like growth factor 1, sarcopenia, and mortality in very old community-dwelling men and women: the Framingham Heart Study. *Am J Med.* 2003;115:429-435.
87. Janssen I, Heymsfield S, Ross R. Low relative skeletal muscle mass (sarcopenia) in older people is associated with functional impairment and physical disability. *J Am Geriatr Soc.* 2002;50:889-896.
88. Fiatarone M, O'Neill E, Ryan ND, et al. Exercise training and nutritional supplementation for physical frailty in very elderly people. *N Engl J Med.* 1994;330(25):1769-1775.
89. de Jong N, Paw M, de Groot L, Hiddink G, van Staveren W. Dietary supplements and physical exercise affecting bone and body composition in frail elderly persons. *Am J Public Health.* 2000;90(6):947-954.
90. Campell AJ, Robertson MC, Gardner M, Norton R, Tilyard M, Buchner D. Randomised controlled trial of a general practice programme of home based exercise to prevent falls in elderly women. *BMJ.* 1997;315(7115):1065-1069.
91. McCartney N, Hicks A, Martin J, Webber C. Long-term resistance training in the elderly: effects of dynamic strength, exercise capacity, muscle, and bone. *J Gerontol.* 1995;50(2):B97-104.
92. Vincent K, Braith R, Feldman R, Kallas H, Lowenthal D. Improved cardiorespiratory endurance following 6 months of resistance exercise in elderly men and women. *Arch Int Med.* 2002;162(6):673-678.
93. Castaneda C, Layne J, Munoz-Orians L, et al. A randomized controlled trial of resistance exercise training to improve glycemic control in older adults with type 2 diabetes. *Diabetes Care.* 2002;25(12):2335-2341.
94. Nelson M, Fiatarone M, Morganti C, Trice I, Greenberg R, Evans W. Effects of high-intensity strength training on multiple risk factors for osteoporotic fractures: a randomized controlled trial. *JAMA.* 1994;272(24):1909-1914.
95. Singh N, Clements K, Fiatarone M. A randomized controlled trial of progressive resistance training in depressed elders. *J Gerontol.* 1997;52:27-35.
96. Singh K, Clements K, Fiatarone M. Sleep, sleep deprivation, and daytime activities: a randomized controlled trial of the effect of exercise on sleep. *Sleep.* 1997;20:95-101.
97. Latham N, Anderson C, Lee A, Bennett D, Moseley A, Cameron I. A randomized, controlled trial of quadriceps resistance exercise and vitamin D in frail older people: the Frailty Interventions Trial in Elderly Subjects (FITNESS). *J Am Geriatr Soc.* 2003;51(3):291-299.
98. Wouters-Wesseling W, Van Hooijdonk C, Wagenaar L, Bindels J, de Groot L, van Staveren W. The effect of a liquid nutrition supplement on body composition and physical functioning in elderly people. *Clin Nutr.* 2003;22(4):371-377.

99. Castaneda C, Charnley J, Evans W, Crim M. Elderly women accomodate to a low-protein diet with losses of body cell mass, muscle function, and immune response. *Am J Clin Nutr.* 1995;62(1):30-39.
100. Castaneda C, Gordon P, Fielding R, Evans W, Crim M. Marginal protein intake results in reduced plasma IGF-1 levels and skeletal muscle fiber atrophy in elderly women. *J Nutr Health Aging.* 2000;4(2):85-90.
101. Gruenewald DA, Matsumoto AM. Testosterone supplementation therapy for older men: potential benefits and risks. *J Am Geriatr Soc.* 2003;51(1):101-115.
102. Diamond P, Cusan L, Gomez J, Belanger A, Labrie F. Metabolic effects of 12-month percutaneous dehydroepiandrosterone replacement therapy in postmenopausal women. *J Endocrinol.* 1996;150 Suppl:S43-50.
103. Kenny A, Dawson L, Kleppinger A, Iannuzzi-Sucich M, Judge J. Prevalence of sarcopenia and predictors of skeletal muscle mass in nonobese women who are long-term users of estrogen-replacement therapy. *J Gerontol.* 2003;58(5):M436-440.
104. Blackman M, Sorkin J, Munzer T, et al. Growth hormone and sex steroid administration in healthy aged women and men: a randomized controlled trial. *JAMA.* 2002;288(18):2282-2292.
105. Rossouw J, Anderson G, Prentice R, et al. Risks and benefits of estrogen plus progestin in healthy postmenopausal women: principal results from the Women's Health Initiative randomized controlled trial. *JAMA.* 2002;288(3):321-333.
106. Davison KK, Ford ES, Cogswell M, Dietz W. Percentage of body fat and body mass index are associated with mobility limitations in people aged 70 and older from NHANES III. *J Am Geriatr Soc.* 2002;50:1802-1809.
107. Inelmen E, Sergi G, Coin A, Miotto F, Peruzza S, Enzi G. Can obesity be a risk factor in elderly people? *Obes Rev.* 2003;4(3):147-155.
108. Whelton P, Appel L, Espeland M, et al. Sodium reduction and weight loss in the treatment of hypertension in older persons: a randomized controlled trial of nonpharmacologic interventions in the elderly (TONE). *JAMA.* 1998;279(11):839-846.
109. Abu-Abeid S, Keidar A, Szoid A. Resolution of chronic medical conditions after laparoscopic adjustable silicone gastric banding for the treatment of morbid obesity in the elderly. *Surg Endosc.* 2001;15(2):132-134.
110. Piers L, Soares M, McCormack L, O'Dea K. Is there evidence for an age-related reduction in metabolic rate? *J Appl Physiol.* 1998;85:2196-2204.
111. Fukagawa N, Bandini L, Young J. Effect of age on body composition and resting metabolic rate. *Am J Physiol.* 1990;259:E233-238.
112. Visser M, Deurenberg P, van Staveren W, Hautvast J. Resting metabolic rate and diet-induced thermogenesis in young and elderly subjects: relationship with body composition, fat distribution, and physical activity level. *Am J Clin Nutr.* 1995;61(4):772-778.
113. Vaughan L, Zurlo F, Ravussin E. Aging and energy expenditure. *Am J Clin Nutr.* 1991;53:821-825.
114. Bosy-Westphal A, Eichhorn C, Kutzner D, Illner K, Heller M, Muller M. The age-related decline in resting energy expenditure in humans is due to the loss of fat-free mass and to alterations in its metabolically active components. *J Nutr.* 2003;133:2356-2362.
115. Roberts SB, Fuss P, Heyman MB, Young VR. Influence of age on energy requirements. *Am J Clin Nutr.* 1995;62:1053S-1058S.
116. Harris J, Benedict F. *A Biometric Study of Basal Metabolism in Man.* Washington, DC: Carnegie Institution of Washington; 1919.
117. Schofield W, Schofield C, James W. Basal metabolic rate review and prediction, together with an annotated bibliography of source material. *Hum Nutr Clin Nutr.* 1985;39C (Supp I).
118. WHO. Energy and protein requirements. Report of a joint FAO/WHO/UNU expert consultation. Geneva: World Health Organization; 1985.
119. Roza A, Shizgal H. The Harris Benedict equation reevaluated: resting energy requirements and the body cell mass. *Am J Clin Nutr.* 1984;40(1):168-182.
120. Ahmad A, Duerksen D, Munroe S, Bistrian B. An evaluation of resting energy expenditure in hospitalized, severely underweight patients. *Nutrition.* 1999;15(5):384-388.
121. Roberts SB. Energy requirements of older individuals. *Eur J Clin Nutr.* 1996;50(Suppl 1):S112-117.
122. Lührmann P, Herbert B, Krems C, Neuhauser-Berthold M. A new equation especially developed for predicting resting metabolic rate in the elderly for easy use in practice. *Eur J Nutr.* 2002;41(108-13).
123. DRI. Dietary reference intakes for energy, carbohydrate, fiber, fat, fatty acids, cholesterol, protein, and amino acids. Washington, DC: National Academies Press; 2002.
124. Gersovitz M, Motil K, Munro H, Scrimshaw N, Young V. Human protein requirements; assessment of the adequacy of the current Recommended Dietary Allowance for dietary protein in elderly men and women. *Am J Clin Nutr.* 1982;35(1):6-14.
125. Morse M, Haub M, Evans W, Campbell W. Protein requirement of elderly women: nitrogen balance responses to three levels of protein intake. *J Gerontol.* 2001;56(11):M724-730.
126. Campbell W, Trappe T, Wolfe R, Evans W. The Recommended Dietary Allowance for protein may not be adequate for older people to maintain skeletal muscle. *J Gerontol.* 2001;56:M373-380.
127. World Health Organization/Tufts University School of Nutrition and Policy. *Keep Fit for Life: Meeting the Nutritional Needs of Older Persons.* Geneva, Switzerland: World Health Organization/Tufts University School of Nutrition and Policy; 2002.
128. Dietary Reference Intakes. *Dietary Reference Intakes for Thiamine, Riboflavin, Niacin, Vitamin B_6, Folate, Vitamin B_{12}, Pantothenic Acid, Biotin, and Choline.* Washington, DC: National Academies Press; 1998.
129. Dietary Reference Intakes. *Dietary Reference Intakes for Vitamin C, Vitamin E, Selenium, and Carotenoids.* Washington, DC: National Academies Press; 2000.
130. Dietary Reference Intakes. *Dietary Reference Intakes for Vitamin A, Vitamin K, Arsenic, Boron, Chromium, Copper, Iodine, Iron, Manganese, Molybdenum, Nickel, Silicon, Vanadium, and Zinc.* Washington, DC: National Academies Press; 2001.
131. Krasinki S, Cohn J, Schaefer E, Russell R. Postprandial plasma retinyl ester response is greater in older subjects compared with younger subjects. Evidence for delayed plasma clearance of intestinal lipoproteins. *J Clin Invest.* 1990;85(3):883-892.
132. Hallfrisch J, Muller D, Singh V. Vitamin A and E intakes and plasma concentrations of retinol, beta-carotene, and alpha-tocopherol in men and women of the Baltimore Longitudinal Study of Aging. *Am J Clin Nutr.* 1994;60(2):176-182.
133. Dwyer JT. *Screening Older Americans' Nutritional Health: Current Practices and Future Possibilities.* Washington, DC: Nutrition Screening Initiative; 1991.
134. Vellas B, Guigoz Y, Baumgartner M, Garry PJ, Lauque S, Albarede J. Relationships between nutritional markers and the mini-nutritional assessment in 155 older persons. *J Am Geriatr Soc.* 2000;48(10):1300-1309.
135. Van Nes M-C, Herrmann F, Gold G, Michel J-P, Rizzoli R. Does the Mini Nutritional Assessment predict hospitalization outcomes in older people? *Age Ageing.* 2001;30:221-226.
136. Persson M, Brismar K, Katzarski K, Nordenstrom J, Cederholm T. Nutritional status using Mini Nutritional Assessment and Subjective Global Assessment predict mortality in geriatric patients. *J Am Geriatr Soc.* 2002;50(12):1996-2002.
137. Detsky A, McLaughlin J, Baker J, et al. What is subjective global assessment of nutritional status? *JPEN J Parenter Enteral Nutr.* 1987;11(1):8-13.
138. Hirsch S, de Obaldia N, Petermann M, et al. Subjective global assessment of nutritional status: further validation. *Nutrition.* 1991;7(1):35-37.
139. Sacks G, Dearman K, Replogle W, Cora V, Meeks M, Canada T. Use of subjective global assessment to identify nutrition-associated complications and death in geriatric long-term care facility residents. *J Am Coll Nutr.* 2000;19(5):570-577.

140. Thoresen L, Fjeldstad I, Krogstad K, Kaasa S, Falkmer U. Nutritional status of patients with advanced cancer: the value of using the subjective global assessment of nutritional status as a screening tool. *Palliat Med.* 2002;16(1):33-42.
141. Enia G, Sicuso C, Alati G, Zoccali C. Subjective global assessment of nutrition in dialysis patients. *Nephrol Dial Transplant.* 1993;8(10):1094-1098.
142. NSI. *Report of Nutrition Screening 1: Toward a Common View. Executive Summary.* Washington, DC: Nutrition Screening Initiative; 1991.
143. McKay D, Perrone G, Rasmussen H, et al. The effects of a multivitamin/mineral supplement on micronutrient status, antioxidant capacity and cytokine production in healthy older adults consuming a fortified diet. *J Am Coll Nutr.* 2000;19(5):613-621.
144. Baik H, Russell R. Vitamin B_{12} deficiency in the elderly. *Ann Rev Nutr.* 1999;19:357-377.
145. Potter J, Roberts M, McColl J, Reilly J. Protein energy supplements in unwell elderly patients--a randomised controlled trial. *JPEN J Parenter Enteral Nutr.* 2001;25(6):323-329.
146. Wilson M-M, Purushothaman R, Morley JE. Effect of liquid dietary supplements on energy intake in the elderly. *Am J Clin Nutr.* 2002;75(5):944-947.
147. Fay D, Poplausky M, Gruber M, Lance P. Long-term enteral feeding: a retrospective comparison of delivery via percutaneous endoscopic gastrostomy and nasoenteric tubes. *Am J Gastr.* 1991;86(11):1604-1609.
148. Park R, Allison M, Lang J, et al. Randomised comparison of percutaneous endoscopic gastrostomy and nasogastric tube feeding in patients with persisting neurological dysphagia. *BMJ.* 1992;304:1406-1409.
149. Weltz C, Morris J, Mullen J. Surgical jejunostomy in aspiration risk patients. *Ann Surg.* 1992;215(2):140-145.
150. Cogen R, Weinryb J, Pomerantz C, Fenstemacher P. Complications of jejunostomy tube feeding in nursing facility patients. *Am J Gastr.* 1991;86(11):1610-1613.
151. Kadakia S, Sullivan H, Starnes E. Percutaneous endoscopic gastrostomy or jejunostomy and the incidence of aspiration in 79 patients. *Am J Surg.* 1992;164(2):114-118.
152. Larson D, Burton D, Schroeder K, DiMagno E. Percutaneous endoscopic gastrostomy: indications, success, complications, and mortality in 314 consecutive patients. *Gastroenterology.* 1987;93:48-52.
153. Petersen T, Kruse A. Complications of percutaneous endoscopic gastrostomy. *Eur J Surg.* 1997;163(5):351-356.
154. Lockett M, Templeton M, Byrne T, Norcross E. Percutaneous endoscopic gastrostomy complications in a tertiary-care center. *Amer Surg.* 2002;68(2):117-120.
155. Finucane T, Bynum J. Use of tube feeding to prevent aspiration pneumonia. *Lancet.* 1996;348(9039):1421-1424.
156. Strong R, Condon S, Solinger M, Namihas B, Ito-Wong L, Leuty J. Equal aspiration rates from postpylorus and intragastric-placed small-bore nasoenteric feeding tubes: a randomized, prospective study. *JPEN J Parenter Enteral Nutr.* 1992;16(1):59-63.
157. Esparza J, Boivin M, Hartshorne M, Levy H. Equal aspiration rates in gastrically and transpylorically fed critically ill patients. *Intensive Care Med.* 2001;27:660-664.
158. Bastow M, Rawlings J, Allison S. Benefits of supplementary tube feeding after fractured neck of femur: a randomised controlled trial. *Br Med J.* 1983;287(6405):1589-1592.
159. Akkersdijk W, van Bergeijk J, van Egmond T, et al. Percutaneous endoscopic gastrostomy (PEG): comparison of push and pull methods and evaluation of antibiotic prophylaxis. *Endoscopy.* 1995;27(4):313-316.
160. Gossner L, Keymling J, Hahn E, Ell C. Antibiotic prophylaxis in percutaneous endoscopic gastrostomy (PEG): a prospective randomized clinical trial. *Endoscopy.* 1999;31(2):119-124.
161. Ahmad A, Mouncher A, Abdoolah A, et al. Antibiotic prophylaxis for percutaneous endoscopic gastrostomy--a prospective, randomised, double-blind trial. *Aliment Pharmacol Ther.* 2003;18(2):209-215.
162. Kulling D, Sonenberg A, Fried M, Bauerfeind P. Cost analysis of antibiotic prophylaxis for PEG. *Gastrointest Endosc.* 2000;51(2):152-156.
163. Al-Jaouni R, Schneider S, Rampal P, Hebuterne X. Effect of age on substrate oxidation during total parenteral nutrition. *Nutrition.* 2002;18(1):20-25.
164. Finucane T, Christmas C, Travis K. Tube feeding in patients with advanced dementia: a review of the evidence. *JAMA.* 1999;282(14):1365-1370.
165. Weaver J, Odell P, Nelson C. Evaluation of the benefits of gastric tube feeding in an elderly population. *Arch Fam Med.* 1993;2:953-956.
166. Carmel S. Life-sustaining treatments: what doctors do, what they want for themselves and what elderly persons want. *Soc Sci Med.* 1999;49(10):1401-1408.

Chapter 15

NUTRITION AND ALCOHOLISM

Charles S. Lieber, MD, MACP, FACG

Nutritional Status of the Alcoholic

Alcoholics hospitalized for medical complications of alcoholism were found to have inadequate dietary protein intake[1] with signs of protein malnutrition[2,3] and anthropomorphic measurements indicative of impaired nutrition: reduced muscle mass estimated by the creatinine-height index[3,4] and thin tricep skin folds.[3-5] Continued drinking resulted in weight loss, whereas abstinence resulted in weight gain. Many patients who drink to excess are either not malnourished or are less malnourished than the group hospitalized for medical problems. Alcohol consumption, especially when accompanied by high fat intake and sedentary behavior,[6] favors truncal obesity, particularly in women.[7] Those with moderate alcohol intake[8]—even those admitted to a hospital for alcohol rehabilitation rather than for medical problems[9]—often barely differ nutritionally from controls (matched for socioeconomic status and health history). The wide range in nutritional status of the alcoholic population reflects, in part, differences in what they eat. Moderate alcohol intake—accounting for 16% of total calories (alcohol included)—is associated with slightly increased total energy intake.[10] Such alcohol consumption and even slightly higher levels (23%)[11] are associated with a substitution of alcohol for dietary carbohydrates. In those individuals consuming more than 30% of total calories as alcohol, there is also a significant decrease in protein and fat intake, and consumption of vitamins A, C and thiamin may descend below the recommended daily allowances.[10] Calcium, iron, and fiber intake are also decreased.[11]

The mechanisms of the altered food intake are not well known. Suppression of appetite has been postulated[12] but has not been much assessed. The decreased food intake is partly explained by depressed consciousness during inebriation and hangover and by the gastroduodenitis caused by ethanol. In addition, ethanol and nutrients interact at almost every level of the gastrointestinal (GI) tract. Ethanol alters the storage, mobilization, activation, and metabolism of nutrients and it is toxic to many tissues. In the United States, alcoholism remains one of the major causes of nutritional deficiency; alcohol-related illness is an enormous medical burden and often requires complex nutritional therapy.

Nutritional Value of Alcoholic Beverages

Alcoholic beverages contain water, ethanol, variable amounts of carbohydrate, and little else of nutritive value. The carbohydrate content varies greatly: whiskey, cognac, and vodka have virtually none; red and dry white wines have 2 to 10 g/L; beer and dry sherry, 30 g/L; and sweetened white and port wines, as much as 120 g/L. The protein, vitamin, and mineral content of these beverages is extremely low.

Alcoholic beverages differ in their alcohol content. Regular beer contains about 4% alcohol. Light beers have nearly as much alcohol (3%) but contain fewer calories. Wine coolers are low in alcohol content (3.5% to 6%) compared to regular wine (11% to 12%) but are high in calories. The alcohol content of distilled spirits such as whiskey, rum, gin, or brandy is more variable. It

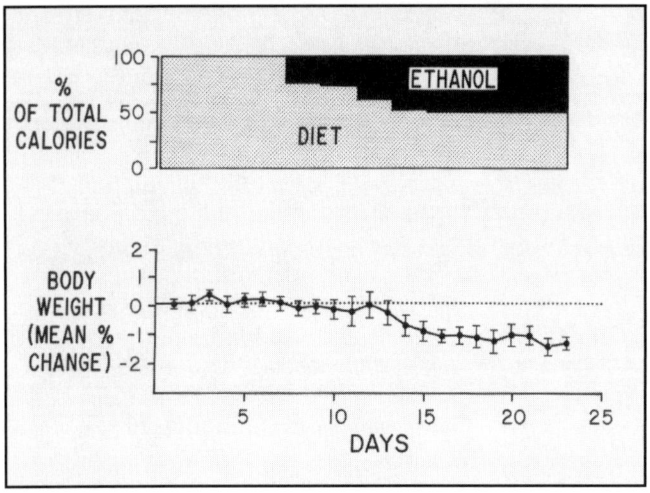

Figure 15-1. Effect of the isocaloric substitution of carbohydrate by ethanol on body weight in man. Substitution of ethanol up to 50% of total calories resulted in body weight loss. From Pirola RC, Lieber CS. The energy cost of the metabolism of drugs, including ethanol. *Pharmacology.* 1972;7:185-96.

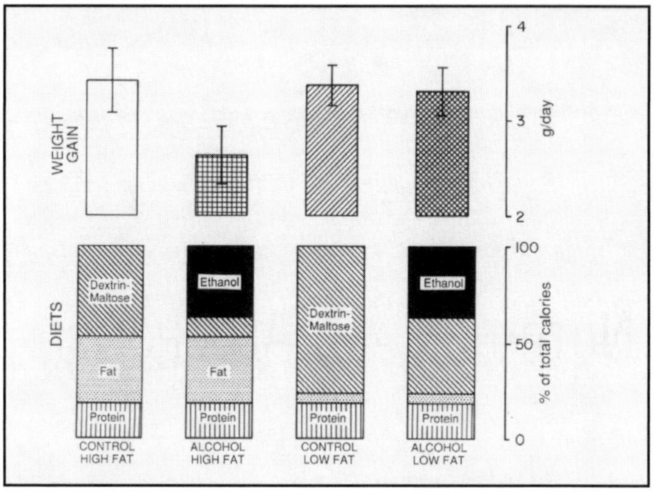

Figure 15-2. Effects of ethanol and/or dietary fat on body weight gain in rats. The ethanol-induced deficit in weight gain was not observed in the presence of a very-low-fat diet (5% of energy). From Lieber CS. Perspectives: Do alcohol calories count? *Am J Clin Nutr.* 1991;54:976-82.

is measured in "proof," and in the United States, 1 proof equals 0.5% alcohol. Based on national consumption data, the estimated contribution of alcohol to the average American diet is 4.5% of total calories.

Combustion of ethanol in a bomb calorimeter yields 7.1 kcal/g; however, its biologic value appears to be less. Lowered body weight in alcohol drinkers compared to nondrinkers is especially apparent in women.[13] When volunteer subjects were given additional calories as alcohol under metabolic ward conditions, they did not gain weight[14,15] and isocaloric substitution of ethanol for carbohydrate, as 50% of total calories (in a balanced diet) resulted in a decline in body weight (Figure 15-1).

There is evidence that ethanol increases the metabolic rate, which could explain, at least part, its reduced biologic energy value. Indeed, ethanol increases oxygen consumption in normal subjects and also, but to a greater degree, in alcoholics.[16] Substitution of ethanol for carbohydrates increased the metabolic rate and the diet-induced thermogenesis in humans and rodents.[17] Resting energy expenditure also increased in humans.[18] Only a small portion of the energy deficit in rats could be attributed to brown fat thermogenesis.[19] It was postulated that energy waste during ethanol consumption might occur via oxidation without phosphorylation by the microsomal ethanol oxidizing system (MEOS).[15] The MEOS is inducible by chronic ethanol consumption, which aggravates energy waste.[20,21] The MEOS is not solely responsible for energy wastage from ethanol. Even when the MEOS is induced, much of the ethanol is metabolized by alcohol dehydrogenase to acetaldehyde, and much of the energy from ethanol is produced by the oxidation of acetaldehyde to carbon dioxide and water. Acetaldehyde may contribute to energy wastage by promoting catecholamine release and by impairing various mitochondrial shuttles and mitochondrial oxidative phosphorylation. Acetate, the next product in the oxidation of ethanol, is also associated with several energy consuming features. Acetate was found to increase myocardial contractility, coronary blood flow, and cardiac output. Hepatic damage itself, secondary to ethanol, decreases energy utilization, particularly from fat.[21] Indeed, it was observed that the damage is greater when the alcohol is associated with a diet rich in fat.[22-24] The damage comprised striking alternations of the liver mitochondria, demonstrated by electron microscopy, both in humans[25] and in rats,[26] which probably explains why the alcohol effect on body weight is striking only in association with a diet containing substantial amounts of fat (Figure 15-2).

In any event, impairment of the activities of the respiratory chain, the citric acid cycle, or both may explain the decreases in oxygen uptake and in carbon dioxide production from citric acid cycle intermediates and fatty acids, as well as the increase in ketone-body production, found for instance in mitochondria from ethanol-fed rats.[27] Evidence for increased ketone production was also obtained in vivo, in experimental animals as well as in humans, in studies carried out under metabolic-ward conditions.[28] Thus, not only does ethanol, when present, become a preferred fuel and displace other fuels (such as fats,[29-31] carbohydrates, and proteins[31]), but it also impairs the energy utilization derived from the oxidation of these other substrates—particularly fats—most likely because of the mitochondrial impairment associated with alcohol abuse (vide supra).

Effects of Ethanol on Digestion and Absorption in the Gastrointestinal Tract

Alcohol injures most tissues in the body, with the GI tract and the liver being predominantly affected (Figure 15-3). Diarrhea is common in alcoholics. In the heavy drinker, diarrhea may occur for a variety of reasons, including ethanol-exacerbated lactase deficiency, especially in Afro-Americans.[32] Alcohol consumption is also

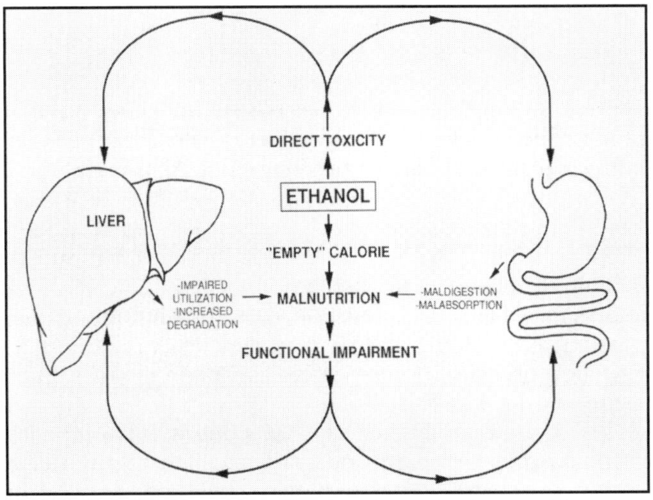

Figure 15-3. Interaction of direct toxicity of ethanol with malnutrition from primary or secondary deficiencies. Secondary malnutrition may be caused by either maldigestion and malabsorption or impaired utilization (decreased activation and/or increased inactivation) of nutrients. Both direct toxicity of ethanol and malnutrition (whether primary or secondary) may affect function and structure of liver and gut. From Lieber CS, ed. *Medical Disorders of Alcoholism: Pathogenesis and Treatment*. Philadelphia: WB Saunders; 1982.

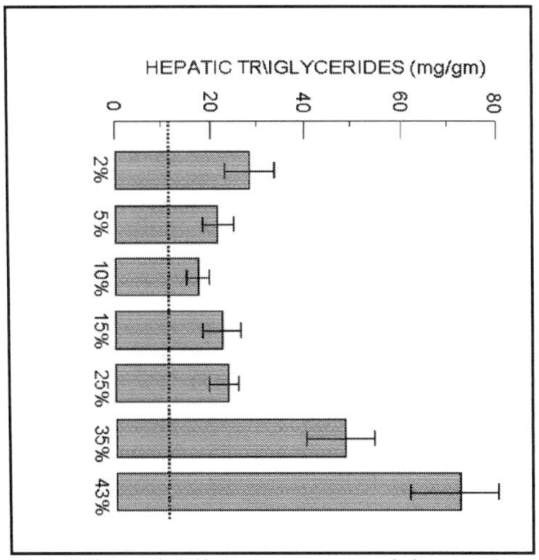

Figure 15-4. Effect of different amounts of dietary fat on hepatic triglycerides. These were measured in seven groups of rats given ethanol (36% of calories) and a diet with normal protein (18% of calories). Average hepatic triglyceride concentration in the control animals is indicated by a dotted line. From Lieber CS, DeCarli LM. Quantitative relationship between the amount of dietary fat and the severity of the alcoholic fatty liver. *Am J Clin Nutr.* 1970;23:474-8.

associated with motility changes. In the jejunum, ethanol decreases type I (impeding) waves, while in the ileum it increases type III (propulsive) waves. Another major complication is alcoholic pancreatitis. Intestinal malabsorption may also be secondary to folic acid deficiency.

Steatorrhea is commonly caused by folic acid and luminal bile salt deficiencies. Intraluminal bile salts are decreased by acute ethanol administration.[33] In rodents, long-term ethanol administration delays the excretion of cholic and chenodeoxycholic acids by decreasing the daily excretion and expanding the pool size slightly.[34] Alcoholic cirrhotic patients may have bile low in deoxycholic acid, possibly because of impaired conversion of cholate to deoxycholate by bacteria.[35]

Hospitalized alcoholics were reported to have impaired thiamin absorption compared to absorption of control patients when tested by radioactive thiamin excretion,[36] a test also affected by steps not related to absorption. Folic acid deficiency was not adequately excluded as a cause of thiamin malabsorption in these studies. Refined testing revealed reduced thiamin absorption caused by alcohol in a minority of subjects.[37] Jejunal perfusion studies did not show an effect of 5% alcohol on thiamin absorption in man.[38] Thus, whereas thiamin absorption may not be much affected by alcohol in humans, it is clearly impaired in rodents.

Alcohol also interferes with riboflavin absorption in rodents, but this has not been studied in humans. Alcohol impairs folic acid absorption in malnourished humans, but the mechanism is unclear. In any event, this may result in increased serum homocysteine. Other alterations in the GI tract are discussed in detail in Chapters 17 to 23, which are dedicated to the discussion of nutrition in regard to different GI diseases.

Respective Roles of Nutrition and Alcohol on Organ Damage in the Alcoholic

Liver

Malnutrition contributes to the development of alcoholic fatty liver: fatty liver is present in protein deficiency, particularly in children with kwashiorkor. A "skid row" subset of alcoholics with fatty liver is also malnourished. Furthermore, rodents subjected to diets deficient in lipotropes (such as choline and methionine) readily develop fatty livers. However, current understanding is that alcohol, given in sufficient quantities, can cause fatty liver in man (and lower animals), despite the presence of an otherwise adequate diet.[39] The lipid and protein composition of the diet have modulating effects on the amount and types of fat that accumulate in the liver. Reduction of dietary fat to 10% of total calories (but not lower) greatly lessens, but does not completely eliminate, hepatic fat accumulation (Figure 15-4). Furthermore, provision of higher than the recommended dietary protein (25% of total calories) will not eliminate hepatic fat accumulation. The amount of fat accumulating in the ethanol-induced fatty liver is but one parameter of damage and must be considered along with organelle dysfunctions.

Alcoholic cirrhosis has been directly linked to the overall ethanol consumption by its drop in the United States during the Prohibition Era and in Europe during World War II when alcoholic beverages were rationed.[40] The studies of Lelbach[41] also showed the direct influence of cumulative alcohol consumption (g/kg/day X years) on the incidence of chronic liver disease in patients admitted to alcohol rehabilitation spas in Europe. Neither the beverage source of ethanol nor concomitant malnutrition was noted to have an influence. These findings have been confirmed in France[42] and the direct effect of ethanol in causing hepatic fibrosis and cirrhosis has been demonstrated in the baboon model of hepatic injury.[43]

The direct hepatotoxic effect of ethanol has also been shown histologically (by light and electron microscopy) and biochemically in both alcoholics and non-alcoholics, regardless of dietary variation in fat, protein, vitamins, and lipotropes.[14,25,44]

As already discussed, the aggregate evidence indicates that acute liver damage consistently occurs if sufficient alcohol is consumed and is not preventable by a nutritious diet, females being more susceptible than males.[45,46]

Stroke

Moderate to heavy alcohol consumption—over 45 g/day—has been identified as an independent predictor of stroke after the increased risk due to hypertension and cigarette smoking were accounted for.[47] A review of most of the English language literature concludes that alcohol intake of less than 60 g/day has a complex association with ischemic stroke in white populations: very low levels are possibly protective and higher levels are definitely deleterious. There is little, if any, such association in Japanese populations. By contrast, such drinking increases hemorrhagic stroke (intracerebral and subarachoid hemorrhage) in diverse populations.[48] Alcohol consumption may contribute to stroke by raising blood pressure to hypertensive levels as shown by most[49,50] but not all[51] studies. Sodium and phosphorus intake were also positively identified as nutrient predictors of hypertension.[49]

Heart

The acute effects of even small amounts of hard liquor (several ounces) include measurable myocardial depression,[52] dose-dependent impairment of left ventricular emptying at rest,[53] and electrophysiologic effects such as slight delay in atrial conduction and shortening of both the atrioventricular conduction time and the effective ventricular myocardial refractory period.[54] These usually are not clinically apparent in people with normal hearts, especially because the impaired left ventricular emptying disappears with exercise.[53] Patients with angina pectoris, even with congestive failure, have responses in left ventricular performance similar to those seen in controls at blood alcohol levels of 100 mg/dl.[55] Patients with myocardial ischemia may experience an unfavorable distribution of coronary blood flow away from ischemic areas.[56] Thus, the result of alcohol intake is not always predictable because it depends on the relative influence of alcohol on peripheral vasodilatation, coronary blood flow, direct myocardial depression, electrophysiologic changes, and the extent of underlying cardiac reserve.[57] Patients with chronic alcoholism or heart disease[57] and even normal non-alcoholic subjects may develop atrial arrhythmias after substantial acute alcohol ingestion.[58]

Chronic alcohol consumption may result in heart disease by its association with hypertension, as discussed above in relation to stroke or by its association with severe thiamin deficiency in the beriberi heart syndrome. Alcohol intake may cause an elevation of serum homocysteine, possibly associated with folic acid deficiency (vide supra). Elevation of serum homocysteine has been linked to premature vascular disease.

The question whether alcohol consumption reduces coronary artery disease and cardiac death rate is still a matter of debate.[59] Epidemiological evidence in favor of the beneficial effects of alcohol on coronary complication and overall mortality have been reported but some of these beneficial effects were associated with amounts of alcoholic beverages that are negligible. For instance, some of the studies that were interpreted to demonstrate beneficial effects of 1 to 2 drinks/day also revealed a reduction of mortality for occasional drinking[60]—as little as 1 drink a week. The possibility of a greater beneficial effect with wine was also challenged when the data revealed a benefit for as little as 1 glass of wine a month.[61] Obviously, such an amount is too small to be effective, and attributing the associated improved outcome only to the alcohol is not plausible. Confounding factors (such as lifestyle) are more likely responsible. Indeed, the Copenhagen Heart study found not only a reduction in relative risk for coronary artery disease in wine drinkers but also that the wine drinkers in this study also consumed twice as much fruit and vegetables.[61] Furthermore, Mortensen et al[62] demonstrated that wine drinking is a general indicator of optimal social, cognitive, and personality development. Consequently, the association between drinking habits and social and psychological characteristics may explain, in large part, the apparent health benefits of wine. This is also the interpretation of others, including the National Institute of Alcohol Abuse and Alcoholism.[63] In any event, contrary to some of the positive studies cited above, in a 21-year follow-up of 5,766 Scottish men aged 35 to 64 years, Hart et al[64] found no cardiovascular or any other evidence that alcohol consumption reduced mortality for light and moderate drinkers. Furthermore, higher levels of intake (≥3 drinks per day) were associated with increased mortality in men with previous myocardial infarction.[65]

A characteristic syndrome known as alcoholic cardiomyopathy has been described in a subset of individuals with alcoholism and heart disease. It is a congestive cardiomyopathy seen typically in men aged 30 to 55 years who have been drinking 30% to 50% of calories as alcohol for 10 to 15 years.[57] Arrhythmias are frequent. Coronary artery disease, hypertension, valvular abnormalities, and congenital heart disease can be contributory.

Blood and Bone Marrow

In addition to the anemias due to blood loss and folic acid deficiency (discussed above), alcohol has direct and partially unexplained hematologic effects. Alcohol consumption is associated with vacuolization of erythroid precursors, which is not prevented by an adequate diet and pharmacologic doses of folic acid.[66] Alcohol intake also causes granulocytopenia, probably mediated by nutritional inadequacy,[66] thrombocytopenia, and impairment of platelet function,[67,68] which are partly attributed to direct toxic effects of alcohol.

Effect of Alcohol on Nutrient Activation and/or Degradation

Thiamine and Pyridoxine

Thiamine deficiency in alcoholics causes Wernicke-Korsakoff syndrome and beriberi heart disease and probably contributes to polyneuropathy. It was once claimed that there is an inborn error of transketolase affinity for the cofactor thiamine pyrophosphate in Wernicke-Korsakoff syndrome, but a number of other pathogenic possibilities exist.[69]

Neurologic, hematologic, and dermatologic disorders can be caused in part by pyridoxine deficiency. Pyridoxine deficiency, as measured by low plasma pyridoxal-5′-phosphate (PLP), was reported in over 50% of alcoholics without hematologic findings or abnormal liver function tests.[70,71] Inadequate intake may partly explain low PLP, but increased destruction and reduced formation may also contribute. PLP is more rapidly destroyed in erythrocytes in the presence of acetaldehyde, the product of ethanol oxidation, perhaps by displacement of PLP from protein and consequent exposure to phosphatase.[70,72] Studies showed that chronic ethanol feeding lowered hepatic content of PLP by decreasing net synthesis from pyridoxine.[73-75] The acetaldehyde produced by alcohol oxidation was hypothesized to enhance hydrolysis of PLP by cellular phosphatases.[70]

Methionine and S-Adenosylmethionine

Methionine deficiency has been described and its supplementation has been considered for the treatment of liver diseases, especially the alcoholic variety; however, excess methionine was shown to have some adverse effects,[76] including a decrease in hepatic ATP.[77] Furthermore, whereas in some patients with alcoholic liver disease, circulating methionine levels are normal,[78] in others elevated levels were observed.[79-81] Kinsell et al[82] found a delay in the clearance of plasma methionine after its systemic administration to patients with liver damage. Similarly, Horowitz et al[83] reported that the blood clearance of methionine after an oral load of this amino acid was slowed. Because about half of the methionine is metabolized by the liver, these observations suggest impaired hepatic metabolism of this amino acid in patients with alcoholic liver disease. Indeed, for most of its functions, methionine must be activated to S-adenosylmethionine (SAMe). In cirrhotic livers, Duce et al[84] reported a decrease in the activity of SAMe synthetase, the enzyme involved, which is also called methionine adenosyltransferase (Figure 15-5).

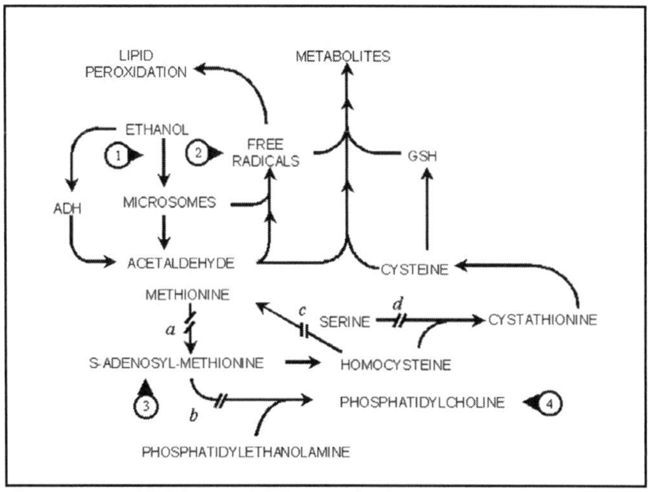

Figure 15-5. Lipid peroxidation and other consequences of alcoholic liver disease and/or increased free radical generation and acetaldehyde production by ethanol-induced microsomes, with sites of possible therapeutic interventions. Metabolic blocks caused by liver disease (*a*,*b*), folate (*c*), B12 (*c*) or B6 (*d*) deficiencies are illustrated, with corresponding depletions in S-adenosylmethionine, phosphatidylcholine, and gluthathione (GSH). New therapeutic approaches include: 1) downregulation of microsomal enzyme induction especially of CYP2E1, 2) decrease of free radicals with antioxidants, 3) replenishment of S-adenosylmethionine, and 4) phosphatidylcholine.

Various mechanisms of inactivation of SAMe synthetase have been incriminated.[85] One factor that may have contributed to the defect is relative hypoxia, with nitric oxide mediated inactivation and transcriptional arrest.[86] In addition, long-term alcohol consumption was found to be associated with enhanced methionine utilization and depletion.[87] As a consequence, SAMe depletion as well as its decreased availability could be expected and, indeed, long-term ethanol consumption under controlled conditions by non-human primates was associated with a significant depletion of hepatic SAMe.[88] Potentially, such SAMe depletion may have a number of adverse effects. SAMe is the principal methylating agent in various transmethylation reactions, which are important to nucleic acid and protein synthesis. Hirata and Axelrod[89] and Hirata et al[90] also demonstrated the importance of methylation for cell membrane function with regard to membrane fluidity and the transport of metabolites and transmission of signals across membranes. Thus, depletion of SAMe, by impairing methyltransferase activity, may promote the membrane injury, which has been documented in alcohol-induced liver damage.[91] Furthermore, SAMe plays a key role in the synthesis of polyamines and provides a source of cysteine for glutathione production (see Figure 15-5). Thus, the deficiency in methionine activation and in SAMe production resulting from the decrease in the activity of the corresponding synthetase results in a number of adverse effects, including inadequate cysteine and GSH production, especially when aggravated by associated folate, B_6, or B12 deficiencies (Figure 15-5). The consequences of this enzymic defect can be alleviated by the provision of SAMe, the product of the reaction. SAMe is unstable, but the synthesis of a stable salt allowed for replenishment of SAMe through ingestion of this compound: blood levels of SAMe increased after oral administration in rodents[92] and in man.[93] It has been claimed that the liver does not take up SAMe from the bloodstream,[94] but results in baboons clearly showed hepatic uptake of exogenous SAMe.[88] The effective use of SAMe for transmethylation and transsulfuration has also been demonstrated in vivo.[95]

Clinical trials revealed that SAMe treatment is beneficial in intrahepatic cholestasis[96] including recurrent intrahepatic cholestasis and jaundice caused by androgens or estrogens. It was also used successfully in severe cholestasis of pregnancy[97] with few, if any, untoward effects. Oral administration of 1200 mg/day of SAMe for 6 months also resulted in a significant increase of hepatic GSH in patients with alcoholic as well as non-alcoholic liver disease.[98]

A therapeutic success was achieved in a long-term randomized, placebo-controlled, double-blind, multicenter clinical trial of SAMe in patients with alcoholic liver cirrhosis in whom SAMe significantly improved survival or delayed liver transplantation.[99]

Phosphatidylcholine

In the presence of liver disease, the activity of phosphatidylethanolamine methyltransferase is depressed,[84] with significant pathologic effects. This enzymatic block can be bypassed through the administration of the product of that reaction, in this case phosphatidylcholine (PC)[100] (Figure 15-5). This is emerging as a potentially important approach to the treatment of liver disease. Indeed, feeding of a mixture rich in polyunsaturated PCs, namely polyenylphosphatidycholine (PPC), including dilinoleoylphosphatidylcholine (DLPC), which has a high bioavailability, exerted a remarkable protection against alcohol-induced fibrosis and cirrhosis in the baboon.[101]

PPC contains choline, but choline, in amounts present in PPC, had no protective action against the fibrogenic effects of ethanol in the baboon.[102] In primates, choline plays a lesser role as a dietary nutrient than in rodents, in part because of lesser choline oxidase activity. In fact, as reviewed by Zeisel and Busztajn,[103] choline becomes essential for human nutrition only in severely restricted feeding situations. The decreased phospholipid methyltransferase activity in cirrhotic livers[84] is not simply secondary to the cirrhosis but may, in fact, be a primary defect related to alcohol, as suggested by the observation that the enzyme activity is already decreased prior to the development of cirrhosis.[101] Another mechanism whereby ethanol may affect phospholipids is increased lipid peroxidation, as reflected by increased F2-isoprostanes,[100] which could explain the associated decrease of arachidonic acid in phospholipids.[104]

One concern was that PPC and DLPC, because of their polyunsaturated nature, may aggravate the oxidative stress, but the opposite was found, both in vitro and in vivo. In alcohol-fed baboons, PPC not only prevented septal fibrosis and cirrhosis,[101] but it also resulted in a total protection against oxidative stress, as determined by normalization of 4-hydroxynonenal, F2-isoprostanes, and GSH levels.[105] In patients with hepatitis C, PPC improved the transaminase levels, but the effect on liver fibrosis was not assessed.[106] However, a clinical trial on alcoholic fibrosis showed beneficial effects in some subgroups,[107] and a hepatitis C study revealed beneficial effects on fibrosis.[108]

References

1. Patek AJ Jr, Toth IG, Saunders MG, Castro GA, Engel JJ. Alcohol and dietary factors in cirrhosis. An epidemiological study of 304 alcoholic patients. *Arch Intern Med.* 1975;135:1053-7.
2. Iber FL. In alcoholism, the liver sets the pace. *Nutr Today.* 1971;6:2-9.
3. Mendenhall C, Bongiovanni G, Goldberg S, et al. VA Cooperative Study on Alcoholic Hepatitis. III: Changes in protein-calorie malnutrition associated with 30 days of hospitalization with and without enternal nutritional therapy. *J Parenter Enteral Nutr.* 1985;9:590-6.
4. Morgan MY. Enternal nutrition in chronic liver disease. *Acta Chir Scand.* 1981;507:81-90.
5. Simko V, Connell AM, Banks B. Nutritional status in alcoholics with and without liver disease. *Am J Clin Nutr.* 1982;3:197-203.
6. Armellini F, Zamboni M, Frigo L, et al. Alcohol consumption, smoking habits and body fat distribution in Italian men and women aged 20-60 years. *Eur J Clin Nutr.* 1993;47:52-60.
7. Tremblay A, Buemann B, Theriault G, Bouchard C. Body fatness in active individuals reporting low lipid and alcohol intake. *Eur J Clin Nutr.* 1995;49:824-31.
8. Bebb HT, Houser HB, Witschi JC, Littell AS, Fuller RK. Calorie and nutrient contribution of alcoholic beverages to the usual diets of 155 adults. *Am J Clin Nutr.* 1971;24:1042-52.
9. Neville JN, Eagles JA, Samson G, Olson RE. Nutritional status of alcoholics. *Am J Clin Nutr.* 1968;21:1329-40.
10. Gruchow HW, Sobociaski KA, Barboriak JJ. Scheller JG. Alcohol consumption, nutrient intake and relative body weight among US adults. *Am J Clin Nutr.* 1985;42:289-95.
11. Hillers VN, Massey LK. Interrelationships of moderate and high school consumption with diet and health status. *Am J Clin Nutr.* 1985;41:356-62.
12. Westerfeld WW, Schulman MP. Metabolism and caloric value of alcohol. *JAMA.* 1959;170:197-203.
13. Williamson DF, Forman MR, Binkin NJ, Gentry EM, Remington PL, Trowbridge FL. Alcohol and body weight in United States adults. *Am J Public Health.* 1987;77:1324-30.
14. Lieber CS, Jones DP, DeCarli LM. Effects of prolonged ethanol intake: Production of fatty liver despite adequate diets. *J Clin Invest.* 1965;44:1009-21.
15. Pirola RC, Lieber CS. The energy cost of the metabolism of drugs, including ethanol. *Pharmacology.* 1972;7:185-96.
16. Tremolieres J, Carre L. Etudes sur les modalites d'oxydation de l'alcool chez l'homme normal et alcoolique. *Rev Alcoolisme.* 1961;7:202-27.
17. Stock MJ, Stuart JA. Thermic effects of ethanol in the rat and man. *Nutr Metabol.* 1974;17:297-305.
18. Klesges RC, Mealer CZ, Kesges LM. Effects of alcohol intake on resting energy expenditure in young women social drinkers. *Am J Clin Nutr.* 1994;59:805-9.
19. Rothwell NJ, Stock MJ. Influence of alcohol and sucrose consumption on energy balance and brown fat activity in the rat. *Metabolism.* 1984;33:768-71.
20. Pirola RC, Lieber CS. Energy wastage in rats given drugs that induce microsomal enzymes. *J Nutr.* 1975;105:1544-8.
21. Lieber CS. Perspectives: Do alcohol calories count? *Am J Clin Nutr.* 1991;54:976-82.
22. Lieber CS, Spritz N, DeCarli LM. Role of dietary, adipose and endogenously synthesized fatty acids in the pathogenesis of the alcoholic fatty liver. *J Clin Invest.* 1966;45:51-62.
23. Lieber CS, Spritz N. Effects of prolonged ethanol intake in man: Role of dietary, adipose, and endogenously synthesized fatty acids in the pathogenesis of the alcoholic fatty liver. *J Clin Invest.* 1966;45:1400-11.
24. Lieber CS, DeCarli LM. Quantitative relationship between the amount of dietary fat and the severity of the alcoholic fatty liver. *Am J Clin Nutr.* 1970;23:474-8.

25. Lane BP, Lieber CS. Ultrastructural alterations in human hepatocytes following ingestion of ethanol with adequate diets. *Am J Path.* 1966;49:593-603.
26. Iseri OA, Lieber CS, Gottlieb LS. The ultrastructure of fatty liver induced by prolonged ethanol ingestion. *Am J Path.* 1966;48:535-55.
27. Cederbaum AI, Lieber CS, Rubin E. Effect of chronic ethanol consumption and acetaldehyde on partial reactions of oxidative phosphorylation and CO2 production from citric acid cycle intermediates. *Arch Biochem Biophys.* 1976;176:525-38.
28. Lefevre A, Adler H, Lieber CS. Effect of ethanol on ketone metabolism. *J Clin Invest.* 1970;49:1775-82.
29. Lieber CS, Lefevre A, Spritz N, Feinman L, DeCarli LM. Difference in hepatic metabolism of long and medium-chain fatty acids: The role of fatty acid chain length in the production of the alcoholic fatty liver. *J Clin Invest.* 1967;46:1451-60.
30. Lieber CS, Schmid R. The effect of ethanol on fatty acid metabolism: Stimulation of hepatic fatty acid synthesis in vitro. *J Clin Invest.* 1961;40:394-9.
31. Shelmet JJ, Reichard GA, Skutches CL, Hoeldtke RD, Owen OE, Boden G. Ethanol causes acute inhibition of carbohydrate, fat and protein oxidation and insulin resistance. *J Clin Invest.* 1988;81:1137-45.
32. Perlow W, Baraona E, Lieber CS. Symptomatic intestinal disaccharidase deficiency in alcoholics. *Gastroenterology.* 1977;72:680-4.
33. Marin GA, Ward NL, Fischer R. Effect of ethanol on pancreatic and biliary secretions in humans. Am J Dig Dis 1973;18:825-33.
34. Lefevre A, DeCarli LM, Lieber CS. Effect of ethanol on cholesterol and bile acid metabolism. *J Lipid Res.* 1972:13:48-55.
35. Knodell RG, Kinsey D, Boedeker EC, Collin D. Deoxycholate metabolism in alcoholic cirrhosis. *Gastroenterology.* 1976;71:196-201.
36. Thomson AD, Majumdar SK. The influence of ethanol on intestinal absorption and utilization of nutrients. *Clin Gastroenterol.* 1981;10:263-93.
37. Breen KJ, Buttigieg R, Iossifidis S, Lourensz C, Wood B. Jejunal uptake of thiamin hydrochloride in man: influence of alcoholism and alcohol. *Am J Clin Nutr.* 1985;42:121-6.
38. Katz D, Metz J, van der Westhuyzen J. Intestinal absorption of thiamin from yeast-containing sorghum beer. *Am J Clin Nutr.* 1985;42:666-70.
39. Lieber CS, Leo MA. Alcohol and the Liver. In: *Medical and Nutritional Complications of Alcoholism. Mechanisms and Management.* Plenum Publishing; 1992:185-239.
40. Lederman S. *Alcohol, alcoholisme, alcoholisation.* Paris, Institut national d'études demographiques, travaux, et documents. Cahier No. 41, Presses Universitaires de France, 1964.
41. Lelbach WK. Liver damage in chronic alcoholism. Results of a clinical, clinical-chemical and bioptic-histologic study of 526 alcoholic patients during withdrawal treatment in a public hospital for alcoholics. 3. Bioptic-histologic findings. *Acta Hepatosplenol.* (Stuttgart) 1967;14:9-39.
42. Tuyns AJ, Esteban J, Pequignot G. Ethanol is cirrhogenic, whatever the beverage. *Br J Addict.* 1984;79:389-93.
43. Lieber CS, DeCarli LM. An experimental model of alcohol feeding and liver injury in the baboon. *J Med Primatol.* 1974;3:153-63.
44. Lieber CS, Rubin E. Alcoholic fatty liver in man on a high protein and low fat diet. *Am J Med.* 1968;44:200-6.
45. Frezza M, DiPadova C, Pozzato G, Terpin M, Baraona E, Lieber CS. High blood alcohol levels in women: Role of decreased gastric alcohol dehydrogenase activity and first pass metabolism. *N Engl J Med.* 1990;322:95-9.
46. Baraona E, Abittan CS, Dohmen K, et al. Gender differences in pharmacokinetics of alcohol. *Alcohol: Clin Exp Res.* 2001;25:502-507.
47. Gill JS, Zezulka AV, Shipley MJ, Gill SK, Beevers DG. Stroke and alcohol consumption. *N Engl J Med.* 1986;315;1041-6.
48. Camargo CA Jr. Moderate alcohol consumption and stroke. The epidemiologic evidence. *Stroke.* 1989;20:1611-26.
49. Gruchow HW, Sobovinski KA, Barboriak JJ. Alcohol, nutrient intake, and hypertension in US adults. *JAMA.* 1985;15:1567-70.
50. Witteman JC, Willett WC, Stampfer MJ, et al. Relation of moderate alcohol consumption and risk of systemic hypertension in women. *Am J Cardiol.* 1990;65:633-7.
51. Coates RA, Corey PN, Ashley MJ, Steele CA. Alcohol consumption and blood pressure: analysis of data from the Canada Health Survey. *Preventive Medicine.* 1985;14:1-14.
52. Lang RM, Borow KM, Neumann A, Feldman T. Adverse cardiac effects of acute alcohol ingestion in young adults. *Ann Intern Med.* 1985;102:742-7.
53. Kelbaek H. Acute effects of alcohol and food intake on cardiac performance. *Prog Cardiovasc Dis.* 1990;32:347-64.
54. Gould L, Reddy CV, Becker W, Oh KC, Kim SG. Electronphysiologic properties of alcohol in man. *J Electrocardiology.* 1978;11:219-26.
55. Kupari M. Reproducibility of M-mode echocardiographic assessment of left ventricular function. Significance of the temporal range of measurements. *Eur Heart J.* 1984;5:412-8.
56. Friedman HS. Acute effects of ethanol on myocardial blood flow in the nonischemic and ischemic heart. *Am J Cardio.* 1981;47:61-7.
57. Segel LD, Klausner SC, Gnadt JT, Amsterdam EA. Alcohol and the heart. *Med Clin North Am.* 1984;68:147-61.
58. Thornton JR. Atrial fibrillation in healthy non-alcoholic people after an alcoholic binge. *Lancet.* 1984;2:1013-5.
59. Lieber CS. Alcohol and Health: A drink a day won't keep the doctor away. *Cleveland Journal of Medicine.* 2003;70:945-953.
60. Boffeta P, Garfinkel L. Alcohol drinking and mortality among men enrolled in an American Cancer Society prospective study. *Epidemiology.* 1990;1:342-348.
61. Gronbaek M, Deis A, Sorensen TIA, Becker U, Schnohr P, Jensen G. Mortality associated with moderate intakes of wine, beer or spirits. *Br Med J.* 1995;310:1165-1169.
62. Mortensen EL, Jensen HH, Sanders SA, Reinisch JM. Better psychological functioning and higher social status may largely explain the apparent health benefits of wine. *Arch Intern Med.* 2001;161:1844-1848.
63. National Institute of Alcohol Abuse and Alcoholism. Alcohol and Coronary Heart Disease. *Alcohol Alert.* 1999;45.
64. Hart CL, Smith GD, Hole DJ, Hawthorne VM. Alcohol consumption and mortality from all causes, coronary heart disease, and stroke: results from a prospective cohort study of Scottish men with 21 years of follow up. *Br Med J.* 1999;318:1725-1729.
65. Shaper AG, Wannamethee SG. Alcohol intake and mortality in middle aged men with diagnosed coronary heart disease. *Heart.* 2000;83:394-399.
66. Lindenbaum J, Lieber CS. Hematologic effects of alcohol in man in the absence of nutritional deficiency. *N Engl J Med.* 1969;281:333-8.
67. Haut MJ, Cowan DH. The effect of ethanol on hemostatic properties of human blood platelets. *Am J Med.* 1974;56:22-33.
68. Lindenbaum J, Hargrove RL. Thrombocytopenia in alcoholics. *Ann Intern Med.* 1968;68:526-32.
69. Victor M. The effects of alcohol on the nervous system: clinical features, pathogenesis, and treatment. In: *Medical and Nutritional Complications of Alcoholism: Mechanisms and Management.* Plenum Publishing; 1992: 413-557.
70. Lumeng L, Li T-K. Vitamin B6 metabolism in chronic alcohol abuse. Pyridoxal phosphate levels in plasma and the effects of acetaldehyde on pyridoxal phosphate synthesis and degradation in human erythrocytes. *J Clin Invest.* 1974;53:693-704.
71. Fonda ML, Brown SG, Pendleton MW. Concentration of vitamin B6 and activities of enzymes of B6 metabolism in the blood of alcoholic and nonalcoholic men. *Alcohol: Clin Exp Res.* 1989;3:804-9.
72. Lumeng LJ. The role of acetaldehyde in mediating the deleterious effect of ethanol on pyridoxal 5'-phosphate metabolism. *J Clin Invest.* 1978;62:286-93.

73. Veech RL, Lumeng L, Li TK. Vitamin B6 metabolism in chronic alcohol abuse. The effect of ethanol oxidation on hepatic pyridoxal 5'-phosphate metabolism. *J Clin Invest*. 1975;55:1026-32.
74. Parker TH, Marshall JP 2nd, Roberts RK, Wang S, Schiff ER, Wilkinson GR, Schenker S. Effect of acute alcohol ingestion on plasma pyridoxal 5'-phosphate. *Am J Clin Nutr*. 1979;32:1246-52.
75. Lumeng L, Schenker S, Li TK, Brashear RE, Compton MC. Clearance and metabolism of plasma pyridoxal 5'-phosphate in the dog. *J Lab Clin Med*. 1984;103:59-64.
76. Finkelstein JD, Martin JJ. Methionine metabolism in mammals. Adaptation to methionine excess. *J Biol Chem*. 1986;261:1582-87.
77. Hardwick DF, Applegarth DA, Cockcroft DM, Ross PM, Cder RJ. Pathogenesis of methionine-induced toxicity. *Metabolism*. 1970;19:381-91.
78. Iob V, Coon WW, Sloan W. Free amino acids in liver, plasma, and muscle of patients with cirrhosis of the liver. *J Surgical Res*. 1967;7:41-3.
79. Fischer JE, Yoshimura N, Aguirre A, et al. Plasma amino acids in patients with hepatic encephalopathy. *Am J Surg*. 1974;127:40-7.
80. Iber FL, Rosen H, Levenson SM, Chalmers TC. The plasma amino acids in patients with liver failure. *J Lab Clin Med*. 1957;50:417-25.
81. Montanari A, Simoni I, Vallisa D, et al. Free amino acids in plasma and skeletal muscle of patients with liver cirrhosis. *Hepatology*. 1988;8:1034-39.
82. Kinsell L, Harper HA, Barton HC, Michaels GD, Weiss HA. Rate of disapperance from plasma of intravenously administrated methionine in patients with liver damage. *Science*. 1947;106:589-94.
83. Horowitz JH, Rypins EB, Henderson JM, et al. Evidence for impairment of transsulfuration pathway in cirrhosis. *Gastroenterology*. 1981;81:668-75.
84. Duce AM, Ortiz P, Cabrero C, Mato JM. S-adenosyl-L-methionine synthetase and phospholipid methyltransferase are inhibited in human cirrhosis. *Hepatology*. 1988;8:65-8.
85. Lu SC. Methionine adenosyltransferase and liver disease: it's all about SAMe. *Gastroenterology*. 1998;114:403-7.
86. Avila MA, Carretero MV, Rodriguez EN, Mato JM. Regulation by hypoxia of methionine adenosyltransferase activity and gene expression in rat hepatocytes. *Gastroenterology*. 1998;114:364-71.
87. Finkelstein JD, Cello FP, Kyle WE. Ethanol-induced changes in methionine metabolism in rat liver. *Biochem Biophys Res Commun*. 1974;61:475-81.
88. Lieber CS, Casini A, DeCarli LM, et al. S-adenosyl-L-methionine attenuates alcohol-induced liver injury in the baboon. *Hepatology*. 1990;11:165-72.
89. Hirata F, Axelrod J. Phospholipid methylation and biological signal transmission. *Science*. 1980;209:1082-90.
90. Hirata F, Viveros OH, Diliberto EJ Jr., Alexrod J. Identification and properties of two methyltransferases in conversion of phosphatidylethanolamine to phosphatidylcholine. *Proc Nat Acad Sci*. 1978;75:1718-21.
91. Yamada S, Mak KM, Lieber CS. Chronic ethanol consumption alters rat liver plasma membranes and potentiates release of alkaline phosphatase. *Gastroenterology*. 1985;88:1799-806.
92. Stramentinoli G, Gualano M, Galli-Kienle G. Intestinal absorption of S-adenosyl-L-methionine. *J Pharmacol Exp Ther*. 1979;209:323-26.
93. Bornbardieri G, Pappalardo G, Bernardi L, Barra D, Di Palma A, Castrini G. Intestinal absorption of S-adenosyl-L-methionine in humans. *Int J Clin Pharmacol, Therapy Toxicol*. 1983;21:186-8.
94. Hoffinan DR, Marion DW, Cornatzer WE, Duerra JA. S-adenosylmethionine and S-adenosylhomocysteine metabolism in isolated rat liver. *J Biol Chem*. 1980; 255:10822-7.
95. Giulidori P. Stramentinoli G. A radioenzymatic method for S-adenosyl-L-methionine determination in biological fluids. *Anal Biochem*. 1984;137:217-20.
96. Giudici GA, Le Grazie C, Di Padova C. The use of ademethionine (SAMe) in the treatment of cholestatic liver disorders: meta-analysis of clinical trials. In: Mato JM, Lieber C, Kaplowitz N, Caballero A, eds. *Methionine Metabolism: Molecular Mechanism and Clinical Implications*. Madrid: CSIC Press; 1992: 67-79.
97. Frezza M, Pozzato G, Chiesa L, Stramentinoli G, Di Padova C. Reversal of intrahepatic cholestasis of pregnancy in women after high dose S-adenosyl-L-methionine administration. *Hepatology*. 1984;4:274-8.
98. Vendemiale G, Altomare E, Trizio T, et al. Effect of oral S-adenosyl-L-methionine on hepatic glutathione in patients with liver disease. *Scand J Gastroenterology*. 1989;24:407-15.
99. Mato JM, Cámara J, Fernández de Paz J, et al. S-Adenosylmethionine in alcoholic liver cirrhosis: A randomized, placebo-controlled, double-blind, multicentre clinical trial. *J Hepatology*. 1999;30:1081-9.
100. Lieber CS, Robins SJ, Leo MA. Hepatic phosphatidylethanolamine methyltransferase activity is decreased by ethanol and increased by phosphatidylcholine. *Alcohol: Clin Exp Res*. 1994;18:592-5.
101. Lieber CS, Robins SJ, Li J, et al. Phosphatidylcholine protects against fibrosis and cirrhosis in the baboon. *Gastroenterology*. 1994;106:152-9.
102. Lieber CS, Leo MA, Mak KM, DeCarli LM, Sato S. Choline fails to prevent liver fibrosis in ethanol-fed baboons but causes toxicity. *Hepatology*. 1985;5:561-72.
103. Zeisel S, Busztajn JL. Choline and human nutrition. *Ann Rev Nutr*. 1994;14:269-96.
104. Arai M, Gordon ER, Lieber CS. Decreased cytochrome oxidase activity in hepatic mitochondria after chronic ethanol consumption and the possible role of decreased cytochrome aa3 content and changes in phospholipids. *Biochim Biophys Acta*. 1984;797:320-7.
105. Lieber CS, Leo MA, Aleynik SI, Aleynik MK, DeCarli LM. Polyenyl phosphatidylcholine decreases alcohol-induced oxidative stress in the baboon. *Alcoholism: Clin Exp Res*. 1997;21:375-9.
106. Niederau C, Strohmeyer G, Heinges T, Peter K, Gopfert E, Leich study Group. Polyunsaturated phosphatidyl-choline and interferon alpha for treatment of chronic hepatitis B and C: a multicenter, randomized, double blind, placebo-controlled trial. *Hepato Gastroenterol*. 1998;45:797-804.
107. Lieber CS, Weiss DG, Groszmann R, Paronetto F, Schenker S, for the VA Cooperative Study 391. II. VA Cooperative study of polyenylphosphatidylcholine in alcoholic liver disease. *Alcohol: Clin Exp Res*. 2003;27:1765-72.
108. Lieber CS, Anand B, Bini EJ, et al. Polyenylphosphatidylcholine (PPC) is beneficial for the treatment of hepatitis C patients. *Hepatol*. 2005;42:695A.
109. Lieber CS, ed. *Medical disorders of alcoholism: pathogenesis and treatment*. Philadelphia: WB Saunders; 1982.

Chapter 16

Nutrition and Diabetes Mellitus

Daniel L. Hurley, MD; M. Molly McMahon, MD; and Michelle Papaconstandinou

Introduction

Hyperglycemia occurs commonly in the hospital setting. Diabetes mellitus is caused by either an absolute (type 1 diabetes; previously called insulin-dependent diabetes) or a relative (type 2 diabetes; previously called non-insulin-dependent diabetes) lack of insulin. Type 1 diabetes is associated with earlier age of onset, potential for ketoacidosis, and absolute dependency on insulin for glucose control. Type 2 diabetes, by far the more common type, is associated with adult onset, abdominal adiposity, peripheral tissue insulin resistance, and larger insulin requirements for glucose control.

Even patients without a previous diagnosis of diabetes can develop stress-induced hyperglycemia during severe illness. For all persons admitted to an urban general hospital, one-third were reported to have either fasting glucose levels exceeding 126 mg/dL or random glucose levels exceeding 200 mg/dL on two or more occasions. Indeed, one-third of these patients with hyperglycemia did not have a prior diagnosis of diabetes.[1] Because of the high prevalence of diabetes and stress-induced hyperglycemia, gastroenterologists will frequently manage hyperglycemia in hospitalized patients. Many of these patients may also require enteral nutrition (EN) or parenteral nutrition (PN) support. This chapter will discuss the interaction between EN and PN administration and hyperglycemia, the increased comorbidity for hospitalized patients with hyperglycemia, and guidelines for glycemic control.

Classification System of Diabetes Mellitus

The diagnosis of diabetes is based on the following: 1) finding any one of three abnormalities—symptoms of diabetes plus a random plasma glucose of ≥200 mg/dL, a fasting plasma glucose ≥126 mg/dL, or a 2-hour plasma glucose level ≥200 mg/dL during an oral glucose tolerance test—and 2) documenting any one of these three abnormalities again by repeat testing on another day.[2] This degree of hyperglycemia has been shown to be associated with serious metabolic complications. For instance, at this level of hyperglycemia, the prevalence of microvascular complications considered specific for diabetes increases dramatically. The previous diagnosis of impaired glucose tolerance has been retained under the term "impaired fasting hyperglycemia." The diagnostic criterion for impaired fasting hyperglycemia is an elevated fasting plasma glucose of 101 to 125 mg/dL.

Pathophysiology

The homeostatic mechanisms present in non-diabetic subjects that maintain fasting euglycemia and limit the postprandial glucose increase are impaired in individuals with diabetes. Patients with diabetes have decreased insulin secretion and/or action resulting in preprandial and postprandial hyperglycemia. This absolute (decreased pancreas insulin production) or relative (decreased peripheral tissue insulin action, ie, insulin resistance) lack of insulin results in hyperglycemia via increased hepatic glucose production and decreased glucose uptake.

Severe physiologic stress can cause hyperglycemia in patients without a prior diagnosis of diabetes. Physiologic stress, as during serious illness, is accompanied by increases in plasma counter-regulatory hormones (ie, glucagon, epinephrine, cortisol, and growth hormone) and cytokines, both of which increase hepatic glucose release and decrease skeletal muscle glucose uptake.[3] Stress causes significant derangement in glucose metabolism in diabetic patients because insulin secretion cannot increase adequately to compensate for the hyperglycemia, as in non-diabetics. The exaggerated glucose response observed following counter-regulatory hormone infusion in healthy diabetic subjects compared with non-diabetic subjects helps to explain why glucose control frequently deteriorates in ill diabetic patients.[4]

Hyperglycemia

In-vitro studies report that hyperglycemia impairs leukocyte function and is associated with abnormalities in granulocyte adhesion, chemotaxis, phagocytosis, respiratory burst, superoxide formation, and intracellular killing. Hyperglycemia can also impair complement activity. All of these abnormalities improve with glucose control. For hospitalized patients with hyperglycemia, poor glucose control can adversely affect fluid balance (via glycosuria and dehydration), immune function,[5-10] inflammation, and medical outcome.

Observational studies indicate that hyperglycemia is a risk factor for adverse outcomes during an acute illness, even in patients without an antecedent diagnosis of diabetes. Two meta-analyses of observational studies quantified the impact of hyperglycemia on the prognosis of non-diabetic patients following myocardial infarction and stroke.[11,12] Immediately following myocardial infarction, patient glucose values in excess of 110 to 144 mg/dL were associated with a higher risk of heart failure and a three-fold increased mortality (odds ratio 3.9, 95% confidence interval 2.9 to 5.4).[11] After an ischemic stroke, patient glucose values in excess of 108 to 144 mg/dL were also associated with a three-fold increased mortality (odds ratio 3.1, 95% confidence interval 2.5 to 3.8) and appeared related to the degree of permanent disability.[12] Similarly, observational studies in patients with diabetes revealed an increased risk of adverse medical outcomes.[1,11-15]

Randomized trials in critically ill patients have also documented an association between hyperglycemia and adverse outcomes. The Veteran Administration Cooperative Study was designed to test the hypothesis that perioperative PN would prevent serious complications following major surgery.[16] In this study, although patients administered PN had fewer noninfectious complications, total infections were doubled compared to those experienced by control subjects. This reported higher infection rate was associated with severe hyperglycemia and provision of excess calories. A serum glucose concentration >300 mg/dL occurred in 20% of patients receiving PN but only in 1% of the control group. Indeed, more than one-half of the patients receiving PN were hyperglycemic. A meta-analysis of patient outcomes during perioperative nutrition reported 61% greater infections during PN compared with enterally fed patients, although the data was confounded by differences in serum glucose within the first 5 postoperative days (180 mg/dL versus 150 mg/dL).[17] In a recent randomized trial of EN and PN, parenterally fed patients with average maximum serum glucose levels of 160 mg/dL had 42% more infections than did the enterally fed group, with an average maximum glucose of 144 mg/dL.[18] Two randomized trials of growth hormone versus placebo in patients in the intensive care unit (ICU) after surgery, trauma, or acute respiratory failure reported a 49% and 57% increased risk of mortality in the respective growth hormone treatment groups. Mortality differences were confounded by higher glucose values of 18 mg/dL and 45 mg/dL in the growth hormone treatment groups.[19] In the last decade, attention by healthcare providers to prevent overfeeding has resulted in more similar glucose values in hospitalized patients receiving EN and PN. As a result, patients receiving similar calories (while avoiding excess calorie provision) from either EN or PN have had similar reported infection rates.

Control of hyperglycemia during acute illness has been associated with improved patient medical outcomes. In an observational study, the implementation of an insulin infusion to maintain glucose levels between 150 to 200 mg/dL decreased by 58% the risk of sternal wound infections following coronary artery bypass surgery.[20] Each sternal wound infection prevented saved $21,000 in hospital charges and resulted in 16 fewer days of hospitalization. These estimates may not be accurate and should not be generalized, because they do not include all costs to the patient and society. However, they do represent hospital charges at a single institution before and after implementation of a glycemic control policy without accounting for trends in practice and costs over time. In a subsequent study, these same investigators compared insulin infusion with subcutaneous insulin administration in diabetic patients requiring coronary artery bypass surgery. Insulin infusion resulted in improved glucose control and a 57% decrease in mortality.[21]

Malmberg et al conducted a randomized trial of intensive insulin therapy (from hospital admission to 3 months following dismissal) in diabetic patients after myocardial infarction. This study, known as the DIGAMI trial, reported a 29% lower 1-year mortality during intensive insulin therapy compared with the standard diabetes treatment group.[22] Van den Berghe et al conducted a randomized trial of intensive glycemic control (glucose goal 80 to 110 mg/dL) compared with usual care in a surgical ICU. Patients received intravenous dextrose during day one and then either EN, PN, or combined PN and EN. All patients received nutrition support providing a mean caloric intake of approximately 19 kcal/kg (non-protein) of body weight. At the end of the study period, patients with an average blood glucose concentration of 103 mg/dL experienced a 44% lower mortality than did patients with an average blood glucose concentration of 153 mg/dL.[23] However, intensive insulin therapy did result in a 60% increase in hypoglycemia, defined in this study as a glucose concentration <40 mg/dL.

An entire body of evidence strongly suggests that hyperglycemia in the hospital setting is associated with adverse patient outcomes (particularly infections, disability after acute cardiovascular events, and death) and that improvement in outcomes can be achieved with glycemic control and infusion of short-acting insulin. Notably, this appears to be true for patients with or without a diagnosis of diabetes. Intensive insulin therapy for treatment of hyperglycemia has been reported to decrease inflammation.[24] It also has been shown to reduce bloodstream infections, acute renal failure requiring dialysis or hemofiltration, median number of red-cell transfusions, and critical illness related polyneuropathy.[25] However, researchers have not elucidated whether these benefits are caused by glucose control or to the correction of relative insulin deficiency.[26]

Hypoglycemia

Avoiding or minimizing the degree of hypoglycemia (defined as a plasma glucose ≤60 mg/dL) is important. Hypoglycemia can cause adrenergic or neuroglycopenic symptoms. The most common adrenergic symptoms are sweating, palpitations, anxiety, tachycardia, and hunger. Neuroglycopenic symptoms include headache, visual changes, seizures, and confusion. However, symptoms of hypoglycemia can be difficult to identify in severely ill patients who are sedated or dependent upon mechanical ventilation. In addition, patients with long-standing diabetes may have hypoglycemic unawareness, defined as the inability to recognize, treat, and report the warning symptoms of hypoglycemia.

Hyperglycemia and Hypoglycemia

Common Causes

Physicians should be familiar with the cause(s) of hyperglycemia and hypoglycemia to minimize both the severity of events and the frequency of recurrence.[27,28] Illness, infection, overfeeding (via nutrition support, dextrose-containing crystalloid, dextrose absorption during peritoneal dialysis, and medications formulated in fat emulsion, such as propofol), medications (eg, corticosteroids, sympathomimetic infusions, or immunosuppressants), insufficient insulin administration, and/or volume depletion may all cause or aggravate hyperglycemia. In the setting of unexplained or worsening hyperglycemia, all intravenous catheters (eg, peripherally inserted central catheters) should be considered as a potential source of infection. Gastroenterologists should be aware that hyperglycemia has been reported in 40% to 90% of patients admitted to hospital with acute pancreatitis, with up to 81% requiring insulin therapy.[29]

Causes of hypoglycemia, during insulin therapy, include excess insulin administration, unanticipated discontinuation of nutrition support during insulin therapy, resolution of severe stress, discontinued or decreased doses of corticosteroids or sympathomimetic agents, renal dysfunction, severe hepatitis, sepsis, and diabetic gastroparesis.

Glucose Goals

There are limited data in hospitalized ICU and ward patients to support "ideal" glucose goals. In an effort to balance potential benefits and risks derived by preventing hyperglycemic while avoiding hypoglycemia for ICU patients, the recommended glucose goal is 80 to 120 mg/dL. The authors aim for a glucose goal between 100 and 150 mg/dL in noncritically ill ward patients because achieving both lower and safer glucose goals using subcutaneous insulin regimens is difficult, because of potential for increased hypoglycemia risk. In addition, studies reporting improved medical outcome with tight glucose control did not include non-ICU patients. Additional studies will be required to establish the benefits, risks, and glycemic goals for different subsets of hospitalized patients.

Nutritional Assessment

The nutritional assessment, indications for nutrition support, and estimate of nutritional requirements for critically ill diabetic patients are generally similar to those of non-diabetic patients.[30] These standards are presented in detail in Chapter 1.

Diabetes can affect the entire GI tract. Significant diabetic gastroparesis is typically observed in patients with longstanding type 1 diabetes. While the term "gastroparesis diabeticorum" implies gastric atony, symptoms of gastroparesis may include dysmotility of both the stomach and small bowel. As many as 30% to 60% of patients with type 1 and type 2 diabetes have radiographic evidence of gastroparesis, yet report no difference in GI symptoms compared to control subjects.[31,32] Impaired visceroception is one explanation for this finding. The cause of gastroparesis is believed to be autonomic (sympathetic vagal nerve dysfunction) and enteric (intrinsic) neuropathy.[31,32]

Common manifestations of diabetic enteropathy include heartburn, dysphagia, nausea, early satiety, post-prandial vomiting (especially partially digested food retained from earlier meals), and epigastric pain. Markedly delayed gastric emptying may result in wide fluctuations of glucose with frequent hyperglycemia and/or hypoglycemia. Hyperglycemia itself may compound the delay in gastric emptying, a generally accepted notion.[33] Hypoglycemia may develop in diabetic subjects who take their usual pre-meal insulin doses but have delayed transit of food or ingest less than usual amount of food because of symptoms of gastroparesis while eating.

The diagnosis of diabetic gastroparesis should be strongly suspected from the patient's history and requires excluding other factors capable of slowing gut motility. Review of the patient's medication profile can identify commonly prescribed drugs with potential to delay gastric motility, including anticholinergics, antidepressants, alpha-2 adrenergic agonists, calcium channel blockers, and opiates. Esophagogastroduodenoscopy can exclude anatomic causes of gastric atony and impaired food transit. Demonstration of a delay in gastric emptying establishes the diagnosis of gastroparesis. Standard barium roentgeno-

TABLE 16-1.

Insulin Preparation Pharmacokinetics

Insulin	*Route*	*Onset*	*Peak*	*Effective Duration*
Rapid-Acting	SQ†			
Lispro		5 to 15 min	30 to 90 min	5 hr
Aspart		5 to 15 min	30 to 90 min	5 hr
Short-acting	SQ	30 to 60 min	2 to 3 hr	5 to 8 hr
Regular	IV‡		0.1 hr	3 to 5 hr
Intermediate-acting	SQ			
NPH		2 to 4 hr	4 to 10 hr	10 to 16 hr
Lente		2 to 4 hr	4 to 10 hr	10 to 16 hr
Long-acting	SQ			
Ultralente		6 to 10 hr	10 to 16 hr	18 to 24 hr
Glargine		2 to 4 hr	No peak	20 to 24 hr

† subcutaneous
‡ intravenous

graphic studies generally demonstrate gastric dilatation and retained solid residue even after a prolonged fast. Follow-up films reveal a marked delay of emptying, with >50% of contrast remaining in the stomach after 30 minutes. However, because gastric emptying of liquids (eg, barium) may be normal, even in the presence of moderately severe symptoms of gastroparesis, scintigraphic assessment of gastric motility with solids has become the preferred diagnostic test. Making an accurate diagnosis of diabetic gastroparesis will avoid the pitfall of attributing the patient's GI symptoms to administration of tube feedings.

Type 2 diabetes is often associated with peripheral insulin resistance in patients who are overweight or obese, and avoidance of overfeeding hospitalized patients is paramount. Administration of excess calories can dramatically exacerbate hyperglycemia. Most hospitalized subjects can be adequately fed by provision of 100% (ICU patients) to 120% (ward patients) of basal caloric needs, as estimated by the Harris-Benedict equation.[34-37] It is our practice to provide 1.0-1.5 g of protein per kilogram body weight; the higher end of the spectrum for more stressed (eg, ICU and critically-ill) patients. Fat is administered as 20% to 30% of the total daily caloric content.

The enteral tube feeds or parenteral lipid emulsion should be tapered appropriately in patients receiving propofol. Propofol is a short-acting anesthetic agent formulated as a lipid emulsion and provides the same calories as an identical volume of 10% fat emulsion. After determining the provision of protein and fat, the patient's remaining daily caloric needs are provided as carbohydrate. However, for patients receiving PN, data addressing optimal dextrose infusion rates are limited.

Consensus guidelines are lacking on how to feed obese hospitalized patients. Outcome data for critically ill obese patients is also limited. For obese patients (eg, body mass index ≥30), we recommend providing calories as 75% of the Harris-Benedict estimate of energy needs based upon current weight and provision of 1.5 g of protein per kilogram of estimated ideal weight.

Management of Patients With Hyperglycemia Receiving Enteral Tube Feeding

Glycemic control can be difficult to obtain in hospitalized patients who are receiving enteral tube feedings. The authors monitor glucose levels by reflectance meter because the results are rapidly obtained and the need for venipuncture is avoided. When using reflectance-meter glucose monitoring, a control program must be established to ensure accuracy of results including meter calibration, personnel training, and comparison measurements.

For patients with hyperglycemia but without prior diagnosis of diabetes and no prior use of insulin or oral diabetic agents, the authors recommend treatment with short-acting regular insulin (versus rapid-acting Aspart or Lispro insulin, see Table 16-1) during tube feeding initiation because of its long history of use and familiarity among providers in the hospital setting. Regular insulin use will also minimize the risk of hypoglycemia, which may result from continued subcutaneous (SQ) absorption of intermediate-acting insulin (NPH isophane or Lente zinc suspensions) following unexpected discontinuation of early tube feeding. Once the tube feeding infusion rate has reached 30 to 40 ml/hour, the use of intermediate-acting NPH or Lente insulin is generally safe.

Oral diabetic agents may be continued in the hospital setting and administered by feeding tube for medically stable diabetic patients with good glucose control and normal renal and hepatic function. However, metformin

TABLE 16-2.

Guidelines for Subcutaneous (SQ) Regular Insulin Supplementation

Glucose, mg/dL	SQ Regular Insulin Dose, Units		
	Algorithm 1	Algorithm 2	Algorithm 3
150–200	1	2	(_)
201–250	2	4	(_)
251–300	3	6	(_)
301–350	4	8	(_)
> 350	5	10	(_)

- Choice of treatment algorithm 1–3 will reflect differences in treatment goals and response to insulin. Response to insulin will vary for differences in insulin resistance (eg, patient weight, medications, physiologic stress) and renal/hepatic function.
- Initiate insulin supplementation if two consecutive glucose values exceed 150 mg/dL for ward patients or 120 mg/dL for ICU patients. Insulin should not be administered more than every 4 to 6 hours.
- Initiate algorithm 1 or 2, depending on anticipated insulin needs to achieve glucose goal. Consider initiating algorithm 1 for type 1 diabetics with previous low-dose insulin requirements, and algorithm 2 for most patients with stress-induced hyperglycemia or type 2 diabetes. Use the next higher treatment algorithm if glucose goal is not met within 24 hours.
- A reflectance meter glucose (RMG) measurement is recommended every 4 to 6 hours during SQ regular insulin supplementation. Insulin infusion should be considered if RMG goal is not achieved with the SQ insulin algorithm.

should be discontinued in hospitalized patients because of a major potential risk of lactic acidosis, especially during compromised hepatic or renal function, dehydration, and decreased tissue perfusion. For diabetic patients with previous oral diabetic agent use and poor glucose control or with hepatic or renal compromise, the authors recommend discontinuation of these diabetic medications during tube feedings and use of insulin as described above. If appropriate for glucose control, oral diabetic agents may be prescribed when the patient resumes an oral diet.

Glucose management is more complex for diabetic patients receiving insulin therapy. For fasting, hospitalized diabetic subjects treated with once or twice daily SQ intermediate-acting insulin (with or without short-acting insulin), begin by providing one-half of the patient's total preadmission morning insulin as a morning intermediate-acting insulin SQ dose. Similarly, one-half of the patient's total preadmission evening insulin may be provided as an evening intermediate-acting insulin SQ dose. For type 1 diabetic subjects treated with long-acting insulin (Glargine or Ultralente insulin) for basal insulin needs, continue their long-acting SQ insulin at the same preadmission dose. The authors adhere to the regular insulin SQ algorithm (Table 16-2) for management of hyperglycemia above the patient's glucose goal range. Non-PN intravenous dextrose hydration solutions should contain 0.2 units regular insulin per gram of dextrose infused (eg, 10 units insulin per liter 5% (50 g) dextrose solution), unless renal function is severely compromised. The following day's insulin needs of intermediate-acting and short-acting insulin are adjusted according to the patient's physiologic stress, daily nutrition provision, insulin doses administered, and glycemic control. Onset of tube feedings, or increases in the tube feeding infusion rate, should be avoided until adequate glucose control has been achieved by appropriate insulin management.

An insulin infusion should be initiated for severe hyperglycemia or if glucose goals cannot be achieved with SQ insulin. The rate of insulin infusion prescribed should depend on the individual patients recent glycemic control (via hemoglobin A1c level), the degree of physiologic stress, and the level of hyperglycemia. The ICU insulin infusion algorithm is more labor intensive than that for ward patients (Tables 16-3 and 16-4), but both require close management for patient safety. In addition, as discussed earlier, outcome studies based on glycemic control have not included hospital ward patients. Discontinuing the insulin infusion before the onset of SQ insulin administration is a common treatment error for patients who require insulin for their diabetes management. Regular insulin administered intravenously has a very short half-life (minutes) and requires continuous infusion for glucose control. Without a SQ depot of insulin, cessation of insulin infusion will result in a rapid rise in glucose with significant hyperglycemia and potential morbidity until SQ insulin delivery is sufficient for glycemic control. To avoid rebound hyperglycemia following discontinuation of insulin infusions, SQ insulin should be administered well before the infusion is discontinued. Patients previously treated with combined intermediate and short-acting insulin can receive a small amount of SQ "basal" insulin (eg, once or twice daily intermediate-acting NPH or Lente insulin), combined with small amounts of short-acting insulin. The dose of SQ insulin is increased daily, and the insulin infusion dose will decrease accordingly per the insulin infusion algorithm. Thus, a smooth and rapid transition from intravenous to SQ insulin can occur in the presence of relatively stable glucose control. The final goal is to establish a glucose management program best suited to the patient's individual needs following hospital dismissal.

If tube feedings are provided by gravity administration, the glucose concentration should be checked immediately before each feeding and no sooner than 4 hours after the end of the prior feeding. For this reason, the use of three versus four daily gastric tube feedings may provide a more

Table 16-3.

Intravenous Insulin Infusion Algorithm for ICU or Intermediate Care Unit Patients

Column 1		Column 2		Column 3		Column 4	
Bedside Glucose (mg/dL)	Insulin Infusion Rate (Units/hr)	Bedside Glucose (mg/dL)	Insulin Infusion Rate (Units/hr)	Bedside Glucose (mg/dL)	Insulin Infusion Rate (Units/hr)	Bedside Glucose (mg/dL)	Insulin Infusion Rate (Units/hr)
> 400	8	≥ 360	12	≥ 360	16	≥ 270	20
351 to 400	6	330 to 359	8	330 to 359	14	240 to 269	16
301 to 350	4	300 to 329	7	300 to 329	12	210 to 239	12
251 to 300	3	270 to 299	6	270 to 299	10	180 to 209	8
200 to 250	2.5	240–269	5	240 to 269	8	150 to 179	4
150 to 199	2	210 to 239	4	210 to 239	6	120 to 149	2
120 to 149	1.5	180 to 209	3	180 to 209	4	100 to 119	1
100 to 119	1	150 to 179	2	150 to 179	3	< 100	Off
< 100	Off	120 to 149	1.5	120 to 149	2		
		100 to 119	1	100 to 119	1		
		< 100	Off	< 100	Off		

- Glucose goals should be individually determined for each patient. For critically-ill patients, RMG values of 80 to 120 mg/dL are appropriate. The algorithm is designed for an average 70-kg patient and may require modification for smaller or larger patients. The algorithm is not appropriate for the treatment of diabetic ketoacidosis or hyperosmolar states.
- Choose the appropriate column for insulin infusion. Follow the column protocol for two hours and, if reflectance meter glucose (RMG) values remain > 120 mg/dL or are not decreasing, proceed to the next higher column. If the RMG's are < 120 mg/dL for 4 hours using column 3 or 4, proceed to the next lower column.
- Initial insulin titration guidelines (Use if any of the criteria listed for each column are met):
- – Column 1: Initial RMG 120 to 200 mg/dL; no corticosteroids or sympathomimetic infusion.
- – Column 2: Initial RMG > 200 mg/dL; oral or IV corticosteroid use (excludes inhaled and ophthalmic steroids); sympathomimetic infusion; RMG remains > 120 mg/dL after 2 hours using Column 1 algorithm.
- – Column 3: RMG remains > 120 mg/dL after 2 hours using Column 2 algorithm.
- – Column 4: RMG remains > 120 mg/dL after 2 hours using Column 3 algorithm.
- RMG's should be measured hourly until glucose levels have stabilized for 4 hours in the desired goal range. RMG monitoring may then be decreased to every 2 hours. Return to hourly monitoring with any of the following: change in nutritional status; RMG < 100 mg/dL or above goal for 2 consecutive measurements; change in clinical status or Column algorithm.

TABLE 16-4.

Intravenous Insulin Infusion Algorithm for Hospital Ward Patients

Glucose (mg/dL)	IV Infusion Rate (mL/hr)	Insulin Infusion Rate (Units/hr)
> 400	8	8
351 to 400	6	6
301 to 350	4	4
250 to 300	3	3
200 to 249	2.5	2.5
150 to 199	2	2
120 to 149	1.5	1.5
100 to 119	1	1
80 to 99	0	0
< 80	0	0

- Glucose goals should be individually determined for each patient. For hospital ward patients, RMG values of 100 to 150 mg/dL are appropriate. The algorithm is designed for an average 70-kg patient and may require modification for smaller or larger patients. The algorithm is not appropriate for treatment of diabetic ketoacidosis or hyperosmolar states.
- RMG's should be measured hourly until glucose concentrations have stabilized for 4 hours in the desired goal range. RMG monitoring may then be decreased to every 2 hours, and once glucose control remains stable, to every 4 hours.
- If RMG's are > 200 mg/dL and do not decrease by at least 50 mg/dL over 2 hours, increase the insulin infusion by 50% increments for each glucose range > 150 mg/dL. Make similar infusion adjustments if the RMG is < 200 mg/dL (but > 150 mg/dL) and does not decrease by at least 25 mg/dL over 2 hours. Risk of hypoglycemia may be greater when the insulin algorithm is increased for RMG values < 150 mg/dL.
- At time of conversion from IV to SQ insulin therapy, continue infusion for three hours following administration of first SQ insulin dose.

accurate assessment of preprandial glucose and glycemic control. This approach may be aided by using a calorie-dense (1.5 kcal/cc) enteral product, versus that of standard formulas (1 kcal/cc), when a larger volume of tube feeding is required. In this setting, choose tube feedings with an osmolarity closest to that of the iso-osmolar standard formulas. Although some patients receiving gravity feedings can be managed with once or twice daily intermediate-acting insulin alone, others will need combined intermediate and short-acting insulin therapy.

Gravity tube feeding may not be initially tolerated in gastric-fed patients and should not be administered to patients requiring jejunal-enteral nutrition. Diabetic patients receiving 12-hour daytime or nocturnal tube feedings may require only a once-daily administration of intermediate-acting insulin prior to the onset of tube feeding. Glucose goals prior to intermittent (gravity) or continuous (12- to 24-hour) tube feedings are similar to those described earlier for ICU and ward patients. In the setting of continuous tube feeding nutrient provision, a reasonable glucose goal would be 100 to 150 mg/dL. Twice-daily administration of intermediate-acting insulin may be required if tube feedings are administered continuously over 24 hours. Alternatively, and if intermittent hypoglycemia occurs during continuous tube feedings and intermediate-acting insulin therapy, once-daily administration of a long-acting insulin (eg, Glargine and Ultralente insulin) may provide a more evenly matched nutrient infusion and insulin delivery. While there are theoretic reasons for using a long-acting insulin in stable patients with hyperglycemia, such as a constant basal insulin profile, outcome studies in hospitalized patients are limited.

Gastric stasis or gastric outlet obstruction may make tube-feeding tolerance more difficult, and aspiration pneumonia is one of the most feared complications of gastric tube feedings in the ICU. Daily measurement of gastric residual volume is recommended during gastric tube feeds, finding an elevated gastric residual should not lead to abandonment of tube feeding, as it has been reported to be an isolated event approximately 80% of the time.38 McClave et al reported that stopping tube feedings at gastric residuals of ≤150 ml would have discontinued EN in 50% of ICU patients (and 30% of normal subjects) who were clinically tolerant of the tube feedings.[39] These authors suggested tube feeding continuance up to gastric residuals of 200 ml. Indeed, a randomized trial of head injury patients found gastric residuals alone associated with catecholamine use, sedation, and reduced tube feedings but not significantly correlated with pneumonia, ICU mortality, or hospital mortality unless in the presence of vomiting.[40]

An oral gastroparesis diet uses smaller meal portions, low residue, and reduced-fat content (meal fat can delay gastric emptying). If nausea or abdominal pain limit oral intake, liquid enteral drinks may be well tolerated (liquids empty quicker than solids), or tube feedings may be required. Drug therapy for gastroparesis is outlined in Table 16-5.

Patients with diabetic gastroparesis or acute pancreatitis (Chapter 22) should be monitored closely for GI tolerance during tube feedings. Approximately 80% of patients with acute pancreatitis recover within 5 to 7 days and do not require nutritional support. However, 5% to 15% of these patients will develop necrotizing severe pancreatitis, and

TABLE 16-5.

Drug Therapy for Gastroparesis

Prokinetic	*Oral Dose*	*Comments*
Metoclopramide	5 to 20 mg QID	Antiemetic and prokinetic (stimulates acetyl-choline receptors). Start at low dose and titrate upward. Adverse effects in up to 20% of patients. Can use IV.
Tegaserod	2 to 6 mg BID-TID	Newest promotility agent. Approved for irritable-bowel syndrome. Gastroparesis outcome studies pending. Diarrhea adverse effect.
Erythromycin	125 to 250 mg QID	Strong prokinetic agent with short-term use. Tachyphylaxis develops with longer-term use. Can use IV.
Domperidone	10 to 30 mg QID	Better adverse event profile than metoclopramide. Not available for use in the United States.
Cisapride	10 to 20 mg QID	Adverse cardiac events (Torsades) and banned by FDA. Adult dose should not exceed 1 mg/kg/day.

Antiemetic

1. No single drug or class of drugs appears superior:
    - Metaclopromide (also prokinetic)
    - Scopolamine patch
    - Low-dose tricyclic antidepressants (affects visceral sensation)
    - Acupuncture wrist bands
2. Avoid constipation.

TABLE 16-6.

A.S.P.E.N. Board of Directors and Clinical Task Force Guidelines for Nutrition Support in Patients With Acute Pancreatitis

1. Patients with pancreatitis are at nutritional risk and should undergo nutritional screening.
2. Specialized nutrition support should not be used routinely in patients with mild to moderate acute pancreatitis.
3. Specialized nutrition support should be used in patients with acute or chronic pancreatitis to prevent or treat malnutrition when oral energy intake is anticipated to be inadequate for 5 to 7 days.
4. Enteral nutrition (EN) is the preferred route of specialized nutrition support in patients with pancreatitis and should be initiated before parenteral nutrition (PN).
5. PN should be used in patients with pancreatitis if specialized nutrition support is indicated and EN is not tolerated.
6. Intravenous PN lipid emulsions are safe in acute pancreatitis provided serum triglyceride levels are monitored and remain below 400 mg/dL.

a significant percent of these patients develop gastric stasis or outlet obstruction due to pancreatic edema and/or pseudocyst formation and may require gastric decompression. When nutrition support is needed, tube feedings in patients with acute, non-necrotizing pancreatitis may be safely tolerated,[41] especially when administered in the jejunum.

Enteral elemental formulas contain a higher percent of dipeptides and medium chain triglycerides and have been shown to decrease pancreatic enzyme secretion by 50% compared to more complex standard enteral feedings.[42] Table 16-6 outlines the American Society for Parenteral and Enteral Nutrition Board of Directors and Clinical Task Force guidelines for nutrition support in patients with acute pancreatitis based on an evidence-based literature review.[43] In the authors' experience, most patients with diabetic gastroparesis intolerant of gastric feedings are able to tolerate iso-osmolar jejunal tube feedings when initiated at a low rate (eg, 20 mL/hour) and advanced slowly (eg, 10 to 20 ml rate increase every 12 hours). PN should be used only if patients fail a reasonable trial of nasoenteric tube feeding.

Hypoglycemia may occur during treatment with SQ insulin because of either delayed nutrient absorption from gastroparesis or unexpected discontinuation of tube feedings. Table 16-7 outlines a protocol developed by these authors to treat hypoglycemia in hospitalized patients.

TABLE 16-7.

Treatment of Hypoglycemia in Hospitalized Adult Patients Requiring Insulin or Oral Diabetic Agents

Presumed symptomatic hypoglycemia should be treated without waiting to check plasma or blood glucose levelIf the patient is able to swallow safely, administer ~15 grams of carbohydrate in one of the following forms:

1. 5 sugar packets dissolved in 4 ounces (1/2 cup) of water.
2. 4 ounces (1/2 cup) of fruit juice.
3. Glucose Oral Gel (Glutose 15). 15 grams must be used for patients taking Acarbose (Precose) or Miglitol (Glyset).

If a functioning feeding tube is present, administer one of the following by feeding tube:

1. 1.4 ounces (½ cup) of fruit juice (not orange juice or other pulp-containing juice).
2. 2.5 sugar packets dissolved in 4 ounces (1/2 cup) of water.

If the patient is not able to take oral or tube feeding safely or is NPO:

1. If intravenous access is available, administer 25 mL D50W (12.5 grams dextrose) intravenously.
2. If no intravenous access is present, administer Glucagon 1 mg by subcutaneous injection. Following Glucagon treatment, for those patients who are not NPO, provide a snack to prevent subsequent hypoglycemia.

Contact either the Primary Service or the Diabetes Consulting Service, whichever is responsible for the patient's diabetes management.
For treatment of asymptomatic hypoglycemia (glucose ≤ 60 mg/dL) follow steps A through C above.
Glucose monitoring following treatment:
Measure a reflectance meter glucose (RMG) within 15 minutes. If the RMG is not > 80 mg/dL, repeat the treatment outlined above. Recheck the RMG within 15 minutes. Repeat further treatment and RMG checks at 15 minutes intervals until the glucose is > 80 mg/dL.

Management of Patients With Hyperglycemia Receiving Parenteral Nutrition

The approach used to achieve glucose control in patients with diabetes and stress-induced hyperglycemia receiving nutrition support can be varied among hospitals and medical centers. These authors' approach has evolved to meet the needs of an institution in which many clinicians prescribe EN and PN.

During PN support, the provider measures glucose by reflectance meter because results are rapidly obtained without the need for venipuncture. A glucose level should be measured before initiation of PN, and hyperglycemia should be controlled prior to the onset of PN. Overfeeding is avoided and PN dextrose is limited to approximately 200 g during thc first day of nutrition support. The frequency of reflectance-meter glucose monitoring should be individualized. Measure glucose levels the first and second morning following implementation of PN in all patients. For patients with established diabetes or significant hyperglycemia, glucose levels are measured 2 to 4 times daily until treatment returns values to within the patient's glucose goal range. Thereafter, reflectance-meter glucose frequency is individualized but obtained at least once to twice daily. If daily glucose values rise suddenly without change in PN admixture, one should consider a significant increase in physiologic stress (eg, inflammation, infection, etc.).

While these providers do not initiate long-acting SQ insulin in hospitalized patients with hyperglycemia, they recommend continuing basal doses of long-acting insulin for diabetic subjects with a prior established multiple daily insulin program when admitted to the ICU and hospital ward (see Table 16-1). The majority of diabetic patients receiving PN dextrose require insulin for glucose control. For patients with two consecutive glucose values >120 mg/dL in the ICU or >150 mg/dL in the hospital ward, the authors initially add 0.1 units of regular insulin per gram of dextrose [eg, 20 units insulin per liter of 20% (200 g) dextrose solution]. If the patient's subsequent daily glucose values remain above goal, the PN insulin can be increased to 0.15 to 0.2 units of regular insulin per gram of dextrose [eg, 30 to 40 units insulin respectively per liter of 20% (200 g) dextrose solution]. A PN regular insulin concentration of 0.2 units/g of dextrose is the maximal dose recommended. This ratio of insulin to dextrose is unlikely to be associated with hypoglycemia either during or after infusion of PN. The PN dextrose content should not be increased until the glucose values of the previous 24-hour period are in the desired goal range. If hyperglycemia persists despite PN insulin, as outlined above, supplemental SQ short-acting insulin is initiated according to the supplemental insulin algorithm (see Table 16-2). The PN insulin concentration should be proportionally increased or decreased when the PN dextrose content is changed, in keeping with the stated recommended guidelines for insulin to dextrose ratio.

If hyperglycemia persists despite use of SQ insulin therapy, an insulin infusion may be required for effective

TABLE 16-8.

Guidelines for Considering Nutrition Consultation in Hospitalized Patients

I. Nutrition Assessment
   A. Assistance in designing an enteral or parenteral nutrition plan and timing of administration to meet patient energy and macronutrient (e.g., protein, lipid and carbohydrate) needs without overfeeding.
   B. Special need patients (eg, patients with diabetes and difficult glycemic control, renal or hepatic insufficiency, obesity, volume restricted and/or bodily fluid excess).

II. Intolerance to EN tube feeding
   A. Diarrhea
   B. Malabsorption
   C. Elevated gastric residuals, clinical gastric stasis, or gastroparesis
   D. Pancreatitis

and safe glycemic control. The authors designed hospital protocol order forms to standardize the use and monitoring of insulin infusion (see Tables 16-3 and 16-4). As previously noted, outcome studies testing tight glucose control did not include hospital ward patients. In addition, studies testing varied insulin infusion protocols to achieve desired glucose goal ranges are limited. Thus, different insulin infusion management algorithms are used for ICU versus ward patients. If two consecutive glucose values in ICU or critically ill patients exceed 120 mg/dL, it is reasonable to initiate an insulin infusion. For hospital ward patients, data are limited, and guidelines for initiating an insulin infusion are less clear. Many ward patients with hyperglycemia can be adequately treated with a more aggressive SQ short-acting insulin regimen (see Table 16-2), thereby avoiding the use of insulin infusion therapy. The authors typically continue the recommended maximal PN insulin dose for patients requiring either SQ insulin or insulin infusion for treatment of hyperglycemia. Conversely, if goal glucose levels are maintained, insulin infusion and SQ insulin should be discontinued prior to PN insulin taper. However, if the patient's glucose decreases below goal range during PN insulin administration only, a substantial (~50%) reduction of insulin in the subsequent PN admixture should decrease the risk of hypoglycemia. If a hospitalized patient develops hypoglycemia, dextrose should be administered as outlined in Table 16-5. For patients receiving PN insulin only, the incidence of symptomatic hypoglycemia after sudden discontinuation of PN is uncommon if the patient has not received excess calories.

Conclusion

Hyperglycemia is a common occurrence in the hospital setting. Because of the high prevalence of diabetes and stress-induced hyperglycemia, gastroenterologists will frequently manage hospitalized patients with hyperglycemia. Guidelines for glycemic control for ICU and hospital ward patients have been established, and nutrition/endocrine consultation may be helpful for patients receiving EN or PN (Table 16-8) who have persistent hyperglycemia or recurring hypoglycemia (Table 16-9). Physicians caring for these patients will need to be mindful of the interaction between EN and PN administration and hyperglycemia, the increased patient morbidity with associated hyperglycemia in the hospital setting, and thus the importance for glycemic control.

Acknowledgment

The authors would like to acknowledge Michelle Papaconstandinou for her assistance in the preparation of this chapter.

Table 16-9.

Guidelines for Considering Endocrine Consultation in Hospitalized Patients

I. During enteral nutrition (EN) and parenteral nutrition (PN) therapy
  A. Hyperglycemia above patient goal
    1. Before initiating EN or PN
    2. During continuous (infusion pump)or intermittent (gravity) EN tube feeding
    3. During PN maximal insulin concentration (eg, 0.2 units Regular insulin per gram of PN dextrose)

II. During subcutaneous (SQ) insulin and insulin infusion (IV) therapy
  A. Frequent hyperglycemia or hypoglycemia above patient goal
  B. Electrolyte or mineral abnormalities before or during SQ or IV insulin
  C. Designing a post-hospital SQ insulin regimen
    1. Education and management of insulin use and reflectance meter glucose monitoring
    a. Patients new to insulin therapy
    b. Insulin treated patients with poor glycemic control
    2. Follow-up health care appointments
    a. Assessment of glucose monitoring, insulin management, and glucose control for the patient's defined goal range
    b. Compliance with the American Diabetes Association national guidelines for monitoring and care of diabetes-related complications (eg, retinopathy, nephropathy, neuropathy) and blood pressure
    c. Compliance with the National Cholesterol Education Program Adult Treatment Panel III (NCEP ATP III) guidelines for lipid management

III. Hypertriglyceridemia
  A. Serum triglycerides > 400 mg/dL before or during EN or PN administration

References

1. Umpierrez GE, Isaacs SD, Bazargan N, et al. Hyperglycemia: an independent marker of in-hospital mortality in patients with undiagnosed diabetes [see comment]. *J Clin Endocrinol Metab.* 2002;87(3):978-82.
2. Report of the Expert Committee on the Diagnosis and Classification of Diabetes Mellitus. *Diabetes Care.* 1997;20(7):1183-97.
3. Shamoon H, Hendler R, Sherwin RS. Synergistic interactions among antiinsulin hormones in the pathogenesis of stress hyperglycemia in humans. *J Clin Endocrinol Metab.* 1981;52(6):1235-41.
4. Shamoon H, Hendler R, Sherwin RS. Altered responsiveness to cortisol, epinephrine, and glucagon in insulin-infused juvenile-onset diabetics. A mechanism for diabetic instability. *Diabetes.* 29:(4):284-91, 1980.
5. Bistrian BR. Hyperglycemia and infection: which is the chicken and which is the egg? *J Parenter Enteral Nutr.* 2001;25:(4):180-1.
6. Hostetter MK. Handicaps to host defense. Effects of hyperglycemia on C3 and Candida albicans. *Diabetes.* 1990;39(3):271-275.
7. Gustafson KS, Vercellotti GM, Bendel CM, Hostetter MK. Molecular mimicry in Candida albicans. Role of an integrin analogue in adhesion of the yeast to human endothelium. *J Clin Invest.* 1991;87(6):1896-1902.
8. Hostetter MK. The third component of complement: new functions for an old friend. *J Lab Clin Med.* 1993;122:(5):491-496.
9. McCowen KC, Malhotra A, Bistrian BR. Stress-induced hyperglycemia. *Crit Care Clin.* 2001;17(1):107-124.
10. McMahon MM, Bistrian BR. Host defenses and susceptibility to infection in patients with diabetes mellitus. In: Eliopoulos GM, ed. *Infectious Disease Clinics of North America.* Philadelphia: Saunders; 1995.
11. Capes SE, Hunt D, Malmberg K, Gerstein HC. Stress hyperglycaemia and increased risk of death after myocardial infarction in patients with and without diabetes: a systematic overview. *Lancet.* 2000;355(9206):773-778.
12. Capes SE, Hunt D, Malmberg K, Pathak P, Gerstein HC. Stress hyperglycemia and prognosis of stroke in nondiabetic and diabetic patients: a systematic overview. *Stroke.* 2001;32(10):2426-2432.
13. Pomposelli JJ, Baxter JK, 3rd, Babineau TJ, et al. Early postoperative glucose control predicts nosocomial infection rate in diabetic patients. *J Parenter Enteral Nutr.* 1998;22(2):77-81.
14. Golden SH, Peart-Vigilance C, Kao WH, Brancati FL. Perioperative glycemic control and the risk of infectious complications in a cohort of adults with diabetes. *Diabetes Care.* 1999;22(9):1408-1414.
15. Latham R, Lancaster AD, Covington JF, Pirolo JS, Thomas CS. The association of diabetes and glucose control with surgical-site infections among cardiothoracic surgery patients. *Infect Control Hosp Epidemiol.* 22:(10):607-12, 2001.
16. The Veterans Affairs Total Parenteral Nutrition Cooperative Study Group. Perioperative total parenteral nutrition in surgical patients. *N Engl J Med.* 1991;325(8):525-532.
17. Moore FA, Feliciano DV, Andrassy RJ, et al. Early enteral feeding, compared with parenteral, reduces postoperative septic complications. The results of a meta-analysis. *Ann Surg.* 1992;216(2):172-183.
18. Kudsk KA, Laulederkind A, Hanna MK. Most infectious complications in parenterally fed trauma patients are not due to elevated blood glucose levels. *J Parenter Enteral Nutr.* 2001;25(4):174-179.
19. Takala J, Ruokonen E, Webster NR, et al. Increased mortality associated with growth hormone treatment in critically ill adults. *N Engl J Med.* 1999;341(11):785-92.
20. Furnary AP, Zerr KJ, Grunkemeier GL, Starr A. Continuous intravenous insulin infusion reduces the incidence of deep sternal wound infection in diabetic patients after cardiac surgical procedures. *Ann Thorac Surg.* 1999;67:(2):352-60.
21. Furnary AP, Gao G, Grunkemeier GL, et al. Continuous insulin infusion reduces mortality in patients with diabetes undergoing coronary artery bypass grafting. *J Thorac Cardiovasc Surg.* 2003;125(5):1007-1021.

22. Malmberg K. Prospective randomised study of intensive insulin treatment on long term survival after acute myocardial infarction in patients with diabetes mellitus. DIGAMI (Diabetes Mellitus, Insulin Glucose Infusion in Acute Myocardial Infarction) Study Group. *BMJ.* 1997;314:(7093):1512-1515.
23. Van den Berghe G, Wouters P, Weekers F, et al. Intensive insulin therapy in the critically-ill patients. *N Engl J Med.* 2001;345:(19):1359-1367.
24. Hansen TK, Thiel S, Wouters PJ, Christiansen JS, Van den Berghe G. Intensive insulin therapy exerts anti-inflammatory effects in critically-ill patients and counteracts the adverse effect of low mannose-binding lectin levels. *J Clin Endocrinol Metab.* 2003;88(3):1082-1088.
25. Ferrando AA, Chinkes DL, Wolf SE, et al. A submaximal dose of insulin promotes net skeletal muscle protein synthesis in patients with severe burns. *Ann Surg.* 1999;229(1):11-8.
26. vom Dahl J, Herman WH, Hicks RJ, et al. Myocardial glucose uptake in patients with insulin-dependent diabetes mellitus assessed quantitatively by dynamic positron emission tomography. *Circulation.* 1993;88(2):395-404.
27. McMahon MM, Rizza RA. Nutrition support in hospitalized patients with diabetes mellitus. *Mayo Clin Proc.* 1996;71(6):587-94.
28. Montori VM, Bistrian BR, McMahon MM. Hyperglycemia in acutely ill patients. *JAMA.* 2002;288(17):2167-2169.
29. Havala T, Shronts E, and Cerra F. Nutritional support in acute pancreatitis. *Gastroenterol Clin North Am.* 1989;18(3):525-542.
30. Hurley DL, Neven A, McMahon MM. Diabetes mellitus. In: Gottschlich MM, ed. *The Science and Practice of Nutrition Support: A Case-Based Core Curriculum.* Dubuque: Kendall/Hunt Publishing Company; 2001: 663-75.
31. Camilleri M. Advances in diabetic gastroparesis. *Rev Gastroenterol Disord.* 2002;2(2):47-56.
32. Stacher G. Diabetes mellitus and the stomach. *Diabetologia.* 2001;44(9):1080-1093.
33. Hebbard GS, Sun WM, Dent J, Horowitz M. Hyperglycaemia affects proximal gastric motor and sensory function in normal subjects. *Eur J Gastroenterol Hepatol.* 1996;8(3):211-217.
34. McMahon MM, Farnell MB, Murray MJ. Nutritional support of critically-ill patients. *Mayo Clin Proc.* 1993;68(9):911-920.
35. Hunter DC, Jaksic T, Lewis D, et al. Resting energy expenditure in the critically ill: estimations versus measurement. *Br J Surg.* 1988;75(9):875-878.
36. Paauw JD, McCamish MA, Dean RE, Ouellette TR. Assessment of caloric needs in stressed patients. *J Am Coll Nutr.* 1984;3(1):51-59.
37. Mann S, Westenskow DR, Houtchens BA. Measured and predicted caloric expenditure in the acutely ill. *Crit Care Med.* 1985;13(3):173-177.
38. McClave SA, Sexton LK, Spain DA, et al. Enteral tube feeding in the intensive care unit: factors impeding adequate delivery. *Crit Care Med.* 1999;27(7):1252-1256.
39. McClave SA, Snider HL, Lowen CC, et al. Use of residual volume as a marker for enteral feeding intolerance: prospective blinded comparison with physical examination and radiographic findings. *J Parenter Enteral Nutr.* 1992;16(2):99-105.
40. Taylor SJ, Fettes SB, Jewkes C, Nelson RJ. Prospective, randomized, controlled trial to determine the effect of early enhanced enteral nutrition on clinical outcome in mechanically ventilated patients suffering head injury. *Crit Care Med.* 1999;27(11):2525-2531.
41. Eatock FC, Brombacher GD, Steven A, et al. Nasogastric feeding in severe acute pancreatitis may be practical and safe. *Int J Pancreatol.* 2000;28(1):23-29.
42. O'Keefe SJ, Lee RB, Anderson FP, et al. Physiological effects of enteral and parenteral feeding on pancreaticobiliary secretion in humans. *Am J Physiol Gastrointest Liver Physiol.* 2003;284(1):G27-36.
43. A.S.P.E.N. Board of Directors and Clinical Guidelines Task Force. Guidelines for the use of enteral and parenteral nutrition in adult and pediatric patients: Pancreatitis. *J Parenter Enteral Nutr.* 2002;26:(suppl):68SA-70SA.

Section III

Nutrition in Gastrointestinal Disease

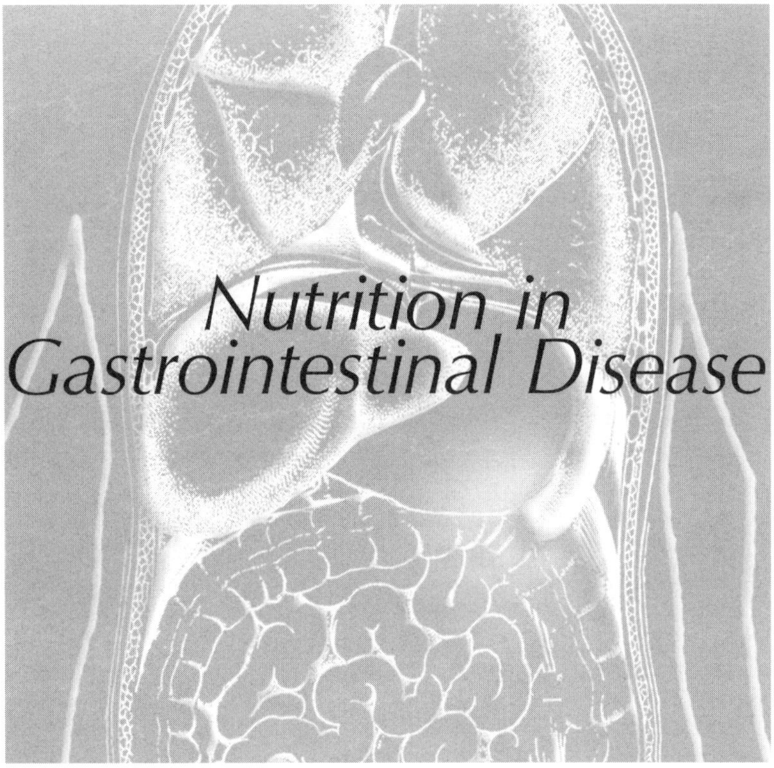

Chapter 17

NUTRITION AND COLORECTAL CANCER

Young-In Kim, MD, FRCP(C)

Introduction

The development of colorectal cancer (CRC) is thought to be the result of an intimate, and yet poorly understood, interplay between environmental and genetic factors. CRC incidence rates vary approximately 10- to 200-fold across different geographic locations around the world, with the highest observed in the developed, westernized, industrialized, and urbanized parts of the world.[1] The international differences, migrant data, and recent rapid increases in incidence rates in the same geographic location with previously low CRC incidence rates over time collectively suggest that environmental factors play a major role in the development of CRC.[1]

Dietary and lifestyle factors are among the most important environmental factors implicated in the development of CRC. For instance, in 1981, Doll and Peto estimated that about 35% (10% to 70%) of all cancers in the United States might be attributable to dietary factors and that up to 90% of CRC in the United States may be preventable through dietary modifications.[2] More recently, it was estimated that one-third of 500,000 cancer deaths that occur in the United States each year are due to dietary factors.[3] Similar estimates were made by the European School of Oncology Task Force on Diet, Nutrition, and Cancer in 1994,[4] and by the World Cancer Research Fund and the American Institute for Cancer Research in 1997.[1] These provocative epidemiologic estimations were supported by a recent study involving 44,788 pairs of twins in Scandinavian countries; findings suggest that 58%, 65%, and 73% of prostate, colorectal, and breast cancers (3 of the 4 most common cancers in the United States), respectively, are attributable to environmental factors.[5]

Much effort has been directed toward defining the relationship between dietary and lifestyle factors and the development of cancer, as well as toward the prevention of cancer through dietary and lifestyle modifications.[1] In this regard, there is evidence that dietary modifications have possibly contributed to a 29% reduction in the CRC mortality in the US White population from 1950 through 1990, with a more pronounced decrease in women than in men.[6]

Consumption of red meat, animal and saturated fat, refined carbohydrates, and alcohol, as well as total caloric (energy) intake, is generally considered to be positively related to the risk of developing CRC[1,7-8] (Table 17-1). On the other hand, the intake of dietary fiber, vegetables, fruits, antioxidant vitamins, calcium, and folate is believed to be negatively associated with the risk of developing CRC[1,7-8] (see Table 17-1). However, a cause-and-effect relationship between dietary factors and cancer, including CRC, is difficult to establish. Because of inherent limitations associated with study design, the results from epidemiological, animal, and interventional studies examining this relationship have often been conflicting. The precise nature of the relationship of cancer with each nutrient and the actual magnitude of the relationship are not clear. Traditionally, correlation, case-control, and prospective epidemiologic studies and intervention trials have been considered to represent a spectrum of increasing weight of evidence for or against a relationship between dietary factors and cancer risk in nutritional epidemiology. Thus, general conclusions and recommendations regarding the effect of dietary factors on cancer risk have relied heavily on data from large prospective studies and randomized, controlled intervention human trials. For example, an internal panel of experts from the Word Cancer Research Fund, in asso-

TABLE 17-1.

Dietary, Lifestyle, and Other Factors That May Modulate Colorectal Cancer Risk

Positive Association	*Inverse Association*
Energy intake	Fiber
Total, saturated, and animal fats	Vegetables and fruits
Red meat	Calcium
Protein	Vitamin D
Simple sugars	Antioxidant vitamins (A, C, E, and ß-carotene)
Alcohol	Selenium
Smoking	Folate
Iron	Fish oil (omega-3 fatty acid)
Body mass index	Physical activity
	Hormonal replacement therapy
	Aspirin, nonsteroidal anti-inflammatory drugs

TABLE 17-2.

Summary of Evidence for the Role of Dietary and Lifestyle Factors in the Development of Colorectal Cancer*

Evidence	*Decreased Risk*	*No Association*	*Increased Risk*
Convincing	Physical activity Vegetables		
Probable			Red meat Alcohol
Possible	Nonstarch polysaccharides/ Fiber Starch Carotenoids	Calcium Selenium Fish	High body mass index Adult height Frequent eating Sugar Total fat Saturated/animal fat Processed meat Eggs Heavily cooked meat
Insufficient	Resistant starch Vitamins C, D, E Folate, methionine Cereal Coffee		Iron

*Presented by the World Cancer Research Fund/American Institute for Cancer Research in 1997.

ciation with the American Institute for Cancer Research, concluded that the dietary constituents and related factors, the foods and drinks, and the methods of food processing listed in Table 17-2 modify the risk of CRC based on the strength of evidence from observational epidemiologic and intervention studies that was available to the panel in 1997.[1]

This traditional approach to grading epidemiologic evidence concerning the relationship between dietary factors and CRC risk has recently been challenged.[9] It has been argued that drawing a definitive conclusion concerning the effect of dietary factors on CRC risk mainly from large prospective studies and randomized, controlled intervention human trials is probably not the right paradigm of nutritional epidemiology.[9] Rather, it has been articulated that the totality or "portfolio" of evidence from observational and intervention studies as well as animal and in vitro experiments must be analyzed for this purpose because definitive answers to questions about diet and CRC are probably beyond the reach of both observational epidemiologic studies and randomized controlled trials.[9] Epidemiologic and experimental evidence indicating a causal association between a dietary factor and CRC is strengthened when a biologic pathway or mechanism by which colorectal carcinogenesis may be modified is identified and when this mechanism is biologically plausible.[9] It can be argued that epidemiologic data, however strong and consistent, are an inadequate basis for any definite judgment of causality unless supported by mechanistic evidence.[9] Although earlier investigations to elucidate potential anticarcinogenic mechanisms associated with dietary factors have focused on physical properties of these factors, more recent work has expanded into physiological functions and molecular mechanisms. A better mechanistic understanding of how dietary factors can modulate carcinogenesis can lead to a more rational strategy using dietary supplementation to prevent cancer in humans.

Recent advances in molecular epidemiology have added another dimension to the already complex field of nutrition and cancer. Recently identified and characterized single nucleotide polymorphisms and other genetic and epigenetic variants of genes that are involved in absorption, transport, metabolism, and excretion of nutrients have been shown not only to modify CRC risk but also to significantly modulate the effect of nutrients and related compounds on CRC risk.[10] This emerging important topic in the field of nutrition and CRC, termed "gene-nutrient interactions" in colorectal carcinogenesis, has a very significant implication in designing and interpreting data from observational epidemiologic and intervention studies. Although individuals are subjected to the same level of nutritional exposure, systemic and target tissue bioavailability of nutrients and their metabolites, as well as their functional effects in the target tissue, might be vastly different because of genetic and epigenetic variations. Genetic and epigenetic susceptibility to CRC and their interaction with diets and other environmental exposures have not been incorporated into the study design of and interpretation of data from previously published epidemiologic and intervention studies. The precise nature and magnitude of gene-nutrient interactions in colorectal carcinogenesis are yet to be clearly defined.

Given these considerations, the objective of this chapter is a critical analysis of currently available data from epidemiologic and intervention studies in humans of effects of nutritional factors on colorectal carcinogenesis. A comprehensive review of the entire field of nutrition and CRC including biological mechanisms of nutritional modulation of CRC risk is beyond the scope of this chapter, and the readers are referred to several recent comprehensive reviews on this topic.[1,7-8,11]

Primer of Nutritional Epidemiology

Probably the most challenging problem encountered in nutritional epidemiological studies that examine the relationship between dietary factors and CRC risk is the difficulty of accurately assessing intakes of dietary factors.[12] Also, qualitative data on food preparation methods, cooking and chewing, and other dietary habits, which can alter the physiological properties of dietary factors, are often lacking. In addition, it is often difficult to determine the exact intake of nutritional supplements because of the availability of hundreds of different products, both over the counter and by prescription.[12] Another difficulty in assessing supplement use is that many individuals take supplements inconsistently and in patterns that are hard to characterize.[12]

Four types of human epidemiologic studies and animal studies are used to study the relationship between dietary factors and CRC risk.[1,8] Broadly, epidemiologic studies are divided into observational (correlation, case-control, and prospective) and intervention studies.[1,8]

Correlation Studies

Correlation studies examine the relationship between the per capita consumption of a dietary factor and the prevalence of, incidence of, or mortality from CRC in the population. Correlation studies can examine this relationship among populations residing in different countries or among different groups within a country either at a given time or over a certain time (ie, a time-trend analysis). These studies provide provocative initial evidence that a particular dietary factor plays a role in the development of CRC and hence is considered worthy only of hypothesis formation. The limitations with the interpretations of data generated from these correlation studies are several, including the inaccuracy with which dietary intake is assessed. Correlation studies often fail to correct for unmeasured confounding factors that may be responsible for the observed association. Correlation studies also do not control for other dietary variables or for any of the other known risk factors associated with CRC.

Case-Control Studies

Case-control studies compare prior consumption of a dietary factor by subjects with CRC with that by matched control subjects without CRC. Many of the weaknesses of correlation studies can be avoided in case-control studies. Known or suspected potential confounding factors can be controlled or eliminated in the study design or controlled in the data analysis. With regard to dietary factors, the most serious limitation in retrospective studies is the accuracy with which intake of dietary factors or supplementation can be established. Case-control studies often fail to incorporated qualitative data on dietary habits and cooking methods into the nutrient estimation. Also, some individual aspects of diet, especially nutrient content, may not vary greatly within a population, so case-control studies may not show wide ranges of CRC risk within that population. Other common problems are the lack of appropriate controls and selection bias because of the absence of patients who do not survive long enough to be enrolled in the study. Another problem is that it is difficult to adequately control or correct potential confounders in retrospective analyses. Lastly, it is difficult to delineate the effect associated with a dietary factor from other potential anti-carcinogens present in the diet in case-control studies. Although inherent problems associated with retrospective analyses often limit the interpretation of results from case-control studies, valuable information can be gathered from well-designed case-control studies in a time- and cost-effective manner.

Prospective Studies

Prospective (or cohort) studies assess the diets of a large group of healthy individuals and follow the participants over time, during which a number of cohort members will develop CRC. The relationship of CRC to specific characteristics of individuals' diets is then analyzed. Prospective studies avoid most of the methodological problems of crude observational and retrospective epidemiologic studies and can control and correct confounding factors more adequately than can correlation and case-control studies. Also, because of the prospective design—with diet being assessed before the occurrence of cancer—there is little likelihood of selection or recording bias in cohort studies.

One of the weaknesses associated with prospective studies is that they correlate dietary consumption of a nutritional factor at baseline to subsequent incidence of CRC. In other words, the dietary intake at baseline is assumed to reflect past and subsequent consumption. Whether the subjects in these studies change their diet during the follow-up period and how this might affect the study outcome cannot be deduced. However, recent prospective studies obtained repeated assessments of diet at regular intervals, which improves the accuracy of individual dietary assessment. A vast majority of prospective studies are limited by the relatively short follow-up. This issue is important because of the uncertainty regarding the biologically relevant period of exposure before the development of CRC.

Another potential shortcoming that limits the interpretation of results from prospective studies relates to imprecise estimation of dietary intake (as in other types of epidemiological studies), as well as the lack data on food preparation methods, cooking, and chewing, which can alter the physiological properties of dietary factors. Some of prospective studies have selected cohorts with relatively homogeneous lifestyle and dietary habits and, therefore, may be quite unrepresentative of the general population. Therefore, the applicability of the observations made in these cohorts to the general population is uncertain. Another problem is that the range of dietary intake of a nutritional factor under investigation may be narrow, so that the factor's effects may not be observed.

Intervention Studies

In theory, randomized intervention studies in humans should provide definitive support for the purported cause-and-effect relationship between a dietary factor and CRC. However, intervention studies are often exceedingly difficult to carry out because of the slowly progressive nature of neoplastic transformation and the large number of subjects necessary to achieve an adequate statistical power. The major weaknesses associated with the majority of published intervention studies are short follow-up periods, small numbers of subjects, poor compliance with dietary interventions, high dropout rates, and use of surrogate end point biomarkers (SEPB) of CRC as the outcome instead of using occurrence or recurrence of CRC.[13] All SEPBs have limitations, and most have not been conclusively validated in clinical studies.[13] Furthermore, except for few biomarkers (eg, adenomas[14-15]), modulating any of these SEPBs has not yet clearly lead to a reduction in CRC occurrence and mortality.[13] Even with adenomas, only a very small portion of adenomas progress to adenocarcinoma, depending on the number, size, and histological features.[14-15] Therefore, using the recurrence of all adenomas as the endpoint of intervention trials may not be most appropriate; rather, advanced adenomas (defined as those >1 cm in diameter or those with either a villous component or high-grade dysplasia) that have been shown to possess a high degree of neoplastic transformation potential might be a better SEPB for this purpose.[14,15]

Another problem is that intervention studies attempt to intervene in incompletely understood biological pathways in special populations of adults at high risk of developing CRC who therefore may be at a late, although preclinical, stage of carcinogenesis or have precancerous lesions. In non-blind studies of foods, individuals in the control group may adopt the dietary behavior of the treatment group if they think the treatment diet is beneficial, which could obscure a real benefit of treatment. In addition, the time between the change in the level of a dietary factor and any expected change in the incidence of CRC (ie, relevant induction time) is usually uncertain and may be decades long. Trials should, therefore, be of a long duration.

Another potential problem lies with uncertainty regarding what constitutes biologically relevant doses of dietary intervention that may modulate colorectal carcinogenesis. Also, people who agree to participate in trials tend to be relatively health conscious and highly motivated; people who are at high potential risk on the basis of dietary intake, and thus susceptible to intervention, are liable to be underrepresented. Hence, the validity of generalizing the results is limited.

In general, observational epidemiologic studies suggest a stronger association between a dietary factor and CRC risk than do intervention studies.[1,8] Findings from randomized controlled intervention trials often do not confirm the relationships between nutrients and CRC risk that have been suggested by observational studies (eg, low-fat, high-fiber, high-vegetables/fruits and colorectal adenoma recurrence[16]; high-fiber and colorectal adenoma recurrence[17]; low-fat, high-fiber and colorectal adenoma recurrence[18]; and antioxidant vitamins and colorectal adenoma recurrence[19]). In some studies, only a modest degree of CRC risk reduction, significantly less than that previously suggested by observations studies, has been demonstrated (eg, low-fat, high-fiber and colorectal adenoma recurrence,[20] and calcium and colorectal adenoma recurrence[21]). In some cases, trials have even demonstrated that high doses of nutrients previously believed to be beneficial could have unexpected harmful effects (eg, ß-carotene and lung cancer[22,23]). Some intervention studies have uncovered beneficial effects of nutrients on CRC that were not hypothesized a priori as the primary endpoints (eg, selenium and CRC[24]).

It has recently been suggested that intervention studies should not be considered as an epidemiological "gold standard."[25] According to Byers, controlled trials in which intervention shows beneficial effects are good evidence that the agents used are protective.[25] Studies in which intervention shows no effect, or even a detrimental effect,

TABLE 17-3.

Possible Anticarcinogenic Mechanisms of Dietary Fiber

Increased Stool Bulk

Dilution of potential carcinogens
Decrease in transit time (less contact time for carcinogens)

Binding With Potential Carcinogens/Binding with Bile Acids

Decrease in fecal bile acid concentrations
Prevention of the conversion of primary to secondary bile acids

Lower Fecal pH

Reduced solubility of free bile acids
Inhibition of 7α-dehydroxylase, which converts primary to secondary bile acids
Inhibition of bacterial degradation of normal fecal constituents to potential carcinogens

Alteration of Colonic Microflora

Inhibition of microbial enzymes involved in carcinogen activation
Changes in bacterial species
Stimulation of bacterial growth, which increases fecal bulk

Fermentation by Fecal Floral to Short-Chain Fatty Acids

Inhibition of cell growth and proliferation
Induction of differentiation
Induction of apoptosis
Modulation of gene expression
Prevention/reduction of insulin resistance and hyperinsulemia

however, do not show that the agents used are irrelevant or harmful in the context of whole diets or among normal, healthy populations.[25] Byers argues that the results of intervention studies should not be treated as a refutation of evidence from other types of epidemiologic study, especially when such other evidence is backed by data from animal studies and identification of plausible biological pathways.[25]

ANIMAL STUDIES

Studies utilizing laboratory animals provide for greater control of variables, enable interventions to be used that would not be feasible in humans, and they are often less expensive than human trials. Furthermore, potential biological pathways or mechanisms by which colorectal carcinogenesis may be modified by dietary factors can be investigated in a time- and cost-efficient manner. However, animal studies lack uniform protocols in terms of carcinogen, route of administration, and dose as well as the species, strain, and age of the animals. Most importantly, they suffer from their inherent differences from human CRC, precluding direct extrapolation of observations from animal studies to humans.

Specific Dietary Factors Implicated in Colorectal Carcinogenesis

FIBER

The role of dietary fiber in the development of CRC was first recognized in the early 1970s, when Burkitt noted the rarity of CRC in most African populations with high intake of fiber and low intake of refined carbohydrates.[26] There exist several biologically plausible physiological, cellular, and molecular mechanisms by which dietary fiber can protect against the development of CRC as outlined in Table 17-3.[27] Most of the published correlation and case-control studies show either a strong or a moderate protective effect of dietary fiber or "fiber-rich foods" or show equivocal results that were nevertheless consistent with the fiber hypothesis.[27] Three analyses of case-control studies, conducted in combined analysis or meta-analysis formats, suggest, on average, a 50% reduction in the risk of CRC in individuals with the highest dietary fiber intake, compared with those with the lowest fiber intake.[28-30] Most of the positive case-control studies and one combined analysis of case-control studies show a significant inverse dose-dependent relationship between dietary fiber intake and CRC risk.[27-30] The strongest argument for the fiber hypothesis that can be made from case-control studies is the remarkable consistency of the protective effect of dietary fiber among studies conducted in populations with different patterns of diet and CRC.[27,29]

By contrast, published large prospective studies have produced equivocal findings. The Second Cancer Prevention Study of the American Cancer Society, involving more than 1 million subjects, showed a significant inverse relationship with a 30% reduction of CRC mortality in subjects consuming the highest amount of dietary fiber compared with those consuming the lowest amount.[31] Three large prospective studies conducted in the United States—the Nurses' Health Study (n=88,757; follow-up=6 to 16 years),[32,33] the Iowa Women's Health Study (n=35,216; follow-up=4 years),[34] and the Health Professionals Follow-up Study (n=47,949; follow-up=6 years)[35]—have shown no significant association between dietary fiber intake and CRC incidence in men and women. These studies, however, have shown a significant protective effect of dietary fiber against distal colon and rectal adenomas in men (35% to 63% reduction in the risk),[36-37] but not in women.[33] The Finnish Alpha-Tocopherol, Beta-Carotene Cancer Prevention Study found no fiber-CRC association after following more than 27,000 male smokers for 8 years.[38] Two most recent prospective studies, however, have demonstrated a significant protective effect of fiber on CRC.[39,40] The European Prospective Investigation into Cancer and Nutrition (EPIC), involving 519,978 adults recruited from 10 European countries, showed a significant inverse relationship between fiber intake and CRC risk after 4.5 years of follow-up.[39] Those in the highest quintile of fiber intake (32 g/day in women and 36 g/day in men) had a significant 40% reduction in CRC risk compared with the lowest quintile (12.6 g/day in women and 12.8 g/day in men) [relative risk=0.58, 95% confidence interval (CI), 0.41 to 0.85).[39] However, no food source of fiber was significantly more protective than others.[39] Another study in 43,611 participants in a multi-center, randomized trial designed to investigate methods for early detection of cancer (the Prostate, Lung, Colorectal, and Ovarian [PLCO] Cancer Screening Trial) in the United States found a significant dose-responsive inverse association between the fiber and intake colorectal adenoma risk.[40] Those in the highest quintile of fiber intake were 27% less likely to have adenoma than were those in the lowest quintile (odds ratio=0.73; 95% CI, 0.62 to 0.86).[40] The inverse association was significant for fiber from grains and cereals and from fruits but not fiber from legumes and vegetables.[40] The conflicting results from these well-designed and well-conducted large prospective studies naturally beg for possible explanations. The observed differences might be partially explained by different sources, types, and amounts of dietary fiber in different populations studied and by methods used for the analysis of dietary fiber.[41]

Although earlier small pilot trials showed the beneficial effect of fiber supplement on adenoma recurrence or regression and on SEPBs of CRC,[27] more recent, larger placebo-controlled randomized trials have generally shown no beneficial effect associated with dietary fiber supplementation, either alone or in combination with other dietary strategies, on adenoma recurrence (Table 17-4).[16-18,20] Of particular importance is the null effect of dietary fiber from the two largest trials published to date (see Table 17-4).[16-17] The Polyp Prevention Trial, a multi-institutional intervention study in the United States, was designed to test the ability of a low-fat (20% of total calories), high-fiber (18 g/1000 kcal daily) diet enriched with vegetables and fruits (3.5 servings/1000 kcal daily) to decrease the recurrence rate of colorectal adenomas in patients previously treated for colorectal adenomas.[16] After 4 years of follow-up, no significant difference in adenoma recurrence was observed between the treatment and placebo groups among the 1905 subjects who completed the trial.[16] The Wheat Bran Fiber trial, a multi-center study from the Phoenix, Arizona, randomized 1429 subjects with colorectal adenomas after polypectomy to receive dietary supplementation with either high (13.5 g/day) or low (2 g/day) amount of wheat bran fiber for 3 years.[17] This study demonstrated no significant protective effect of high fiber supplementation on adenoma recurrence.[17] One recently published trial, the European Cancer Prevention Organisation Intervention Study (n=665; 3 years of follow-up),[42] indicated that fiber supplementation (3.5 g ispaghula husk) was associated with a significant 67% increase in adenoma recurrence (see Table 17-4). A recent meta-analysis of the randomized controlled trial data (5 studies, n=4349) found no evidence that increased dietary fiber reduces either incidence or recurrence of adenomas within a 2- to 4-year period.[43]

As discussed in the previous section, randomized intervention trials utilizing fiber supplementation are limited by several factors: 1) uncertainty concerning the optimal timing, duration, and dose of fiber intervention; 2) use of SEPBs; 3) a small number of subjects; 4) possibility of over- and under-reporting of dietary fiber consumption by study participants; and 5) lack of incorporation of genetic variability in metabolism of fiber into the study design. Therefore, randomized intervention trials cannot definitively rule out the beneficial effect of dietary fiber that has been shown to be associated with a lower risk of CRC in observational studies.

The relationship between dietary fiber and CRC risk provides an excellent case study in nutrition and CRC and highlight inherent, probably unresolvable, limitations of currently available tools to detect a real effect associated with dietary fiber. In summary, currently available evidence from observational epidemiological and intervention studies does not unequivocally support the protective role of fiber against the development of CRC. However, when the portfolio of evidence from these studies is analyzed critically, the overall conclusion supports an inverse association between dietary fiber intake and CRC risk. The magnitude of CRC risk reduction and threshold level above which dietary fiber is associated with a significant degree of CRC risk reduction are not clearly defined. The duration and timing of fiber supplementation, as well as which specific target groups would benefit most from fiber supplementation, are not well established.

Vegetables and Fruits

Among dietary factors implicated in the development of CRC, the inverse relationship between vegetable and fruit consumption and CRC risk has long been considered to represent the strongest epidemiologic evidence. Despite

TABLE 17-4.

Summary of Recent Fiber Colorectal Cancer Chemoprevention Trials

Study (Reference)	Subjects (N)	Intervention	Duration	Endpoint	Outcome
Toronto Polyp Prevention Group[18]	Adenoma (201)	20% fat calories/day 50 g fiber/day vs placebo	2 years	Adenoma recurrence	No effect
Australian Polyp Prevention Project[20]	Adenoma (424)	2 x 2 x 2 factorial <25% fat calories/day 25 g wheat bran/day 20 mg ß-carotene/day	4 years	Adenoma recurrence	Fiber alone no effect Fiber with low fat protective against >10 mm adenomas
Wheat Bran Fiber Trial[17]	Adenoma (1429)	Wheat bran fiber 13.5/day vs 2.0 g/day	3 years	Adenoma recurrence	No effect
Polyp Prevention Trial[16]	Adenoma (1905)	20% fat calories/day 18 g fiber/100 kcal/day 3.5 servings of fruits & vegetables/1000 kcal/day vs placebo	4 years	Adenoma recurrence	No effect
European Cancer Prevention Organisation Intervention Study[42]	Adenoma (665)	2 g calcium/day 2.5 g ispaghula husk/day vs placebo	3 years	Adenoma recurrence	67% increase in adenoma recurrence (P=0.042)

the paucity of supporting data from randomized studies, an international panel of experts from the World Cancer Research Fund concluded that "evidence that diets rich in vegetables protect against cancers of the colon and rectum is convincing. The data on fruit are more limited and inconsistent; no judgment is possible."[1] This strong endorsement for the purported protective role of vegetable consumption in CRC was based on observational epidemiologic evidence that was available to the panel in 1997. The overwhelming majority of the published correlation and case-control studies suggest the protective effect of high consumption of vegetables and fruits on the risk of CRC and adenomas; the effect is more pronounced for vegetables than for fruits.[1,7,8,44,45] A meta-analysis of six case-control studies of vegetables and colon cancer reported a 52% reduction in the risk of colon cancer associated with the highest consumption of vegetables compared with the lowest consumption.[28]

Large prospective studies published before 1997 also generally support the protective role of high vegetable and fruit consumption in colorectal carcinogenesis. The study of Seventh-Day Adventists (n=25,943) reported a 30% reduction in the risk of fatal colon cancer in women consuming ≥7 servings of green salad/week compared to that in those consuming <4 servings/week.[46] In the Second Cancer Prevention Study of the American Cancer Society, a statistically significant inverse association between vegetable consumption and the risk of fatal colon cancer was observed in both men and women with a 25% to 38% reduction in the risk of fatal colon cancer in subjects consuming the highest amount of vegetables compared with those consuming the lowest.[31]

In a US cohort of elderly persons (the Leisure World Study; n=11,580), a significantly reduced risk of colon cancer was noted for combined intake of all vegetables and fruits and for fruit intake alone in women but not in men.[47] In the Iowa Women's Health Study involving 98,030 postmenopausal women, the total intake of both vegetables and fruits did not significantly reduce the risk of CRC.[34] When each vegetable or fruit item was independently analyzed, it was shown that individuals consuming more than 1 garlic per week had a 32% reduction in the risk of CRC compared to those not eating any garlic.[34] The protective effect of garlic on CRC risk has recently been supported by a meta-analysis of 7 case-control and prospective studies that showed that high garlic consumption (>28.8 g/week) was associated with a significant 30% reduction in CRC risk compared with low consumption (<3.5 g/week) (relative risk [RR]), 0.69; 95% CI, 0.55-0.89).[48] One study of colorectal adenomas in men (the Health Professionals Follow-Up Study) reported an approximate 50% reduction of colorectal adenoma risk associated with high intake of vegetables and fruits.[36]

However, large prospective studies published after 1997 with conflicting results have dampened the enthusiasm for the protective role of vegetable and fruit consumption

TABLE 17-5.

Potential Anticarcinogens in Vegetables and Fruits

Carotenoids	Dithiothiones
Ascrobate	Glucosinolate/indoles
Tocopherols	Isothiocyanates/thiocyanates
Selenium	Allium compounds
Folate	Plant sterols
Dietary fiber	Isoflavones
	Protease inhibitors
	Coumarins

in colorectal carcinogenesis. The Health professionals' Follow-up Study (n=47,325, 10 years of follow-up) and the Nurses' Health Study (n=88,764, 16 years of follow-up) reported that consumption of vegetables and fruits does not confer protection against CRC in men and women.[49] There was no appreciable benefit from any of the specific subgroup fruits and vegetables considered.[49] The only exception was prune consumption; the RR of colon cancer associated with a 1-serving-per-day higher prune consumption was 1.46 (95% CI, 0.93 to 2.31) among women and 1.73 (95% CI, 1.20 to 2.50) among men.[49] By contrast, a prospective study of a population-based cohort of 61,463 Swedish women (ages 40 to 74 years, 9.6 years of follow-up), who had been on a mammography screening program, reported a significant dose-dependent inverse relationship between consumption of vegetables and fruits and CRC risk 50. Total consumption of >5 servings of vegetables and fruits per day was associated with a 27% reduction in the risk of CRC (RR, 0.73; 95% CI, 0.56 to 0.96), compared with risk of those whose total consumption was <2.5 servings per day.[50] Subanalyses showed that this association was due largely to fruit consumption and was stronger for rectal cancer than for colon cancer 50. This study also showed a significant dose-dependent inverse association between consumption of vegetables and fruits and CRC risk among individuals taking less than 2.5 servings per day (P=0.001).[50] Total vegetable and fruit consumption <1.5 servings per day was associated with a 65% increase in CRC risk compared with consumption of >2.5 servings per day (RR, 1.65; 95% CI, 1.23 to 2.20).[50]

In the Netherlands Cohort Study on Diet and Cancer (n=120,852; 6.3 years of follow-up), no significant associations with total vegetable intake or total fruit intake for colon cancer.[51] However, among women, an inverse association was observed with vegetables and fruits combined [for the highest consumption versus the lowest, RR was 0.66 (95% CI, 0.44 to 1.01).[51] Brassica vegetables and cooked leafy vegetables showed inverse associations for both men and women.[51] For rectal cancer, no significant associations were found for vegetable consumption or fruit consumption or for specific groups of vegetables and fruits.[51] The Breast Cancer Detection Demonstration Project (n=45,490 women; 9 years of follow-up) reported no significant associations between vegetable and fruit intake and the risk of CRC.[52]

To date, only one randomized intervention human trial that used high consumption of vegetables and fruits as a dietary strategy has been reported.[16] In the Polyp Prevention Trial, a low-fat (20% of total calories), high-fiber (18 g/1000 kcal daily) diet enriched with vegetables and fruits (3.5 servings/1000 kcal daily) did not significantly reduce colorectal adenoma recurrence compared with placebo.[16]

In summary, in contrast to the strong endorsement for the protective role of vegetables in colorectal carcinogenesis by the World Cancer Research Fund,[1] currently available evidence from epidemiologic and intervention studies is conflicting with regard to the association between vegetable and fruit consumption and CRC risk. Again, this conflict is likely due to limitations of currently available tools to detect a real effect associated with vegetables and fruits, as discussed earlier. Vegetables and fruits contain a large number of substances that possess anticarcinogenic properties (Table 17-5).[7,53-54] These compounds have both complementary and overlapping mechanisms of action, including the induction of detoxification enzymes, inhibition of nitrosamine formation, provision of substrate for formation of antineoplastic agents, dilution, and binding of carcinogens in the digestive tract, alteration of hormone metabolism, antioxidant activity, stimulation of the immune system, and others mechanisms.[1,53-54] The existence of plausible anticarcinogenic mechanisms and the portfolio of epidemiologic evidence generally support the inverse association between vegetable and fruit consumption and CRC risk. Collectively, observational epidemiological studies suggest decreased CRC risk particularly with raw vegetables, green vegetables, and cruciferous vegetables.[7-9,44-45] Furthermore, garlic consumption [34,48], as discussed earlier, and consumption of tomatoes, tomato-based products, and lycopene,[55] as recent evidence indicates, appear to be particularly protective against CRC development.

FAT AND CHOLESTEROL

The majority of correlation and case-control studies suggest a positive association between dietary fat intake and CRC incidence and mortality.[1,7-8] However, a number of these studies failed to adjust for total energy intake, another possible risk factor for CRC.[1,7-8] In this regard, a recent combined analysis of 13 case-control studies of CRC involving 5,287 cases and 10,478 controls from various populations with differing cancer rates and dietary practices demonstrated no evidence of any increased risk with higher dietary fat after adjustment for total energy intake.[56] There were no statistically significant associations for any type of fat (ie, total, saturated, monounsaturated, and polyunsaturated fats) in sub-group analyses.[56] Four large, prospective studies—the Iowa Women's Study,[57] the Health Professionals Follow-up Study[35] and the Netherlands Cohort Study on Diet and Cancer[58,59]—did not find any significant association between total fat intake and CRC risk. However, in the Nurses' Health Study, the highest intake of total fat was associated with a significant 2-fold increase in the risk for colon cancer compared with the lowest intake of total fat.[32] The Nurses' Health Study[32] and the Netherlands Cohort Study[58] demonstrated that a high intake of animal and saturated fat was associated with a significantly increased risk of CRC in women, whereas the other three prospective studies did not show appreciable association.[35,57,59] Of the four prospective studies that examined the risk of CRC in association with intakes of monounsaturated fatty acids,[32,35,57-58] only the Nurses' Health Study reported a significantly increased risk.[32] Three prospective studies[35,57-58] have demonstrated a weakly decreased risk of CRC with high intake of polyunsaturated fat. Therefore, there is evidence, albeit not entirely consistent and convincing, that high intakes of animal and saturated fat are associated with increased CRC risk. Evidence for intakes of total fat, monounsaturated and polyunsaturated fatty acids are inconsistent.

Three randomized intervention studies have been published concerning the effect of low-fat diet on colorectal adenoma recurrence. In the trial reported by the Toronto Polyp Prevention Group from Canada,[18] a diet low in fat (<50 g/day or 20% of energy) and high in fiber (50 g/day) did not significantly reduce colorectal adenoma recurrence compared with placebo after 2 years of intervention. In the Australian Polyp Prevention Project,[20] neither low-fat intervention (<25% of energy) nor high-fiber intake (25 g wheat bran supplement per day) significantly reduced the rate of colorectal adenoma recurrence. However, the low-fat diet combined with wheat bran supplementation significantly reduced the recurrence rate of large adenomas (>10 mm) after 4 years of follow-up.[20] The largest randomized study published to date, the Polyp Prevention Trial, demonstrated no protective effect of a low-fat diet (20% of total calories) in conjunction with high-fiber (18 g/1000 kcal daily) and high intakes of vegetables and fruits (3.5 servings/1000 kcal daily) on the recurrence rate of colorectal adenomas after 4 years of intervention.[16]

Another randomized intervention study utilizing a low-fat component for the nutritional chemoprevention of CRC is currently underway in the United States. The Women's Health Initiative is an ongoing, multi-center clinical trial that will include approximately 64,500 postmenopausal women (age 50 to 79 years) in a 3x2x2 factorial intervention involving hormones, calcium, vitamin D, and a low-fat dietary plan 60. The primary end points of this trial are incident colorectal and breast cancer, coronary heart disease and other cardiovascular disease, and hip and other fractures.

The evidence is conflicting for the effects of cholesterol on CRC and adenoma incidence and mortality. Earlier case-control and prospective studies including the Framingham Study, the Multiple Risk Factor Intervention Trial (MRFIT), and the Honolulu Japanese-Hawaiian Study suggested an inverse association between cholesterol levels and CRC incidence and mortality.[1] Other prospective studies did not confirm this purported inverse relationship, and some found a positive association between serum cholesterol levels and CRC risk.[1] It was suggested that the inverse association might be caused by the metabolic effects of undiagnosed cancer on serum cholesterol levels.[1] In a combined analysis of 13 case-control studies of CRC, which involved 5,287 cases and 10,478 controls, a weak, albeit significant, increase (of 30%) in risk with higher dietary cholesterol was reported.[56] Two most recent, large prospective studies (the Iowa Women's Study[57] and the Health Professionals Follow-up Study[35]), however, found no significant relationship between dietary cholesterol intake and the risk of CRC.

MEAT

The majority of correlation and case-control studies suggest a positive association between meat intake and CRC risk.[1,7,8] However, the evidence from large prospective studies is conflicting. The Iowa Women's Study,[57] the Second Cancer Prevention Study of the American Cancer Society,[31] the Netherlands Cohort Study on Diet and Cancer,[58] the Finnish study,[61] and the New York University Women's Health Study[62] suggest no association between meat intakes and CRC incidence and mortality. In contrast, the Nurses' Health Study[32] reported that women who consumed red meat frequently had a 2.5-fold increased risk of colon cancer than the risk in those who rarely consumed red meat. The Health Professionals Follow-up Study[35] also reported that men who consumed 5 or more servings per week of beef, pork, or lamb had a 1.7-fold increased risk of colon cancer, compared with men who consumed these products less than once per month.

It is difficult to accurately assess dietary intake of meat because of variable preparation time (eg, rare, medium, well done), cooking methods (eg, charcoal, barbecue, frying), and fat content in meat and uncertainty whether fat was removed prior to cooking.[1,8] It is also difficult to rule out the confounding effects of other potential carcinogens present in red meat (eg, iron). Several case-control studies as well as large prospective studies using the First National Health and Nutrition Examination Survey in the United States have suggested a positive association between body iron stores and CRC.[1,63-64]

Another potential confounder is protein present in red meat. However, large prospective studies[35,57-59] do not support a positive association between animal protein intake and CRC risk as suggested by observations from some case-control studies.[1,7]

Generally, observational studies, including the Iowa Women's Health Study[57] and the Health Professionals Follow-up Study,[35] suggest no appreciable relationship between poultry consumption and CRC risk.[1,7] In the Nurses' Health Study,[32] however, consumption of chicken without skin, at least 5 times per week was associated with a statistically significant decreased risk of colon cancer compared with consumption less than once per month.

For meat and fat, there exist a number of biological plausible anticarcinogenic mechanisms. Cooked meat, especially high in fat and cooked at high temperature, produces carcinogens such as heterocyclic amines, polycyclic aromatic hydrocarbons, and nitrosamines, which

TABLE 17-6.

Summary of Antioxidant Colorectal Cancer Chemoprevention Trials

Study (Reference)	Subjects (N)	Intervention	Duration	Endpoint	Outcome
Toronto Polyp Prevention Group[18]	Adenomas (137)	Vitamins C (400 mg/day) + E (400 mg/day) vs placebo	2 years	Adenoma recurrence	No effect
Roncucci L, et al[74]	Adenomas (255)	Vitamins A (30,000 IU/day) + C (1000 mg/day) + E (400 mg/day) vs lactulose vs placebo	18 months	Adenoma recurrence	Vitamin mixture protective; Lactulose also protective
Australian Polyp Prevention Project[20]	Adenomas (424)	2 x 2 x 2 factorial <25% fat calories/day 25 g wheat bran/day 20 mg ß-carotene/day	4 years	Adenoma recurrence	ß-carotene—no effect
Antioxidant Polyp Prevention Study[19]	Adenomas (864)	25 mg ß-carotene/day vs 1000 mg ascorbic acid/day vs 1000 mg ascorbic acid/day + 400 mg α-tocopherol/day vs placebo	4 years	Adenoma recurrence	No effect; ß-carotene reduced the risk of recurrence by 44% in nonsmokers and nondrinkers (RR=0.56; 95% CI, 0.35 to 0.89) but increased the risk by 2-fold in smokers and drinkers (RR=2.07; 95% CI, 1.39 to 3.08)[75]

can potentially induce DNA adduct formation, DNA damage, and mutations.[7] Dietary fat also enhances cholesterol and bile acid synthesis by the liver, increasing the amount of these sterols in the colonic lumen. Colonic bacteria convert these compounds to secondary bile acids, cholesterol metabolites, and other potentially toxic metabolic compounds.[7] These compounds are known to damage the colonic mucosa, increase the proliferative activity of the epithelium, activate secondary cellular transduction signals, alter membrane fluidity, and alter prostaglandins metabolism.[7] More recently, polymorphisms of several genes encoding detoxifying enzymes—including P450, N-acetyltransferase (NAT), and glutathione-S-transferase (GSH), which handle toxic compounds resulting from cooking meat and fat—have been observed to modify CRC risk associated with high dietary fat and meat consumption.[7]

ANTIOXIDANT VITAMINS

The antioxidant micronutrients—including vitamin A, carotenoids, vitamin C, vitamin E, selenium, zinc, copper, iron, and manganese—are part of the body's defense against free radicals and reactive oxygen species. These antioxidants are thought to convey protection via a host of different mechanisms including trapping and neutralization of free radicals and reactive oxygen species, protection against lipid peroxidation in cell membranes, potentiation of immune responses, reduction in mutation rates, antiproliferation, and inhibition of nitrosamine and nitrosamide formation.[65]

Relatively few epidemiological studies have addressed dietary antioxidant intake and the risk of CRC. Reported studies are plagued by problems of inaccuracy in determining dietary or blood levels of antioxidant vitamins.[65] The Iowa Women's Health Study[66] reported no significant association between intakes of vitamins A and C and CRC risk. However, total vitamin E intake (dietary plus supplemental) and supplemental vitamin E intake, but not dietary vitamin E intake, were inversely associated with CRC risk in this study.[66] The Nurses' Health study, however, did not show a significant association between vitamin E intake and colon cancer risk.[32] In a US cohort of elderly persons (the Leisure World Study; n=11,580), a significantly reduced risk of colon cancer was noted for intake of dietary vitamin C and for supplemental use of vitamins A and C in women but not in men.[47] The Second Cancer Prevention Study of the American Cancer Society involving 711,891 men and women followed for 14 years did not find a substantial effect of vitamin C or E supplement use on overall CRC mortality.[67] In the same cohort, multivitamin use alone or in combination with vitamin A, C, or E had minimal effect on cancer mortality overall, although mortality from all cancers combined was increased among male current smokers but decreased in male who had never or formerly smoked.[68] Other large prospective studies (the Nurses' Health Study, the Health Professionals Follow-up Study, and the Second Cancer Prevention Study of the American Cancer Society) have suggested a long-term use of multivitamins (>10 to 15 years) containing antioxidants and folic acid reduces CRC incidence and mortality.[69-72] It is unclear, however, which components of multivitamin preparations have played a major role in CRC prevention in these studies.

Five small pilot trials studies suggested that antioxidant vitamins, either alone or in combination, improve proliferation labeling indices,[73] but these studies are severely limited by study design. As shown in Table 17-6, more recent and larger well-designed and conducted randomized human trials (the Toronto Polyp Prevention Study, the Australian Polyp Prevention Project, and the Antioxidant Polyp Prevention Study) do not support the protective role of antioxidant vitamins on colorectal carcinogenesis.[18-20] One exception is the Italian trial that reported a significant protective effect of the combination of vitamins A, C, and E on the rate of colorectal adenoma recurrence after 18 months of intervention (see Table 17-6).[74] However, this study was not a real randomized trial.

Of particular importance is the Antioxidant Polyp Prevention Study that randomized 864 patients into four groups using a factorial design: 1) placebo, 2) ß-carotene (25 mg/day), 3) vitamins C (ascorbic acid; 1000 mg/day) and E (α-tocopherol; 400 mg/day), and 4) ß-carotene plus vitamin C.[19] After 4 years of follow-up, this study showed no beneficial effect on adenoma recurrence from the antioxidant vitamins. A recent subgroup analysis of this trial demonstrated a very interesting interaction between ß-carotene and smoking and alcohol.[75] Among subjects who neither smoked cigarettes nor drank alcohol, ß-carotene was associated with a marked decrease in the risk of recurrent adenomas (RR, 0.56; 95% CI, 0.35 to 0.89), but ß-carotene supplementation conferred a modest increase in the risk of recurrence among those who smoked (RR, 1.36; 95% CI, 0.70 to 2.62) or drank (RR, 1.13; 95% CI, 0.89 to 1.43). For those who smoked cigarettes and also drank more than one alcohol drink per day, ß-carotene doubled the risk of adenoma recurrence (RR, 2.07; 95% CI, 1.39 to 3.08). This analysis therefore suggests that ß-carotene may have both proneoplastic and antineoplastic effects depending on smoking and alcohol status.

Four large trials that adopted ß-carotene supplementation as a preventive strategy for cardiovascular disease and cancer have produced either disappointing or alarming results. The Finnish Alpha-Tocopherol, Beta-Carotene (ATBC) Study (male smokers; ages 50 to 69 years; n=29,133; follow-up= 5 to 8 years) found that ß-carotene (20 mg/day) increased the risk of lung cancer (by 18%) and total mortality compared with placebo.[22] The American Beta-Carotene and Retinol Efficacy Trial (CARET; smokers; ages 45-74 years; n=18,314; follow-up=4 years) reported that ß-carotene (30 mg/day) administered with retinol (25,000 IU/day) increased the risk of lung cancer by 28% and total mortality.[23]

By contrast, two large trials—the Physicians' Health Study (22,071 male physicians; 40 to 84 years of age; 12 years of follow-up) 76 and the Women's Health Study (39,876 healthy female health professionals 2.1 years' treatment plus another 2.0 years' follow-up) 77—found no benefit or harm from ß-carotene supplementation (50 mg/day) on the incidence of cancer. These 2 latter studies recruited healthy male and female physicians who had a low prevalence of smoking. These findings collectively suggest that ß-carotene likely has no appreciable protective effect on cancer but can increase cancer risk in cigarette smokers. Also, some of these trials (the ATBC and the CARET) suggested that alcohol consumption increases lung cancer risk among ß-carotene-supplemented subjects.[78-79] In none of these trials did ß-carotene supplementation increase the risk of CRC, even among subjects who smoked or drank alcohol.[78-81]

It is evident from the above discussion that antioxidant vitamins should not be routinely used as a chemopreventive agent against CRC. As a matter of fact, the US Preventive Services Task Force (USPSTF) has recently concluded that the evidence is insufficient to recommend for or against the use of supplements of vitamins A, C, or E; multivitamins with folic acid; or antioxidant combinations for the prevention of cancer or cardiovascular disease.[82-83] For ß-carotene, the USPSTF concluded that ß-carotene supplements, either alone or in combination, are unlikely to provide important benefits in the prevention of cancer or cardiovascular disease and might cause harm in some groups.[82-83]

FOLATE

Folate is a water-soluble B vitamin that appears to play an important role in the pathogenesis of several disorders in humans including anemia, cardiovascular disease, neural tube defects, neuropsychiatric disorders and cancer.[84-85] Folic acid is the fully oxidized monoglutamyl form of this vitamin that is used commercially in supplements and in fortified foods. An accumulating body of evidence over the past decade suggests that folate status (assessed by dietary intake or by the measurement of blood folate levels) is inversely related to the risk of sporadic and ulcerative colitis-associated CRC or its precursor, adenomas.[84-87]

Collectively, over 20 case-control studies suggest an approximately 40% reduction in the risk of colorectal adenomas and cancer in individuals with the highest dietary intake and/or blood concentrations of folate compared with those with the lowest intake and/or blood concentrations.[84-87] Several large prospective studies (the Health Professionals Follow-up Study, the Nurses' Health Study, the First National Health and Nutrition Examination Survey Epidemiologic Follow-up Study, the Iowa Women's Health Study, and the Netherlands Cohort Study on Diet and Cancer) also suggest a 40% reduction in the risk of colorectal adenomas and cancer in those with the highest intake of folate compared with those with the lowest intake.[69,88-93] A recent meta-analysis of 11 prospective studies from the United States, Canada, the Netherlands, and Sweden including over 500,000 male and female subjects demonstrated a significant inverse association between folate intake (dietary and supplemental) and the risk of CRC (David Hunter, presented at the 2003 Environmental Mutagen Society Colon Cancer Conference, Miami Beach, FL, May 14 to 16, 2003). This meta-analysis also showed a 20% reduction in the risk of CRC in subjects with the highest folate intake compared with those with the lowest intake. Some epidemiologic studies have shown a beneficial effect of multivitamin supplements containing ≥400 µg folic acid for ≥15 years on CRC risk and mortality.[69-71] In some epidemiologic studies, the observed inverse association between folate status and CRC risk was further modified by the intake of alcohol, a known folate antagonist 94, and other methyl group donors (eg, methionine, vitamins B6 and B12) that are involved in the folate metabolic pathway.[84-87] The role of folate in colorectal carcinogenesis has been further

TABLE 17-7.

Potential Mechanisms of the Folate Deficiency-Mediated Colorectal Carcinogenesis

DNA damage, uracil misincorporation, impaired DNA repair
Increased mutagenesis
Aberrant genomic and site-specific DNA methylation
Hyperproliferation
Abnormal apoptosis
Polymorphisms of genes involved in the folate metabolic pathway and related gene-nutrient interactions

strengthened by the observations that genetic polymorphisms in the folate metabolic pathway (eg, the methylenetetrahydrofolate reductase C677T polymorphism) modify CRC risk.[95,96]

Although there is no definitive evidence supporting the protective effect of folate supplementation on colorectal carcinogenesis from human experiments at present, several small intervention studies have demonstrated that folate supplementation can improve or reverse SEPBs of CRC.[84,85] The data from animal studies generally support a causal relationship between folate depletion and CRC risk and an inhibitory effect of modest levels of folate supplementation on colorectal carcinogenesis.[85] However, animal studies have also shown that folate supplementation may increase CRC risk and accelerate CRC progression if too much is given or if it is provided after neoplastic foci are established in the colorectum.[85]

In summary, a growing body of observational epidemiologic studies has suggested that folate deficiency increases whereas folate supplementation decreases the risk of CRC. Although the results from these studies are not uniformly consistent, the portfolio of evidence strongly supports the inverse association between folate status and CRC risk. Several potential mechanisms relating to the disruption of the known biochemical function of folate (mediating the transfer of 1-carbon moieties and consequent DNA synthesis and methylation) exist to support the role of folate in colorectal carcinogenesis (Table 17-7).[84,94,97-98]

ALCOHOL

Most correlation and case-control studies that have examined alcohol consumption suggest a positive association between alcohol intake and colorectal neoplasia.[1,7-8,73,99] Some studies have suggested greater risks in the rectum than in the colon and with beer consumption than with other types of liquor.[1,7-8,73,99] Also, these studies have shown a more consistently elevated risk among men than among women, perhaps because of the generally lower consumption of alcohol among women.[1,7-8,73,99] None of 6 prospective studies that compared the cancer mortality of alcoholics with that of the general population found significant associations with CRC.[1,73] Interestingly, the Copenhagen Center for Prospective Population Studies with approximately 25,000 participants reported that wine drinkers had significantly lower mortality from cancer than did non wine drinkers (P=0.004).[100] Most of the published large prospective studies in the general population have found significant positive associations between alcohol consumption and the risk of CRC and adenomas.[1,73,99] A meta-analysis involving a total of 22 studies (6 prospective and 16 case-control) showed that alcohol consumption significantly increases the risk of CRC (pooled RR [95% CI]: 1.08 [1.06 to 1.10] for alcohol intake of 25 g/day; 1.18 [1.14 to 1.22] for 50 g/day; and 1.38 [1.29 to 1.49] for 100 g/day).[101] A recently published pooled analysis of 8 cohort studies (the Alpha-Tocopherol Beta-Carotene Cancer Prevention Study, the Canadian national Breast Screening Study, the Health Professionals Follow-up Study, the Iowa Women's Health Study, the Netherlands Cohort Study, the New York State Cohort Study, the Nurses' Health Study, and the Swedish Mammography Cohort Study) demonstrated a significant positive association between alcohol consumption and CRC risk.[102] Compared with nondrinkers, the pooled multivariate relative risks were 1.16 (95% CI, 0.99 to 1.36) fro those who consumed 30 to <45 g alcohol/day and 1.41 (95% CI, 1.16 to 1.72) for those who consumed ≥45 g/day.[102] The association was evident for all sites of CRC and no clear difference in relative risks was found among specific alcoholic beverages.[102] The international panel of experts from the World Cancer Research Fund concluded that "high alcohol consumption probably increases the risk of cancers of the colon and rectum. The effect generally seems to be related to total ethanol intake, irrespective of the type of drink."[1]

The mechanisms by which alcohol consumption may contribute to colorectal carcinogenesis appear to relate to the breakdown of alcohol to acetaldehyde, which exerts either a direct or an indirect toxic effect on the colonic epithelium.[103-104] Acetaldehyde is a portent adduct former, and is known to inhibit DNA repair.[103-104] Alcohol may exert its carcinogenic effects through associated deficiencies in nutrients, particularly folate.[103-104] Alcohol has also been also shown to induce genomic DNA hypomethylation,[103-104] which, in turn, may increase genomic instability, mutations, expression of protooncogenes.[103-104]

Calcium and Vitamin D

Results from correlation and case-control studies generally suggest an inverse association between calcium intake and CRC risk.[73] Although earlier prospective studies reported an inverse association between calcium intake and CRC risk, more recent and larger prospective studies, including the Nurses' Health Study, the Health Professionals Follow-up Study, and the Iowa Women's Study, have failed to demonstrate beneficial effects of calcium on the risk of CRC and adenomas after multivariate adjustment.[105] A systemic review published in 1998 of 15 case-control and 8 prospective studies that reported results for the association between calcium and CRC suggests that calcium intake is not associated with a substantially lower risk of CRC.[105] In particular, findings from large prospective studies were notably consistent in finding weak and nonsignificant inverse associations.[105]

A meta-analysis published in 1996 that included 24 case-control and prospective studies did not find a substantial protective effect of calcium on CRC or adenoma risk.[106] The summary relative risk of developing CRC and adenomas in those with the highest intake of calcium compared with those with the lowest intake was 0.89 (95% CI, 0.79 to 1.01), 0.90 (95% CI, 0.78 to 1.05), and 0.88 (95% CI, 0.73 to 1.04) for combined, prospective, and case-control studies, respectively.[106] For adenomas and CRC, relatives risks were 1.13 (95% CI, 0.91 to 1.39) and 0.86 (95% CI, 0.74 to 0.98).[106] Subsequently, a fairly consistent modest inverse association (risk reductions in the range of 15% to 40% for the highest versus the lowest intake categories) has emerged from several prospective studies (the Nurses' Health Study, the Health Professionals Follow-up Study, the Iowa Women's Study, and the Second Cancer Prevention Study Nutrition Cohort)[107-110] as well as large case-control studies with some 2000 colon cancer cases.[111]

Almost all of the uncontrolled intervention trials have demonstrated a protective effect of calcium supplementation on proliferation SEPBs of CRC.[73,112] However, less than one-third of the published small, placebo-controlled, randomized human trials have confirmed this protective effect of calcium on proliferation markers.[73,112] One published report on a larger US multicenter study (n=333) reported no significant protective effect of calcium supplementation (1200 mg elemental calcium for 6 to 9 months) on proliferation biomarkers compared with placebo.[113] Another randomized trial showed that calcium supplementation (1 to 2 mg elemental calcium for 6 months) normalized the distribution of proliferating cells without affecting the overall proliferation rate in the colorectal mucosa.[114]

Three placebo-controlled, randomized trials that investigated the effect of calcium supplementation on adenoma recurrence have been published. A small study involved 116 polyp-bearing patients who received a daily mixture of ß-carotene (15 mg), vitamin C (150 mg), vitamin E (75 mg), selenium (101 µg), and calcium carbonate (4 g or 1.6 g elemental calcium) or placebo for 3 years.[115] The adenoma recurrence reduction (but no adenoma growth) was statistically significant in this trial, but a separate calcium effect could not be discerned because the intervention combined calcium and antioxidant vitamins 115. The European Cancer Prevention Organisation Intervention Study (n=665; 3 years of follow-up) reported a 34% reduction in the recurrence of adenoma associated with 2 g calcium supplementation/day but this reduction did not attain statistical significance (P=0.16).[42] The Calcium Polyp Prevention Study (n=930) showed that calcium supplementation (3 g calcium carbonate [1200 mg of elemental calcium] daily) significantly reduced the recurrence rate of colorectal adenomas by 15% after 4 years of intervention.[21] A further analysis of this trial demonstrated that vitamin D status strongly modified the effect of calcium supplementation on adenoma recurrence.[116] Calcium supplements significantly lowered adenoma risk (by 30%) only among subjects with 25 hydroxyvitamin D [25(OH) D] levels above the overall median (29.1 ng/mL) 116. Similarly, 25(OH) D was associated with a reduced risk only among subjects randomly assigned to received calcium 116. The Calcium Polyp Prevention Study has recently reported results from another analysis.[117] This analysis suggests that calcium supplementation has a more profound effect on the risk of recurrence of "histologically advanced neoplasms", which possess a higher potential for progressing to adenocarcinoma, (RR, 0.65; 95% CI, 0.46 to 0.93) compared with that for tubular adenomas, which are associate with a lower potential to progress to adenocarcinoma, (RR, 0.89; 95% CI, 0.77 to 1.03).[117] The Women's Health Initiative is underway to determine the effect of hormones, calcium, vitamin D and a low-fat dietary plan on CRC risk in 64,500 postmenopausal women (50 to 79 years of age).[60]

The role of vitamin D in colorectal carcinogenesis has not been unequivocally established in epidemiological studies. Correlation and case-control studies have reported conflicting results.[1,73,105] Although large prospective studies (the Western Electric Workers Study, the Nurses' Health Study, the Health Professionals Follow-up Study, the Iowa Women's Study, and the Second Cancer Prevention Study Nutrition Cohort) have suggested a weak inverse association between vitamin D intake and CRC and adenoma risk, only few studies attained statistical significance.[1,73,105]

In summary, the portfolio of observational epidemiologic studies and results from intervention trials generally support the modest protective effect of calcium supplementation on CRC risk. Also, there is evidence that the chemopreventive effect of calcium supplementation may be enhanced by the concomitant use of vitamin D. The case for calcium as a potential chemopreventive agent against CRC is further strengthened by the existence of several plausible physiological and molecular mechanisms as outlined in Table 17-8.[118-119] In contrast, given the scarcity of data, additional studies are needed to investigate the relationship between vitamin D and CRC risk in more detail. Mechanistically, however, the physiologically most active molecular form of vitamin D, 1,25dihydroxyvitamin D_3, has been shown to restrain cell proliferation and induces differentiation and apoptosis in a large variety of normal and tumor cells, including cells of the colon.[119]

Selenium

Descriptive epidemiological studies, including many prospective studies, have suggested that dietary intake and/or serum and toenail levels of selenium are inversely related to overall cancer risk.[1,7-8,73] Although most case-

Table 17-8.

Potential Anticarcinogenic Mechanisms of Calcium

Calcium binds free bile acids and fatty acids, forming insoluble calcium soaps, thereby reducing their carcinogenic effects on the colonic epithelium.
Calcium suppresses proliferation and promotes apoptosis of the colonic epithelium.
Calcium reduces or suppresses molecular alterations implicated in colorectal carcinogenesis such as k-ras mutations, c-myc protooncogene expression, and ß-catenin transcriptional activation.
Calcium suppresses the activation of secondary transduction signals such as protein kinase C and alters intracellular calcium regulation.
Calcium activates a calcium-sensing receptor, which results in increased levels of intracellular calcium inducing a wide range of biological effects, some of which restrain the growth and promote the differentiation of transformed colon cells.
Calcium decreases luminal cytotoxic surfactant concentrations and thus inhibits luminal cytolytic activity.

control and earlier prospective studies reported a weak inverse association between serum levels of selenium and CRC risk,[1,7-8,73] a subsequent large prospective study in the Finnish cohort participating in the Social Insurance Institution's Mobile Clinic Health Examination Survey in Finland (n=39,268 men and women; 10 years of follow-up) failed to confirm this relationship.[120] More recent large prospective studies (the Netherlands Cohort Study on Diet and Cancer[121] and the Nurses' Health Study[122]) using toenail selenium, an indicator of long-term selenium status, found no significant association between selenium status and CRC risk. In fact, the Nurses' Health Study found nonsignificant positive associations between selenium status and CRC, lung cancer, and melanoma.[122] Another large prospective study from Italy reported a 3.9-fold increase in melanoma incidence in 2065 individuals who consumed high levels of inorganic selenium in tap water for 11 years compared with unexposed controls,[123] raising alarm regarding the role of selenium in cancer chemoprevention.

The Nutritional Prevention of Cancer Trial in the southeastern United States randomized 1312 patients with a history of basal cell or squamous cell carcinomas of the skin to either selenium as selenized yeast (200 µg/day) or placebo to determine the effect of selenium on the incidence of nonmelanoma skin cancers.[24] Although no significant effect of selenium on these primary endpoints were observed, selenium supplementation significantly reduced total cancer incidence (by 37%), and incidence of lung (by 46%), colorectal (by 58%), and prostate (by 63%) cancers compared with placebo during the 6.4 years of follow-up.[24] A recent report that extends follow-up of the participants of this trial to over 10 years showed that selenium supplementation significantly increased the risk of squamous cell carcinoma (by 25%) and total nonmelanoma skin cancer (by 17%).[124]

Although potential biologically plausible chemopreventive mechanisms do exist for selenium,[125] the portfolio of evidence from observational and intervention studies does not support the role of selenium in chemoprevention of CRC at present.

Unifying Hypothesis—Insulin Resistance

There tends to be agreement among epidemiological studies regarding the risk of CRC and its relationship with overall diet.[126] However, when many of the findings are examined closely and correlations between CRC and individual dietary factors are sought, the relationship tends to be less convincing.[126] These observations suggest that overall diet, rather than individual factors, play the more important role, thus underscoring the importance of as yet undetermined interactions among dietary components in the development of cancer. This conclusion has lead to several intervention trials in humans that examined combinations of dietary and lifestyle modifications in the prevention of CRC (eg, The Polyp Prevention Trial[16] and the Women's Health Initiative[60]).

Furthermore, McKeown-Eyssen[127] and Giovannucci[128] proposed a unifying hypothesis that may explain how obesity, physical inactivity, alcohol consumption, and a typical Western diet (low in fruits, vegetables, and fiber and high in animal and saturated fat, refined carbohydrates, and extensively processed foods) increase colorectal cancer risk. This hypothesis suggests that the putative dietary and lifestyle factors associated with CRC risk causes insulin resistance and hyperinsulinemia and that hyperinsulinemia, in turn, may stimulate the growth of colorectal tumors.[127-128] Although it remains unproven whether insulin stimulates the growth of colon tumors in humans, several lines of evidence from animal and in vitro studies support the role of insulin in tumor promotion via the insulin and insulin-like growth factor (IGF) axes.[129] Another indirect line of evidence comes from the observations that subjects with acromegaly, characterized by chronic growth hormone and IGF-1 hypersecretion, have an increased risk of developing CRC.[130]

Although case-control and earlier prospective epidemiologic studies that examined the relationship between diabetes mellitus and CRC risk did not consistently support this hypothesis,[131] more recent large prospective studies generally indicate a significant increase in CRC risk in subjects with type 2 diabetes compared with risk in non-diabetic controls. A population-based cohort study from Sweden (n=153,852) has demonstrated that subjects with diabetes have on average 40% increased risk of developing colon cancer and a 60% increased risk of dying from colon cancer compared with the general population.[132] The First Cancer Prevention Study of the American Cancer Society,[133] with more than 1 million participants showed that diabetic men had a significant 30% increased risk of developing CRC compared with nondiabetic men during a 13-year follow-up period. The Nurses' Health Study (n=118,403; 18 years of follow-up) also reported that type 2 diabetic women had a significant 43% increase in CRC risk than did non-diabetic women.[134] The Norwegian National Health Screen Service Study (n=75,219; 12 years of follow-up) showed that a history of type 2 diabetes was associated with a 55% increase in CRC risk in women (no men) compared to that in women without diabetes 135. The European Prospective Investigation into Cancer —Norfolk Study has recently reported a significant 3-fold increase in CRC risk in diabetic subjects compared with nondiabetic controls.[136] In this study, concentrations of glycated hemoglobin (HbA1c), which is an integrated indicator of average blood glucose concentrations over the preceding 3 months, were continuously related to incident CRC risk, with lowest rates observed in those with HBA1c below 5%. The relative risk of incident CRC per 1% absolute increase in HbA1c was 1.34 (95% CI, 1.12 to 1.59).[136] Large prospective studies (the Cardiovascular Health Study, the New York University Women's Health Study, the Physicians' Health Study) have also reported a significantly increased CRC risk in individuals with higher levels of fasting glucose and insulin, with higher levels of glucose and insulin 2 hours after oral glucose challenge, with higher levels of C-peptide (a marker of pancreatic insulin secretion), and with higher circulating levels of IGFs.[137-140]

These epidemiologic observations have been supported by animal experimental studies[141-145] that demonstrate growth promoting effects of exogenous insulin and dietary-induced hyperinsulinemia on CRC and aberrant crypt foci, a putative precursor of colon cancer. Therefore, the recently proposed hypothesis linking insulin resistance and hyperinsulinemia with CRC risk provides a very attractive unifying mechanism by which a majority of dietary and lifestyle factors promote the development of CRC.

Conclusion

Currently available evidence from epidemiological, laboratory animal, and intervention studies does not unequivocally support the role of dietary factors in the development of CRC. However, when the whole body or portfolio of evidence from these studies is analyzed critically, the overall conclusion supports that dietary factors play a major role in the development of CRC. The precise nature of the relationship to each nutrient and the actual magnitude of the relationship are, however, not clear at present. Disappointingly, recent, large, placebo-controlled randomized intervention trials in humans have not supported the protective role of some of the diets and nutritional supplements thought to lower the risk of CRC.

As discussed in this chapter, several inherent limitations are associated with nutritional epidemiological and intervention studies that are designed to elucidate the relationship between dietary factors and CRC risk. Therefore, definitive answers to questions about diet and CRC are probably beyond the reach of both observational epidemiologic studies and randomized controlled trials. However, it appears that overall diet, rather than individual factors, plays the more important role in the development of CRC, thus underscoring the importance of as yet undetermined interactions among dietary components in the development of CRC.

Recent advances in molecular and cell biology have greatly increased the potential for understanding the mechanistic roles that nutrients play in the development of CRC at the molecular and cellular levels. Also, the topic of nutrient-gene interactions in carcinogenesis, which modifies CRC risk conferred by genetic susceptibility and dietary habits, has just begun to emerge. Identifying and understanding biologically plausible mechanisms by which dietary factors modulate CRC risk further strengthens epidemiological and experimental evidence.

It is difficult to advise the public with absolute confidence given the insufficient scientific evidence currently available. It is important that the recommendation for prevention of CRC include modifications of overall dietary and lifestyle factors considered to be associated with an increased risk of CRC. These include decreasing consumption of fat (total, animal, and saturated fat) and red meat, increasing consumption of vegetables, fruits, and all sources and types of fiber-rich foods, avoiding obesity, curtailing alcohol consumption to minimal to moderate amounts, quitting smoking, and engaging in daily physical activity. These dietary recommendations can not only potentially protect against CRC but also provide other health benefits including decreased cholesterol levels, improved insulin resistance, reduced blood pressure, and prevention of cardiovascular disease.

Among individual dietary factors considered in this chapter, calcium supplementation may confer a modest protective effect on CRC risk. It is clear that antioxidants supplementation should not be recommended for this purpose. Although folic acid and selenium appear to be promising, there are some concerns that these agents may exert procarcinogenic effects depending on the timing and dose of intervention. Over-all dietary and lifestyle modifications to reduce insulin resistance appear to be one of the most promising and rational chemopreventive strategies against CRC.

References

1. World Cancer Research Fund/American Institute for Cancer. *Food, nutrition, and the prevention of cancer: a global perspective.* Washington, DC: American Institute for Cancer Research; 1997.
2. Doll R, Peto R. The causes of cancer: quantitative estimates of avoidable risks of cancer in the United States today. *J Natl Cancer Inst.* 1981;66(6):1191-1308.
3. McGinnis JM, Foege WH. Actual causes of death in the United States. *JAMA.* 1993;270(18):2207-2212.

4. Miller AB, Berrino F, Hill M, Pietinen P, Riboli E, Wahrendorf J. Diet in the aetiology of cancer: a review. *Eur J Cancer.* 1994;30A(2):207-220; discussion 220-208.
5. Lichtenstein P, Holm NV, Verkasalo PK, et al. Environmental and heritable factors in the causation of cancer--analyses of cohorts of twins from Sweden, Denmark, and Finland. *N Engl J Med.* 2000;343(2):78-85.
6. Chu KC, Tarone RE, Chow WH, Hankey BF, Ries LA. Temporal patterns in colorectal cancer incidence, survival, and mortality from 1950 through 1990. *J Natl Cancer Inst.* 1994;86(13):997-1006.
7. Potter JD. Colorectal cancer: molecules and populations. *J Natl Cancer Inst.* 1999;91(11):916-932.
8. Kim YI. Nutrition and cancer. In: Bowman BA, Russell RM, eds. *Present knowledge in nutrition.* 8th ed. Washington, D.C.: International life Science Institute; 2001:573-689.
9. Kim YI. Vegetables, fruits, and colorectal cancer risk: what should we believe? *Nutr Rev.* Dec 2001;59(12):394-398.
10. Rebbeck TR, Ambrosone CB, Bell DA, et al. SNPs, haplotypes, and cancer: applications in molecular epidemiology. *Cancer Epidemiol Biomarkers Prev.* 2004;13(5):681-687.
11. Courtney ED, Melville DM, Leicester RJ. Review article: chemoprevention of colorectal cancer. *Aliment Pharmacol Ther.* 2004;19(1):1-24.
12. Thompson FE, Byers T. Dietary assessment resource manual. *J Nutr.* 1994;124(11 Suppl):2245S-2317S.
13. Schatzkin A, Gail M. The promise and peril of surrogate end points in cancer research. *Nat Rev Cancer.* 2002;2(1):19-27.
14. Winawer SJ, Fletcher RH, Miller L, et al. Colorectal cancer screening: clinical guidelines and rationale. *Gastroenterology.* 1997;112(2):594-642.
15. Winawer S, Fletcher R, Rex D, et al. Colorectal cancer screening and surveillance: clinical guidelines and rationale-Update based on new evidence. *Gastroenterology.* 2003;124(2):544-560.
16. Schatzkin A, Lanza E, Corle D, et al. Lack of effect of a low-fat, high-fiber diet on the recurrence of colorectal adenomas. Polyp Prevention Trial Study Group. *N Engl J Med.* 2000;342(16):1149-1155.
17. Alberts DS, Martinez ME, Roe DJ, et al. Lack of effect of a high-fiber cereal supplement on the recurrence of colorectal adenomas. Phoenix Colon Cancer Prevention Physicians' Network. *N Engl J Med.* 2000;342(16):1156-1162.
18. McKeown-Eyssen GE, Bright-See E, Bruce WR, et al. A randomized trial of a low fat high fibre diet in the recurrence of colorectal polyps. Toronto Polyp Prevention Group. *J Clin Epidemiol.* 1994;47(5):525-536.
19. Greenberg ER, Baron JA, Tosteson TD, et al. A clinical trial of antioxidant vitamins to prevent colorectal adenoma. Polyp Prevention Study Group. *N Engl J Med.* 1994;331(3):141-147.
20. MacLennan R, Macrae F, Bain C, et al. Randomized trial of intake of fat, fiber, and beta carotene to prevent colorectal adenomas. The Australian Polyp Prevention Project. *J Natl Cancer Inst.* 1995;87(23):1760-1766.
21. Baron JA, Beach M, Mandel JS, et al. Calcium supplements for the prevention of colorectal adenomas. Calcium Polyp Prevention Study Group. *N Engl J Med.* 1999;340(2):101-107.
22. The Alpha-Tocopherol, Beta Carotene Cancer Prevention Study Group. The effect of vitamin E and beta carotene on the incidence of lung cancer and other cancers in male smokers. *N Engl J Med.* 1994;330(15):1029-1035.
23. Omenn GS, Goodman GE, Thornquist MD, et al. Effects of a combination of beta carotene and vitamin A on lung cancer and cardiovascular disease. *N Engl J Med.* 1996;334(18):1150-1155.
24. Clark LC, Combs GF, Jr., Turnbull BW, et al. Effects of selenium supplementation for cancer prevention in patients with carcinoma of the skin. A randomized controlled trial. Nutritional Prevention of Cancer Study Group. *JAMA.* 1996;276(24):1957-1963.
25. Byers T. What can randomized controlled trials tell us about nutrition and cancer prevention? *CA Cancer J Clin.* 1999;49(6):353-361.
26. Burkitt DP. Relationship as a clue to causation. *Lancet.* 1970;2(7685):1237-1240.
27. Kim YI. AGA technical review: impact of dietary fiber on colon cancer occurrence. *Gastroenterology.* 2000;118(6):1235-1257.
28. Trock B, Lanza E, Greenwald P. Dietary fiber, vegetables, and colon cancer: critical review and meta-analyses of the epidemiologic evidence. *J Natl Cancer Inst.* 1990;82(8):650-661.
29. Howe GR, Benito E, Castelleto R, et al. Dietary intake of fiber and decreased risk of cancers of the colon and rectum: evidence from the combined analysis of 13 case-control studies. *J Natl Cancer Inst.* 1992;84(24):1887-1896.
30. Friedenreich CM, Brant RF, Riboli E. Influence of methodologic factors in a pooled analysis of 13 case-control studies of colorectal cancer and dietary fiber. *Epidemiology.* 1994;5(1):66-79.
31. Thun MJ, Calle EE, Namboodiri MM, et al. Risk factors for fatal colon cancer in a large prospective study. *J Natl Cancer Inst.* 1992;84(19):1491-1500.
32. Willett WC, Stampfer MJ, Colditz GA, Rosner BA, Speizer FE. Relation of meat, fat, and fiber intake to the risk of colon cancer in a prospective study among women. *N Engl J Med.* 1990;323(24):1664-1672.
33. Fuchs CS, Giovannucci EL, Colditz GA, et al. Dietary fiber and the risk of colorectal cancer and adenoma in women. *N Engl J Med.* 1999;340(3):169-176.
34. Steinmetz KA, Kushi LH, Bostick RM, Folsom AR, Potter JD. Vegetables, fruit, and colon cancer in the Iowa Women's Health Study. *Am J Epidemiol.* 1994;139(1):1-15.
35. Giovannucci E, Rimm EB, Stampfer MJ, Colditz GA, Ascherio A, Willett WC. Intake of fat, meat, and fiber in relation to risk of colon cancer in men. *Cancer Res.* 1994;54(9):2390-2397.
36. Giovannucci E, Stampfer MJ, Colditz G, Rimm EB, Willett WC. Relationship of diet to risk of colorectal adenoma in men. *J Natl Cancer Inst.* 1992;84(2):91-98.
37. Platz EA, Giovannucci E, Rimm EB, et al. Dietary fiber and distal colorectal adenoma in men. *Cancer Epidemiol Biomarkers Prev.* 1997;6(9):661-670.
38. Pietinen P, Malila N, Virtanen M, et al. Diet and risk of colorectal cancer in a cohort of Finnish men. *Cancer Causes Control.* 1999;10(5):387-396.
39. Bingham SA, Day NE, Luben R, et al. Dietary fibre in food and protection against colorectal cancer in the European Prospective Investigation into Cancer and Nutrition (EPIC): an observational study. *Lancet.* 2003;361(9368):1496-1501.
40. Peters U, Sinha R, Chatterjee N, et al. Dietary fibre and colorectal adenoma in a colorectal cancer early detection programme. *Lancet.* 2003;361(9368):1491-1495.
41. Ferguson LR, Harris PJ. The dietary fibre debate: more food for thought. *Lancet.* 2003;361(9368):1487-1488.
42. Bonithon-Kopp C, Kronborg O, Giacosa A, Rath U, Faivre J. Calcium and fibre supplementation in prevention of colorectal adenoma recurrence: a randomised intervention trial. European Cancer Prevention Organisation Study Group. *Lancet.* 2000;356(9238):1300-1306.
43. Asano TK, McLeod RS. Dietary fibre for the prevention of colorectal adenomas and carcinoams (Cochrane Review). *The Cochrane Library. Vol 2.* Chichester, UK: John Wiley & Sons; 2004.
44. Steinmetz KA, Potter JD. Vegetables, fruit, and cancer prevention: a review. *J Am Diet Assoc.* 1996;96(10):1027-1039.
45. Steinmetz KA, Potter JD. Vegetables, fruit, and cancer. I. Epidemiology. *Cancer Causes Control.* 1991;2(5):325-357.
46. Phillips RL, Snowdon DA. Dietary relationships with fatal colorectal cancer among Seventh-Day Adventists. *J Natl Cancer Inst.* 1985;74(2):307-317.
47. Shibata A, Paganini-Hill A, Ross RK, Henderson BE. Intake of vegetables, fruits, beta-carotene, vitamin C and vitamin supplements and cancer incidence among the elderly: a prospective study. *Br J Cancer.* 1992;66(4):673-679.

48. Fleischauer AT, Poole C, Arab L. Garlic consumption and cancer prevention: meta-analyses of colorectal and stomach cancers. *Am J Clin Nutr.* 2000;72(4):1047-1052.
49. Michels KB, Edward G, Joshipura KJ, et al. Prospective study of fruit and vegetable consumption and incidence of colon and rectal cancers. *J Natl Cancer Inst.* 2000;92(21):1740-1752.
50. Terry P, Giovannucci E, Michels KB, et al. Fruit, vegetables, dietary fiber, and risk of colorectal cancer. *J Natl Cancer Inst.* 2001;93(7): 525-533.
51. Voorrips LE, Goldbohm RA, van Poppel G, Sturmans F, Hermus RJ, van den Brandt PA. Vegetable and fruit consumption and risks of colon and rectal cancer in a prospective cohort study: The Netherlands Cohort Study on Diet and Cancer. *Am J Epidemiol.* 2000;152(11):1081-1092.
52. Flood A, Velie EM, Chaterjee N, et al. Fruit and vegetable intakes and the risk of colorectal cancer in the Breast Cancer Detection Demonstration Project follow-up cohort. *Am J Clin Nutr.* 2002; 75(5):936-943.
53. Steinmetz KA, Potter JD. Vegetables, fruit, and cancer. II. Mechanisms. *Cancer Causes Control.* 1991;2(6):427-442.
54. Lampe JW. Health effects of vegetables and fruit: assessing mechanisms of action in human experimental studies. *Am J Clin Nutr.* 1999;70(3 Suppl):475S-490S.
55. Giovannucci E. Tomatoes, tomato-based products, lycopene, and cancer: review of the epidemiologic literature. *J Natl Cancer Inst.* 1999;91(4):317-331.
56. Howe GR, Aronson KJ, Benito E, et al. The relationship between dietary fat intake and risk of colorectal cancer: evidence from the combined analysis of 13 case-control studies. *Cancer Causes Control.* 1997;8(2):215-228.
57. Bostick RM, Potter JD, Kushi LH, et al. Sugar, meat, and fat intake, and non-dietary risk factors for colon cancer incidence in Iowa women (United States). *Cancer Causes Control.* 1994;5(1):38-52.
58. Goldbohm RA, van den Brandt PA, van 't Veer P, et al. A prospective cohort study on the relation between meat consumption and the risk of colon cancer. *Cancer Res.* 1994;54(3):718-723.
59. Kampman E, Verhoeven D, Sloots L, van 't Veer P. Vegetable and animal products as determinants of colon cancer risk in Dutch men and women. *Cancer Causes Control.* 1995;6(3):225-234.
60. The Women's Health Initiative Study Group. Design of the Women's Health Initiative clinical trial and observational study. *Control Clin Trials.* 1998;19(1):61-109.
61. Knekt P, Steineck G, Jarvinen R, Hakulinen T, Aromaa A. Intake of fried meat and risk of cancer: a follow-up study in Finland. *Int J Cancer.* 1994;59(6):756-760.
62. Kato I, Akhmedkhanov A, Koenig K, Toniolo PG, Shore RE, Riboli E. Prospective study of diet and female colorectal cancer: the New York University Women's Health Study. *Nutr Cancer.* 1997;28(3):276-281.
63. Stevens RG, Jones DY, Micozzi MS, Taylor PR. Body iron stores and the risk of cancer. *N Engl J Med.* 1988;319(16):1047-1052.
64. Wurzelmann JI, Silver A, Schreinemachers DM, Sandler RS, Everson RB. Iron intake and the risk of colorectal cancer. *Cancer Epidemiol Biomarkers Prev.* 1996;5(7):503-507.
65. Dorgan JF, Schatzkin A. Antioxidant micronutrients in cancer prevention. *Hematol Oncol Clin North Am.* 1991;5(1):43-68.
66. Bostick RM, Potter JD, McKenzie DR, et al. Reduced risk of colon cancer with high intake of vitamin E: the Iowa Women's Health Study. *Cancer Res.* 1993;53(18):4230-4237.
67. Jacobs EJ, Connell CJ, Patel AV, et al. Vitamin C and vitamin E supplement use and colorectal cancer mortality in a large American Cancer Society cohort. *Cancer Epidemiol Biomarkers Prev.* 2001; 10(1):17-23.
68. Watkins ML, Erickson JD, Thun MJ, Mulinare J, Heath CW, Jr. Multivitamin use and mortality in a large prospective study. *Am J Epidemiol.* 2000;152(2):149-162.
69. Giovannucci E, Rimm EB, Ascherio A, Stampfer MJ, Colditz GA, Willett WC. Alcohol, low-methionine--low-folate diets, and risk of colon cancer in men. *J Natl Cancer Inst.* 1995;87(4):265-273.
70. Giovannucci E, Stampfer MJ, Colditz GA, et al. Multivitamin use, folate, and colon cancer in women in the Nurses' Health Study. *Ann Intern Med.* 1998;129(7):517-524.
71. Jacobs EJ, Connell CJ, Patel AV, et al. Multivitamin use and colon cancer mortality in the Cancer Prevention Study II cohort (United States). *Cancer Causes Control.* 2001;12(10):927-934.
72. Jacobs EJ, Connell CJ, Chao A, et al. Multivitamin use and colorectal cancer incidence in a US cohort: does timing matter? *Am J Epidemiol.* 2003;158(7):621-628.
73. Kim YI, Mason JB. Nutrition chemoprevention of gastrointestinal cancers: a critical review. *Nutr Rev.* 1996;54(9):259-279.
74. Roncucci L, Di Donato P, Carati L, et al. Antioxidant vitamins or lactulose for the prevention of the recurrence of colorectal adenomas. Colorectal Cancer Study Group of the University of Modena and the Health Care District 16. *Dis Colon Rectum.* 1993; 36(3):227-234.
75. Baron JA, Cole BF, Mott L, et al. Neoplastic and antineoplastic effects of beta-carotene on colorectal adenoma recurrence: results of a randomized trial. *J Natl Cancer Inst.* 2003;95(10):717-722.
76. Hennekens CH, Buring JE, Manson JE, et al. Lack of effect of long-term supplementation with beta carotene on the incidence of malignant neoplasms and cardiovascular disease. *N Engl J Med.* 1996;334(18):1145-1149.
77. Lee IM, Cook NR, Manson JE, Buring JE, Hennekens CH. Beta-carotene supplementation and incidence of cancer and cardiovascular disease: the Women's Health Study. *J Natl Cancer Inst.* 1999; 91(24):2102-2106.
78. Albanes D, Heinonen OP, Taylor PR, et al. Alpha-Tocopherol and beta-carotene supplements and lung cancer incidence in the alpha-tocopherol, beta-carotene cancer prevention study: effects of base-line characteristics and study compliance. *J Natl Cancer Inst.* 1996;88(21):1560-1570.
79. Omenn GS, Goodman GE, Thornquist MD, et al. Risk factors for lung cancer and for intervention effects in CARET, the Beta-Carotene and Retinol Efficacy Trial. *J Natl Cancer Inst.* 1996; 88(21):1550-1559.
80. Albanes D, Malila N, Taylor PR, et al. Effects of supplemental alpha-tocopherol and beta-carotene on colorectal cancer: results from a controlled trial (Finland). *Cancer Causes Control.* 2000; 11(3):197-205.
81. Cook NR, Le IM, Manson JE, Buring JE, Hennekens CH. Effects of beta-carotene supplementation on cancer incidence by baseline characteristics in the Physicians' Health Study (United States). *Cancer Causes Control.* 2000;11(7):617-626.
82. Routine vitamin supplementation to prevent cancer and cardiovascular disease: recommendations and rationale. *Ann Intern Med.* 2003;139(1):51-55.
83. Morris CD, Carson S. Routine vitamin supplementation to prevent cardiovascular disease: a summary of the evidence for the U.S. Preventive Services Task Force. *Ann Intern Med.* 2003;139(1):56-70.
84. Kim YI. Folate and carcinogenesis: evidence, mechanisms, and implications. *J Nutr Biochem.* 1999;10:66-88.
85. Kim YI. Role of folate in colon cancer development and progression. *J Nutr.* 2003;133(11 Suppl 1):3731S-3739S.
86. Bailey LB, Rampersaud GC, Kauwell GP. Folic acid supplements and fortification affect the risk for neural tube defects, vascular disease and cancer: evolving science. *J Nutr.* 2003;133(6):1961S-1968S.
87. Giovannucci E. Epidemiologic studies of folate and colorectal neoplasia: a review. *J Nutr.* 2002;132(8 Suppl):2350S-2355S.
88. Giovannucci E, Stampfer MJ, Colditz GA, et al. Folate, methionine, and alcohol intake and risk of colorectal adenoma. *J Natl Cancer Inst.* 1993;85(11):875-884.
89. Fuchs CS, Willett WC, Colditz GA, et al. The influence of folate and multivitamin use on the familial risk of colon cancer in women. *Cancer Epidemiol Biomarkers Prev.* 2002;11(3):227-234.
90. Wei EK, Giovannucci E, Wu K, et al. Comparison of risk factors for colon and rectal cancer. *Int J Cancer.* 2004;108(3):433-442.

91. Su LJ, Arab L. Nutritional status of folate and colon cancer risk: evidence from NHANES I epidemiologic follow-up study. *Ann Epidemiol.* 2001;11(1):65-72.
92. Harnack L, Jacobs DR, Jr., Nicodemus K, Lazovich D, Anderson K, Folsom AR. Relationship of folate, vitamin B-6, vitamin B-12, and methionine intake to incidence of colorectal cancers. *Nutr Cancer.* 2002;43(2):152-158.
93. Konings EJ, Goldbohm RA, Brants HA, Saris WH, van den Brandt PA. Intake of dietary folate vitamers and risk of colorectal carcinoma: results from The Netherlands Cohort Study. *Cancer.* 2002;95(7):1421-1433.
94. Hillman RS, Steinberg SE. The effects of alcohol on folate metabolism. *Annu Rev Med.* 1982;33:345-354.
95. Potter JD. Methyl supply, methyl metabolizing enzymes and colorectal neoplasia. *J Nutr.* 2002;132(8 Suppl):2410S-2412S.
96. Sharp L, Little J. Polymorphisms in Genes Involved in Folate Metabolism and Colorectal Neoplasia: A HuGE Review. *Am J Epidemiol.* 2004;159(5):423-443.
97. Kim YI. Folate, colorectal carcinogenesis, and DNA methylation: Lessons from animal studies. *Environ Mol Mutagen.* 2004;44(1):10-25.
98. Kim YI. Folate and DNA methylation: a mechanistic link between folate deficiency and colorectal cancer? *Cancer Epidemiol Biomarkers Prev.* 2004;13(4):511-519.
99. Kune GA, Vitetta L. Alcohol consumption and the etiology of colorectal cancer: a review of the scientific evidence from 1957 to 1991. *Nutr Cancer.* 1992;18(2):97-111.
100. Gronbaek M, Becker U, Johansen D, et al. Type of alcohol consumed and mortality from all causes, coronary heart disease, and cancer. *Ann Intern Med.* 2000;133(6):411-419.
101. Bagnardi V, Blangiardo M, La Vecchia C, Corrao G. A meta-analysis of alcohol drinking and cancer risk. *Br J Cancer.* 2001;85(11):1700-1705.
102. Cho E, Smith-Warner SA, Ritz J, et al. Alcohol intake and colorectal cancer: a pooled analysis of 8 cohort studies. *Ann Intern Med.* 2004;140(8):603-613.
103. Garro AJ, Lieber CS. Alcohol and cancer. *Annu Rev Pharmacol Toxicol.* 1990;30:219-249.
104. Seitz HK, Matsuzaki S, Yokoyama A, Homann N, Vakevainen S, Wang XD. Alcohol and cancer. *Alcohol Clin Exp Res.* 2001;25(5 Suppl ISBRA):137S-143S.
105. Martinez ME, Willett WC. Calcium, vitamin D, and colorectal cancer: a review of the epidemiologic evidence. *Cancer Epidemiol Biomarkers Prev.* 1998;7(2):163-168.
106. Bergsma-Kadijk JA, van 't Veer P, Kampman E, Burema J. Calcium does not protect against colorectal neoplasia. *Epidemiology.* 1996; 7(6):590-597.
107. Zheng W, Anderson KE, Kushi LH, et al. A prospective cohort study of intake of calcium, vitamin D, and other micronutrients in relation to incidence of rectal cancer among postmenopausal women. *Cancer Epidemiol Biomarkers Prev.* 1998;7(3):221-225.
108. Wu K, Willett WC, Fuchs CS, Colditz GA, Giovannucci EL. Calcium intake and risk of colon cancer in women and men. *J Natl Cancer Inst.* 2002;94(6):437-446.
109. McCullough ML, Robertson AS, Rodriguez C, et al. Calcium, vitamin D, dairy products, and risk of colorectal cancer in the Cancer Prevention Study II Nutrition Cohort (United States). *Cancer Causes Control.* Feb 2003;14(1):1-12.
110. Sellers TA, Bazyk AE, Bostick RM, et al. Diet and risk of colon cancer in a large prospective study of older women: an analysis stratified on family history (Iowa, United States). *Cancer Causes Control.* 1998;9(4):357-367.
111. Kampman E, Slattery ML, Caan B, Potter JD. Calcium, vitamin D, sunshine exposure, dairy products and colon cancer risk (United States). *Cancer Causes Control.* 2000;11(5):459-466.
112. Bostick RM. Human studies of calcium supplementation and colorectal epithelial cell proliferation. *Cancer Epidemiol Biomarkers Prev.* 1997;6(11):971-980.
113. Baron JA, Tosteson TD, Wargovich MJ, et al. Calcium supplementation and rectal mucosal proliferation: a randomized controlled trial. *J Natl Cancer Inst.* 1995;87(17):1303-1307.
114. Bostick RM, Fosdick L, Wood JR, et al. Calcium and colorectal epithelial cell proliferation in sporadic adenoma patients: a randomized, double-blinded, placebo-controlled clinical trial. *J Natl Cancer Inst.* 1995;87(17):1307-1315.
115. Hofstad B, Almendingen K, Vatn M, et al. Growth and recurrence of colorectal polyps: a double-blind 3-year intervention with calcium and antioxidants. *Digestion.* 1998;59(2):148-156.
116. Grau MV, Baron JA, Sandler RS, et al. Vitamin D, calcium supplementation, and colorectal adenomas: results of a randomized trial. *J Natl Cancer Inst.* 2003;95(23):1765-1771.
117. Wallace K, Baron JA, Cole BF, et al. Effect of calcium supplementation on the risk of large bowel polyps. *J Natl Cancer Inst.* 2004; 96(12):921-925.
118. Pence BC. Role of calcium in colon cancer prevention: experimental and clinical studies. *Mutat Res.* 1993;290(1):87-95.
119. Lamprecht SA, Lipkin M. Chemoprevention of colon cancer by calcium, vitamin D and folate: molecular mechanisms. *Nat Rev Cancer.* Aug 2003;3(8):601-614.
120. Knekt P, Aromaa A, Maatela J, et al. Serum selenium and subsequent risk of cancer among Finnish men and women. *J Natl Cancer Inst.* 1990;82(10):864-868.
121. van den Brandt PA, Goldbohm RA, van 't Veer P, et al. A prospective cohort study on toenail selenium levels and risk of gastrointestinal cancer. *J Natl Cancer Inst.* 1993;85(3):224-229.
122. Garland M, Morris JS, Stampfer MJ, et al. Prospective study of toenail selenium levels and cancer among women. *J Natl Cancer Inst.* Apr 5 1995;87(7):497-505.
123. Vinceti M, Rothman KJ, Bergomi M, Borciani N, Serra L, Vivoli G. Excess melanoma incidence in a cohort exposed to high levels of environmental selenium. *Cancer Epidemiol Biomarkers Prev.* 1998;7(10):853-856.
124. Duffield-Lillico AJ, Slate EH, Reid ME, et al. Selenium supplementation and secondary prevention of nonmelanoma skin cancer in a randomized trial. *J Natl Cancer Inst.* 2003;95(19):1477-1481.
125. Ip C. Lessons from basic research in selenium and cancer prevention. *J Nutr.* 1998;128(11):1845-1854.
126. Helzlsouer KJ, Block G, Blumberg J, et al. Summary of the round table discussion on strategies for cancer prevention: diet, food, additives, supplements, and drugs. *Cancer Res.* 1994;54(7 Suppl): 2044s-2051s.
127. McKeown-Eyssen G. Epidemiology of colorectal cancer revisited: are serum triglycerides and/or plasma glucose associated with risk? *Cancer Epidemiol Biomarkers Prev.* 1994;3(8):687-695.
128. Giovannucci E. Insulin and colon cancer. *Cancer Causes Control.* 1995;6(2):164-179.
129. Sandhu MS, Dunger DB, Giovannucci EL. Insulin, insulin-like growth factor-I (IGF-I), IGF binding proteins, their biologic interactions, and colorectal cancer. *J Natl Cancer Inst.* 2002;94(13):972-980.
130. Ritter MM, Richter WO, Schwandt P. Acromegaly and colon cancer. *Ann Intern Med.* 1987;106(4):636-637.
131. Kim YI. Diet, lifestyle, and colorectal cancer: is hyperinsulinemia the missing link? *Nutr Rev.* 1998;56(9):275-279.
132. Weiderpass E, Gridley G, Nyren O, Ekbom A, Persson I, Adami HO. Diabetes mellitus and risk of large bowel cancer. *J Natl Cancer Inst.* 1997;89(9):660-661.
133. Will JC, Galuska DA, Vinicor F, Calle EE. Colorectal cancer: another complication of diabetes mellitus? *Am J Epidemiol.* 1998; 147(9):816-825.
134. Hu FB, Manson JE, Liu S, et al. Prospective study of adult onset diabetes mellitus (type 2) and risk of colorectal cancer in women. *J Natl Cancer Inst.* 1999;91(6):542-547.
135. Nilsen TI, Vatten LJ. Prospective study of colorectal cancer risk and physical activity, diabetes, blood glucose and BMI: exploring the hyperinsulinaemia hypothesis. *Br J Cancer.* 2001;84(3):417-422.
136. Khaw KT, Wareham N, Bingham S, Luben R, Welch A, Day N. Preliminary communication: glycated hemoglobin, diabetes, and incident colorectal cancer in men and women: a prospective analysis from the European prospective investigation into cancer-norfolk study. *Cancer Epidemiol Biomarkers Prev.* 2004;13(6):915-919.

137. Schoen RE, Tangen CM, Kuller LH, et al. Increased blood glucose and insulin, body size, and incident colorectal cancer. *J Natl Cancer Inst.* 1999;91(13):1147-1154.
138. Kaaks R, Toniolo P, Akhmedkhanov A, et al. Serum C-peptide, insulin-like growth factor (IGF)-I, IGF-binding proteins, and colorectal cancer risk in women. *J Natl Cancer Inst.* 2000;92(19):1592-1600.
139. Ma J, Pollak MN, Giovannucci E, et al. Prospective study of colorectal cancer risk in men and plasma levels of insulin-like growth factor (IGF)-I and IGF-binding protein-3. *J Natl Cancer Inst.* 1999;91(7):620-625.
140. Ma J, Giovannucci E, Pollak M, et al. A prospective study of plasma C-peptide and colorectal cancer risk in men. *J Natl Cancer Inst.* 2004;96(7):546-553.
141. Tran TT, Medline A, Bruce WR. Insulin promotion of colon tumors in rats. *Cancer Epidemiol Biomarkers Prev.* 1996;5(12):1013-1015.
142. Corpet DE, Jacquinet C, Peiffer G, Tache S. Insulin injections promote the growth of aberrant crypt foci in the colon of rats. *Nutr Cancer.* 1997;27(3):316-320.
143. Koohestani N, Tran TT, Lee W, Wolever TM, Bruce WR. Insulin resistance and promotion of aberrant crypt foci in the colons of rats on a high-fat diet. *Nutr Cancer.* 1997;29(1):69-76.
144. Koohestani N, Chia MC, Pham NA, et al. Aberrant crypt focus promotion and glucose intolerance: correlation in the rat across diets differing in fat, n-3 fatty acids and energy. *Carcinogenesis.* 1998;19(9):1679-1684.
145. Tran TT, Gupta N, Goh T, et al. Direct measure of insulin sensitivity with the hyperinsulinemic-euglycemic clamp and surrogate measures of insulin sensitivity with the oral glucose tolerance test: correlations with aberrant crypt foci promotion in rats. *Cancer Epidemiol Biomarkers Prev.* 2003;12(1):47-56.

Chapter 18

Nutritional Support in Inflammatory Bowel Disease

Alan L. Buchman, MD, MSPH
and James S. Scolapio, MD

Nutritional Assessment

The nutritional management of a patient with inflammatory bowel disease (IBD) first begins with appropriate nutritional assessment (Chapter 1). Multiple factors contribute to malnutrition in both Crohn's disease and ulcerative colitis. It is reported that nutritional deficiencies are greater in Crohn's disease than in ulcerative colitis. It is estimated that as many as 75% of hospitalized Crohn's patients are malnourished.[1]

Reduced intake of food secondary to abdominal cramps, nausea, and diarrhea is a major cause of weight loss in IBD patients. Intestinal malabsorption also contributes to malnutrition in patients with active IBD. Extensive mucosal disease, bacterial overgrowth, and surgical resection all contribute to malabsorption and subsequent weight loss. Increased energy expenditure, as seen with fever, abscess, or sepsis, can also result in weight loss. Nutrient deficiency can result in altered cellular immunity with increased risk of infection, delayed wound healing, and (in children) growth retardation. Therefore, it is important to identify those patients who are at potential risk of malnutrition. Management goals should then include correction of nutritional deficits.

There is no gold standard or one laboratory test for measuring the malnutrition of a patient. All current assessment methods may be affected by the underlying illness and not necessary reflect the nutritional reserve of the patient. For example, serum albumin and prealbumin can be reduced in all inflammatory disorders including IBD without a history of weight loss or other micronutrient deficiency, as hepatic protein synthesis shifts to that of acute phase reactants. Likewise, extracellular fluid shifts can result in low serum albumin and prealbumin concentrations without a clinical history to suggest weight loss or malnutrition. Also delayed cutaneous hypersensitivity is an unreliable marker of malnutrition because medications used in the treatment of IBD, including prednisone and immunosuppressants, can affect results.

A history and physical examination (Chapter 1) is the best tool to access the gross nutritional status of an individual patient (Table 18-1). Patients that have lost significant weight (defined as >10%) and have had reduced oral caloric intake over a 2- to 24-week period are at risk for both macronutrient and micronutrient deficiencies. In addition to an accurate weight, data collected in a comprehensive physical examination includes loss of subcutaneous fat, muscle wasting, dependent edema, and ascites. The subjective global assessment (SGA) is a clinical method for evaluating nutritional status that includes historical, symptomatic and physical parameters of patients.[2] (Information for the SGA is presented in Chapter 1, with a sample assessment in Table 1-2.) The use of the SGA has been shown to give reproducible results with more than 80% agreement.[2]

When to begin nutritional support and by which method are discussed in the following sections of this chapter.

Specific Nutrient Deficiencies

Deficiencies of vitamins, minerals, and trace elements may result from either inadequate intake or increased intestinal losses. Deficiencies are more common in Crohn's disease than they are in ulcerative colitis, given that the majority of micronutrients are absorbed in the

TABLE 18-1.

Nutritional Assessment

History	Unusual dietary habits, medication/vitamin or mineral supplements, change in hair color or texture, poor night vision, dysguesia, dysphagia/odynophagia, abdominal pain/distention, diarrhea, bone pain, muscle pain/cramps/twitching, numbness/parathesias, fatigue, diminished mental activity, weakness
Physical examination	Hair loss/texture, keratomalacia, cheilosis, glossitis, red tongue, parotid enlargement, dentition, skin rash/petechia/bruising, muscle wasting, hepatomegaly, edema, peripheral neuropathy
Anthropometrics	
IBW	Males: 48kg + 2.3kg for each in >60 Females: 45kg + 2.7kg for each in >60 Calculate % IBW: >5% weight loss in 1 month, >7.5% in 2 mos, or >10% in 6 mos are significant "Preferred" Body Weight for obese (Hamwi Formula) = (ABW-IBW)(0.25) + IBW* ABW* for amputation: entire arm (-6.5%); upper arm (-3.5%); hand (-0.8%); forearm with hand (-3.1%); forearm without hand (-2.5%); entire leg (-18.6%); foot (-1.8%)
Muscle function	Handgrip strength, peak insp pressure
Midarm circumference Triceps skin fold thickness	Assess skeletal mass and fat stores†
Laboratory measurements	
Nitrogen balance	N intake = grams protein/6.25 Balance = N intake - UUN + 4‡
Indirect calorimetry	
Visceral proteins	Albumin, pre-albumin, transferrin, retinol-binding protein§
Immune function	Total lymphocyte count Delayed hypersensitivity skin tests§

* Used clinically but not validated (ABW = actual body weight).
† Operator-dependent variability, unreliable to assess short-term responses.
‡ Requires sufficient calories as well as protein; UUN = 24-hour urine urea nitrogen.
§ Affected by many non-nutritional conditions.

small intestine. (See Chapter 3 for additional information on nutrient deficiencies.)

Folic acid and vitamin B12 are the two most common water-soluble vitamin deficiencies that can occur. Deficiency of other water-soluble vitamins is rare. Folate deficiency may result from intestinal malabsorption when proximal jejunal disease is present as can interaction with sulfasalazine, which inhibits folate uptake. Approximately 30% of Crohn's patients have been reported to have low serum folate.[3] Replacement can be given with oral folic acid at a dose of 1.0 mg daily. Vitamin B12 absorption can be impaired if the distal 60 cm of the ileum is diseased or resected, which can occur with Crohn's disease.[4] Also, bacterial overgrowth in the small intestine can reduce vitamin B12 absorption. Patients at risk should receive 1000 ug monthly of subcutaneous vitamin B12.

Vitamin D is the most common fat-soluble vitamin (A, D, E, K) that is reported deficient in patients with IBD. Fat-soluble vitamin deficiency results from malabsorption secondary to a reduced bile salt pool, which results from terminal ileal disease or resection. The combination of both vitamin D and calcium malabsorption and corticosteroid use can result in significant metabolic bone disease (Chapter 13). Corticosteroids cause both decreased intestinal absorption and increased urinary excretion of calcium. Patients at risk should receive 1500 mg of elemental calcium daily. Measurement of bone density using dual-energy x-ray absorptiometry should be performed early after the diagnosis of IBD. Supplementation with 1000 IU of daily vitamin D has been reported to prevent bone loss in patients with Crohn's disease.[5] Sixteen percent of patients with IBD may also have low serum vitamin A and E concentrations.[6] One study reported a consistent relationship between low vitamin A and E concentrations and disease activity.[6]

Iron deficiency is common in both active Crohn's disease and ulcerative colitis. Iron deficiency has been reported in 20% to 40% of IBD patients and usually results from blood loss from the gastrointestinal (GI) tract. Iron deficiency is more common in patients whose disease is limited to the colon. Low serum ferritin concentration is the most reliable marker of reduced iron stores, although, as an acute phase reactant, serum ferritin may be elevated in the presence of systemic inflammation. Anemia in IBD, however, is usually the result of the chronic disease rather than of iron deficiency. Zinc deficiency may also occur, especially in patients with significant diarrhea and intestinal fistulas. Zinc deficiency has been reported in about 40% of patients with Crohn's disease.[7] A combination of low serum and urinary zinc concentrations is highly suggestive of zinc deficiency. Zinc can be replaced using 220 mg twice daily of oral zinc sulfate. Magnesium and potassium are electrolytes that may need to be replaced, especially in those patients who have had partial small bowel resections or who have significant diarrhea. Oral magnesium supplements can worsen diarrhea; therefore, intramuscular or intravenous replacement is often necessary.

General Dietary Measures

For most nonhospitalized patients, the most important advice is for patients to consume a diet liberal in protein, with sufficient calories to maintain weight. Oral intake of 25 to 35 kcal/kg of ideal body weight (IBW) per day (40 kcal/kg/day for weight gain) and 1.0 to 1.5 g/kg of protein will meet the requirements of most adults who are normally nourished. In regard to the specifics of a diet, controlled studies have not shown benefit of low-residue diets except in those patients with intestinal obstruction. There is limited data to support the use high fiber diets to maintain remission in patients with ulcerative colitis.[8] Soluble fiber is metabolized by colonic bacteria to short chain fatty acids. One of these, butyrate, is the preferred fuel for the colonocyte and may be useful in the healing process.

Lactose intolerance is not a problem in all patients with IBD, as lactase is present in the proximal intestine, uncommonly involved with Crohn's disease. Dietary lactose should only be restricted if patients have symptoms associated with diary intake and for those in whom lactose intolerance can be demonstrated by breath hydrogen testing; many patients with symptoms of lactose intolerance are not really lactose intolerant.[9] Lactose-containing foods are an excellent source of dietary calcium. Furthermore, there is no consistent epidemiological data supporting milk as a cause of IBD.

A low oxalate diet may be required for those patients who have had their terminal ileum resected or who have significant fat malabsorption and still have part of their colon remaining. These patients have a propensity for oxalate kidney stones.

Liquid dietary supplements, such as Ensure (Ross, Columbus, OH) and Boost (Novartis, Minneapolis, MN), may help some patients who otherwise are unable to consume sufficient energy. Most supplements are lactose free and well tolerated.

Initial studies with fish oil supplements (n-3 fatty acids) in ulcerative colitis showed decreased disease activity in patients who received these formulas, but randomized trials in Crohn's disease have failed to show consistent results.[10,11] Fish oil may have anti-inflammatory activity because n-3 fatty acids are thought to compete in the substrate pool of the lipoxygenase pathway, thus reducing the production of inflammatory leukotrienes.[12] A study by Belluzzi et al found 2.7 g of n-3 fatty acids administered as an enteric-coated fish oil preparation maintained 59% of Crohn's patients in remission after 1 year compared to 26% in the placebo group ($p<0.05$).[10] Another study by Lorenz-Meyer failed to show a difference in remission rates compared to those in patients taking a placebo.[11] In each study, large amounts were given, which is unpalatable for most people. Studies have not shown any benefit of glutamine supplementation in patients with either Crohn's disease or ulcerative colitis.

When Is Nutritional Support Necessary?

Nutritional support refers to the use of either intravenous or enteral tube feeding and is usually administered to hospitalized patients. Nutritional support of the hospitalized patient should be instituted promptly when it has been determined from daily calorie counts that a patient is not taking sufficient oral intake of food for 7 or more days. After approximately 7 to 10 days of nil per os (npo), negative nitrogen balance occurs, which increases the risk of infection and interferes with wound healing. Nutritional support may also be considered an adjunctive therapy in malnourished patients for whom sufficient oral intake to promote nutritional repletion is not immediately achievable. Therefore, for both active Crohn's disease and ulcerative colitis, nutritional therapy has a significant supportive role.

The role for nutritional support as primary therapy for IBD is limited as discussed below. The use of preoperative parenteral nutrition (PN) has been suggested to improve surgical outcome and limit bowel resection in Crohn's patients undergoing small bowel resections but not those undergoing large bowel resections.[13] Most of the reports are retrospective and uncontrolled. The analysis of the data showed positive changes in nutritional parameters that were not accompanied by reduced postoperative complications. Therefore, 7 to 10 days of preoperative PN in Crohn's disease should be restricted to seriously malnourished patients (SGA "C") who are not candidates for enteral nutrition (EN), usually because of bowel obstruction. For patients who are significantly nutritionally depleted, longer term nutritional support may be required to improve postoperative morbidity.

In the majority of patients, surgery should not be delayed because of the administration of nutritional support. Delaying surgery often leads to a further decline in the nutritional reserve of a patient. Nutritional support should be continued or started postoperatively if the patient is considered moderately (SGA "B") or severely malnourished (SGA "C") preoperatively. Patients are usually unable to take sufficient oral nutrition for at least 5 days following intestinal resection as a result of postoperative ileus.

Parenteral Nutrition

Once nutritional support is deemed necessary, which route—PN versus EN—should be used? Indications for PN usually include small bowel obstruction, which may develop in Crohn's disease because of adhesions related to prior surgery, severe edema with luminal compromise during an acute flare, or chronic, fibrotic scar tissue; severe diarrhea and malabsorption during active disease; small bowel ileus; GI hemorrhage; treatment for entero-cutaneous or entero-enteric fistulae; and as supportive care in patients who are severely malnourished (SGA "C") or who have active disease with compromised absorptive surface. PN may also be indicated in a patient with ulcerative colitis and toxic mega colon in which EN is not possible. PN is not generally indicated in patients who have a nonobstructive GI tract or when the duration of nutritional support is expected to be less than 7 days.

It is thought that the gut "atrophies" in the absence of EN. While this may be the case in animal studies, the data in humans fails to support this concept. It is commonly thought that in the absence of EN, bacteria will translocate across the intestinal epithelium, to the mesenteric lymph nodes, and into the systemic circulation, resulting in sepsis and multi-organ failure. Although this has been reported in the rat model, it rarely occurs in humans.[14] When bacterial translocation does occur in humans, it is usually in the setting of small bowel obstruction, is unrelated to the route of feeding, and is usually clinically inconsequential.[14]

It is controversial whether the combination of complete bowel rest and PN can be used successfully as primary therapy in patients with acute IBD with or without the addition of other medical therapy including diet. The consensus of the literature would suggest that patients with Crohn's enteritis might be placed into clinical remission with the combination of bowel rest and PN alone.[15-20] The composite results suggest npo and PN for 3 to 6 weeks will achieve a clinical response rate of 64% in patients with acute Crohn's disease.[20] However, in most studies, prednisone was given simultaneously with PN, which makes it difficult to discern whether the positive effects observed are totally the result of bowel rest and PN or the combined effects of prednisone. On the other hand, the consensus of the literature would suggest that patients with Crohn's colitis and idiopathic ulcerative colitis do not respond any better to PN and bowel rest (with or without prednisone) than do patients treated with prednisone and diet.[21-23] Also reported in many of these reports is a 10% risk of complications associated with PN, including pneumothorax from central catheter placement, catheter sepsis, and various metabolic complications. Therefore, before administrating a therapy with questionable benefit, the potential risk of therapy should be considered. PN is generally reserved for supportive therapy to maintain nutritional reserve rather than as primary treatment.

Intestinal fistula is one circumstance in which npo and bowel rest may serve as primary treatment. A 38% of fistula closure rate has been reported in Crohn's patients.[24] However, the reported studies lack a non-PN control group and there generally was no long-term follow-up reported. In the opinion of these authors, if closure is not obvious after 3 months, surgery is usually required. For Medicare reimbursement, 3 months or longer of PN is usually required and distal EN has to be documented as not possible.

With newer medications, such as infliximab, PN and bowel rest may serve less of a role in the treatment of fistulas. A randomized study comparing PN plus bowel rest to infliximab in addition to an oral diet is needed. Octreotide should only be used in patients with high output proximal fistulas. Octreotide is not compatible in PN and therefore should not be mixed. The role of EN is discussed in following sections of this chapter.

Choosing the Route for Parenteral Nutrition Delivery

Once it has been determined that PN is indicated for a particular patient, a route for delivery must be selected. PN can be delivered via a peripheral or a central vein. Peripheral PN is generally used when short-term nutritional support is required (eg, <7 to 10 days). The peripheral access can sometimes be used to supply total nutritional needs (30 to 40 kcal/day), especially if a lipid emulsion is used. Lipid emulsions are isotonic. Because of the hypertonicity of the dextrose, thrombophlebitis is a significant risk when concentrations above 10% are used. The amino acid concentration in the PN solution should also be <3.5% to ensure the solution has <900 mOsm. Heparin (1000 units/l) and hydrocortisone (10 mg/l) will reduce the risk of thrombophlebitis. Central parenteral nutrition (CPN), more typically referred to as PN, is infused into a large central vein. Large veins such as the superior vena cava (SVC) or the inferior vena cava (IVC) can tolerate a greater solution osmolarity (up to 1800 mOsm, typically 35% dextrose and 5% amino acids).

It is important that the catheter tip reside in either the SVC or IVC. Should the tip be located in a smaller vessel, catheter thrombosis could result when the hypertonic PN solution is infused. Catheter location within the right atrium may increase the risk of cardiac arrhythmia. A catheter useful for PN may include a percutaneously inserted central catheter (PICC) that is typically inserted via the brachial (although occasionally the antecubital) vein and advance to the SVC. The risk of a pneumothorax can be avoided with this method and therefore should be the choice of access, in the authors' opinion. A triple, double, or single lumen (preferably) catheter inserted into the subclavian, internal jugular, or femoral vain may also be used, provided the catheter tip is located within the SVC or IVC. For longer-term use, it is typical that a single lumen Hickman, Broviac, or Groshong catheter or a subcutaneous infusion port be inserted. Regardless of the catheter type, it is critical that a catheter lumen be reserved for the exclusive use of PN to minimize infection risk.

(Routes of administration for PN and EN are the topics of Chapters 35 and 41.)

Writing the Parenteral-Nutrition Prescription: How Much is Necessary?

A number of studies have investigated energy expenditure and nitrogen excretion in patients with both active and inactive disease.[25] Patients with inactive disease do not differ from normal controls whereas patients with active disease may require 1.2 to 1.5 times additional calories above resting energy expenditure. For most adult patients, 30 to 40 kcal/kg of IBW per day and 1 to 1.5 g/kg of IBW of protein is usually sufficient. Most hospitalized patients only require nutritional support for 2 weeks or less.

IBW can be calculated using the following equations: 48 kg + 2.7(x) in males and 45 kg + 2.3(x) in females, with "x" being the number of inches over 60 inches in the patient's height. Caloric measurement using indirect calorimetry is usually not needed. A minimum of 200 g of dextrose is necessary daily to meet the needs of brain metabolism. The carbohydrate used in PN solutions is dextrose monohydrate, which contains between 3.4 kcal/ml.

Intravenous fat emulsion is typically used to supply 20% to 40% of the daily calories. Only 6% of daily calories are needed as lipid emulsion to prevent essential fatty acid deficiency. Fat emulsions supply either 1.1 or 2.0 kcal/ml, depending upon whether a 10% or 20% emulsion is selected. Fluid requirements can usually be met by using 1 ml/kcal or a 1.5- to 2.0-L PN formula. Patients with cardiac or renal insufficiency may require less and patients with significant diarrhea or fistula losses may require more.

Depending upon the specific order form used, one can order PN either in terms of absolute amounts of macromolecules (ie, dextrose, lipid, and protein) or by indicating a total volume and final concentration of these PN constituents. Electrolytes, minerals, trace elements, and vitamins can be written for using "standard " amounts—ie, multi-trace metals and multiple vitamin solutions—unless the addition of a specific nutrient is required to correct or prevent a deficiency or withholding of a specific ingredient is necessary to avoid potential toxicity. For example, a 70-kg male who requires 25 kcal/kg/day and 1.0 g/kg/day of protein for maintenance might receive the following formula: 2 L of 20% dextrose (400 g, providing 1360 kcal) + 200 ml of 20% lipid emulsion (400 kcal) with 3.5% amino acids (700 g). Again, depending upon the formulation capabilities of the hospital pharmacy, the complete solution can be provided as a 3-in-1 emulsion (3 being dextrose, lipid, and amino acids) or as a 2-in-1 solution (2 being dextrose and amino acids) with the lipid emulsion hung in a "piggybacked" fashion. Initially, the PN rate should be relatively slow (eg, 40 ml/hour) and even slower in the malnourished patient. The rate can be advanced as rapidly as every 8 hours in a normally nourished individual without diabetes mellitus as long as the blood glucose is <160 mg/dl. During continuous CPN, the blood glucose should be determined every 6 hours.

Monitoring Parenteral Nutrition

Safety

If used inappropriately or not monitored appropriately, PN will not have any value to the patient and may even become a life-threatening therapy rather than life saving. It is generally recommended to consult the services of a multidisciplinary nutritional support team in the hospital to assist in writing the PN prescription, monitoring the therapy, and making adjustments as required. However, it is imperative the responsible physician understand the importance of appropriate monitoring, especially in the absence of a nutritional support team.

Patients should be weighed daily, and accurate inputs and outputs should be recorded. If weight gain is planned, anything more than 1 to 2 kg/week indicates fluid retention. This may occur in the first week or two of PN; decreasing the rate of PN is usually sufficient, although occasionally diuretic therapy becomes necessary.

In general, electrolytes should be monitored daily during the first few days of PN and then at least twice weekly. Acid base disturbances can often be managed by increasing or decreasing acetate or chloride in the solution. Metabolic acidosis may be caused by diarrhea and can usually be corrected by a slight increase of potassium acetate to the solution. Hypochloremic metabolic alkalosis may result from nasogastric suction in the absence of adequate replacement fluid. Elevated BUN may result because of the provision of insufficient fluid, excessive amino acid infusion, or renal insufficiency.

Mild elevations in the hepatic aminotransferases (ALT, AST), as well as the alkaline phosphatase, are often observed within 2 to 14 days of initiating PN and should be determined at baseline and subsequently on a weekly basis.[26] These elevations are generally transient. More persistent elevation in ALT and/or AST may result from hepatic steatosis from overfeeding or choline deficiency.[26,28] Persistently elevated alkaline phosphatase may signify the development of biliary sludge, which will occur in virtually 100% of patients on PN that are npo. It is usual to see a rise in serum bilirubin as a direct result of PN. A rise in bilirubin is a concern and other causes besides PN should be evaluated. A low alkaline phosphatase, especially in the Crohn's patient with chronic diarrhea, may be a sign of zinc deficiency.[29]

The serum triglyceride concentration should be monitored twice weekly during the first week and weekly thereafter to ascertain adequate clearance of the lipid emulsion. It should be obtained 4 to 6 hours after infusion of the lipid emulsion has been completed. Although there is no clear evidence of the deleterious effects of a serum triglyceride concentration <1000 mg/dl, it is generally recommended to decrease the infusion rate and/or volume of the lipid emulsion if the triglyceride concentration is greater than 400-500 mg/dl; a concentration of >1000 mg/dl may be associated with the development of pancreatitis.[30]

The human body adapts to starvation and weight loss by decreasing resting energy expenditure. When massive amounts of carbohydrate are supplied to a malnourished patient in an overzealous attempt to renourish them, refeeding syndrome may result.[31] This potentially life-threatening complication of either PN or EN therapy occurs when carbohydrate intake stimulates pancreatic insulin release, which results in the flow of potassium and magnesium to the intercellular space, which may result in cardiac arrhythmias. In addition, the demand for phosphate to produce ATP from the infused carbohydrate may result in hypophosphatemia with subsequent hemolytic anemia, seizures, rhabdomyolysis, and/or respiratory muscle dysfunction. In rare cases, respiratory failure may ensue. Prevention of refeeding syndrome can be prevented by the slow introduction of carbohydrate, use of protein (amino acids), and lipid. Small amounts of supplemental potassium phosphate and magnesium may be helpful. Serum potassium, magnesium, and phosphate concentrations should be determined daily or more frequently if necessary until the goal caloric support and a stable electrolyte pattern in the normal range can be achieved. (See chapter 46 for a detailed discussion of refeeding syndrome.)

Infectious complications are also common in PN-treated patients and must be treated promptly to ensure the patient's safety.[32-34] Infections and other complications related to PN are discussed in detail in Chapter 38.

Efficacy

There is no gold standard or specific laboratory test to measure the efficacy of nutritional support with either PN or EN. Weight gain in the hospital during a 1- to 2-week course of nutritional support is usually the result of fluid and not lean body mass. Serum visceral proteins, such as prealbumin, can be measured and followed during the course of therapy if desired. The half-life of prealbumin is 2 days, whereas the half-life of albumin at 21 days, which is too long to be useful in the inpatient setting. The serum concentrations of all visceral proteins, including prealbumin, may be affected by many non-nutritional factors including intra- and extravascular fluid shifts in the postoperative patient; may be depressed because of the protein losing enteropathy seen in active IBD; or may be depressed because of decreased synthesis as the liver turns towards increased production of acute phase proteins during active disease. Although serum concentration of visceral proteins may guide nutritional therapy, they should be interpreted with the caveats described above. Also, normal visceral protein synthesis cannot occur in the absence of sufficient energy intake because skeletal muscle will be catabolized as a fuel source. Serum transferrin will be low in the face of iron-deficient anemia, and, as such, is often not useful in patients with IBD.

The nitrogen balance can also be determined if one has a laboratory to perform accurate measurements. A 24-hour urine collection is required. Total urine nitrogen (TUN) is measured and subtracted from the nitrogen intake from PN (or EN, for that matter). An additional 2 g is subtracted to account for stool, sweat, and other insensible losses. It is assumed some 95% of nitrogen is generally absorbed and that the average amino acid or protein is 16% nitrogen. Therefore, to derive the nitrogen intake, the grams of amino acids (or protein in the case of enteral feeding) are divided by 6.25. If the TUN is not readily available, the urine urea nitrogen can be measured. If that is the case, 4 g should be added to the measured nitrogen excretion in order to account for insensible losses and urinary nitrogen losses than are not in the form of urea. Similar to visceral proteins, a positive nitrogen balance requires not only greater nitrogen intake than excretion, but also an energy intake at least equal to energy expenditure. Maintaining a patient in positive nitrogen balance has been associated with better outcome and lower mortality.

Home Parenteral Nutrition

Patients may require home parenteral nutrition (HPN) because they have developed short bowel syndrome from multiple bowel resections for Crohn's disease, have chronically draining entero-enteric or enterocutaneous fistulae, or have become severely malnourished in the face of active disease. Such therapy requires assessment of the home environment for appropriateness and safety and proper training of either the patient or a responsible adult, especially in aseptic catheter care.

The patient should be metabolically stable prior to discharge. It is appropriate to cycle the PN to a 10- to 12-hour nocturnal infusion prior to discharge. IBD is the most common group of patients treated with long-term HPN at most centers. Catheter infection is the most common complication associated with HPN use. Catheter infection is no greater in the IBD group than in other patients receiving HPN. Patients with IBD have a better-estimated 5-year survival than do other groups of patients treated with HPN.[35] HPN is discussed in detail in Chapter 40.

Enteral Nutrition

In the absence of bowel obstruction, fistula, or toxic mega colon, EN is the preferred form of nutritional support provided the patient will consent to having a nasogastric tube placed. Occasionally, patients are too ill or refuse to have a tube placed in their nose. In general, EN in the patient with IBD will take place via a nasogastric tube. A small bore, 8- to 10-Fr feeding tube should be used rather than a larger tube used for gastric decompression. Complications (discussed in Chapter 38) are generally fewer with such a tube. The risk of aspiration is not necessarily decreased with post pyloric feeding and hence such feeding is rarely necessary in this population. However, because of postoperative gastro paresis, jejunal feeding may be preferred in those individuals.

Tube placement should be verified radiologically prior to beginning feeding because physical examination, namely ausculatory confirmation, is often inaccurate for determining tube position. In general, feeding is begun at a relatively slow rate (typically 40 ml/hour) and advanced every 8 hours until the goal rate is achieved and if gastric residuals are <200 ml prior to each rate increase. However, if a small bore feeding tube is used or if jejunal feeding is undertaken, it may be difficult to aspirate and to determine an accurate gastric residual volume. In these patients, abdominal pain, distention, and tenderness are used to determine enteral feeding tolerance.

In malnourished patients, the formula infusion rate should be increased more gradually to avoid refeeding syndrome. (See above and, for more detail, see Chapter 45.) In addition, jejunal feeding in postoperative patients should be started at as little as 10 ml/hour, although this can often be accomplished in the immediate postoperative phase and advanced as tolerated. Most isotonic formulas are 1.0 to 1.5 kcal/ml and include the protein content in this calculation.

The protein content varies among formulas, and formulas for EN are discussed in Chapter 42. No formula provides sufficient free water to meet the daily fluid requirement. Therefore, it is important that patients with normal or increased fluid requirements receive at least the equivalent of 25% of the formula's volume as free water.

To prevent aspiration the patient's head and shoulders should be elevated to 30° to 45° at all times. Gastric residuals should also be checked every 4 hours and, if <200 ml, the aspirated formula should be returned to the tube as a bolus. The tube should be flushed with 30 ml of water after aspiration. Accurate input and outputs should be recorded and the patient should be weighted at least three times weekly.

Occasionally the nasogastric feeding tube may become clogged despite proper flushing as described. Often this is related to protein precipitates. Sugar-free, decaffeinated soda is often useful for dislodging this type of occlusion. Sometimes, meat tenderizer (papain) is necessary. One teaspoon of non-potato flake papain meat tenderizer can be mixed in the smallest amount of tap water (to dissolve it) and instilled in the catheter. The specific pancreatic enzyme preparations Pancrease (Ortho-McNeil, Raritan, NJ) or Viokase (Axscan Scandipharm, Birmingham, AL) can be mixed with one crushed 324-mg sodium bicarbonate tablet in 5 ml of tap water and instilled into the feeding tube. It may be necessary to repeat the procedure. Some medications are not compatible with EN; therefore, compatibility should be determined prior to using the feeding tube for instillation.

Other complications of tube feeding include esophagitis, esophageal and/or gastric erosions or ulceration, or esophageal stricture or mucosal bridge formation. Esophageal or gastric erosions may be evident within a week, although longer-term use is generally required before clinically significant disease, including GI hemorrhage, may occur. In addition, nasal erosions and nasal cartilage sloughing may result from excessive pressure on the nasal alae and cartilage, and, therefore, nasogastric feeding should be undertaken via the same nares for a maximum of 4 to 6 weeks. Complications of EN are discussed in detail in Chapter 39.

Regarding the formula to use (Chapter 42), a defined formula given either orally or via feeding tube may have potential benefit as primary treatment in Crohn's patients.[36-39] The composite data suggest that the administration of either an elemental, peptide-based, or polymeric diet for 3 to 6 weeks will achieve a remission rate of approximately 68%, which is similar to the remission rate reported with PN and bowel rest. The reason patients with active Crohn's disease may respond to polymeric EN but not an ad-lib regular oral diet is unclear but may be related to the lipid composition of the enteral formula. Diets high in long-chain triglycerides and polyunsaturated fats may be risk factors for the relapse of Crohn's disease.[40]

References

1. Seidman EG. Nutritional management of inflammatory bowel disease. *Gastroenterology Clinics of North Am.* 1989;18:129-155.
2. Detsky AS, McLaughlin JR, Baker JP, et al. What is subjective global assessment of nutritional status? *JPEN.* 1987:8-13.
3. Franklin JL, Rosenberg IH. Impaired folic acid absorption in inflammatory bowel disease: effects of salicylazosulfapyridine. *Gastroenterology.* 1973;64:517-525.
4. Behrend C, Jeppesen PB, Mortensen PB. Vitamin B-12 absorption after ileorectal anastomosis for Crohn's disease: effect of ileal resection and time span after surgery. *Eur J Gastroenterol Hepatol.* 1995;7:397-400.
5. Vogelsang H, Ferenci P, Resch H, et al. Prevention of bone mineral loss in patients with Crohn's disease by long term oral vitamin D supplementation. *Eur J Gastroenterology Hepatol.* 1995;7:609-614.
6. Bousvaros A, Zurakowski D, Duggan C, et al. Vitamins A and E serum levels in children and young adults with inflammatory bowel disease: effect of disease activity. *J Ped Gastro Nutr.* 1999;26:129-134.
7. Valberg LS, Flanagan PR, Kertesz A, et al. Zinc absorption in inflammatory bowel disease. *Dig Dis Sci.* 1986;31:724-731.
8. Fernandez-Banares F, Hinojosa J, Sanchez-Lombrana JL, et al. Randomized clinical trial of Plantago ovata seeds (dietary fiber) as compared with mesalamine in maintaining remission in ulcerative colitis. *Am J Gastroenterol.* 1999; 94:427-433.
9. Suarez FL, Savaiano DA, Levitt MD. A comparison of symptoms after the consumption of milk or lactose-hydrolyzed milk by people with self-reported severe lactose intolerance. New Engl J Med 1995; 333:1-4.
10. Belluzzi A, Brignola C, Campieri M, et al. Effect of enteric coated fish oil preparations on relapses in Crohn's disease. NEJM 1996;334:1557-1560.
11. Lorenz-Meyer H, Nicolay C, Schulz B, et al. Omega 3 fatty acids and low carbohydrate diet for maintenance of remission in Crohn's disease: a randomized controlled multicenter trial. *Scand J Gastroenterol.* 1996;31:778-785.
12. Caughey GE, Mantzioris E, Gibson RA, et al. The effect on human tumor necrosis factor alpha and interleukin 1B production of diets enriched in n-3 fatty acids from vegetable oil or fish. *Am J Clin Nutr.* 1996;63:116-122.
13. Lashner BA, Evans AA, Hanauer SB. Preoperative total parenteral nutrition for bowel resection in Crohn's disease. *Dig Dis Sci.* 1989;34:741-746.
14. Sedman PC, MacFie J, Palmer MD, et al. Preoperative total parenteral nutrition is not associated with mucosal atrophy or bacterial translocation in humans. *Br J Surg.* 1995; 82:1663-1667.
15. Ostro MJ, Greenberg GR, Jeejeebhoy KN. Total parenteral nutrition and complete bowel rest in the management of Crohn's disease. *JPEN.* 1985;9:280-287.
16. Reilly J, Ryan JA, Stole W, et al. Hyperalimentation in inflammatory bowel disease. *Am J Surg.* 1976;131:192-200.
17. Mullen JL, Hargrove WC, Dudrick SJ, et al. Ten years experience with intravenous hyperalimentation and inflammatory bowel disease. *Ann Surg.* 1978;187:523-529.
18. Greenberg GR, Fleming CR, Jeejeebhoy KN. Controlled trial of bowel rest and nutritional support in the management of Crohn's disease. *Gut.* 1988;29:1309-1315.
19. Lochs SH, Meryn S, Marosi L, et al. Has total bowel rest have a beneficial effect in the treatment of Crohn's disease. *Clin Nutr.* 1983;2:61-64.
20. Greenberg GR. Nutritional management of inflammatory bowel disease. *Semin Gastrointest Dis.* 1993;4:69-86.
21. Dickinson RJ, Ashton MG, Axon AT, et al. Controlled trial of intravenous hyperalimentation and bowel rest as an adjunct to routine therapy of acute colitis. *Gastroenterology.* 1980; 79:1199-1204.
22. McIntyre PB, Powell-Tuck J, Wood SR. Controlled trial of bowel rest in the treatment of severe acute colitis. *Gut.* 1986;27:481-5.
23. Sitzmann JV, Converse RL, Bayless TM. Favorable response to parenteral nutrition and medical therapy in Crohn's colitis. *Gastroenterology.* 1990;99:1647-52.
24. Afonso JJ, Rombeau JL. Nutritional care for patients with Crohn's disease. *Hepato-gastroenterol.* 1990;37:32-41.
25. Chan ATH, Fleming CR, O'Fallon WM, et al. Estimated versus measured basal energy requirements in patients with Crohn's disease. *Gastroenterology.* 1986;91:75-78.
26. Buchman AL, Ament ME. Liver disease and total parenteral nutrition. In: Zakim D, Boyer TD, eds. *Textbook of Liver Disease.* 3rd ed. Philadelphia: WB Saunders; 1996: 1812-1821.

27. Buchman AL. *Handbook of Nutritional Support*. Baltimore: Williams and Wilkins; 1997.
28. Buchman AL, Sohel M, Dubin M, Jenden DJ, Roch M. Choline deficiency causes reversible hepatic abnormalities in patients during parenteral nutrition: proof of a human choline requirement; a placebo-controlled trial. *JPEN.* 2001; 25:260-268.
29. Samman S, Soto C, Cooke L, et al. Is erythrocyte alkaline phosphatase activity a marker of serum zinc status in humans? *Biol Trace Elem Res.* 1996; 51:285-291.
30. Toskes PP. Hyperlipidemic pancreatitis. *Gastroenterol Clin N Am.* 1990;19:783-791.
31. Solomon SM, Kirby DF. The refeeding syndrome: a review. *JPEN.* 1990;14:90-97.
32. Buchman AL, Moukarzel A, Goodson B, et al. Catheter-related infections associated with home parenteral nutrition and predictive factors for the need for catheter removal in their treatment. *JPEN.* 1994; 18:297-302.
33. Messing B, Peitra-Cohen S, Debure A, et al. Antibiotic-lock technique: a new approach to optimal therapy for catheter-related sepsis in home-parenteral nutrition patients. *JPEN.* 1988;12:185-189.
34. Atkinson JB, Bagnall HA, Gomperts E. Investigational use of tissue plasminogen activator (t-PA) for occluded central venous catheters. *JPEN.* 1990;14:310-311.
35. Scolapio JS, Fleming CR, Kelly DG, et al. Survival of home parenteral nutrition treated patients: 20 year experience at the Mayo Clinic. *Mayo Clinic Proc.* 1999;74:217-222.
36. O'Morain C, Segal AW, Levi AJ, et al. Elemental diet as primary treatment of acute Crohn's disease: a controlled trial. *BMJ.* 1984;288:1859-62.
37. Jones VA. Comparison of total parenteral nutrition and elemental diet in induction of remission of Crohn's disease. *Dig Dis Sci.* 1987;32:100-7.
38. Gonzalez-Huix F, de Leon R, Fernandez-Banares F, et al. Polymeric enteral diets as primary treatment of active Crohn's disease: a prospective steroid controlled trial. *Gut.* 1993;34:778-82.
39. Rigaud D., Cosnes J, Le Quintree Y, et al. Controlled trial comparing two types of enteral nutrition in treatment of active Crohn's disease: elemental v polymeric diet. *Gut.* 1991;32:1492-7.
40. Miura S, Tsuzuki Y, Hokari R, Ishii H. Modulation of intestinal immune system by dietary fat intake: relevance to Crohn's disease. *J Gastroenterol Hepatol.* 1998; 13:1183-1190.

Chapter 19

Celiac Disease

Darlene G. Kelly, MD, PhD, and
Vandana Nehra, MD

Introduction

Celiac disease—also known as celiac sprue, nontropical sprue, or gluten-sensitive enteropathy—is intimately related to diet and nutrition from the aspects of etiology and clinical manifestations and as the sole treatment modality. The disease was first described in ancient times, although its relationship to gluten was not identified until 1950, when Dicke reported it in a doctoral thesis.[1] Celiac disease can be defined as a pathological intolerance of the intestinal mucosa to prolamins, which are the storage proteins in cereal grains, that occurs in genetically predisposed individuals.

Epidemiology

Celiac disease was thought to be primarily a disease of certain regions in the world, especially Ireland and Italy. However, recent studies based on both histological and immune markers of celiac disease have identified celiac disease as one of the most prevalent chronic diseases across Europe.[2] In Switzerland, researchers found a prevalence of 1 in 132 adolescents, representing a 10-fold increase compared to similar studies reported 20 years previously.[3] A population study of a small area of Saharan west Africa found celiac disease to affect 1 in 20 children.[4] South American studies have reported prevalences that are similar.[5,6] A recent study of the population of Olmsted County, Minnesota, found that the incidence of diagnosis of celiac disease had increased by nearly 12-fold over the past 4 decades.[7] This apparent increase is, at least in part, likely to be the result of increased awareness of the latent form of the disease and the availability of better screening tests. Clearly, many of those affected with celiac disease have been given other diagnoses, such as irritable bowel syndrome. Overall, prevalence of celiac disease among Caucasians in Europe and North America has been estimated at 1 in 200,[8] and the disease appears to be decreasing in children while it is increasing in older individuals.[2] Women are more commonly affected than men with a ratio of 2:1.[9]

Pathogenesis: Genes, Peptides, and Immune Response

Celiac disease has been observed to cluster in families, suggesting a genetic link to the disease. The disease is polygenic, but it is also multi-factorial in that it requires triggering by the environment in the form of gluten.[10] Human leukocyte antigens (HLA) DQ2 and DQ8 have been found to be risk factors for the disease.[11] These genes are expressed on the surface of B cells, T cells, and macrophages where they code for a class II MHC molecule that has the function of presenting short peptide antigens to receptor on CD4+ (helper) T cells.

Fasano et al[12] have proposed that histological damage seen in celiac disease is mediated by the upregulation of zonulin, a protein in the mucosa responsible for altering gut permeability. Normally, the tight junctions of the intestine regulate passage of molecules of varying sizes. In celiac disease, the disruption of this controlled transit of larger molecules may allow the antigenic peptide components of gluten to pass into the lamina propria, where they are recognized by the inflammatory cells containing DQ2 or DQ8 genes, thus setting up an autoimmune reaction and the resulting immune-mediated tissue damage.[13]

The antigenic motifs consist of amino acid segments containing proline and glutamine within the structure and are found within the α-gliadin peptides of gluten. These motifs require deamidation of glutamine residue(s) by tissue transglutaminase 2 (tTG) to alter the domain for binding with the HLA-DQ2 molecule.[14] The α-gliadin–specific CD4+ cells that produce γ-interferon are responsible for the characteristic villous atrophy and crypt hyperplasia within the mucosa of the small bowel. These CD4+ cells can be isolated from biopsies of the duodenum from individuals with celiac disease but not from those of normal individuals.[15]

Up to 95% of cases of celiac disease are associated with HLA-DQ2 and 5% to 10% with HLA-DQ8.[16] Meanwhile, 20% to 30% of normal individuals express these haplotypes.[17] Those lacking DQ2 or DQ8 are rarely affected by celiac disease. Studies in monozygotic twins demonstrated concordance rates for celiac disease to be 75%, and for dizygotic twins it was 11%.[18] The fact that individuals with genetic predisposition do not develop the disease suggests that a yet-unrecognized additional factor(s) is responsible for homeostatic tolerance to gluten or conversely is the trigger(s) for the breakdown of the mechanisms responsible for the expression of celiac disease. There is evidence from epidemiological studies that breast-feeding offers an independent protective effect against celiac disease if it occurs when gluten was introduced into the diet.[19]

Clinical Presentation

In children, the onset of celiac disease is usually within the first to third year of life, when gluten is introduced into their diet. There may be a latent period of months to years, however. Children with the disease may present with symptoms of chronic diarrhea, failure to thrive, muscle wasting, abdominal distention, vomiting, and abdominal pain. If the diagnosis is delayed, it may result in severe malnutrition and ataxia. In some children, constipation, pseudo-obstruction, and intussusception may be seen. It has been estimated that 2% to 8% of children with unexplained short stature may have celiac disease.[20] Dental enamel defects involving secondary dentition as well as neurological syndrome and epilepsy with intracranial calcification have also been reported in children with celiac disease.

Initially, celiac disease was believed only to present in younger age groups. However, in recent years celiac disease has also been recognized to present in a latent or so-called silent form, with a mean age at diagnosis of 45 years and the age range extending into the tenth decade.[7] This form of the disease has been estimated to be 7 to 15 times more prevalent than classical celiac disease.[21]

In adults, celiac disease may be overt in presentation, with classic symptoms of diarrhea, weight loss, and abdominal pain. The presence of diarrhea and steatorrhea, which occurs in about 50% of patients, indicates severe disease and malabsorption. The symptoms of abdominal discomfort and bloating often lead to a mistaken diagnosis of irritable bowel syndrome.

Celiac disease may primarily present with nongastrointestinal (GI) symptoms such as anemia, abnormal liver tests, osteopenic bone disease, neurological symptoms, or menstrual abnormalities. Anemia is common in both children and adults with celiac disease and may be secondary to iron deficiency, folate deficiency, or a combination of the two. Iron deficiency is frequently associated with celiac disease.[22] When evaluated by upper endoscopy, 6% to 10% of the patients with unexplained iron deficiency anemia were noted to have celiac disease based on small bowel biopsies.[23,24]

The finding of unexplained elevated serum transaminases (ALT, AST) should also raise the suspicion of undiagnosed celiac disease, even in those without GI symptoms, making measurement of immune markers an important part of workup of hypertransaminasemia. Up to 9% of adults with unexplained elevated serum transaminases have been diagnosed with celiac disease based on serological testing or small bowel biopsy.[25] Liver biopsies in these individuals may show reactive hepatitis. In this setting, adherence to a gluten-free diet results in improvement or normalization of the liver enzyme levels.[26]

Patients with untreated celiac disease are at increased risk for the development of osteoporosis and low bone mineral density[27] (Chapter 13). A variety of mechanisms predispose to the development of bone disease in patients with celiac disease; these include malabsorption of calcium and vitamin D (because of impaired absorption of calcium secondary to impaired transport by the diseased small bowel) as well as precipitation of the ingested calcium with unabsorbed intraluminal fats to form insoluble soaps that are then excreted in the stool. Untreated, patients with celiac disease have been observed to have increased bone turnover and elevated levels of 1,25 dihydroxy cholecalciferol because of secondary hyperparathyroidism that helps maintain a positive calcium balance.[28] This results in diminished bone densities associated with increased risk fractures in patients with classical celiac disease. Moreno et al[29] reported that 34% of their study population with celiac disease had fractures in the peripheral skeleton. For those with classical celiac symptoms, the odds ratio for fracture was 5.2 compared to those without celiac disease. Those with subclinical or silent celiac disease were no different than healthy controls. Although the reduced bone mineral density improves on a gluten-free diet, adults with celiac sprue are at increased risk for the development of bone fractures.[30]

Infertility and recurrent spontaneous abortions have been reported in women with celiac disease.[31] Male infertility has also been observed in patients with untreated celiac disease.[32] Reversal of infertility both in males and females has been observed following treatment with a strict gluten-free diet.[33]

Patients with celiac disease may also present with neurological symptoms such as ataxia, muscle weakness, paresthesias, sensory loss, epilepsy, and bilateral parietoccipital calcification. Researchers in the United Kingdom reported that 30% of patients with celiac disease followed in their clinics had neurological and psychiatric conditions, the most common of which were depression, epilepsy, and migraine.[34]

Associated Disorders

Dermatitis Herpetiformis

Dermatitis herpetiformis is characterized by an extremely pruritic papulovesicular eruption that usually occurs symmetrically on the elbows, knees, buttocks, and back. About 80% of patients with dermatitis herpetiformis have small intestine histology indistinguishable from celiac sprue.[35] The diagnosis is established by skin biopsy demonstrating granular IgA deposits in areas of normal-appearing skin.[36] A majority of patients with the skin lesion who undergo small bowel biopsy have intestinal mucosal changes of celiac disease. The skin lesions, as well as small bowel histology, improve on a gluten-free diet.[37] Dapsone is an effective short-term treatment for dermatitis herpetiformis; however, it does not have any impact on management of small bowel enteropathy. Those with dermatitis herpetiformis who are not compliant with the gluten-free diet are at higher risk for malignancy, as are those with celiac disease.

Diabetes Mellitus

Celiac disease has also been associated with other autoimmune as well as nonautoimmune disorders. It has been reported that the longer there is exposure to gluten in patients with celiac disease, the greater the occurrence of other autoimmune diseases.[38] There is evidence for strong association between type 1 diabetes mellitus and celiac disease. Screening studies of type 1 diabetics have identified a prevalence of celiac disease ranging from 0.97% to 16.4% with an average of 4.5%.[39] The highest prevalence among diabetic children was found in children from the Sahara where 5% to 6% of children have celiac disease, although the coexistence of these diseases is the same as the overall prevalence rate for celiac disease in that population.[4]

When the two diseases coexist, 90% have the diagnosis of diabetes before that of celiac disease.[39] This observation may be related to the fact that diabetes is a very common disease, and, until recently, celiac disease was considered quite rare. The possible diagnosis of concurrent celiac disease may be considered when treatment of the diabetes fails to resolve the symptom array. Sometimes, the GI symptoms are only recognized retrospectively.[39] Among the symptoms that may be suggestive of coexisting celiac disease, in addition to those considered classical for celiac disease, are delayed puberty, hypertransaminasemia, anemia, iron deficiency, arthralgias, dental enamel defects, hypoglycemia, and unexplained reduction in insulin requirements.[39,40] Treatment with a gluten-free diet may actually improve diabetic control and decrease the occurrence hypoglycemia episodes.[41,40]

There is also a strong association between selective IgA deficiency occurring in 2% to 3% of patients with celiac disease.[42,43] This must be considered in diagnostic testing.

Down Syndrome

There is a strong association between Down syndrome and celiac disease. Individuals with Down syndrome and celiac disease more commonly have GI manifestations such as intermittent diarrhea, failure to thrive, anemia, and low serum iron and calcium. The prevalence of celiac disease in patients with Down syndrome varies between 5% and 12%.[44,45]

Liver Disease

There have been associations reported with many liver diseases, but predominant among these have been diseases with an immune basis. Associations between celiac disease and primary biliary cirrhosis (PBC) have been described for many years. British investigators found a prevalence of PBC in 3% of their patients with celiac disease and celiac disease in 6% of their patients with PBC.[46] Hay and coworkers[47] identified an association between primary sclerosing cholangitis (PSC) and celiac disease. A prevalence of celiac in approximately 3% of patients with PSC was subsequently reported by Volta et al.[48] These authors also found that in autoimmune hepatitis there was a 4% prevalence in celiac disease, and this was at least 8 times greater than the prevalence in the general population.[49]

Diagnosis of Celiac Disease

Small bowel biopsy remains the gold standard for diagnosis of celiac disease. Based on the 1990 revised criteria[50] of the European Society of Paediatric Gastroenterology and Nutrition, the diagnosis of celiac sprue can be made with a diagnostic small bowel biopsy in a patient with highly suggestive clinical symptoms, followed by a favorable clinical and serologic response to a gluten-free diet. The original criteria requiring a series of three biopsies—ie, first to confirm the diagnosis, second for demonstration of response to gluten-free diet, and the third for deterioration after gluten challenge—is no longer required. Endoscopic biopsies from the distal duodenum are preferable because the presence of Brunner glands in the duodenal bulb and second portion of the duodenum may affect histologic interpretation.[51,52]

Classical endoscopic features in patients with celiac disease include scalloped folds, absence of folds, and visible submucosal blood vessels. However, Oxentenko et al recently found that these endoscopic features are remarkably unreliable in diagnosing celiac disease.[53] Characteristic histologic changes described are partial or total villus atrophy, elongation of crypts, a decreased villous:crypt ratio, and increased intraepithelial lymphocytes (>30 per 100 enterocytes) (Figure 19-1). Marsh proposed a classification for the spectrum of histologic changes ranging from increased intraepithelial lymphocytes, termed Marsh I, to total villous atrophy, crypt hyperplasia, and intraepithelial lymphocytosis in Marsh IIIC.[54] In addition, Marsh described a fourth lesion—irreversible hypoplastic or aplastic lesions—that could develop malignant transformation. Wahab and colleagues[55] reported that a 30-g daily gluten challenge given to 12 of 38 patients with intraepithelial lymphocytes only (Marsh I) had progression of their mucosal changes to crypt hyperplasia and either partial or subtotal villus atrophy. A gluten-free diet subsequently reversed malabsorption and symptoms and reversed the changes seen in the biopsies. These

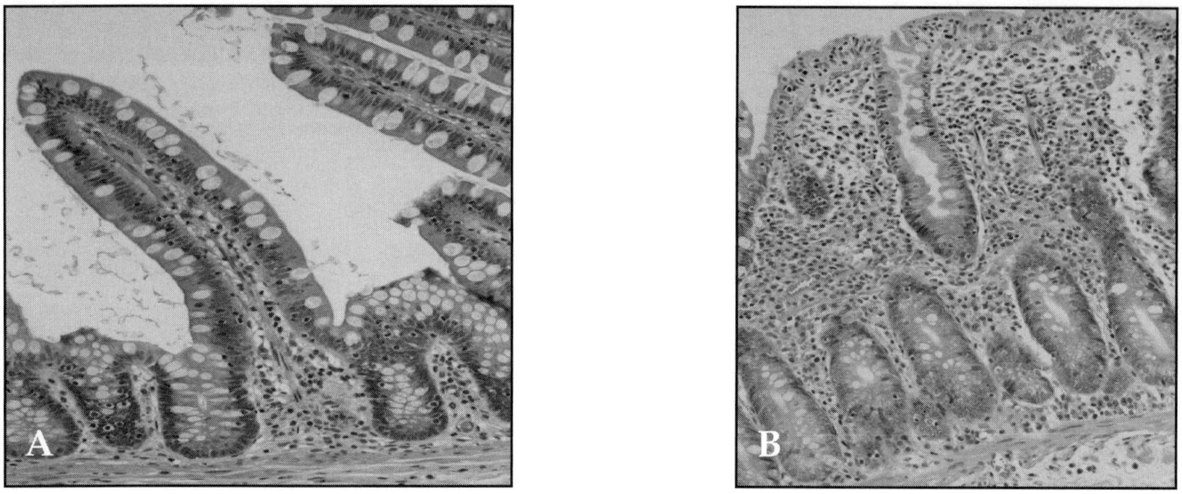

Figure 19-1. Small bowel biopsies comparing (A) a normal mucosa and (B) celiac disease demonstrating total villous atrophy, elongation of crypts, a decreased villous:crypt ratio, and increased intraepithelial lymphocytes. Images courtesy of Thomas Smyrk, MD, Mayo Clinic Rochester.

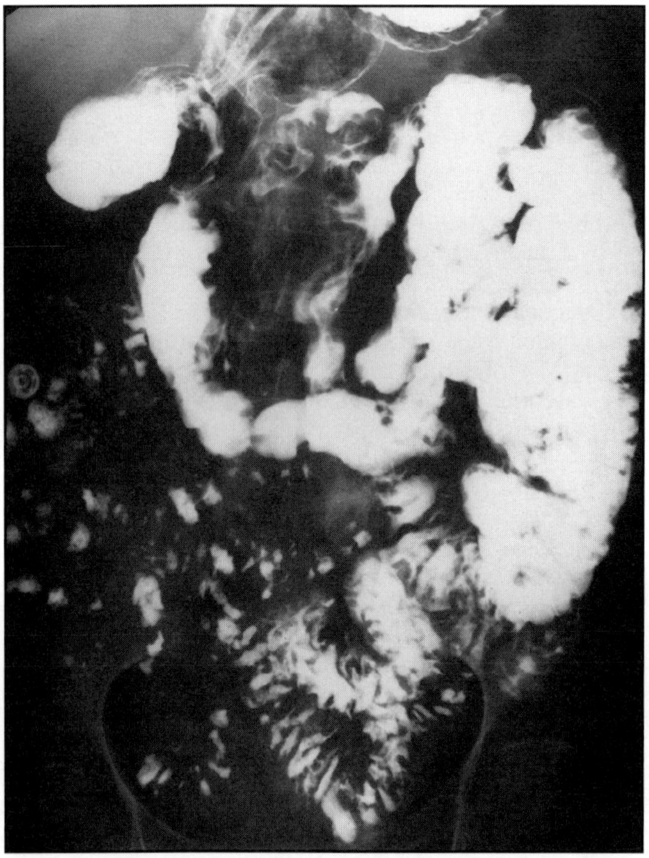

Figure 19-2. Small bowel X-ray showing findings of flocculation and segmentation of barium representing excessive fluid secretion in the lumen of the small intestine, thickened mucosal folds, and dilation of the small intestine. These are non-specific. Mayo Clinic Gastrointestinal Imaging (in press). Reprinted with permission of Mayo Foundation.

studies appear to lend credence to celiac disease playing a role in the cases of some individuals with lymphocytic enteritis and possibly even with lymphocytic colitis. Using response to a gluten-free diet without either serologic studies or biopsy is discouraged.[56]

The role of radiological studies in the initial diagnosis of celiac sprue is limited. The findings of flocculation and segmentation of barium representing excessive fluid secretion in the lumen of the small intestine, thickened mucosal folds, and dilation of the small intestine are nonspecific (Figure 19-2). Computerized tomography (CT) techniques may be useful in diagnosing the complications of celiac sprue, such as development of lymphoma, malignancy, hyposplenism, or cavitating mesenteric lymphadenopathy. CT enterography techniques are currently under investigation and may become an accepted diagnostic test in the future.

Serological tests have been used to test individuals with suggestive symptoms and to screen high-risk groups who may or may not have signs of disease and may ultimately undergo small bowel biopsy. The high-risk groups include first degree relatives of confirmed case of celiac disease, those with type 1 diabetes, Down syndrome, Turner's syndrome, unexplained dental enamel deficits, and children with unexplained short stature in childhood. Serological tests are also used to monitor progress after diagnosis as well as to use in prevalence studies in unselected populations. The serological tests utilized in current clinical practice include the endomysial antibody, tissue transglutaminase antibody, and the antigliadin antibodies (IgA and IgG).

The antigliadin antibodies are found in the intestinal secretions as well as serum of patients with untreated celiac disease. An enzyme-linked immunosorbent assay (ELISA) for both the IgA and IgG subclass of antibodies to gliadin has been used for the diagnosis of celiac disease. Their role in diagnosis is limited because of their moderate sensitivity and specificity. These antibodies are found in a variety of autoimmune disorders including rheumatoid arthritis, Sjogren's syndrome, sarcoidosis, inflammatory

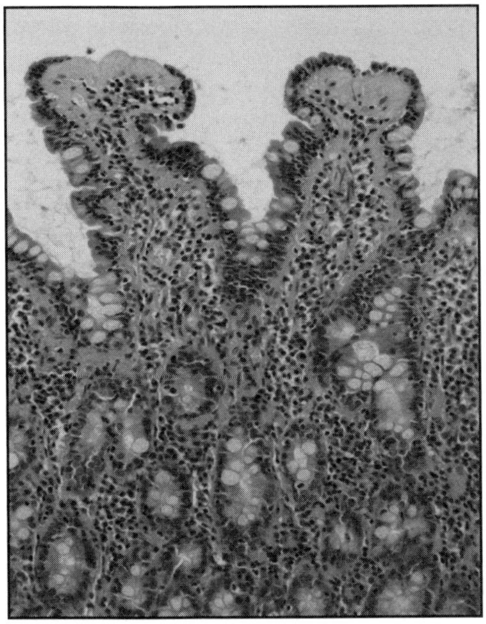

Figure 19-3. Collagenous celiac disease on small intestinal biopsy is characterized by a layer of collagen underlying the villous changes of celiac disease. Image courtesy of Thomas Smyrk, MD, Mayo Clinic Rochester.

bowel disease, and cow's milk protein intolerance. IgA antigliadin antibodies have sensitivity of 75% to 90% and specificity of 82% to 95%. Although the IgG antigliadin antibodies range in sensitivity from 69% to 85% and have specificity of 73% to 90%,[57] they are useful in diagnosis of celiac patients with IgA deficiency.

The IgA antiendomysial antibody (EMA) assay directed against the connective tissue protein found in the collagenous matrix of human and monkey tissue is both highly sensitive and specific. This test is based on immunofluorescence techniques using monkey esophagus or human umbilical cord as a substrate. Though highly sensitive (85% to 98%)[58] and specific (97% to 100%),[59] it has several limitations including false negative results, which may be evident in 2% to 3% of patients with celiac disease who have selective IgA deficiency. Other factors that have an impact on sensitivity and specificity of this test are laboratory variations and disease severity. In a study 60 of 101 patients with untreated celiac disease, the sensitivity of the endomysial antibody in those with total villous atrophy was excellent (100%) but decreased remarkably (31%) in patients with partial villous atrophy.

Tissue transglutaminase (tTG) is a cytosolic protein released by damaged epithelial cells. This is the autoantigen recognized by the endomysial antibody indirect immunofluorescence assay in patients with celiac disease.[61] The advantage of this test is that it is performed using ELISA techniques, which makes it easier to perform, widely available, and less costly. It eliminated the use of monkey esophagus as well as the subjective interpretation of immunofluorescence analysis of the endomysial antibody test.[8] Although the tTG test is comparable to EMA in sensitivity, there is loss of specificity in patients with autoimmune disorders;[62] hence, it is important to confirm the diagnosis with small intestine biopsy.

Complications of Celiac Disease

Nonresponsive and Refractory Sprue

Nonresponsive celiac disease has been described as a lack of clinical response to a gluten-free diet or the recurrence of symptoms despite maintenance of a gluten-free diet in a patient who initially responded. The most common cause of nonresponsive sprue is continued exposure to gluten intake. Evaluation should include confirmation of the initial diagnosis by reviewing the original small bowel biopsies, as well as review of dietary history by an experienced dietitian. Other diagnostic considerations include exclusion of other causes of malabsorption (Chapter 5), such as bacterial overgrowth,[63] pancreatic insufficiency,[64,65] lymphocytic colitis,[66] collagenous colitis,[67] lymphoma, ulcerative jejunitis, autoimmune,[68] and inflammatory bowel disease.[69,70]

The diagnosis of refractory sprue is considered when compliance with a gluten-free diet is definite and all causes of malabsorption associated with villous atrophy have been excluded. Refractory sprue is defined as primary when the patient has no response to gluten-free diet after initial diagnosis, or secondary when the patient has an initial response to gluten-free diet but symptoms recur despite strict adherence to gluten-free diet. Once diagnosis has been established, consideration needs to be given for treatment with steroids or other immunosuppressive agents, such as cyclosporine.[71]

Collagenous celiac disease, considered by many to be a variant of classical celiac disease, has a characteristic layer of collagen underlying the mucosa (Figure 19-3). It tends to be refractory to standard treatment and in some patients requires institution of long-term parenteral nutrition to prevent malnutrition.

Ulcerative Jejunitis

Ulcerative jejunitis is characterized by ulcers affecting the jejunum and the ileum. The clinical presentation is characterized by severe malabsorption and may present with the complications of bleeding, perforation, obstruction, and a high mortality.[72,73,74] Mills[75] has described four different groups of patients with ulcerative jejunitis: those with known celiac disease, those with villous atrophy unresponsive to gluten-free diet, those with normal intervening mucosa, and those with enteropathy-associated T-cell lymphoma. The diagnosis is generally achieved with an extended endoscopy, small bowel enteroscopy, capsule endoscopy, or laparotomy if the patient has presented with the complication of perforation or obstruction. Prognosis is generally poor, though steroids and azathioprine may induce remission.[76]

Lymphoma and Other Malignancies

Patients with celiac disease are at a greater risk than the general population for the development of malignant neoplasms, including lymphomas.[77,78] These T-cell lymphomas develop either in patients with known celiac disease who initially responded to a gluten-free diet but deteriorated with onset of lymphoma or in those with villous atrophy without a prior diagnosis of celiac disease. These are now termed enteropathy-type intestinal T-cell lymphoma. They usually present in fifth to seventh decades of life with weight loss, worsening diarrhea, abdominal pain, lymphadenopathy, abdominal mass, bleeding, obstruction, or perforation. Lesions are commonly in the jejunum but may occur throughout the small intestine. Diagnosis is based on clinical suspicion, small bowel biopsy, small bowel radiography, or CT[79] or at laparotomy.[80] The prognosis of these lymphomas is worse than that for primary GI lymphomas.[81] In most patients, the lymphoma is widespread at the time of diagnosis, with few surviving more than a year after diagnosis.[80,82]

Other tumors of the GI tract—including those of the mouth, pharynx, esophagus, and small intestine—as well as primary liver cancers occur with increased frequency in patients with either celiac sprue or dermatitis.[83] This increased risk of cancer disappears after 5 years on a strict gluten-free diet but not in those on a normal or reduced-gluten diet, thus suggesting the protective role of a gluten-free diet in celiac disease.[84]

Therapy

Since the identification of gluten as the major etiology for celiac disease in those who are genetically prone to express the disease, elimination of this inciting factor has been the only effective treatment. Gluten is present in many cereal grains, primarily wheat, barley, and rye. The question of whether oats also contain gluten has been debated in the literature for years.

Gluten is part of a group of prolamines that are storage proteins in cereal grains. It consists of proteins with a high content of glutamine (~35 mol%), proline (15 mol%), and hydrophobic amino acids (19 mol%) that contribute a rubbery structure to bread products.[85] It consists of two major protein fractions, gliadin, and glutenin with gliadin being the soluble component. Gliadin has been shown to be highly toxic in celiac disease, while glutenin has been shown to be contaminated by gliadins and possibly contributing to its purported toxicity.

The grains in the Triticeae group (including wheat, rye, and barley) all contain the amino acid sequences of peptides that are responsible for toxicity in celiac disease. The storage proteins of maize, rice, millet, sorghum, and buckwheat are not harmful to those with celiac disease. The prolamin in oats, avenin, has been tested with variable outcomes, but two short-term studies suggest that oats are nontoxic in celiac disease.[86,87] More recently, Janatuinen et al extended their study to 5 years, allowing oats to be used freely in a group of randomized adults with celiac disease.[88] Those receiving oats were not different from those on a strict gluten-free diet with respect to either antibodies or histology. Hogberg and colleagues reported that children with newly diagnosed celiac disease who were randomized to ingest moderate amounts of oats daily for 1 year had IgA antigliadin or antiendomysial antibody levels that were not different from those on a strict gluten-free diet, and biopsy specimens recovered to normal in both groups.[89] A recent review indicated that the risk with respect to oats is likely contamination with gluten arising in the milling process and not to antigens arising directly from the oats.[90]

Acid hydrolysis renders gliadin nontoxic in those with celiac disease, as does deamidation of the glutamine side chains.[85] However, digestion with pepsin, trypsin, or pancreatic juice does not alter toxicity of gluten or gliadin.

Wheat starch-based gluten-free flour products have been used in diets for celiac disease, but there are trace amounts of residual gluten in these products. It has been reported that up to 6% of foods labeled as gluten-free contain more than 30 mg of gliadin/100 g (300 ppm).[91] Additionally, many medications and other products, not typically thought of as foods, may contain significant amounts of gluten. Therefore, dietitians who are very experienced with celiac disease and others who are responsible for educating patients on the intricacies of the gluten-free diet must be well educated on products that may inadvertently introduce gliadin into the patient's intake, including many medications that contain gluten.

Dietary compliance is an issue, as a lifelong, strict, gluten-free diet is the only treatment available at this time. It has been reported that compliance is better in those diagnosed in early childhood.[92] Clearly, regular reinforcement of the importance of dietary compliance should be a part of any clinician's interaction with patients who have celiac disease.

Murray and coworkers[7] reported the response of GI symptoms to a gluten-free diet in a large group of patients with celiac disease in the US Midwest. Diarrhea responded to diet within days to weeks, with a mean time to resolution of 4 weeks. Among patients with alternating diarrhea and constipation, there was also resolution with a gluten-free diet. Fecal incontinence was also resolved. Although two-thirds of patients had lost weight prior to diagnosis, 23% had a body mass index (Chapters 2 and 47) greater than 25 and 11% above 30. Interestingly, after institution of a gluten-free diet, about 36% of patients actually lost weight. Of the 79% who had abdominal pain (most commonly lower abdominal or diffuse), nearly one-half fulfilled the Rome II criteria for irritable bowel syndrome. More than 95% of these individuals had relief of pain, typically within days of starting a gluten-free diet. Bloating was a common complaint in these patients, and this, too, responded to the gluten-free diet.

Another issue is whether there is tolerance to very small amounts of gluten in some patients. There is no conclusive evidence about the amount of gluten that can be tolerated by all patients with celiac disease.

New proposals for treatment have surfaced as the interactions of gluten and the cascade of inflammation has been better recognized. Genetically engineered grains to delete toxic potential may offer one approach to therapy.[21] Another proposed treatment option could interfere with HLA-DQ binding and T-cell activation.[21] Maiuri and colleagues have suggested that blockage of signals from interleukin-15 might offer an alternative treatment for the disease.[93] Additionally, there has been a suggestion of using a bacterial endoprotease to cleave gliadin peptides that are not digested within the intestinal lumen.[94] However, all of these approaches will be years in coming. Overall, these options may eventually offer an opportunity for those with celiac disease to stop their very restricted diet.

Conclusion

Celiac disease is a very common genetic disease that results in destruction of the small intestinal mucosa because of the toxicity of gluten. Gluten is widely found as a component of many cereal grains. The pathophysiology of the disease has been largely described within the last decade. The manifestations of celiac disease were initially thought to be expressed in childhood as a GI malabsorptive disease; however, recent observations have identified a wide range of severity of disease and even disease presenting without GI symptoms. Serious complications may occur, especially in the setting of untreated disease. The only treatment available at this time is a diet devoid of gluten.

References

1. Dicke WK, Weijers HA, Van De Kamer JH. Coeliac disease. II. The presence in wheat of a factor having a deleterious effect in cases of coeliac disease. *Acta Paediatr.* 1953;42:34-42
2. Schapira M, Maisin JM, Ghilain JM, et al. Epidemiology of coeliac disease. *Acta Gastroenterol Belg.* 2003;66:234-236.
3. Rutz R, Ritzler E, Fierz W, Herzog D. Prevalence of asymptomatic celiac disease in adolescents of eastern Switzerland. *Swiss Medical Weekly.* 2002;132:43-47.
4. Catassi C, Doloretta Macis M, Ratsch IM, et al. The distribution of DQ genes in the Saharawi population provides only a partial explanation for the high celiac disease prevalence. *Tissue Antigens.* 2001;58:402-406.
5. Pratesi R, Gandolfi L, Garcia SG, et al. Prevalence of coeliac disease: unexplained age-related variation in the same population. *Scand J of Gastroenterol.* 2003;38:747-750.
6. Gomez JC, Selvaggio GS, Viola M, et al. Prevalence of celiac disease in Argentina: screening of an adult population in the La Plata area. *Amer J of Gastroenterol.* 2001;96:2700-2704.
7. Murray JA, Van Dyke C, Plevak MF, et al. Trends in the identification and clinical features of celiac disease in a North American community, 1950-2001. *Clin Gastroenterol Hepatol.* 2003;1:19-27.
8. Fasano A, Catassi C. Current approaches to diagnosis and treatment of celiac disease: an evolving spectrum. *Gastroenterology.* 2001;120:636-651.
9. Oxentenko AS, Murray JA. Celiac disease and dermatitis herpetiformis: the spectrum of gluten-sensitive enteropathy. International Journal of Dermatology. 2003;42:585-587.
10. Louka AS, Sollid LM. HLA in coeliac disease: unravelling the complex genetics of a complex disorder. *Tissue Antigens.* 2003;61:105-117.
11. Sollid LM, Thorsby E: HLA susceptibility genes in celiac disease: genetic mapping and role in pathogenesis. *Gastroenterology.* 1993;105:910-922.
12. Fasano A, Not T, Wang W, et al. Zonulin, a newly discovered modulator of intestinal permeability, and its expression in coeliac disease. *Lancet.* 2000;355:1518-1519.
13. Schuppan D. Current concepts of celiac disease pathogenesis. *Gastroenterology.* 2000;119:234-242.
14. Mowat AM. Coeliac disease--a meeting point for genetics, immunology, and protein chemistry. *Lancet.* 2003;361:1290-1292.
15. Nilsen EM, Lundin KE, Krajci P, Scott H, Sollid LM, Brandtzaeg P. Gluten specific, HLA-DQ restricted T cells from coeliac mucosa produce cytokines with Th1 or Th0 profile dominated by interferon gamma. *Gut.* 1995;37:766-776.
16. Fasano A. Celiac disease--how to handle a clinical chameleon. *N Engl J of Med.* 2003;348:2568-2570.
17. Branski D, Troncone R. Celiac disease: a reappraisal. *J Pediatr.* 1998;133:181-187.
18. Greco L, Romino R, Coto I, et al. The first large population based twin study of coeliac disease. *Gut.* 2002;50:624-628.
19. Persson LA, Ivarsson A, Hernell O. Breast-feeding protects against celiac disease in childhood--epidemiological evidence. *Adv Exp Med Biol.* 2002;503:115-123.
20. Tumer L, Hasanoglu A, Aybay C. Endomysium antibodies in the diagnosis of celiac disease in short-statured children with no gastrointestinal symptoms. *Pediatr Int.* 2001;43:71-73.
21. Cerf-Bensussan N, Cellier C, Heyman M, Brousse N, Schmitz J. Coeliac disease: an update on facts and questions based on the 10th International Symposium on Coeliac Disease. *J Pediatr Gastroenterol Nutr.* 2003;37:412-421.
22. Delco F, El-Serag HB, Sonnenberg A. Celiac sprue among US military veterans: associated disorders and clinical manifestations. *Dig Dis Sci.* 1999;44:966-972.
23. Ackerman Z, Eliakim R, Stalnikowicz R, Rachmilewitz D. Role of small bowel biopsy in the endoscopic evaluation of adults with iron deficiency anemia. *Amer J Gastroenterol.* 1996;91:2099-2102.
24. Carroccio A, Iannitto E, Cavataio F, et al. Sideropenic anemia and celiac disease: one study, two points of view. *Dig Dis Sci.* 1998;43:673-678.
25. Volta U, De Franceschi L, Lari F, et al. Coeliac disease hidden by cryptogenic hypertransaminasaemia. *Lancet.* 1998;352:26-29.
26. Abdo A, Meddings J, Swain M. Liver abnormalities in celiac disease. *Clin Gastroenterol Hepatol.* 2004;2:107-112.
27. Kemppainen T, Kroger H, Janatuinen E, et al. Osteoporosis in adult patients with celiac disease. *Bone.* 1999;24:249-255.
28. Corazza GR, Di Sario A, Cecchetti L, et al. Bone mass and metabolism in patients with celiac disease. *Gastroenterol.* 1995;109:122-128.
29. Moreno ML, Vazquez H, Mazure R, et al. Stratification of bone fracture risk in patients with celiac disease. *Clin Gastroenterol Hepatol.* 2004;2:127-134.
30. Vasquez H, Mazure R, Gonzalez D, et al. Risk of fractures in celiac disease patients: a cross-sectional, case-control study. *Amer J Gastroenterology.* 2000;95:183-189.
31. Molteni N, Bardella MT, Bianchi PA. Obstetric and gynecological problems in women with untreated celiac sprue. *J Clin Gastroenterol.* 1990;12:37-39.
32. Farthing MJ, Rees LH, Edwards CR, Dawson AM. Male gonadal function in coeliac disease: 2. Sex hormones. *Gut.* 1983;24:127-135.
33. Baker PG, Read AE. Reversible infertility in male coeliac patients. *Br Med J.* 1975;2:316-317.
34. Pengiran Tengah DS, Wills AJ, Holmes GK. Neurological complications of coeliac disease. *Postgrad Med J.* 2002;78:393-398.
35. Gawkrodger DJ, McDonald C, O'Mahony S, Ferguson A. Small intestinal function and dietary status in dermatitis herpetiformis. *Gut.* 1991;32:377-382.
36. Otley C, Hall RP III. Dermatitis herpetiformis. *Dermatol Clin.* 1990;8:759-769.
37. Andersson H, Mobacken H. Dietary treatment of dermatitis herpetiformis. *Eur J Clin Nutr.* 1992;46:309-315.
38. Ventura A, Magazzu G, Greco L. Duration of exposure to gluten and risk for autoimmune disorders in patients with celiac disease. SIGEP Study Group for Autoimmune Disorders in Celiac Disease. *Gastroenterology.* 1999;117:297-303.
39. Holmes GK. Screening for coeliac disease in type 1 diabetes. *Arch Disease Child.* 2002;87:495-498.

40. Iafusco D, Rea F, Prisco F. Hypoglycemia and reduction of the insulin requirement as a sign of celiac disease in children with IDDM. *Diabetes Care.* 1998;21:1379-1381.
41. Calero P, Ribes-Koninckx C, Albiach V, Carles C, Ferrer J. IgA antigliadin antibodies as a screening method for nonovert celiac disease in children with insulin-dependent diabetes mellitus. *J Pediatr Gastroenterol Nutr.* 1996;23:29-33.
42. Cataldo F, Marino V, Ventura A, Bottaro G, Corazza GR. Prevalence and clinical features of selective immunoglobulin A deficiency in coeliac disease: an Italian multicentre study. Italian Society of Paediatric Gastroenterology and Hepatology (SIGEP) and "Club del Tenue" Working Groups on Coeliac Disease. *Gut.* 1998;42:362-365.
43. Heneghan MA, Stevens FM, Cryan EM, Warner RH, McCarthy CF. Celiac sprue and immunodeficiency states: a 25-year review. *J Clin Gastroenterol.* 1997;25:421-425.
44. Book L, Hart A, Black J, Feolo M, Zone JJ, Neuhausen SL. Prevalence and clinical characteristics of celiac disease in Downs syndrome in a US study. *Amer J Med Genet.* 2001;98:70-74.
45. Zachor DA, Mroczek-Musulman E, Brown P. Prevalence of celiac disease in Down syndrome in the United States. *J Pediatr Gastroenterol Nutr.* 2000;31:275-279.
46. Kingham JG, Parker DR. The association between primary biliary cirrhosis and coeliac disease: a study of relative prevalences. *Gut.* 1998;42:120-122.
47. Hay JE, Wiesner RH, Shorter RG, LaRusso NF, Baldus WP. Primary sclerosing cholangitis and celiac disease. A novel association. *Ann Intern Med.* 1988;109:713-717.
48. Volta U, Rodrigo L, Granito A, et al. Celiac disease in autoimmune cholestatic liver disorders. *Amer J Gastroenterol.* 2002;97:2609-2613.
49. Volta U, De Franceschi L, Molinaro N, et al. Frequency and significance of anti-gliadin and anti-endomysial antibodies in autoimmune hepatitis. *Dig Dis Sci.* 1998;43:2190-2105.
50. Walker-Smith JA. Management of infantile gastroenteritis. *Archives of Disease in Childhood.* 1990;65:917-918.
51. Dandalides SM, Carey WD, Petras R, Achkar E. Endoscopic small bowel mucosal biopsy: a controlled trial evaluating forceps size and biopsy location in the diagnosis of normal and abnormal mucosal architecture. *Gastrointestinal Endoscopy.* 1989;35:197-200.
52. Vogelsang H, Hanel S, Steiner B, Oberhuber G. Diagnostic duodenal bulb biopsy in celiac disease. *Endoscopy.* 2001;33:336-340.
53. Oxentenko AS, Grisolano SW, Murray JA, et al. The insensitivity of endoscopic markers in celiac disease. *Amer J Gastroenterol.* 2002;97:933-938.
54. Marsh MN. Gluten, major histocompatibility complex, and the small intestine. A molecular and immunobiologic approach to the spectrum of gluten sensitivity ('celiac sprue'). *Gastroenterology.* 1992;102:330-354.
55. Wahab PJ, Meijer JW, Goerres MS, Mulder CJ. Coeliac disease: changing views on gluten-sensitive enteropathy. *Scand J Gastroenterol.* 2002;Suppl:60-65.
56. Abdulkarim AS, Murray JA. Review article: The diagnosis of coeliac disease. *Aliment Pharmacol Ther.* 2003;17:987-995.
57. Farrell RJ, Kelly CP. Diagnosis of celiac sprue. *Amer J Gastroenterology.* 2001;96:3237-3246.
58. Ferreira M, Davies SL, Butler M, et al. Endomysial antibody: is it the best screening test for coeliac disease? *Gut.* 1992;33:1633-1637.
59. Grodzinsky E, Hed J, Skogh T. IgA antiendomysium antibodies have a high positive predictive value for celiac disease in asymptomatic patients. *Allergy.* 1994;49:593-597.
60. Rostami K, Kerckhaert J, Tiemessen R, et al. Sensitivity of antiendomysium and antigliadin antibodies in untreated celiac disease: disappointing in clinical practice. *Amer J Gastroenterol.* 1999;94:888-894.
61. Dieterich W, Laag E, Schopper H, et al. Autoantibodies to tissue transglutaminase as predictors of celiac disease. *Gastroenterology.* 1998;115:1317-1321.
62. Reeves GE, Burns C, Hall ST, et al. The measurement of IgA and IgG transglutaminase antibodies in celiac disease: a comparison with current diagnostic methods. *Pathology.* 2000;32:181-185.
63. Spiller RC, Lee YC, Edge C, et al. Delayed mouth-caecum transit of a lactulose labelled liquid test meal in patients with steatorrhoea caused by partially treated coeliac disease. *Gut.* 1987;28:1275-1282.
64. Gomez JC, Moran CE, Maurino EC, Bai JC. Exocrine pancreatic insufficiency in celiac disease. *Gastroenterology.* 1998;114:621-623.
65. Carroccio A, Iacono G, Lerro P, et al. Role of pancreatic impairment in growth recovery during gluten-free diet in childhood celiac disease. *Gastroenterology.* 1997;112:1839-1844.
66. DuBois RN, Lazenby AJ, Yardley JH, et al. Lymphocytic enterocolitis in patients with 'refractory sprue'. *Jama.* 1989;262:935-937.
67. McCashland TM, Donovan JP, Strobach RS, et al. Collagenous enterocolitis: a manifestation of gluten-sensitive enteropathy. *J Clin Gastroenterol.* 1992;15:45-51.
68. Corazza GR, Biagi F, Volta U, et al. Autoimmune enteropathy and villous atrophy in adults. *Lancet.* 1997;350:106-109.
69. Fine KD, Meyer RL, Lee EL. The prevalence and causes of chronic diarrhea in patients with celiac sprue treated with a gluten-free diet. 1998 Feb;114(2):424-5]. *Gastroenterology.* 1997;112:1830-1838.
70. Kitis G, Holmes GK, Cooper BT, et al. Association of coeliac disease and inflammatory bowel disease. *Gut.* 1980;21:636-641.
71. Longstreth GF. Successful treatment of refractory sprue with cyclosporine. Ann Intern Med. 1993;119:1014-1016.
72. Robertson DA, Dixon MF, Scott BB, et al. Small intestinal ulceration: diagnostic difficulties in relation to coeliac disease. *Gut.* 1983;24:565-574.
73. Isaacson P, Wright DH. Malignant histiocytosis of the intestine. Its relationship to malabsorption and ulcerative jejunitis. *Human Pathology.* 1978;9:661-677.
74. Baer AN, Bayless TM, Yardley JH. Intestinal ulceration and malabsorption syndromes. *Gastroenterology.* 1980;79:754-765.
75. Mills PR: Small Intestine Ucleration. *Curr Opin Gastroenterol.* 1985;1:254-256.
76. Mills PR, Brown IL, Watkinson G: Idiopathic chronic ulcerative enteritis. Report of five cases and review of the literature. *Q J Med.* 1980;49:133-149.
77. Holmes GK, Stokes PL, Sorahan TM, et al. Coeliac disease, gluten-free diet, and malignancy. *Gut.* 1976;17:612-619.
78. Swinson CM, Slavin G, Coles EC, Booth CC. Coeliac disease and malignancy. *Lancet.* 1983;1:111-115.
79. Loberant N, Cohen I, Noi I, Herskovits M, Szvalb S. Enteropathy-associated T-cell lymphoma: a case report with radiographic and computed tomography appearance. *J Surg Oncol.* 1997;65:50-54.
80. Cooper BT, Holmes GK, Ferguson R, Cooke WT. Celiac disease and malignancy. *Medicine.* 1980;59:249-261.
81. Egan LJ, Walsh SV, Stevens FM, et al. Celiac-associated lymphoma. A single institution experience of 30 cases in the combination chemotherapy era. Journal of Clinical Gastroenterology. 1995;21:123-129.
82. Gale J, Simmonds PD, Mead GM, Sweetenham JW, Wright DH. Enteropathy-type intestinal T-cell lymphoma: clinical features and treatment of 31 patients in a single center. *J Clin Oncol.* 2000;18:795-803.
83. Askling J, Linet M, Gridley G, Halstensen TS, Ekstrom K, Ekbom A. Cancer incidence in a population-based cohort of individuals hospitalized with celiac disease or dermatitis herpetiformis. *Gastroenterology.* 2002;123:1428-1435.
84. Holmes GK, Prior P, Lane MR, Pope D, Allan RN. Malignancy in coeliac disease--effect of a gluten free diet. *Gut.* 1989;30:333-338.
85. Stern M, Ciclitira PJ, van Eckert R, et al. Analysis and clinical effects of gluten in coeliac disease. *Eur J Gastroenterol Hepatol.* 2001;13:741-747.

86. Janatuinen EK, Pikkarainen PH, Kemppainen TA, et al. A comparison of diets with and without oats in adults with celiac disease. *N Engl J Med*. 1995;333:1033-1037.
87. Srinivasan U, Weir DG, Feighery C, O'Farrelly C. Emergence of classic enteropathy after longstanding gluten sensitive oral ulceration. *Bmj*. 1998;316:206-207.
88. Janatuinen EK, Kemppainen TA, Julkunen RJ, et al. No harm from five year ingestion of oats in coeliac disease. *Gut*. 2002;50:332-335.
89. Hogberg L, Laurin P, Falth-Magnusson K, et al. Oats to children with newly diagnosed coeliac disease: a randomised double blind study. *Gut*. 2004;53:649-654.
90. Thompson T: Oats and the gluten-free diet. *J Amer Diet Assoc*. 2003;103:376-379.
91. Ciacci C, Mazzacca G. Unintentional gluten ingestion in celiac patients. *Gastroenterology*. 1998;115:243.
92. Hogberg L, Grodzinsky E, Stenhammar L. Better dietary compliance in patients with coeliac disease diagnosed in early childhood. *Scand J Gastroenterol*. 2003;38:751-754.
93. Maiuri L, Ciacci C, Ricciardelli I, et al. Association between innate response to gliadin and activation of pathogenic T cells in coeliac disease. *Lancet*. 2003;362:30-37.
94. Shan L, Molberg O, Parrot I, et al. Structural basis for gluten intolerance in celiac sprue. *Science*. 2002;297:2275-2279.

Chapter 20

Nutrition and Liver Disease

Marwan Ghabril, MD, and
Jaime Aranda-Michel, MD

Introduction

The liver is the largest metabolic organ in the human body, fulfilling critical roles in the metabolism of a variety of nutrients that are essential to maintaining the integrity and adequate physiologic function of multiple organ systems and the body as a whole. Severe hepatic impairment leads to a broad spectrum of metabolic derangements, which lead to protein-energy malnutrition, which significantly impacts clinical outcomes. Better recognition of this correlation has led to an increased interest in better delineating the relationship, establishing a recognized standard of measuring malnutrition, and improving nutritional status in patients with liver disease. These standards, however, as well as the specifics of modalities and duration of treatment, remain ill defined at present.

Prevalence

Protein-energy malnutrition (PEM) is defined as "a condition resulting from long-term inadequate intake of protein and energy that can lead to wasting of body tissues and increased susceptibility to infection." It is a distinct entity under the International Classification of Disease code, carrying a code ICD-9 263,[1] and is considered a treatable component of associated disease states. Patients with severe liver disease can develop kwashiorkor, a state of visceral protein deficiency, which is frequently superimposed on a state of severe calorie deficiency or marasmus.[2] These patients are better characterized as having combined PEM.

The true prevalence of malnutrition in patients with liver disease is difficult to ascertain and is influenced by the severity of liver disease, patient population, and the acuity of liver disease. Most of the early data are on malnutrition and liver disease related to alcoholic liver disease in general and to hospitalized patients with alcoholic hepatitis in particular, where it is almost universal. Though it was thought that malnutrition was more prevalent and severe in alcoholic liver disease,[3] recent data reflect similar prevalence rates in all patients with chronic liver disease, regardless of etiology.[4]

PEM is a common finding in patients with advanced chronic liver disease and is found in 100% of patients at the time of liver transplantation.[5] It is also important to recognize PEM in early or compensated cirrhosis,[6] where it can be found in 20% of patients, without the easily recognized signs of muscle wasting and loss of subcutaneous fat stores. Acute liver diseases have more variable presentations, where malnutrition is generally not a feature at the outset, but can progress to fulminant liver failure, where nutritional support is an integral component of care.

Prognosis

PEM is associated with worse outcomes in alcoholic liver disease[7] and in end-stage liver disease (ESLD) and orthotopic liver transplantation (OLT).[8] PEM has also been found to be an independent risk factor for esophageal variceal bleeding.[9] In addition, features of malnutrition in ESLD, such as high metabolic rates and low lean body weights or body cell mass, are also associated with shorter mean survival post OLT.[10,11] Some of these factors may be modified with aggressive nutritional support. Therefore, it is crucial to identify these high-risk patients so that morbidity and mortality may improve with focused therapy. There is limited data from prospective studies to support intervention at earlier stages of disease, rather than in advanced ESLD in hospitalized patients.[12]

Etiology

The etiology of malnutrition in chronic liver disease is multifactorial and can generally be attributed to impairments in dietary intake, absorption and metabolism, and increased nutritional losses.

Decreased Dietary Intake

Patients with severe liver disease frequently have decreased caloric intake because of a variety of factors and limitations.[13,14] They typically suffer from poor appetites relating to alterations in taste, early satiety, side effects of medications, and psychological and neurological impairment, among other complications. Factors such as zinc deficiency[15] and hyperinsulinemia appear to add to appetite suppression. There may also be an anorexic effect of proinflammatory cytokines[16] and leptin,[17,18] which are increased in chronic liver disease. It is difficult to ascertain to what degree each of these factors contribute to poor caloric intake, but it is not always evident to patients that they are not receiving adequate nutrition. A dietary journal with formal calorie counts by a dietitian is necessary to assess both the total number and nutritional value of all calories. Additionally, this population is at risk for recurrent episodes of acute decompensation such as gastrointestinal (GI) bleeding and portosystemic encephalopathy, during which there is further set backs in terms of nutritional intake. The concern for precipitating encephalopathy and worsening fluid retention often lead to excessive restriction of protein and fluid intake, exacerbating general illness, and negative nitrogen balance. This is discussed in more detail in relation to protein metabolism in ESLD.

Impaired Intestinal Absorption

Patients with chronic liver disease may have malabsorption, particularly in the presence of cholestasis. These patients often have fat, fat-soluble vitamin, and mineral malabsorption, even in the early stages of disease (Chapter 5). Alteration in bowel flora with illness or iatrogenically through medications such as neomycin or lactulose can also affect absorption. Diarrhea and decreased transit time through the small intestine may also play a role. Associated conditions such as chronic pancreatitis (Chapter 21) and pancreatic insufficiency with alcoholic liver disease are recognized factors in poor absorption of nutrients.

Excessive Losses

Negative nitrogen balance is generally caused by an altered metabolic state in patients with advanced liver disease. This negative balance can be exacerbated by losses of protein and electrolytes with repeated large volume paracentesis in the face of diuretic refractory ascites. Interestingly, large volume paracentesis may transiently reduce sympathetic tone and basal metabolic rate,[19] but the net effect on nutritional status is still regarded as unfavorable.

Altered Metabolism

Patients with ESLD have metabolic processes that mirror those seen in states of starvation.[20] These include a relatively increased metabolism that can predate the development of fat and muscle loss that are seen with progressive malnutrition.[21,22] Metabolic derangements in ESLD involve those of carbohydrate, protein, lipid, and energy, with alterations in preferential substrate use in the nonprandial state.

Carbohydrate Metabolism

A significant number of patients with ESLD are glucose intolerant, with associated insulin resistance and hyperinsulinemia. Glucose intolerance is noted in over 70% of cirrhotics, and frank diabetes mellitus can develop in up to 37% of patients.[23] Interestingly, despite the high prevalence of diabetes, these patients do not appear to carry a significantly increased risk of microvascular and cardiovascular complications. The mechanisms of this intolerance include decreased hepatic circulation and extraction of insulin, decreased hepatic sensitivity to insulin, and decreased production and storage of glycogen in muscles. As a consequence of decreased glycogen stores, fat is preferentially utilized as the main substrate for energy[24] similar to a state of starvation, even with only moderate periods of fasting.[20] The resulting metabolic profile leads to an "accelerated starvation" phenomenon, with increased gluconeogensis, lipid oxidation, and protein catabolism.

Fat Metabolism

As noted above, fat is preferentially metabolized in the setting of ESLD, with a lower respiratory quotient, even after overnight fasting as measured by indirect calorimetry. Though total free fatty acids are increased in ESLD, polyunsaturated and essential fatty acid levels are reduced, and this reduction may correlate with the degree of both malnutrition and liver dysfunction.[25] Polyunsaturated fatty acids such as arachidonic acid are necessary for prostaglandin and leukotriene synthesis, as well as cell membrane function. Arachidonic acid supplementation in cirrhotics may represent a novel approach to managing patients with ESLD.[26]

Protein Metabolism

Protein is also an alternate energy substrate for patients with ESLD and the "accelerated starvation" state, combined with limited protein intake result in negative nitrogen balance in early cirrhosis.[6] The ensuing muscle wasting becomes more marked with progression of liver disease. Studies on amino acid metabolism, typically performed on stable cirrhotic patients, would suggest increased protein degradation in the face of variable amino acid oxidation. Leucine oxidation is decreased in ESLD, particularly when assessed in relation to body cell mass instead of total body weight.[27,28] The increased proteolysis relative to lean body mass can be a prominent feature of ESLD, where patients may not suppress endogenous protein breakdown in response to refeeding or amino acid administration.[29] This phenomenon may contribute to the loss of body cell mass and fat stores commonly observed in cirrhosis. Despite this, it is possible for some patients with stable ESLD to maintain neutral or positive nitrogen balance through adequate dietary intake and supplementation. Assessment of cirrhotic patient's nitrogen balance is useful in identifying those at risk for PEM, in an effort to maximize nutritional therapy. Based on isotope amino acid studies, the dietary protein requirements of patients with stable ESLD appear to match those of normal controls.[28]

Though basal protein requirements are approximately 0.8 to 1 g/kg/day, these may approach 2 g/kg/day during periods of stress. Dietary protein restriction is often routinely imposed on ambulatory and hospitalized patients, in fear of exacerbating portosystemic encephalopathy. However, refeeding experiments over prolonged periods on patients with compensated liver disease have yielded positive nitrogen balance without inducing encephalopathy.[29,30] Levels of dietary protein close to 1.8 g/kg/day are well tolerated. Therefore, PEM in the setting of stable cirrhosis is potentially amenable to nutritional therapy, and avoidance of protein restriction should be the default approach, except in uncommon cases of encephalopathy that is refractory to aggressive therapies. Additionally, avoidance of a fasting state, with frequent meals, may play an equally important role in favorably shifting the balance of protein synthesis and degradation.

Branched-chain amino acid (BCAA) supplementation in patients with ESLD can theoretically fulfill protein requirements while playing a beneficial role in hepatic encephalopathy. The exact mechanisms of hepatic encephalopathy and the nature of the effect of amino acids on the central nervous system are not known. Imbalances in the ratio of plasma BCAA and aromatic amino acids (AAA)—normally 3.5 but dropping to 1.0 in cirrhotic patients—may result in increased AAA uptake in the central nervous system. Central nervous system metabolism of AAA to false neurotransmitters is a hypothesized mechanism of hepatic encephalopathy. Liver disease can result in lower plasma BCAA by a number of theoretical processes, which may include increased catabolism in skeletal muscle and the kidneys. Decreased hepatic deamination may also play a role in increasing plasma AAA levels. Improvement in regional cerebral blood flow after treatment with BCAA has been described in cirrhotic patients and may be a mechanism by which it may exert a beneficial effect in resolution of encephalopathy.[31]

Energy Expenditure

Energy expenditure can be quite variable in patients with ESLD,[32] where resting energy expenditure (REE) can be difficult to predict with the commonly utilized Harris-Benedict equation: Men: 66.5 [13.8 weight (kg)] [5.0 height (cm)] – 6.8 Age (year) = kcal/day. Women: 655.1 [9.6 weight (kg)] [1.8 height (cm)] – 4.7 Age (year) = kcal/day. In a review of cirrhotic patients, 70% had measured REE that differed from the predicted values.[33] REE was found to closely relate to fat-free or lean body mass, age, gender, and increased beta-adrenergic activity, which explained some of the variability.[33,34] However, the demonstrated variability in REE in this group, in which 18% were hypermetabolic and 31% were hypometabolic, did not consistently correlate with the cause, duration, or the severity of cirrhosis,[33] suggesting that hypermetabolism may be an extrahepatic manifestation of liver disease.[34]

The differentiation between total body mass and body cell mass is also very important. Body cell mass is the active metabolic compartment of the body and is directly responsible for basal energy expenditure (BEE). Though total energy consumption in patients with ESLD is, on average, similar to that of control subjects, energy expenditure relative to body cell mass is more reflective of true BEE and patient physiology. In prospective studies, low body cell mass and hypermetabolism, with high REE, correlated with a poorer prognosis after liver transplantation, irrespective of degree of ascites or Childs-Pugh score.[10] Moreover, hypermetabolism appears to persist after transplantation, further supporting the notion of hypermetabolism as an extrahepatic manifestation of ESLD.

Energy requirements in stable cirrhosis (without ascites) may not exceed 30 to 40 kcal/kg/day; however, superimposed illnesses, decompensation, or malnutrition will increase the requirements.

Assessment of Malnutrition

Improved accuracy in measuring basal energy requirements and body cell mass in patients with ESLD is vital to better identification of at-risk individuals and possibly more reliable evaluation of therapeutic intervention. This is particularly relevant to this heterogeneous patient population, where a state of physiologic malnutrition may exist in the absence of obvious stigmata of cirrhosis. Moreover, the lack of a standardized definition of PEM in patients with stable or decompensated liver disease adds to the challenge of universally classifying degrees of malnutrition, nutritional therapy, and effects of intervention.

Nevertheless, a systematic approach to assessing nutritional status and needs in patients with liver disease is helpful and recommended.[3] This includes basic clinical assessment, anthropometric measurements, and specialized testing.

Nutritional assessment—including information about the medical history, nutritional assessment, and physical examination—is discussed in detail in Chapter 1.

Body composition analysis and information specific to the assessment tools below are discussed in Chapter 2.

Clinical Assessment

A full medical history should be supplemented with a complete dietary history, ideally with the guidance of an experienced dietitian. Though patients may feel and report subjectively adequate food intake, their caloric intake is often suboptimal. It is useful to ask specific questions regarding the loss of appetite, altered sense of taste, postprandial fullness, weight loss, and chronic diarrhea.

Though loss of more than 10% of body weight or involuntary weight loss is a clear indicator of malnutrition, it is important to remember that patients with chronic liver disease develop fluid retention with ascites and edema. Hence, patients may maintain or gain weight despite loss of fat and muscle stores, such that body weight alone is an inadequate measure of malnutrition.

A complete physical examination should be performed and can yield subtle signs of nutrient deficiencies by changes in skin, hair, and mucosa, in addition to obvious signs of muscle and fat wasting. Glossitis may develop because of multiple nutrient deficiencies and may impair taste and appetite. Zinc deficiency is common in patients with ESLD and has been associated with changes in smell, taste, protein metabolism, and encephalopathy.[35] Patients with cholestatic liver disease frequently have malabsorption and deficiencies of the fat-soluble vitamins A, D, E, and K and of magnesium, though clinical signs may be absent.[36] This can result in loss of bone density, which is prevalent in patients undergoing liver transplantation, particularly in patients with cholestatic liver disease.[37] Magnesium deficiency can be seen frequently in the setting of alcoholic liver disease.[38]

Anthropometric Measurements

Anthropometric measurements are specific and may reflect nutritional reserves. The most commonly used measurements in clinical practice are triceps skin fold and mid arm muscle circumference. Although fluid retention can involve the upper arms and alter these measurements, these parameters are still a useful way to assess subcutaneous fat and muscle mass. Additionally, they can be combined with other variables in assessing nutritional status.

Subjective Global Assessment

The Subjective Global Assessment (SGA) is a general nutritional evaluation that is based on a patient's weight, height, nutritional history, changes on physical examination that include anthropometric measurements, and existing medical conditions. The SGA has been modified to evaluate nutritional status in patients undergoing liver transplantation.

Patients are classified by the SGA as being well nourished, or having mild, moderate, or severe malnutrition, with 80% reproducibility of classification by different raters.[39] Although this test has been reported to be highly specific (96%), it was also found to be very insensitive (22%) in diagnosing malnutrition in patients with alcoholic liver disease.[40]

Indirect Measurement of Body Cell Mass

Muscle mass is thought to be more reliable and important than fat-free mass for determining PEM. Accurate measurement of fat-free mass is not accurate in patients with ESLD with fluid retention.[6] Therefore, body cell mass rather than fat-free mass should be the ideal measured mass, as it represents the true metabolic compartment of the body.

A number of tests and assays have been used to measure body cell mass, which include 24-hour urinary creatinine excretion, total body potassium, and bioelectrical impedance analysis (BIA). These measurements are discussed briefly below and are presented with detail in Chapter 2.

24-Hour Urinary Creatinine Excretion

A 24-hour urinary creatinine excretion has been used and validated for assessing muscle mass, as well as body cell mass, in patients with ESLD.[41] Importantly, however, the reliability of this assay is significantly impaired in the setting of renal dysfunction. In fact, creatinine clearance predicted from body cell mass (when known) and plasma creatinine may be a better indicator of renal function than is measured 24-hour creatinine clearance.[42]

Total Body Potassium

Total body potassium has been found to correlate with skeletal muscle mass[43] and body cell mass; however, this correlation has not been validated in adult patients with ESLD.

Bioelectrical Impedance Analysis

BIA is a simple, inexpensive, and noninvasive test that yields immediate results in determining body cell mass. The test measures body electrical conductivity and resistance or impedance. In principle, fat offers resistance, while water conducts electric current. The comparison of conductivity and resistance can reflect lean body weight and fat mass. Fluid retention in ESLD may represent a major limitation of this technique in the measurement of body cell mass.[44,45] However, there is conflicting data regarding the validity of BIA in assessing body composition in patients with ESLD. Recent reports suggest that BIA is a reliable tool for the determination of body cell mass in cirrhotic patients with and without ascites.[46] Some data suggest that bioimpedance indices might be superior to derived body composition as a prognostic indicator.[47] Further studies are needed to validate this technique in patients with varying degrees of edema or ascites and for comparison with other techniques for measuring body composition.

Dual-Energy X-Ray Absorptiometry

Dual-energy x-ray absorptiometry (DEXA) can be used to measure total body bone mineral, fat, and fat-free soft tissue mass. Although very accurate in assessing body composition in healthy individuals, DEXA has not been validated in patients with ESLD. This test is also influenced by fluid retention. In cirrhotic patients without overt fluid retention, DEXA has shown accuracy in assessing percentage of body fat.[48]

Indirect Calorimetry

Assessment of energy expenditure through indirect calorimetry has, through technological advances, become a simple and reproducible test. REE should be measured in cirrhotic patients, not predicted by using the most common mathematical formulas such as the Harris-Benedict, Schofield, Mifflin, Cunningham, and Owen formulae, and the disease-specific Muller formula. These predictions vary widely from measured values.[49] The main application of indirect calorimetry is in assessing metabolic rates and respiratory quotients, which can be inferred from oxygen consumption and carbon dioxide production at steady state. Carbohydrates, protein, and fat have unique respiratory quotients (1.0, 0.8, and 0.7, respectively). In addition to prognostic value,[11] preferential substrate use may be identified in patients with ESLD for more targeted therapy. If indirect calorimetry is not available, the Harris-Benedict equation may be used, employing ideal body weight as opposed to measured weight, which is influenced by excess fluid weight (ie, ascites and edema). Hypermetabolic patients are at higher risk of rapid nutritional compromise. As a general rule, the total amount of calories provided should be at least 1.2 times the BEE, approximately 30 to 35 kcal/kg/day. Under periods of stress such as infection or GI bleeding, requirements may approach 50 kcal/kg/day.

Treatment of Malnutrition

In light of the prognostic significance of PEM in ESLD, prompt diagnosis and aggressive management may provide a unique opportunity to improve outcomes both pre and post liver transplantation. General guidelines on nutritional support in patients with ESLD have been reviewed in the literature;[50] however, despite great interest in PEM as an independent risk factor for mortality and morbidity in patients with ESLD, there are a limited number of prospective randomized clinical trials assessing the impact of nutritional therapy in this patient population.[51,52] These studies have focused on outcomes in liver transplantation with enteral nutrition (EN) and parenteral nutritional (PN) support with improvements in nitrogen balance but no proven alteration of posttransplant survival.[53] These modalities have also been used extensively in treatment of severe acute alcoholic hepatitis, with equivocal results.[7] Most post liver transplant nutritional support, however, is commonly provided at transplant centers, and increasing attention to pre transplant nutritional status may lead to an expanded database of evidence for efficacy of early treatment.

Though there has been some interest in the role that vitamin E may play in patients with nonalcoholic steatohepatitis or in psychomotor function in primary biliary cirrhosis (PBC), there is insufficient evidence for a proven therapeutic role. However, vitamin E appears to be well tolerated, and supplementation for measured deficient states with standardized formulations may currently be the ideal approach.

Vitamin K deficiency may be encountered in both cholestatic and noncholestatic liver disease, secondary to poor intake or malabsorption. Supplementation with vitamin K is a mainstay of support for patients with liver disease and is generally safe. Patients with liver disease can be vitamin K deficient with little or no obvious markers of malnutrition, and supplementation over a defined period may partially correct the coagulopathy arising from vitamin K dependant clotting factor deficiency.

Adequate vitamin D supplementation is an important component of managing those patients with bone density loss or cholestatic liver disease, where endogenous production, intestinal absorption, and 25 hydroxylation of vitamin may be impaired. There are no proven antifracture benefits to vitamin D and calcium supplementation in liver disease, although the rate of bone mineral density loss was noted to be slower in supplemented patients with cirrhosis.[54]

Vitamin A levels can be decreased in liver disease and have been studied in the setting of PBC. Though deficiency can be associated with altered night vision, there is no proven role for aggressive supplementation, particularly as impaired hepatic release may be as important as deficiency or malabsorption in etiology. There may also be an antagonistic effect of vitamin A on intestinal calcium response to vitamin K.[55] Thus, supplementation with standard formulations in the setting of deficiency may be the most prudent approach.

Lipid supplementation in ESLD is typically encountered in the setting of PN. It is thought that medium chain triglycerides (MCT) are more readily utilized than are long chain triglycerides (LCT). However, animal studies have shown increased hepatic fat deposition with overfeeding with MCT alone, and a mixture of MCT and LCT is believed to be a more reasonable approach.[56] Other animal studies suggest a possible protective role against fibrosis in alcohol-induced hepatic injury, but there is no support for use of both MCT and LCT in humans for indications other than those dictated by nutritional status and requirements. Prospective clinical trials indicate that the elimination of MCT and LCT is not altered in chronic liver disease, and these may be suitable for use in PN.[57]

A general approach to management of nutritional deficiency in patients with ESLD is summarized in Table 20-1.[50] It is important to have a cohesive, communicative, and responsive multidisciplinary team that includes patients and their caregivers, dedicated registered dietitians, nurses and transplant coordinators, and physicians. After a detailed systematic assessment, specific aspects of an individual's nutritional profile can be addressed. For example, some reversible causes of anorexia may be identified and corrected (eg, zinc deficiency). A daily multivitamin is a safe and easy mainstay of therapy (Chapter 10). Malabsorption and maldigestion (Chapter 5) should be suspected in patients with cholestatic liver disease or coexisting pancreatic insufficiency with alcoholic liver disease. Fat-soluble vitamin and minerals should be supplemented as needed. Consideration can also be given to oral supplements of MCT where malabsorption is identified and pancreatic enzyme supplements where indicated.

Prospective dietary journals should be kept regularly and reviewed by a full-time dietitian, with attention to calorie counts, calorie sources, and patterns of meals and fasting. The pathophysiology of hypermetabolism and accelerated starvation in patients with ESLD is such that these patients should be encouraged to eat frequent meals. Five to seven meals taken throughout the day with a snack at bedtime is important to minimize the consumption of muscle tissue and fat stores during the nonprandial state.

Close monitoring for bacterial infections and GI bleeding, which increase BEE requirements, is important in this relatively immune-compromised population. Bacterial infections such as spontaneous bacterial peritonitis and urinary and respiratory tract infections are common in patients with decompensated liver disease who await OLT.

Once energy requirements are defined for individual patients, aggressive nutritional support should be instituted

Table 20-1.

General Guidelines for Nutritional Support in Patients With End-Stage Liver Disease

- Patients with ESLD have protein-energy malnutrition until proven otherwise.
- Look for cause of hypermetabolism, such as infections, ascites, and encephalopathy.
- Exclude malabsorption and maldigestion in patients with cholestatic liver disease.
- Perform frequent nutritional assessment, including anthropometrics, changes in body weight, 24-hour creatinine excretion, and 24-hour urinary urea nitrogen in patients awaiting liver transplantation.
- BEE can be predicted in patients with absence of decompensated liver disease and measured using indirect calorimetry in patients with decompensated liver disease.
- Multiple meals (5-7) should be encouraged, especially at bedtime to decrease gluconeogenesis.
- Portosystemic encephalopathy should be treated aggressively before protein restriction is instituted.
- Branched-chain amino acids should be restricted to patients with refractory encephalopathy.
- Progressive increments of protein supplementation should be given up to 1.8 to 2.0 g/kg/day, as tolerated.
- Sodium restriction (2 g/d) is advised in the presence of ascites/peripheral edema.
- Do not restrict to fluid unless serum sodium is 120 mmol/L.
- All patients with ESLD should receive multivitamins; rule out deficiency of fat-soluble vitamins (A, D, E, K).
- Remember that patients with ESLD have higher incidence of osteoporosis; use folic acid in patients with alcoholic liver disease and zinc sulfate in patients with changes in taste and/or smell and encephalopathy.
- Give aggressive oral supplementation and low threshold to place a nasoenteric feeding tube in patients awaiting OLT.
- Total parenteral nutrition should be considered only in patients with contraindications for enteral feeding.
- Physical therapy should be provided for hospitalized patients awaiting liver transplantation.
- After liver transplantation, indirect calorimetry should be performed regularly to avoid under- and overfeeding.
- Close monitoring of patients after OLT is important; particular attention should be given to the development of obesity, hyperlipidemia, osteoporosis, and hypertension.

BEE=basal energy expenditure; ESLD=end-stage liver disease; OLT=orthotopic liver transplantation.

From Aranda-Michel J. Nutrition in hepatic failure and liver transplantation. *Current Gastroenterology Reports.* 2001;3:362-370.

in those who are unable to meet their daily requirements. Dietary supplementations with oral supplements and/or EN through a nasoenteric feeding tube are the most common means of augmenting nutritional intake. (EN is discussed in Chapters 34, 39, 41, and 42.) Nasoenteric tubes, despite concerns of some, do not increase the risk of GI bleeding, though there may be some increased risk of sinusitis, gastroesophageal reflux, and aspiration pneumonia. Oral intake is always preferred and encouraged, even while nasoenteric feeding is being used. Administration of tube feedings overnight offers dual advantages of allowing normal daily activity during waking hours and minimizing accelerated starvation physiology during sleeping hours.

Protein and fluid restriction are often routinely recommended to patients with a history of portosystemic encephalopathy, ascites, and edema. These complications of cirrhosis can generally be adequately treated without a need to resort to nutritional restriction. Portosystemic encephalopathy should be treated aggressively with standard therapy before protein restriction is instituted. In fact, patients with ESLD can safely tolerate protein intakes of up to 1.8 to 2 g/kg/day. Hence, in patients with PEM, protein intake of 1 g/kg/day as a starting point can be initiated and titrated per response, guided by 24-hour urinary creatinine.

Standard amino acid formulas are effective and well tolerated, even in patients with advanced liver disease. When encephalopathy becomes truly refractory, however, BCAA should be considered. As previously discussed, there is no consensus on whether BCAA supplementation has a significant beneficial effect in patients with chronic hepatic encephalopathy;[58] however, a recent prospective randomized trial performed comparing BCAA to standard preparations in patients with advanced cirrhosis did show an advantage in reduced rates of death and hospitalization. There were also improvements in nutritional parameters and Child-Pugh scores.[59] There are no studies assessing the use and effectiveness of BCAA for hepatic encephalopathy in patients with acute liver failure.

In a comprehensive meta-analysis, no convincing evidence was found for clinical or survival benefit in use of BCAA in patients with ESLD and hepatic encephalopathy. However, the heterogeneity of the reviewed studies, with respect to treatment regimens, duration of therapy, and patient populations, may have limited the beneficial effects of selective BCAA therapy. There was some data that

TABLE 20-2.

Branched-Chain Amino Acid Formulations

NutriHep Enteral Nutrition	Hepatic-Aid II Instant Drink	HepatAmine (8% amino acid)
Nestle, Deerfield, Ill	B. Braun McGaw, Irvine, Calif	B. Braun McGaw
Enteral	Dietary supplement	Parenteral
1.5 kcal/mL	1.2 kcal/mL	0.32 kcal/mL
Fat (12%)	Fat (28%)	Fat free
MCT (66%)	No MCT	No MCT
Protein	Protein	Protein
50% BCAA	46% BCAA	36% BCAA
50% aromatic AA	low methionine	low aromatic AA
Carbohydrate 77%	Carbohydrate 58%	Carbohydrate adjusted
RDI 100%	Vitamin and electrolyte free	Vitamin and electrolyte free
Gluten free, lactose free		

AA=amino acid; BCAA=branched-chain amino acid; MCT=medium-chain triglyceride; RDI=recommended daily intake.

From Aranda-Michel J. Nutrition in hepatic failure and liver transplantation. *Current Gastroenterology Reports.* 2001;3:362-370.

suggested a benefit in encephalopathy using parenteral BCAA in acute hepatic encephalopathy and enteral BCAA in chronic hepatic encephalopathy.[58] Randomized controlled trials are needed to better define a role for BCAA in patients with decompensated liver disease.

It is important, however, to note that there are a number of preparations of BCAA-enriched supplements available on the market (Table 20-2). These formulations are often vitamin- and electrolyte-free and are designed as supplements to nutritional therapy rather than as mainstay treatments. The exact duration of BCAA-enriched supplement therapy is not well established but it is reasonable to use nutritional stability and control of the encephalopathy as a clinical marker for conversion to standard amino acid formulas.

In patients with fluid retention (ie, ascites and edema) only sodium restriction is needed. Free water should not be restricted unless the serum sodium is less than 120 mmol/L. Daily weights can be most useful in short-term monitoring of fluid balance. In cases of refractory ascites, the impact of frequent paracentesis on nutritional status is undefined. In cirrhotic patients with refractory ascites, resolution of the ascites after transjugular intrahepatic portosystemic shunt placement resulted in improvement of several nutritional parameters, notably for body composition.[60] Although there can be significant loss of protein and electrolytes, there is a potential benefit from neurohormonal effects of large paracentesis. A potential benefit of decreased early satiety with large volume paracentesis in patients with ESLD has been refuted.[61]

Patients with ESLD, particularly those with cholestatic disease, have a higher incidence of osteopenia, which can be a major cause of morbidity before and after OLT.[37,62] Osteopenic patients should be placed on calcium supplementation, and bisphosphonate therapy should be considered for severe osteopenia and osteoporosis (Chapter 13). Adequate vitamin D supplementation is an important component of managing those patients with bone density loss or cholestatic liver disease, where endogenous production, intestinal absorption, and 25 hydroxylation of vitamin may be impaired.

The effectiveness of arginine, ornithine-aspartate, or ornithine alpha-glutarate in lowering ammonia levels and improving nutritional status in patients with ESLD is unproven. There is insufficient data to recommend nutrient supplementation such as arginine, glutamine, and omega-3 fatty acids or routine use of androgenic and anabolic steroids, and insulin growth factor-1.

Parenteral Nutrition and Liver Disease

PN is not commonly indicated in patients with ESLD and is generally well tolerated when used. However, PN itself is commonly associated with a wide range of hepatic injuries. Although it is unclear if this relates to direct toxicity versus deficiency of nutrients, both patient and nutritional factors are likely involved. In adults, the earliest injury pattern is hepatocellular with steatosis, typically reflected by mild liver enzyme and bilirubin elevations (>1.5 times the upper normal limit). In the pediatric population, a cholestatic pattern is more common. These biochemical abnormalities can appear within 1 to 2 weeks of therapy, are initially transient, and are fully reversible by cessation of PN. A second peak in liver enzymes can follow and may represent the early manifestation of chronic hepatotoxicity (duration >6 months), usually in the setting of home parenteral nutrition (HPN). Chronic hepatotoxicity with HPN is common, particularly in the setting of intestinal failure, with a prevalence rate of 46% to 50% after 6 years of therapy.[63,64] Outcomes are variable, but mortality rates of 7% to 15% have been reported.[64,65] Identified risk factors include short bowel syndrome, inflammatory diseases, excess lipid infusion, and independent risks for liver dysfunction. In patients with short bowel syndrome and chronic liver injury on HPN, early referral for combined liver and small bowel transplantation is important because mortality rates on the waiting list are particularly high.[66] Early cycling of PN may limit hepatic function deterioration in patients with jaundice and persistent need for PN.[67]

The histopathology of PN-associated liver injury can vary from initial periportal steatosis or cholestasis to pan-lobular steatohepatitis, fibrosis, and micronodular cirrhosis. Cirrhotic stage disease is usually accompanied by portal hypertension. The exact mechanisms of hepatic injury with PN are not fully understood, but a number of hypotheses and associated therapeutic interventions have been studied.

Imbalances of insulin and glucagon, aluminum toxicity, deficiencies of amino acids and essential fatty acids, and caloric excess have been implicated. There has been a great deal of interest in a possible hepatoprotective effect of the gluconeogenic amino acid glutamine.[68] However, a clinical role for glutamine supplementation remains unproven.[69] Essential fatty acid supplementation may alleviate hepatic triglyceride accumulation and impaired lipoprotein synthesis. Oral lecithin and parenteral choline supplementation have been shown to reduce hepatic steatosis in patients on long-term PN.[70]

In the absence of enteral stimulation, bacterial overgrowth, intestinal atrophy and impaired immunity may increase hepatotoxic bile acid formation. These toxins and associated endotoxins may, in turn, induce a cytokine- and macrophage-mediated injury to the biliary tree, mimicking the presumed mechanism of sepsis-induced cholestasis. Antibiotic (metronidazole) and bile acid (ursodiol) therapy targeting these mechanisms may improve biochemical injury profile, but a benefit in hepatic function or outcomes is unproven.[71]

Sludge and/or stone formation can develop quite rapidly in patients receiving PN, and a high index of suspicion should be maintained. Bile stasis in the absence of enteral stimulation of cholecystokinin may significantly contribute to sludge formation, gallstone disease, and acalculous cholecystitis.[72] This can develop in as little as 2 weeks and may be considered universal when parenteral feeding is maintained for longer than 3 months. Caution should be exercised with mineral supplementation with PN in patients with cholestatic liver disease, as they are at risk for Manganese deposition in the basal ganglia, with resulting movement disorders.

Conclusion

PEM in patients with stable or decompensated ESLD is a common finding. It is multifaceted in etiology and is associated with significant mortality and morbidity in this group of patients. Early detection of the presence of PEM is the first step in allowing a multidisciplinary team to effect a positive change in nutritional status and possibly outcomes. Data on treatment of PEM pre liver transplant is limited, and there is a need for randomized controlled studies in this and other areas relating to malnutrition and liver disease. There is an increasing interest in understanding and further delineating the pathophysiology of PEM in ESLD, as it is becoming a more distinctly recognized component of advanced liver disease.

References

1. The International Classification of Disease, Ninth Revision, Clinical Modification (ICD-9 CM), Practice Management Information Corporation. Hyattsville, MD: National Center for Health Statistics; 1998.
2. Lautz HU, Selberg O, Korber J, et al. Protein-calorie malnutrition in liver cirrhosis. *Clin Invest.* 1992;70:478-486.
3. Italian Multicentre Cooperative Project on Nutrition in Liver Cirrhosis: Nutritional status in cirrhosis. *J Hepatol.* 1994;21:317-325.
4. McCullough AJ, Bugianesi E, et al. Protein calorie malnutrition and the etiology of cirrhosis. *Am J Gastroenterol.* 1997;92:734-738.
5. DiCecco SR, Wieners EJ, Wiesner RH. Assessment of nutritional status of patients with end-stage liver disease undergoing liver transplantation. *Mayo Clin Proc.* 1989;64:95-102.
6. Prijatmoko D, Strauss BJ, Lambert JR, et al. Early detection of protein depletion in alcoholic cirrhosis: role of body composition analysis. *Gastroenterology.* 1993;105:1839-1845.
7. Mendenhall CL, Moritz TE, Roselle GA, et al. Protein energy malnutrition in severe alcoholic hepatitis: diagnosis and response to treatment. The VA Cooperative Study Group 275. *JPEN J Parenter Enteral Nutr.* 1995;19:258-265.
8. Merli M, Riggio O, Dally L. Does malnutrition affect survival in cirrhosis? PINC (Policentrica Italiana Nutrizione Cirrosi). *Hepatology.* 1996;23:1041-1046.
9. Moller S, Bendtsen F, Christensen E, Henriksen JH. Prognostic variables in patients with cirrhosis and oesophageal varices without prior bleeding. *J Hepatol.* 1994;21:940-946.
10. Selberg O, Bottcher J, Tusch G, et al. Identification of high- and low-risk patients before liver transplantation: a prospective cohort study of nutritional and metabolic parameters in 150 patients. *Hepatology.* 1997;25:652-657.
11. Tajika M, Kato M, Mohri H, et al. Prognostic value of energy metabolism in patients with viral liver cirrhosis. *Nutrition.* 2002;18(3):229-234.
12. Campillo B, Richardet JP, Scherman E, Bories PN. Evaluation of nutritional practice in hospitalized cirrhotic patients: results of a prospective study. *Nutrition.* 2003;19(6):515-521.
13. Davidson HI, Richardson R, Sutherland D, Garden OJ. Macronutrient preference, dietary intake, and substrate oxidation among stable cirrhotic patients. *Hepatology.* 1999;29(5):1380-1386.
14. Richardson RA, Davidson HI, Hinds A. Influence of the metabolic sequelae of liver cirrhosis on nutritional intake. *Am J Clin Nutr.* 1999;69:331-337.
15. Prasad AS. The role of zinc in gastrointestinal and liver disease. *Clin Gastroenterol.* 1983;12(3):713-741.
16. Miki C, Iriyama K, Mayer AD. Energy storage and cytokine response in patients undergoing liver transplantation. *Cytokine.* 1999;11:244-248.
17. Testa R, Franceschini R, Giannini E et al. Serum leptin levels in patients with viral chronic hepatitis or liver cirrhosis. *J Hepatol.* 2000;33:33-37.
18. McCullough AJ, Bugianesi E, Marchesini G, Kalhan SC. Gender-dependent alterations in serum leptin in alcoholic cirrhosis. *Gastroenterology.* 1998;115:9479-9453.
19. Dolz C, Raurich JM, Ibanez J, Obrador A, Marse P, Gaya J. Ascites increases the resting energy expenditure in liver cirrhosis. *Gastroenterology.* 1991;100(3):738-744.
20. Yamanaka H, Genjida K, Yokota K, et al. Daily pattern of energy metabolism in cirrhosis. *Nutrition.* 1999;15(10):749-754.
21. Greco AV, Mingrone G, Benedetti G. Daily energy and substrate metabolism in patients with cirrhosis. *Hepatology.* 1998;27:346-350.
22. Merli M, Riggio O, Romiti A, et al. Basal energy production rate and substrate use in stable cirrhotic patients. *Hepatology.* 1990;12(1):106-112.
23. Muller MJ, Pirlich M, Balks HJ, Selberg O. Glucose intolerance in liver cirrhosis: role of hepatic and non-hepatic influences. *Eur J Clin Chem Clin Biochem.* 1994;32:749-758.

24. Riggio O, Angeloni S, Ciuffa L, et al. Malnutrition is not related to alterations in energy balance in patients with stable liver cirrhosis. *Clinical Nutrition.* 2003;22(6):553-559.
25. Cabre E, Abad-Lacruz A, Nunez MC, et al. The relationship of plasma polyunsaturated fatty acid deficiency with survival in advanced liver cirrhosis: multivariate analysis. *Am J Gastroenterol.* 1993;88:718-722.
26. Pantaleo P, Marra F, Vizzutti F, et al. Effects of dietary supplementation with arachidonic acid on platelet and renal function in patients with cirrhosis. *Clin Sci (Lond).* 2004;106(1):27-34.
27. McCullough AJ, Mullen KD, Kalhan SC. Defective non-oxidative leucine degradation and endogenous leucine flux in cirrhosis during an amino acid infusion. *Hepatology.* 1998;28:1357-1364.
28. Mullen KD, Denne SC, McCullough AJ, et al. Leucine metabolism in stable cirrhosis. *Hepatology.* 1986;6:622-630.
29. Kondrup J, Nielsen K, Juul A. Effect of long-term refeeding on protein metabolism in patients with cirrhosis of the liver. *Br J Nutr.* 1997;77:197-212.
30. Nielsen K, Kondrup J, Martinsen L, et al. Long-term oral refeeding of patients with cirrhosis of the liver. *Br J Nutr.* 1995;74:557-567.
31. Iwasa M, Matsumura K, Watanabe Y, et al. Improvement of regional cerebral blood flow after treatment with branched-chain amino acid solutions in patients with cirrhosis. *Eur J Gastroenterol Hepatol.* 2003;15:733-737.
32. McCullough AJ, Raguso C. Effect of cirrhosis on energy expenditure. *Am J Clin Nutr.* 1999;69:1066-1068.
33. Muller MJ, Lautz HU, Plogmann B, et al. Energy expenditure and substrate oxidation in patients with cirrhosis: the impact of cause, clinical staging and nutritional state. *Hepatology.* 1992;15:782-794.
34. Muller MJ, Bottcher J, Selberg O. Hypermetabolism in clinically stable patients with liver cirrhosis. *Am J Clin Nutr.* 1999;69:1194-1201.
35. Marchesini G, Fabbri A, Bianchi G, et al. Zinc supplementation and amino acid-nitrogen metabolism in patients with advanced cirrhosis. *Hepatology.* 1996;23:1084-1092.
36. Floreani A, Baragiotta A, Martines D, et al. Plasma antioxidant levels in chronic cholestatic liver diseases. *Aliment Pharmacol Ther.* 2000;14:353-358.
37. Trautwein C, Possienke M, Schlitt HJ, et al. Bone density and metabolism in patients with viral hepatitis and cholestatic liver diseases before and after liver transplantation. *Am J Gastroenterol.* 2000;95:2343-2351.
38. Koivisto M, Valta P, Hockerstedt K, Lindgren L. Magnesium depletion in chronic terminal liver cirrhosis. *Clin Transplant.* 2002;16(5):325-328.
39. Hasse J, Strong S, Gorman MA, Liepa G. Subjective global assessment: alternative nutrition-assessment technique for liver-transplant candidates. *Nutrition.* 1993;9:339-343.
40. Naveau S, Belda E, Borotto E, et al. Comparison of clinical judgment and anthropometric parameters for evaluating nutritional status in patients with alcoholic liver disease. *J Hepatol.* 1995;23:234-235.
41. Pirlich M, Selberg O, Boker K, et al. The creatinine approach to estimate skeletal muscle mass in patients with cirrhosis. *Hepatology.* 1996;24:1422-1427.
42. Donadio C, Lucchesi A, Tramonti G, Bianchi C. Creatinine clearance predicted from body cell mass is a good indicator of renal function. *Kidney Int Suppl.* 1997;63:S166-S168.
43. Wang Z, Zhu S, Wang J, Pierson RN Jr, Heymsfield SB. Whole-body skeletal muscle mass: development and validation of total-body potassium prediction models. *Am J Clin Nutr.* 2003;77(1):76-82.
44. Schloerb PR, Forster J, Delcore R, Kindscher JD. Bioelectrical impedance in the clinical evaluation of liver disease. *Am J Clin Nutr.* 1996;64(Suppl 3):510S-514S.
45. Zillikens MC, van den Berg JW, Wilson JH, Swart GR. Whole-body and segmental bioelectrical-impedance analysis in patients with cirrhosis of the liver: changes after treatment of ascites. *Am J Clin Nutr.* 1992;55:621-625.
46. Pirlich M, Schutz T, Spachos T, et al. Bioelectrical impedance analysis is a useful bedside technique to assess malnutrition in cirrhotic patients with and without ascites. *Hepatology.* 2000;32:1208-1215.
47. Selberg O, Selberg D. Norms and correlates of bioimpedance phase angle in healthy human subjects, hospitalized patients, and patients with liver cirrhosis. *Eur J Appl Physiol.* 2002;86(6):509-516. Epub 2002 Jan 31.
48. Fiore P, Merli M, Andreoli A, et al. A comparison of skinfold anthropometry and dual-energy X-ray absorptiometry for the evaluation of body fat in cirrhotic patients. *Clin Nutr.* 1999;18:349-351.
49. Madden AM, Morgan MY. Resting energy expenditure should be measured in patients with cirrhosis, not predicted. *Hepatology.* 1999;30(3):655-664.
50. Aranda-Michel J. Nutrition in hepatic failure and liver transplantation. *Curr Gastroenterol Rep.* 2001;3:362-370.
51. Cabre E, Gonzalez-Huix F, Abad-Lacruz A, et al. Effect of total enteral nutrition on the short-term outcome of severely malnourished cirrhotics: a randomized controlled trial. *Gastroenterology.* 1990;98:715-720.
52. Hasse JM, Blue LS, Liepa GU, et al. Early enteral nutrition support in patients undergoing liver transplantation. *JPEN J Parenter Enteral Nutr.* 1995;19:437-443.
53. Wicks C, Somasundaram S, Bjarnason I, et al. Comparison of enteral feeding and total parenteral nutrition after liver transplantation. *Lancet.* 1994;24:837-840.
54. Shiomi S, Masaki K, Habu D, et al. Calcitriol for bone disease in patients with cirrhosis of the liver. *J Gastroenterol Hepatol.* 1999;14960:547-552.
55. Johansson S, Melhus H. Vitamin A antagonizes calcium response to vitamin D in man. *J Bone Miner Res.* 2001;169(10):1899-1905.
56. Fan ST. Review: nutritional support for patients with cirrhosis. *J Gastroenterol Hepatol.* 1997;12(4):282-286.
57. Druml W, Fischer M, Pidlich J, Lenz K. Fat elimination in chronic hepatic failure: long-chain vs medium-chain triglycerides. *Am J Clin Nutr.* 1995;61(4):812-817.
58. Als-Nielsen B, Koretz RL, Kjaergard LL, Gluud C. Branched-chain amino acids for hepatic encephalopathy. Cochrane Database Syst Rev. 2003;(2):CD001939.
59. Marchesini G, Bianchi G, Merli M, et al. Italian BCAA Study Group. Nutritional supplementation with branched-chain amino acids in advanced cirrhosis: a double-blind, randomized trial. *Gastroenterology.* 2003;124(7):1792-1801.
60. Allard JP, Chau J, Sandokji K, Blendis LM, Wong F. Effects of ascites resolution after successful TIPS on nutrition in cirrhotic patients with refractory ascites. *Am J Gastroenterol.* 2001;96(8):2442-2447.
61. Scolapio JS, Ukleja A, McGreevy K, Burnett OL, O'Brien PC. Nutritional problems in end-stage liver disease: contribution of impaired gastric emptying and ascites. *J Clin Gastroenterol.* 2002;34(1):89-93.
62. Heathcote J. Osteoporosis in chronic liver disease. *Curr Gastroenterol Rep.* 1999;1:455-458.
63. Luman W, Shaffer JL. Prevalence, outcome and associated factors of deranged liver function tests in patients on home parenteral nutrition. *Clin Nutr.* 2002;21(4):337-343.
64. Cavicchi M, Beau P, Crenn P, et al. Prevalence of liver disease and contributing factors in patients receiving home parenteral nutrition for permanent intestinal failure. *Ann Intern Med.* 2000;132(7):525-532.
65. Chan S, McCowen KC, Bistrian BR, et al. Incidence, prognosis, and etiology of end-stage liver disease in patients receiving home total parenteral nutrition. *Surgery.* 1999;126(1):28-34.
66. Fryer J, Pellar S, Ormond D, et al. Mortality in candidates waiting for combined liver-intestine transplants exceeds that for other candidates waiting for liver transplants. *Liver Transpl.* 2003;9(7):748-753.

67. Hwang TL, Lue MC, Chen LL. Early use of cyclic TPN prevents further deterioration of liver functions for the TPN patients with impaired liver function. *Hepatogastroenterology*. 2000;47(35):1347-1350.
68. Kudsk KA, Wu Y, Fukatsu K, et al. Glutamine-enriched total parenteral nutrition maintains intestinal interleukin-4 and mucosal immunoglobulin A levels. *JPEN J Parenter Enteral Nutr.* 2000;24(5):270-4; discussion 274-275.
69. Buchman AL. Glutamine: commercially essential or conditionally essential? A critical appraisal of the human data. *Am J Clin Nutr.* 2001;74(1):25-32.
70. Buchman AL, Dubin M, Jenden D, et al. Lecithin increases plasma free choline and decreases hepatic steatosis in long-term total parenteral nutrition patients. *Gastroenterology*. 1992;102(4[Pt 1]):1363-1370.
71. Gunsar C, Melek M, Karaka I, et al. The biochemical and histopathological effects of ursodeoxycholic acid and metronidazole on total parenteral nutrition-associated hepatic dysfunction: an experimental study. *Hepatogastroenterology*. 2002;49(44):497-500.
72. Messing B, Bories C, Kunstlinger F, Bernier JJ. Does total parenteral nutrition induce gallbladder sludge formation and lithiasis? *Gastroenterology*. 1983;84(5[Pt 1]):1012-1019.

Chapter 21

Nutrition in Chronic Pancreatitis

William B. Evans, MD, and
Stephen A. McClave, MD

Introduction

Chronic pancreatitis produces a prolonged inflammatory state, resulting in a steadily progressive destruction of the pancreatic gland. A multitude of factors, ranging from poor oral intake and hypermetabolism to malassimilation and endocrine dysfunction, predispose the patient with chronic pancreatitis to protein energy malnutrition (PEM). (Chapter 20 also discusses PEM.) The success of nutritional therapy is dependent on abstinence from alcohol and control of abdominal pain. Nutritional support varies depending on disease severity, from diet restriction with continued oral intake to provision of artificial enteral or parenteral nutrients. Supplementation with pancreatic enzymes helps control pain and improve maldigestion. Specific vitamin deficiencies should be anticipated and treated appropriately. Careful assessment, design of the proper nutritional regimen, and documentation of response to therapy are all required to reduce the morbidity from this disease process.

Clinical Manifestations

Chronic pancreatitis is a persistent inflammatory condition of the pancreas characterized by progressive, irreversible damage to the pancreas, leading to extensive fibrosis and the destruction of both exocrine and endocrine tissue. In several retrospective studies, the annual incidence ranges from 3.5 to 10 cases per 100,000.[1]

There are multiple etiologies involved in the pathogenesis of chronic pancreatitis, the incidence of which depends on geographic location. In Western countries, alcohol consumption is the main cause in 70% to 90% of cases.[2-6] For the disease process to develop, consumption of 150 to 175 grams of alcohol per day is required for a duration ranging from as short as 5 years in either sex up to 18 years for men and up to 11 years for women.[7] At this level of consumption, however, only 10% to 15% of patients will develop chronic pancreatitis. Other etiologies range from metabolic, genetic, and autoimmune disorders to processes involving disruption of the pancreatic duct (Table 21-1).

The most common clinical presentation in these patients is abdominal pain, diarrhea, and weight loss. Most patients present with a variable course of intermittent acute flares of abdominal pain that become constant as the disease evolves. With destruction of the gland, diarrhea due to fat malabsorption develops, leading to progressive weight loss. The natural history of the disease and the prognosis in these patients is somewhat variable, being associated with a high morbidity rate and a mortality rate of up to 50% over 20 years.[8] Patients who continue to consume alcohol are more likely to develop complications, such as acute episodes of pancreatitis, formation of pseudocysts, duodenal obstruction, splenic vein thrombosis, and biliary strictures. These complications lead to surgical intervention in approximately 50% of patients.[2] At the end-stage of disease, diabetes mellitus and malnutrition are common.

Factors Precipitating Protein Energy Malnutrition

Malnutrition in chronic pancreatitis patients is a multifactorial process and a common late manifestation of disease. Destruction of the gland occurs, leading to maldigestion. (Malabsorption and maldigestion are also

Table 21-1.

Causes of Chronic Pancreatitis

Cause	
Alcohol	
Pancreatic duct disruption	
	Pancreas divisum
	Post-traumatic duct stricture
	Sphincter of Oddi dysfunction
	Papillary stenosis
Metabolic	
	Hypercalcemia
	Hypertriglyceridemia
Genetic	
	Hereditary pancreatitis
	Cystic fibrosis
Autoimmune	
	Isolated autoimmune pancreatitis
	Part of other systemic diseases (PSC, PBC, Sjögren's syndrome)
Idiopathic	
Tropical calcific pancreatitis	

discussed in Chapter 5.) The chronic underlying inflammatory process causes abdominal pain, an aversion to food, and a hypermetabolic state. There is step-wise deterioration as the disease progresses, leading to PEM.[10] The major factors that lead to malnutrition include poor oral intake, maldigestion resulting in malabsorption, hypermetabolism, and endocrine dysfunction.

The main reason for poor oral intake is persistent epigastric abdominal pain, which is exacerbated by eating and often accompanied by nausea and vomiting. Approximately 90% of patients with chronic pancreatitis have persistent pain, which leads to anorexia, sitophobia, and weight loss.[11] The exact cause of the pain is unknown. It is theorized that oral intake stimulates exocrine secretion of pancreatic juices released through scarred abnormal ducts, which in turn causes an increase in ductal pressure, a decrease in blood flow, and possible ischemic injury to the gland. Poor outflow of digestive enzymes may trigger autodigestion of pancreatic tissue and subsequent inflammation. Poor nutritional intake may also be related to continued ethanol consumption in the majority of these patients, who even without pancreatitis are often malnourished. Investigations into alternative reasons for poor oral intake, other than inflammation, have suggested gastric dysmotility as a cause for symptoms. One study showed that 44% of patients with exocrine insufficiency due to small-duct chronic pancreatitis in fact had gastroparesis, diagnosed by an abnormal gastric emptying scan.[12] There is a subset of patients, usually with more advanced disease, who may develop anatomic obstruction. A large pseudocyst or diffuse inflammation of the pancreatic head may cause gastric outlet obstruction, resulting in nausea and vomiting.

Another component of malnutrition in these patients results from advanced destruction of the pancreas with scarring of the exocrine tissue. Over 90% of the exocrine portion of parenchymal tissue must be destroyed before this process clinically manifests as diarrhea, steatorrhea, and malassimilation. This late complication, estimated to occur in 25% to 45% of patients (mean 33%),[10,13-16] presents as maldigestion of fat, protein, and carbohydrates. Most patients with maldigestion present with steatorrhea, an excessive amount of fat in the stool (>7 g/day on a 100-g fat diet), which is due to a lack of lipase secreted into the small bowel. Fat malabsorption is the initial presentation in most patients with chronic pancreatitis for several reasons. Digestion of fat is more dependent on pancreatic lipase and colipase (80%) than on gastric lipase (20%). Pancreatic lipase output decreases earlier in the course of disease, and lipase is more susceptible to destruction from gastric acid than from other pancreatic enzymes.

Patients with steatorrhea present clinically with diarrhea and usually some degree of significant weight loss. Patients usually have 3 to 4 loose, bulky, greasy, foul-smelling stools per day and often give a history of oil droplets present in the stools, which are difficult to flush. Symptoms differ from those of patients with a classic malabsorptive process, which in contrast is typically characterized by watery diarrhea, abdominal bloating, and cramping. This difference in symptomatology is due to better preservation of carbohydrate absorption in patients with maldigestion from chronic pancreatitis. It has been shown that protein malabsorption is corrected to a greater extent than fat malabsorption because trypsin is less vulnerable to acid destruction than lipase.[17]

The exocrine pancreas also produces bicarbonate, which is secreted with digestive enzymes in response to a meal. The bicarbonate helps neutralize gastric acid in the duodenum, which would otherwise cause breakdown of pancreatic enzymes and bile salts. Without bicarbonate present, both bile salts and enzymes are inactivated by the gastric acid, which serves to worsen maldigestion.[18]

The presence of steatorrhea, due to pancreatic exocrine insufficiency, can be assessed by either a quantitative or qualitative stool collection. Both methods require adherence to a strict diet of 100 g of fat per day starting 3 days prior to the study. The quantitative method is the gold standard to estimate stool fat. Stool is collected for 72 hours, an abnormal result being the presence of >7 g of fat (or >7% of the ingested dose) per day. The qualitative method involves collection of one stool specimen, then staining for fat with Sudan III stain. Observation of greater than 6 fat globules per high power field is considered to be abnormal. Both tests have disadvantages because of the strict dietary measures required. The qualitative test requires significant steatorrhea for a positive test. The quantitative test involves a long, cumbersome stool collection, which often results in patient noncompliance and an insufficient volume collected. (Testing for malabsorption is discussed in Chapter 5.)

Patients with chronic pancreatitis and maldigestion are at risk for deficiencies of vitamins and trace elements. Vitamin B12 deficiency may occur because of a lack of a proteolytic enzyme that normally cleaves the protein-binding competitor to intrinsic factor. Low levels of the vitamin are present in an estimated 10% to 15% of patients with chronic pancreatitis, but hematologic and neurologic complications are rare.[19] When present, the deficiency may be corrected either by supplementing B12 with monthly injections or by administrating pancreatic enzymes. Theoretically, patients with chronic pancreatitis are at significant risk for malabsorption of fat-soluble vitamins (A, D, E, and K); however, very rarely does clinical evidence for a specific vitamin deficiency occur.

Compared to a healthy control population, these patients have been shown to have lower plasma levels of antioxidants, such as selenium, vitamins A and E, xanthine, beta-carotene, betacryptoxanthine, and lycopene.[20,21] The overall clinical significance of vitamins A and E deficiency is unknown. Hemorrhagic complications from vitamin K deficiency are sporadic. Once thought to be insignificant, vitamin D malabsorption leading to secondary hyperparathyroidism and either osteomalacia or osteoporosis has been documented in 20% of patients with chronic pancreatitis.[16] A study by Haaber et al showed that approximately one-half of patients with chronic pancreatitis and up to 69% of those with documented steatorrhea, had bone-mineral density Z-scores <1, with mean 25 hydroxyvitamin D and 1,25 dihydroxyvitamin D3 serum levels below normal.[22]

Chronic persistent pancreatic inflammation causes a continuous hypermetabolic state that plays a role in the development of malnutrition in these patients. Up to one-third of patients with uncomplicated disease demonstrated hypermetabolism with a resting energy expenditure (REE) above that predicted by the Harris-Benedict equation.[23] Results from an intricate study by Hebuterne et al found that hypermetabolism (with an REE >110%) was present in 65% of patients with alcohol-induced chronic pancreatitis who were underweight versus 20% in those patients who were of normal weight.[24] Such hypermetabolism was associated with up to a 10% to 20% loss of body weight. This study suggests that the hypermetabolic effect from chronic inflammation seen in these patients compounds their poor nutritional intake and malabsorptive process, resulting in further weight loss and exacerbation of their malnourished state.

What causes hypermetabolism in this group of patients is not clear. Although Hebuterne's study showed no increase in hypermetabolism in active drinkers, other studies have shown that alcohol intake does increase energy expenditure.[24,25] Still other studies suggest that a hypermetabolic state is attributable to elevated levels of circulating cytokines and catabolic hormones.[26,27] The release of these agents leads to an imbalance between pro-oxidant and antioxidant substances, creating a continued state of increased oxidative stress and serving as a confounding factor in the progression of damage and destruction to pancreatic tissue.[28] The damage oxidative stress induces on the pancreas is mediated by pro-inflammatory cytokines, which have been found in the serum, blood monocytes, pancreatic juices, and glandular tissue of patients with both acute and chronic pancreatitis.[29-32] Evidence for such a process has led to studies evaluating a role for antioxidant therapy in patients with chronic pancreatitis, a topic to be discussed later in this chapter.

Endocrine dysfunction manifesting as type 1 diabetes can occur on average 7 to 15 years after the diagnosis is made. Over 90% of the insulin-producing beta cells must be destroyed before this complication manifests. Along with the destruction of beta cells is the loss of glucagon-producing alpha cells. As a result of this combined defect, 20% to 30% of these patients become "brittle," insulin-dependent diabetics who are difficult to manage, with labile blood glucose levels and frequent hypoglycemic episodes.[33,34] Wide swings in the blood glucose levels and continued abnormalities in carbohydrate metabolism may contribute to delayed gastric emptying, all of which exacerbates a malnourished state. (Nutrition and diabetes are discussed in Chapter 16.)

Nutritional Therapy

Nutritional therapy plays an important role in the management of patients with chronic pancreatitis. Reversing malnutrition alone may change the overall disease course and ultimate clinical outcome. Although a number of means exists by which to provide nutritional support to these patients, success depends on attention to two specific strategies that must be used in conjunction with nutritional therapy.

First, absolute abstinence from alcohol is of utmost importance. Those patients with chronic pancreatitis who continue to abuse alcohol do worse clinically than nonalcoholic patients. Studies have shown that symptoms did not progress as rapidly once patients stop drinking.[35] Outside the setting of pancreatitis, alcohol alone has been shown to cause an increase in REE when compared to levels of nondrinking controls. Although alcohol has greater caloric density than carbohydrate or protein at 7 kcal/g, the calories are considered "empty," containing minimal protein and little nutrient value. These factors may contribute to deterioration of nutritional status. Additionally, cessation of alcohol is more likely to result in pain relief, occurring in one study in up to 75% of patients with chronic pancreatitis.[36]

Second, controlling abdominal pain is also an important strategy for correcting malnutrition in patients with chronic pancreatitis. Control of pain may stimulate increased appetite and nutritional intake. Controlling abdominal pain requires putting the pancreas to rest through reduction in stimulation of pancreatic exocrine secretion. An understanding of the physiologic gastropancreatic and enteropancreatic secretory mechanisms involved is needed to achieve optimal nutritional support. Pancreatic stimulation is under both neural and hormonal influences.

In response to food entering the stomach and duodenum, cholecystokinin (CCK) and secretin are released. These hormones stimulate secretion of digestive enzymes and bicarbonate. CCK-releasing factor (CCK-RF) is a trypsin-sensitive protein that regulates pancreatic exocrine secretion. In the fasting state, a basal output of trypsin and other proteases degrades CCK-RF, thereby reducing further secretion of digestive enzymes. In the fed state, proteases bind to protein in digested food that has entered the duodenum. The increased amount of luminal unbound CCK-RF that results serves to increase CCK levels and promote further enzyme secretion. This natural feedback mechanism is a cause for postprandial abdominal pain in patients with acute and chronic pancreatitis. In patients with pancreatitis and chronic inflammation, pancreatic stimulation is thought to cause elevated pancreatic ductal pressure, resulting from distorted ductal anatomy. The increased ductal pressure may, in turn, compromise blood flow to the parenchyma, producing ischemia and worsening abdominal pain. Obstruction to flow through the pancreatic duct may force enzymes into the parenchyma, resulting in autodigestion of pancreatic tissue.[37]

Although different options of nutritional support exist for these patients, all attempts should be made to provide nutrition while inhibiting this key feedback mechanism, to decrease the likelihood for postprandial abdominal pain. Nutritional therapy may utilize the traditional oral route with a restrictive diet designed to reduce stimulation of the pancreas, with or without supplemental enzymes (that suppress the feedback mechanism). Other routes include providing nutrition directly into the small bowel by nasoenteric or percutaneous feeding tubes or by parenteral infusion (thereby nearly eliminating pancreatic secretion).

Upon initiating nutritional support in patients with chronic pancreatitis, a proper assessment should be performed to evaluate risk of malnutrition. Subjective global assessment, described by Detsky, is one measure that can be used to screen for significant nutritional risk.[38] (The SGA is discussed in detail in Chapter 2.) Other data collected during the history and physical exam should include body mass index, amount of weight loss, and anthropometric measurements. Laboratory data (basic chemistry panel, CBC, serum calcium) and vitamin D levels should be obtained. Assessing risk in these patients helps dictate how aggressive one needs to be in providing nutritional support. (Nutritional assessment is covered in Chapter 1.)

Some patients with chronic pancreatitis with signs of mild malnutrition may be able to consume adequate calories through an oral diet without exacerbation of abdominal pain. Specific recommendations may be given to these patients, allowing full oral nutritional support and yet minimal secretion, thereby decreasing the likelihood of postprandial abdominal pain. Studies have shown that different diet compositions may be associated with varying degrees of pancreatic exocrine secretion. High fat diets are associated with more amylase and lipase secretion than high carbohydrate diets. While protein may be a stronger stimulant than carbohydrates, one study showed that varying the protein content from 10% to 40% of calories failed to show a difference in pancreatic enzyme secretion.[39] An optimal diet described for patients with chronic pancreatitis would include high calories (35 kcal/kg/day), high protein (1.0 to 1.5 g/kg/day), increased carbohydrates, and a moderate amount of fat (0.7 to 1.0 g/kg/day).[40] Vegetable fats are thought to be better tolerated than animal fats because of less pancreatic secretion.

Patients with continued weight loss and poor response to oral pancreatic enzymes (see below) may gain sufficient calories from supplemental formulas containing medium-chain triglyceride (MCT) oil. MCT oil minimizes pancreatic secretion because of its direct absorption by the intestinal mucosa into the portal venous system, in the absence of lipase, colipase, or bile salts. In comparison to long-chain fat, MCT oil has been shown to have greater and more efficient absorption.[40,41] In healthy volunteers, mean peak CCK levels were lower with the administration of formula composed of hydrolyzed peptides and MCT oil, compared to levels seen in response to an oral high-fat meal. In a 10-week pilot study of 8 patients with chronic pancreatitis and postprandial pain, daily provision of 3 to 4 cans of a small peptide formula with MCT oil improved pain scores in 62%.[42] Larger trials are needed to see whether such formulas can be tolerated and reproduce the same results over the long-term.

Approximately 80% to 85% of patients with chronic pancreatitis can be managed with dietary recommendations and/or enzyme supplementation. For those 10% to 15% of patients who are intolerant or unable to sustain adequate nutritional intake with a low-fat diet and pancreatic enzyme supplementation, two other more invasive methods for nutritional therapy may be required during the course of their disease process.[40] Either parenteral nutrition (PN) or enteral nutrition (EN) can provide adequate nutritional support while minimally stimulating the pancreas, reducing abdominal pain, and decreasing the likelihood for complications associated with chronic pancreatitis.

PN has been used in the past to rest the pancreas, halt inflammation, and promote relief of abdominal pain. Most trials have evaluated its use in acute pancreatitis. There are no reported prospective randomized trials of PN in patients with chronic pancreatitis. However, anecdotally, PN has been used to provide pancreatic rest in those patients with overly painful symptomatic flares. Studies evaluating the effects of parenterally infused nutrients on pancreatic secretion have shown no significant increase in pancreatic exocrine secretion in a wide variety of subjects, ranging from healthy volunteers to patients with pancreatic disease.[43-50] The few reports of an exacerbation of pancreatitis in patients receiving intravenous fat infusions[51,52] have been attributed to an associated hypercalcemia or hypertriglyceridemia. Disadvantages and complications from use of PN include increased cost (compared to EN), greater risk of catheter-related sepsis and thrombosis, and a higher incidence of hyperglycemia and other metabolic derangements. These PN-related complications occurred in 35% of patients in one study.[53] In general, PN should only be used in patients with chronic pancreatitis in whom signs of small bowel dysmotility develop or enteral access to the small bowel is not available.

Enteral feeding low enough in the small bowel can simultaneously rest the pancreas and decrease secretion while providing aggressive nutritional supplementation. Oral or gastric feedings are more likely to stimulate pancreatic exocrine secretion, but jejunal infusions result in subclinical increases of volume, bicarbonate, and protease levels in most canine and human studies.[54,55] Significantly reduced degrees of stimulation of pancreatic enzyme secretion occur as the level at which nutrients are infused descends the GI tract.[56-58]

There have been only a few studies, mostly uncontrolled and retrospective, which have evaluated use of EN in patients with chronic pancreatitis. Overall, they have shown that EN is superior to PN. In a group of patients with necrotizing exacerbations of chronic pancreatitis, those on nasojejunal feedings had less complications, required fewer surgical interventions, and demonstrated improved healing compared to those patients on PN.[59] In a separate study in patients with refractory acute pancreatitis, those patients sent home on jejunal feeds were less likely to be rehospitalized than were those patients who remained on an oral diet.[60] Enteral feedings maintain gut integrity,[61] which in turn, reduces the levels of pro-inflammatory cytokines generated by the gut that contribute to hypermetabolism.

Several different approaches are available by which to obtain access for postpyloric enteral feeding in patients with chronic pancreatitis. Nasojejunal or percutaneous gastrojejunostomy tubes may be placed by a radiologist using fluoroscopic or ultrasonographic guidance. If the patient has pancreatic surgery for intractable pain or a long-term complication from chronic pancreatitis, a surgically placed jejunostomy may be performed at the time of the operation. Unfortunately, local expertise is variable from one institution to the next, and there are no controlled studies available providing outcome data on radiologically or surgically placed jejunal feeding tubes in patients with chronic pancreatitis. An endoscopic approach to jejunal tube placement is minimally invasive and readily performed. A percutaneous endoscopic gastrojejunostomy (PEGJ) is an 8-12 French jejunal tube endoscopically placed into the small bowel through an existing percutaneous endoscopic gastrostomy (PEG).[62] While this procedure is of only moderate technical difficulty, PEGJ tubes have a high rate of tube malfunction due to migration back into the stomach, kinking, or tube clogging (requiring repeat procedures and tube replacement) in 39% to 55% of patients.[63-66] Direct percutaneous endoscopic jejunostomy (DPEJ) is similar to PEG placement except that a small bowel enteroscope or pediatric colonoscope is used to advance into the small bowel beyond the Ligament of Treitz, and the feeding tube is placed directly into the proximal jejunum. The DPEJ procedure is technically more difficult than the PEGJ, with lower reported success rates ranging from 72% to 88%.[67-69] Those major complications associated with PEGJ tube placement that require surgical intervention (such as bleeding, abdominal wall abscess, and colonic perforation) are usually low in frequency. Minor complications seen in patients with long-term PEGJ tubes include infections in 7%, ulcers in 5%, and peristomal leakage in 8%.[67-69] Although technically more challenging, DPEJ is associated with fewer minor complications and requires less reinterventions than PEGJ. For more permanent postpyloric enteral access, DPEJ is recommended over PEGJ.

The most common indication for percutaneous placement of an enteral access device is the need for prolonged (>30 days) jejunal feeding to manage chronic pancreatitis and its complications. Other indications include refractory pain that leads to anorexia and severe malnutrition or preoperative nutritional therapy for the malnourished patient with chronic pancreatitis who requires surgical intervention. Complications—such as pseudocyst, ascites, and fistula—are not a contraindication to jejunal feeding. Table 21-2 lists the main indications for postpyloric enteral feeding in patients with chronic pancreatitis. For those patients in whom permanent enteral access is anticipated, preliminary placement of a nasojejunal tube is recommended to see if the patient tolerates postpyloric feedings. Contraindications to DPEJ placement include inability to transilluminate due to large body habitus and continued pain or worsening clinical outcome in response to jejunal feedings. (EN complications, routes, and formulas are discussed in Chapters 39, 41, and 42, respectively.)

Adjunctive Medical Therapy for Malnutrition

The two goals of treatment with pancreatic enzyme supplements are control of malabsorption and achievement of pain relief. Pancreatic enzyme supplementation is warranted in any patient with chronic pancreatitis who demonstrates evidence of steatorrhea. The supplements provide proteases and lipases that are no longer produced by the pancreas to facilitate digestion and absorption of nutrients. Enzyme supplements also have a role in pain management in that subset of patients with chronic pancreatitis who suffer from constant, intermittent, or postprandial abdominal pain.

Enzyme supplements are given with meals and snacks and sometimes at bedtime. There are two types of enzyme preparations: enteric-coated (Creon, Ultrase) and nonenteric-coated (Viokase) (Table 21-3). The coated forms are designed to resist inactivation by gastric acid as the medication passes through the stomach. Once in the proximal small bowel, the increase in pH causes dissolution of the enteric coating and the active enzymes are released.

Because lipase can be destroyed by gastric acid with pH <4, the nonenteric coated forms should be given with simultaneous acid suppression (using either proton pump inhibitor or histamine-2 receptor antagonist agents).[19,70,71] Acid-suppressive medications should not be used with the enteric-coated preparations because the elevated

Table 21-2.

Main Indications for Postpyloric Enteral Nutrition

Malnutrition leading to progressive weight loss due to:
- Abdominal pain from oral intake
- Intolerance of pancreatic enzyme supplementation
- Intolerance of oral supplemental nutritional formulas

Acute complications of chronic pancreatitis:
- Acute bout of pancreatitis
- Pseudocyst formation
- Ascites
- Fistula formation

Prepancreatic and postpancreatic surgery

intragastric pH will cause premature enzyme release in the stomach. Enteric-coated supplements may not be effective if the microsphere size is too big to empty from the stomach in synchrony with food or if the enzymes are released too far distally in the GI tract to effectively aid in digestion and absorption. Studies have shown that these two general types of enzyme preparations (enteric-coated and nonenteric coated) are equally effective.[71]

While conventional pancreatic enzyme supplements are derived from porcine preparations, alternative forms are derived using bacterial lipase. Studies involving Burkholderia plantarii have shown that the bacterial lipase produced by this organism survives longer in gastric and duodenal juice than does porcine lipase, which is currently used in conventional supplements.[72] In studies using an animal model, dogs with exocrine insufficiency placed on a high-fat, high-calorie diet, provision of this bacterial lipase resulted in complete correction of steatorrhea.[73,74] This lipase preparation needs further investigation before its use can be applied to clinical practice.

To treat steatorrhea, approximately 10% of the volume of lipase normally produced by the pancreas should be delivered to the duodenum, timed to be present when the food is passing through the proximal small bowel.[75] This amount of enzyme has been shown to be equivalent to approximately 30,000 IU of lipase per meal,[76] thus requiring 4 to 8 tablets at each meal and at bedtime and 2 to 3 tablets with snacks. One study showed steatorrhea to be significantly reduced from 24 g to 10 g fat/day with appropriate enzyme therapy.[77] Current pancreatic enzyme supplements and their contents are listed in Table 21-3.

Documenting a favorable response to treatment does not necessarily require repeat stool collection but may be ascertained by a clinical improvement in stool consistency, loss of visible fat in the stool, relief of diarrhea, and weight gain.[75] A key clinical problem is coordinating the release of active enzymes into the duodenum or proximal jejunum at the correct time that food is also present. This problem is compounded by the fact that acid inactivates lipase, food empties from the stomach faster than the enzymes, and lipase seems to be inactivated to a greater extent in the small bowel than proteases.[75] With correct dosing, there is usually improvement in symptoms, but steatorrhea may not necessarily be totally corrected. Tolerance of the enzyme supplements may be a problem in some patients due to nausea, bloating, cramping, constipation, or diarrhea. Rarely, patients experience allergic reactions. Fibrosing colonopathy, possibly leading to colonic strictures, has been reported in patients with cystic fibrosis and high pancreatic enzyme supplements (>6000 lipase IU/kg/meal).[78] Failure of therapy most commonly is due to inadequate dosing, patient noncompliance, or improper use of acid suppressive medications. Changing to a different preparation, decreasing daily fat intake to <60 g, or increasing dosage to >30,000 IU of lipase per meal may improve symptomatic response. If these measures fail to resolve symptoms, then other causes of malabsorption, such as small bowel bacterial overgrowth, should investigated (Chapter 5). Intestinal bacterial overgrowth was found in approximately one-third of patients with pancreatic exocrine insufficiency from chronic pancreatitis in one study.[79]

Pancreatic enzyme therapy can also be used for the management of abdominal pain. The mechanism of pain relief from the enzyme preparations may involve suppressing the feedback mechanism of CCK-induced pancreatic secretion that was previously described. Preparations high in trypsin content (>50,000 IU) should be used. Surprisingly, two trials using nonenteric-coated preparations reported relief of pain, whereas four other trials using enteric-coated preparations were not effective in relieving pain.[80] Results from the two studies reporting a favorable response indicated that patients with less advanced or "small duct" disease, in which the etiology was nonalcohol related, were more likely to show improvement in pain.[81,82] A recent consensus review recommended a trial of pancreatic enzymes for pain, particularly in patients with less advanced disease who have failed other treatments.[80]

Some evidence supports the use of antioxidants to help reduce the amount of oxidative stress, created by elevated pro-inflammatory cytokines and the associated hypermetabolic rate. Studies using a combination of vitamins E and C with selenium and other trace elements have shown favorable clinical outcomes, with a decrease in pain and reduced number of admissions to the hospital[83,84]. A larger retrospective study showed patients on antioxidant therapy had a decrease in need for surgical intervention,

TABLE 21-3.

Comparison of Pancreatic Enzyme Supplements

Product	Enteric-coated	Lipase USP units	Protease USP units	Amylase USP units	Initial adult dose with meals, snacks	Distributor
Creon 5	yes	5,000	18,750	16,600	2 to 4 pills	Solvary (Marietta, GA)
Creon 10	yes	10,000	37,500	33,200	1 to 2 pills	Solvary
Creon 20	yes	20,000	75,000	66,400	1 pill	Solvary
Ultrase	yes	4,500	25,000	20,000	1 to 2 pills	Axcan Scandipharm (Birmingham, AL)
Ultrase MT12	yes	12,500	39,000	39,000	1 to 2 pills	Axcan Scandipharm
Ultrase MT18	yes	18,000	58,500	58,500	1 pill	Axcan Scandipharm
Ultrase MT20	yes	20,000	65,000	65,000	1 pill	Axcan Scandipharm-
Viokase 8	no	8,000	30,000	30,000	1 to 4 tablet(s)	Axcan Scandipharm-
Viokase 16	no	16,000	60,000	60,000	1 to 2 tablet(s)	Axcan Scandipharm-
Viokase powder	no	16,800	70,000	70,000	0.7 g/0.25 tsp	Axcan Scandipharm

Data from *Physician's Desk Reference.* 58th ed. Montvale, NJ: Thomson PDR; 2004.

the number and intensity of painful attacks, and fewer absences from work.[85] These encouraging results should generate larger placebo-controlled trials in patients with chronic pancreatitis.

Studies indicate that in pancreatic exocrine insufficiency, malabsorption of vitamin D is most likely to result in deficiency, in turn leading to osteomalacia and osteoporosis (Chapter 13). Thus, patients with advanced disease should be placed on vitamin D supplementation. The 25-hydroxylated form of vitamin D, Calcifediol (Calderol®), is more readily absorbed than vitamin D2 (calciferol). Adult dosing starts at 20 mcg/day, with maintenance dosing ranging from 20 to 100 mcg/day. Close monitoring of calcium levels is needed to avoid hypercalcemia.

Conclusion

Chronic pancreatitis is a progressive disease that increases risk of PEM and raises the potential for long-term complications. Successful management of the patient's poor nutritional state requires abstinence from alcohol and good control of abdominal pain. An accurate nutritional assessment must be obtained (Chapter 1) and an evaluation of the severity of malabsorption is needed to decide on the course of treatment (Chapter 3).

All patients with steatorrhea due to significant exocrine insufficiency should be given pancreatic enzymes and assessed for osteomalacia. If present, supplementation with Calderol is needed. For those patients with severe malnourishment, life-threatening complications, or need for preoperative strengthening, more invasive nutritional support is warranted. Because of the complications, increased cost, and deterioration of gut mucosa, PN is usually a second alternative choice after postpyloric enteral feedings have been attempted. If technically feasible, DPEJ is the optimum choice for prolonged jejunal feeding. More trials are needed, but there appears to be a potential role for antioxidant combinations to treat this chronic inflammatory process.

References

1. Etemad B, Whitcomb DC. Chronic pancreatitis: diagnosis, classification, and new genetic developments. *Gastroenterology.* 2001;120:682-707.
2. Copenhagen Pancreatitis Study: An interim report from a prospective epidemiological multicentre study. *Scand J Gastroenterol.* 1981;16:305.
3. Everhart JE, Go VLW. Pancreatitis. In: Everhart JE, eds. *Digestive Diseases in the United States: Epidemiology and Impact.* US Department of Health and Human Services, Public Health Service, National Institutes of Health. NIH Publication No 94-1447. Washington, DC: US Government Printing Office; 2004:691.
4. Lankisch PG, Lohr-Happe A, Otto J, et al. Natural course in chronic pancreatitis. *Digestion.* 1993;54:148.
5. Layer P, Yamamoto H, Katloff L, et al. The different courses of early- and late-onset idiopathic and alcoholic pancreatitis. *Gastroenterology.* 1994;107:1481.
6. Worning H. Alcoholic chronic pancreatitis. In: Berger HG, Warshaw AL, Buchler MW, et al, eds. *The Pancreas.* Malden, Mass: Blackwell Science; 1998:672.
7. Steer ML, Waxman I, Freedman S. Chronic pancreatitis. *N Engl J Med.* 1995;332:1482-1490.
8. Lowenfels AB, Maisonneuve P, Cavallini G, et al. Prognosis of chronic pancreatitis: an international multicenter study. International Pancreatitis Study Group. *Am J Gastroenterol.* 1994;89:1467-1471.
9. Ammann RW, Akovbiantz A, Largiader F, et al. Course and outcome of chronic pancreatitis. *Gastroenterology.* 1984;86:820-829.
10. Scolapio JS, Malhi-Chowla N, Ukleja A. Nutrition supplementation in patients with acute and chronic pancreatitis. *Gastroenterol Clin North Am.* 1999;28:695-707.
11. Ammann RW, Muellhaupt B. The natural history of pain in alcoholic chronic pancreatitis. *Gastroenterology.* 1999;116:1132-1140.
12. Chowdhury RS, Forsmark CE, Davis RH, et al. Prevalence of gastroparesis in patients with small duct chronic pancreatitis. *Pancreas.* 2003;26:235-238.
13. Apte MV, Keogh GW, Wilson JS. Chronic pancreatitis: complications and management. *J Clin Gastroenterol.* 1999;29:225-240.
14. DiMagno ER, Go VLW, Summerskil WHJ. Relationship between pancreatic enzyme outputs and malabsorption in severe pancreatic insufficiency. *N Engl J Med.* 1973;288:813-815.
15. Nakamura T, Tando Y, Yamada N, et al. Study on pancreatic insufficiency (chronic pancreatitis) and steatorrhea in Japanese patients with low fat intake. *Digestion.* 1999;60:93-96.
16. Twersky Y, Bank S. Nutritional deficiencies in chronic pancreatitis. *Gastroenterol Clin North Am.* 1989;18:543-565.
17. Layer P, Go VL, DiMagno EP. Fate of pancreatic enzymes during small intestinal aboral transit in humans. *Am J Physiol.* 1986;251: G475-G480 (abstract).
18. Petersoen JM, Forsmark CE. Chronic pancreatitis and maldigestion. *Semin Gastrointest Dis.* 2002;13:191-199.
19. Taubin HL, Spiro HM. Nutritional aspects of chronic pancreatitis. *Am J Clin Nutr.* 1973;26:367-373.
20. Mathew P, Wyllie F, Steffan RM, et al. Antioxidants in hereditary pancreatitis. *Am J Gastroenterol.* 1996;91:1558-1562.
21. Morris-Stiff GJ, Bowrey DJ, Oleesky D, et al. The antioxidant profiles of patients with acute and chronic pancreatitis. *Am J Gastroenterol.* 1999;94:2135-2140.
22. Haaber AB, Rosenfalck AM, Hansen B, et al. Bone mineral metabolism, bone mineral density, and body composition in patients with chronic pancreatitis and pancreatic exocrine insufficiency. *Int J Pancreatol.* 2000;27:21.
23. Dickerson RN, Vehe KL, Mullen JL, et al. Resting energy expenditure in patients with pancreatitis. *Crit Care Med.* 1991;19:484-490.
24. Hebuterne X, Hastier P, Peroux JL, et al. Resting energy expenditure in patients with alcoholic chronic pancreatitis. *Dig Dis Sci.* 1996;41:533-539.
25. Suter PM, Schutz Y, Jequier E. The effect of ethanol on fat storage in healthy subjects. *N Engl J Med.* 1992;326:983-987.
26. Bessey PQ, Watters JM, Aoki TT, Wilmore DW. Combined hormonal infusion stimulates the metabolic response to injury. *Ann Surg.* 1984;200:264-281.
27. Evans RD, Argiles JM, Williamson DH. Metabolic effects of tumor necrosis factor-alpha (cachectin) and interleukin-1. *Clin Sci.* 1989;37:357-364.
28. McCloy R. Chronic pancreatitis at Manchester, UK. Focus on antioxidant therapy. *Digestion.* 1998;59(suppl 4):36-48.
29. Gukovskaya AS, Gukovsky I, Zaninovic V, et al. Pancreatic acinar cells produce, release, and respond to tumor necrosis factor-alpha. Role in regulating cell death and pancreatitis. *J Clin Invest.* 1997;100:1853-1862.
30. Krueger KJ, Fortunato F, Cender CJ, et al. Cytokines in human pancreatic juice: different profiles for acute and chronic pancreatitis. *Gastroenterology.* 2000;118:A3689.
31. McKay CJ, Gallagher G, Brooks B, et al. Increased monocyte cytokine production in association with systemic complications in acute pancreatitis. *Br J Surg.* 1996;83:919-923.
32. Simovic MO, Bonham MJ, Abu-Zidan FM, et al. Anti-inflammatory cytokine response and clinical outcome in acute pancreatitis. *Crit Care Med.* 1999;27:2662-2665.
33. Holt S. Chronic pancreatitis. *South Med J.* 1993;86:201-207.
34. Latifi R, McIntosh JK, Dudrick SJ. Nutritonal management of acute and chronic pancreatitis. *Surg Clin North Am.* 1991;71:579-595.
35. Marks IN, Louw JH, Girdwood AH, et al. The prognosis of alcohol-induced calcified pancreatitis. *S Afr Med J.* 1980;57:640-643.
36. Trapnell JE. Chronic relapsing pancreatitis: a review of 64 cases. *Br J Surg.* 1979;66:471-475.
37. Owyang C. Negative feedback control of exocrine pancreatic secretion: role of cholecystokinin and cholinergic pathway. *J Nutr.* 1994;124:1321S-1326S.
38. Detsky AS, McLaughlin JR, Baker JP, et al. What is subjective global assessment of nutritional status? *J Parenter Enteral Nutr.* 1987;11:8-13.
39. Boivin M, Lanspa SJ, Zinsmeister AR, et al. Are diets associated with different rates of human interdigestive and postprandial pancreatic enzyme secretion? *Gastroenterology.* 1990;99:1763-1771.
40. Meier R. Nutrition in chronic pancreatitis. In: Buchler M, Friess H, Uhl W, eds. *Chronic Pancreatitis.* Berlin, Germany: Blackwell; 2002:421-427.
41. Symersky T, Vu MK, Frölich M, et al. The effect of equicaloric medium-chain and long-chain triglycerides on pancreas enzyme secretion. *Clin Physiol Funct Imaging.* 2002;22:307-311.
42. Shea JC, Bishop MD, Parker EM, et al. An enteral therapy containing medium-chain triglycerides and hydrolyzed peptides reduces post-prandial pain associated with chronic pancreatitis. *Pancreatology.* 2003;3:36-40.
43. Bivins BA, Bell RM, Rapp RP. Pancreatic exocrine response to parenteral nutrition. *JPEN J Parenter Enternal Nutr.* 1984;8:34-36.
44. Buch A, Buch J, Carlsen A, et al. Hyperlipidemia and pancreatitis. *World J Surg.* 1980;4:307-314.
45. Edelman K, Valenzuela JE. Effect of intravenous lipid on human pancreatic secretion. *Gastroenterology.* 1983;85:1063-1066.
46. Grant JP, James S, Grabowski V, et al. Total parenteral nutrition in pancreatic disease. *Ann Surg.* 1984;200:627-631.
47. Grundfest S, Steiger E, Selinkoff P, et al. The effect of intravenous fat emulsions in patients with pancreatic fistula. *JPEN J Parenter Enternal Nutr.* 1980;4:27-31.
48. Niederau G, Sonnenberg A, Erkhenbrecht J. Effects of intravenous infusion of amino acids, or glucose on unstimulated pancreatic secretion in healthy humans. *Dig Dis Sci.* 1995;90:446-55.

49. Silberman H, Dixon NP, Eisenberg D. The safety and efficacy of a lipid-based system of parenteral nutrition in acute pancreatitis. *Am J Gastroenterol.* 1982;77:494-497.
50. Stabile BE, Borzatta M, Stubbs RS, et al. Intravenous mixed amino acids and fats do not stimulate exocrine pancreatic secretion. *Am J Physiol.* 1984;246:G274-G280.
51. Havala T, Shronts E, Cerra F. Nutritional support in acute pancreatitis. *Gastroenterol Clin North Am* 1989;18:525-542.
52. Marulendra S, Kirby DF. Nutrition support in pancreatitis. *Nutr Clin Pract.* 1995;10:45-53.
53. Shahrudin MD, Noori SM. Pancreatic pseudocyst: the controversial value of total parenteral nutrition. *Hepatogastroenterology.* 1997;44:559-563.
54. Bodoky G, Harsanyi L, Pap A, et al. Effect of enteral nutrition on exocrine pancreatic function. *Am J Surg.* 1991;161:144-148.
55. Harsanyi L, Bodoky G, Pap A. The effect of jejunal nutrition on pancreatic exocrine function. *Acta Chir Hung.* 1992;33:13-21.
56. DiMagno EP, Gov L, Summerskill HJ. Intraluminal and postabsorptive effects of amino acids on pancreatic enzyme secretion. *J Lab Clin Med.* 1971;82:241-248.
57. Ertan A, Brooks FP, Ostrow, et al. Effect of jejunal amino acid perfusion and exogeneous cholecystokinin on the exocrine pancreatic and biliary secretions in man. *Gastroenterology.* 1971;61:686-692.
58. Vison N, Hecketsweiler P, Butel J, et al. Effect of continuous jejunal perfusion of elemental and complex nutritional solutions on pancreatic enzyme secretion in human subjects. *Gut.* 1978;19:194.
59. Hamvas J, Schwab R, Pap A. Jejunal feeding in chronic panj creatitis with severe necrosis. *Journal of the Pancreas.* 2001;2:112-116.
60. Gonzalez C, Silverman W. The impact of prolonged nasojejunal tube feeding in patients with refractory pancreatitis and abdominal pain: a five year retrospective review. *Gastroenterology.* 2003;124: A401.
61. DeWitt RC, Kudsk KA. The gut's role in metabolism, mucosal barrier function, and gut immunology. *Infect Dis Clin North Am.* 1999;13:465-481.
62. Ponsky JL, Aszodi A. Percutaneous endoscopic jejunostomy. *Am J Gastroenterol.* 1984;79:113-116.
63. Duckworth PF, Kirby DF, McHenry L, et al. Percutaneous endoscopic gastrojejunostomy made easy: a new over-the-wire technique. *Gastrointest Endosc.* 1994;40:350-353.
64. Fan AC, Baron TH, Rumalla A, Harewood GC. Comparison of direct percutaneous endoscopic jejunostomy and PEG with jejunal extension. *Gastrointest Endosc.* 2002;56:890-894.
65. Leichus LS, Patel R, Johlin F. Percutaneous endoscopic gastrostomy/jejunostomy (PEG/PEJ) tube placement, A novel approach. *Gastrointest Endosc.* 1997;96;45:79-81.
66. Wolfsen HC, Kozarek RA, Ball TJ, et al. Tube dysfunction following percutaneous endoscopic gastrostomy and jejunostomy. *Gastrointest Endosc.* 1990;36:261-263.
67. Mellert J, Naruhn MB, Grund KE, Becker HD. Direct endoscopic percutaneous jejunostomy (EPJ). *Surg Endosc.* 1994;8:867-869.
68. Rumalla A, Baron TH. Results of direct percutaneous endoscopic jejunostomy, an alternative method for providing jejunal feeding. *Mayo Clin Proc.* 2000;75:807-810.
69. Shike M, Latkany L, Gerdes H, Bloch AS. Direct percutaneous endoscopic jejunostomies for enteral feeding. *Gastrointest Endosc.* 1996;44:536-540.
70. Heijerman HG, Lamers CB, Bakker W. Omeprazole enhances the efficacy of pancreatin (pancrease) in cystic fibrosis. *Ann Intern Med.* 1991;114:200-201.
71. Regan PT, Malagelada JR, DiMagno EP, et al. Comparative effects of antacids, cimetidine, and enteric coating on the therapeutic response to oral enzymes in severe pancreatic insufficiency. *N Engl J Med.* 1977;297:854-858.
72. Raimondo M, DiMagno EP. Lipolytic activity of bacterial lipase survives better than that of porcine lipase in human gastric and duodenal content. *Gastroenterology.* 1994;107:231-235.
73. Suzuki A, Mizumoto A, Rerknimitr R, et al. Effect of bacterial or porcine lipase with low- and high-fat diets on nutrient absorption in pancreatic-insufficient dogs. *Gastroenterology.* 1999;116:431-437.
74. Suzuki A, Mizumoto A, Sarr MG, et al. Bacterial lipase and high-fat diets in canine exocrine pancreatic insufficiency: a new therapy of steatorrhea? *Gastroenterology.* 1997;112:2048-2055.
75. Forsmark CE. Chronic pancreatitis. In: Feldman M, Friedman LS, Sleisenger MH, eds. *Sleisenger and Fordtran's Gastrointestinal and Liver Disease: Pathophysiology/Diagnosis/Management.* 7th ed. Philadelphia, Pa: Saunders; 2002:943-969.
76. DiMagno EP, Malagelada JR, Go VL. Relationship between alcoholism and pancreatic insufficiency. *Ann NY Acad Sci.* 1975;252: 200-207.
77. Halgreen H, Pedersen NT, Worning H. Symptomatic effect of pancreatic enzyme therapy in patients with chronic pancreatitis. *Scand J Gastroenterol.* 1986;21:104-108.
78. Smyth RL, van Velzen D, Smyth AR, et al. Strictures of the ascending colon in cystic fibrosis and high-strength pancreatic enzymes. *Lancet.* 1994;343:85-86.
79. Trespi E, Ferrieri A. Intestinal bacterial overgrowth during chronic pancreatitis. *Curr Med Res Opin.* 1999;15:47-52.
80. Warshaw AL, Banks PA, Fernandez-Del Castillo C: AGA technical review: treatment of pain in chronic pancreatitis. *Gastroenterology.* 1998;115:765-776.
81. Isaksson G, Ihse I. Pain reduction by an oral pancreatic enzyme preparation in chronic pancreatitis. *Dig Dis Sci.* 1983;28:97-102.
82. Slaff J, Jacobson D, Tillman CR, et al. Protease-specific suppression of pancreatic exocrine secretion. *Gastroenterology.* 1984;87:44-52.
83. De Las Heras Castano G, Garcia de la Paz A, Fernandez MD, et al. Use of antioxidants to treat pain in chronic pancreatitis. *Rev Esp Enferm Dig.* 2000;92:375-385.
84. Uden S, Bilton D, Nathan L, et al. Antioxidant therapy for recurrent pancreatitis: placebo-controlled trial. *Aliment Pharmacol Ther.* 1990;4:357-371.
85. Whiteley G, Kienle A, Lee S, et al. Micronutrient antioxidant therapy in the non-surgical management of painful chronic pancreatitis: long term observations. *Pancreas.* 1994;9:A807.

Chapter 22

Nutritional Support In Acute Pancreatitis

Stephen J.D. O'Keefe, MD, MSc, FRCP

Background and Rationale

Pathophysiology of Acute Pancreatitis

It is essential to understand how acute pancreatitis occurs before attempts at nutritional support are conducted. Compelling evidence now exists that the root cause of acute pancreatitis is premature activation of trypsinogen within the acinar cell of the pancreas.[1] Normally, proteolytic enzymes, such as trypsinogen, are stored within the acinar cells in an inactive form as zymogens. Following stimulation of the pancreas by the consumption of food, the trypsinogen is released from the cell and travels via the duct system into the intestine (Figure 22-1). Only once within the lumen is the trypsinogen lyzed into active trypsin by enterokinase, another proteolytic enzyme released from the intestine.

Once free trypsin is formed, it then auto-activates further trypsinogen to trypsin. The trypsin then commences digestion of the ingested food and protein to form free amino acids suitable for absorption across the mucosal cells. The mucosa is protected from auto-digestion by the trypsin by a layer of mucous. In acute pancreatitis, this tightly orchestrated process is disrupted with premature activation of the trypsinogen to trypsin within the acinar cell. As there is little protection from the proteolytic effects of trypsin in the cytoplasm, auto-digestion of cell content commences.

Intracellular injury results in degeneration of a cascade of pro-inflammatory cytokines such as interleukin-(IL) lb, TNF-alpha, IL-17, IL-18 via activation of periacinar myofibrocytic NF kappa B and mitogen-activating protein kinase. This, in turn, stimulates the release of IL-6 and the cyto-attraction of neutrophils, which in turn leads to further cytokine generation. The intense inflammatory response results in the arterial constriction with resultant apoptosis and necrosis. If the inflammation were contained within the pancreatic bed, the disease process would be far less serious. Unfortunately, the cytokines are released into the circulation and, 48 hours later, a secondary response commences that leads to the generation of prostaglandin,[2] thromboxane, leukotriene B4, and oxygen-derived free radicals within the bronchial and intestinal mucosa. The result is cytotoxic injury.

The situation is compounded further by the release of proteolytic enzymes—such as trypsin, elastase, phospholipase, and caspase I—into the circulation, which leads to amplification of cell injury within the lung ('2nd hit') and gastrointestinal (GI) tract and resulting acute respiratory distress syndrome (ARDS), intestinal ischemia, bacterial translocation, and the well-recognized systemic inflammatory response syndrome (SIRS) (Figure 22-2). These complications account for the high mortality rates, which can approach 30% to 40% in severe necrotizing pancreatitis.

An understanding of these events will enable the practicing physician to understand how feedings should be given and what complications may be anticipated. For example, in the early stages, pancreatic stimulation should be avoided to minimize the synthesis of new proteolytic enzymes by the pancreas and thereby reduce the risk of exacerbation of the auto-digestion and inflammatory responses. Also, severe hypovolemia can result from the intense inflammatory response leading to hemoconcentration and reduced renal perfusion. The development of lung injury and ARDS could mislead the physician into believing that the patient was

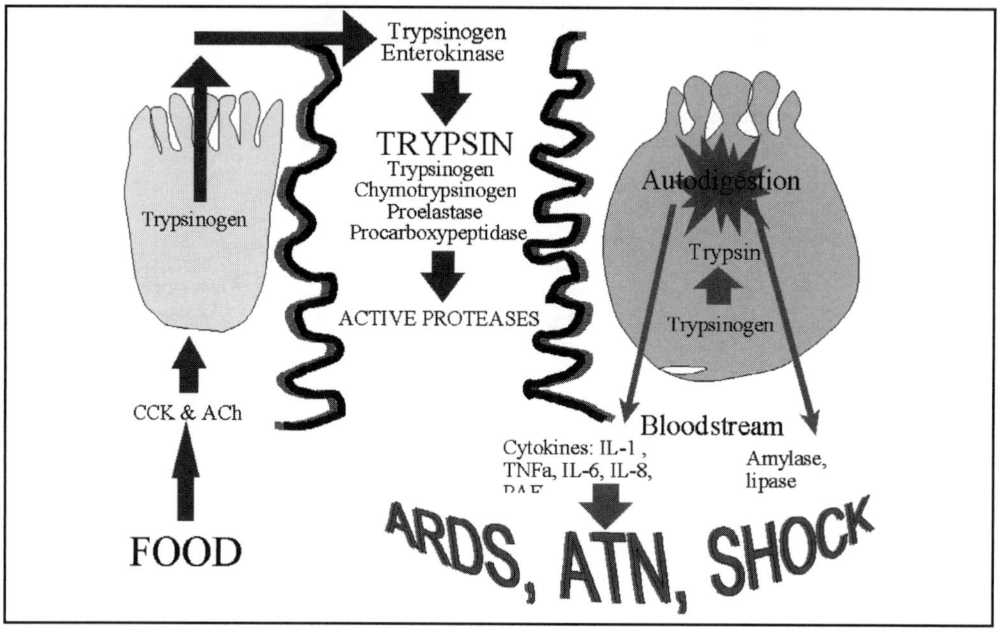

Figure 22-1. The pathophysiology of acute pancreatitis.

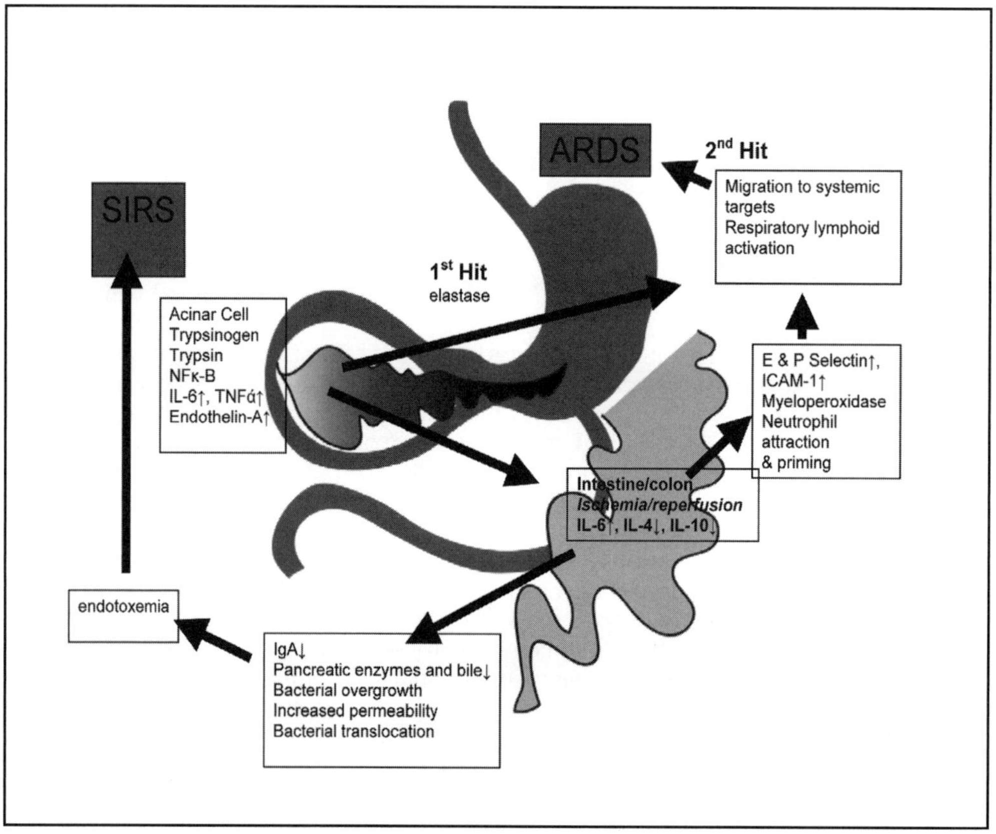

Figure 22-2. Generation of the systemic inflammatory response (SIRS) and acute respiratory distress syndrome (ARDS) by acute pancreatitis.

fluid overloaded. This would be extremely dangerous, as restriction of intravenous fluid resuscitation leads to renal failure and multiple organ failure, which is associated with high mortality rates. Consequently, patients who develop the systemic inflammatory response should be moved as soon as possible to the intensive care unit, where central venous pressures can be monitored and intravenous fluids are administered rigorously.

A further factor that influences the administration of nutritional support is the fact that acute pancreatitis affects not only the exocrine but also the endocrine pancreas, which results in impairment of insulin production. If this is taken in conjunction with the acute stress response that arises from acute inflammation and necrosis, counter-regulatory hormones will impair the function of what insulin is produced, making hyperglycemia inevitable during feeding. On this account, gram for gram, the infusion of glucose by vein produces a higher glycemic response than if it is given intravenously[2] (Figure 22-3).

Consequently, patients given total parenteral nutrition (TPN) are at an even greater risk of developing hyperglycemia than patients on enteral feeding. Furthermore, in

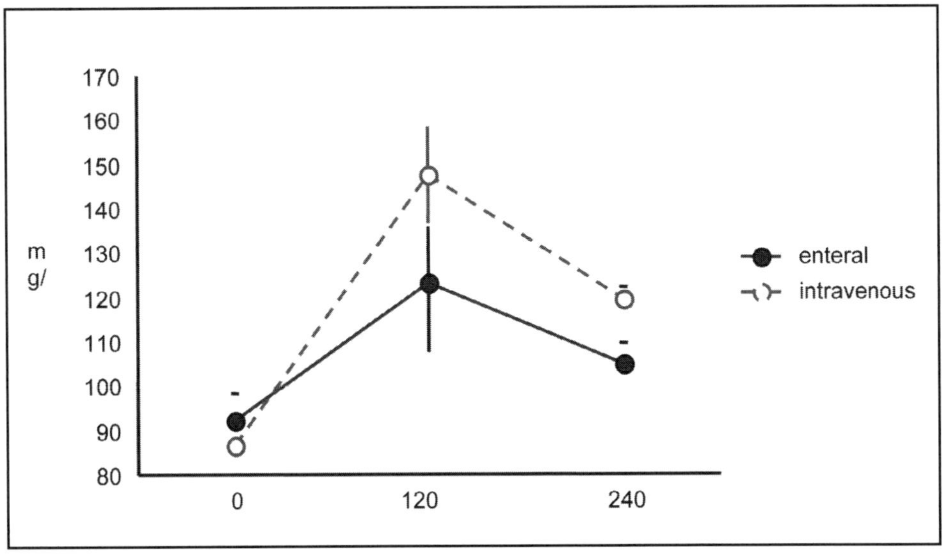

Figure 22-3. The relative glycemic response to glucose infused IV and enterally: the response is higher by IV route. Reprinted from O'Keefe SJD, Lee RB, Anderson FP, et al. The physiological effects of enteral and parenteral feeding on pancreatic enzyme secretion in humans. *Am J Physiol.* 2003;284:27-36.

clinical practice, a patient receives more of the prescribed nutrition given intravenously than in enteral form; this fact accounts for the almost universal finding of hyperglycemia in patients given intravenous feeding.[3]

Evaluation of Enteral and Parenteral Nutrition in the Management of Acute Pancreatitis

An appreciation of the pathobiological response to acute pancreatitis raises a number of concerns regarding the use of nutritional support. First, the rates of expenditure of energy and protein are increased[4] and, therefore, so are nutritional requirements. However, there is concern that providing these increased requirements might exacerbate the disease. The consumption of food can be expected to stimulate the pancreas and to exacerbate the auto-digestion and inflammatory response within the pancreas. Second, the inflammatory mass within the pancreas commonly compresses the duodenum, resulting in obstruction to the outflow from the stomach and subsequent nausea and vomiting[5] (Figure 22-4). The associated systemic inflammatory response might also lead to partial ileus. Together, these factors make enteral feeding difficult. Third, the metabolic tolerance of nutrients is reduced by pancreatic endocrine damage and relative hypoinsulinemia. Fourth, as intravenous feeding has a higher glycemic response than enteral feeding, the use of intravenous feeding almost certainly results in hyperglycemia unless intensive insulin therapy is used. Fifth, intestinal ischemia, ileus, and bowel rest results in hypomotility and bacterial overgrowth, which results in increased risk of infection and endotoxemia from enteric organisms. The systemic inflammatory response, insulin deficiency, and hyperglycemia result in immunoparesis, which increases the risk of bacterial infections and septicemia, particularly in patients with central lines.

Enteral Versus Parenteral

(Enteral nutrition is discussed in Chapters 34, 39, and 41 through 44. Parenteral nutrition is covered in Chapters 34 to 38 and 40.)

In every other critical illness, controlled studies of enteral versus parenteral feeding have demonstrated that early enteral feeding is preferable[6] and that TPN should only be used in patients with absolute obstruction. For many years, acute pancreatitis was considered different because of fears that enteral feeding would stimulate the pancreas. However, as predicted above, it was soon realized that the complications associated with TPN outweighed the potential benefits of maintaining nutrition.

In an early study by Sax and colleagues on 54 patients with relatively mild disease, a controlled study was performed between TPN and simple intravenous fluids.[7] Interestingly, those participants given TPN fared worse: the length of stay was an average of 16 days as compared to only 10 days in those given no nutrition. Secondly, catheter sepsis was significantly higher, with 11 patients in the TPN group and only two in the non-nutritional group developing septicemia. The average Ranson's criteria in this study was only 1, and it is doubtful if any of these patients really needed nutritional support, as patients with mild pancreatitis usually settle after 48 hours of bowel rest and intravenous fluids. This study illustrates that TPN should only be used in those patients who are nutritionally depleted and, therefore, can be expected to accrue some benefit from nutritional support; otherwise, only complications arise.

The results of Sax et al's studies led to the search for alternative methods of nutritional support. McClave and

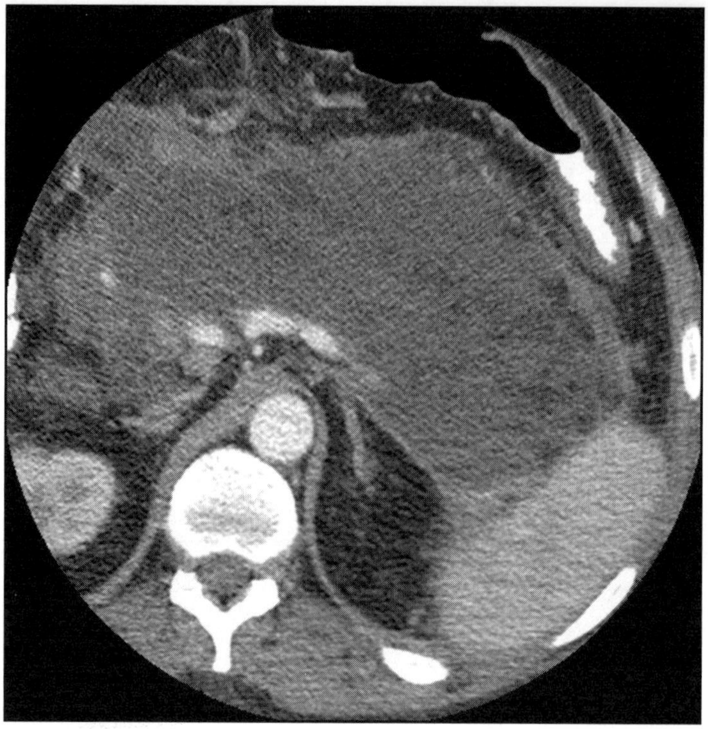

Figure 22-4. Patient with necrotizing pancreatitis with the liquefied mass compressing the stomach resulting in gastric outlet obstruction and vomiting. (Photo kindly provided by Dr. John Martin, Division of Gastroenterology, Feinberg School of Medicine, Northwestern University, Chicago, IL.)

colleagues were one of the first to perform a randomized control trial of enteral versus parenteral feeding in acute pancreatitis.[8] In an attempt to minimize pancreatic stimulation, they used jejunal feeding with an elemental diet, in comparison to parenteral nutrition after 48 hours of observation. Unfortunately, their trial was not analyzed on an intention-to-treat basis; nonetheless, they found that stress-related hyperglycemia was more common in those randomized to TPN, and the cost of enteral feeding was considerably cheaper. Importantly, they excluded eight patients for tube-feeding failure, patients who should have been included to illustrate the practical value of tube feeding. Another criticism of the study is that the investigators included a majority of patients who had mild disease (average Ranson's criteria 1.3, range 0 to 5) and, again, many of their patients did not need nutritional support. However, it was a landmark study in demonstrating that some patients with severe disease could be fed by enteral route.

This author performed a randomized controlled trial of enteral versus parenteral feeding.[3] Over 200 patients with acute pancreatitis were screened over an 18-month period. All were initially treated with 48 hours of simple intravenous fluids, bowel rest, and analgesics. They were then re-evaluated. Those who had become progressively worse were randomized to enteral or parenteral feeding. Twenty-six received jejunal feeding with an elemental diet, and the other 27 received TPN and bowel rest. It is important to note that 75% of the patients improved without nutritional support and were discharged within 5 days.

In general terms, patients given enteral feeding fared considerably better. The average duration of feeding in the enteral group was significantly lower (6.7 versus 10.8 days, $P < .05$), and length of stay in the hospital was shorter. Considered with the fact that enteral diets are cheaper, this resulted in considerable cost savings: the use of enteral feeding in comparison to TPN saved $2362 per patient fed. Complications were again more common in those given TPN, with significantly more patients developing hyperglycemia requiring insulin (14 versus 4, $P = 0.03$) and catheter-associated septicemia (9 versus 1, $P < .01$). Median blood glucose concentrations were also significantly higher during feeding in TPN patients, at 180 mg/dL versus 139 mg/dL ($P < .05$). A novel finding was that the tolerance to restarting oral feeding was considerably better in those given enteral feeding, presumably because of maintained GI function. Tube intolerance was rare: only one patient could not tolerate tube feeding. Another interesting observation was that the lower rates of hyperglycemia might have been explained in part by the lower quantities of nutrition received by those randomized to enteral feeding. Average protein and caloric intakes were less than 50% of estimated requirement levels in those given enteral feeding, whereas those given parenteral feeding received approximately 85% of estimated requirements ($P < .005$). This pattern has been observed by others worldwide and can be explained by logistical problems with enteral feeding. In practice, it is much easier to turn up intravenous infusion rates than it is to maintain enteral infusion rates. Feeding pumps are frequently turned off during transportation, investigations, and procedures.

A further controlled trial between enteral and parenteral feeding was reported by Windsor and colleagues.[9] This was a small study including only 34 patients, 16 randomized to enteral and 18 to parenteral feeding. The study protocol was also complex, with only six of the patients receiving jejunal feeding; the remaining 28 received oral feeding. Regardless of size, the study corresponded with those of other studies. Their study focused on the effect of feeding on the inflammatory response. They noticed that endotoxin antibodies increased during the TPN feed-

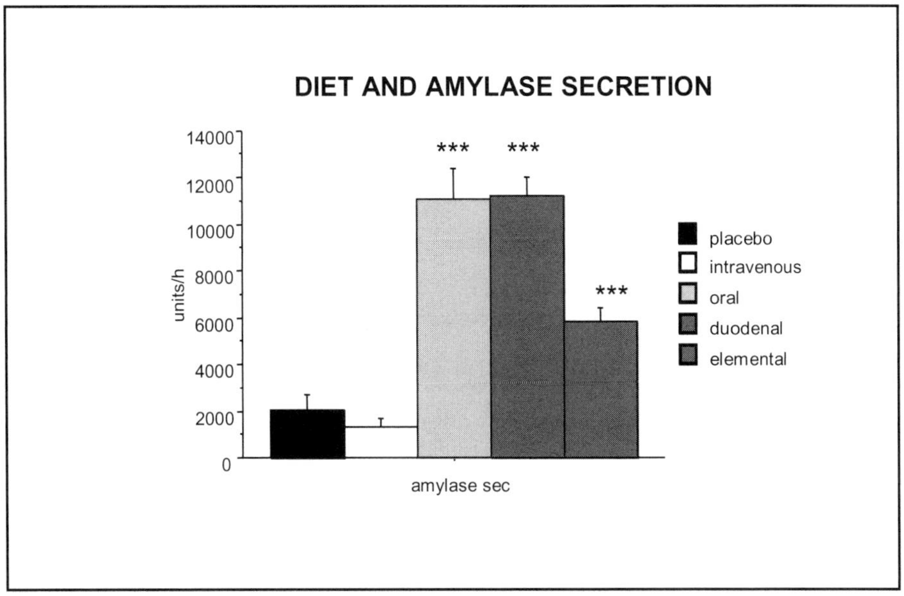

Figure 22-5. Relative stimulatory effects of various forms of conventional feeding techniques on pancreatic secretion in healthy volunteers. Reprinted from O'Keefe SJD, Lee RB, Anderson FP, et al. The physiological effects of enteral and parenteral feeding on pancreatic enzyme secretion in humans. *Am J Physiol.* 2003;284:27-36.

ing but not with enteral; that multiple organ failure was only observed in patients given parenteral feeding (five patients); that intra-abdominal sepsis was again only seen in patients receiving TPN (three patients); and that none of the patients given enteral feeding needed intensive care unit management. Consistent with these findings was their observation that markers of the inflammatory response—C-reactive protein (CRP) and APACHE 11 scores—decreased only in those patients given enteral feeding.

Since this study was reported, a number of others have investigated the role of enteral feeding in suppressing the systemic inflammatory response. An interesting controlled study in healthy volunteers reported by Fong et al tested the response to intravenous endotoxin injection in healthy volunteers after 7 days of either enteral feeding or parenteral feeding.[10] The reaction was significantly higher in those given parenteral feeding. For example, they found that TNF-α levels and CRP responses were higher in those given TPN, that the epinephrine levels were higher, and that protein catabolism was accelerated in the TPN group but not in the enteral group.

Finally, there was concern that, although enteral feeding might be a safe alternative in patients with mild pancreatitis, it might still be contraindicated in those with severe or necrotizing disease. Consequently, the results of the randomized, comparative study reported by Kalfarentzos et al in 40 patients with necrotizing pancreatitis were of great interest.[11] It should be noted that necrotizing pancreatitis is a rare disease and it took them 5 years to accrue 40 patients. However, their overall finding was that, although nitrogen balance could be achieved by enteral or parenteral feeding, septic (10 versus 5, $P < .01$) and total (15 versus 8, $P < .05$) complications were significantly higher in those given TPN. Furthermore, the cost was three times higher in the TPN group. They were unable to document any exacerbation of the acute pancreatitis during enteral feeding.

Why Enteral Feeding Is Better Than TPN for Patients With Pancreatitis

Enteral feeding is better than TPN. The explanation may involve the beneficial effects of enteral feeding or the adverse effects of parenteral feeding. It is extremely important to note that to date no controlled trial has been performed between enteral feeding and no nutrition; therefore, it is not proven that enteral feeding does not exacerbate pancreatitis. This author's concern is that physiological studies in healthy volunteers demonstrated that enteral feeding, as it is normally performed in clinical practice and in the studies quoted above (ie, jejunal elemental feeding), continues to stimulate the pancreas and only parenteral feeding avoids pancreatic stimulation.[2] Although the use of an elemental formulation reduces the secretory response by 50%, the response is still 70% above the unstimulated state (Figure 22-5).

It, therefore, remains possible that enteral feeding may, in certain subjects, perpetuate the disease activity. Although intolerance has rarely been described, it is difficult to detect in someone who is already critically ill with a systemic inflammatory response. This author and others,[8] however, have noticed an exacerbation of symptoms in some patients. A recent case report demonstrated that the commencement of enteral feeding in necrotizing pancreatitis was associated with an increase in pancreatic secretion and at the same time a worsening of symptoms and signs on computed tomography scanning (CT scan)[5] (Figure 22-6). Following withdrawal of enteral feeding and implementation of TPN, patient symptoms promptly resolved with a decrease in white cell count from 35,000 to 9000 within 3 days. This has led to this physician's use of distal jejunal feeding, as physiological studies in volunteers[12,13] demonstrate that, if the feeding tube is placed 60

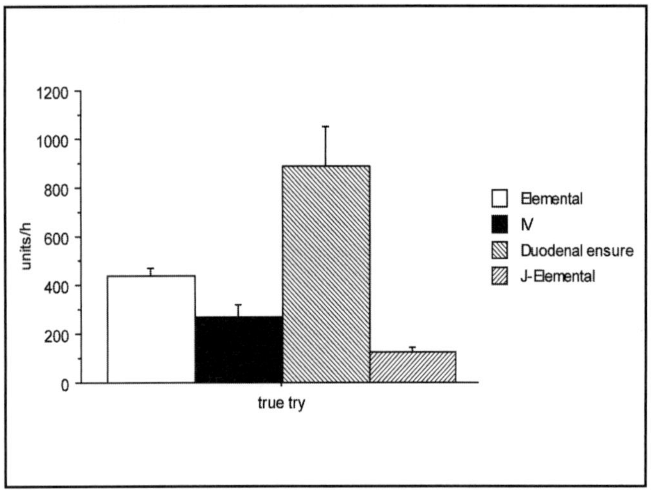

Figure 22-6. (Group mean[SE]) shows that pancreatic enzyme secretion rate was significantly lower in the group that received distal jejunal elemental feeding (J-Elemental group) compared with proximal jejunal elemental feeding (Elemental group) ($p<0.05$).

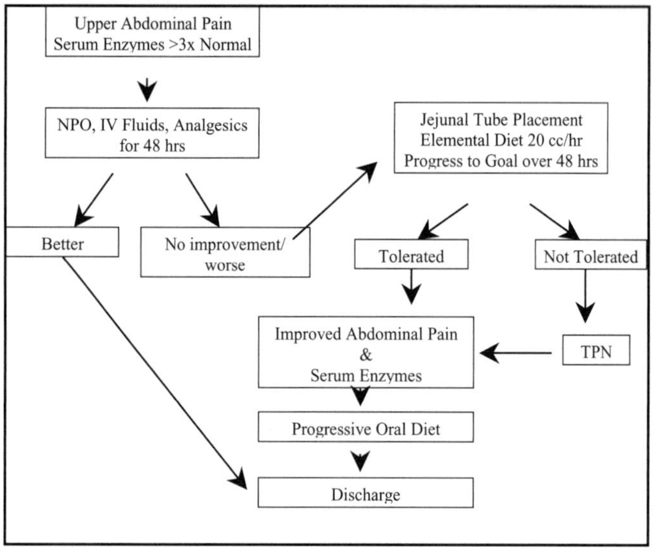

Figure 22-7. Practical management algorithm.

to 80 cm beyond the ligament of Trietz, the stimulation of the pancreas is negligible. In this way, patients receive the benefits of enteral feeding and avoid the risks of septic and metabolic complications associated with TPN.

The provision of minimally stimulatory enteral feeding can arrest many of the pathways that lead to SIRS and ARDS, as illustrated in Figure 22-2. Reduced pancreatic stimulation will reduce trypsin activation within the acinar cells and therefore the initiating event in the inflammatory cascade. Reduced systemic elastase will remove the 'first hit' on the lungs. The infusion of enteral nutrients stimulates nitric oxide production and counteracts endothelin-1 and 2,[12] thereby preventing intestinal ischemia[14] and necrosis.[15] Enteral nutrients maintain CD4:CD8 balance, innate immunity, and secretory IgA production, thus suppressing neutrophil activation and inflammatory cytokine production.[16] This prevents lymphocyte priming and respiratory lymphoid activation, or the "2nd hit", thus preventing ARDS. The combination of nutrient-stimulated mucosal blood flow, motility, and secretion of bile acids prevent bacterial overgrowth and prevent endotoxemia and bacterial translocation, thereby attenuating the SIRS. The importance of maintaining the stability of the gut flora was evidenced by a recent controlled clinical trial that demonstrated that outcome from acute pancreatitis was improved when a prebiotic (wheat bran) and a probiotic (lactobacillus) (= synbiotic) were added to enteral feed.[17] (Prebiotics and Probiotics are discussed in Chapter 11.) Finally, physiological studies demonstrate a massive increase in the splanchnic flux of amino acids during acute pancreatitis and compartmentation between the splanchnic and systemic circulations, such that enteral feeding would be far better positioned than would parenteral feeding to provide substrate for the increased metabolic needs.[18]

Practical Management

Based on the above rationale, suggested management is outlined in the algorithm (Figure 22-7) and explained below.

First, on admission, monitor the patient's serial serum lipase concentrations, blood glucose, and liver-function tests. Second, insert a peripheral line and feed the patient only with intravenous fluids for 48 hours. Provide analgesics as necessary. After 48 hours, review progress. Patients with worsening symptoms of abdominal pain and complications such as renal failure or respiratory distress should receive a contrast enhanced CT scan.

The next step is to insert a nasojejunal feeding tube. In patients with nausea and vomiting amd with evidence of gastric outlet obstruction, use a double lumen gastric-decompression jejunal-feeding tube system (eg, Kendal Sherwood Tyco). The best way to place these tubes is by transnasal endoscopy allowing intubation of the compressed jejunal loop and deployment of a guide wire beyond the ligament of Trietz.[19] The transnasal endoscope is then withdrawn leaving the guidewire in position, which allows passage of the feeding tube over the guide wire. Final position is checked by repeat endoscopy or fluoroscopy; the tip of the feeding tube should be as far down the jejunum as possible (preferably 40 cm distal to the ligament of Treitz). It is imperative to avoid coils of guidewire within the stomach before the tube is placed in position; otherwise, the tube may simply recoil back into the stomach. Commence gastric decompression at low negative pressure (50 mm of mercury) and jejunal feeding at 20 cc/hour for 24 hours. Then, advance feeding rates by 10 to 20 cc/hour over the next 3 days towards a caloric infusion rate of approximately 20 kcal/kg/day, based on the patient's ideal body weight. It is imperative to control hyperglycemia during the advance of tube feeding to decrease the risk of infective complications (20). Intolerance to this form of tube feeding should lead to the use of TPN but again, intensive insulin cover will be required to maintain blood sugar levels below 110 mg/dL. It is also extremely important to avoid overfeeding.

Following resolution of symptoms (ie, abdominal pain, general well being), attempts at reintroducing oral feeding should be commenced. It is important to maintain the jejunal feeding until a trial of oral liquids has been successful. Patients will then be advanced to a low fat (20 g/day) diet and finally discharged home on a normal balanced diet. Remarkably, few patients, even those following necrotizing pancreatitis, require pancreatic enzyme supplements, but some may. It is always important to check for stool function following the reintroduction of normal feeding.

References

1. Steer ML. The early intracellular cell events which occurred during acute pancreatitis. *Pancreas.* 1988;17(1):31-37.
2. O'Keefe SJD, Lee RB, Anderson FP, et al. The physiological effects of enteral and parenteral feeding on pancreatic enzyme secretion in humans. *Am J Physiol.* 2003;284:27-36.
3. Abou-Assi S, Craig K, O'Keefe SJD. Hypocaloric jejunal feeding is better than total parenteral nutrition in acute pancreatitis: results of a randomized comparative study. *Am J Gastroenterol.* 2002;97(9):2255-2262.
4. Abou-Assi SA, O'Keefe SJD. Nutrition in acute pancreatitis. *J Clin Gastroenterol.* 2001;32(3):203-209.
5. O'Keefe SJD, Broderick T, Turner M, Stevens S, O'Keefe JS. Nutrition in the management of necrotizing pancreatitis. *Clin Gastroenterol Hepatol.* 2003;1:315-321.
6. Kudsk KA, Croce MA, Fabian TC, et al. Enteral versus parenteral feeding. *Ann Surg.* 1992;215(5):503-513.
7. Sax HC, Warner BW, Talamini MA, et al. Early total parenteral nutrition in acute pancreatitis: lack of beneficial effects. *Am J Surg.* 1987;153:117-124.
8. McClave SA, Greene LM, Snider HL, et al. Comparison of the safety of early enteral versus parenteral nutrition in mild acute pancreatitis. *JPEN J Parenter Enteral Nutr.* 1997;21:14-20.
9. Windsor AC, Kanwar S, Li AG, et al. Compared with parenteral nutrition, enteral feeding attenuates the acute phase response and improves disease severity in acute pancreatitis. *Gut.* 1998;42:431-435.
10. Fong YM, Marano MA, Barber A, et al. Total parenteral nutrition and bowel rest modify the metabolic response to endotoxin in humans. *Ann Surg.* 1989;210:449-456.
11. Kalfarentzos F, Kehagias J, Mead N, et al. Enteral nutrition is superior to parenteral nutrition in severe acute pancreatitis: results of a randomized prospective trial. *Br J Surg.* 1997;84:1665-1669.
12. Kaushik N, Pietraszewski M, Zhou W, Ng B, O'Keefe SJD. Elemental feeding into the distal jejunum but not the proximal jejunum avoids pancreatic stimulation. *DDW.* 2004.
13. Vu MK, Van Der Veek P, Frolich M, et al. Does jejunal feeding activate exocrine pancreatic secretion? *Eur J Clin Invest.* 1999;29(12):1053-1059.
14. Plusczyk T, Witzel B, Menger MD, Schilling M. ETA and ETB receptor function in pancreatitis-associated microciculatory failure, inflammation and parenchymal injury. *Am J Physiol.* 2003;285: G145-G153.
15. Hirota M, Inoue K, Kimura Y, et al. Non-occlusive mesenteric ischemia and its associated intestinal gangrene in acute pancreatitis. *Pancreatology.* 2003;3(4):316-322.
16. Kudsk KA. Effect of route and type of nutrition on intestine-derived inflammatory responses. *Am J Surg.* 2003;185(1):16-21.
17. Olah A, Belagyi T, Issekutz A, Gamal ME, Bengmark S. Randomized clinical trial of specific lactobacillus and fibre supplement to early enteral nutrition in patients with acute pancreatitis. *Br J Surg.* 2002;89:1103-1107.
18. O'Keefe SJD, Lee RB, Clore J. Enteral feeding during acute pancreatitis is associated with preserved trypsin synthesis and increased splanchnic protein metabolism. *Gastroenterology.* 2004;126(4): 696.
19. O'Keefe SJD, Foody W, Gill S. Transnasal endoscopic placement of feeding tubes in the intensive care unit. *JPEN J Parenter Enteral Nutr.* 2003;27(5):349-354.
20. Van den Berghe G, Wouters P, Weekers F, et al. Intensive insulin therapy in critically ill patients. *N Engl J Med.* 2001;345:1359-1367.

Chapter 23

NUTRITION AND GASTROINTESTINAL MOTILITY IN HEALTH AND DISEASE

Gregg W. Van Citters, PhD, and
Henry C. Lin, MD

Introduction

Digestion and absorption are time-demanding events. To achieve optimal nutrition, the movement of the meal through the gastrointestinal (GI) tract is controlled by nutrient-triggered inhibitory feedback that slows gastric emptying and intestinal transit. This chapter focuses on the physiology of the control of the transit of a meal through the gut and the information needed for nutritional management when such controls are impaired. Each section begins with a review of the normal controls that govern meal transit through each section of the gut and then provides an example of disordered motility to discuss nutritional management strategies.

In reading each section, the reader must consider a few important issues. First, symptoms arising from dysmotility may result from transit that is either too fast or too slow, and often the presenting complaints are similar. It is important to understand whether transit is too fast or too slow because inappropriate treatment will exacerbate the problem. For example, giving a prokinetic agent to a patient complaining of postprandial bloating and early satiety would be inappropriate if the patient was experiencing these symptoms from rapid transit. Second, the most critical step is identifying and treating the reversible component of the abnormality. For example, a diabetic patient may have reversible delayed gastric emptying associated with hyperglycemia (Chapter 16).

Although GI transit normally serves to facilitate nutrition, in disease states, problems moving food to the right place may serve as barriers to adequate nutrition. The first potential barrier is getting food through the pharynx and esophagus into the stomach, which is exemplified by the dysphagic patient. The second potential barrier is getting the gastric content expelled into the intestine in an orderly fashion, which is exemplified by the patient with delayed gastric emptying. The third potential barrier is retaining food in the small intestine long enough to properly assimilate the nutrients, which is exemplified by the patient with rapid intestinal transit. The final potential barrier is getting the available nutrients across the absorptive mucosa, which is exemplified by the patient with small intestinal bacterial overgrowth (SIBO).

Nutrient assimilation consists of the time-demanding events of digestion and absorption. When there is not adequate time for digestion and absorption, nutrients appear in the waste stream rather than the bloodstream. Transit of a meal is therefore meticulously controlled to ensure adequate time for nutrient assimilation. The GI tract is equipped with nutrient sensors along its entire length. These sensors respond to type and quantity of nutrients to generate the neuropeptidergic feedback signals that slow transit in order to optimize nutrient digestion and absorption. Rapid movement of a meal through the GI tract limits contact time with digestive enzymes and reduces hydrolytic capacity to result in maldigestion. Similarly, rapid movement of a meal impairs nutrient transport to result in malabsorption. Malabsorption can then occur in the setting of rapid transit even when the meal is well-digested[1] and the absorptive surface is entirely normal. (Maldigestion and malabsorption are discussed in Chapter 5.) To illustrate the importance of adequate time for assimilation, the chapter will "follow" a bolus of food through the GI tract and assess the impact of nutrient-triggered inhibitory feedback on transit of the bolus.

Mouth and Esophagus

Although the thought or act of chewing food stimulates release of salivary enzymes, a meal bolus is seldom retained in the oral cavity long enough for extensive hydrolysis of nutrients to occur. The oropharynx and larynx work together to propel the bolus out of the mouth into the esophagus without compromising the airway. Once in the esophagus, deglutition triggers the primary esophageal peristalsis that moves the bolus aborally to the stomach. The bolus is also not retained in the esophagus long enough for substantial nutrient hydrolysis to occur.

Dysphagias

Difficulty swallowing (dysphagia) occurs at the rate of 6% to 22% in the general population, reaching a 60% prevalence in nursing homes.[2] Food must move from the mouth through the pharynx and esophagus to begin digestion in the stomach. This process can be disrupted by a mechanical obstruction (eg, stricture) or by a neuromuscular dysfunction (eg, stroke). Oropharyngeal or transfer dysphagia describes difficulty moving a bolus from the mouth into the esophagus, as in the stroke patient. Esophageal dysphagia describes difficulty moving a bolus through the esophagus, as in the scleroderma patient or the patient with a lumen-obstructing esophageal tumor or stricture. Thus, it is important to determine whether the patient's dysphagia is transfer or esophageal in type, and if the cause is a mechanical or neuromuscular (motility) problem.

A history of drooling, coughing, or choking while swallowing, or nasal regurgitation, would suggest transfer dysphagia. A history of substernal discomfort after swallowing, food getting stuck after the bolus clears the mouth, or delayed regurgitation would suggest esophageal dysphagia. For esophageal dysphagia, whether anatomic or neuromuscular in nature, symptoms are typically worse with solids. However, because gravity assists movement of liquids, symptoms resulting from a mechanical cause of dysphagia may be especially noticeable with solids. With further narrowing of the lumen by an obstruction, the dysphagia may progressively worsen to involve both liquids and solids. However, a neuromuscular or motility dysfunction is classically associated with dysphagia to both solids and liquids right from the start. In contrast to the "every meal" timing of mechanical obstruction, the timing of a dysmotility-related dysphagia may be a episodic.[2]

Imaging studies help pinpoint the underlying cause. A video swallowing study coupled with a barium esophagram will detect dysphagia occurring on both short (oropharyngeal) and long (esophageal) time scales. Radiological imaging studies (ie, computed tomography [CT], magnetic resonance imaging [MRI]) are helpful in detecting stroke and tumors, particularly in the oropharynx.[2] Further confirmation with endoscopy and biopsy may often be required. If mechanical causes have been ruled out, esophageal manometry studies may reveal the site and nature of the motility dysfunction, permitting the diagnosis of such conditions as achalasia, diffuse esophageal spasm, and esophageal hypomotility. The abnormality accounting for the dysphagia may only be elicited with swallowing of solids rather than the standard water bolus. In the case of obstructive dysphagia, the patient must be nutritionally supported until therapy succeeds in removing or palliating the lesion. Nasogastric feeding may be needed early in the course of obstructive dysphagia. If long-term nutritional support is required, a percutaneous endoscopic gastrostomy (PEG) tube may be needed. In the case of esophageal dysmotility, efforts are directed at correction of the abnormality, eg, surgical and nonsurgical treatment of achalasia.

Oropharyngeal (Transfer) Dysphagia Secondary to Stroke

Stroke patients typically have impairment of the pharyngeal muscles on the side opposite that of the brain hemisphere in which the stroke occurred. Diagnosis typically involves performing a video swallowing study with barium esophagram.[2,3] The radiologist should evaluate the risk of airway penetration using a variety of liquids and solids. Once the impairment is understood, a swallow therapist will often work with the patient on compensatory swallowing techniques.[2] In addition, the physical form of the diet can be altered to facilitate swallowing. Switching from flat to carbonated liquids may help some patients. Thickened liquids may be used to avoid aspiration if airway penetration is reduced with a more viscous liquid.

Esophageal Dysphagia Secondary to Scleroderma

Systemic scleroderma is associated with progressive impairment of the motor function of the entire GI tract.[4,5] Dysphagia secondary to esophageal dysmotility is a hallmark of this condition. Hypomotility of the esophagus leading to impaired bolus propulsion is a characteristic finding of esophageal manometry. Prokinetics may be useful early on[6] but will not work in advanced stages of the disease when the smooth muscles responsible for esophageal peristalsis are gradually replaced with sclerodermatous collagen. Switching from regular meals to liquid enteral formulas (Chapter 42) may help, with PEG tube placement for long-term therapy as the disease progresses (Chapter 41).

Gastroesophageal Reflux Disease

Gastroesophageal reflux disease (GERD) is one of the most common albeit under-reported medical complaints.[7] Nutrient-triggered changes in esophageal and lower esophageal sphincter (LES) motility are important determinants of reflux of the gastric content into the esophagus. LES pressure is decreased by fat in the proximal intestine[8,9] and by the by-products of colonic fermentation of nondigestible carbohydrates,[10,11] while proteins[9,12,13] and to a lesser extent carbohydrates[9] increase LES tone. Accordingly, a fatty meal often precipitates an episode of symptomatic acid reflux. When the Bernstein (esophageal acid infusion) test was performed in GERD patients, acid sensitivity was increased by concurrent perfusion of the duodenum with a fat emulsion at the rate of 8 g/hour.[14] This may be explained in part by intestino-esophageal feedback generated by fat that contributes to acidic reflux, both directly by relaxing the LES[8] and indirectly by lowering the sensory threshold to acid. While these physiologic responses to nutrients are commonly experienced, when symptoms become more than occasional, the physician must work with the patient to find an acceptable combination of dietary modifications and/or antisecretory agents (eg, omeprazole) to manage the GERD. Among the dietary components that are known to reduce LES pressure, fatty foods, chocolate, caffeine, ethanol, and carminatives (mints) are commonly avoided by the patient with GERD[15].

Stomach

Although intragastric digestion optimizes nutrition by preparing chyme for digestion and absorption in the small intestine, this step is equally important in making available the end products of nutrient digestion that are required to activate control of transit through the GI tract. By liberating these end products—mono- and oligo-saccharides, oligo-peptides and amino acids, and fatty acids—early in the postprandial period, intestino-gastric inhibitory feedback would be activated in time to slow the movement of a meal out of the stomach and ensure adequate time for digestion and absorption.

Physical Fragmentation, Gastric Sieving, and Peristalsis

Efficient digestion of food particles by hydrolytic enzymes requires a large surface area-to-mass ratio. Physical fragmentation (trituration) of the bolus begins with chewing and is completed in the stomach as gastric motility converts from the fasted to fed state in response to meal stimuli including cholinergic neural input and peptides such as gastrin.[16] The stimulated stomach generates contractions that produce a ring-like peristaltic wave that moves the bolus toward the pylorus. As the lumen-obliterating contractions of the terminal antrum encounter the closure of the pylorus, solids are fragmented to small particles to increase the surface area available for digestion.[17]

As the peristaltic wave moves toward the pylorus, gastric fluid and solids suspended in the fluid acquire forward velocity and behave like a laminar flow, with fluid and the smallest particles concentrated in the center of the flow and moving most rapidly. With the pyloric opening positioned to receive the center of the flow, only the smallest solid particles and liquids are ejected from the stomach, while the larger chunks of solids are retained and fall to the side for further fragmentation by the next set of antral contractions. This size selection property of the fed motility state, known as gastric sieving, prevents digestible solids larger than approximately 0.1 mm from entering the small intestine.[18,19] The time required to fragment solids down to this small size accounts for the lag phase of the gastric emptying time course for digestible solids. In contrast, the liquid component of a meal empties rapidly and linearly because liquids need not be fragmented before expulsion from the stomach.

Chemical Hydrolysis

Release of end products of nutrient digestion in the stomach is critically important for proper regulation of gastric emptying. Gastric proteolytic zymogens are secreted in response to feeding and activated by the acidic environment of the stomach.[20] Up to 20% of total protein digestion occurs in the stomach but is reduced by the use of antisecretory agents that diminish both acid and pepsin secretion from the stomach. More time would then be needed to fragment digestible solids; therefore, the lag phase of gastric emptying may be prolonged, often leading to the incorrect diagnosis of gastroparesis. Because gastric emptying may lengthen beyond the normal range, salivary amylase contained in the food bolus retains activity in the stomach and can account for up to 60% of starch hydrolysis by the time the bolus exits the stomach.[21,22] Gastric lipase, secreted by the fundus in response to feeding, is responsible for up to 30% of total triglyceride hydrolysis.[23,24] Gastric lipolysis in conjunction with physiological duodeno-gastric bile reflux[25] enhances emulsification of the fatty contents of the meal[26] to provide micellar substrate for pancreatic lipase.[27-29] Most importantly, gastric lipolysis provides the fatty acids that serve as the trigger of the inhibitory feedback that tightly controls gastric emptying. Early availability of some end products of lipid digestion in the intestinal lumen inhibits gastric emptying to regulate the movement of the meal through the remainder of the GI tract. The processes of chemical hydrolysis of chyme are more thoroughly discussed in Chapter 8 in this book.

Gastric Emptying

A volume of liquid devoid of nutrient empties rapidly at first then slows to approximate an exponential decay[30] because the rate of gastric emptying of such liquid depends on its volume in the stomach (ie, first order kinetics of emptying). In contrast, a solid meal empties from the stomach in two phases: lag and linear. During the lag phase, larger food particles are triturated into smaller particles to increase surface area available for digestion. Gastric sieving is the property of the stomach for size selection. Under gastric sieving, only fine particles and liquids (chyme) are allowed to exit the stomach during the initial linear phase. Because the emptying of solids is rate-limited by the time-demanding step of trituration, the amount emptied from the stomach per unit time is fixed and independent of the volume of food in the stomach (ie, zero order kinetics of emptying). Even with gastric sieving, assimilation of particles of solids is time demanding. Accordingly, the gut optimizes digestion and absorption by limiting the delivery rate of chyme into the small intestine to prevent the capacity of the small intestine from being overwhelmed.

Nutrient- and Load-Dependence of Gastric Emptying

Gastric emptying is controlled by the physical and chemical natures of the meal, including its physical phase, osmolarity, acidity, type of nutrient, and nutrient load.[31-35] Increased lumenal osmolarity, such as that seen in the setting of maldigestion and malabsorption[36] (Chapter 5), stimulates nonpropagative duodenal motility to increase outflow resistance and delay gastric emptying.[37] This is an example of how feedback inhibition of gastric emptying can be generated without altering gastric motility.

The response of the GI tract to nutrients depends on the load (amount) of nutrients presented to the intestine.[38] As the amount of nutrients increase, a longer length of the intestine must participate in absorption. As a result, the higher nutrient load generates greater inhibitory feedback as more nutrient sensors are stimulated. Just as the rate of gastric emptying decreases as the nutrient load increases to extend time for assimilation,[39,40] other digestive functions such as pancreatic exocrine secretion increase in response to increasing nutrient load in order to optimize digestion of the meal. These feedback responses depend on nutrient saturation of absorptive mucosal surface recruitment of a greater number of nutrient sensors along a longer length of gut and the spilling of nutrients to more distal portions of the intestine.[41,42]

The magnitude of inhibition of gastric emptying also depends on the type of nutrient. For example, exposure of nutrient sensors in the small intestine to 1000 mM glucose maximally inhibits gastric emptying,[38] but only 27 mM oleate is needed to achieve the same effect.[43] Because assimilation of fat is slower than assimilation of carbohydrate, oleate must spread along a greater length of small intestine before it is removed from absorption compared to rapidly absorbed glucose. In this setting, more inhibitory feedback sensors are recruited to account for the greater potency of fat in the inhibition of gastric emptying.

Early in the meal, there are no nutrients in the small intestine to generate intestino-gastric inhibitory feedback. During that initial period, the meal surges out of the stomach to spill nutrients along a longer length of small intestine. This initial surge of nutrients sets the intensity of the inhibitory feedback to control transit of the rest of the meal.[38,43] Any change in motility or digestive and absorptive capacity would then have a significant impact on the intensity of the feedback response. For example, after a vagotomy and antrectomy, gastric sieving is impaired, so large chunks of food nearing their original swallowed size enter the small intestine. These poorly triturated food chunks would resist assimilation to travel further and expose an abnormally long length of small intestine to nutrients. An exaggerated inhibitory feedback results.

Delayed Emptying and Gastric Residual Volume

To illustrate the importance of accounting for nutrient-triggered inhibitory feedback or gastric emptying, one must consider the issue of gastric residual volume (GRV), or the amount of a meal that remains in the stomach after a defined unit of time. Currently, enteral feeding is often arbitrarily stopped when the GRV exceeds a threshold volume, such as 150 or 200 mL. GRV is the net difference between gastric input volume meal (endogenous secretions) and gastric output (primarily determined by the ratio of gastric emptying controlled by nutrient-triggered inhibitory feedback). The capacity of a normal adult stomach is 4000 to 6000 mL,[44] with a normal postprandial capacity in excess of 3000 mL.[45] In the case of enteral feeding, endogenous secretions account for volume of input about 125 mL/hour in a healthy, normally fed adult human[45] and the delivery of the enteral formula itself adds another 25 to 125 mL/hour[46] to the total input volume. Gastric emptying rates commonly range from approximately 20%/hour to 30% to 50%/hour under maximal inhibitory feedback by nutrients for a typical iso-osmolar load of nutrients.[38,43] Accordingly, the GRV will not continue to rise but rather reaches a plateau. Under these input and output conditions, equilibrium is reached. As long as input equals output and the GRV reaches a plateau, it should not matter whether GRV is 300, 600, or 900 mL, because these volumes are normally encountered after meals.

Delayed Gastric Emptying and Hyperglycemia

In the setting of delayed gastric emptying, associated with hyperglycemia in patients with diabetes mellitus, the treatment strategy is directed at correcting the reversible impairment of gastric motility. That is, the gastric dysmotility may resolve completely to refute the idea of permanent pump failure, as implied by the diagnosis gastroparesis associated with hyperglycemia. By normalizing blood glucose, any remaining irreversible component may be addressed by modifying the meal. A true pump failure patient would benefit from a meal that minimizes the need for the rate-limiting steps of fragmentation by the stomach, such as substituting ground meats for whole steak. Diabetic patients with severe nausea and vomiting may need continuous post-pyloric tube feeding to normalize their blood glucose because insulin therapy alone is inadequate to overcome the erratic rate of emptying. (Nutrition and diabetes are discussed in Chapter 16.)

Accelerated Emptying and Fat Intolerance

The presenting complaints of delayed gastric emptying are often indistinguishable from those of accelerated gastric emptying. Even so, early satiety and postprandial pain, distention, nausea, and vomiting are often assumed to be secondary to "gastroparesis" or abnormally delayed gastric emptying. The role of the small intestine in generating symptoms is illustrated by the nausea that is induced with infusion of triglycerides into the proximal small intestine of healthy volunteers[47] and by symptoms of the patients with postgastrectomy dumping syndrome, which is known to be secondary to accelerated gastric emptying.[48] Gastric emptying is normally regulated to deliver fat to the intestine at a rate below the physiological maximum for assimilation, which is approximately 6.6 g fat/hour.[49] As delivery of nutrients to the small intestine exceeds this limit, load-dependent inhibitory feedback becomes exaggerated to precipitate symptoms of postprandial bloating, pain, nausea, and vomiting.

Patients complaining of fat intolerance frequently present with symptoms of early satiety and nausea, suggesting gastroparesis. However, gastric emptying in these patients is actually accelerated.[50] They are symptomatic because of exaggerated feedback from the entry of too much fat per unit time into the small intestine. Thus, patients who complain of early satiety and nausea should have gastric emptying studies performed to determine whether the problem is too fast or too slow emptying.

When gastroparesis is suspected, a prokinetic agent such as the motilin-mimicking drug erythromycin is commonly prescribed. However, instead of inducing the normal gastric emptying of the fed state, erythromycin accelerates gastric emptying by inducing a pattern of powerful lumen-obliterating sweeping contraction (intestine "housekeeper" wave) that is normally seen only in the fasted state. Such contractions would expel the content of the stomach without adequate gastric sieving. Erythromycin thus causes an effect similar to that of antrectomy, wherein food is allowed entry into the small intestine without size selection. Because these chunks of food are inadequately triturated, the small intestine cannot properly assimilate them and the undigested food is presented to an excessively long section of intestine, resulting in exaggerated inhibitory feedback.

In this setting of accelerated gastric emptying, the treatment strategy is to increase the latency of emptying. Once again, this is easily accomplished with meal modification by extending the rate-limiting steps of fragmentation by the stomach and gastric sieving while minimizing the intensity of nutrient-triggered inhibitory feedback. For example, eliminating or severely limiting liquid forms of fat and substituting solid foods in a slowly digested matrix that require fragmentation such as steak or chicken extend gastric emptying time to relieve symptoms. Lowering the overall fat content by trimming excess fat from the meat also reduces fat-triggered inhibitory feedback.

Small Intestine

In addition to control of gastric emptying, the end products of digestion liberated by intragastric digestion also regulate transit of the meal through the small intestine. Cholecystokinin and secretin are stimulated by these end products of gastric fat digestion[51] to further promote assimilation through stimulation of pancreatic and biliary secretions. Biliary and pancreatic exocrine secretions mix with the chyme entering the duodenum. Thus, when the end products of gastric digestion are unavailable,[52] digestion may be further impaired.

As with the control of gastric emptying, intestinal transit depends on the nutrient composition and load of the chyme. Using protein assimilation as an example, intestinal transit time increases in proportion to the protein content of a meal.[53] This allows more protein to be assimilated. Similar to fat and carbohydrates, the intensity of inhibitory feedback on transit depends on contact with the intestinal nutrient sensors that respond to proteolytic by-products. A meal of hydrolyzed protein is rapidly assimilated, limiting the number of sensors exposed to the lumenal content. A smaller inhibitory response is then generated when compared to a meal of intact protein[54] that remains available in the lumen longer to trigger greater feedback. Assimilation of the intact protein requires more time; therefore, the greater inhibitory feedback matches workload with time available for digestion as assumption. About 10% of ingested starch escapes assimilation by the small intestine. By accessing distal glucose-sensitive inhibitory mechanisms, gastric emptying and intestinal transit are slowed.[16,45]

Examples

Delayed Transit and Postoperative Ileus

The decision to resume oral or enteral feeding following surgery is commonly made on the resumption of bowel sounds and/or passing of flatus, a process that is linked to return of colonic motility and one that may take a week or more.[55] However, postoperative feeding can safely begin much sooner. Postanesthesia recovery time for the small intestine is most rapid, occurring within 4 to 8 hours, and for the stomach within 24 to 48 hours.[55] As such, even though bowel sounds and passage of flatus may not have returned, direct feeding into the small intestine is possible without delay. Thus, food may be presented to the small intestine on the same day as surgery. In early enteral feeding, the stomach may be bypassed by placement of a jejunal feeding tube during the surgery and removal of that tube after the remainder of the GI tract resumes normal motility. This strategy is safe and well tolerated[56] and avoids sepsis and other complications of parenteral nutrition (PN) (Chapter 38).[57] The use of elemental formulas allows for enteral feeding even if postoperative ileus is protracted.

Delayed Transit and Scleroderma

As with esophageal motility, small bowel motility is frequently impaired in the patient with scleroderma, which leads to disabling postprandial symptoms.[6,58] These symptoms arise directly via motor impairment [eg, reduced frequency and disorganization of the interdigestive motility pattern known as the Migrating Motor Complex (MMC)] early in the course of the disease,[59] or indirectly via SIBO as a complication of impaired motility. These patients are often labeled with the diagnosis of pseudo-obstruction to account for the abnormal motility and intestinal stasis.[6] Regardless of the implications of the term "pseudo-obstruction," a great deal of patient symptoms are secondary to SIBO because symptoms, as well as digestion and absorption, can be markedly improved by eradicating the SIBO, followed by treatment with prokinetic agents that normalize gut motility to restore the MMC.[6] For example, treatment with subcutaneous injections of the somatostatin analog octreotide induces the housekeeper wave and relieves symptoms of nausea, vomiting, bloating, and pain.[59]

The Ileal Brake

Throughout the course of intestinal lipolysis, increasing amounts of the end products of fat digestion are liberated to trigger slowing of gastric emptying and intestinal transit by activating transit controls located in the proximal and distal small intestine. The distal transit control mechanism was first described as the "ileal brake" by Spiller et al[60] and Read et al.[61] Both groups concurrently described slowing of intestinal transit by perfusion of distal gut with fat emulsions. Read's group demonstrated that Intralipid triglyceride emulsion but not saline perfused into the ileum 205 cm from the teeth slowed orocecal transit time of an indigestible carbohydrate marker or a solid meal.[61] Spiller and colleagues showed that partially hydrolyzed Intralipid (approximately 60 mM free fatty acids) perfused 170 cm from the teeth decreased jejunal motility.[60]

The Jejunal Brake

Clinical observations made around the same time as the experiments by Spiller et al and Read et al could not be explained if transit control depended solely on the ileal brake. Woolf et al reported unchanged excretion of fat in patients lacking an ileum, even after fat intake was tripled.[62] Because a larger fat load would require longer assimilation time, the constant stool fat output in the setting of three-fold greater fat intake would require slowing of transit. There is indeed a more proximally located transit control a "jejunal brake."[63] This proximally located brake relies on end products of digestion. For fat, fatty acids serve as the trigger. Although a putative duodenal brake that slowed gastric emptying was described in the early 1970s,[64,65] in those experiments the slowing of gastric emptying may have been secondary to triggering of the jejunal and/or ileal brakes.

Importance of Nutrient-Regulated Intestinal Motility

The ileal brake is more potent than the jejunal brake,[66] allowing for proximal-to-distal graded inhibitory feedback on intestinal transit. After a large meal, nutrients empty from the stomach and spill far down the intestine, activating not only proximal but also distal braking mechanisms. By spreading a large load of nutrients down a long length of intestine, more transit-slowing inhibitory feedback is activated to increase time available for digestion and absorption, which minimizes potential loss of nutrients. Any nutrients that are not assimilated in the proximal gut enter the distal gut to trigger the more potent ileal brake. In the setting of extensive ileal resection, the jejunal brake is of primary importance as the sole remaining transit control mechanism. This importance is also because of its physical position, which allows for an immediate response to chyme emptying out of the stomach. When the distal half of the small intestine is resected[67] or taken out of continuity with the proximal gut,[68] recovery of fat in the feces rises from the normal 8%-to-10% range to 80% to 90%. The loss of nutrients is far lower in the setting of extensive (50% to 70%) proximal gut resection, which limits recovery of fat in the stool to 15% to 24%.[68] The severe adverse effect of removing the distal half of the small intestine can be explained by the loss of controlled intestinal transit with resection of the ileal brake. Massive steatorrhea with nearly complete loss of ingested fat results when transit becomes so rapid that there is no time for assimilation.

Patients with rapid transit from loss of control are symptomatic with chronic postprandial diarrhea. Narcotics are often used to treat this symptom. Narcotics alter intestinal motility patterns from propagative to nonpropagative, effectively slowing intestinal transit to increase contact time of the intestinal content with the absorptive mucosa[69] and reducing diarrhea.[70] However, these agents often fail and are accompanied by serious side effects. As an alternative, it is now possible to exploit nutrients as physiologic triggers of intestinal brakes to achieve even more potent slowing of transit to optimize digestion and absorption.

Accelerated Transit and Enteral Feeding

Rather than reducing formula delivery rates, and therefore calories delivered, high-fiber enteral formulas are now commonly used to avoid flow-dependent acceleration of intestinal transit and the resultant diarrhea[71,72] that affects up to 68% of patients receiving enteral nutritional (EN) support.[73,74] The use of so-called soluble fiber in enteral formulas improves bowel function and extends intestinal transit time,[75] suggesting that nutrient-triggered inhibitory feedback on intestinal transit may be important in this setting. Water-soluble fiber increases the viscosity of the lumenal content and thickens the unstirred water layer, to decrease the rate of nutrient uptake.[76] This change leaves a greater load of unabsorbed nutrients available to spread further down the small intestine to contact more nutrient sensors, and to trigger more potent distal braking mechanisms.[37]

Small Intestinal Bacterial Overgrowth

In the setting of ileocecal resection, ileal disease, or loss of phase III of the MMC,[77-80] colonic bacteria may expand into the small intestine, which is normally inhabited by low concentrations of bacteria.[81] In the absence of the normal stripping motions, intestinal housekeeper waves last only about 7 to 9 minutes,[16] and the colonic bacterial flora expand proximally into the small intestine to result in SIBO. In this setting, any ingested food becomes substrate for bacterial fermentation. Gases are formed to distend the gut, which accelerates intestinal transit to overwhelm nutrient-triggered inhibitory feedback.[82,83] Pain, bloating, nausea, and diarrhea may result. For many patients with chronic diarrhea, the identification and eradication of SIBO may reverse many of the symptoms.[82,83] (Overgrowth is also addressed in Chapter 5.)

Accelerated Transit and Short Bowel Syndrome

The term short bowel syndrome (SBS) is applied to those patients with less than 100 cm of small bowel, a limit cited at times as incompatible with survival without PN. In these SBS patients, the problem is not limited to the reduced absorptive surface area. The loss of the ileocecal valve and the loss of the ileal brake from resection of the distal small intestinal would accelerate the transit of a meal throughout the entire GI tract. Because digestion and absorption cannot be completed without adequate time, these patients chronically face postprandial symptoms of diarrhea, bloating, nausea, and abdominal pain with malnutrition and the possibility of lifetime dependence on PN. Their problems may be exacerbated by the complication of SIBO that further accelerates transit and worsens digestion. Although for some patients with SBS, it may not be possible to nutritionally maintain the patient with EN alone, it is often possible to identify bacterial overgrowth as a treatable complication.

In addition to antibiotics, it may be possible to eradicate SIBO by putting the patient on an elemental diet exclusively for 2 weeks.[84] This treatment simultaneously targets the problems of SIBO and malnutrition. However, rapid intestinal transit may remain after bacterial overgrowth is treated, and the remaining jejunal brake may not be able to slow transit because of unavailability of the end products of digestion, as there is no time available for digestion. To jump-start the jejunal brake, fatty acid may be administered before a meal as a potent trigger of physiologic inhibitory intestinal feedback. This approach may be used to slow transit through the upper gut in patients with chronic diarrhea from a variety of causes, including SBS.[85] GI transit time increases in a dose-dependent manner, more than doubling the transit time in most patients with just 3.2 mL of oleic acid. When patients continued to take the oleic acid pre-meal, they reported decreased stool frequency and volume.

The provider must also counsel the SBS patient on meal consumption patterns that can help slow transit. For example, volume-induced acceleration of transit can be limited by shifting fluid intake to the interdigestive period. As with rapid gastric emptying, slowing intestinal transit relies on sustained delivery of nutrient triggers throughout a meal. To achieve this effect, patients should consume foods that are not easily triturated (eg, steak or chicken) to permit nutrient-rich food to enter the small intestine continuously over a prolonged period of time.

Colon

The Ileocecal Junction

Meal constituents that remain unabsorbed by the small intestine are normally held for a period in the terminal ileum by the ileocecal valve. Loss of the ileocecal junction by resection[81,86] speeds orocecal transit and promotes SIBO. As expected, loss of distal intestine in addition to the ileocecal junction further accelerates transit because nutrient sensors are most densely distributed in the ileum.

The Colonic Brake

As unabsorbed nutrients enter the colon, the colonic brake[87,88] responds by delaying gastric emptying and slowing intestinal transit.[87,89] This response, similar to the jejunal and ileal brake, is mediated by the distal gut peptide YY (PYY)[88-90] and, to a lesser extent, glucagon-like peptide 1 (also called GLP-1).[88] When the colon is taken out of continuity with the small intestine, as in the setting of jejunostomy, no nutrient triggers of inhibitory feedback are presented to the distal gut. However, nutrient-triggered inhibitory feedback via PYY is still possible via a proximal-to-distal gut link.[91-94] The dependence on PYY may explain the difficulty in providing adequate EN support to patients lacking both ileum and colon.

Unassimilated nutrients that enter the colon are subject to bacterial fermentation by the indigenous flora, including as much as 20% of ingested starches[95] and 80% to 100% of various dietary fibers.[96,97] Colonic fermentation produces a mixture of gases including hydrogen, methane, and carbon dioxide, in addition to short chain fatty acids (SCFA)—mainly propionate and butyrate.[96-98] Gastric emptying[50,51] and lower esophageal sphincter function[10] in the setting of undigested carbohydrate and SCFA in the colon may be inhibited by fermentation byproducts.

Conclusion

Delivery of adequate nutrition in the setting of abnormal GI motility demands understanding of the interplay of motility and food. Motility determines how effectively EN can be delivered to the sites of digestion and absorption. The nutrients in a meal, in turn, determine the motility response that dictates efficacy of digestion and absorption.

Barriers to proper nutrition include impaired swallowing, gastric emptying, and transit of a meal through the small intestine. For dysphagia, treatment may require circumventing the esophagus and delivering nutrients directly into the stomach or small intestine. For gastric emptying disorders, treatment involves correction of either accelerated or delayed emptying and by altering the physical form or nutrient content of the meal. For abnormal small intestinal transit, treatment is similar to that for gastric emptying, with particular emphasis on using nutrient-triggered inhibitory feedback to slow transit.

For the patient with a motility disorder, it is critical to determine not only the location of the dysfunction but also whether symptoms are caused by motility that is too fast or too slow. With fat intolerance, motility is actually accelerated although the presenting complaints may suggest delayed gastric emptying to the clinician. Providing prokinetic agents in this setting would (and frequently does) exacerbate symptoms. What is actually required is modification of the physical and nutrient composition of the meal to avoid excessively rapid entry of fat into the small intestine.

For all patients, the most effective therapeutic strategy is the accurate identification of a reversible mechanism from which the symptoms arise. Although abnormal motility may be the primary defect, patients are often primarily symptomatic from a secondary, reversible problem, such as the SIBO seen in the short bowel syndrome. In this setting, the appropriate therapy is to address bacterial overgrowth before providing motility altering agents. Improved nutrition is only possible by addressing the mechanisms that are responsible for the malnutrition (Chapter 5). A motility defect may also arise from a primary, reversible problem such as delayed gastric emptying caused by hyperglycemia. In that setting, delayed gastric emptying is not caused by paralysis of the stomach or gastroparesis but, rather, as a reversible complication of hyperglycemia. The patient's delayed gastric emptying can be improved by administering hypoglycemic agents and by prescribing meals that do not provoke great fluctuations of blood glucose.

Adequate nutritional support for the patient with symptoms suggestive of abnormal motility requires accurate diagnosis of the site of the problem, understanding of the true nature of the altered transit (too fast versus too slow), and the identification of reversible cause of symptoms. Only then can a successful nutritional treatment regimen be envisioned, planned, and implemented.

Acknowledgment

Dr. Lin's research is supported by the Jill and Tom Barad Family Fund.

References

1. Holgate AM, Read NW. Can a rapid small bowel transit limit absorption? *Gut.* 1982;23:A912.
2. Lind CD. Dysphagia: evaluation and treatment. *Gastroenterol Clin N Am.* 2003;32:553-575.
3. Hila A, Castell JA, Castell DO. Pharyngeal and upper esophageal sphincter manometry in the evaluation of dysphagia. *J Clin Gastroenterol.* 2001;33:355-361.
4. Clements PJ, Becvar R, Drosos AA, Ghattas L, Gabrielli A. Assessment of gastrointestinal involvement. *Clin Exp Rheumatol.* 2003;21:S15-S18.
5. Henry MA, Harbermann MC, Rocha OM. Esophageal motor disturbances in progressive systemic sclerosis. *Dis Esophagus.* 1999;12:51-53.
6. Rose S, Young MA, Reynolds JC. Gastrointestinal manifestations of scleroderma. *Gastroenterol Clin North Am.* 1998;27:563-594.
7. Shaheen N, Provenzale D. The epidemiology of gastroesophageal reflux disease. *Am J Med Sci.* 2003;326:264-273.
8. Becker DJ, Sinclair J, Castell DO, Wu WC. A comparison of high and low fat meals on postprandial esophageal acid exposure. *Am J Gastroenterol.* 1989;84:782-786.
9. Nebel OT, Castell DO. Lower esophageal sphincter pressure changes after food ingestion. *Gastroenterology.* 1972;63:778-783.
10. Piche T, Zerbib F, Varannes SB, et al. Modulation by colonic fermentation of LES function in humans. *Am J Physiol Gastrointest Liver Physiol.* 2000;278:G578-G584.
11. Piche T, des Varannes SB, Sacher-Huvelin S, Holst JJ, Cuber JC, Galmiche JP. Colonic fermentation influences lower esophageal sphincter function in gastroesophageal reflux disease. *Gastroenterology.* 2003;124:894-902.
12. Babka JC, Castell DO. On the genesis of heartburn. The effects of specific foods on the lower esophageal sphincter. *Am J Dig Dis.* 1973;18:391-397.
13. Lepsien G, Dietrich K. Peptone stimulation of the lower esophageal sphincter in patients with reflux disease. *Zeitschrift für Gastroenterol.* 1988;26:209-216.
14. Meyer JH, Lembo A, Elashoff JD, Fass R, Mayer EA. Duodenal fat intensifies the perception of heartburn. *Gut.* 2001;49:624-628.
15. Castell DO. Diet and the lower esophageal sphincter. *Am J Clin Nutr.* 1975;28:1296-1298.
16. Bueno L, Fioramonti J. Neurohormonal control of intestinal transit. *Reprod Nutr Dev.* 1994;34:513-525.
17. Meyer JH. The physiology of gastric motility and gastric emptying. In: Yamada T, ed. *Textbook of Gastroenterology.* Philadelphia, Pa: Lippincott; 1991:137-158.
18. Mayer EA, Thomson JB, Jehn D, et al. Gastric emptying and sieving of solid food and pancreatic and biliary secretions after solid meals in patients with nonresective ulcer surgery. *Gastroenterology.* 1984;87:1264-1271.
19. Meyer JH, Thomson JB, Cohen MB, Shadchehr A, Mandiola SA. Sieving of solid food by the canine stomach and sieving after gastric surgery. *Gastroenterology.* 1979;76:804-813.
20. Richter C, Tanaka T, Yada RY. Mechanism of activation of the gastric aspartic proteinases: pepsinogen, progastricsin and prochymosin. *Biochem J.* 1998;335:481-490.
21. James AH. The nature of the gastric contents in man. In: James AH, ed. *The Physiology of Gastric Digestion.* London: Edward Arnold; 1957:1-24.
22. Murray RD, Kerzner B, Sloan HR, et al. The contribution of salivary amylase to glucose polymer hydrolysis in premature infants. *Pediatr Re.* 1986;20:186-191.
23. Carriere F, Barrowman JA, Verger R, Laugier R. Secretion and contribution to lipolysis of gastric and pancreatic lipases during a test meal in humans. *Gastroenterology.* 1993;105:876-888.
24. Pafumi Y, Lairon D, de la Porte PL, et al. Mechanisms of inhibition of triacylglycerol hydrolysis by human gastric lipase. *J Biol Chem.* 2002;277:28070-28079.
25. Sonnenberg A, Muller-Lissner SA, Weiser HF, Muller-Duysing W, Heinzel F, Blum AL. Effect of liquid meals on duodenogastric reflux in humans. *Am J Physiol.* 1982;243:G42-G47.
26. Armand M, Borel P, Dubois C, et al. Characterization of emulsions and lipolysis of dietary lipids in the human stomach. *Am J Physiol.* 1994;266:G372-G381.
27. Bernback S, Blackberg L, Hernell O. Fatty acids generated by gastric lipase promote human milk triacylglycerol digestion by pancreatic colipase-dependent lipase. *Biochim Biophys Acta.* 1989;1001:286-293.
28. Bernback S, Blackberg L, Hernell O. The complete digestion of human milk triacylglycerol in vitro requires gastric lipase, pancreatic colipase-dependent lipase, and bile salt-stimulated lipase. *J Clin Investigation.* 1990;85:1221-1226.
29. Gargouri Y, Pieroni G, Riviere C, et al. Importance of human gastric lipase for intestinal lipolysis: an in vitro study. *Biochimica et Biophysica Acta.* 1986;879:419-423.
30. Dubois A, Natelson BH, van Eerdewegh P, Gardner JD. Gastric emptying and secretion in the rhesus monkey. *Am J Physiol.* 1977;232:E186-E192.
31. Guyton AC, Hall JE. *Textbook of Medical Physiology.* 10th ed. Philadelphia, Pa: WB Saunders Co; 2000.
32. Phan CT, Tso P. Intestinal lipid absorption and transport. *Frontiers in Bioscience.* 2001;6:D299-D319.
33. Reuss L. One-hundred years of inquiry: the mechanism of glucose absorption in the intestine. *Ann Rev Physiol.* 2000;62:939-946.
34. Thomson AB, Keelan M, Thiesen A, Clandinin MT, Ropeleski M, Wild GE. Small bowel review: normal physiology part 1. *Dig Dis Sci.* 2001;46:2567-2587.
35. Wright EM, Loo DD. Coupling between Na+, sugar, and water transport across the intestine. *Ann NY Acad Sci.* 2000;915:54-66.
36. Binder HJ. Pathophysiology of acute diarrhea. *Am J Med.* 1990;88:2S-4S.
37. Lin HC, Elashoff JD, Kwok GM, Gu YG, Meyer JH. Stimulation of duodenal motility by hyperosmolar mannitol depends on local osmoreceptor control. *Am J Physiol.* 1994;266:G940-G943.
38. Lin HC, Doty JE, Reedy TJ, Meyer JH. Inhibition of gastric emptying by glucose depends on length of intestine exposed to nutrient. *Am J Physiol.* 1989;256:G404-G411.
39. McHugh PR, Moran TH. Calories and gastric emptying: a regulatory capacity with implications for feeding. *Am J Physiol.* 1979;236:R254-R260.
40. Williams NS, Elashoff J, Meyer JH. Gastric emptying of liquids in normal subjects and patients with healed duodenal ulcer disease. *Dig Dis Sci.* 1986;31:943-952.
41. Meyer JH, Kelly GA. Canine pancreatic responses to intestinally perfused proteins and protein digests. *Am J Physiol.* 1976;231:682-691.
42. Meyer JH, Kelly GA, Jones RS. Canine pancreatic response to intestinally perfused oligopeptides. *Am J Physiol.* 1976;231:678-681.
43. Lin HC, Doty JE, Reedy TJ, Meyer JH. Inhibition of gastric emptying by sodium oleate depends on length of intestine exposed to nutrient. *Am J Physiol.* 1990;259:G1031-G1036.
44. Spiro HM. *Clinical Gastroenterology.* 3rd ed. New York, NY: Macmillan Publishing Company; 1983.
45. Ganong WF. *Review of Medical Physiology.* 20th ed. Stamford, Conn: Appleton & Lange, 2001.

46. Kohn CL, Keithley JK. Enteral nutrition. Potential complications and patient monitoring. *Nurs Clin N Am.* 1989;24:339-353.
47. Hebbard GS, Samson M, Andrews JM, et al. Hyperglycemia affects gastric electrical rhythm and nausea during intraduodenal triglyceride infusion. *Dig Dis Sci.* 1997;42:568-575.
48. Machella TE. Mechanism of the post-gastrectomy dumping syndrome. *Gastroenterology.* 1968;54 (Suppl 2):721-722.
49. Meyer JH, Elashoff JD, Lake R. Gastric emptying of indigestible versus digestible oils and solid fats in normal humans. *Dig Dis Sci.* 1999;44:1076-1082.
50. Lin HC, Van Citters GW, Zhao XT, Waxman. Fat intolerance depends on rapid gastric emptying. *Dig Dis Sci.* 1999;44:330-335.
51. Hildebrand P, Beglinger C, Gyr K, et al. Effects of a cholecystokinin receptor antagonist on intestinal phase of pancreatic and biliary responses in man. *J Clin Invest.* 1990;85:640-646.
52. Czako L, Hajnal F, Nemeth J, Takacs T, Lonovics J. Effect of a liquid meal given as a bolus into the jejunum on human pancreatic secretion. *Pancreas.* 1999;18:197-202.
53. Zhao XT, Miller RH, McCamish MA, Wang L, Lin HC. Protein absorption depends on load-dependent inhibition of intestinal transit in dogs. *Am J Clin Nutr.* 1996;64:319-323.
54. Zhao XT, McCamish MA, Miller RH, Wang L, Lin HC. Intestinal transit and absorption of soy protein in dogs depend on load and degree of protein hydrolysis. *J Nutr.* 1997;127:2350-2356.
55. Kehlet H, Holte K. Review of postoperative ileus. *Am J Surg.* 2001;182:3S-10S.
56. Reissman P, Teoh TA, Cohen SM, Weiss EG, Nogueras JJ, Wexner SD. Is early oral feeding safe after elective colorectal surgery? A prospective randomized trial. *Ann Surg.* 1995;222:73-77.
57. Braga M, Gianotti L, Vignali A, et al. Artificial nutrition after major abdominal surgery: impact of route of administration and composition of the diet. *Crit Care Med.* 1998;26:24-30.
58. Lock G, Holstege A, Lang B, Scholmerich J. Gastrointestinal manifestations of progressive systemic sclerosis. *Am J Gastroenterol.* 1997;92:763-771.
59. Soudah HC, Hasler WL, Owyang C. Effect of octreotide on intestinal motility and bacterial overgrowth in scleroderma. *N Engl J Med.* 1991;325:1461-1467.
60. Spiller RC, Trotman IF, Higgins BE, et al. The ileal brake--inhibition of jejunal motility after ileal fat perfusion in man. *Gut.* 1984;25:365-374.
61. Read NW, McFarlane A, Kinsman RI, et al. Effect of infusion of nutrient solutions into the ileum on gastrointestinal transit and plasma levels of neurotensin and enteroglucagon. *Gastroenterology.* 1984;86:274-280.
62. Woolf GM, Miller C, Kurian R, Jeejeebhoy KN. Diet for patients with a short bowel: high fat or high carbohydrate? *Gastroenterology.* 1983;84:823-828.
63. Lin HC, Zhao XT, Wang L. Jejunal brake: inhibition of intestinal transit by fat in the proximal small intestine. *Dig Dis Sci.* 1996;41:326-329.
64. Shahidullah M, Kennedy TL, Parks TG. Proceedings: the duodenal brake—hormonal or vagal?. *Br J Surg.* 1973;60:912-913.
65. Shahidullah M, Kennedy TL, Parks TG. The vagus, the duodenal brake, and gastric emptying. *Gut.* 1975;16:331-336.
66. Lin HC, Zhao XT, Wang L. Intestinal transit is more potently inhibited by fat in the distal (ileal brake) than in the proximal (jejunal brake) gut. *Dig Dis Sci.* 1997;42:19-25.
67. Reynell PC, Spray GH. Small intestinal function in the rat after massive resections. *Gastroenterology.* 1956;31:361-368.
68. Kremen AJ, Linner JH, Nelson CH. An experimental evaluation of the nutritional importance of proximal and distal small intestine. *Ann Surg.* 1954;140:439-448.
69. Barrett KE, Dharmsathaphorn K. Pharmacological aspects of therapy in inflammatory bowel diseases: antidiarrheal agents. *J Clin Gastroenterol.* 1988;10:57-63.
70. Chang EB, Sitrin MD, Black DD. *Gastrointestinal, Hepatobiliary, and Nutritional Physiology.* Philadelphia, Pa: Lippincott-Raven Publishers; 1996.
71. Homann HH, Kemen M, Fuessenich C, Senkal M, Zumtobel V. Reduction in diarrhea incidence by soluble fiber in patients receiving total or supplemental enteral nutrition. *JPEN J Parenter Enteral Nutr.* 1994;18:486-490.
72. Shankardass K, Chuchmach S, Chelswick K, et al. Bowel function of long-term tube-fed patients consuming formulae with and without dietary fiber. *JPEN J Parenter Enteral Nutr.* 1990;14:508-512.
73. Eisenberg P. An overview of diarrhea in the patient receiving enteral nutrition. *Gastroenterol Nurs.* 2002;25:95-104.
74. Mobarhan S, DeMeo M. Diarrhea induced by enteral feeding. *Nutr Rev.* 1995;53:67-70.
75. Meier R, Beglinger C, Schneider H, Rowedder A, Gyr K. Effect of a liquid diet with and without soluble fiber supplementation on intestinal transit and cholecystokinin release in volunteers. *JPEN J Parenter Enteral Nutr.* 1993;17:231-235.
76. Fuse K, Bamba T, Hosoda S. Effects of pectin on fatty acid and glucose absorption and on thickness of unstirred water layer in rat and human intestine. *Dig Dis Sci.* 1989;34:1109-1116.
77. Lifshitz F, Wapnir RA, Wehman HJ, Diaz-bensussen S, Pergolizzi R. The effects of small intestinal colonization by fecal and colonic bacteria on intestinal function in rats. *J Nutr.* 1978;108:1913-1923.
78. Pimentel M, Chow EJ, Lin HC. Eradication of small intestinal bacterial overgrowth reduces symptoms of irritable bowel syndrome. *Am J Gastroenterol.* 2000;95:3503-3506.
79. Pimentel M, Soffer EE, Chow EJ, Kong Y, Lin HC. Lower frequency of MMC is found in IBS subjects with abnormal lactulose breath test, suggesting bacterial overgrowth. *Dig Dis Sci.* 2002;47:2639-2643.
80. Stotzer PO, Bjornsson ES, Abrahamsson H. Interdigestive and postprandial motility in small-intestinal bacterial overgrowth. *Scand J Gastroenterol.* 1996;31:875-880.
81. Thompson JS, Quigley EM, Adrian TE, Path FR. Role of the ileocecal junction in the motor response to intestinal resection. *J Gastrointest Surg.* 1998;2:174-185.
82. Caldarella MP, Serra J, Azpiroz F, Malagelada JR. Prokinetic effects in patients with intestinal gas retention. *Gastroenterology.* 2002;122:1748-1755.
83. Lasser RB, Bond JH, Levitt MD. The role of intestinal gas in functional abdominal pain. *N Engl J Med.* 1975;293:524-526.
84. Pimentel M, Constantino T, Kong Y, Bajwa M, Rezaei A, Park S. A 14-day elemental diet is highly effective in normalizing the lactulose breath test. *Dig Dis Sci.* 2004;49:73-77.
85. Lin HC, Van Citters GW, Heimer F, Bonorris G. Slowing of gastrointestinal transit by oleic acid: a preliminary report of a novel, nutrient-based treatment in humans. *Dig Dis Sci.* 2001;46:223-229.
86. Fallingborg J, Pedersen P, Jacobsen BA. Small intestinal transit time and intraluminal pH in ileocecal resected patients with Crohn's disease. *Dig Dis Sci.* 1998;43:702-705.
87. Nightingale JM, Kamm MA, van der Sijp JR, et al. Disturbed gastric emptying in the short bowel syndrome. Evidence for a 'colonic brake'. *Gut.* 1993;34:1171-1176.
88. Wen J, Phillips SF, Sarr MG, Kost LJ, Holst JJ. PYY and GLP-1 contribute to feedback inhibition from the canine ileum and colon. *Am J Physiol.* 1995;269:G945-G952.
89. Nightingale JM, Kamm MA, van der Sijp JR, Ghatei MA, Bloom SR, Lennard-Jones JE. Gastrointestinal hormones in short bowel syndrome. Peptide YY may be the 'colonic brake' to gastric emptying. *Gut.* 1996;39:267-272.
90. Wen J, Luque-de Leon E, Kost LJ, Sarr MG, Phillips SF. Duodenal motility in fasting dogs: humoral and neural pathways mediating the colonic brake. *Am J Physiol.* 1998;274:G192-G195.
91. Lin HC, Chey WY. Cholecystokinin and peptide YY are released by fat in either proximal or distal small intestine in dogs. *Regulatory Peptides.* 2003;114:131-135.
92. Lin HC, Zaidel O, Hum S. Intestinal transit of fat depends on accelerating effect of cholecystokinin and slowing effect of an opioid pathway. *Dig Dis Sci.* 2002;47:2217-2221.

93. Lin HC, Chey WY, Zhao X. Release of distal gut peptide YY (PYY) by fat in proximal gut depends on CCK. *Peptides.* 2000;21:1561-1563.
94. Lin HC, Taylor IL. Release of Peptide YY by fat in the proximal but not distal gut depends on an atropine-sensitive cholinergic pathway. *Regulatory Peptides.* 2004;117:73-76.
95. Stephen AM, Haddad AC, Phillips SF. Passage of carbohydrate into the colon. Direct measurements in humans. *Gastroenterology.* 1983;85:589-595.
96. Koruda MJ. Dietary fiber and gastrointestinal disease. *Surg Gynecol Obstetr.* 1993;177:209-214.
97. Topping DL. Soluble fiber polysaccharides: effects on plasma cholesterol and colonic fermentation. *Nutr Rev.* 1991;49:195-203.
98. Jenkins DJ, Jenkins AL, Wolever TM, Rao AV, Thompson LU. Fiber and starchy foods: gut function and implications in disease. *Am J Gastroenterol.* 1986;81:920-930.

Chapter 24

Inborn Errors of Metabolism for the Gastroenterologist

Charles P. Venditti, MD, PhD and
Gerard T. Berry, MD

Introduction

Inborn errors of metabolism, especially those that feature perturbations of small molecules, may be difficult to diagnose. In some instances, the presenting symptom complex may not be classical. Specialized metabolic laboratory studies are also usually more likely to be informative in the face of intercurrent illness or acute decompensation. This is the case with fatty acid oxidation defects and organic acidemias. Such situations can be life-threatening for the patient, and attempts to obtain diagnostic metabolic studies can be difficult under emergency circumstances. The co-occurrence of developmental delay, poor feeding and/or failure to thrive, multisystemic organ involvement, and, in some disorders, congenital malformations can further complicate diagnostic evaluations.

Relatively few inborn errors are linked with direct pathological effects in the gastrointestinal (GI) tract. The manifestations of these disorders include chronic diarrhea, malabsorption, and a protein-losing enteropathy.

This chapter reviews common inborn errors of metabolism that can feature hepatobiliary involvement and primary disorders of the gastrointestinal (GI) tract. The reader is referred to more specialized sources for a deeper discussion of the diagnostic subtleties and management of affected patients.[1]

Inborn Errors of Metabolism

The liver plays a central role in body metabolism. Hepatocytes, functionally heterogeneous in their spatial distribution along the tracts from the periportal to the centrilobular zones, are the principal players in a complex process that involves: 1) transport of water and solutes across membrane bilayers; 2) biosynthesis of small and complex molecules, the latter of which are largely destined for export; 3) interconversion of metabolites assimilated from ingested food such as amino acids; 4) catabolism of decaying macromolecules; 5) oxidation of fuels such as fatty acids, the most important energy source for hepatocytes; and 6) export plus synthesis of glucose, as well as its storage form, glycogen.

Many inborn errors of metabolism affect the liver. In some of these biochemical genetic disorders, such as phenylketonuria (PKU), the enzyme function in the hepatocyte is defective but the complications related to accumulation of phenylalanine metabolites are extrahepatic. Other disease types globally affect the hepatocyte or damage one or more organelles. In addition to hepatocytes, the liver contains other cell populations, such as the Kupffer cells, which can also be affected; this may lead to alterations in hepatic function or size. Mechanisms of hepatic injury, including discrete involvement of organelles (as evidenced by biochemical or pathologic findings) are discussed for selected disorders of amino acid, ammonia, organic acid, carbohydrate, glycogen, fatty acid, complex lipid, cholesterol, bile salt, glycosaminoglycan, glycoprotein, and metal metabolism.

Timing of the Presentation of Inborn Errors of Metabolism

Inborn errors of metabolism are most commonly thought of as being the so-called small molecule diseases, in which the pathophysiology is usually a result of either the presence of a toxic intermediate or the absence of a necessary substrate, as well as the large molecule or complex macromolecule disorders, often termed storage diseases. This division is artificial in that all of the biochemical genetic diseases arise as a result of abnormalities in protein structure or enzymatic function. In turn, these abnormalities are caused by alterations in nuclear or mitochondrial genes and their expression.

Most disorders of intermediary metabolism may not show signs in the fetus. The placenta and maternal circulation provide a constant supply of calories, which reduces the metabolic stress on the affected pathway of the fetus. Maternal hepatic function is also a means of elimination of many of the toxic metabolites that would otherwise cause symptoms. The free exchange of metabolites from the affected fetus to the maternal circulation has been demonstrated in a number of disorders. However, a metabolic toxicity syndrome featuring maternal liver disease can be seen when the fetus is affected with one of several disorders. The best-described syndrome is when the fetus is affected with long-chain hydroxylacyl-CoA dehydrogenase (LCHAD) deficiency.[2] Other inborn errors in which this can be seen include carnitine palmitoyl transferase type I (CPT I) deficiency[3] and short-chain acyl-CoA dehydrogenase (SCAD) deficiency.[4] A history of maternal illness during pregnancy should always be sought when evaluating patients for metabolic disease.

Prenatal effects can be seen in several different classes of inborn errors. Lesions of the electron transport chain can feature multiple antenatal effects such as intrauterine growth retardation, cardiac abnormalities, and malformations.[5] Other disorders of energy metabolism—such as deficiencies of pyruvate carboxylase, pyruvate dehydrogenase, and fumarase deficiency—can feature central nervous system (CNS) dysgenesis and aberrant migration in the form of corpus colossal defects, nodular heterotopias, and polymicrogyria.[6] Renal cystic changes are seen in multiple acyl-CoA dehydrogenase deficiency,[7] the neonatal variant of carnitine palmitoyl transferase II (CPT II) deficiency,[8] and in the congenital disorders of glycosylation (CDG).[9] Peroxisomal disorders may have a combination of dysmorphic features and hepatocellular involvement by birth.[10] A number of sterol synthetic defects—including Smith-Lemli-Opitz syndrome, lathosterolosis, desmosterolosis, and Conradi-Hunerman syndrome—can feature multiple malformations.[11] These patients can develop cholestatic liver disease and may secrete inadequate quantities of normal bile acids. More specifically, hepatobiliary malformations and developmental defects have been noted to also occur in the setting of hereditary metabolic disease such as ductal plate malformations, which is seen in phosphomannose isomerase deficiency;[12] a CDG; and biliary atresia, which has been documented in one set of siblings with Niemann-Pick type C disease[13] and one patient with deficiency of the mitochondrial trifunctional protein.[14] These examples heighten the indication to initiate a metabolic evaluation in the setting of prenatal manifestations and/or aberrant development.

A few storage disorders may appear with prenatal or peripartum clues caused by the accumulation of normal cellular materials as the result of a block at one or more steps of their degradation. Examples in which the disease may be evident at birth include several lysosomal storage disorders, glycogen storage disease (GSD) type IV, CDG type Ik, and Niemann-Pick type C.[15] In such cases, it is imperative to obtain the placenta and send it for pathological examination. The recognition of accumulated material in the liver and in other tissues, or the secondary alteration of the somatic structure as a result of the perturbations in metabolism, may take months to occur.

Each inborn error of metabolism can arise as the result of more than one DNA mutation within the gene. Each mutation can have different effects on the phenotype because of varying levels of residual function of the affected protein. In the case of multimeric proteins, the net activity of the complex may be different based on the structure of the altered subunits. The residual activity, the net metabolic stress on the body (in the case of catabolic errors in intermediary metabolism), and the amount of substrate combine to determine the timing of the recognition of the altered phenotype. Epigenetic or nongenic factors also can influence the phenotype seen in recessive enzymopathies in a less predictable fashion, best evidenced in the intrafamilial variability seen in cystic fibrosis.

Categories of Inborn Errors of Metabolism Involving the Liver and Gastrointestinal Tract

Table 24-1 outlines many of the disorders that have a known disturbance in the structure or function of the liver and GI tract as a result of inborn errors of metabolism in the pediatric population. Selected examples of these disorders are discussed briefly in the subsection on mechanisms of pathogenesis.

A few examples of metabolic diseases in which the liver serves the primary role in maintaining normal extrahepatic concentrations of metabolites and in which the signs are exclusively extrahepatic should be mentioned. A prime example of the importance of hepatic metabolism as it relates to central nervous system (CNS) effects is PKU due to defects in phenylalanine hydroxylase. The enzymatic blockage prevents the conversion of phenylalanine to tyrosine. Consequences of the increased phenylalanine and lowered tyrosine concentrations include alterations in the transport of neutral aromatic amino acids into the brain and the production of neurotransmitters. As a result, mental retardation and seizures can occur. By lowering the blood phenylalanine concentration, many of the effects on cognition can be prevented or reversed. Hepatic size, synthetic functions, and laboratory tests are normal.

Nonketotic hyperglycinemia (NKH) is due to defects in the glycine cleavage system. Although the system is found in the brain and kidney, the vast majority of the activity is expressed in the liver. Except in the atypical form, the failure of the cleavage system results in the accumulation of glycine in all tissues; however, the pathophysiology is due to elevated glycine levels in the CNS. Unlike PKU, in which no symptoms are seen in the early neonatal period, infants with NKH may present with intractable seizures within hours of birth. Glycine levels are massively elevated in the cerebrospinal fluid in the neonatal period, implying that intrauterine elevations are a feature of this disorder. The liver in these patients is unremarkable.

TABLE 24-1.

Selected Inborn Errors of Metabolism That Feature Gastrointestinal Dysfunction

Class of Disorder	*Enzyme Defect*	*Management Strategies/Comments*
Carbohydrate Metabolism		
Galactosemia	Galactose-1-phosphate uridyltransferase	Remove lactose and galactose from diet
Hereditary fructose intolerance	Fructose 1-phosphate aldolase	Remove sucrose, fructose, and sorbitol from diet
Fructose 1,6-bisphosphatase deficiency	Fructose 1,6-bisphosphatase	Avoidance of fasting; Remove sucrose, fructose, and sorbitol from diet
Glycogen synthase defect	Glycogen synthase	Avoidance of fasting
Glycogen storage disease (GSD), type I	Glucose-6-phosphatase	Continuous calories, nocturnal cornstarch feedings. Liver transplantation?
GSD, type III	Amylo-1,6-glucosidase (debrancher enzyme)	High carbohydrate diet, frequent feedings may be needed
GSD, type IV	Amylo 1,4 ->1,6 transglucosidase (brancher enzyme)	Patient may need liver transplantation
GSD, type VI	Liver phosphorylase	Therapy depends on symptoms
Phosphorylase kinase def.	Phosphorylase kinase	Therapy depends on symptoms
Fanconi Bickel Syndrome	GLUT2	Patients always have a renal Fanconi syndrome
Transaldolase deficiency[32]	Transaldolase	One patient had cirrhosis and rock-hard hepatomegaly
Amino- and Organic Acid Disorders		
Tyrosinemia, type I	Fumarylacetoacetate hydrolase	NTBC, dietary tyrosine restriction Eventual need for liver transplantation
Maple syrup urine disease	Branch chain oxoacid dehydrogenase	Leucine restriction; isoleucine and valine supplementation usually needed Thiamine in responders Liver transplantation?
Propionic acidemia	Propionyl-coenzyme A carboxylase A, B	Branched chain amino acid restriction, carnitine supplementation Liver transplantation?
Methylmalonic acidemia	L-Methylmalonyl coenzyme A mutase (mut class) MMAA (cblA class) MMAB (cblB class)	Branched chain amino acid restriction, carnitine supplementation, hydroxylcobalamin IM (not all patients respond) Liver transplantation?
Urea Cycle and Related Disorders		
Carbamyl phosphate synthase deficiency	Carbamyl phosphate synthetase	Stringent dietary protein restriction Sodium benzoate and/or Sodium phenylbutyrate, L-citrulline

continued

TABLE 24-1, CONTINUED

Selected Inborn Errors of Metabolism That Feature Gastrointestinal Dysfunction

Ornithine transcarbamylase (OTC) deficiency	Ornithine transcarbamylase	Stringent dietary protein restriction Sodium benzoate and/or Sodium phenylbutyrate L-citrulline Liver transplantation?
Citrullinemia	Argininosuccinate synthase	Stringent dietary protein restriction Sodium benzoate and/or Sodium phenylbutyrate L- arginine Liver transplantation?
Argininosuccinic acidemia	Argininosuccinate lyase	Stringent dietary protein restriction Sodium benzoate and/or Sodium phenylbutyrate L-arginine Liver transplantation?
N-Acetyl glutamate synthase deficiency	N-acetyl glutamate synthetase	Stringent dietary protein restriction Sodium benzoate and/or Sodium phenylbutyrate L- citrulline N-carbamyl glutamate Liver transplantation?
Hyperornithinemia-hyperammonemia -homocitrullinuria (HHH) syndrome	ORNT1 mitochondrial ornithine transporter	Stringent dietary protein restriction Sodium benzoate and/or Sodium phenylbutyrate L- citrulline
Lysinuric protein intolerance	SLC7A7	Stringent dietary protein restriction L-citrulline, HSM
Fatty Acid Oxidation Defects		
Carnitine palmitoyltransferase-I (CPT-I) deficiency	Carnitine palmitoyltransferase-I	Avoidance of fasting Carnitine may be useful Can be associated with maternal HELLP syndrome
Carnitine palmitoyltransferase-II (CPT-II) deficiency	Carnitine palmitoyltransferase-II	Avoidance of fasting Carnitine may be useful Can be associated with dysplastic kidneys and brain malformations
Carnitine-acylcarnitine translocase deficiency	Carnitine-acylcarnitine translocase	Neonatal lethality in most cases
Very long chain acyl-CoA dehydrogenase (VLCAD) deficiency	Very long chain acyl-CoA dehydrogenase	Avoidance of fasting Carnitine may be useful
Long chain 3-hydroxyl acyl-CoA dehydrogenase (LCHAD) deficiency	Long chain 3-hydroxy acyl-CoA dehydrogenase	Avoidance of fasting Carnitine therapy may promote dysrythmias Can be associated with maternal HELLP syndrome

TABLE 24-1, CONTINUED

Selected Inborn Errors of Metabolism That Feature Gastrointestinal Dysfunction

Medium chain acyl-CoA dehydrogenase deficiency	Medium chain acyl-CoA dehydrogenase	Avoidance of fasting Carnitine may be useful
Short chain acyl-CoA (SCAD) dehydrogenase deficiency	Short chain acyl-CoA dehydrogenase	Can be associated with maternal HELLP syndrome
HMG-CoA lyase deficiency	3-hydroxy-3-methylglutaryl-CoA lyase	Avoidance of fasting
Multiple Acyl-CoA dehydrogenase deficiency	ETFA, ETFB, ETFDH	Can be associated with congenital anomalies
Mitochondrial Energy Production/Primary Lactic Acidosis Syndromes		
Electron transport chain (ETC) deficiencies	Complexes I, II, III, IV (Cytochrome c oxidase), V (ATPase) of the ETC	Clinically heterogeneous, Can have prenatal manifestations
GRACILE syndrome	BCS1L gene defect	Neonatal lethality
Pyruvate carboxylase deficiency	Pyruvate carboxylase	Features neurodegeneration
PEPCK deficiency	Phosphoenolpyruvate carboxykinase	Extremely rare, may be associated with cirrhosis
Storage Disorders		
Gaucher, type II	Beta-glucosidase	Can feature nonimmune hydrops fetalis
Niemann Pick, type A	Acid sphingomyelinase	
Niemann Pick, type C	NPC1, NPC2	Can feature nonimmune hydrops fetalis
Sialidosis, type II	Neuraminidase	Can feature nonimmune hydrops fetalis
Galactosialidosis	Protective protein deficiency	Can feature nonimmune hydrops fetalis
Sialic acid transport disorder (infantile free sialic acid storage disease)	SLC17A5	Can feature nonimmune hydrops fetalis
I-cell disease	N-acetylglucosaminyl-1-phosphotransferase	Can feature nonimmune hydrops fetalis
GM1 gangliosidosis	B-galactosidase	Can feature nonimmune hydrops fetalis
Multiple sulfatase deficiency	SUMF1 (sulfatase-modifying factor-1 gene)	
Wolman disease	Acid lipase	Can feature nonimmune hydrops fetalis
Farber Disease type I	Ceramidase	Can feature nonimmune hydrops fetalis
Mucopolysaccharidosis, type VII	B-glucuronidase	Can feature nonimmune hydrops fetalis

TABLE 24-1, CONTINUED

Selected Inborn Errors of Metabolism That Feature Gastrointestinal Dysfunction

Congenital Disorders of Glycosylation		
	Multiple enzymopathies; phosphomannomutase (type I), N-acetylglucosaminyl-transferase II (type II), GDP-Man:GlcNAc2-PP-dolicholmannosyltransferase	Can feature hyperinsulinism, protein-losing enteropathy, nonimmune hydrops fetalis Oral mannose for phosphomannomutase deficiency
Sterol Synthesis Defects		
Smith-Lemli-Opitz syndrome	7-dehydrocholesterol reductase	Malformation syndrome
Lathosterolosis	3B-hydroxy steroid-delta-5 desaturase	Malformation syndrome
Desmosterolosis	24-dehydrocholesterol reductase	Malformation syndrome
Conradi-Hunermann syndrome	3B-hydroxysteroid-8,7-isomerase, others	Malformation syndrome
Mevalonic acidemia	Mevalonate kinase	Dysmorphic features, HSM
Peroxisomal Biosynthesis and Function		
Zellweger disease	Peroxisomal biogenesis defects	Dysmorphic features, malformations
Infantile Refsum disease	Peroxisomal biogenesis defects	Dysmorphic features
Bile salt metabolic defects	Delta(4)-3-oxosteroid 5β reductase, 3 β-hydroxy-Δ steroid dehydrogenase-isomerase, Oxysterol 7α-hydroxylase	Cholestatic liver disease treat first two with chenodeoxycholic acid +/- cholic acid
Metal Metabolism		
Neonatal iron storage disease/ perinatal hemochromatosis	Defect(s) uncertain	Prenatal and neonatal lethality Liver transplantation?
Juvenile hemochromatosis	hemojuvelin; hepcidin antimicrobial peptide	
Hemochromatosis, other	HFE 3 (transferrin receptor-2) HFE4 (ferroportin) Atransferrinemia Aceruloplasminemia	 Autosomal dominant inheritance Neurological syndrome
Wilson disease	ATP7B	Penicillamine
Indian childhood cirrhosis	Defect(s) uncertain	
Idiopathic copper toxicosis	Defect(s) uncertain	
Other Disorders		
Glycine-N-methyltransferase	Glycine-N-methyltransferase	A cause of hypermethionemia
Progressive Familial Intrahepatic Cholestasis Syndromes (PFIC1-4), including Byler disease (PFIC1)	ATP8B1, ABCB11, ABCB4; 3-beta-hydroxy-delta-5-C27-steroid oxidoreductase	PFIC1-3 may encode transporter proteins

Another example of an inborn error of metabolism where the liver is responsible for whole body metabolism is hyperoxalosis type I, a disorder of glyoxyalate metabolism. It is caused by a deficiency of alanine-glyoxylate aminotransferase, which is due to either a mutant protein or a mistargeting event whereby the enzyme localizes to the mitochondria in lieu of the peroxisomes, where it normally participates in glyoxyalate metabolism. Patients with this disorder progressively deposit calcium oxalate crystals throughout the body because of increased production of oxalate by the liver. The liver is spared, but many other organs—including the kidneys, heart, skin, retina, peripheral nerves, arteries, and skeleton—are not. Nephrocalcinosis eventually leads to end-stage renal failure and ultimately death. Liver or combined liver-kidney transplantation is needed to treat this disorder, depending on the duration and magnitude of the blood oxalate elevation. A liver is transplanted to stop the production of oxalate and provide a reserve for the defective enzyme, and in patients with coexisting renal failure, kidney transplantation is also required to provide essential functions and ensure adequate oxalate clearance.

The last group of metabolic disorders includes those in which the signs and symptoms can be hepatic and extrahepatic. Included are a large number of conditions, such as the urea cycle, fatty acid oxidation, and organic acid disorders, as well as others that affect storage and transport. Liver transplantation has been employed as a treatment modality in some of these diseases with variable success.[16]

Hepatic Injury

The metabolic processes within the hepatocyte, as in any cell, are closely regulated and interactive; they are responsive to external as well as internal stimuli. Central to the well-being of any cell are adequate stores of energy or the means to produce energy from readily available substrates as needed. With this energy, the cell maintains its homeostasis, grows, synthesizes material for export, exports, transports, and recycles unneeded or decaying materials. All of these processes are affected by one or more biochemical genetic disorders.

Compartmentalization of cellular functions is a necessary part of the synthetic and degradative pathways, as well as being essential for the production and maintenance of electrochemical gradients in energy production. Hepatic metabolism is quantitatively and even qualitatively different in the periportal inflow zone compared to the perivenous outflow area. Periportal cells are responsible for the majority of gluconeogenesis, glycogen synthesis by the indirect pathway, urea synthesis, and fatty acid oxidation. This regionalization may allow for discontinuous histopathologic findings during acute and less than massive metabolic insult. As the degree of hepatic injury becomes more severe, or as the duration of repeat injury increases and fibrosis occurs, the distinctions become less obvious.

Pathophysiology

For many of the biochemical genetic disorders, common histologic appearance and laboratory perturbations exist, precluding exact diagnosis without the use of extraordinary testing. The common pathways of hepatic pathophysiology include inflammation, necrosis, and cholestasis as the result of alterations in homeostasis; steatosis as the result of the accumulation of intermediates and the response to metabolic stress; and the accumulation of relatively nontoxic macromolecules, which usually alter cellular function on the basis of mass effects rather than chemical composition. It is also clear that the pathophysiology in some instances is different with many metabolic diseases if the patient is a newborn infant rather than a child or an adult. A factor that can confound diagnosis of a metabolic disorder is the nonspecific malhandling of metabolites by a diseased liver, particularly methionine and tyrosine.

Cholestasis and Hepatobiliary Disease

Cholestasis can result from multiple groups of metabolic disorders. Defects in bile acid metabolism; absence of peroxisomes; and disorders of amino acid, lipid, carbohydrate, or complex molecule degradation; metal metabolism; and transport can lead to the recognition of cholestasis.

Cystic fibrosis, an extremely common autosomal recessive disease, is due to defects in the cystic fibrosis transmembrane conductance regulator (CFTR), whose gene is located on chromosome 7q31.2. Although respiratory disease, pancreatic exocrine insufficiency, and failure to thrive are easily recognized as components of the clinical spectrum, hepatobiliary disease may be seen in very early infancy with impaired intrahepatic and extrahepatic biliary drainage. CFTR is localized to the intrahepatic biliary epithelium and is a regulator of cholangiocellular bile production. Cholestasis is believed to be secondary to defective chloride transport across this epithelium. Focal biliary cirrhosis can occur early with later evidence of steatosis and fibrosis. In a minority of patients, prolonged neonatal jaundice with cirrhotic change is seen. In rare instances, liver transplantation may be required.

Other transport system defects can also cause a cholestatic change in the liver. A series of disorders—the progressive familial intrahepatic cholestasis syndromes—feature mutations in a variety of proteins likely involved in cannilicular transport. Four distinct genetic loci exist, and mutations have been demonstrated in patients from diverse backgrounds, including the Old Order Amish[17] and an Eskimo isolate from Greenland.[18] Three of the genes appear to encode transport-related proteins while the fourth encodes a steroid oxidoreductase.[19-21]

Bile acid synthetic defects can present with cholestatic liver disease and progress to cirrhosis.[22] A number of these rare enzymopathies are known to exist and it is likely that others remain to be discovered. Cheondeoxycholic acid and cholic acid can be used to treat patients with these disorders, in some instances, with great efficacy.

The genetic basis of other cholestatic syndromes, such as North American Indian childhood cirrhosis, appears to involve novel proteins and illustrates that the current understanding of the mechanisms of cholestasis are far from complete.[23]

Hepatocellular Necrosis

Hepatocellular necrosis manifesting with jaundice, edema, ascites, hepatic synthetic failure, or hepatic encephalopathy is a major common pathology due to catabolic errors. The laboratory studies show variable degrees of elevation of serum transaminases, hypoglycemia, hyperammonemia, hypofibrinogenemia, and hypoprothrombinemia. The clinical picture is similar to that of sepsis, and the laboratory findings can be indistinguishable from those of a severe viral hepatitis.

Galactosemia is a typical example of a disorder in this group. Classic galactosemia is due to a severe deficiency of hepatic galactose-1-phosphate uridyl transferase (GALT) activity. As a result of significant impairment of the function of the enzyme, a syndrome of neonatal-onset toxicity occurs when the at-risk infant is exposed to significant amounts of dietary lactose or galactose. The toxic metabolites are galactose-1-phosphate (a substrate of the enzyme) and galactitol (the result of aldose reductase activity on the sugar). Because there is trapping of cellular phosphate as galactose-1-phosphate, hepatic intracellular adenosine triphosphate/adenosine diphosphate ratios may be altered. Interference with other enzymatic systems has been postulated. Both mechanisms can lead to severe acute hepatocellular damage, which is reversible if treated immediately. The acute manifestations of the disease in the extended neonatal period often are noted within a few days of the onset of milk feedings. Vomiting and diarrhea are common. Most patients present with jaundice caused by an unconjugated hyperbilirubinemia. Severe hemolysis occurs in some patients so that the clinical presentation resembles erythroblastosis fetalis. Ascites has been a prominent early finding. With the progression of hepatic disease, bile stasis, pseudoacinar formation, and portal fibrosis are seen. An end-stage cirrhotic liver can result whose histology is indistinguishable from that of other metabolic etiologies. Laboratory findings include derangements of hepatic function, albuminuria, hyperaminoaciduria, hyperchloremic metabolic acidosis, hypergalactosuria, and elevated blood galactose concentrations. There is increased production and elimination of galactitol and the presence of increased concentrations of tissue galactose-1-phosphate. In the untreated state, alterations in carbohydrate composition of glycoproteins can be seen paralleling the congenital disorders of glycosylation.

The other affected organ systems in the neonate include the lens of the eye, the CNS, the immune system, and the renal tubules. Increased synthesis of galactitol in the lens is associated with cataract formation. CNS findings in the infant include alterations in the level of consciousness and hypotonia. Cerebral edema and increased intracranial pressure can occur. A high frequency of *Escherichia coli* sepsis has been noted with fulminant courses. With prompt supportive therapy and the elimination of lactose and galactose from the diet, the acute toxicity syndrome resolves. Chronic, or long-term, effects of GALT deficiency occur in the CNS and ovary.

Hereditary fructose intolerance (HFI) usually presents with vomiting, diarrhea, and sometimes hypoglycemia. Symptoms are related to the ingestion of fructose or sucrose. The pathophysiology includes phosphate trapping, with resultant similar intrahepatic pathologic progression in the face of additional carbohydrate, and, as in galactosemia, there is renal tubular dysfunction. Beneficial effects from the withdrawal of the offending carbohydrates are seen in 2 to 3 days. Older patients characteristically avoid sucrose and have an unusual history of not having any dental caries. Two common mutations are known in the Caucasian population and molecular diagnosis is possible in some cases.

Neonatal iron storage disease, or perinatal hemochromatosis, is a disorder resulting from severe prenatal hepatic disease. There is no single etiology for the disease; nor is there a clear genetic link to any single enzymatic defect, although a recessive pattern of inheritance seems likely. The liver shows diffuse fibrosis with hepatocellular nodular regeneration and ductal transformation. Siderosis in the apical cytoplasm of the tubular hepatocytes is typical. Some patients have had Down syndrome. A newer entity, GRACILE, reported in Finish infants, presents with growth retardation, lactic acidemia, anemia, and hemochromatosis.[24] The defect is in the BCS1L gene, involved in the assembly of complex III of the respiratory chain, and has been mapped to a locus on 2q33.37 and cloned. Other conditions may feature neonatal hemochromatosis, such as the tricho-hepato-enteric syndrome.[25] The neonatal onset cases, regardless of distinct etiology, all seem to share severe affectation and a difficult clinical course.

Juvenile hemochromatosis, another form of primary hemochromatosis, can be caused by mutations in hemojuvelin[26] or the gene encoding hepcidin antimicrobial peptide.[27] This condition, like the more commonly seen adult variant caused by mutations in the HFE gene, can feature severe iron overload with hepatocytic iron deposition, liver fibrosis, hypogonadotrophic hypogonadism, and cardiac involvement. Two other genetic forms of primary hemochromatosis are also known. HFE3 is caused by mutations in the gene encoding transferrin receptor-2 and is intermediate in severity.[28] HFE4, the only documented autosomal dominant form of the disease, is caused by a mutant ferroportin gene.[29]

Other inborn errors of metabolisms can feature hepatocytic iron deposition by unclear mechanisms. Atransferrinemia, caused by mutation in the structural gene for transferrin, produces a syndrome of microcytic anemia and iron overload and is treated by plasma infusions to provide functional transferrin. Aceruloplasminemia produces a syndrome of hepatic and CNS iron deposition. The basal ganglia seem to be most affected and the syndrome is dominated by neurological signs. Ceruloplasmin is low, as is serum iron, but excessive iron deposition is seen in the liver, brain, and pancreas.

Disorders of copper metabolism are another group of important metal metabolic diseases. The prototype is Wilson disease, an autosomal recessive disorder characterized by intracellular hepatic copper accumulation, cirrhosis, and, in a sizable number of patients, neurologic abnormalities. The primary defect resides in the ATP7B gene, which encodes a polypeptide that acts as a membrane copper-transport protein. The protein likely plays a role in intracellular copper delivery as well as release of copper into the bile. Like galactosemia and hereditary fructose intolerance, patients with Wilson disease can have a renal tubulopathy featuring aminoaciduria and phosphaturia. Neurological and psychiatric presentations are well described. Chelation therapy can be used to enhance copper excretion. Some patients with hepatic failure will need liver transplantation. Another group of less well-characterized disorders of copper overload exist; these include Indian childhood cirrhosis and idiopathic copper toxicosis. The exact basis of these disorders is not known at present.

Urea cycle enzyme disorders may appear as early as 1 to 3 days of age. Infants show combinations of vomiting, lethargy, increased respiratory drive, and CNS dysfunction that may progress to seizure activity. Their glucose concentrations are normal, with normal or slightly alkalotic blood pHs. Markedly elevated plasma ammonium concentrations are a common feature. Blood urea nitrogen concentrations may be low. The common pathogenesis is an inability to detoxify ammonia, which is produced as the result of the catabolism of amino acids. Thus, either protein ingestion or catabolic stress can trigger hyperammonemia. The presentation of the individual disorders is nonspecific, and specialized laboratory testing such as quantitative plasma amino acid analysis and measurement of urinary orotic acid concentration is used to separate the diseases. The enzymes of ureagenesis are present in intestinal, renal, and hepatic compartments, but only in the liver are the full complement of activities of the urea cycle present to enable the conversion of NH3 to urea. In the liver, only the proximal enzymes N-acetyl glutamate synthase, carbamoylphosphate synthetase, and ornithine transcarbamylase are localized within the mitochondrial matrix. In biopsied material examined by electron microscopy, pleomorphic mitochondria with swollen cristae and electron-dense matrices are seen. Other hepatocellular changes include alterations in the appearance of the endoplasmic reticulum. Chronic injury, as the result of either prolonged hyperammonemia or repeated episodes of metabolic crisis, may cause portal fibrosis. Synthetic function of the liver is normal, although elevations in serum transaminases can occur. Such elevations may be present between episodes of hyperammonemia and despite the use of ammonia-trapping agents and enhancers of alternative nitrogen metabolic pathways. In the acute hyperammonemic crisis, detoxification by hemodialysis or hemofiltration may be essential.

In alpha1-antitrypsin deficiency due to the PI ZZ phenotype, the protein has a lysine residue instead of a glutamic acid at position 342. The altered protein is not secreted, because the reactive loop center of one molecule is inserted into the beta-pleated sheet structure of a second molecule. This protein is retained within the endoplasmic reticulum, as is reflected by the accumulation of periodic acid–Schiff (PAS)–positive diastase-resistant material. In some susceptible individuals, the accumulation of the abnormal protein damages the endoplasmic reticulum or Golgi membranes, leading to hepatocellular damage and cirrhosis. Liver transplantation is required in some instances.

Tyrosinemia Type I can present in early infancy with varying degrees of hepatomegaly and a mild elevation of serum transaminases. The biochemical lesion is a defect in fumarylacetoacetate hydrolase. Common features also include abnormalities of coagulation, with clotting factors often markedly reduced. Vitamin K does not correct the disorder. Renal dysfunction is usually evident. A porphyuric presentation with neuropathy due to increased succinylacetone can be seen in the acute setting. Specialized testing (ie, quantitive analysis of plasma amino acids by anion exchange chromatography) usually reveals hypertyrosinemia, an increased urinary excretion of succinylacetone, and an elevated serum alpha-fetoprotein concentration. The hepatic disease is progressive and advances from microscopic cirrhosis, which can be seen in the first weeks of life, to macronodular cirrhosis with regenerating nodules. Hepatocellular carcinomas are frequent. In this disorder, biochemical abnormalities may be seen prenatally. The molecular mechanism of the hepatic and renal damage is not known, although the intracellular compartmentalization of toxic metabolites has been proposed to induce local damage. The inhibition of 4-hydroxyphenylpyruvate dioxygenase by fumarylacetoacetate is a major factor in the recognized biochemical abnormalities, and treatment with 2-(nitro-4-trifluoromethylbenzoyl)-1,3-cyclohexanedione (NTBC) corrects these but does not always prevent the progression to hepatocellular carcinoma.

Steatosis

Steatosis can be associated at some point in the natural history of a number of the organic acidopathies that result from enzymatic defects in the metabolism of branched-chain amino acids or odd-chain fatty acids. Propionic acidemia, due to defects in either subunit of the heterodimeric propionyl coenzyme A carboxylase, is a prototype for these diseases. Affected infants present with severe metabolic acidosis, refusal to feed, vomiting, and alterations in CNS function. Hepatomegaly is found in a fraction of the patients. The livers at autopsy have shown fatty infiltration and necrosis, and the reticuloendothelial cells may have increased iron deposits. The exact mechanism of the fat deposition is unknown but may relate to an imbalance between the rate of fat synthesis and the rate of export of lipoproteins. Laboratory findings of a metabolic ketoacidosis with hyperammonemia and hyperglycinemia are characteristic during the initial presentation and subsequent metabolic crises.

Almost all the disorders of beta-oxidation of fatty acids from defects in carnitine palmitoyltransferase I, carnitine/acylcarnitine translocase, and carnitine palmitoyltransferase II through to the utilization of hydroxy-, medium-chain or short-chain fatty acids have been associated with some degree of hepatic dysfunction and fat accumulation. In the majority of cases when histology has been performed, the accumulation occurs as macrovesicular lipid storage. Hypothetical mechanisms of fat accumulation in these disorders include effects of a constant supply of fatty acids with a block in their utilization, increased availability of glycerol, and net intracellular accumulation.

Hepatic Pathology Resulting From Peroxisomal Disease

The absence of hepatocyte organelles and their functions can result in recognized hepatic disease in late fetal or early infant life. The best characterized group of these disorders includes those due to the peroxisomal diseases, which comprise a group of disorders with effects on multiple viscera, skeletal development, and the CNS. Zellweger disease, the paradigm for peroxisomal disorders, is caused by biosynthetic defects in the formation of the peroxisome. As a result, more than 50 enzymes involved in multiple pathways can be perturbed. The peroxisomes are responsible for the oxidation of amino acids, alcohols, dicarboxylic acids, pipecolic acid, and phytanic acid, as well as very long chain fatty acids. They are also essential for the synthesis of bile acids, ether-phospholipids such as the plasmalogens, and cholesterol, and they are a major reservoir of the hydrogen peroxide–degrading enzyme, catalase. Zellweger disease was also called cerebrohepatorenal disease because of the organ systems involved in the neonate. The infants have distinct dysmorphic features, an enlarged fontanelle, profound hypotonia, hepatomegaly, and neurodegeneration. Neuronal migratory defects are often seen. The liver has micronodular cirrhosis and fibrosis on examination. The laboratory abnormalities are explained by the missing multiple enzyme functions. Diagnosis can be strongly suspected by the constellation of physical findings and is confirmed by the abnormalities in very long chain fatty acid metabolism. The dysmorphia varies with the severity of the defect. For example, infantile Refsum disease, considered to be a milder phenotype of the peroxisomal biogenesis disorders, generally presents with failure to thrive and milder degrees of hepatocellular dysfunction in older infants or toddlers with dysmorphic facial features.

Hepatic Disease Due to Glycosylation Defect

Disorders of glycosylation result from various defects in the formation or processing of the carbohydrate residues attached by N- or O-linkages of peptides. These disorders can be considered prelysosomal storage disorders, as improperly glycosylated proteins initially accumulate in the endoplasmic reticulum. This may, in turn, lead to cellular dysfunction via the unfolded peptide response. The most common hepatic pathology is steatosis, but hydrops and severe hepatocellular dysfunction have been reported. Common clinical manifestations include failure to thrive, GI dysfunction or dysmotility, hypotonia, cognitive delays, and alterations in fat distribution.

Hepatic Disease Due to Mitochondrial Dysfunction

Multiple reports have described infants with severe or fatal hepatic disease of early onset due to a mitochondrial depletion syndrome. In some cases, increased fat has been seen histologically; however, ultrastructural examination of other patients' tissues has shown increased numbers of mitochondria with morphologic abnormalities, and even glycogen storage within the mitochondria. Focal biliary necrosis has been reported, but fibrosis is a later finding. Lactic acidosis, hypoglycemia, and synthetic defects have also been reported. In all cases, activities of the electron transport chain complexes with subunits encoded by mitochondrial DNA have been reduced. The amount of mitochondrial DNA has been reduced to less than 10% of normal. Mutations in the deoxyguanosine kinase gene have been identified in some patients.

Hepatic Disease Due to Storage Disorders

Material either synthesized within the cell or accumulated through endocytic processes as part of the body's recycling of macromolecules is the sine qua non of the heterogeneous storage disorders. In the GSDs type I, III, or IV presenting in early infancy, there is accumulation of glycogen as well as fat. GSD type I should also be thought of as a steatosis disorder. In Niemann-Pick type A, sphingomyelin accumulates in hepatocytes, as well as in the reticuloendothelial elements, but in Niemann-Pick type C, the accumulated material includes both sphingomyelin and cholesterol. In the latter disorder, hepatocellular necrosis and a progression to fibrosis can also occur, blurring the distinctions made here about disorders primarily associated with hepatocytic dysfunction or storage with minimally altered hepatocytes. The accumulation and storage of glucocerebroside in Kupffer cells in Gaucher disease and of glycolipids and complex lipids in other disorders leads to liver enlargement but relatively little hepatocellular functional abnormality. In many cases, the histopathology and histochemical staining patterns can identify the disorder.

Hepatic Disease Due to Porphyrias

The heme biosynthetic pathway begins in the mitochondria with a condensation reaction of glycine and succinyl-CoA and ends with the production of heme, which is then used for hemoglobin formation in the bone marrow and, of equal importance, for cytochrome formation. Defects in any of the steps in this pathway represent a group of eight disorders that can feature cutaneous, psychiatric, neurologic, and hepatic symptoms. One disorder of this group, protoporphyria, can be associated with severe liver disease that can require liver transplantation. A detailed discussion of these conditions is beyond the scope of this chapter.

Other Disorders With Primary Gastrointestinal Disturbances

Chronic diarrhea can be a manifestation of a number of inborn errors of metabolism, including lactase and sucrase-isomaltase deficiencies, glucose-galactose malabsorption, congenital chloride diarrhea, and congenital secretory diarrhea due to defective sodium/hydrogen exchange. Diarrhea, malabsorption, and protein-losing enteropathy can also be features of other disorders discussed in this chapter, such as cystic fibrosis, lysinergic protein intolerance, and phosphomannose isomerase deficiency. Selective vitamin malabsorption disorders, such as congenital folate malabsorption, the intestinal biotin transporter defect,[30] and Imerslund-Grasbeck disease[31] might also be included as metabolic disorders where the primary defect lies in the GI tract.

Conclusion

A wide variety of catabolic, anabolic, and transport defects affecting the GI tract can be recognized. The age of presentation ranges from mid-gestation to adulthood and encompasses a wide range of symptoms and signs, some of which are nonspecific. For some disorders, the pathophysiology has been delineated and molecular determinants characterized, but in the majority only the broader features are currently comprehended. Increased awareness of inborn errors of metabolism, in particular with the goal of earlier diagnosis, is a constant challenge for providers. A low threshold for biochemical genetic evaluation in patients presenting with symptoms suggestive of hereditary metabolic disease is desirable.

References

1. Scriver CR, Beaudet AL, Sly WS, et al. *The Metabolic and Molecular Bases of Inherited Disease*. New York, NY: McGraw-Hill; 2001:2165-2192.
2. Ibdah JA, Bennett MJ, Rinaldo P, et al. A fetal fatty-acid oxidation disorder as a cause of liver disease in pregnant women. *N Engl J Med.* 1999;340(22):1723-1731.
3. Innes AM, Seargeant LE, Balachandra K, et al. Hepatic carnitine palmitoyltransferase I deficiency presenting as maternal illness in pregnancy. *Pediatr Res.* 2000;47(1):43-45.
4. Matern D, Hart P, Murtha AP, et al. Acute fatty liver of pregnancy associated with short-chain acyl-coenzyme A dehydrogenase deficiency. *J Pediatr.* 2001;138(4):585-588.
5. von Kleist-Retzow JC, Cormier-Daire V, Viot G, et al. Antenatal manifestations of mitochondrial respiratory chain deficiency. *J Pediatr.* 2003;143(2):208-212.
6. Kerrigan JF, Aleck KA, Tarby TJ, Bird CR, Heidenreich RA. Fumaric aciduria: clinical and imaging features. *Ann Neurol.* 2000;47(5):583-588.
7. Chisholm CA, Vavelidis F, Lovell MA, et al. Prenatal diagnosis of multiple acyl-CoA dehydrogenase deficiency: association with elevated alpha-fetoprotein and cystic renal changes. *Prenat Diagn.* 2001;21(10):856-859.
8. Strom EH, Stromme P, Westvik J, Pedersen SJ. Renal cysts in the carbohydrate-deficient glycoprotein syndrome. *Pediatr Nephrol.* 1993;7(3):253-255.
9. Wanders RJ. Metabolic and molecular basis of peroxisomal disorders: a review. *Am J Med Genet A.* 2004;126(4):355-375.
10. Elpeleg ON, Hammerman C, Saada A, et al. Antenatal presentation of carnitine palmitoyltransferase II deficiency. *Am J Med Genet.* 2001;102(2):183-187.
11. Kelley RI, Herman GE. Inborn errors of sterol biosynthesis. *Annu Rev Genomics Hum Genet.* 2001;2:299-341.
12. de Koning TJ, Nikkels PG, Dorland L, et al. Congenital hepatic fibrosis in 3 siblings with phosphomannose isomerase deficiency. *Virchows Arch.* 2000;437(1):101-105.
13. Adam G, Brereton RJ, Agrawal M, Lake BD. Biliary atresia and meconium ileus associated with Niemann-Pick disease. *J Pediatr Gastroenterol Nutr.* 1988;7(1):128-131.
14. Matthews RP, Russo P, Berry GT, Piccoli DA, Rand EB. Biliary atresia associated with a fatty acid oxidation defect. *J Pediatr Gastroenterol Nutr.* 2002;35(5):624-628.
15. Stone DL, Sidransky E. Hydrops fetalis: lysosomal storage disorders in extremis. *Adv Pediatr.* 1999;46:409-440.
16. Leonard JV, Walter JH, McKiernan PJ. The management of organic acidaemias: the role of transplantation. *J Inherit Metab Dis.* 2001;24(2):309-311.
17. Bull LN, van Eijk MJ, Pawlikowska L, et al. A gene encoding a P-type ATPase mutated in two forms of hereditary cholestasis. *Nature Genet.* 1998;18:219-224.
18. Klomp LW, Bull LN, Knisely AS, et al. A missense mutation in FIC1 is associated with Greenland familial cholestasis. *Hepatology.* 2000;32(6):1337-1341.
19. Schwarz M, Wright AC, Davis DL, Nazer H, Bjorkhem I, Russell DW. The bile acid synthetic gene 3-beta-hydroxy-delta-5-C27-steroid oxidoreductase is mutated in progressive intrahepatic cholestasis. *J Clin Invest.* 2000;106:1175-1184.
20. Strautnieks SS, Bull LN, Knisely AS, et al. A gene encoding a liver-specific ABC transporter is mutated in progressive familial intrahepatic cholestasis. *Nat Genet.* 1998;20(3):233-238.
21. de Vree JM, Jacquemin E, Sturm E, et al. Mutations in the MDR3 gene cause progressive familial intrahepatic cholestasis. *Proc Natl Acad Sci USA.* 1998;95(1):282-287.
22. Bove KE, Heubi JE, Balistreri WF, Setchell KD. Bile acid synthetic defects and liver disease: a comprehensive review. *Pediatr Dev Pathol.* 2004;7(4):315-334.
23. Chagnon P, Michaud J, Mitchell G, et al. A missense mutation (R565W) in cirhin (FLJ14728) in North American Indian childhood cirrhosis. *Am J Hum Genet.* 2002;71(6):1443-1449.
24. Visapaa I, Fellman V, Vesa J, et al. GRACILE syndrome, a lethal metabolic disorder with iron overload, is caused by a point mutation in BCS1L. *Am J Hum Genet.* 2002;71(4):863-876.
25. Verloes A, Lombet J, Lambert Y, et al. Tricho-hepato-enteric syndrome: further delineation of a distinct syndrome with neonatal hemochromatosis phenotype, intractable diarrhea, and hair anomalies. *Am J Med Genet.* 1997;68(4):391-395.
26. Papanikolaou G, Samuels ME, Ludwig EH, et al. Mutations in HFE2 cause iron overload in chromosome 1q-linked juvenile hemochromatosis. *Nat Genet.* 2004;36(1):77-82.
27. Roetto A, Papanikolaou G, Politou M, et al. Mutant antimicrobial peptide hepcidin is associated with severe juvenile hemochromatosis. *Nat Genet.* 2003;33(1):21-22.
28. Camaschella C, Roetto A, Cali A, et al. The gene TFR2 is mutated in a new type of haemochromatosis mapping to 7q22. *Nat Genet.* 2000;25:14-15.
29. Njajou OT, Vaessen N, Joosse M, et al. A mutation in SLC11A3 is associated with autosomal dominant hemochromatosis. *Nat Genet.* 2001;28(3):213-214.
30. Mardach R, Zempleni J, Wolf B, et al. Biotin dependency due to a defect in biotin transport. *J Clin Invest.* 2002;109(12):1617-1623.
31. Aminoff M, Carter JE, Chadwick RB, et al. Mutations in CUBN, encoding the intrinsic factor-vitamin B12 receptor, cubilin, cause hereditary megaloblastic anaemia 1. *Nat Genet.* 1999;21(3):309-313.
32. Verhoeven NM, Huck JH, Roos B, et al. Transaldolase deficiency: liver cirrhosis associated with a new inborn error in the pentose phosphate pathway. *Am J Hum Genet.* 2001;68(5):1086-1092.

Chapter 25

Nutrition and Cystic Fibrosis

Elisabeth Luder, PhD

Introduction

Cystic fibrosis (CF) is the most frequent lethal genetic disorder among Caucasians. The disease is caused by alterations of the CF transmembrane regulator (CFTR) protein, a cAMP-activated chloride channel located in the apical membrane of most secretory cells.[1] Classic (severe) CF reflects two loss-of-function mutations in the CFTR gene and is characterized by chronic bacterial infection of the airways and sinuses, fat maldigestion due to pancreatic exocrine insufficiency, infertility in males due to obstructive azoospermia, and elevated concentration of chloride (90 to 100 mmol/L) in sweat[1,2] (Table 25-1). Patients with nonclassic (mild) CF have at least one copy of a mutant gene that confers partial function of the CFTR protein, and such patients usually have no overt signs of maldigestion because some pancreatic exocrine function is preserved and the sweat chloride concentration is usually lower (60 to 90 mmol/L). Some CFTR mutations that result in residual CFTR function have been linked to disease of one organ, such as late-onset pulmonary disease, congenital bilateral disease of the vas deferens, or idiopatic pancreatitis.[1,2] Many of these complications can interfere with nutrient intake, assimilation, or utilization. This chapter will discuss the recent development regarding the pathogenesis of this disorder, its nutritional complications, and management of these complications.

Pathogenesis of Cystic Fibrosis

Major advances in the understanding of the pathogenesis of the disease have included the discovery of the CF gene and demonstration of impaired epithelial chloride transport. More than 1000 mutations have been discovered since 1989, when investigators described the most common CFTR allele known as ΔF508.[1,2] Although CF is primarily a disease of Caucasians, the incidence of CF has been described in virtually every race and varies, depending on region, ancestry, and CFTR allele prevalence in reproducing populations. In the United States, the incidence is one CF homozygote or compound heterozygote patient for every 3500 live births, which reflects a predicted CF heterozygote frequency of 1 in 30. In the nonwhite US populations, the incidence has been calculated at 1:12163, predicting a heterozygote frequency of 1 in 65 African Americans and 1 in 46 Hispanic Americans.[3]

The survival of CF patients has been increasing during the past four decades. The report from the US Cystic Fibrosis Foundation (CFF) patient registry for 2001 included 22,732 patients ranging in age from 1 month to 74 years and showed a medial survival of 33.4 years. In 2001, approximately 40% of patients were older than 18 years. It should be emphasized that the CFF-registered patients reflect the diagnostic and therapeutic modes of the past several decades and the majority of the older patients did not have access as children to recent advances in nutritional and respiratory care.[4] In contrast, patients diagnosed early through newborn screening show a relative flat survival curve, leading to longevity estimates exceeding 50 years.[5]

Genotype and Phenotype Correlations in Cystic Fibrosis

The most common disease-causing mutation, accounting for approximately 66% to 70% of CF chromosomes worldwide, gives rise to a deletion of a single amino acid, phenylalanine, at position 508 (ΔF508) of the CFTR product.[1] Although more than 1000 other mutations have been described, most of them are rare. The

TABLE 25-1.

Classic and Nonclassic Cystic Fibrosis

Classic Cystic Fibrosis (no functional CFTR protein)	*Nonclassic Cystic Fibrosis (some functional CFTR protein, providing survival advantage)*
Chronic sinusitis	Chronic sinusitis
Severe chronic bacterial infection of airways	Chronic bacterial infection of airways (later onset, but variable)
Severe hepatobiliary disease (5% to 10% of cases)	
Pancreatic exocrine insufficiency	Adequate pancreatic exocrine function (usually); pancreatitis (5% to 20% of cases)
Meconium ileus at birth (15% to 20% of cases)	
Sweat chloride value usually 90 to 110 mmol/L; sometimes 60 to 90 mmol/L	Sweat chloride value usually 60 to 90 mmol/L; sometimes normal (<40 mmol/L)
Obstructive ozoospermia	Obstructive ozoospermia

Reprinted from Knowles MR, Durie PR. What is cystic fibrosis? *N Engl J Med.* 2002;347:439-442.

type of genetic mutation is not always predictive of CFTR function. As increasing numbers of mutations have been identified, there have been attempts to classify the different mutations into five classes according to the functional properties of the encoded gene product with respect to chloride regulation in the apical membrane of epithelial cells.[6,7]

Class I represents gene mutations for which the intact CFTR protein product is not found. Class II represents the forms of mutant CFTR that fail to reach the apical membrane under physiologic conditions. Class III mutant CFTR proteins include those that are inserted into the apical cell membrane but fail to respond to stimulation by cAMP. Class IV mutants produce proteins that reach the apical membrane and generate cAMP-regulated apical membrane chloride current but have altered channel properties resulting in a reduction in the amount of current. Class V mutations result in reduced synthesis of normally functioning CFTR because of defective processing or aberrant splicing of alternative sites. The Class IV and Class V mutations have a strong association with the pancreatic sufficient phenotype.[6,7]

Major Clinical Problems in Cystic Fibrosis

PULMONARY DISEASE IN CYSTIC FIBROSIS

The large number of CFTR mutations, the variable impact of these mutations on the protein, and the wide spectrum of phenotypic expression of the disease prompted the search for a correlation between the molecular defect of the CFTR gene and the clinical heterogeneity of the disease.[1,2] Respiratory disorders account for about 95% of mortality in CF patients, but the severity of respiratory expression is highly heterogenous among CF patients. Mucous obstruction and infections are the typical causes of the respiratory phenotype. The hypersecretion of dense mucous and its accumulation in conducting airways gradually obstructs the small airways. The altered composition of the mucous and the consequent reduced mucocilliary clearance and possible alteration of local defense mechanisms give rise to colonization of the airways by opportunistic bacteria—ie, *Staphylococcous aureus* (particularly in the first two years of life), *Pseudomonas* (P) *aeroginosa, Burkholderia* (B) *cepacia*, and *Haemophilus influenzae*. Associated with chronic infection is inflammation, a process thought to lead to destruction of the airways.[8]

In affected patients, pulmonary function tests typically show a reduction in forced expiratory volume (FEV) and in forced vital capacity, but the magnitude of alteration varies greatly among CF patients.[9] Links between pulmonary expression and CFTR genotype are debatable. Several findings suggest that the pulmonary phenotype is directly related to the CFTR genotype or that genetic factors, inherited independently of CFTR, could modulate pulmonary expression.[10] Studies of "mild" or nonclassic CF describe that these patients have better nutritional status and better overall survival. Although the lung disease is variable, patients with nonclassic CF usually have late-onset or more slowly progressive lung disease.[2,11]

Appropriate antibiotic therapy directed against bacterial pathogens isolated from the respiratory tract is an essential component in the management of CF lung disease. Most clinicians prescribe antibiotic therapies in three distinct clinical settings during the lifespan of an individual with CF. First, during early lung disease, patients may receive

TABLE 25-2.

Gastrointestinal/Hepatic Complications of Cystic Fibrosis

Esophagus	Gastroesophageal reflux Esophagitis ± strictures
Gastroduodenum	Peptic ulcers
Small intestine	Neonatal meconium ileus Distal intestinal obstruction syndrome Intussusception Appendiceal disease Crohn's disease Ileal carcinoma
Large intestine	Fecal impaction Rectal prolapse Crohn's disease Colonic strictures
Pancreas	Pancreatic insufficiency Cystic fibrosis related diabetes (CFRD) Pancreatitis (in pancreatic sufficient patients) Pancreatic adenocarcinoma
Liver	Steatosis Focal biliary cirrhosis Multilobular cirrhosis Portal hypertension Liver failure
Biliary tract	Micro/nonfunctioning gallbladder Cholelithiasis Distal common bile duct stenosis Cholangiocarcinoma

Adapted from Borowitz D, Baker RD, Stallings V. Consensus report on nutrition for pediatric patients with cystic fibrosis. *J Pediatr Gastroenterol Nutr.* 2002;35:246-259; Rudolph CD, Mazur LJ, Liptak GS, et al. Guidelines for evaluation and treatment of gastroesophageal reflux in infants and children:recommendations of the North American Society for Pediatric Gastroenterology and Nutrition. *J Pediatr Gastroenterol Nutr.* 2001;32 (Suppl 2):S1-S31; Sokol RJ, Durie PR. Recommendations for management of liver and biliary tract disease in cystic fibrosis. Cystic Fibrosis Foundation Hepatobiliary Disease Consensus Group. *J Pediatr Gastroenterol.* Nutr. 1999;28 (Suppl 1):S1-S13.

antibiotics to delay the onset of chronic colonization with *Pseudomonas* (P) *aeruginosa*. Second, once patients are colonized with pathogens, chronic maintenance antibiotics are administered to slow decline in pulmonary function and reduce frequency and morbidity of pulmonary exacerbation. Third, at the time of periodic exacerbations in pulmonary symptoms, intensive antibiotic regimens (intravenous) are frequently administered to relieve symptomatology and restore pulmonary function to baseline values.[8]

The progression of lung disease and frequent exacerbation of chronic infections may lead to anorexia and decreased nutrient and caloric intake and may adversely affect the nutritional status of the patients. The prevention of malnutrition is associated with increased survival.[12] The evidence supporting aggressive nutrition intervention in severely malnourished patients in an effort to improve prognosis is less clear.[13]

Gastrointestinal Disease in Cystic Fibrosis

There is a wide spectrum of gastrointestinal (GI) diseases in CF (Table 25-2). Many of these problems interfere with nutritional intake and assimilation and therefore need to be considered when investigating the cause of malnutrition in CF.[14,15] Esophagitis may produce severe symptoms of heartburn and nausea but commonly can present with anorexia alone. The exact extent of these problems is unknown, but gastroesophageal reflux disease (GERD) occurs with increased frequency in patients with CF of all ages and can cause pulmonary symptoms and poor growth, and a large percent of these patients may develop esophagitis.[16,17] Given this high incidence, patients with persistent anorexia should be investigated for GERD and esophagitis and treated appropriately.[14,15]

Meconium Ileus

Meconium ileus is one of the earliest intestinal manifestations of CF. It affects up to 15% of CF neonates and is a disease seen in infants with pancreatic insufficiency. Patients classically present soon after birth with symptoms of bowel obstruction due to inspissated meconium in the distal small intestine. Gastro graffin enemas have been used extensively as diagnostic and therapeutic tools for the management of uncomplicated meconium ileus.[18] Complicated meconium ileus, requiring operative intervention, carries a higher early mortality rate and a higher incidence of distal intestinal obstruction syndrome (DIOS) and surgical complications.[19] Studies in the past reported that the overall outcome for these patients in terms of survival appears to be similar to that of CF patients who do not suffer from meconium ileus. However, two large epidemiological studies demonstrated that patients with meconium ileus experience more severe malnutrition, greater risk of acquiring *P aeruginosa* and having poor lung function, and greater mortality risk compared with patients without meconium.[20,21] A multicenter study on 197 pairs of CF siblings described a CF modifier locus for meconium ileus on chromosome,[19] which gives some insight as to why meconium ileus occurs in only a small proportion of patients with pancreatic insufficiency and CF.[22]

Distal Intestinal Obstruction Syndrome

From the age of 5 to 15 years and onward, DIOS has an estimated prevalence of 15%. It presents as recurrent, crampy, abdominal pain with distension, occasional vomiting, and decreased stooling suggestive of bowel obstruction. DIOS results from inspissation and impact of fecal material in the terminal ileum and cecum, which can be palpated as a tender mass in the right lower quadrant. In evaluating a patient with CF who has abdominal pain, in addition to DIOS, a wide range of possibilities should be considered including intussusception, fibrosing colonopathy, and appendicitis.[23,24] Thus, in patients with suspected DIOS who fail to respond to the administration of a large volume polyethylene glycal-balanced electrolyte solution given orally or nasogastrically,[25] further studies may be required to differentiate the disorder.[24]

Liver and Biliary Tract Disease in Cystic Fibrosis

The prevalence of significant liver disease in children with CF is estimated to be 17% to 25%,[26] but the true prevalence might be higher.[27] The difficulty lies in the spectrum of liver disease that includes neonatal cholestasis, hepatomegaly, and persistent enzyme elevation, to the more classical focal biliary cirrhosis. It may be that CF-associated liver disease represents a heterogeneous group of liver pathology and is not simply a result of bile ductular inspissation and damage.[27] Potentially, these complications can interfere with appetite or absorption and therefore contribute to the presence of malnutrition. The reader is referred to the Consensus Conference on liver and biliary disease in CF.[27]

Pancreatic Disease in Cystic Fibrosis

Endocrine Disease—Cystic Fibrosis-Related Diabetes Mellitis

Cystic fibrosis related diabetes (CFRD) is a distinct form of diabetes mellitus seen in pancreatic-insufficient CF patients. CFRD differs from type 1 or type 2 diabetes, with respect to both etiology and clinical presentation. (Diabetes is discussed in Chapter 16.) It is speculated that glucose intolerance is caused by a deficiency of insulin as a reduction in the beta cell mass in pancreatic islets.[28] Supporting this supposition is the age-related increase in the prevalence of CFRD, together with its strong association with the pancreatic insufficiency status. CFRD is an important complication of CF that needs to be screened for and managed appropriately as it is associated with detrimental effects on the nutritional status, including derangements in protein metabolism. Furthermore, patients with uncontrolled CFRD are at risk of developing complications, including nephropathy, neuropathy, and hypertension.[29,30]

Diagnostic criteria for CFRD are similar to those for other forms of diabetes:[30,31]

1. Fasting plasma glucose >126 mg/dL (7.0 mM) on two or more occasions
2. Fasting plasma glucose >126 mg/dL (7.0 mM) plus a casual glucose level of 200 mg/dL (11.1 mM)
3. Casual glucose level >200 mg/dL (11.1 mM) on two or more occasions with symptoms; and
4. Two-hour plasma glucose >200 mg/dL (11.0 mM) during a standard 75 g OGTT.

Once identified, the care of CFRD should be focused on providing a high energy intake, with 35% to 40% of calories from fat, to ensure normal weight gain, growth, and development in children and adolescents and normal weight gain in adults. Caloric restriction is never an appropriate means of glycemic control in individuals with CFRD. Flexibility in meal planning is important to optimize intake and to allow for normal eating patterns. Self-monitoring of blood glucose levels is recommended. The patient should be taught to recognize glucose patterns related to insulin dose, diet, and activity.[30] Patients with CFRD should be cared for by a multidisciplinary medical team experienced in their management. Furthermore, to enhance adherence to the treatment plan, family participation in the care plan is encouraged.[30]

Exocrine Pancreatic Disease—Pancreatic Insufficiency

Exocrine pancreatic insufficiency is the most common GI complication of CF and is present in 85% to 90% of patients. From the pathophysiologic perspective, exocrine pancreatic disease in CF develops because of deficient ductal fluid secretion, which is caused by reduced chloride and bicarbonate secretion. As a result, the protein concentration in the duct increases, and the high protein

TABLE 25-3.

Pancreatic Function and Mutations

Pancreatic-Sufficient Dominant CF Mutations	*Variable Pancreatic-Sufficient CF Mutations*
G551S	G85E
P574H	R347P
R117H	3849 + 10kb C → T
R334W	A455E
R347H	2789 5G → A
R352Q	
T3381	

Adapted with permission from Consensus Conference on Pediatric Nutrition for Patients with Cystic Fibrosis, Cystic Fibrosis Foundation; 2001.

concentration increases susceptibility to precipitation and obstruction of duct lumina.[32,33] The obstruction of pancreatic ducts by these dense secretions leads to the gradual development of fibrosis that causes pancreatic insufficiency.[32,33] Only 1% to 2% of residual colipase and lipase secretion is required to prevent steatorrhea. The reduced secretion of pancreatic enzymes in the small intestine impedes digestion of protein and fat and therefore causes steatorrhea.[2,33] As a consequence, growth failure and signs and symptoms of maldigestion (Chapter 5) and hypo-albuminemia, with or without pulmonary symptoms, are the frequent hallmarks of this condition in infancy and young children.[21,34] Unlike other manifestations of CF disease, pancreatic exocrine involvement is closely related to the CFTR genotype.[35] This was known before the CFTR gene was cloned and was confirmed by the familial concordance of pancreatic status in CF families, CF siblings, and monozygotic twins.[36-38] Soon after the CFTR gene was cloned, the concordance for pancreatic insufficiency was found in practically all of the CF patients homozygous for the ΔF508 mutation reported, confirming the close relationship between pancreatic status and the CFTR genotype.[39,40] In general, all mutations classified as nonsense, frame shift, and amino acid deletions and some missence and splice site mutations will be considered classic or "severe" and therefore confer the pancreatic insufficient phenotype (Classes I, II, III).[2,6,7,40] A series of mutations usually associated with pancreatic sufficiency have been identified and defined as nonclassic or "mild" (Classes IV, V) with reference to the pancreatic status (see Table 25-1).[2,40] Furthermore, some missense mutations and splice site defects may be associated with pancreatic sufficiency.

Nonclassic mutations have a dominant effect because they are associated with residual exocrine function and pancreatic sufficiency, even in patients bearing a severe mutation on the other allele (Table 25-3).[2,40] The association of well-known mutations with pancreatic sufficiency is a useful guide for therapy because pancreatic insufficiency can be corrected by the assumption of pancreatic enzyme supplements. A small subset of patients carrying classic CFTR gene mutations may be pancreatic sufficient initially, and then develop pancreatic insufficiency. This is observed mostly at an early age, especially if patients are diagnosed by neonatal screening.[41] In the 10% to 15% of patients who possess sufficient pancreatic exocrine function for normal digestion, relentless progression of pancreatic disease either does not occur or seems to be retarded for many decades. The pancreatic functional status plays a significant role in determining overall prognosis. Those with pancreatic sufficiency are diagnosed at a later age and experience milder symptoms and, as a group, far superior overall prognosis than do patients with pancreatic insufficiency.[39,40] Specifically, patients with CF with pancreatic sufficiency have lower mean sweat chloride concentration, maintain better pulmonary function with age, and are less likely to have chronic pulmonary colonization with *P aeruginosa* or *B cepacia* infections. This subgroup of patients grow normally in childhood and very seldom experience nutritional difficulties in adulthood. Survival is far superior to those with pancreatic insufficiency.[2,9] However, acute recurrent pancreatitis is a relatively common clinical complication for patients with pancreatic sufficiency.[42,43]

(Nutrition for patients with chronic and acute pancreatitis is discussed in Chapters 21 and 22, respectively.)

Malabsorption

When the diagnosis of CF has been established, pancreatic insufficiency is often inferred by clinical symptoms such as frequent, malodorous, greasy stools; the presence of meconium ileus; or distal intestinal obstruction syndrome. Tests to document pancreatic insufficiency include 1) duodenal intubations with stimulation; 2) immunoreactive trypsinogen after 8 years of age; and 3) other markers as they become more widely available, such as fecal elastase-1 and fecal chymotrypsin determinations.[44] The 72-hour fat balance study, which determines fat losses as percentage of daily fat intake, is still regarded as the "gold" standard test for fat malabsorption in many CF centers. In normal individuals, stool fat output is less than 7% of fat intake (coefficient of fat absorption more than 93%) in children and adults, and 15% for infants younger than 6 months of age.[44]

Exocrine pancreatic insufficiency leads to intestinal malabsorption of fats, fat-soluble vitamins, proteins, and to a lesser extent, carbohydrates (Chapter 5). Mean fecal fat excretion is 38% of intake but may range as high as 80% in some patients.[45] Clinical consequences include poor or absent weight gain; abdominal distention; crampy abdominal pain; flatulence; deficiency of subcutaneous fat and muscle tissue; frequent passage of pale, bulky, malodorous and often oily stools; and rectal prolapse. Biochemical consequences include deficiency of fat-soluble vitamins (A, D, E, K), essential fatty acids, and albumin.[14,24] (Deficiencies of these and other micronutrients are discussed in Chapter 3.)

Pancreatic-Enzyme Replacement Therapy

Patients with exocrine pancreatic insufficiency require life-long replacement therapy with pancreatic-enzyme supplements. Enzymes are given with all foods and food products containing fat and protein, including breast milk and predigested formulas. Medium chain triglycerides (MCT) require less lipase activity than do long-chain fats for efficient absorption, although lipase is still needed.[14,46] Microsphere or microtablet preparations are preferable to powder because the acid-resistant enteric coating prevents acid-inactivation of the enzymes and are not associated with mouth and/or perianal excoriation. Decreased pancreatic bicarbonate secretion combined with gastric acid may cause the duodenum and proximal jejunum to remain acidic, preventing dissolution of the protective coating until the capsules have bypassed a significant amount of intestinal absorptive surface. This can be treated by the administration of a histamine-2 receptor blocker or a proton pump inhibitor.[47,48] Enzymes should be taken before each meal and snack. For prolonged meal events, such as at a buffet or party, the enzymes may be more efficient if distributed throughout the meal.[14] (Enzyme supplementation is also addressed in Chapter 21.)

Pancreatic enzyme replacement has long been considered a safe, well-tolerated treatment for pancreatic insufficiency in CF. However, in 1994, fibrosing colonopathy was recognized as an iatrogenic complication, and its strong association with high doses of pancreatic enzymes has led to the reevaluation of this assumption.[23,49] Current consensus committee guidelines recommend that the daily dose of pancreatic enzymes for most patients remain below 2500 units of lipase/kg/meal, 10,000 units/kg/day, and that higher doses should be used with caution and only if quantitative measures demonstrate substantially improved absorption with such treatment.[23,49] The adequacy of enzyme therapy can be assessed subjectively by following growth parameters and stool patterns.[23] At present, the best objective test available is a 72-hour fecal fat collection with calculation of a coefficient of fat absorption.[23] (Fecal fat assessment is discussed in Chapter 5.)

Nutrition in Cystic Fibrosis

Achieving and maintaining age-appropriate growth and weight gain remains one of the most important challenges in treating patients with CF. The key concepts for nutritional management include proper assessment of nutritional requirements, taking into consideration age, height, weight, severity of lung disease, pancreatic status (genotype), and CFRD.[2,9-10] By providing effective care, medical, nutritional, and behavioral factors should always be considered in the patient who fails to gain weight [12-14] (Figure 25-1).

Growth

Monitoring of growth and nutritional status every 3 months is an essential part of the management of patients with CF, commencing at the time of diagnosis and throughout the life of the patient. For adult patients, the body mass index (BMI) is used to assess appropriate weight, calculated as weight in kilograms divided by height in square meters. In adults, a BMI of 22 for women and 23 for men is desirable. In pediatric patients the BMI percentile should be used.[14] (BMI is discussed in Chapter 2.)

Just as with percentile height and weight charts, an individual BMI percentile value reflects genetic as well as health factors. Plotted sequential values indicate problems when the pattern varies from a consistent percentile. If the patient is losing weight or a child appears to develop a weight plateau and the BMI is between the 10th and 25th BMI percentile, the child is at risk for nutritional insufficiency. Some but not all patients in this category are at risk for nutritional failure. Nutritional failure occurs when weight plateaus for more than 3 months in children younger than 5 years or for more than 6 months in children older than 5 years or the BMI is less than 10th percentile.[14] When poor growth is identified, patients should be seen more frequently than every 3 months and evaluated as outlined in Figure 25-1. Although frequent height and weight and other anthropometric measurements (Chapter 2) remain a core part of the nutritional assessment (Chapter 1), evaluation of nutrient absorption (72-hour fecal fat study) and monitoring lab values reflecting nutritional status should be conducted annually.[13,14]

Recommendations for Energy and Nutrient Intake

Nutrient requirements vary considerably with age and from one individual to another. Therefore, it is most important for each patient to receive dietary counseling at regular intervals. An optional diet requires a caloric intake of 120% to 140% (in some patients >140%) of the recommended daily allowance for energy (Chapter 6). This can be accomplished by a well-balanced diet with a fat intake (35% to 40%) as a source of energy. Patients with CF are advised to take in a high salt diet. This recommendation should be emphasized during the summer months and for those who live in hot climates. Recommendations for surveillance and replacement of macro and micronutrients for CF patients are shown in Tables 25-4 and 25-5.[14,50]

Infants can be breast fed; however, if steatorrhea is present, they will require pancreatic enzyme supplements and sodium chloride supplementation (1/8 teaspoon of table salt per day or 10 mEq sodium chloride solutions available through pharmacies), especially during the summer. Close monitoring of weight gain is indicated.[14,24] Most infants show adequate growth on standard formula feedings, which can be concentrated to maximize caloric

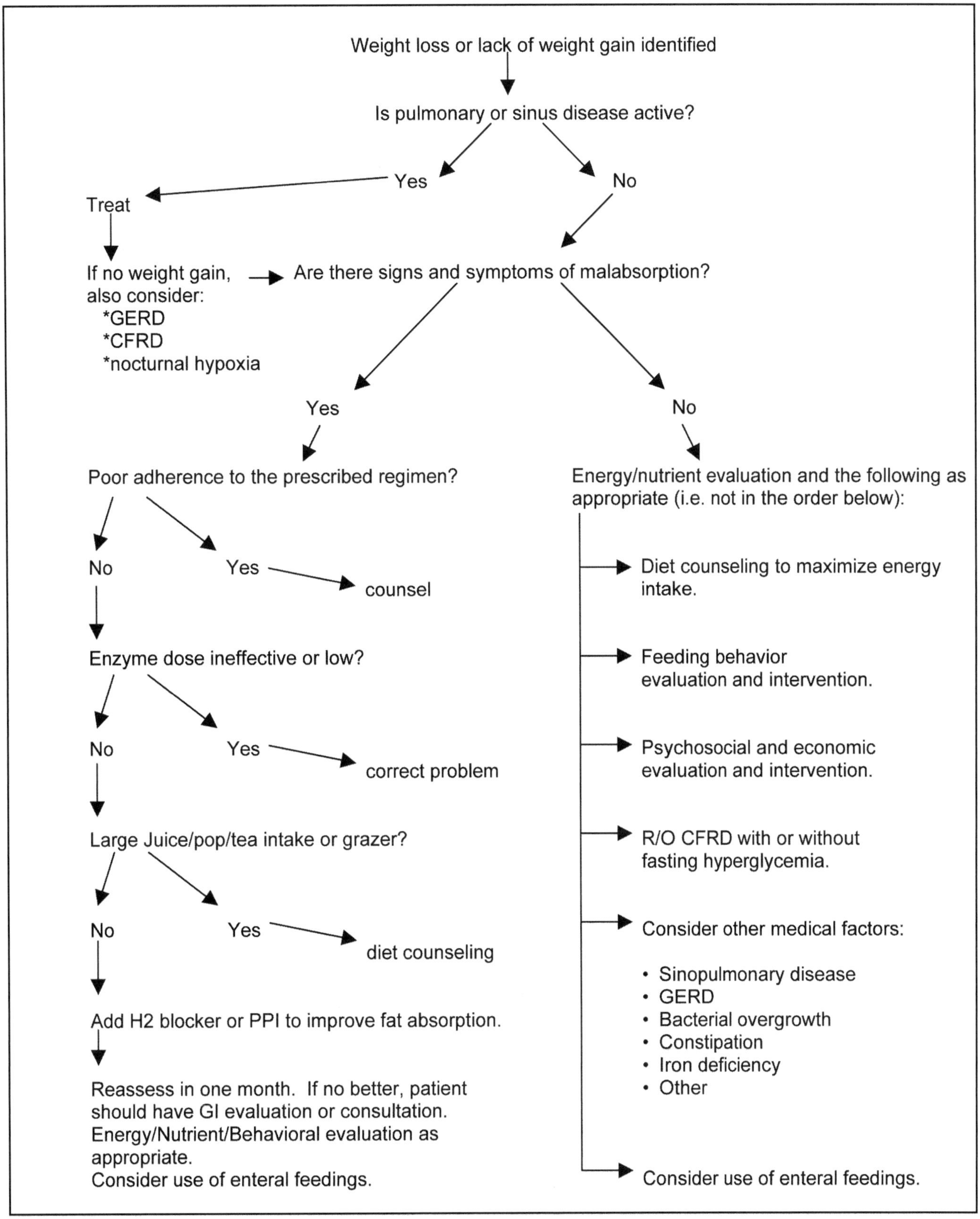

Figure 25-1. Algorithm for CF patients with weight loss or lack of weight gain. Adapted with permission from Consensus Conference on Pediatric Nutrition for Patients with Cystic Fibrosis, Cystic Fibrosis Foundation, 2001.

TABLE 25-4.

Laboratory Monitoring of Nutritional Status

	How Often to Monitor			
	At Diagnosis	**Annually**	**Other**	**Tests**
β-carotene			At physician's discretion	Serum levels
Vitamin A	X[1]	X		Vitamin A (retinol)
Vitamin D	X[1]	X		25-OH-D
Vitamin E	X[1]	X		α-tocopherol
Vitamin K	X[1]		If patient has hemoptysis or hematemesis; in patients with liver disease	PIVKA-II (preferably) or prothrombin time
Essential Fatty Acids			Consider checking in infants or those with FTT	Triene:tetraene
Calcium/Bone status			age >8 years if risk factors are present (see text)	Calcium, phosphorus, ionized PTH, DEXA scan
Iron	X	X	Consider in-depth evaluation for patients with poor appetite	Hemoglobin, hematocrit
Zinc			Consider 6 month supplementation trial and follow growth	No acceptable measurement
Sodium			Consider checking if exposed to heat stress and becomes dehydrated	Serum sodium; spot urine sodium if total body sodium depletion suspected
Protein Stores	X	X	Check in patients with nutritional failure or those at risk	Albumin

[1]Patients diagnosed by neonatal screening do not need these measured.

Adapted with permission from Consensus Conference on Pediatric Nutrition for Patients with Cystic Fibrosis, Cystic Fibrosis Foundation, 2001.

TABLE 25-5.

Recommendations for Vitamin Supplementation for Cystic Fibrosis Patients

In addition to a standard, age appropriate dose of nonfat-soluble multivitamins, the following should be given:

Individual Vitamin Daily Supplementation

	Vitamin A (IU)	**Vitamin E (IU)**	**Vitamin D (IU)**	**Vitamin K(mg)**
0 to 12 months	1500	40 to 50	400	0.3 to 0.5
1 to 3 years	5000	80 to 150	400 to 800	0.3 to 0.5
4 to 8 years	5,000 to 10,000	100 to 200	400 to 800	0.3 to 0.5
> 8 years	10,000	200 to 400	400 to 800	0.3 to 0.5

Adapted with permission from Consensus Conference on Pediatric Nutrition for Patients with Cystic Fibrosis, Cystic Fibrosis Foundation; 2001.

and nutrient intake. Predigested formulas containing MCT may be recommended for infants with liver involvement, persistent steatorrhea, or short gut syndrome. MCTs also require pancreatic enzymes for optional digestion and absorption.[13-15,27]

Commercially available high-energy liquid dietary supplements are often prescribed for adolescents and adults with poor eating habits. However, very often, oral supplements fail to improve nutritional status.[13,14] Respiratory problems usually cause restricted oral intake due to anorexia, which results in acute weight loss. With improvement in respiratory symptoms, patients with mild pulmonary disease can be expected to show a rapid catch-up in weight. As the lung disease progresses, patients may not be able to consume adequate calories to maintain a steady rate of weight gain. For these patients, caloric supplementation through enteral feeding techniques (tubefeeding) may be indicated.[13,14] (Different aspects of enteral nutrition are discussed in Chapters 34, 39, 41, and 42.) The nocturnal infusion of a high-calorie formula through a nasogastric, gastrostomy, or jejeunostomy tube can provide 40% to 50% of total energy needs. Nocturnal supplemental feedings, while reducing voluntary caloric intake from food by about 20%, result in significant increase in total daily energy intake, catch-up growth, and weight gain.[13,14]

Recommendations for Specific Nutrients

In patients with CF, fat malabsorption can lead to the loss of vitamins that are aggregated with fat. Bile acids and pancreatic enzymes are necessary for absorption of fat and fat-soluble vitamins.[14,50] Patients with CF who have liver disease or interruption of the enterohepatic bile acid circulation are at even higher risk for fat-soluble vitamin malabsorption.[14,27,50] Recommendations for surveillance and replacement of these substances for patients with CF are given in Tables 25-4 and 25-5. (Chapter 8 includes information on the absorption and metabolism of macronutrients. General information regarding vitamins and minerals and the signs of deficiency is presented in Chapter 3.)

Beta-Carotene

Beta- (β) carotene is a precursor of vitamin A and may also function as an antioxidant. Studies have documented low serum levels of β-carotene in patients with CF that, with oral supplementation can be corrected and lead to decreased number of days on antibiotics[51] or to improved lung function.[52]

Vitamin A

Vitamin A is important for vision, epithelial cell integrity, epithelial proliferation, and immunity. Pancreatic lipase is required to digest retinyl esters before absorption. Studies indicate that 15% to 40% of patients with CF are vitamin A deficient.[50,53] Vitamin A is a negative acute phase reactant; therefore, levels measured during acute illness may yield misleading low results.[54]

Vitamin D

Vitamin D functions to increase calcium absorption. Vitamin D nutriture takes on added importance because of the prevalence of osteoporosis and bone fractures among patients with CF.[14] (Metabolic bone disease is discussed in Chapter 13.) Ten percent to 40% of patients with CF have documented vitamin D deficiency.[50] Older children and adults and those residing in northern latitude are more likely to have inadequate 25-hydroxy vitamin D levels, because of limited exposure to sunlight.[14]

Vitamin E

Vitamin E (alpha tocopherol) is an antioxidant. Deficiency states lead to hemolytic anemia, neuromuscular degeneration, and retinal deficit. Vitamin E has been reported to be low in patients with CF, even in those taking pancreatic enzymes and multivitamins, and symptomatic deficiency states have been reported.[14,27,52]

Vitamin K

Vitamin K (phylloquinone, menaquinone) functions in the biosynthesis of clotting factors and with osteocalcin, as well as in GLA protein hydroxylation. Measurement of serum vitamin K levels is not practical; therefore, plasma prothrombin concentration has been used as a surrogate. Although it is not widely available, PIVKA-II (proteins induced by vitamin K absence or antagonism) is a more sensitive measure of vitamin K adequacy.[14]

Colonic bacteria are a source of vitamin K. Disruption of the enteric flora by antibiotic use can reduce vitamin K levels.[50] In adults with CF who were taking oral antibiotics, vitamin K at doses of 5 mg four times a week was not sufficient to correct PIVKA-II levels.[55] In a recent review, no adverse effects have been reported at any dosage level of vitamin K.[56] The consensus report[14] recommends that patients with CF receive 0.3 to 0.5 mg vitamin K per day.

Essential Fatty Acids

Essential fatty acids are polyunsaturated fats that can be metabolized to linoleic (n-6 series) and alpha-linolenic acid (n-3 series). Linoleic acid is further metabolized to arachidonic acid, and alpha-linolenic acid is metabolized to docosahexaenoic acid (DHA).

Patients with CF have altered levels of plasma fatty acids. Research has shown that humans with mutations in the CFTR gene have a similar fatty acid defect in tissues expressing CFTR to those reported in CF-knockout mice. Freedman et al[57] showed that the ratio of arachidonic acid to DHA was significantly increased in mucosal and submucosal nasal-biopsy and rectal-biopsy specimen from subjects with CF with pancreatic sufficiency and pancreatic insufficiency as compared with values in healthy control subjects. This fatty acid abnormality may be caused by abnormal or mutant CFTR and not by abnormal intestinal absorption of fat caused by pancreatic insufficiency.[57] Although the mechanism by which CFTR regulates fatty acid metabolism is unknown, the low DHA levels may be important in the excessive host inflammatory response in cystic fibrosis.[57] This study shows that the biologic effects of fatty acids depend not only on the absolute levels of a particular fatty acid but also on the ratio of n-6 to n-3 fatty acids.[58] A high linoleic acid intake may depress the synthesis of DHA. Whether DHA supplementation is indicated in patients with CF is the subject of research and no recommendations can be made at the present time. Vegetable oils such as flax, canola, soy, and walnut, as well as cold-water marine fish are rich in linolenic acid (n-3). These products are also a good source of energy and can be recommended.[59] Human breast milk contains DHA and should be encouraged for infants.[14]

Another area of CF lipid research is the role antioxidants (vitamin E, β-carotene, and selenium) have in reducing oxidative stress in CF, thereby decreasing lung deterioration and improving clinical status. Fats, specifically polyunsaturated fats, complicate this issue because they are an integral part of the high fat diet recommended to maintain weight, but their double bonds are particularly susceptible to oxidative damage. Although increased fatty acid concentrations via dietary supplementation have been associated with increased oxidative stress (quantified by plasma 8-iso-PGF2a), they were also associated with improved pulmonary function (quantified by $\Delta\%FEV_1$).[52] Ciabattoni et al also measured urinary 8-iso-PGF_{2a} (oxidative stress marker) and TXB_2 (indicator of platelet activation) in CF patients and control subjects. They found that vitamin E supplementation decreased the level of 8-iso-PGF_{2a} and TBX_2 and concluded that lipid peroxidation likely contributes to CF pathogenesis.[60] These results provide a rationale for reassessing the adequacy of antioxidant supplementation in patients with CF.[51,52,60]

Special Considerations

The Adult Patient With Cystic Fibrosis

Advances in medical treatment and nutrition have markedly improved the prognosis of patients with CF. The 2001 CFF patient reports show that approximately 40% of patients with CF were ≥18 years of age.[4] The treatment necessary to reach this milestone requires attention to wide range of issues involving multiple organ systems, nutritional changes, developmental problems, social issues, and other considerations. These are usually best met by well-coordinated multidisciplinary teams. The CFF recommends that adult patients with CF should transition to physicians specializing in adult patient care sometime between the age of 18 and 21 years, depending on the medical condition, the emotional maturity of the patient, and the readiness of the family.[61]

Although adult patients with CF suffer from the same problems recognized in the pediatric population, the symptoms might be more severe. As a group, adults have more severe pulmonary disease than children and are at increased risk for serious complications.[61] From adolescence into adulthood, there is a progressive increase in the incidence of CF-related diabetes, osteopenia, and osteoporosis. Adult patients who are malnourished (BMI <19) or are losing weight may require nocturnal supplemental feedings. These patients should be evaluated and treated as described in consensus documents for pediatric and adult patients.[14,61] Gall bladder disease, peptic ulcer disease, pancreatitis, and cirrhosis with portal hypertension are more common in adults than in children. Increasingly, adult CF patients will require evaluation for potential malignancies of the digestive tract and evaluation for liver disease or other complications that will necessitate the specialized attention of a gastroenterologist.[61]

Enteral Nutrition/Gastrostomy Feeding

Patients with advanced cystic fibrosis are often unable to meet their rapidly increasing energy requirements. If diet counseling and/or voluntary supplements are not effective, the patient should be evaluated for long-term gastrostomy feeding. A recent study of 37 patients with CF describes that 11 patients died during 2 years on feeding, reflecting the advanced disease state of the cohort. Survival was worse in females. Malnutrition as indicated by WAZ-score more than 2 standard deviations below the population mean, and advanced lung disease, FEV_1 level less than 50% predicted at time of gastrostomy placement, were significantly associated with poor clinical outcome.[62] Therefore, evaluation for enteral feeding should take place before nutritional failure is present. It includes both a family and a social evaluation and a medical/nutritional assessment.

Once the CF multidisciplinary team has considered the factors for and against nutritional intervention, the patient and family are brought into the decision-making process.[13,14] Enteral feedings should be presented as a positive treatment, a supportive therapy to improve the quality of life and not as a threat or "the beginning of the end". CF caregivers should provide the patient and family concrete information on the types of feeding tubes (Chapter 41) and formulas (Chapter 42), and explain how feeding systems work.

Standard formulas with complete protein and long-chain fatty acids are well tolerated by most patients. Calorically dense formulas (1.5 to 2.0 kcal/mL) might be necessary for provision of adequate calories. Nocturnal infusion is encouraged to promote normal eating patterns during the day. Initially, 30% to 50% of estimated energy requirements should be provided overnight. In malnourished infants, a caloric goal of 120 to 150 kcal/kg/day may be needed to achieve catch-up growth and promote optimal lung growth. For all patients on tube feedings, the amount of calories delivered should be titrated based on the rate of weight gain and growth.[13,14]

There are inadequate data on the appropriate dosing of pancreatic enzymes with overnight feedings. The Consensus Committee[14] recommends that pancreatic enzyme supplements be taken orally in the usual premeal dose before nocturnal enteral feedings. Additional doses may need to be given at the end of the feeding. Complications such as carbohydrate intolerance, excessive bloating, or local skin breakdown may be associated with enteral feeding (Chapter 38).

Once the full caloric goal has been achieved, blood sugars should be evaluated 2 to 3 hours into the feeding and at the end of the feeding on two separate nights. Insulin should be added if these blood sugars are >180 mg/dL. This schedule of blood sugar monitoring should be repeated when a patient is ill, receiving steroids, or if the patient is not gaining weight.[13,14] (For in-depth information on EN, see Section VI, Nutritional Support.)

Bone Health/Disease

Bone health is of increasing interest for patients with CF, as several studies have demonstrated bone fragility in children and adults with CF.[14,61,63] Peak bone mass is one of the major determinants of life-long bone health and is attained by early adulthood.[64] The prevalence of bone disease in patients with CF depends on the health status of the individual, including severity of lung disease and nutritional status. CF with pancreatic insufficiency poses many potential risk factors for poor bone health: failure to thrive; malabsorption of calcium, magnesium, and vitamins D and K; hepatobiliary disease; and reduced weight-bearing physical activity. Chronic use of corticosteroid medications for lung disease is also a risk factor for poor bone health and may decrease calcium absorption and suppress linear growth.[64,65] Bone health can be evaluated by history (atraumatic bone fracture), physical examination (poor growth, back pain), and radiologic and laboratory assessment.[14,64,65] In individuals with CF from Australia, with high level of sun exposure, bone mineral density was normal before the onset of puberty in a well-nourished population with preserved lung function. However, low bone mineral density was identified in adolescents and adults with CF, despite the fact that the majority had vitamin D sufficiency, supporting the findings of abnormal bone histomorphology not consistent with osteomalacia in CF individuals.[65-67]

Current treatment of osteopenia or osteoporosis in children, adolescents, and adults includes optimizing nutritional status by supplying adequate calories, vitamin D and K intake to normalize blood levels, and calcium intake that meets the recommendation for age (upper level 1300 mg/day) and by fostering weight-bearing physical activity as tolerated.[14,57,61,63] Antiresorptive drug therapy may be used in lung transplant patients and may prove appropriate for patients with a history of low-impact bone fractures.[14,61,63] Metabolic bone disease in those with GI disease is discussed in detail in Chapter 13.

Pregnancy

As the survival of patients with CF has increased, more women reach reproductive age and wish to become pregnant. Pregnancy in women with CF should be considered a high-risk pregnancy.[61] An evaluation on 33 pregnancies showed that the most frequent complication, preterm delivery, occurred in 24% of cases. Those with preterm delivery had significantly lower lung function, were most likely to have diabetes, asthma or liver disease, and the weight gain was significantly lower than in those delivering at term. As for the total group, lung function did not deteriorate during pregnancy and average weight gain was 10.3 kg.[68] A study in women who were enrolled in the CFF from 1985 to 1997 showed that 680 of 8136 women in the cohort became pregnant. At entry into the cohort, the women who became pregnant had significantly higher lung function values and higher weight status (52.9 kg versus 46.4 kg). The 10-year survival rate in pregnant women was higher than in those who did not become pregnant (77% versus 58%). In this cohort, pregnancy was not harmful in any subgroup including patients with low lung function values (FEV_1 <40%) or diabetes.[69] Therefore, women with CF with mild to moderate disease may safely go through pregnancy but require close monitoring by a team of specialists.[61]

Substantial evidence indicates that optimal birthweight is influenced by gestational weight gain. A female with a prepregnancy BMI <20 should aim for a weight gain of 12.5 kg. A weight gain of 0.300 kg/week is recommended during the second and third trimesters. To achieve this weight gain, an additional 300 kcal/day may be required, which can be achieved through the consumption of frequent snacks or high calorie drinks.

Improving Survival

Survival rates of the US patients with CF have improved remarkably since 1985. However, most of the improvement was limited to patients 2 to 15 years old. Although both genders benefitted from this trend, female patients have had consistently poorer survival rates than males in the age range of 2 to 20 years, and this gender gap did not narrow throughout time. Furthermore, adult patients with CF had little improvement in survival rate.[70] In an effort to improve the survival rate in patients with CF, several studies have described that the degree of disease severity, morbidity, and mortality in individual patients is determined by multiple, interrelated factors. These factors may include specific mutations of the CFTR gene and phenotypic presentations, for example, meconium ileus[22] and pancreatic status,[2,71] but also demographic characteristics, the well-described gender gap[70,72] and socioeconomic status.[73] Early diagnosis of CF neonatal screening combined with aggressive nutritional therapy resulted in significantly enhanced long-term nutritional status,[74] but neonatal screening did not positively affect *P aeruginosa* acquisition.[75] Lai et al[21] studied whether the mode of diagnosis and initial disease presentation influences long-term survival. The study population included 27703 patients reported to the 1986 to 2000 Cystic Fibrosis Foundation Registry. The researchers found that patients who were diagnosed with meconium ileus, or patients presenting at diagnosis with combined respiratory and GI symptoms, followed by respiratory or GI symptoms alone, had the greatest risks of shortened survival when compared to patients who were diagnosed by prenatal or neonatal screening.[21]

A study by Konstan et al[76] demonstrated that in a cohort of 931 children with CF, lower indexes of growth and nutrition at age 3 years were highly associated with lower pulmonary function age 6 years. Signs and symptoms of lung disease at age 3 were also associated with lower pulmonary function at age 6 years. Nevertheless, indexes of growth and nutrition at age 3 years were strong predictors of pulmonary function at age 6 years even when controlling for clinical indexes of lung disease at age 3. Furthermore, relative weight loss between age 3 and 6 was associated with worse pulmonary function at age 6, and relative weight gain was associated with better pulmonary function at age 6.[76]

In a two-year prospective study on 319 children with CF, age 6 to 8 years, Peterson et al[77] established that children who weigh more and who gain weight at an appropriate and uninterrupted rate have a better lung function (FEV_1) trajectory. Aggressive nutritional support to maintain growth in these children may therefore improve FEV_1, which can be surrogate for better lung health and may ultimately lead to better survival.[77]

Conclusion

Classic CF is a recessive genetic disease with heterogeneous pathobiologic features that reflect mutations in the CFTR gene. Classic CF, which is the severest form of the disease, reflects two losses of function mutations in the CFTR gene. These patients are diagnosed at a very early age, with variable multi-organ manifestations involving the bronchopulmonary system, the exocrine pancreas, intestine, and hepatobiliary system. Patients with nonclassic CF have at least one copy of a mutant gene that confers partial function of the CFTR protein. These patients usually have no overt symptoms of maldigestion because sufficient exocrine pancreatic function is preserved. The diagnosis of patients with nonclassic CF generally occurs at an older age, in adolescence or adulthood. At diagnosis, patients with classic CF are frequently malnourished and/or stunted. Even infants diagnosed by neonatal screening have evidence of nutritional deficiencies. In contrast, nonclassic CF patients are less likely to be malnourished at diagnosis.[2,13,71]

In patients with classic CF, complex related or nonrelated factors carry the risk of creating energy imbalance at any stage in life. The effect on growth potential may vary from patient to patient and is influenced by the severity of phenotypic expression in specific organs, modifier gene effects, the environment, and age-related manifestation of the disease. Highly susceptible to disorders of malnutrition would be the neonate following surgery for complicated meconium ileus; the adolescent or adult, who develops CF-related diabetes, is at great risk of energy losses and protein catabolism. Significant negative influences may be caused by social and developmental factors. Poor compliance with medical/drug prescription in adolescence, clinical depression, and denial of disease are common consequences of patients with chronic life-shortening disorders and are impacting on the health and nutritional status of patients with CF. As median survival of patients with CF has improved, poorly understood clinical factors including fatty acid abnormalities, micro- and macronutrient deficiencies, osteoporosis, or overall health status of women with CF require considerable attention.

We know that CF is a complex disease, affecting multiple organs with diverse clinical manifestations ranging from pulmonary infections and malabsorption to malnutrition and bowel obstructions. We also know that the best therapy for patients with CF includes treatment for all of these complications, which enables attack of the disease from many different angles. Regardless of whether CFTR mutations alone or modifier genes produce abnormalities in CF, diet is one of the most important environmental factors in CF pathogenesis. As healthcare providers learn more about abnormalities specific to CF and how they influence disease manifestation, the providers should be able to offer novel therapies, including nutritional therapies, thereby enhancing the quality of life and increase the survival of patients with CF.

References

1. Welsh MJ, Ramsey BW, Accurso FJ, Cutting GR. Cystic fibrosis. In: Scriver CR, Beaudet Al, Sly WS, Valle D, eds. *The Metabolic and Molecular Bases of Inherited Disease.* 8th ed. New York, NY: McGraw-Hill; 2001:5121-5188.
2. Knowles MR, Durie PR. What is cystic fibrosis? *N Engl J Med.* 2002; 347: 439-442.
3. Kosorok MR, Wei WH, Farrell PM. The incidence of cystic fibrosis. *Stat Med.* 1996;15:449-462.
4. Cystic Fibrosis Foundation. *Cystic Fibrosis Foundation Patient Registry Annual Data Report, 2001.* Bethesda, Md: Cystic Fibrosis Foundation; 2001.
5. Merelle ME, Schouten JP, Gerritsen J, Dankert-Roelse JE. Influence of neonatal screening and centralized treatment of long-term clinical outcome and survival of CF patients. *Eur Respir J.* 2001;18:306-315.
6. Cystic Fibrosis Mutation Data Base. The Chromosome 7 Project. http://www.genet.sickkids.on.ca. Accessed:
7. Zielenski J, Tsui LC. Cystic fibrosis: genotypic and phenotypic variations. *Annu Rev Genet.* 1995;29:777-807.
8. Gibson RL, Burns JL, Ramsey BW. Pathophysiology and management of pulmonary infections in cystic fibrosis. *Am J Respir Crit Care Med.* 2003;168:918-951.
9. Corey M, Edwards L, Levison H, Knowles M. Longitudinal analysis of pulmonary function decline in patients with cystic fibrosis. *J Pediatr.* 1997;131:809-814.
10. Salvatore F, Scudiero O, Castaldo G. Genotype-phenotype correlation in cystic fibrosis: the role of modifier genes. *Am J Med Genet.* 2002;111:88-95.
11. Noone PG, Knowles MR. CFTR-opathies: disease phenotypes associated with cystic fibrosis transmembrane regulator gene mutations. *Respir Res.* 2001;2:328-332.
12. Corey M, McLaughlin FJ, Williams M, Levison H. A comparison of survival, growth and pulmonary function in patients with cystic fibrosis in Boston and Toronto. *J Clin Epidemiol.* 1988;41:588-591.
13. Pencharz PB, Durie PR. Pathogenesis of malnutrition in cystic fibrosis and its treatment. *Clin Nutr.* 2000;19:387-394.
14. Borowitz D, Baker RD, Stallings V. Consensus report on nutrition for pediatric patients with cystic fibrosis. *J Pediatr Gastroenterol Nutr.* 2002;35:246-259.
15. Rudolph CD, Mazur LJ, Liptak GS, et al. Guidelines for evaluation and treatment of gastroesophageal reflux in infants and children: recommendations of the North American Society for Pediatric Gastroenterology and Nutrition. *J Pediatr Gastroenterol Nutr.* 2001;32 (Suppl 2):S1-S31.
16. Malfroot A, Dab I. New insights on gastroesophageal reflux in cystic fibrosis by longitudinal followup. *Arch Dis Child.* 1991;66:1339-1345.
17. Scott RB, O'Loughlin EV, Gall DG. Gastroesophageal reflux in patients with cystic fibrosis. *J Pediatr.* 1985;106:223-227.
18. Mak GZ, Harberg FJ, Hiatt P, et al. T-tube ileostomy for meconium ileus: four decades of experience. *J Pediatr Surg.* 2000;35:349-352.
19. Coutts JA, Docherty JG, Carachi R, Evans TJ. Clinical course of patients with cystic fibrosis presenting with meconium ileus. *Br J Surg.* 1997;84:555-556.
20. Lai HC, Kosorok MR, Laxova A, Davis LA, FitzSimmon SC, Farrell PM. Nutritional status of patients with cystic fibrosis with meconium ileus: a comparison with patients without meconium ileus and diagnosed early through neonatal screening. *Pediatrics.* 2000;105:53-61.

21. Lai HC, Cheng Y, Cho H, Kosorok MR, Farrell PM. Association between initial disease presentation, lung disease outcomes, and survival in patients with cystic fibrosis. *Am J Epidemiol.* 2004;159:537-546.
22. Zielenski J, Corey M, Rozmahel R, et al. Detection of a cystic fibrosis modifier locus for meconium ileus on human chromosome 19q13. *Nat Genetics.* 1999;22:128-129.
23. FitzSimmons SC, Burkhart GA, Borowitz D, et al. High-dose pancreatic-enzyme supplements and fibrosing colonopathy in children with cystic fibrosis. *N Engl J Med.* 1998;336:1283-1289.
24. Orenstein D, Rosenstein B, Stern R. *Cystic Fibrosis: Medical Care.* Philadelphia, Pa: Lippincott Williams & Wilkins; 2000:93-145.
25. Koletzko S, Stringer DA, Cleghorn GJ, Durie PR. Lavage treatment of distal intestinal obstruction syndrome in children with cystic fibrosis. *Pediatrics.* 1989;83:727-733.
26. Feranchak AP, Sokol RJ. Cholangrocyte biology and cystic fibrosis liver disease. *Semin Liver Dis.* 2001;21:471-488.
27. Sokol RJ, Durie PR. Recommendations for management of liver and biliary tract disease in cystic fibrosis. Cystic Fibrosis Foundation Hepatobiliary Disease Consensus Group. *J Pediatr Gastroenterol.* Nutr. 1999;28 (Suppl 1):S1-S13.
28. Soejima K, Landing BH. Pancreatic islets in older patients with cystic fibrosis with and without diabetes mellitus: morphometric and immunocytologic studies. *Pediatr Pathol.* 1986;6:25-46.
29. Lanng S, Thorsteinsson B, Nerup J, Koch C. Influence of the development of diabetes mellitus on clinical status in patients with cystic fibrosis. *Eur J Pediatr.* 1992;151:684-687.
30. Moran A, Hardin D, Rodman D, et al. Diagnosis, screening and management of cystic fibrosis related diabetes mellitus: a consensus report. *Diabetes Res Clin Pract.* 1999;45:61-73.
31. American Diabetes Association. Clinical practice recommendations. Diabetes Care S1; 1998.
32. Kopelman H, Corey M, Gaskin KJ, Durie P, Weizman Z, Forstner GG. Impaired chloride secretion, as well as bicarbonate secretion, underlies the fluid secretory defect in the cystic fibrosis pancreas. *Gastroenterology.* 1988;95:349-355.
33. Kopelman H, Forstner G, Durie P, Corey M. Origins of chloride and bicarbonate secretory defect in the cystic fibrosis pancreas, as suggested by pancreatic function studies in control and CF subjects with preserved pancreatic function. *Clin Invest Med.* 1989;12:207-211.
34. Bronstein MN, Sokol RJ, Abman SH, et al. Pancreatic insufficiency, growth, and nutrition in infants identified by newborn screening as having cystic fibrosis. *J Pediatr.* 1992;120:533-540.
35. Cystic Fibrosis Genotype-Phenotype Consortium. Correlation between genotype and phenotype in patients with cystic fibrosis. *N Engl J Med.* 1993;18:1308-1313.
36. Corey M, Durie PR, Moore D, Forstner G, Levison H. Familial concordance of pancreatic function in cystic fibrosis. *J Pediatr.* 1989;115:274-277.
37. Kerem BS, Buchanan JA, Durie P, et al. DNA marker haplotype association with pancreatic sufficiency in cystic fibrosis. *Am J Hum Genet.* 1989;44:827-834.
38. Santis G, Osborne L, Knight R, Smith M, Davison T, Hudson M. Genotype-Phenotype relationship in cystic fibrosis results from the study of monozygotic and dizygotic twins with cystic fibrosis. *Pediatr Pulmonol.* 1992;(Suppl 8):239-240.
39. Kerem E, Corey M, Kerem BS, et al. The relation between genotype and phenotype in cystic fibrosis analysis of the most common mutation (delta F508). *N Engl J Med.* 1990;323:1517-1522.
40. Kristidis P, Bozon D, Corey M, et al. Genetic determination of pancreatic function in cystic fibrosis. *Am J Hum Genet.* 1992;50:1178-1184.
41. Waters DL, Dorney SF, Gaskin KJ, et al. Pancreatic function in infants identified as having cystic fibrosis in a neonatal screening program. *N Engl J Med.* 1990;322:303-308.
42. Weizman Z, Durie PR. Acute pancreatitis in childhood. *J Pediatr.* 1988;113 (1 [Pt 1]):24-29.
43. Noone PG, Zhou Z, Silverman LM, Jowell PS, Knowles MR, Cohn JA. Cystic fibrosis gene mutations and pancreatitis risk: relation to epithelial ion transport and trypsin inhibitor gene mutations. *Gastroenterology.* 2001;121:1310-1319.
44. Borowitz D. Evidence for the diagnosis of pancreatic sufficiency. *Pediatr Pulmonol.* 2000;29:167-168.
45. Forstner GG, Gall G, Corey M, et al. Digestion and absorption of nutrients in cystic fibrosis. In: Sturgess JM, ed. *Proceedings of the 8th International Congress on CF.* Ontario, Canada: The Imperial Press Ltd; 1980:137.
46. Caliari S, Benini L, Sembenini C, Gregori B, Carnielli V, Vantini I. Medium-chain triglyceride absorption in patients with pancreatic insufficiency. *Scand J Gastroenterol.* 1996;31:90-94.
47. Zentler-Munro PL, Fine DR, Batten JC, Northfield TC. Effect of cimetidine in enzyme inactivation, bile acid precipitation, and lipid solubilisation in pancreatic steatorrhea due to cystic fibrosis. *Gut.* 1985;26:892-901.
48. Heijerman HG, Lamers CB, Bakker W, Dijkman JH. Improvement of fecal fat excretion after addition of omeprazole to pancrease in cystic fibrosis is related to residual exocrine function of the pancreas. *Dig Dis Sci.* 1993;38:1-6.
49. Borowitz D, Grand RJ, Durie PR. Use of pancreatic enzyme supplements for patients with cystic fibrosis in the context of fibrosing colonopathy. *J Pediatr.* 1995;127:681-684.
50. Feranchak AP, Sontag MK, Wagener JS, Hammond KB, Accurson FJ, Sokol RJ. Prospective, long-term study of fat-soluble vitamin status in children with cystic fibrosis identified by newborn screen. *J Pediatr.* 1999;135:601-610.
51. Renner S, Rath R, Rust P, et al. Effects of beta-carotene supplementation for six-months on clinical and laboratory parameters in patients with cystic fibrosis. *Thorax.* 2001;56:48-52.
52. Wood LG, Fitzgerald DA, Lee AK, Garg ML. Improved antioxidant and fatty acid status of patients with cystic fibrosis after antioxidant supplementation is linked to improved lung function. *Am J Clin Nutr.* 2003;77:150-159.
53. Lindblad A, Diczfalusy U, Hultcrantz R, Thorell A, Strandvik B. Vitamin A concentration in the liver decreases with age in patients with cystic fibrosis. *J Pediatr Gastroenterol Nutr.* 1997;24:264-270.
54. Duggan C, Colin AA, Agil A, Higgins L, Riafai N. Vitamin A status in acute exacerbation of cystic fibrosis. *Am J Clin Nutr.* 1996;64:635-639.
55. Wilson DC, Rashid M, Durie PR, et al. Treatment of vitamin K deficiency in cystic fibrosis: effectiveness of a daily fat-soluble vitamin combination. *J Pediatr.* 2001;138:851-855.
56. Dietary Reference Intakes for Vitamin A, Vitamin K, Arsenic, Boron, Chromium, Copper, Iodine, Iron, Manganese, Molybdenum, Nickel, Silicon, Vanadium, and Zinc. Food and Nutrition Board, Institute of Medicine. Washington DC: National Academy Press; 2001.
57. Freedman SD, Blanco PG, Zaman MM, et al. Association of cystic fibrosis with abnormalities in fatty acid metabolism. *N Engl J Med.* 2004;350:560-569.
58. Rubin D, Laposata M. Cellular interactions between n-6 and n-3 fatty acids: a mass analysis of fatty acid elongation/desaturation, distribution among complex lipids and conversion to eicosanoids. *J Lipid Res.* 1992;33:1430-1440.
59. Simopoulous AP. The importance of the ratio of omega-6/omega-3 essential fatty acids. Biomed Pharmacother. 2002;56:365-379.
60. Ciabattoni G, Davi G, Collura M, et al. In vivo lipid peroxidation and platelet activation in cystic fibrosis. *Am J Respir Crit Care Med.* 2000;162:1195-1201.
61. Yankaskas JR, Marshall BC, Sufian B, Simon RH, Rodman D. Cystic fibrosis adult care: consensus conference report. *Chest.* 2004;125:1S-39S.
62. Oliver MR, Heine RG, N CH, Volders E, Olinsky A. Factors affecting clinical outcome in gastrostomy-fed children with cystic fibrosis. *Pediatr Pulmonol.* 2004;37:324-329.

63. Hecker TM, Aris RM. Management of osteoporosis in adults with cystic fibrosis. *Drugs.* 2004;64:133-147.
64. National Institutes of Health Consensus Development Conference Statement: Osteoporosis Prevention, Diagnosis, and Therapy. NIH Consensus Statement, 2000, March 27-29; 17(1):1-36.
65. Lai HC, FitzSimmons SC, Allen DB, et al. Persistent growth impairment in children with cystic fibrosis following treatment of alternate-day prednisone. *N Engl J Med.* 2000;342:851-859.
66. Buntain HM, Greer RM, Schluter PJ, et al. Bone mineral density in Australian children, adolescents and adults with cystic fibrosis: a controlled cross-sectional study. *Thorax.* 2004;59:149-155.
67. Elkin SL, Vedi S, Bord S, Graham NJ, Hodson ME, Compston JE. Histomorphometric analysis of bone biopsies from the iliac crest of adults with cystic fibrosis. *Am J Respir Crit Care Med.* 2002;166:1470-1474.
68. Odegaard I, Stray-Pedersen B, Hallberg K, Haanaes OC, Storrosten OT, Johannesson M. Maternal and fetal morbidity in pregnancies of Norwegian and Swedish women with cystic fibrosis. *Acta Obstet Gynecol Scand.* 2002;81:698-705.
69. Goss CH, Rubenfeld GD, Otto K, Aitken ML. The effect of pregnancy on survival in women with cystic fibrosis. *Chest.* 2003;124:1460-1468.
70. Kulich M, Rosenfeld M, Goss CH, Wilmott R. Improved survival among young patients with cystic fibrosis. *J Pediatr.* 2003;142:631-636.
71. Ahmed N, Corey M, Forstner G, et al. Molecular consequences of cystic fibrosis transmembrane regulator (CFTR) gene mutations in the exocrine pancreas. *Gut.* 2003;52:1159-1164.
72. Rosenfeld M, Davis R, Fitzsimmons S, Pepe M, Ramsey B. Gender gap in cystic fibrosis mortality. *Am J Epidemiol.* 1997;145:794-803.
73. Schechter MS, Shelton BJ, Margolis PA, FitzSimmons SC. The association of socioeconomic status with outcomes in cystic fibrosis patients in the United States. *Am J Respir Crit Care Med.* 2001;163:1331-1337.
74. Farrell PM, Kosorok MR, Rock MJ, et al. Early diagnosis of cystic fibrosis through neonatal screening prevents severe malnutrition and improves long-term growth. *Pediatrics.* 2001;107:1-13.
75. Wang SS, FitzSimmons SC, O'Leary LA, et al. Early diagnosis of cystic fibrosis in the newborn period and risk of Pseudomonas aeruginosa acquisition in the first 10 years of life: a registry-based longitudinal study. *Pediatrics.* 2001;107:274-279.
76. Konstan MW, Butler SM, Wohl ME, et al. Growth and nutritional indexes in early life predict pulmonary function in cystic fibrosis. J Pediatr. 2003;142:624-630.
77. Peterson ML, Jacobs DR Jr, Milla CE. Longitudinal changes in growth parameters are correlated with changes in pulmonary function in cystic fibrosis. *Pediatrics.* 2003;112:588-592.

Chapter 26

Nutrition and Gastrointestinal Oncology

James S. Scolapio, MD
and Alan L. Buchman, MD, MSPH

Dietary and Nutritional Factors

The evidence connecting food to gastrointestinal (GI) cancers are derived from epidemiological studies, case-control studies, and prospective observational studies. However, in many of these studies, it is difficult to determine the independent effects of specific nutrients given the many potential environmental contributors.[1,2]

Esophageal cancer has been linked to low intake of vitamin C, zinc, and selenium, and a protective effect from eating fruits and vegetables have been reported in more than one study. Meat and fish consumption have shown inconsistent associations with esophageal cancer. Despite these positive observations, randomized controlled studies from China have failed to show reduced esophageal cancer mortality in patients treated with multivitamin supplements.[3] As with other malignancies, obesity also appears to be a risk factor.

It has been shown that foods high in salt or that have been preserved with salt (ie, pickled, smoked foods) are associated with an increased risk of gastric cancer. Migration studies from Japan have suggested a strong environmental component to gastric cancer.[4] Preserved foods contain nitrates, which form N-nitroso compounds, including nitrosamines, which may increase the risk of gastric cancer. There is consistent data that fruit and vegetable consumption decreases the risk of gastric cancer. Also, green tea has been shown to be protective against gastric cancer in a number of studies.[5]

Pancreatic cancer has been linked to excess caloric intake and obesity. The intake of fruits and vegetables may be protective.[2]

It is widely believed that dietary fat increases the risk of colon cancer and that fiber has a protective effect. Many case control studies have shown a link with high animal fat and increased total calorie and colon cancer.[6] Fiber may have a protective effect, but it is less strong than once thought. The consumption of fruits and vegetables is strongly associated with a reduced risk of colon cancer. (Nutrition for patients with colon cancer is discussed in detail in Chapter 17.)

The American Cancer Society recommends the following dietary guidelines for cancer prevention: 1) choose most foods from plant sources; 2) eat more than five servings of fruits and vegetables each day; 3) limit intake of high fat foods, particularly from animal sources; 4) achieve and maintain a healthy weight; and 5) limit consumption of alcoholic beverages.[7]

Nutritional Assessment

The nutritional management of a patient with GI cancer begins with appropriate nutritional assessment (Table 26-1). Multiple factors contribute to malnutrition in cancer patients: anorexia from tumor cytokines, intestinal obstruction, taste changes, chemotherapy and radiation side effects, and depression are examples. Intestinal malabsorption also contributes to malnutrition in patients with certain types of GI cancers. Extensive mucosal infiltrative disease, bacterial overgrowth, and surgical resection all contribute to malabsorption (Chapter 5) and subsequent weight loss. Increased energy expenditure has also been reported in patients with cancer.[8] Nutrient deficiency can result in altered cellular immunity with increased risk of infection and delayed wound healing

Table 26-1.
Nutritional Assessment

History and Physical Examination	
History	Unusual dietary habits, medication/vitamin or mineral supplements, change in hair color or texture, poor night vision, dysguesia, dysphagia/odynophagia, abdominal pain/distention, diarrhea, bone pain, muscle pain/cramps/twitching, numbness/parathesias, fatigue, diminished mental activity, weakness
Physical Examination	Hair loss/texture, keratomalacia, cheilosis, glossitis, red tongue, parotid enlargement, dentition, skin rash/petechia/bruising, muscle wasting, hepatomegaly, edema, peripheral neuropathy
Anthropometrics	
Ideal Body Weight	Males: 48 kg + 2.3 kg for each in >60 Females: 45 kg + 2.7 kg for each in >60 Calculate % IBW: >5% weight loss in 1 month, >7.5% in 2 months or >10% in 6 months are significant "Preferred" Body Weight for obese (Hamwi Formula)= (ABW-IBW)(0.25) + IBW (used clinically, but not validated) Adjusted Body Weight for Amputation: Entire Arm (-6.5%) Upper Arm (-3.5%) Hand (-0.8%) Forearm with Hand (-3.1%) Forearm without hand (-2.5%) Entire Leg (-18.6%) Foot (-1.8%)
Muscle Function	Handgrip strength, peak insp pressure
Midarm Circumference Triceps Skin Fold Thickness	Assess Skeletal Mass Assess Fat Stores. Operator-dependent variability, unreliable to assess short-term responses
Laboratory Measurements	
Nitrogen Balance	N intake = grams protein/6.25 Balance = N intake – (24 urine urea nitrogen (UUN) + 4. Requires sufficient calories as well as protein
Indirect Calorimetry	
Visceral Proteins	Albumin, Prealbumin, Transferrin, Retinol- binding protein Affected by many non-nutritional conditions.
Immune Function	Total Lymphocyte Count Delayed Hypersensitivity Skin Tests Affected by many non-nutritional conditions.

following surgery. Therefore, it is important to identify those patients who are at potential risk of malnutrition. Management goals should then include correction of nutritional deficits when possible. Nutritional Assessment is discussed in detail in Chapter 1.

Patients who have lost significant weight (defined as >10%) and have had reduced oral caloric intake over a 2- to 24-week period are at risk of both macronutrient and micronutrient deficiencies (Chapter 3). We know from clinical studies that cancer patients who have lost greater than 10% of their usual weight and have a reduced appetite have a shorter median survival and lower chemotherapy response.[9] The important findings on physical examination, besides an accurate weight, include loss of subcutaneous fat, muscle wasting, dependent edema, and ascites. The subjective global assessment (SGA) is a clinical method for evaluating nutritional status that includes historical, symptomatic, and physical parameters of patients.[10] The findings from a history and physical examination are subjectively weighted to rank patients as being well nourished (see Chapter 1). The use of the SGA has been shown to give reproducible results with more than 80% agreement.[10] This chapter discusses when to begin nutritional support and which method to use in patients with GI cancers.

General Dietary Measures

For most cancer patients, the most important advice is to consume a diet liberal in protein, with sufficient calories to maintain weight. Oral intake of 25 to 35 kcal/kg/day and 1.0 to 1.5 g/kg of protein meet the requirements of most nonwasted cancer patients. For those patients who have lost more than 5% of their usual weight, the addition of 500 kcal/day (above the 25 to 35 kcal/day) will help promote weight gain. Protein should be maximized at a minimum of 1.5 g/kg/day in those patients with signs of muscle wasting. In patients with advanced cancer, the addition of added calories and protein might not improve lean muscle mass given the inflammatory process (ie, cytokines) associated with cancer itself.

Each patient should meet with a registered dietician to determine actual calories consumed. The dietician can also recommend specific foods and supplements of high caloric density. The addition of flavoring to the food may help improve food intake. Liquid oral supplements (eg, Ensure, Boost and Instant Carnation) may provide the additional calories that a patient requires. In those patients unable to consume sufficient oral calories, the addition of an appetite stimulant may be helpful.

Pharmacological Treatment

Cachexia is a common and major complication of cancer. The severe loss of weight and appetite can produce both physical and emotional disabilities. Cancer cells promote the secretion of host-derived cytokines. These cytokines can result in significant lean tissue loss and depressed appetite. Those that have been studied more recently include tumor necrosis factor alpha, interleukin-6, and proteolysis inducing factor.[11] Experimental agents that have been tried to reduce this cytokine cachexia syndrome include pentoxifylline, hydrazine sulfate, melatonin, thalidomide, ibuprofen, and more recently infliximab. These treatments should still be regarded as experimental.

In terms of appetite stimulants, positive results have been reported with dronabinaol, cortiosteroids, and megestrol acetate (Megace, Bristol-Myers Co, New York, NY).[12,13] Of these, Megace has been studied the most extensively in randomized controlled studies. The administration of 400 to 800 mg/day has been shown to increase appetite, weight gain (primary fat mass), and quality of life. Improved morbidity and mortality have not been shown with this treatment.[14] Megace comes in an oral suspension that can be given once per day. The drug may cause adrenal suppression and exacerbate preexisting diabetes mellitus. Thromboembolic events have also been reported in cancer patients treated with 800 mg/day of Megace. Currently, Megace is the most promising agent for the treatment of cancer anorexia. The safest and most efficacious dose is still somewhat controversial; therefore, the drug should be titrated to the lowest effective dose.

Cannabinoids and its derivative dronabinol have been shown to increase weight gain and appetite in cancer and human immunodeficiency virus patients.[12] Dronabinol has been approved by the Food and Drug Association (FDA) for the treatment of nausea and vomiting associated with chemotherapy. The dose used is 2.5 mg orally three times daily 1 hour after meals. Further controlled trails are needed to identify the optimal dose and patient population that may derive the most benefit.

Corticosteroids most likely stimulate appetite by the euphoria they produce. The appetite stimulation effects appear to be short lived and complications from long-term use are well established. Dexamethasone should be only given (0.75 mg four times per day) to terminal cancer patients if increased appetite and quality of life are the short-term goals (ie, weeks).

Cyproheptadine hydrochloride is an antihistamine that presumably increases weight by serotonin antagonism. It has been used primarily in Europe to promote weight gain in cancer patients. A randomized placebo controlled study would suggest lack of benefit of weight gain with this medication.[15]

Perioperative Nutritional Support

Nutritional support refers to the use of either intravenous, also called parenteral nutrition (PN) or enteral tube feeding, also called enteral nutrition (EN), and is usually administered to hospitalized patients. Nutritional support of the hospitalized patient should be instituted promptly when it has been determined from daily calorie counts that a patient is not receiving sufficient oral intake of food for 7 or more days. After a patient has experienced approximately 7 to 10 days of nil per os (npo), negative nitrogen balance occurs, which increases the risk of infection and interferes with wound healing. Nutritional support may also be considered an adjunctive therapy in malnourished patients in whom sufficient oral intake to promote nutritional repletion is not immediately achievable. Perioperative nutrition refers to the use of nutritional support pre and post surgery.

In cancer patients requiring surgery, the health care provider needs to ask if there is a benefit to delaying surgery for repletion of nutrition. The available literature would suggest that cancer patients who are severely malnourished (defined as >10% weight loss of usual weight) benefit from 7 to 10 days of preoperative PN.[16] Although improved mortality has not been reported, a 10% improvement in postoperative complications (ie, reduced postoperative infections) has been reported compared to improvements with placebo. Administering PN to those cancer patients who were not malnourished (ie, <10% weight loss) resulted in increased complications from the PN itself.[17] Therefore, indiscriminate use of preoperative PN should be avoided.

There is a lack of studies evaluating the benefit of total enteral nutrition (TEN) prior to surgery in malnourished cancer patients. The results would most likely be similar and perhaps even better than those with PN. The practicality of giving PN for 7 to 10 days before surgery is difficult. It would be difficult to justify hospitalizing a patient for 10 days prior to surgery to administer PN. Most insurance companies would not approve PN coverage at home for this indication. Administering TEN at home via a nasal gastric feeding tube for 7 to 10 days might be more appropriate. Each clinician needs to decide if delaying surgery for 10 days is worthwhile, given only a 10% decrease in postoperative complications and lack of mortality benefit.

Postoperatively, cancer patients who are severely malnourished prior to surgery or have an anticipated 7 or more days of inadequate caloric intake following surgery appear to benefit from postoperative TEN given within 48 hours of surgery.[16] Results with TEN appear better than those with PN.[18] It is the opinion of these authors that, in high nutrition risk patients (ie, >10% weight loss, extensive upper abdominal surgical resection), a jejunal feeding tube be place at the time of surgery. The feeding tube can be removed during the 4- to 8-week outpatient return visit, once the patient is consuming adequate calories orally.

Nutrition Support of Specific Cancers

Esophageal Cancer

Malnutrition is very common in patients with cancer of the esophagus, primarily because of the severe dysphagia. Average weight loss has been reported to be 10 kg at presentation. Surgery is the primary treatment of choice, with radiation and chemotherapy given preoperatively. Side effects of the chemotherapy and radiation can result in further weight loss. Surgical treatment usually involves total or distal esophagectomy requiring bilateral vagotomy, proximal gastrectomy, and anastomosis of the retained portion of the esophagus to the remaining stomach.

Postoperative regurgitation of food and bloating are common complications following surgery that can result in further weight loss and debilitation. Also, esophageal strictures can occur postoperatively; these often require dilatation for adequate food passage. In those patients who are not surgical candidates and whom have severe dysphagia resulting from esophageal luminal cancer growth, stent placement may be palliative and may improve food and liquid passage.

The data regarding the benefit of perioperative nutrition (discussed earlier) applies to patients with esophageal cancer. Many of these perioperative studies have included patients with esophageal cancer. Liquid nutritional supplements and small frequent meals may help the postoperative patient who is experiencing dumping and bloating. In those patients who have lost significant (>10%) preoperative weight, placing a jejunal feeding tube at the time of surgery is suggested. Iron and vitamin-B12 deficiency may result postoperatively depending on the amount of stomach removed and should therefore be replaced accordingly. (Replacement of these and other deficiencies is discussed in Chapter 3.)

Gastric Cancer

Patients with gastric cancer frequently present with early satiety, postprandial abdominal pain, and weight loss. Surgical resection usually requires a total gastrectomy with an esophagojejunal anastomosis. Dumping, fat malabsorption, iron, calcium, and vitamin-B12 deficiency can all occur in the postoperative setting. To help with the dumping syndrome, small, frequent meals (6 to 8 meals per day) should be encouraged, and protein should be maximized in the diet. Deficiencies of vitamins and minerals can be prevented and treated with adequate oral administration of iron with ascorbic acid and monthly injections of vitamin B12. For patients who continue to lose weight despite dietary adjustments, nocturnal jejunal feeding is usually beneficial to prevent further weight loss and to maintain hydration.

Pancreatic Cancer

Pancreatic cancer can result in significant weight loss, even prior to diagnosis. If patients are surgical candidates, the same data regarding perioperative nutrition (discussed above) will apply. Pancreatic exocrine and endocrine insufficiency can also occur in these patients, and exogenous pancreatic enzyme replacement and insulin should be given as clinically indicated. Nocturnal jejunal feeding can supplement the oral intake and provide needed calories and hydration in those patients who are unable to orally consume adequate calories.

Colorectal Cancer

Patients with colorectal cancer usually present with little or no weight loss. Treatment involves resection of the bowel containing the cancer. If postoperative chemotherapy (5-fluorouracil) is required, it is usually tolerated without significant side effects. If large resections of the right colon are required and the ileocecal valve is compromised, postprandial diarrhea may result. Although cholestyramine may improve bile-salt–induced diarrhea, it can also further deplete the bile salt pool if greater than 100 cm of the terminal ileum has been resected, which results in fat-soluble–vitamin deficiencies. Likewise, if more than 60 cm of the terminal ileum is resected, vitamin-B12 deficiency may result and replacement is thus necessary. (Nutrition supplementation is discussed in Chapter 10.)

Radiation-Treated Cancers

Some cancers, including colorectal cancer, are treated with radiation therapy. Although direct tumor treatment with the radiation is the goal, scatter radiation damage can occur. This is especially a nutritional concern when the small intestine is damaged. Radiation enteritis can be classified as acute or chronic. By definition, "acute" is defined as that occurring within the first 6 weeks of therapy. Acute injury to the small bowel is usually self-limited and presents clinically with nausea and diarrhea. Acute injury does not necessarily predict those patients who will go on to develop chronic radiation injury. Chronic small bowel injury from radiation is marked by inflammation and fibrosis of the small intestine. The fibrosis can result in bowel obstruction and episodic bleeding. Partial small bowel obstruction can result in bacterial overgrowth and diarrhea. Treatment with broad-spectrum antibiotics may be helpful in improving the diarrhea if bacterial overgrowth is the cause. Recurrent bowel obstructions can also result in inadequate oral intake over time, which induces significant weight loss. The primary goal should be to surgically correct the obstruction. Often surgeons are reluctant to operate given the extensive damage of the bowel from the radiation, which is often not appreciated until the time of surgery. Selection of an experienced surgeon in the area of radiation injury (eg, a gynecologic surgeon) is critical in the care of these patients. If patients are not surgical candidates, and they are unable to take sufficient fluids and nutrients orally, then placement of a gastric or jejunal feeding tube may be helpful. Often placing a dual gastric-jejunal tube for gastric venting and jejunal feeding is helpful. There is insufficient data to recommend elemental formulas or glutamine for these patients. If patients cannot tolerate enteral feeding, then the use of PN may be required and can be used successfully provided patients are monitored closely.[19,20]

Parenteral Nutrition for Cancer Patients

Once nutritional support is deemed necessary for oncologic patients, which route—PN versus EN—should be used? Indications for parenteral feeding usually include small bowel obstruction, which may develop in cancer patients because of tumor growth; severe diarrhea and malabsorption during active disease and treatment; GI hemorrhage; treatment for entero-cutaneous or entero-enteric fistulae; and as supportive care in patients who are severely malnourished (SGA "C"). PN is not generally indicated in patients who have an unobstructed GI tract or when the duration of nutritional support is expected to be less than 7 days.

A number of studies have investigated energy expenditure and nitrogen excretion in patients with cancer. Cancer patients with active disease may require 1.2 to 1.5 X additional calories above resting energy expenditure. For most adult cancer patients, 30 to 40 kcal/kg/day of usual body weight and 1 to 1.5 g/kg of ideal body weight of protein is usually sufficient. Most hospitalized cancer patients only require nutritional support for 2 weeks or less.

If used inappropriately or not monitored appropriately, PN will not have any value to the patient and may even become a life-threatening rather than a life-saving therapy. It is generally recommended to consult the services of a multidisciplinary nutritional support team in the hospital to assist in writing the PN prescription, monitoring the therapy, and making adjustments as required. However, it is imperative that the responsible physician understands the importance of appropriate monitoring, especially in the absence of a nutritional support team.

The human body adapts to starvation and weight loss by decreasing resting energy expenditure. When massive amounts of carbohydrate are supplied to a malnourished cancer patient in an overzealous attempt to renourish them, refeeding syndrome may result.[21] This potentially life-threatening complication of either PN or EN therapy occurs when carbohydrate intake stimulates pancreatic insulin release, which results in the flow of potassium and magnesium to the intercellular space, which may result in cardiac arrhythmias. In addition, the demand for phosphate to produce adenosine triphosphate from the infused carbohydrate may result in hypophosphatemia with subsequent hemolytic anemia, seizures, rhabdomyolysis, and/or respiratory muscle dysfunction. In rare cases, respiratory failure may ensue. Prevention of refeeding syndrome can be prevented by the slow introduction of carbohydrate and byconsumption of protein (amino acids) and lipid. Small amounts of supplemental potassium phosphate and magnesium may be helpful. Serum potassium, magnesium, and phosphate concentrations should be determined daily or more frequently if necessary until the goal caloric support and a stable electrolyte pattern in the normal range can be achieved. (The refeeding syndrome is discussed in detail in Chapter 45.)

There is no gold standard or specific laboratory test to measure the efficacy of nutrition with either PN or enteral feeding. Weight gain in the hospital during a 1- to 2-week course of nutritional support is usually the result of fluid and not of lean body mass. Serum visceral proteins such as prealbumin can be measured and followed during the course of therapy if desired. The half-life of prealbumin is 2 days, whereas the half-life of albumin is 21 days, which is too long to be useful in the inpatient setting. The serum concentrations of all visceral proteins, including prealbumin, may be affected by many non-nutritional factors including intra- and extravascular fluid shifts in the postoperative patient or may be depressed, because of the protein losing enteropathy seen in cancer or because of decreased synthesis as the liver turns towards increased production of acute phase proteins during active disease. Although serum concentration of visceral proteins may guide nutritional therapy, they should be interpreted with the caveats described above. Also, normal visceral protein synthesis cannot occur in the absence of sufficient energy intake because skeletal muscle will be catabolized as a fuel source.

Patients may require home parenteral nutrition (HPN) because they have become severely malnourished in the face of cancer or they have developed short bowel syndrome from multiple bowel resections from cancer, required because of radiation strictures, which have chronically draining entero-enteric or enterocutaneous fistulae.[22] Such therapy requires assessment of the home environment for appropriateness and safety and for proper training of either the patient or a responsible adult (especially for aseptic catheter care). Patients who have a life expectancy of less than 3 months and are not being actively treated with chemotherapy or radiation should not be treated with HPN.

Medicare and most insurance companies have specific guidelines for the reimbursement on HPN. Medicare requires documentation in the medical record that the HPN will be required for at least 3 months and that TEN is not feasible because of complications (ie, bowel obstruction). The case manager should evaluate each potential HPN patient prior to discharge to home. If the patient is determined to be a reasonable candidate for HPN, it is important that the patient be metabolically stable prior to hospital discharge. It is appropriate to cycle the PN to a 10- to 12-hour nocturnal infusion prior to discharge. Nocturnal infusion gives the patient more freedom during the day to ambulate. Nocturnal infusion may also help prevent PN-associated liver disease and encourage eating during the normal day.

Enteral Nutrition for Cancer Patients

In the absence of bowel obstruction, distal fistula, or toxic mega colon, EN is the preferred form of nutritional support for the cancer patient, provided the patient consents to having a nasogastric or percutaneous placed feeding tube. For nasal gastric feeding, a small-bore (8 to 10 Fr) feeding tube should be used rather than a larger tube that is typically used for gastric decompression. Complications (discussed below) are generally fewer with such a tube. Because of postoperative gastroparesis, jejunal feeding may be preferred in specific individuals. Tube placement should be verified radiologically prior to beginning feeding because physical examination, namely ausculatory confirmation, is often inaccurate for determining tube position.

In general, feeding is begun at a relatively slow rate (typically 40 mL/hour) and advanced every 8 hours until the goal rate is achieved and if gastric residuals are <200 mL prior to each rate increase. However, if a small-bore feeding tube is used or if jejunal feeding is undertaken, it may be difficult to aspirate and to determine an accurate gastric residual volume. In these patients, abdominal pain, distention, and tenderness are used to determine enteral feeding tolerance. The presence or absence of bowel sounds may be helpful but actually indicates nothing more than an air-fluid interface, and feeding can often be undertaken in the absence of bowel sounds. In severely malnourished cancer patients, the formula infusion rate should be increased more gradually to avoid refeeding syndrome (discussed above and in Chapter 45). In addition, jejunal feeding in postoperative patients should be started at as little as 10 mL/hour, although this can often be accomplished in the immediate postoperative phase and advanced as tolerated. Most isotonic formulas contain 1.0 to 1.5 kcal/mL and include the protein content in this calculation.

Complications of tube feeding include esophagitis, esophageal and/or gastric erosions or ulceration, or esophageal stricture or mucosal bridge formation. Esophageal or gastric erosions may be evident within a week of commencing enteral feedings, although longer-term use is generally required before clinically significant disease, including GI hemorrhage, may occur. In addition, nasal erosions and nasal cartilage sloughing may result from excessive pressure on the nasal alae and cartilage, and, therefore, nasogastric feeding should be undertaken via the same nares for a maximum of 4 to 6 weeks.

Gastroenterologists may be asked to place a percutaneous endoscopic gastrostomy (PEG) tube prophylactically in patients with head and neck cancer who will be receiving radiation postoperatively. Although the practice of placing a PEG prophylactically is acceptable given the length of time following radiation therapy that patients are unable to take oral nutrients (ie, mean 4 months) and improved quality of life, reports of cancer seeding to the cutaneous skin site have been reported using the traditional pull method of insertion.[23] The endoscopic push or radiology-assisted method, in which the feeding tube does not come into contact with the cancer in the oropharyngeal cavity, is recommended by the authors' in patients with head and neck cancer.

Regarding the formula to use, more recent findings would suggest that immune enhancing formulas containing glutamine, arginine, nucleotides, and omega-3 fatty acids are associated with less postoperative infections, reduced hospital length of stay, reduced overall cost, and improved immune function compared to those of standard formulas.[24] Improved mortality has not been reported with these formulas. At a United States consensus conference, the following recommendations were made regarding the use of immune enhancing formulas: they should be used in moderately to severely malnourished major elective surgical patients (including cancer patients) and those patients who are severely malnourished undergoing lower GI surgery.[24] The immune enhancing formulas were also recommended for patients with torso trauma. For the formulas to have the most beneficial effect, administering 1200 to 1500 mL/day for 5 to 7 days before surgery and 5 to 7 days after surgery was recommended.[24]

References

1. Hensrud DD, Heimburger DC. Diet, nutrients, and gastrointestinal cancer. *Gastroenterol Clin North Am.* 1998;27:325-346.
2. Silverman DT, Swanson CA, Gridley G, et al. Dietary and nutritional factors and pancreatic cancer: a case-control study based on direct interviews. *J Natl Cancer Inst.* 1998;90:1710-1719.
3. Li JY, Taylor PR, Li B, et al. Nutrition intervention trials in Linxian, China: multiple vitamin/mineral supplementation, cancer incidence, and disease-specific mortality among adults with esophageal dysplasia. *J Natl Cancer Inst.* 1993;85:1492-1498.
4. Haenszel W, Kurihara M. Studies of Japanese migrants. I. Mortality from cancer and other diseases among Japanese in the United States. *J Natl Cancer Inst.* 1968;40:43-68.
5. Kono S, Hirohata T. Nutrition and stomach cancer. *Cancer Causes Control.* 1996;7:41-55.
6. Armstrong B, Doll R. Environmental factors and cancer incidence and mortality in different countries, with special reference to dietary practices. *Int J Cancer.* 1975;15:617-631.
7. The American Cancer Society 1996 Advisory Committee on Diet Nutrition, and Cancer Prevention. Guidelines on diet, nutrition, and cancer prevention: reducing the risk of cancer with healthy food choices and physical activity. *CA Cancer J Clin.* 1996;46:325-341.
8. Russell DM, Shike M, Marliss EB, et al. Effects of total parenteral nutrition and chemotherapy on the metabolic derangements in small cell lung cancer. *Cancer Res.* 1984;44:1706-1711.
9. Dewys WD, Begg C, Lavin PT, et al. Prognostic effect of weight loss prior to chemotherapy in cancer patients. Eastern Cooperative Oncology Group. *Am J Med.* 1980;69:491-497.
10. Detsky AS, McLaughlin JR, Baker JP, et al. What is subjective global assessment of nutritional status? *JPEN J Parenter Enteral Nutr.* 1987;11:8-13.
11. Jatoi A Jr, Loprinzi CL. Current management of cancer-associated anorexia and weight loss. *Oncology.* 2001;15:497-502.
12. Heerington AM. *Nutr Clin Pract.* 1997;12:101-113.
13. Loprinzi CL, Bernath AM, Schaid DJ, et al. Phase III evaluation of 4 doses of megestrol acetate as therapy for patients with cancer anorexia and/or cachexia. *Oncology.* 1994;51 (Suppl 1):2-7.
14. Loprinzi CL, Ellison NM, Schaid DJ, et al. Controlled trial of megestrol acetate for the treatment of cancer anorexia and cachexia. *J Natl Cancer Inst.* 1990;82:1127-1132.
15. Kardinal CG, Loprinzi CL, Schaid DJ, et al. A controlled trial of cyproheptadine in cancer patients with anorexia and/or cachexia. *Cancer.* 1990;65:2657-2662.

16. Satyanarayana R, Klein S. Clinical efficacy of perioperative nutrition support. *Curr Opin Clin Nutr Metab Care.* 1998;1:51-58.
17. The Veterans Affairs Total Parenteral Nutrition Cooperative Study Group. Perioperative total parenteral nutrition in surgical patients. *N Engl J Med.* 1991;325:525-532.
18. Bozzetti F. Nutrition and gastrointestinal cancer. *Curr Opin Clin Nutr Metab Care.* 2001;4:541-546.
19. Jain G, Scolapio J, Wasserman E, Floch MH. Chronic radiation enteritis: a ten-year follow-up. *J Clin Gastroenterol.* 2002;35:214-217.
20. Scolapio JS, Ukleja A, Burnes JU, Kelly DG. Outcome of patients with radiation enteritis treated with home parenteral nutrition. *Am J Gastroenterol.* 2002;97:662-666.
21. Solomon SM, Kirby DF. The refeeding syndrome: a review. *JPEN J Parenter Enteral Nutr.* 1990;14:90-97.
22. Scolapio JS, Fleming CR, Kelly DG, Wick DM, Zinsmeister AR. Survival of home parenteral nutrition-treated patients: 20 years of experience at the Mayo Clinic. *Mayo Clin Proc.* 1999;74:217-222.
23. Sinclair JJ, Scolapio JS, Stark ME, Hinder RA. Metastasis of head and neck carcinoma to the site of percutaneous endoscopic gastrostomy: case report and literature review. *JPEN J Parenter Enteral Nutr.* 2001;25:282-285.
24. Proceedings from Summit on Immune-Enhancing Enteral Therapy. May 25-26, 2000, San Diego, California, USA. *JPEN J Parenter Enteral Nutr.* 2001;25:S1-S63.

Section IV

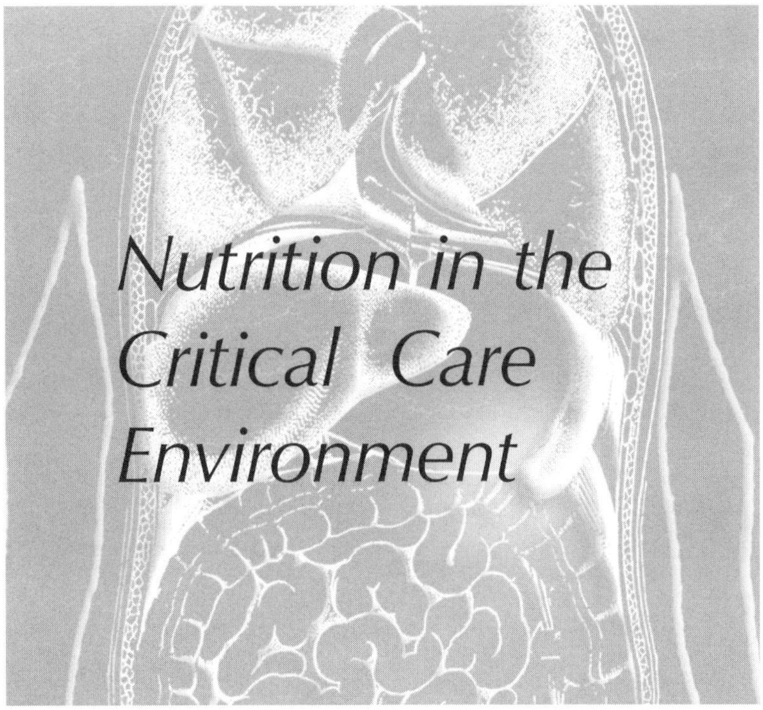

Nutrition in the Critical Care Environment

Chapter 27

The Metabolic Response to Critical Illness

Stephen F. Lowry, MD, and
J. Martin Perez, MD

Introduction

The metabolic response to critical illness is induced by the endogenous production of a variety of humoral and cellular mediators in response to diverse stimuli including trauma, sepsis, ischemia/reperfusion, and other disease states. This state is characterized by progressive severe loss of body protein, alterations in carbohydrate metabolism, increased oxidation of lipid, and increased extracellular volume that may result in organ dysfunction or failure. This state may be mitigated to some degree by nutritional support but can be reversed only by major palliation or cure of the underlying disease process. Prolonged catabolism in the critically ill may contribute to increased morbidity and mortality.

The hypermetabolic response has also evolved to allow substrate mobilization and, with changes in intermediary metabolism, to serve the purpose of healing and resolution of inflammation. Over 50 years ago, Cuthbertson demonstrated a hypermetabolic response in injured patients that was characterized by loss of protein and fat with water and salt retention.[1] Further pioneering work of Campbell and Ingle, established the role of glucocorticoids in the metabolic response to injury and Egdahl delineated the importance of the nervous system in the early endocrine response to injury. Subsequent research has focused on the cellular mechanisms, molecules, and, most recently, the genes that underlie this host metabolic response to injury or disease. Further elucidation of these underlying processes may allow the identification of therapeutic targets to modify the hypercatabolic response. This chapter describes the metabolic response to critical illness, the neuro-immuno-endocrine and cytokine mediators of this response, and the metabolic consequences of prolonged net hypermetabolism to the host. The clinical features of this response in the critically ill, in general, are qualitatively similar, regardless of the nature of the insult.

Utilizing injury as an example of an initial insult leading to critical illness, the temporal sequence of postinjury metabolic events, is well known from the careful evaluation of many investigators. In patients with long-bone fractures, Cuthbertson noted marked elevated urinary excretion of nitrogen, potassium, and phosphorous similar to the composition of muscle and concluded that muscle was the ultimate source of these losses.[1] In the 1940s and 1950s, Campbell and Ingle demonstrated that in adrenalectomized rats nitrogen loss following femoral shaft fracture was obliterated as compared to controls.[2] Egdahl demonstrated in a canine model—in which he disconnected the limb from the body leaving only the sciatic nerve and vessels—that subsequent traumatic injury to the limb where the sciatic had been divided failed to produce a rise in glucocorticoids.[3] Isotopic dilution studies by Moore characterized the "ebb and flow phases" of the postinjury response.[4] The early ebb phase occurs immediately post insult and is characterized by hemodynamic instability with decreased cardiac output and oxygen consumption, low core temperature, and elevated glucagon, catecholamine, and free fatty acid levels. This phase typically lasts from 12 to 24 hours and is modified to some degree by the extent and adequacy of fluid resuscitation.

The subsequent flow phase is fundamentally a metabolic response mediated by cytokines, reactive oxygen species, arachidonic acid metabolites, and nitric oxide that alters energy and protein use to preserve critical organ function and to repair damaged tissue. Total body oxygen consumption, metabolic rate, and amino

TABLE 27-1.

Metabolic Alterations Following Critical Illness

Ebb Phase	*Flow Phase*
Increased blood glucose	Normal/slightly elevated blood glucose
Increased circulating free fatty acids	Normal/slightly increased free fatty acids
Decreased insulin	Normal/increased insulin
Increased catecholamines	Increased catecholamines
Decreased cardiac output	Increased cardiac output
Decreased oxygen consumption	Increased oxygen consumption
Decreased core temperature	Elevated core temperature

acid efflux from peripheral muscle stores all increase; counter-regulatory hormone concentrations are elevated; glucose metabolism is altered; and lactate production, urinary nitrogen losses, and tissue protein catabolism all increase[5] (Table 27-1). The recovery phase of the metabolic response serves to enhance survival in times of stress and provides a mechanism of mobilizing energy stores and building blocks such as amino acids for new tissue growth and for acute phase reactants. With the resolution of the inciting event, a period of recuperative anabolism ensues in which metabolic homeostasis is reestablished in concert with replenishment of fat and muscle stores. The discussion below focuses on the elements that comprise the flow phase response and the endogenous mediators that regulate this response.

Energy Expenditure: Critical Illness

During the post insult flow phase, there is increased energy expenditure by the body as well as an increased metabolic rate. Total body oxygen consumption increases in concert with increased oxidation of fuel sources (carbohydrates, amino acids, and lipids). To some extent, the elevation of the metabolic rate correlates with the cause and/or the severity of the initial injury. Energy expenditure may increase minimally with mild injury[6], 15% to 25% following long-bone fractures[1], and as much as double with burn injury over more than 40% of total body surface.[7] The physiologic consequences of the flow phase insult serve as the basis for modern critical care medicine in which key features—such as support of adequate cardiac hemodynamics, optimized ventilation strategies, fluid administration, monitoring of organ function, and nutrition—are supported in the critically ill patient.

The increased metabolic rate requires mobilizing the body's nutrient stores to provide substrates for the increased energy demand. The body's stores of carbohydrates, primarily glycogen, are quickly depleted in the first 24 hours post injury. Thereafter, fat and protein serve as the main energy sources. In the hypermetabolic state, there is an obligatory net protein loss that partly serves to provide substrates for gluconeogenesis and amino acids for increased synthesis of acute phase proteins. Nitrogen is used as a surrogate marker of protein loss because of the fixed relation between the two substances (eg, protein in grams/6.25 = nitrogen in grams). Following an inciting event, an increase occurs in urinary nitrogen excretion, which is generally related to the magnitude of the injury and adequacy of insult resolution. The nitrogen loss is primarily in the form of urea but other contributing losses are in the form of creatinine, ammonia, uric acid, and amino acids excreted in urine. Skeletal muscle represents the majority of protein containing tissues and the net protein loss characteristic of the catabolic response results in loss of lean muscle mass. Stored triglycerides are also mobilized and oxidized to provide substrates for the hypermetabolic state but are unable to prevent protein catabolism.

During this state, there is also a marked rise in the counter-regulatory hormones: glucocorticoids, catecholamines, and glucagon mediated in large part by the central nervous system (CNS) and at the level of individual tissues. These hormones promote a variety of metabolic effects, as discussed below. Also important in the response to injury are cytokines, whose effects are mediated by both endocrine and paracrine mechanisms. These acute alterations in metabolic and hormonal responses serve to maintain tissue functions.

Protein Metabolism: Critical Illness

Protein represents a large reserve of body fuel. In response to the increased energy demands after injury or critical illness, skeletal muscle stores are mobilized. This leads to increased amino acid efflux from peripheral stores and increased urinary nitrogen excretion. The extent of urinary nitrogen loss correlates with the severity of the insult. The result is a net negative nitrogen balance as protein catabolism exceeds protein synthesis by the liver. This acceleration of protein catabolism generally parallels the increase in oxygen consumption and represents a constant fraction of total oxidation following injury.[6] If allowed to proceed unabated, this net protein catabolism leads to loss of lean muscle mass and, in turn, contributes to organ dysfunction or failure.[8]

The mechanism of muscle catabolism during sepsis, for example, involves increased protein breakdown in a fashion similar to injury, especially myofibrillar protein, as well as reduced protein synthesis and inhibition of amino acid uptake by muscle.[9-11] In animal models, important mediators of this catabolism during sepsis include glucocorticoids as well as certain cytokines, particularly tumor necrosis factor (TNF) and interleukin (IL) -1.[12] The current understanding of cytokine function in muscle homeostasis including muscle catabolism, anabolism, and links between other intermediaries in metabolism remains incomplete. Cytokines appear to have a bi-directional effect on muscle during inflammation with myocytes capable of producing cytokines; expressing cytokine receptors, adhesion molecules, and costimulatory molecules; and influencing the course of inflammation itself.[13]

Cytokines that effect muscle homeostasis can be produced by the myocyte and by nonmyocytes cells (ie, macrophages), either at the site of injury or from a distance. Cytokines, therefore, can exert their effects in an endocrine, autocrine, or paracrine manner, depending upon the nature of the injury and the particular cytokine.[14] The principal sources of extrinsic cytokine production appear to be neutrophils and macrophages resident in muscle.[15] Intrinsic muscle cytokines appear to include IL-1β, IL-6, IL-8, and transforming growth factor beta. GM-CSF production by myoblasts appears to be induced by exposure to IL-1α, IL-1β, and TNF-α.[16]

The relevance of cytokines in pathologic conditions such as injury and sepsis remains incompletely characterized despite extensive studies searching for putative mediators in muscle protein breakdown. The body of literature does indicate a complex network including, but not limited to, TNF-α, IL-1β, IL-6, gp130 proteins, interferons, and growth/differentiation factor-8 involved in the regulation of muscle protein homeostasis. Individual cytokine contributions to the overall milieu remain difficult to elucidate. Certainly, data exist that would argue against the hypothesis that cytokines alone are responsible for all the metabolic changes seen in injury and infection. First, cytokines have not been found to be uniformly elevated in all injured patients. Second, the effects of intravenously administered cytokines appear to be temporally limited. Third, some evidence exists that cytokines do not appear to have a direct effect on muscle protein breakdown.[17]

The intracellular mechanisms involved in muscle protein breakdown in sepsis and injury are not clearly defined; however, animal studies indicate that sepsis induces a nonlysosomal, energy-dependent proteolysis.[18] This involves activation of the ubiquitin-proteasome-dependent pathway that increases mRNAs encoding ubiquitin and proteasomes in muscle. In this pathway, proteins destined for degradation are ligated to the polypeptide ubiquitin and then degraded by a protease that acts on ubiquinated proteins.[19-21] The ubiquitination of proteins destined to undergo proteolysis by the proteasome is regulated by ubiquitin ligases as well as other enzymes. Recent studies have demonstrated E2 (14k) and E3alpha, ubiquitin ligases, to be involved in increased breakdown of proteins in atrophying muscle.[22] Other studies indicated that the mRNA for ubiquitin increases during glucocorticoid excess and acidosis and may occur in septic states.[23] In rats, endotoxemia can induce increased ubiquitin mRNA, IL-6, TNF-α, and net release of 3-methylhistidine, a marker of protein breakdown.[24] Studies have also demonstrated that the ubiquitin-proteasome system does not break down the complexes of proteins contained in actomyosin or myofibrils, which constitute the bulk of muscle protein.[25] Additional proteases such as caspase-3 may release constituent proteins of actomyosin prior to ubiquitin-proteasome system activation.[26] It is likely that the ubiquitin pathway is important in proteolysis in sepsis and in other catabolic conditions, but further studies are needed to delineate the mechanisms leading to ubiquitin-proteasome system activation.

The increased amino acids efflux from peripheral stores postinjury provides substrates for enhanced hepatic gluconeogenesis and acute-phase protein synthesis. It also allows new protein tissue in wounds and proliferation of cellular components involved in the inflammatory response. There is increased splanchnic uptake of glucogenic amino acids, particularly alanine and glutamine. This increase in uptake in burn patients corresponds to the quantity and distribution of peripheral tissue amino acid release.[27] The enhanced splanchnic uptake is achieved by increased glutamine uptake in the gut enterocytes, while alanine is released by the gastrointestinal (GI) tract in increasing amounts during stress.[28]

During the postinjury response, alanine and glutamine are also preferentially released from muscle stores. While these amino acids make up approximately 6% of protein in muscle stores, they constitute 60% to 80% of the free amino acids released in response to insult.[29,30] This effect may be influenced by glucocorticoid activity; in a study using canine models both acute and chronic glucocorticoid excess increased glutamine and alanine release.[31] Glutamine availability may become limited during catabolic illness, and mortality in critically ill patients has been associated with low glutamine levels.[32,33] Glutamine supplementation, in some studies, has improved immune function and reduced intestinal permeability.[34,35] Glutamine supplementation has been demonstrated to preserve skeletal muscle and improve nitrogen balance.[36] Given that glutamine is a precursor to glutathione, supplementation results in higher antioxidant capacity mediated in part by glutamine.[37] According to a recent meta-analysis of 14 randomized trials that compared the use of glutamine supplementation in surgical and critically ill patients, glutamine supplementation may be associated, in critically ill patients, with a reduction in complication and mortality rates; greatest benefit was seen with high-dose parenteral glutamine.[38]

Despite net peripheral proteolysis, liver mass is usually preserved during injury, often with an increase in total liver protein, RNA, and DNA.[39] Preservation of liver mass occurs with sustained or increased hepatic capacity for gluconeogenesis and synthesis of acute-phase proteins.[40]

In summary, skeletal protein catabolism may serve three main purposes. First, it provides amino acids that can serve as substrate for protein synthesis by the wound or liver. Second, the released amino acids can be converted to glucose by the liver as an energy source during the hypermetabolic response. Third, it provides a source of glutamine to be used as a fuel source by the gut and possibly by other tissues involved in the metabolic response to stress.

Glucose Metabolism: Critical Illness

Hyperglycemia is a common response to septic or traumatic injury. It results from both increased hepatic gluconeogenesis and decreased glucose uptake by insulin-dependent tissues. In the ebb phase, insulin levels are depressed, but they become normal to elevated during the flow phase, although they remain depressed in relation to the degree of hyperglycemia. The persistent hyperglycemia suggests injury-induced insulin resistance.[5] In addition, studies using hepatic vein cannulations in thermally injured patients demonstrate increased uptake of gluconeogenic amino acids by the splanchnic tissues.[27] These amino acids are then used for gluconeogenesis, resulting in increased splanchnic production of glucose and further contributing to the hyperglycemic state.

Altered glucose metabolism in response to stress results in decreased skeletal muscle uptake of glucose and decreased glucose incorporation into fatty acids by adipocytes.[41] The decreased uptake by skeletal muscle is due to peripheral insulin resistance, which may be mediated in part by excess cortisol and catecholamines.[42,43] Recent evidence also indicates that TNF-α induces insulin resistance.[44] In these stressed patients, hyperglycemia fails to suppress hepatic gluconeogenesis or glycogenolysis; administration of a dextrose infusion suppresses gluconeogenesis less effectively in septic or trauma patients than it does in healthy volunteers.[45] Amino acid infusions are also unable to inhibit gluconeogenesis in trauma patients.[46] This alteration in glucose metabolism maintains glucose availability to noninsulin dependent tissues such as the CNS, kidneys, wound tissue, and hematologic cells, which are vital for survival.

During the stress response, another source of glucose results from the change to anaerobic glycolysis in skeletal muscle and hypoxic tissue (ie, the wound), producing increased amounts of lactate. Lactate can be converted into glucose in the liver via the Cori cycle, which is increased in both burn and trauma patients.[47,48] In burn patients, lactate is the most important gluconeogenic substrate.[49] The resultant lacticacidemia may be mediated in part by both catecholamines and cytokines.[50,51] In critically ill patients, elevated lactate levels may reflect impaired tissue oxygenation; however, elevated lactate levels may persist despite evidence of adequate tissue oxygenation. The higher lactate levels in this circumstance reflects excess production of pyruvate as a consequence of accelerated glycoylysis, which stems from increased glucose uptake and glycogen breakdown rather than from tissue dysoxia.[52]

The efficiency of glucose oxidation is altered by injury[53] and, in postoperative[54] and burn patients,[55] further contributes to the hyperglycemic state. Maximum glucose oxidative capacity appears to be inversely related to severity of the injury. The decrease in oxidation may be due to reduced activity of intracellular enzymatic metabolic pathways, such as pyruvate dehydrogenase.[56]

Lipid Metabolism: Critical Illness

Lipid is a major source of fuel for the body, representing 80% of the body's energy reserves. In response to stress, lipid mobilization and use can potentially preserve proteins. Immediately post insult, there is enhanced lipolysis mediated by sympathetic stimulation of adipose tissue as well as activation of lipase by norepinephrine and glucagon.[57] Leptin, a hormone, also stimulates fatty acid oxidation and is expressed by adipocytes. Leptin is related to cytokines in that it is considered a stress-related hormone. Insulin, insulin-like growth factor 1, thyroid hormones, somatotropin release-inhibiting factor, glucocorticoids, and beta-adrenergic agonists are known to enhance leptin production. Leptin levels correlate with early sepsis, and survivors appear to have higher plasma levels than controls.[58] However, leptin levels are not elevated in patients with sepsis of longer duration and do not predict outcome.[59] The overall net result of these hormones and cytokines is an increase in free fatty acids and glycerol concentration in the circulation.

Several studies have indicated that there may be a preference for oxidation of fat as a source of energy in septic or trauma patients.[60] In the nonstressed condition, the normal respiratory quotient (RQ) is approximately 0.85.[61] In the injured patient, the RQ is lower, which indicates increased lipid oxidation.[7] A decreased RQ is also seen in patients with worsening sepsis, and isotopic studies have corroborated increased fat oxidation in these patients.[62,63] Other studies have demonstrated that, with increased severity of sepsis, oxidation and clearance of lipids from the bloodstream falls, which suggests poor utilization and may account for feeding resistant protein wasting with preservation of fat stores seen in critical illness.[64] Overall, the increased amount of free fatty acids serves as a fuel source for tissues except red blood cells and the CNS.

Mediators of the Hypermetabolic Response

There is a characteristic postinjury neuroendocrine response, with an increase in catecholamines and glucocorticoids. However, despite extensive investigation of the hormonal milieu and response to injury and stress, hormone increases in normal subjects have not been able to reproduce the amount of protein catabolism seen in severe injury. This indicates that hormonal changes alone cannot account for all the metabolic consequences of severe stress and injury. Therefore, increased attention to other possible mediators of hypercatabolic stress mechanisms has largely focused on the role of immunopeptide regulation of host metabolic response to injury. These endogenous mediators of postinjury hypermetabolism—including the humoral mediators of the neuroendocrine system, the autonomic nervous systems, and the cytokines—can integrate and transfer information from the injury site to affect a response beneficial to the host. The next section focuses on the role of these mediators in the postinjury response.

Another recent hypothesis attempts to correlate the amount of protein catabolism observed in the hypermetabolic state with the cellular hydration state.[65] The cell swelling theory argues that cellular volume is the key signal for the metabolic orientation of cell metabolism, namely cellular swelling leads to anabolism whereas cellular shrinkage promotes catabolism.[66] A recent study of sequential changes in intracellular water, total body protein, total body potassium, and intracellular potassium in critically ill patients with blunt trauma or sepsis demonstrated that the loss of protein and potassium is accompanied by progressive cellular dehydration.[67] Cellular dehydration is influenced by many factors, including altered nutrition, hormones, cytokines, and oxygen radicals. Although it proposes an interesting mechanism for the proteolysis observed in critically ill patients, this hypothesis remains to be substantiated in clinical trials.

Neuro-Immuno-Endocrine Response

The neuroendocrine and immune systems are interrelated by sharing, in common, chemical mediators (hormones, cytokines, steroids, neuropeptides, and neurotransmitters) and their associated receptors. These shared chemical mediators and receptors in turn allow for an integrated molecular response to stress, inflammation, and infection. Sensory afferent and postganglionic sympathetic neurons also influence inflammation by secreting proinflammatory or anti-inflammatory neuropeptides, such as substance P and somatostatin, into the site of inflammation.

Early studies by Hume and Egdahl established the importance of an intact CNS in mediating the early response to injury.[68] Their original studies demonstrated that the increase in adrenocorticoid steroids after a burn injury could be blocked by sectioning the peripheral nerve, cervical spinal cord, or medulla oblongata in dogs. Other clinical studies show less adrenocorticotrophic hormone (ACTH) or growth hormone (GH) release in response to minor tissue injury (herniorraphy) in patients receiving spinal anesthesia than those receiving general anesthesia.[69] The CNS also appears to be instrumental in the hypermetabolic response to injury. One study demonstrated that administration of inert gas anesthesia to hypermetabolic burn patients lowered their core temperatures and metabolic rates.[70] In a study of head injury patients who were in barbiturate coma, metabolic rate and nitrogen excretion were reduced to basal levels with administration of a barbiturate.[71]

Afferent signals from the site of injury, baroreceptors sensing hypovolemia, and infection can elicit hypothalamic mechanisms to stimulate the anterior pituitary to secrete prolactin, ACTH, antidiuretic hormone, and GH.[29] ACTH release stimulates an increase in adrenal glucocorticoid secretion. Evidence of increased ACTH secretion has been observed following elective operations, extensive trauma,[72-74] thermal injury,[75,76] and infection.[77,78] Circulating levels of GH are markedly increased immediately postinjury and tend to decrease to normal levels within 24 to 48 hours. However, in protracted critical illness the dominant profile of endocrine response is that of suppression of anterior pituitary hormone secretion. Cortisol appears unaffected and remains high; this effect is potentially mediated by endothelin.[79,80]

Thyroid stimulating hormone (TSH) levels do not appear to be greatly affected by critical illness. However, there is a characteristic pattern of normal T_4, elevated rT_3, and depressed T_3 during prolonged periods of stress, which is related in part to calorie deficiency[81,82] as well as in response to an inflammatory stimulus.[83] In patients exhibiting this euthyroid sick syndrome, proposed mechanisms include impaired responsiveness of the thyroid to TSH, reduced serum binding of thyroid hormones, or reduced peripheral conversion of T_4 to T_3. Glucocorticoids inhibit the enzymatic conversion of T_4 to T_3. Cytokines appear not to inhibit this glucocorticoid-mediated inhibition of the conversion of T_4 to T_3.[84]

Catecholamines

The catecholamines, specifically epinephrine and norepinephrine, are rapidly produced in response to a variety of insults. Elevated levels are most pronounced during the early postinjury period (48 hours) and decrease during recovery.[85,86] Post injury levels of catecholamines correlate to some extent with the severity of initial injury.[87] Mild injury may elicit a moderate increase in catecholamines, whereas more severe injuries may be associated with a prolonged rise in urinary or circulating levels of catecholamines.[5]

The net metabolic influence of catecholamines is to increase energy expenditure, hepatic glycogenolysis, glycolysis, and lipolysis with resultant increase in free fatty acid concentration. Paradoxically, catecholamine excess acutely decreases the efflux of amino acids from peripheral tissue while increasing lactate release from skeletal muscle. This was confirmed by studies in which epinephrine infusion into healthy subjects resulted in increased energy expenditure, hyperglycemia, lactic acidosis, and decreased amino acid efflux.[7,87,88] Although the precise effect of adrenergic stimulation on protein kinetics is controversial, studies indicate that beta-stimulation promotes gluconeogenesis and may limit skeletal muscle nitrogen loss, whereas alpha-adrenergic stimulation leads to protein catabolism.[89,90] A recent study of beta-blockade in severe pediatric burns demonstrated attenuation of hypermetabolism and reversal of muscle-protein catabolism. In this study, propranolol was thought to increase the intracellular recycling of free amino acids resulting in reincorporation into bound protein.[91] Beta-blockade, however, has not been associated with improved survival and has the potential of converting intermediate thickness burn wounds to full thickness if hypoperfusion results. Taken together, these studies indicate appreciable catecholamine influence on extreme changes in protein metabolism that is seen in severe stress and injury.

Cortisol

Glucocorticoid excess promotes negative nitrogen balance but exhibits little influence on overall energy expenditure.[88,89] The lines of evidence indicating glucocorticoid's role in catabolism of muscle tissues are 1) glucocorticoid levels are increased in a number of conditions characterized by muscle atrophy; 2) humans or experimental animals treated with glucocorticoids induce a catabolic response in skeletal muscle; 3) in vitro, cultured muscle cells treated with glucocorticoids exhibit net protein loss; and 4) muscle wasting can be inhibited by adrenalectomy or by treating animals with a glucocorticoid receptor antagonist.[92] Cortisol affects a slight increase in free fatty acid concentration, promotes hepatic gluconeogenesis, and increases peripheral tissue amino acid efflux. In normal subjects, cortisol infusion alone produced the same net sustained nitrogen loss as that produced by combined cortisol, epinephrine, norepinephrine, and glucagon infusion.[88] Also, short-term cortisol infusion in high physiologic concentrations in healthy subjects increased plasma amino acid concentration, particularly the branched-chain amino acids (leucine, isoleucine, and valine).[93] Glucocorticoids mediate muscle catabolic activity in part via the ubiquitin-proteasome-pathway and calcium-dependent protein degradation.[94] During sepsis and other catabolic conditions, glutamine utilization increases with increased glutamine synthetase expression and activity in skeletal muscle and lung. Overall, glutamine levels are reduced in muscle during critical illness and are proposed to be an important mechanism of stimulated muscle breakdown and inhibited protein synthesis.[95,96] Glucocorticoids appear to regulate the expression and activity of glutamine synthetase in skeletal muscle thus possibly playing a role in glutamine-mediated muscle breakdown.[97,98]

Insulin

Insulin levels are initially decreased during the ebb phase after injury but are mildly to markedly increased during the early flow phase. Hyperglycemia and hyperinsulinemia are characteristic of the early stress response. As stated above, the body becomes resistant to insulin in such tissues as adipocytes and skeletal myocytes.[99] The splanchnic tissues also display a relative resistance to insulin, manifested by continued hepatic gluconeogenesis despite elevated glucose levels.[100] Insulin resistance may be mediated in part by cortisol[42] as well as by catecholamines.[43] The role of the characteristic hyperinsulinemia observed in critical illness remains unclear, as critical organs—including the CNS, hematogenous cells, wounds, and the kidney—incorporate glucose in an insulin-independent manner. Nevertheless, continuous infusion of glucose and insulin result in decreased urine urea nitrogen excretion as well as decreased amino acid efflux and decreased 3-methylhistidine excretion (a marker of protein catabolism);[101] therefore, the increase in insulin may serve to decrease protein catabolism during the flow phase. Hyperglycemia and glucose intolerance have long been recognized features of various types of critical illness and injury states to include burns,[48,102] myocardial infarction,[103] and surgery.[104]

Recent studies examining the relationship between insulin, blood glucose, and clinical outcomes in critically ill patients have reported decreased infectious complications,[105] improved skin grafting success in burn patients, and a reduction in morbidity and mortality in patients subjected to an intensive insulin regimen.[106] These results have, for the first time, demonstrated a clinical benefit to insulin therapy; however, the question remains whether the derived benefit is due to the effects of lowered blood glucose, insulin action independent of lowered blood glucose, or both.

Glucagon

Circulating glucagon levels increase during the hypermetabolic postinjury phase and correlate roughly with the severity of injury.[107,108] Glucagon appears to exert little independent influence on peripheral tissue metabolism[109] but is a potent stimulant of the hepatic cyclic AMP system, facilitating hepatic uptake of amino acids[110] and gluconeogenesis.[111] Glucagon is also influenced by the autonomic nervous system.[112]

Cytokines: Proinflammatory Cytokine Peptides

Proinflammatory cytokine peptides were originally studied for their effect on immunologic homeostasis in several areas, but they also exert potent activity toward regulation of hemodynamic and metabolic responses.[113] During early postinjury or infectious conditions, the initial cytokine response to such insults likely mediates beneficial protective signaling of the immune system. Nevertheless, excessive acute production of some cytokines, such as TNF, may promote septic shock. Prolonged production of tissue cytokines sustains some metabolic effects of the hypercatabolic state.

Diverse cell types of both myeloid and nonmyeloid origin produce the proinflammatory cytokine peptides. These proteins may function by autocrine, paracrine, or systemic mechanisms of action. They produce local tissue responses by cell-to-cell interaction at very low concentrations but also may exert systemic effects in higher concentrations. While many cytokines are now well characterized, those exhibiting the more prominent proinflammatory activities include TNF-α, IL-1, IL-6, and interferon-gamma (IFN-γ) have been more widely studied from a metabolic perspective (Table 27-2).

Tumor Necrosis Factor

TNF is a 17-Kda protein primarily secreted from monocytes and macrophages. Although originally isolated as a soluble factor that produced cachexia during infection (as implied by the name) and in vivo necrosis of some solid tumors,[114] this cytokine has been implicated as the initiating signal for a variety of cellular and metabolic events seen in critically ill patients. TNF administration

TABLE 27-2.

Major Cytokines Involved in Hypermetabolic Response

Cytokine	Cell Source	Metabolic Effects
Tumor Necrosis Factor-α	Monocytes/macrophages, lymphocytes, Kupffer cells, glial cells, endothelial cells, natural killer cells, mast cells	Decrease FFA synthesis Increased lipolysis Increased peripheral amino acid loss Increased hepatic amino acid uptake Fever
IL-1	Monocytes/macrophages, neutrophils, lymphocytes, keratinocytes, Kupffer cells	Increased ACTH Increased hepatic acute-phase protein synthesis Fever
IL-6	Monocytes/macrophages, keratinocytes, endothelial cells, fibroblasts, T cells, epithelial cells	Increased acute-phase protein synthesis Fever
IFN-γ	Lymphocytes, pulmonary macrophages	Increased monocyte respiratory burst

to healthy subjects elicits a systemic response resembling that observed during sepsis,[115] including increased stress hormone release, temperature elevation and increased acute-phase protein synthesis.[116] The systemic effects of bacterial liposaccharide (endotoxin) are replicated, if not largely mediated, by TNF.[117] Indeed endotoxin infusion induces a rapid increase in circulating TNF levels, and blocking TNF with antibodies in animal models alleviates many of the toxic effects of endotoxin.[118,119] TNF may circulate predominately as a complex with its soluble receptors, making detection of the bioactive ligand more difficult. Increased levels of these soluble TNF receptors are seen in response to diverse inflammatory stimuli including sepsis, cancer, and acquired immunodeficiency syndrome (AIDS).[119] Nevertheless, elevated TNF levels are detected in many disease states including bacterial infection, infected thermal injury, tumor-bearing states, sepsis, and AIDS.[120]

The metabolic effects of TNF and perhaps also the other proinflammatory cytokines seem to promote redistribution of body protein and lipid stores.[115] The result is a net loss of peripheral tissue protein with a concomitant increase in hepatic uptake. Alterations in fat metabolism elicited by TNF resemble the changes seen in infection. They include promotion of cellular lipolysis and hepatic lipogenesis with decreased free fatty acid synthesis and decreased clearance of extracellular lipids.[120-122] Increased TNF-α levels have been demonstrated in obesity-induced insulin resistance, suggesting a role for TNF-alpha in mediating insulin resistance. Soluble TNF receptors have also been demonstrated to neutralize unbound TNF and inhibit the development of TNF-alpha–induced insulin resistance and adipogenesis.[123]

Interleukin-1

IL-1 is produced by macrophages/monocytes, neutrophils, lymphocytes, and keratinocytes.[113] Its production is stimulated by TNF and endotoxin, and, like TNF, it may represent an early cytokine response to injury. Once released, it exerts multiple immunologic and metabolic effects including stimulation of ACTH[124], induction of fever, hepatic acute-phase protein synthesis, and alteration of energy metabolism.[125] IL-1 also induces anorexia and inhibition of fatty acid synthesis and adipocytes differentiation.[125,126] Like TNF activity, IL-1 activity is regulated by shedding of soluble receptors, as well as by unique, naturally occurring receptor antagonist (IL-1ra).[127] IL-1ra binds to the IL-1 receptor without an agonist influence. IL-1ra–deficient mice exhibit growth retardation, resistance to high-fat-diet induced obesity, reduced activity of lipoprotein lipase, and low insulin levels.[128] In humans, IL-1ra is up-regulated in serum of obese individuals and correlates with insulin resistance.[129]

Interleukin-6

IL-6 is the most frequently detected cytokine in patients with acute infection,[129] injury, and tumor-bearing states[130] and after elective surgical procedures.[131] The biologic actions of this protein include regulation of acute-phase protein synthesis after injury[132,133] and differentiation of lymphocytes.[134] In one study, administration of IL-6 to humans induced modest changes in the kinetics of glucose and protein.[135] IL-6 is produced in large part by adipose tissue and circulating levels correlate with body mass index, insulin sensitivity, and glucose tolerance.

Interferon-gamma

IFN-γ is secreted from lymphocytes and macrophages and exerts antiviral effects as well as protection against bacteria, fungi, and parasites. It enhances TNF production in response to endotoxin[136] and increases the cytotoxicity of monocytes, possibly by increasing their respiratory burst activity.[137] A direct role for IFN-γ in directing altered metabolic processes has not been defined in humans, although its administration does induce cachexia and loss of protein and lipid stores in animals.[138]

Anti-Inflammatory Cytokines

Regulation of the various cytokines produced in response to injury or disease is complex and involves counter-regulation by anti-inflammatory cytokines such as IL-10, which down-regulates secretion of proinflammatory cytokines (ie, TNF and IL-1) as well as suppressing macrophage and T-cell functions. Counterregulatory mechanisms likely are important in maintaining a counterbalance to unopposed systemic inflammation and hypercatabolism and may play a role in restoration of metabolic homeostasis and anabolism.

Neuroendocrine System and Cytokines

The response to injury, infection, and ischemia/reperfusion is associated with concurrent activation of the hypothalamic-pituitary-adrenal axis (HPA). Recent work suggests that organ systems express and respond to a large number of common regulatory and counter-regulatory molecules such as cytokines, neuropeptides, neurotransmitters, and steroids, which provide an integrated and bi-directional molecular response to disturbances induced by injury, infection, or ischemia/reperfusion. The end result is an integration of the nervous, endocrine, and immune systems to these perturbations.[139-142] Cytokines—including IL-1, IL-6, TNF, and leukemia inhibitory factor (LIF)—appear to mediate the complex HPA axis response to stress or inflammation.[143] Cytokines may function like classic endocrine hormones acting locally or may impact a distant target.[144] During stress, cytokines stimulate pituitary corticotroph POMC gene expression and ACTH secretion in the hypothalamus and pituitary.[145] The gp130 cytokine family consisting of LIF, IL-6, IL-11, ciliary neurotrophic factor, and Oncostatin M participate in ACTH regulation and mediate the immuno-neuroendocrine interface.[146,147] Through intracellular signaling systems such as cyclic adenosine monophosphate (c AMP) and the JAK/STAT/SOCS pathway and in synergy with POMC inducers and CRH, cytokines mediate cell proliferation, mature ACTH secretion, and impart negative feedback to the HPA axis.[148]

Glucocorticoid secretion, mediated by ACTH and indirectly through cytokines, is a potent anti-inflammatory mechanism. The α-glucocorticoid receptor (α-GR) binds the steroid hormone, translocates to the nucleus, and binds to the glucocorticoid responsive elements (GRE).[149] Some GREs down-regulate the transcription of other genes (eg, most cytokines) and prevent transcription initiated by transcriptional factors such as nuclear factor (NF) -κB.[150] Glucocorticoids can inhibit production of TNF or IL-6,[133,151,152] and, in the case of TNF, the mechanism appears to include altering transcription of the mRNA.[153] Cortisol infusion attenuates the endogenous TNF response to endotoxin administration.[134,153] Cathecholamine infusion also inhibits endotoxin-induced TNF production while simultaneously increasing release of IL-10.[154] Proinflammatory cytokines such as TNF and IL-1 initiate a cascade of inflammatory responses by activating NF-κB, which in turn stimulates proinflammatory genes. Glucocorticoids bound to GR interact with NF-κB in the nucleus and alter its ability to promote transcription of cytokine-responsive genes.[155] These two opposing regulatory systems are coupled to maintain the homeostatic balance of the inflammatory response. Glucocorticoids, in turn, antagonize the actions of GH and the sex steroids on adipose tissue (lipolysis) and muscle/bone anabolism.[156] Chronic activation of the system would lead to decrease lean body mass through the loss of muscle and bone and suppression of osteoblastic activity.

Hence, the neuro-immuno-endocrine milieu elicited by injury, infection, or other hypermetabolic conditions may serve to alter cytokine mediator activities in a complex manner. It remains to be determined to what extent these parallel signaling pathways direct the human metabolic response.

Systemic and Organ Reactions: Gastrointestinal Tract

The GI tract provides important nutrient absorptive and metabolic functions and recently has emerged as an immunologically important organ. In the late 1960s, parenteral nutritional (PN) support provided a life-saving therapy to progressive hypermetabolism.[156] (PN is discussed in Chapters 34 through 38.) PN administration provided fluids and macro- and micronutrients in sufficient quantity to meet nutritional needs and avoided progressive starvation-induced malnutrition and in turn changed the outcome of patients who would have otherwise died.[158] Subsequent studies have demonstrated that enteral processing of nutrients affected the metabolic response to septic insults and improved host defenses. In a study of randomized severely burned children receiving standard enteral or protein-supplemented diet, those receiving high-protein diets had fewer septic complications and a lower mortality.[159] In vitro evidence also demonstrated that in a rat model of *Escherichia coli* peritonitis, enteral support lowered mortality.[160]

Recent studies have focused on intestinal permeability after injury and translocation of intraluminal bacteria to mesenteric lymph nodes and to the systemic circulation.[161-163] These studies suggest that maintenance of intestinal barrier function is required to reduce permeability to intraluminal organisms. The gut mucosa normally provides a barrier to foreign material such as bacteria, their products, and other ingested particles. Enteral feeding is essential to maintain the integrity of the mucosal barrier.[164,165] In animal studies, bowel rest and PN produce increased translocation of bacteria to intestinal lymphoid tissue.[166] PN and bowel rest are associated with an exaggerated response to injury.[167]

Whether bacterial translocation is an important source of systemic bacteriemia and sepsis during disease states in humans is a matter of debate; however, it may be that stimulation of splanchnic immune cells by foreign antigens that have crossed the mucosal barrier influences systemic immunologic and metabolic processes during disease states. Cytokines secreted by splanchnic cells or lymphocytes or macrophages influence both the immune and hemodynamic responses to injury as well as the metabolic response.[168,169] In this way, the intestine may partially regulate the immune response to injury or disease.

References

1. Cuthbertson D. *Br Med Bull.* 1945;3:96-102.
2. Ingle DJ, Ward EO, Kuizenga MH. The relationship of the adrenal glands to changes in urinary non-protein nitrogen following multiple fractures in the force fed rat. *Am J Physiol.* 1947;149:510.
3. Egdahl RH. Pituitary-adrenal response following trauma to the isolated leg. *Surgery.* 1959;46:9-21
4. Moore F. *Metabolic Care of the Surgical Patient.* Philadelphia, Pa: WB Saunders; 1959.
5. Lowry SF. Host metabolic response to injury. In: Gallin JI, Fauci AS, eds. *Advances in Host Defense Mechanisms.* Vol 6. New York: Raven Press; 1986:169-190.
6. Duke JH, Jorgensen SB, Broell JR, et al. Contribution of protein to caloric expenditure following injury. *Surgery.* 1970;68:168-174.
7. Wilmore DW, Long JM, Mason AD Jr, et al. Catecholamines: mediator of the hypermetabolic response to thermal injury. *Ann Surg.* 1974;180:653-669.
8. Lowry SF. Nutritional support of the trauma patient. In: Shires GT, ed. *Principles of Trauma Care.* Vol 3. New York, NY: McGraw-Hill; 1985: 592-608.
9. Hasselgren PO, James JH, Benson DW, et al. Total and myofibrillar protein breakdown in different types of rat skeletal muscle: effects of sepsis and regulation of insulin. *Metabalism.* 1989;38:634-640.
10. Hummel RP III, Hasselgren PO, James JH, et al. The effect of sepsis in rats on skeletal muscle protein synthesis in vivo and in periphery and central core of incubated muscle preparations in vitro. *Metabolism.* 1988;37:1120-1127.
11. Hasselgren PO, James JH, Fischer JE. Inhibited muscle amino acid uptake in sepsis. *Ann Surg.* 1986;203:360-365.
12. Zamir O, Hasselgren PO, O'Brien W, et al. Muscle protein breakdown during endotoxemia in rats and after treatment with interleukin-1 receptor antagonist (IL-1ra). *Ann Surg.* 1992;216:381-386.
13. Nagaraju K. Immunologic capabilities of skeletal muscle cells. *Acta Physiol Scand.* 2001;171:215-223.
14. Curfs JH, Meis JF, Hoogkamp-Korstanje JA. A primer on cytokines: sources, receptors, effects and inducers. *Clin Microbiol Rev.* 1997;10:742-780.
15. Cannon JG. Cytokines in aging and muscle homeostasis. *J Gerontol A Biol Sci Med Sci.* 1995;50A:120-123.
16. Nagaraju K, Raben N, Merritt G, et al. A variety of cytokines and immunologically relevant surface molecules are expressed by normal human skeletal muscle cells under proinflammatory stimuli. *Clin Exp Immunol.* 1998;113:407-414.
17. Hill AG. Initiators and propagators of the metabolic response to injury. *World J Surg.* 2000;24:624-629.
18. Tiao G, Fagan JM, Samuels N, et al. Sepsis stimulates nonlysosomal, energy-dependent proteolysis and increases ubiquitin mRNA levels in rat skeletal muscle. *J Clin Invest.* 1994;94:2255-2264.
19. Hershko A, Ciechanover A. The ubiquitin system for protein degradation. *Annu Rev Biochem.* 1992;61:761-807.
20. Mitch WE, Goldberg AL. Mechanisms of muscle wasting. The role of the ubiquitin-proteasome pathway. *N Engl J Med.* 1996;335:1897-1905.
21. Price SR. Increased transcription of ubiquitin-proteasome system components: molecular responses associated with muscle atrophy. *Int J Biochem Cell Bio.* 2003;35:617-628.
22. Solomon V, Baracos V, Sarraf P, Goldberg AL. Rates of ubiquitin conjugation increase when muscles atrophy largely through ativation of the N-end rule pathway. *Proc Natl Acad Sci USA.* 1998;13: 12602-12607.
23. Price SR, England BK, Bailey JL, et al. Acidosis and glucocorticoids concomitantly increase ubiquitin and proteasome subunit mRNA in rat muscle. *Am J Physiol.* 1994:267:C955-C960.
24. Chai J, Wu Y, Sheng ZZ. Role of ubiquitin-proteasome pathway in skeletal muscle wasting in rats with endotoxemia. *Crit Care Med.* 2003;31(6);1802-1807.
25. Lecker SH, Solomon V, Mitch WE, Goldberg AL. Muscle protein breakdown and the critical role of the ubiquitin-proteasome pathway in normal and disease states. *J Nutr.* 1999;129:227S-237S.
26. Du J, Wang X, Miereles C, et al. Activation of caspase-3 is an initial step triggering accelerated muscle proteolysis in catabolic conditions. *J Clin Invest.* 2004;113:115-123.
27. Wilmore DW, Goodwin CW, Aulick LH, et al. Effect of injury and infection on visceral metabolism and circulation. *Ann Surg.* 1980;192:491-504.
28. Souba WW, Wilmore DW. Postoperative alteration of arteriovenous exchange of amino acids across the gastrointestinal tract. *Surgery.* 1983;94:342-350.
29. Bessey PQ. Metabolic response to critical illness. In: Wilmore DS, ed. Care of the surgical patient. *Sci Am.* 1994;(Suppl):3-31.
30. Shou J. Glutamine. In: Zaloga GP, ed. *Nutrition in Critical Care.* St. Louis, Mo: CV Mosby; 1994:123-141.
31. Muhlbacher F, Kapadia CR, Colpoys MF, et al. Effects of glucocorticoids on glutamine metabolism in skeletal muscle. *Am J Physiol.* 1984;247:E75-E83.
32. Planas M, Schwartz S, Arbos MA, et al. Plasma glutamine levels in septic patients. *JPEN J Parenter Enteral Nutr.* 1993;17:299-300.
33. Oudemans-Van Straaten HM, Bosman RJ, et al. Plasma glutamine depletion and patient outcome in acute ICU admissions. *Intensive Care Med.* 2001;27:84-90.
34. Zhou YP, Jiang ZM, Sun YH, et al. The effect of supplemental enteral glutamine on plasma levels, gut function, and outcome in severe burns: a randomized, double-blind, controlled clinical trial. *JPEN J Parenter Enteral Nutr.* 2003;27(4):241-245.
35. Ogle CK, Ogle JD, Mao JX, et al. Effect of glutamine on phagocytosis and bacterial killing by normal and pediatric burn patient neutrophils. *JPEN J Parenter Enteral Nutr.* 1994;18:128-133.
36. Hammarqvist F, Wernerman J, Ali R, et al. Addition of glutamine to total parenteral nutrition after elective abdominal surgery spares free glutamine in muscle, counteracts the fall in muscle protein synthesis, and improves nitrogen balance. *Ann Surg.* 1989;209:455-466.
37. Amores-Sanchez MI, Medina MA. Glutamine as a precursor of glutathione and oxidative stress. *Mol Genet Metab.* 1999;67:100-105.
38. Novak F, Heyland DK, Avenell A, et al. Glutamine supplementation in serious illness: a systematic review of the evidence. *Crit Care Med.* 2002;30;2022-2029.
39. Kinney JM, Elwyn DH. Protein metabolism and injury. *Annu Rev Nutr.* 1983;3:433-466.
40. Wannemacher RW Jr, Pekarek RS, Thompson WL, et al. A protein from polymorphonucler leukocytes (LEM) which affects the rate of hepatic amino acid transport and synthesis of acute-phase globulins. *Endocrinology.* 1975;96:651-661.
41. Fong Y, Lowry SF. Metabolic consequences of critical illness. In: Barie PS, Shires GT, eds. *Surgical Intensive Care.* Vol 1. Boston, Mass: Little, Brown & Co.; 1993;893-905.
42. Deibert DC, DeFronzo RA. Epinephrine-induced insulin resistance in man. *J Clin Invest.* 1980;65:717-721.

43. Diethelm AG. Surgical management of complications of steroid therapy. *Ann Surg*. 1977;185:251-263.
44. Tracey KJ, Cerami A. Tumor necrosis factor, other cytokines and disease. *Annu Rev Cell Biol*. 1993;9:317-343.
45. Nelson KM, Long CL, Bailey R, et al. Regulation of glucose kinetics in trauma patients by insulin and glucagons. *Metabolism*. 1992;41:68-75.
46. Long CL, Nelson KM, Geiger JW, et al. Effect of amino acid infusion on glucose production in trauma patients. *J Trauma*. 1996;40:335-341.
47 Wolfe RR, Miller HI, Spitzer JJ. Glucose and lactate kinetics in burn shock. *Am J Physiol*. 1977;232:415-418.
48. Wolfe RR, Herndon DN, Jahoor F, et al. Effect of severe burn injury on substrate cycling by glucose and fatty acids. *N Engl J Med*. 1987;317:403-408.
49. Warren RS, Starnes HF Jr, Gabrilove JL, et al. The acute metabolic effects of tumor necrosis factor administration in humans. *Arch Surg*. 1987;122:1396-1400.
50. Bearn AG, Billing B, Sherlock S. The effect of adrenaline and noradrenaline on hepatic blood flow and splanchnic carbohydrate metabolism in man. *J Physiol*. 1951;115:430-431.
51. Shaw JH, Wolfe RR. An integrated analysis of glucose, fat, and protein metabolism in severely traumatized patients. Studies in the basal state and the response to total parenteral nutrition. *Ann Surg*. 1989;209:63-72.
52. Wolfe RR, Martini WZ. Changes in intermediary metabolism in severe surgical illness. *World J Surg*. 2000;24:639-647.
53. Clowes GH Jr, O'Donnell TF, Blackburn GL, Maki TN. Energy metabolism and proteolysis in traumatized and septic man. *Surg Clin North Am*. 1976;56:1169-1184.
54. Wolfe RR, O'Donnell TF Jr, Stone MD, et al. Investigation of factors determining the optimal glucose infusion rate in total parenteral nutrition. *Metabolism*. 1980;29:892-900.
55. Burke JF, Wolfe RR, Mullany CJ, et al. Glucose requirements following burn injury. Parameters of optimal glucose infusion and possible hepatic and respiratory abnormalities following excessive glucose intake. *Ann Surg*. 1979;190:274-285.
56. Vary TC, Siegel JH, Nakatani T, et al. Effect of sepsis on activity of pyruvate dehydrogenase complex in skeletal muscle and liver. *Am J Physiol*. 1986;250(6 [Pt 1]):E634-E640.
57. Wolfe RR, Bagby GJ. Lipid metabolism in shock. In: Altura BM, Lefer AM, Schumer W, et al, eds. *Handbook of Shock and Trauma*. New York, NY: Raven Press; 1983:199-219.
58. Bornstein SR, Licinio J, Tauchnitz R, et al. Plasma leptin levels are increased in survivors of acute sepsis: associated loss of diurnal rhythm in cortisol and leptin secretion. *J Clin Endocrinol Metab*. 1998;83:280-283.
59. Carlson GL, Saeed M, Little RA, et al. Serum letpin concentrations and their relation to metabolic abnormalities in human sepsis. *Am J Physiol*. 1999;276:E658-E662.
60. Askanazi J, Carpentier YA, Elwyn DH, et al. Influence of total parenteral nutrition on fuel utilization in injury and sepsis. *Ann Surg*. 1980;191:40-46.
61. Wolfe RR, Allsop JR, Burke JF. Glucose metabolism in man: responses to intravenous glucose infusion. *Metabolism*. 1979;28:210-220.
62. Nanni G, Siegel JH, Coleman B, et al. Increased lipid fuel dependence in the critically ill septic patient. *J Trauma*. 1984;24:14-30.
63. Stoner HB, Little RA, Fraynk RN, et al. The effect of sepsis on the oxidation of carbohydrate and fat. *Br J Surg*. 1983;70:32-35.
64. Tissot S, Normand S, Khalfallah Y, et al. Effects of a continuous lipid infusion on glucose metabolism in critically ill patients. *Am J Physiol*. 1995;269:E753-E758.
65. Haussinger D, Roth E, Lang F, et al. Cellular hydration state: an important determinant of protein catabolism in health and disease. *Lancet*. 1993;341:1330-1332.
66. Ritz P, Salle A, Simard G, et al. Effects of changes in water compartments on physiology and metabolism. *Eur J Clin Nutr*. 2003;57: S2-S5.
67. Finn PJ, Plank LD, Clark MA, et al. Progressive cellular dehydration and proteolysis in critically ill patients. *Lancet*. 1996;347:654-656.
68. Hume DM, Egdahl RH. The importance of the brain in the endocrine response to injury. *Ann Surg*. 1959;150:697-712.
69. Newsome HH, Rose JC. The response of human adrenocorticotrophic hormone and growth hormone to surgical stress. *J Clin Endocrinol Metab*. 1971;33:481-487.
70. Taylor JW, Hander EW, Skreen R, et al. The effect of central nervous system narcosis on the sympathetic response to stress. *J Surg Res*. 1976;20:313-320.
71. Dempsey DT, Guenter P, Mullen JL, et al. Energy expenditure in acute trauma to the head with and without barbiturate therapy. *Surg Gynecol Obstet*. 1985;160:128-134.
72. Meguid MM, Brennan MF, Aoki TT, et al. Hormone substrate interrelationships following trauma. *Arch Surg*. 1974;109:776-783.
73. Hume DM, Bell CC, Bartter F. Direct measurement of adrenal secretion during operative trauma and convalescence. *Surgery*. 1962;52:174-187.
74. Carey LC, Cloutier CT, Lowery BD. Growth hormone and adrenal cortical response to shock and trauma in the human. *Ann Surg*. 1971;174:451-460.
75. Popp MB, Srivastava LS, Knowles HC Jr, MacMillan BG. Anterior pituitary function in thermally injured male children and young adults. *Surg Gynecol Obstet*. 1977;145:517-524.
76. Wise L, Margraf HW, Ballinger WF. Adrenal cortical function in severe burns. *Arch Surg*. 1972;105:213-220.
77. Marchuk JB, Finley RJ, Groves AC, et al. Catabolic hormones and substrate patterns in septic patients. *J Surg Res*. 1977;23:177-182.
78. Beisel WR. Magnitude of the host nutritional response to infection. *Am J Clin Nutr*. 1977;30:1236-1247.
79. Van den Berghe G, de Zegher F, Bouillon R. Acute and prolonged critical illness as different neuroendocrine paradigms. *J Clin Endocrinol Metab*. 1998,83:1827-1834.
80. Vermes I , Bieshuizen A, Hampsink RM, Haanen C. Dissociation of plasma adrenocorticotropin and cortisol levels in critically ill patients: possible role of endothelin and atrial natriuretic hormone. *J Clin Endocrinol Metab*. 1995,80:1238-1242.
81. O'Brian JT, Bybee DE, Burman KD, et al. Thyroid hormone-homeostasis in state of relative caloric deprivation. *Metabolism*. 1980;29:721-727.
82. Richmand DA, Molitch ME, O'Donnell TF. Altered thyroid hormone levels in bacterial sepsis: the role of nutritional adequacy. *Metabolism*. 1980;29:936-942.
83. Van der Poll T, Van Zee KJ, Endert E, et al. Interleukin-1 receptor blockade does not affect endotoxin-induced changes in plasma thyroid hormone and thrytropin concentrations in man. *J Clin Endocrinol Metab*. 1995;80:1341-1346.
84. Davies PH, Sheppard MC, Franklyn JA. Inflammatory cytokines and type I 5'-deiodinase expression in phi1 rat liver cells. *Mol Cell Endocrinol*. 1997;129:191-198.
85. Jaattela A, Alho A, Avikainen V, et al. Plasma catecholamines in severely injured patients: a prospective study on 45 patients with multiple injuries. *Br J Surg*. 1975;62:177-181.
86. Davies CL, Newman RJ, Molyneux SG, et al. The relationship between plasma catecholamines and severity of injury in man. *J Trauma*. 1984;24:99-105.
87. Gelfand RA, Matthews DE, Bier DM, Sherwin RS. The role of counterregulatory hormones in the catabolic response to stress. *J Clin Invest*. 1984;74:2238-2248.
88. Fong Y, Albert JD, Tracey K, et al. The influence of substrate background on the acute metabolic response to epinephrine and cortisol. *J Trauma*. 1991;31:1467-1476.
89. Kraenzlin ME, Keller U, Keller A, et al. Elevation of plasma epinephrine concentrations inhibits proteolysis and leucine oxidation in man via beta-adrenergic mechanisms. *J Clin Invest*. 1989;84:388-393.

90. Shaw JH, Holdaway CM, Humberstone DA. Metabolic intervention in surgical patients: the effect of alpha- or beta-blockade on glucose and protein metabolism in surgical patients receving total parenteral nutrition. *Surgery.* 1988;103:520-525.
91. Herndon DN, Hart DW, Wolf SE, et al. Reversal of catabolism by beta-blockade after severe burns. *N Engl J Med.* 2001;345:1223-1229.
92. Hasselgren PO. Glucocorticoids and muscle catabolism. *Curr Opin Clin Nutr Metab Care.* 1999;2(3):9-14.
93. Simmons PS, Miles JM, Gerich JE, Haymond MW. Increased proteolysis. An effect of increases in plasma cortisol within the physiologic range. *J Clin Invest.* 1984;73:412-420.
94. Wang L, Luo GJ, Wang JJ, Hasselgren PO. Dexamethasone stimulates proteasome- and calcium-dependent proteolysis in cultured L6 myotubes. *Shock.* 1998;10:298-306.
95. MacLennan PA, Brown RA, Rennie MJ. A positive relationship between protein synthesis rate and intracellular glutamine concentration in perfused rat skeletal muscle. *FEBS Lett.* 1987;215:187-191.
96. MacLennan PA, Smith K, Weryk B, et al. Inhibition of protein breakdown in perfused rat skeletal muscle. *FEBS Lett.* 1988;237:133-136.
97. Abcouwer SF, Bode BP, Souba WW. Glucocorticoids regulate rat glutamine synthetase expression in tissue-specific manner. *J Surg Res.* 1995;59:59-65.
98. Lukaszewicz GC, Souba WW, Abcouwer SF. Induction of muscle glutamine synthetase gene expression during endotoxemia is adrenal gland dependent. *Shock.* 1997;7:332-338.
99. Porte D Jr, Robertson RP. Control of insulin secretion by catecholamines, stress, and the sympathetic nervous system. *Fed Proc.* 1973;32:1792-1796.
100. Flaim KE, Hutson SM, Lloyd CE, et al. Direct effect of insulin on albumin gene expression in primary cultures of rat hepatocytes. *Am J Physiol.* 1985;249:E447-E453.
101. Inculet RI, Finley RJ, Duff JH, et al. Insulin decreases muscle protein loss after operative trauma in man. *Surgery.* 1986;99:752-758.
102. Yu CC, Hua HA, Tong C. Hyperglycaemia after burn injury. *Burns.* 1989;15:145-146.
103. Ellenberg M, Osserman KE, Pollack H. Hyperglycemia in coronary thrombosis. *Diabetes.* 1952;1:16-21.
104. Ross H, Johnston ID, Welborn TA, Wright AD. Effect of abdominal operation on glucose tolerance and serum levels of insulin, growth hormone, and hydrocortisone. *Lancet.* 1966;2:563-566.
105. Gore DC, Chinkes D, Heggers J, et al. Association of hyperglycemia with increased mortality after severe burn injury. *J Trauma.* 2001;51:540-544.
106. Van den Berghe G, Wouters P, Weekers F, et al. Intensive insulin therapy in critically ill patients. *N Engl J Med.* 2001;19:1359-1367.
107. Alberti KG, Batstone GF, Foster KJ, Johnson DE. Relative role of various hormones in mediating the metabolic response to injury. *JPEN J Parenter Enteral Nutr.* 1980;4:141-146.
108. Wolfe BM, Culebras JM, Aoki TT, et al. The effects of glucagon on protein metabolism in normal man. *Surgery.* 1979;86:248-257.
109. Pozefsky T, Tancredi RG, Moxley RT, et al. Metabolism of forearm tissues in man. Studies with glucagon. *Diabetes.* 1976;25:128-135.
110. Warren RS, Donner DB, Starnes HF Jr, Brennan MF. Modulation of endogenous hormone action by recombinant human tumor necrosis factor. *Proc Natl Acad Sci USA.* 1987;84:8619-8622.
111. Felig P, Wahren J, Hendler R. Influence of physiologic hyperglucagonemia on basal and insulin-inhibited splanchnic glucose output in normal man. *J Clin Invest.* 1976;58:761-765.
112. Iversen J. Adrenergic receptors and the secretion of glucagon and insulin from the isolated, perfused canine pancreas. *J Clin Invest.* 1973;52:2102-2116.
113. Fong Y, Lowry SF. Cytokines and the cellular response to injury and infection. In: Harken AH, Wilmore DW, eds. Care of the surgical patient. *Sci Am.* 1996;(Suppl) 1-21.
114. Carswell EA, Old LJ, Kassel RL, et al. An endotoxin-induced serum factor that causes necrosis of tumors. *Proc Natl Acad Sci USA.* 1975;72:3666-3670.
115. Van der Poll T, Romijn JA, Endert E, et al. Tumor necrosis factor mimics the metabolic response to acute infection in healthy humans. *Am J Physiol.* 1991;261:E457-E465.
116. Michie HR, Spriggs DR, Manogue KR, et al. Tumor necrosis factor and endotoxin induce similar metabolic responses in human beings. *Surgery.* 1988;104:280-286.
117. Van Zee KJ, Kohno T, Fischer E, et al. Tumor necrosis factor soluble receoptors circulate during experimental and clinical inflammation and can protect against excessive tumor necrosis factor alpha in vitro and in vivo. *Proc Natl Acad Sci USA.* 1992;89:4845-4849.
118. Fong Y, Lowry SF. Tumor necrosis factor in the pathophysiology of infection and sepsis. *Clin Immunol Immunopathol.* 1990;55:157-170.
119. Beutler B, Mahoney J, Le Trang N, et al. Purification of cachectin, lipoprotein lipase-suppressing hormone secreted by endotoxin-induced RAW 264.7 cells. *J Exp Med.* 1985;161;984-985.
120. Lahdevirta J, Maury CP, Teppo AM, et al. Elevated levels of circulating cachectin/tumor necrosis factor in patients with acquired immunodeficiency syndrome. *Am J Med.* 1988;85:289-291.
121. Feingold KR, Grunfeld C. Tumor necrosis factor alpha stimulates hepatic lipogenesis in the rat in vivo. *J Clin Invest.* 1987;80:184-190.
122. Zechner R, Newman TC, Sherry B, et al. Recombinant human cachectin/tumor necrosis factor but not interleukin-1 alpha downregulate lipoprotein lipase gene expression at the transcriptional level in mouse 3T3-L1 adipocytes. *Mol Cell Biol.* 1988;8:2394-2401.
123. Fruhbeck G, Gomez-Ambrosi J, Muruzabal FJ, Burrell MA The adipocytes: a model for integration of endocrine and metabolic signaling in energy metabolism regulation. *Am J Physiol Endocrinol Metab.* 2001;280:E827-E847.
124. Tracey KJ, Lowry SF. The role of cytokine mediators in septic shock. *Adv Surg.* 1990;23:21-56.
125. Haddad JJ, Saade NE, Safieh-Garabedian B. Cytokines and neuro-immuno-endocrine interactions: a role for the hypothalamic-pituitary-adrenal revolving axis. *J Neuroimmunol.* 2002;133:1-19.
126. Matsuki T, Horai R, Sudo K, Iwakura Y. IL-1 plays an important role in lipid metabolism by regulating insulin levels under physiological conditions. *J Exp Med.* 2003;198:877-888.
127. Fischer E, Van Zee KJ, Marano MA, et al. Interleukin-1 receptor antagonist circulates in experimental inflammation and in human disease. *Blood.* 1992;79:2196-2200.
128. Juge-Aubry CE, Somm E, Giusti V, et al. Adipose tissue is a major source of interluekin-1 receptor antagonist: upregulation in obesity and inflammation. *Diabetes.* 2003;52:1104-1110.
129. Helfgott DC, Tatter SB, Santhanam U, et al. Multiple forms of IFN-beta 2/IL-6 in serum and body fluids during acute bacterial infection. *J Immunol.* 1989;142:948-953.
130. Gelin J, Moldawer LL, Lonnroth C, et al. Appearance of hybridoma growth factor /interleukin-6 in the serum of mice bearing a methyl cholanthrene-induced sarcoma. *Biochem Biophys Res Commun.* 1988;157:575-579.
131. Shenkin A, Fraser WD, Series J, et al. The serum interleukin-6 response to elective surgery. *Lymphokine Res.* 1989;8:123-127.
132. Ritchie DG, Fuller GM. Hepatocyte-stimulating factor: a monocyte-derived acute-phase regulatory protein. *Ann NY Acad Sci.* 1983;408:490-502.
133. Castell JV, Gomez-Lechon MJ, David M, et al. Interleukin-6 is the major regulator of acute phase protein synthesis in adult human hepatocytes. *FEBS Lett.* 1989;242:237-239.
134. Garman RD, Jacobs KA, Clark SC, Ravlet DH. B-cell-stimulatory factor 2 (beta 2 interferon) functions as a second signal for interleukin 2 production by mature murine T cells. *Proc Natl Acad Sci USA.* 1987;84:7629-7633.

135. Stouthard JM, Romijn JA, Van der Poll T, et al. Endocrinologic and metabolic effects of interleukin-6 in humans. *Am J Physiol.* 1995;268:E813-E819.
136. Luedke CE, Cerami A. Interferon-gamma overcomes glucocorticoid suppression of cachectin/tumor necrosis factor biosynthesis by murine macrophages. *J Clin Invest.* 1990;86:1234-1240.
137. Nathan CF, Murray HW, Wiebe ME, Rubin BY. Identification of interferon-gamma as the lymphokine that activates human macrophage oxidative metabolism and antimicrobial activity. *J Exp Med.* 1983;158:670-689.
138. Matthys P, Dijksman R, Proost P, et al. Severe cachexia in mice inoculated with interferon-gamma-producing tumor cells. *Int J Cancer.* 1991;49:77-82.
139. Chesnokova V, Melmed S. Minireview: Neuro-immuno-endocrine modulation of the hypothalamic-pituitary-adrenal (HPA) axis by gp130 signaling molecules. *Endocrinology.* 2002;143:1571-1574.
140. Wilder RL. Neuroendocrine-immune system interactions and autoimmunity. *Annu Rev Immunol.* 1995;13:307-338.
141. Besedovsky HO, del Rey A. Immune-neuro-endocrine interactions: facts and hypotheses. *Endocr Rev.* 1996;17:64-102.
142. Turnbull AV, Rivier CL. Regulation of the hypothalamic-pituitary-adrenal axis by cytokines: actions and mechanisms of action. *Physiol Rev.* 1999;79:1-71.
143. Tsigos C, Papanicolaou DA, Defensor R, et al. Dose effects of recombinant human interleukin-6 on pituitary hormone secretion and energy expenditure. *Neuroendocrinology.* 1997;66:54-62.
144. Reichlin S. Neuroendocrinology of infection and the innate immune systems. *Recent Prog Horm Res.* 1999;54:133-181.
145. Chrousos G. Stressors, stress, and neuroendocrine integration of the adaptive response. The 1997 Hans Selye Memorial Lecture. *Ann NY Acad Sci.* 1998;851:311-335.
146. Auernhammer CJ, Melmed S. Luekemia-inhibiting factor-neuroimmune modulator of endocrine function. *Endocr Rev.* 2000;21:313-345.
147. Arzt E. gp130 cytokine signaling in the pituitary gland: a paradigm for cytokine-neuro-endocrine pathways. *J Clin Invest.* 2001;108:1729-1733.
148. Chesnokova V, Melmed S. Minireview: Neuro-immuno-endocrine modulation of the hypothalamic-pituitary-adrenal (HPA) axis by gp130 signaling molecules. *Endocrinology.* 2002;143:1571-1574.
149. Annane D, Cavaillon JM. Corticosteroids in sepsis: from bench to bedside? *Shock.* 2003;20:197-207.
150. Scheinman RI, Gualberto A, Jewell CM, et al. Characterization of mechanisms involved in transrepression of NF-kappa B by activated glucocorticoid receptors. *Mol Cell Biol.* 1995;15:943-953.
151. Ray A, LaForge KS, Sehgal PB. On the mechanism for efficient repression of interleukin-6 promoter by glucocorticoids: enhancer, TATA box, and RNA start site (Inr motif) occlusion. *Mol Cell Biol.* 1990;10:5736-5746.
152. Zuckerman SH, Shellhaas J, Butler LD. Differential regulation of lipopolysaccharide-induced interleukin-1 and tumor necrosis factor synthesis: effects of endogenous and exogenous glucocorticoids and the role of the pituitary-adrenal axis. *Eur J Immunol.* 1989;19:301-305.
153. Han J, Thompson P, Beutler B. Dexamethasone and pentoxifylline inhibit endotoxin-induced cachectin/tumor necrosis factor synthesis at separate points in the signaling pathway. *J Exp Med.* 1990;172:391-394.
154. Van der Poll T, Coyle SM, Barbosa K, et al. Epinephrine inhibits tumor necrosis factor-alpha and potentiates interleukin 10 production during human endotoxemia. *J Clin Invest.* 1996;97:713-719.
155. Webster JC, Oakley RH, Jewell CM, Cidlowski JA. Proinflammatory cytokines regulate human glucocorticoid receptor gene expression and lead to the accumulation of the dominant negative beta isoform: a mechanism for the generation of glucocorticoid resistance. *Proc Natl Acad Sci USA.* 2001;98:6865-6870.
156. Chrousos GP. The role of stress and the hypothalamic-pituitary-adrenal axis in the pathogenesis of the metabolic syndrome: neuro-endocrine and target rissue-related causes. *J Obes Relat Metab Disord.* 2000;24(S2);S50-S55.
157. Dudrick SJ, Wilmore DW, Vars HM, Rhoads JE. Can intravenous feeding as the sole means of nutrition support growth in the child and restore weight loss in an adult? An affirmative answer. *Ann Surg.* 1969;70:974-984.
158. Kudsk KA. Current aspects of mucosal immunology and its influence by nutrition. *Am J Surg.* 2002;183:390-398.
159. Alexander JW, Macmillan BG, Stinnett JD, Sheldon GF. Beneficial effects of aggressive protein feeding in severely burned children. *Ann Surg.* 1980;192;505-517.
160. Kudsk KA, Stone JM, Carpenter G, et al. Enteral and parenteral feeding influences mortality after hemoglobin-E.coli peritonitis in normal rats. *J Trauma.* 1983;23:605-609.
161. Ziegler TR, Smith RJ, O'Dwyer ST, et al. Increased intestinal permeability associated with infection in burn patients. *Arch Surg.* 1988;123:1313-1319.
162. Deitch EA. Bacterial translocation of the gut flora. *J Trauma.* 1990;30:S184-S189.
163. Deitch EA, Winterton J, Li M, Berg R. The gut as a portal of entry for bacteremia. Role of protein malnutrition. *Ann Surg.* 1987;205:681-692.
164. Williamson RC. Intestinal adaptation (first of two parts). Structural, functional, and cytokinetic changes. *N Engl J Med.* 1978;298:1393-1402.
165. Streilen JW, Stein-Streilen J, Head J. Regional specialization in antigen presentation. In: Phillips SM, Escobar MR, eds. *The Reticuloendothelial System.* Vol 9. New York, NY: Plenum; 1986:37-94.
166. Alverdy JC, Aoys E, Moss GS. Total parenteral nutrition promotes bacterial translocation from the gut. *Surgery.* 1988;104:185-190.
167. Fong Y, Marano MA, Barber A, et al. Total parenteral nutrition and bowel rest modify the metabolic response to endotoxin in humans. *Ann Surg.* 1989;210:449-456.
168. Fong Y, Lowry SF, Cerami A. Cachectin/TNF: a macrophage protein that induces cachexia and shock. *JPEN J Parenter Enteral Nutr.* 1988;12:72S-77S.
177. Fong Y, Moldawer LL, Marano M, et al. Endotoxemia elicits increased circulating beta 2-IFN/IL-6 in man. *J Immunol.* 1989;142:2321-2324.

Chapter 28

Clinical Implications of Oxidative Stress and Antioxidant Therapy in Gastrointestinal Disease

Gavin Arteel, PhD; Gerald W. Dryden, Jr, MD, MSPH; and Craig J. McClain, MD

Introduction

Oxidative stress is a unifying mechanism of organ injury in many forms of gastrointestinal (GI) diseases. Moreover, antioxidant therapy is increasingly recognized as a form of therapy for many GI diseases. This chapter will provide an overview of oxidative stress and review the role of oxidative stress in liver disease, inflammatory bowel disease (IBD), and pancreatic disease.

Overview of Oxidative Stress

The first study of free radical chemistry is attributed to Henry John Horstman Fenton,[1] who described the classical pathway of iron-catalyzed reduction of H_2O_2 to OH that bears his name (Figure 28-1). Gerschman and Gilbert[2] first proposed that radiation-induced cell killing might be mediated by oxygen free radicals, based on the observation that the pattern of toxicity of radiation was quite similar to that of hyperoxygen in vivo. Another turning point in the concept of prooxidants came with the hypothesis of Harman and the "free radical theory of aging."[3] However, it should be noted that it was generally thought that free radical formation in the cell was limited to either external stimuli (such as radiation) or random events and did not occur under "normal" circumstances. In 1969, when Fridovich and McCord described the function of superoxide dismutase (SOD) as a catalytic reducer of O_2.– to H_2O_2,[4] the concept that oxidants are produced by the cell under normal conditions gained hold.

The discovery of enzymes that normally produce prooxidants (in contrast to electron leakage from other enzyme systems)—such as nicotinamide adenine dinucleotide phosphate (NADPH) oxidases, xanthine oxidases, and myeloperoxidases—further strengthened the concept that prooxidants are regularly found in vivo. Later discoveries of catalytic functions of the glutathione peroxidases, glutaredoxin peroxidases, thioredoxin peroxidases, and reinvestigation of catalase indicated that hydroperoxides are also kept in close check in vivo. It became clear that a balance between prooxidants and antioxidants is critical for both survival and functioning of aerobic organisms. An imbalance favoring prooxidants and/or disfavoring antioxidants, potentially leading to damage, was coined as "oxidative stress" by Sies.[5] While prooxidants can directly damage tissues, their reactions with other molecules can also initiate or alter cellular signaling cascades that can then serve to amplify the oxidant's effect.

Causes of Oxidative Stress In Vivo

One way to tip the balance towards oxidative stress is to increase the production of prooxidants within the cell. Sources can be exogenous (eg, ionizing radiation or toxins) or endogenous. One example of an extrinsic toxin is acetaminophen (paracetamol). A normally minor pathway for metabolizing this drug leads to formation of the prooxidant, N-acetyl-p-benzoquinone imine (NAPQI).[6] Under conditions of increased formation of NAPQI, hepatotoxicity can ensue. In contrast, a disease or ingested compound may not directly form prooxidants but rather stimulate endogenous production of oxidants from enzymes normally designed to create prooxidants or by increasing electron leakage from other enzymes or enzyme systems (eg, CYP isozymes and mitochon-

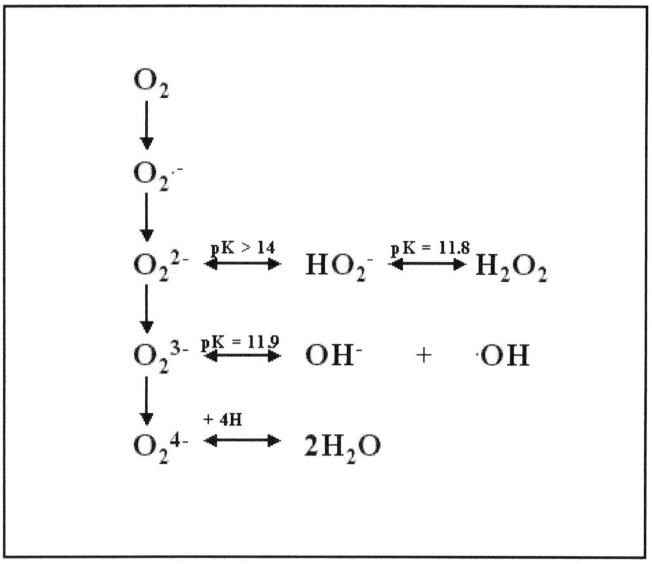

Figure 28-1. Reactive oxygen intermediates formed during the reduction of molecular oxygen to water. During the 4 electron reduction of oxygen (O_2) to water ($2H_2O$), a number of reactive free radicals can be formed. 1 electron reduction leads to the formation of superoxide (O_2.-); 2 electron reduction forms hydrogen peroxide (H_2O_2); 3 electron reduction forms hydroxyl radical (.OH). All three of these reactive oxygen intermediates are hypothesized to be involved in oxidative stress. It is likely for this reason that their formation is kept tightly in check under normal conditions.

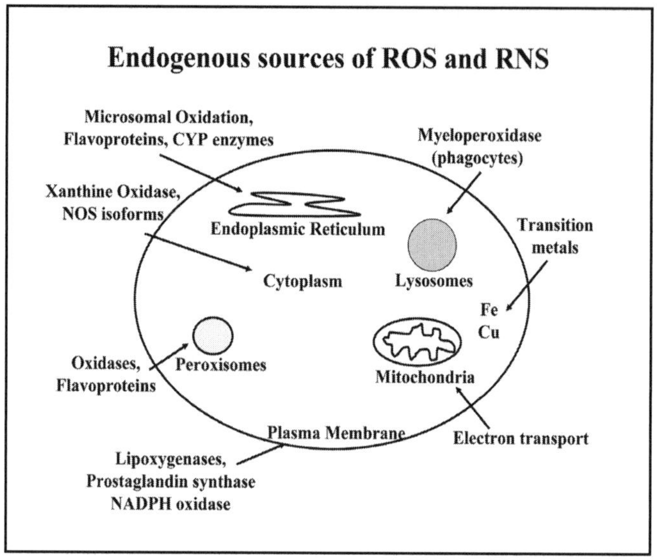

Figure 28-2. Endogenous sources of reactive oxygen and nitrogen species (ROS and RNS) in the cell. ROS and RNS can be formed by electron leakage from normal cellular (eg, mitochondria and CYP isozymes), or can be formed by numerous processes specifically designed to create these products (eg, nitric oxide synthases, NADPH oxidases and myeloperoxidases). Increased formation of ROS/RNS can lead to tipping the cellular homeostasis towards oxidative stress. Furthermore, even in the absence of a net increase in ROS/RNS formation, mobilization of transition metals (Fe and Cu) that catalyze the formation of the potent hydroxyl radical (see Figure 28-1) can also contribute to oxidative stress.

dria). Figure 28-2 is a schematic depiction of some of the proposed sources of endogenous prooxidants within the cell. As can be seen from this scheme, a number of prooxidant enzymes are involved in host immune defense (eg, NADPH oxidases, myeloperoxidases, lipoxygenases). It is therefore not surprising that GI tract diseases of altered/impaired immune responses are often postulated to involve oxidant production from these sources.[7-9]

Oxidative stress can also be created by decreased antioxidant defenses. Lower antioxidant levels due to nutritional deficiencies serve as an example.[10] The mobilization of free iron by some disease processes (eg, hemochromatosis) can also lead to an increase in transition-metal catalysis to potent oxidants (eg, the Fenton reaction).[11] Finally, there exist a host of proteins and systems involved in the "antioxidant network." This family does not directly intercept prooxidants but serves instead as ancillary reductants and maintains the catalytic activity of antioxidant proteins or small molecules.[12,13] These reactions require cellular energy to maintain such cycles. Figure 28-3 is a schematic depiction of this point using the catalytic reduction of hydroperoxides (ROOH) by glutathione peroxidase (GPX) as an example; the maintenance of this reaction is dependent on the supply of NADPH from cytosolic sources by the hexose monophosphate shunt, or by the mitochondrial citrate cycle via the mitochondrial transhydrogenases. Therefore, conditions that alter defenses against prooxidant formation can also lead to increased oxidative stress, even if the net production of prooxidants does not necessarily increase.

Mechanisms by Which Oxidative Stress Mediates Its Effects

One mechanism by which oxidative stress is proposed to cause cellular injury is by chemical modification of biologic molecules, which can then alter and/or interfere with normal processes within the cell. Specifically, chemical alteration of small molecules (eg, glutathione and vitamin E), lipids, proteins (eg, cysteine residues), and DNA (eg, formation of 8-OH-dG residues) are all well-known effects of oxidative stress on the cell (Figure 28-4). However, it is now clear that prooxidants can also mediate and/or amplify their signal by modifying signaling cascades within the cell, even in the absence of robust broad-spectrum chemical damage by oxidants. Many recent reviews have focused on the role of signaling cascades in damage due to oxidative stress.[14-17] Oxidant sensitive signaling cascades include small molecules (eg, intracellular Ca++),[18] stress-activated protein kinases (eg, JNK, ERK 1/2, and p38), transcription factors (eg, AP-1, HIF-1, and NFκB),[19] and modulators of apoptosis signaling (eg, caspases, Bad, and Bcl-2).[20] Via these mechanisms, it is likely that low level oxidative stress (eg, during chronic inflammatory diseases) contributes to tissue damage and disease progression.

Mechanisms of Defense against Oxidative Stress

The physiological and pharmacological strategies for antioxidant defense are organized in three categories:

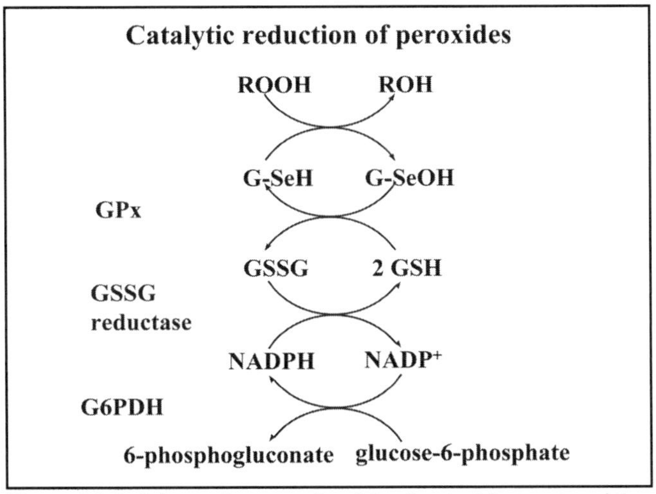

Figure 28-3. Schematic example of the "antioxidant network". Defense against antioxidants comprises not only enzymes or small molecules that directly intercept prooxidants (eg, glutathione peroxidase in figure), but also processes that catalytically maintain this defense. The scheme in this figure shows the transfer electrons from glucose-6-phosphate through to hydroperoxides. Abbreviations: ROOH, hydroperoxide; ROH, alcohol; GPx, glutathione peroxidase; GSSH reductase, glutathione disulfide reductase; G6PDH, glucose-6-phosphate dehydrogenase.

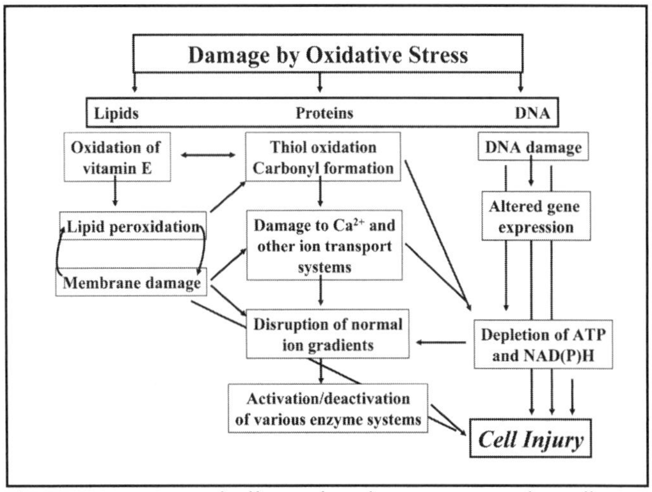

Figure 28-4. Potential effects of oxidative stress on the cell. Oxidative stress can cause damage to multiple types of molecules in the cell, including lipids, proteins, and DNA. This damage can alter cell function/viability directly (eg, altered gene expression) or indirectly (eg, by depleting energy supplies during repair of the damage).

prevention, interception, and repair.[12] Dietary or pharmacologic manipulation of these defenses are important goals to stemming the effects of oxidative stress in vivo.

Prevention

The first line of defense against reactive species is preventing their formation. Prevention against reactive species can be physical or biochemical in nature. Organisms can design barriers to protect sensitive areas from reactive species. Barriers may be molecules (eg, melanin in the skin), cells (eg, intestinal mucosal cells with high turnover rates), or even organs (eg, the 'first pass effect' of liver removing ingested toxins from the portal blood). Biochemical prevention refers to the tight homeostasis of both prooxidant and antioxidant proteins and molecules maintained by an organism. For example, the concentration of free metal ions in the mammalian body is kept in check by metal-binding proteins (eg, ferritin, transferrin and metallothionein). Any therapy that serves to prevent the formation of prooxidants (eg, anti-inflammatory drugs, transition metal chelators), while not antioxidants in their own right, will serve as an antioxidant therapy. Pharmacologic inhibitors of prooxidant enzymes also fall into the category of preventative antioxidants.

Interception

The goal of interception is to prevent a damaging species, once formed, from further activity. In the context of free radical prooxidants, the main point of interception is to make it less reactive. Further, interception often leads to transfer of the prooxidant away from more sensitive compartments of the cell. This is often accomplished by making the prooxidant more water-soluble, thereby sequestering it to the aqueous compartment and away from the hydrophobic compartments of the cell. Most "classical" antioxidants utilized in therapy (eg, polyphenolic extracts, vitamin E) fall into this category of antioxidant defense.

The enhancement of the cell's own intrinsic antioxidant capacity is also an approach to increasing prooxidant interception. Indeed, this is part of the rationale for supplementation with glutathione precursors such as S-adenosylmethionine (SAMe), N-acetyl cysteine (NAC), and oxothiazolidine carboxylate (OTC). A recent advance in our understanding is that some "classical" antioxidants may mediate protection in vivo, not by directly scavenging prooxidants per se but by stimulating intrinsic antioxidant production through activation of the antioxidant response element on genes.[21] Results of experiments along these lines appear promising and should be pursued further. The finding that oxidants may mediate their effects in vivo predominantly through signal transduction cascades is an exciting prospect, as many relatively specific inhibitors of these pathways exist. The clinical utility of targeting such sites is an area of active investigation.

Repair

The effects of oxidative stress can be attenuated by repairing the damage once it has occurred. As prevention and interception processes are not completely effective, damage products could continuously form at low levels during excessive nitric oxide (NO)/peroxynitrite generation and may accumulate. As discussed above, damaged biomolecules include DNA (occurring as modified bases or in the form of single- or double-strand breaks),[22] membranes (occurring as phospholipid oxidation and nitration products), or proteins (occurring as oxidized and nitrated amino acid side-chains). Measurement of these damaged biomolecules is a frequently utilized method of indirectly determining oxidative stress in disease states (see Figure 28-4). There are biological systems involved in DNA repair,[22,23] modified lipid turnover, and proteolysis that are capable of providing the functions of restitution or replenishment. Pharmacologically, targeting these systems deserves further investigation.

Oxidative Stress in Liver Disease

Oxidative stress is an underlying mechanism for the cell injury and ultimate fibrosis in many forms of liver injury. This section will review the role of oxidative stress in the three major forms of liver disease in the United States: alcoholic liver disease, nonalcoholic steatohepatitis (NASH), and hepatitis C, and touch on selected toxin and metabolic forms of liver injury. (Nutrition and liver disease are discussed in Chapter 20, and nutrition and alcoholism are discussed in Chapter 15.)

Alcoholic Liver Disease

Oxidative stress is well documented in alcoholic liver disease using both direct spin-trapping techniques as well as indirect measures of oxidative stress such as lipid peroxidation.[24-27] Human studies in volunteers in a clinical research setting demonstrated a dose-response increase in urinary isoprostane levels following increasing amounts of acute alcohol consumption.[27] Moreover, these same investigators showed that patients with alcoholic hepatitis had very elevated levels of urinary isoprostanes. In animal models of alcoholic liver disease, electron spin resonance has been used to detect free radicals, and multiple indirect markers of oxidative stress, such as T-BARS, 4HNE, and isoprostane levels have been shown to be increased.[25]

The potential cell sources for oxidative stress in liver disease are multiple and include both parenchymal and nonparenchymal cells. Major hepatocyte sources for reactive oxygen species (ROS) include cytochrome P4502E1 and mitochondria.[28,29] Alcohol consumption increases CYP2E1 activity and CYP2E1 colocalizes immunohistochemically in the liver to the most severe areas of injury in alcoholic liver disease. The CYP2E1 system leaks electrons to initiate oxidative stress.[29] Overexpression of CYP2E1 in mice and in HepG2 cells leads to enhanced alcohol hepatotoxicity.[30] Conversely, CYP2E1 knockout mice still develop alcohol-induced liver injury,[31] suggesting that increased CYP2E1 plays a role in alcoholic liver disease but is not the sole factor. In the CYP2E1 knockout mice, other compensatory mechanisms are likely playing a role.

Mitochondria are the major consumers of molecular oxygen and are major generators of reactive oxygen species in alcoholic liver disease. Mitochondrial abnormalities are well documented in alcoholic liver disease, beginning with the megamitochondria observed histologically. Short-term alcohol consumption causes increased superoxide generation in hepatic mitochondria with increased flow of electrons through the respiratory electron transport chain.[32] The decreased ratio between nicotinamide adenine dinucleotide NAD and NAD plus one hydrogen atom (NADH) caused by ethanol intake favors superoxide generation. Because hepatic mitochondria lack catalase, glutathione takes on a critical role in protecting against mitochondrial oxidative stress. Importantly, because mitochondria do not make glutathione, they import it from the cytosol.[33] This transport system is defective in alcoholic liver disease, and selective mitochondrial glutathione depletion is observed.[33] This depressed mitochondrial glutathione sensitizes to tumor necrosis factor (TNF) hepatotoxicity and mitochondrial function is also impaired by TNF.[34] Thus, there is a close interaction between mitochondrial function, TNF, and oxidative stress.[24,29]

Nonparenchymal cells and infiltrating inflammatory cells such as neutrophils also represent major sources of prooxidants in alcoholic liver disease. Enzyme systems for prooxidant production in Kupffer cells include NADPH oxidase and inducible nitric oxide synthetase (iNOS). Mice deficient in NADPH oxidase are resistant to alcohol-induced liver injury, and mice treated with the drug diphenylenelodium sulfate to block this enzyme system are protected against alcohol hepatotoxicity.[35,36] Infiltrating neutrophils use enzyme systems such as myeloperoxidase to generate HOCl and reactive oxygen species.

Increased levels of proinflammatory cytokines are observed in alcoholic liver disease.[37] Their production can be initiated by oxidative stress, and their production also can cause oxidative stress. Dysregulated TNF production was first documented in alcoholic hepatitis with the observation that cultured monocytes (major producers of circulating TNF) spontaneously produced TNF and produced significantly more TNF in response to endotoxin or lipopolysaccharide (LPS) stimulus in alcoholic hepatitis patients compared to normal controls.[38] One stimulus for this cytokine production is LPS; another major stimulus is ROS. ROS can activate the redox-sensitive transcription factor NFkB in Kupffer cells, resulting in the production of certain inflammatory cytokines such as TNF. Increased serum TNF concentrations and concentrations of other cytokines and chemokines such as interleukin (IL) -6, IL-8, and IL-18 were next documented in the sera of alcoholic hepatitis patients, and values correlated either severity of disease/mortality in alcoholic hepatitis.[37,39-41] Studies in rats, mice, and tissue culture further supported a role for cytokines such as TNF in the pathogenesis of alcoholic liver disease. Rats chronically fed alcohol had much higher LPS-stimulated TNF levels than control rats, and liver injury could be attenuated by agents that down-regulate TNF production, such as prostaglandin analogs, or by giving anti-TNF antibody.[42,43] Moreover, studies using the intragastric alcohol feeding model have demonstrated that the development of liver injury coincides with increased TNF mRNA in the liver and in isolated Kupffer cells.[44,45]

Oxidative stress appears to play a role not only in the cell injury in alcoholic liver disease but also in the development of fibrosis. Fibrosis represents a maladaptive wound-healing process in the liver. It is a dynamic state with constant remodeling of scar tissue. Thus, some fibrosis may resolve when alcohol consumption is discontinued. Hepatic stellate cells are a major source of collagen production.[46] They normally exist in a quiescent state; but following activation or stimulation, stellate cells assume a myofibroblast-like contractile phenotype and produce collagen. Cytokines, such as transforming growth factor beta (TGF-β), are one major stimulus for stellate cell activation and collagen production.[46] However, early studies also suggested that oxidative stress plays a critical role in stellate cell activation, and various antioxidants, including vitamin E, inhibited stellate cell activation and subsequent collagen production.[47] Moreover, 4-hydroxynonenal (4HNE) has been shown to act as a profibrotic stimulus in clinically relevant concentrations in human hepatic stellate cells. Thus, 4HNE up-regulated procollagen as well as tissue inhibitor of metalloproteinase-1 (TIMP1) gene expression.[48] Matrix TIMP1 plays an important role in degrading type 1 collagen, and inhibiting this enzyme could shift the balance towards fibrosis in alcoholic liver disease. Importantly, TIMP1 levels are elevated in alcoholic liver disease.

Because of the important mechanistic role of oxidative stress in the development of alcoholic liver disease, multiple studies in mice and rats fed alcohol were devised to determine whether antioxidant therapy was efficacious in experimental alcoholic liver disease. Diverse antioxidants range from green tea polyphenols (GrTP) to glutathione prodrugs to gene therapy overexpressing superoxide dismutases 1 and 2, and all of these strategies blocked or attenuated alcoholic liver disease in rodents.[25] These treatment data strongly support the concept that oxidative stress plays an etiologic role in the development and progression of alcoholic liver disease.

These rodent studies led to subsequent human intervention trials with antioxidant therapy in alcoholic liver disease. Perhaps the most compelling data for antioxidant therapy in human alcoholic liver disease relates to SAMe. SAMe has multiple theoretic benefits in alcoholic liver disease including antioxidant properties, serving as a critical methyl donor, maintaining mitochondrial function, decreasing proinflammatory cytokine production, playing a role in glutathione production, and others.[49] A recent multi-center clinical study from Spain reported that SAMe supplementation (1200 mg/day) significantly improved mortality and decreased the need for liver transplantation in alcoholic liver disease.[50] SAMe has also been used in a variety of other types of clinical liver disease in Europe (especially cholestatic liver disease) and it appears to have a good safety profile.

Silymarin, or milk thistle, also has potent antioxidant properties and has been used in a variety of forms of experimental liver disease, ranging from carbon tetrachloride to mushroom poisoning, with efficacy (Chapter 10).[51] Large clinical trials have been performed in Europe with varying results. Ferenci and coworkers used silymarin (140 mg TID) in evaluating 170 patients with cirrhosis and observed clinical benefits.[52] On the other hand, Pares and coworkers, using a similar dose, did not find statistically-significant positive results.[53] Despite apparently conflicting efficacy data, silymarin has an excellent safety profile and is probably the most widely used form of complementary and alternative medicine in most forms of liver disease, including alcoholic liver disease.

Vitamin E has well-documented antioxidant properties, and vitamin E deficiency, as well as deficiency in many other nutrients, is well documented in alcoholic liver disease, especially in more severe liver disease.[54] Vitamin E has been shown to protect against several types of experimental liver injury and also inhibits stellate cell activation and collagen production.[55] Unfortunately, the major randomized study of vitamin E in alcoholic liver disease did not show significant benefit, possibly because a relatively low dose was used.[56]

Glutathione prodrugs are another potential form of therapy for alcoholic liver disease. Patients with alcoholic liver disease have both low whole blood glutathione levels and depleted mitochondrial glutathione levels. No large randomized studies of glutathione prodrugs have been performed in alcoholic liver disease; however, the glutathione prodrug, procysteine, has been shown to decrease proinflammatory ex vivo cytokine production (TNF and IL-8) from alcoholic cirrhotic monocytes.[56]

Nonalcoholic Fatty Liver Disease and Nonalcoholic Steatohepatitis

Nonalcoholic steatohepatitis (NASH) is an increasingly recognized liver disease that histologically appears identical to alcoholic hepatitis. However, by definition, it only occurs in patients who do not drink and often have the metabolic syndrome, or syndrome X, comprised of obesity, diabetes mellitus, hyperlipidemia, hypertension, and in some instances, other metabolic abnormalities, such as polycystic ovary disease.[57] In NASH, there is underlying fat as well as some component of inflammation and possibly fibrosis or cirrhosis. A broader term is nonalcoholic fatty liver disease (NAFLD), which requires only underlying steatosis. The etiology of NASH remains elusive, but most investigators agree that a baseline of steatosis requires a "second hit" capable of inducing inflammation, necrosis, and fibrosis. There are multiple different postulated "second hits" including dysregulated cytokines, oxidative stress, mitochondrial dysfunction, insulin resistance, and others.[57]

Oxidative stress is well documented in NASH. Obesity itself is a state of increased oxidative stress, and weight loss can decrease oxidative stress, as assessed by markers such as isoprostane levels. In NASH, biomarkers of oxidative stress, such as immunohistochemical staining for nitrotyrosine in the liver, are increased in patients with NASH compared to those with simple steatosis, and steatosis is increased compared to normal liver.[58] Similarly, the oxidative stress inducible thiol-containing antioxidant protein, thioredoxin, is increased in the serum of patients with NASH, and levels directly relate to the severity of disease.[59] Similar to alcoholic liver disease, alterations in cytochrome p450 2E1, mitchondrial dysfunction, and cytokines likely play etiologic oxidative stress roles in human NASH. Increased CYP2E1 levels can occur with obesity. Recent studies by Emery and coworkers demonstrated increased CYP2E1 levels in morbidly obese subjects with NASH, with levels significantly correlating with body mass index. Importantly, levels decreased following gastric bypass surgery and weight reduction.[60] Mitochondrial abnormalities are noted in NASH patients; histologic findings of large mitochondria with paracrystalline inclusions occur in patients with NASH but not in those with simple steatosis.[58] Moreover, patients with NASH have defects in mitochondrial fatty acid metabolism.[60] Lastly, patients with NASH have elevated serum concentrations of the proinflammatory cytokine, TNF, which can induce oxidative stress, and they also have inadequate levels of the anti-inflammatory cytokine, adiponectin.[39,61]

Animal models of NASH also have major evidence of oxidative stress. The most frequently used models are the genetically-obese mice and rats (ob/ob mice and fa/fa rats), which exhibit obesity and insulin-resistant hyperglycemia, hyperlipidemia, and fatty liver, and animal models of nutritionally-induced NASH such as animals fed the methionine-restricted choline-deficient diet (MCD rats).[62,63] Not only do both rats with the nutritionally-induced fatty livers and ob/ob mice have biomarkers of hepatic oxidative stress, such as increased TBARS and 4HNE, but both groups of animals develop markedly-enhanced liver injury following endotoxin injection (which induces oxidative stress). Thus, they are much more susceptible to a second insult.[62,63]

Similar to alcoholic liver disease, there is no FDA-approved therapy for NASH, but antioxidant therapy is highly attractive and widely used. The first form of therapy should be lifestyle modification with weight reduction. Indeed, several studies suggest that both diet-induced weight loss (of even relatively modest amounts) and surgically-induced weight loss following gastric bypass surgery cause a significant improvement in liver enzymes and, in some cases, liver histology.[39,64] (Obesity, medical management of obesity, and gastric bypass surgery are discussed in Section VII of this book.)

Because many patients are unable to lose weight by dietary means, drug therapy represents an important alternative approach. Initial studies by Lavine in 11 obese children showed that vitamin E therapy was associated with a significant improvement in liver enzymes.[65] Importantly, this improvement occurred without weight loss, and selected patients experienced an increase in their liver enzymes following withdrawal of vitamin E. An important study from Japan showed that 300 mg vitamin E per day significantly reduced levels of the profibrotic cytokine, TGF-β, in patients with NASH who had already undergone lifestyle modifications.[66] Some of these patients also showed improved liver histology. Further randomized studies of antioxidant therapy and weight loss are planned by the National Institutes of Health. Lastly, betaine has been used to help correct the abnormalities in methionine metabolism, which can lead to increases in S-adenosyl-homocysteine and homocysteine. Betaine can help decrease these potentially toxic metabolites of methionine by regenerating methionine from homocysteine. A pilot study using betaine in NASH produced significant improvement in liver enzymes.[67] Thus, antioxidant therapy is a promising potential form of therapy for NASH that warrants further investigation.[68]

Hepatitis C

Hepatitis C affects over three million Americans, and there is extensive evidence to document increased oxidative stress in this liver disease. Patients with hepatitis C have increased urinary isoprostane levels, but values are not as high as those seen in alcoholic hepatitis.[27] Serum thioredoxin levels are significantly elevated in hepatitis C patients and levels correlated with the severity of disease, as assessed by histologic quantification of fibrosis.[69] Importantly, patients who became HCV-RNA negative after 14 days of interferon therapy had significantly lower pretreatment thioredoxin levels than those who remained positive, suggesting that oxidative stress may have played a role in the poor interferon response. Oxidative stress has also been documented indirectly by immunohistochemical staining for 8-hydroxydeoxyguanosine in liver biopsy specimens.[70] This serves as an indirect marker of DNA damage induced by oxidative stress, and immunohistochemical staining was present in 71% of patients with hepatitis C, 56% of patients with alcoholic liver disease, and in none of the normal liver biopsies. Oxidative stress has also been measured more directly in liver biopsies of patients with hepatitis C using EPR spin-probe techniques.[71] Lastly, one of the strongest pieces of clinical evidence that HCV infection increases oxidative stress comes from the recognition that HCV is commonly associated with the hepatic disorder of uroporphyrin accumulation, acquired porphyria cutanea tarda, which is a well-documented disorder of hepatic oxidative stress.[72]

Investigation of Hepatitis C–Induced Oxidative Stress

Mechanisms for hepatitis C–induced oxidative stress are under active investigation. Mice expressing certain structural or nonstructural hepatitis C proteins have been shown to develop hepatic steatosis, generate ROS, and express NFkB activation.[73-76] Thus, components of the hepatitis C virus appear to be directly responsible for oxidative stress. Moreover, environmental factors also may play a role. Patients who drink or smoke cigarettes have more rapid progression of hepatitis C, and both behaviors are associated with oxidative stress.[77,78]

Antioxidant therapy could have a theoretic role in hepatitis C in at least two areas: 1) antioxidant treatment in conjunction with standard pegylated interferon plus ribavirin therapy; and 2) antioxidant therapy to attenuate injury and fibrosis in patients nonresponsive to standard antiviral therapy. Only limited studies have been done with antioxidants in conjunction with antiviral therapy, mainly using a glutathione prodrug, N-acetylcysteine. While pilot studies were promising, the largest randomized study was negative. Similarly, antioxidants have the potential to decrease the common complication of ribavirin-induced red blood cell hemolysis, but studies to date have not shown consistent positive results. A study of vitamin E therapy for nonresponders showed significant decrease in liver enzymes; however, long-term studies are required to see if fibrosis and disease progression are reduced.[79]

Toxin/Metabolic Induced Liver Disease

As discussed in the introduction to this chapter, overdose with acetaminophen is a major cause of fulminant hepatic failure in the United States. It is not the parent drug but a metabolite (NAPQI) that causes the hepatotoxicity (Figure 28-5). This reactive metabolite first markedly depletes cellular glutathione pools and mitochondrial dysfunction and then occurs with reduced cellular ATP levels as well as increased generation of superoxide. Superoxide may react with NO to form peroxynitrite. In the face of depleted glutathione stores, peroxynitrite can then cause severe protein oxidation and nitration, which ultimately leads to cell death.[80] This whole process may be blocked by maintaining cellular glutathione stores. This probably presents the most extensively studied experimental and clinical use of antioxidant therapy in liver disease.

The glutathione prodrug, N-acetylcysteine, helps maintain glutathione stores, even in the face of NAPQI generation. In the clinical situation, almost all patients sur-

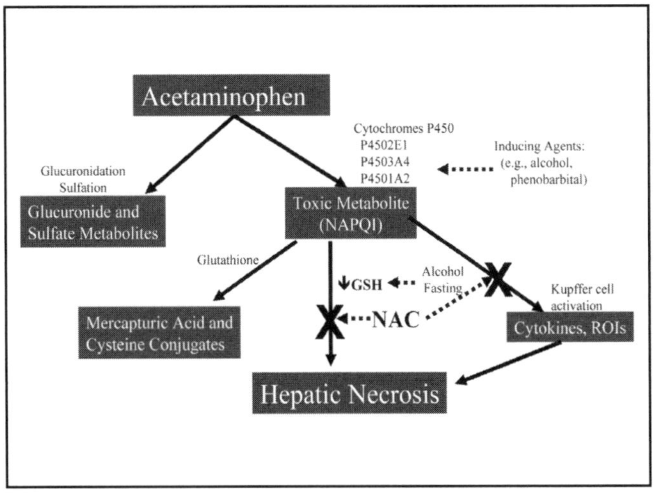

Figure 28-5. Most acetaminophen is metabolized via glucuronidation and sulfation. A small amount is metabolized through the P450 system to generate the toxic metabolite NAPQI. Hepatic glutathione normally binds this toxic metabolite and renders it harmless. However, if the cytochrome P450 system, especially P450 2E1, is induced by agents such as alcohol or if there are inadequate hepatic glutathione stores, the toxic metabolite binds to liver cell macromolecules and causes hepatocyte death. Administration of N-acetylcysteine (NAC) inhibits hepatic glutathione depletion and subsequent liver injury. The toxic metabolite NAPQI or some other metabolic products of acetaminophen cause Kupffer cell activation with subsequent release of cytokines, reactive oxygen intermediates, etc, which can also cause hepatic necrosis. N-acetylcysteine administration can also attenuate this process.

vive suicide attempts with acetaminophen overdose if they are brought to the emergency room early enough (within 12 hours) and are aggressively treated with Mucomyst, which contains N-acetylcysteine (NAC).[9] On the other hand, patients who have therapeutic misadventures with acetaminophen (accidentally take too much of the drug) and who do not come to the emergency room until they have clinical symptoms or evidence of liver failure often die of acetaminophen toxicity.[81,82] They receive limited benefit from NAC therapy because injury has already developed. This form of hepatotoxicity and treatment clearly documents the great potential efficacy of antioxidant therapy in liver diseases.

A variety of metabolic liver diseases also have oxidative stress as a major mechanism of toxicity, such as hemochromatosis (iron overload) and Wilson's disease (copper overload). Patients with Wilson's disease have low plasma ceruloplasmin levels and elevated free copper levels. Damage presumably occurs because of the formation of ROS, catalyzed by the excess copper.[83] Initially, copper accumulates in the cytoplasm and is bound mainly to the metal-binding protein, metallothionein. Once the capacity of metallothionein is exceeded, oxidative damage occurs with resulting cell injury/death. Initial therapy for Wilson's disease was with drugs that chelated copper, such as penicillamine. More recently, a frequently used form of therapy, especially in the initial phases of the disease, is oral zinc supplementation.[84] Zinc has antioxidant properties; it induces intestinal metallothionein, which will decrease copper absorption; and it also induces hepatic metallothionein, which has antioxidant properties and binds copper. The effectiveness of zinc therapy raises the question of whether zinc plus other antioxidants may be even more effective in therapy for Wilson's disease.

In summary, oxidative stress, as determined both directly and indirectly, clearly occurs in the major forms of clinically relevant liver disease and antioxidant therapy, including possible targeted delivery of antioxidants, and holds great promise in the treatment of multiple forms of liver disease.

Oxidative Stress in Inflammatory Bowel Disease

The term "IBD" covers a range of chronic inflammatory conditions that affect the human digestive tract. In most cases, the term refers to two disease states: ulcerative colitis and Crohn's disease (Chapter 18). Our knowledge regarding these disease processes continues to evolve, but definitive causal factors have yet to be identified. Individual susceptibility genes for IBD have been discovered but fail to explain the full extent of abnormalities found in IBD. One current hypothesis states that dysregulated immune cells (mainly T-helper cells) establish and maintain the chronic intestinal inflammation in IBD.[85] A steadily growing list of contributing genetic mutations has been compiled that support this theory. However, abnormalities, such as the NOD2/CARD15 mutations, are not the only variables in the inflammation equation. Increasing evidence points to the importance of mucosal epithelial cells as active contributors to the system responsible for maintaining intestinal homeostasis.

Acting as a physical barrier, the intestinal mucosa minimizes the uncontrolled contact between intestinal antigens from food and luminal bacteria and the intestinal immune system, and a change in the epithelial barrier can cause a continuous stimulation of immune cells.[86] Expanding lines of evidence document that epithelial cells, far from serving merely as a simple barrier, participate fully in modulating the local immune responses.[86] Epithelial cells express a variety of factors, including IL-15 and TGF-β, even before the onset of overt intestinal inflammation.[86] The proximity to luminal contents allows epithelial cells to play the role of mediator, processing luminal antigens and presenting them to the mucosal immune system via the major histocompatability complex I-related MICA and MICB molecules, especially under conditions of stress such as inflammation, cell damage, infection, or transformation.[87] Under-recognized protective functions performed by epithelial cells include detoxification and biotransformation of luminal agents.[88]

Evidence of Oxidative Stress in Inflammatory Bowel Disease

In IBD, oxidative stress plays many roles. Oxidative stress may be a consequence of inflammation but may also play a causative role in some of the symptoms of IBD. By-products of oxidative stress may participate in regulating intestinal inflammation. Lastly, there is evidence that abnormalities in oxidative defense mechanisms may confer susceptibility to IBD.

Glutathione Metabolism

Gluathione, one of the most important components of the antioxidant defense system, is a tripeptide thiol that is synthesized in the cytoplasm of most mammalian cells.[89] Several studies suggest that in ulcerative colitis, glutathione depletion may be related to inflammation, whereas in Crohn's disease, depletion of glutathione appears to be independent of inflammation.[89] Glutathione is replenished by incoming dietary sources and depleted by antioxidant defense. In active Crohn's disease of the ileum, inflammation was associated with decreased glutathione concentrations, when compared to noninflamed ileums and controls. γ-glutamyl synthetase activity was also decreased in the ileum from patients with active Crohn's disease. Glutathione levels were significantly depleted in active ulcerative colitis, compared to levels in control colon or inactive colitis. Gluathione synthetase activity was also decreased in rectal biopsies from active colitis patients.[89] However, glutathione levels in inactive Crohn's colitis cases ranged from normal to undetectable. In a mouse model evaluating the effects of glutathione depletion, acute depletion altered immune cell recruitment, whereas chronic depletion impaired the production of inhibitory nerve cell products compared to controls treated with saline.[89]

Membrane Fluidity/Mucosal Transporter Abnormalities

Excessive ROS production has been postulated to be responsible for the excess electrolyte and water secretion that lead to diarrhea in IBD.[7] The most direct evidence for this comes from McKenzie et al,[7] who showed that oxidation by $HOCl^-$ led to the loss of glyceraldehyde-3-phosphate dehydrogenase enzyme activity in colon epithelial crypt cells harvested from active Crohn's disease and ulcerative colitis lesions. A preliminary study demonstrated that in vitro oxidation of brush border membrane vesicles prompted a marked reduction in rates of glucose transport with a coincidental alteration in membrane fluidity, and when membrane fluidity was restored, glucose transport activity recovered significantly.[90] The loss of transporter function was believed to be dependent upon the lipid bilayer in which the transporter is imbedded and not solely as a consequence of damage to the transport protein.[90] Utilizing a unique membrane fluidity preparation, investigators demonstrated that oxidation-related changes in hemi-leaflet fluidity resulted in impairment of glucose transporters.[90] Oxidized vesicles had lower rates of glucose uptake than did respective controls.[90] The effect seemed to be most strongly related to changes in fluidity of the outer hemi-leaflet.

Altered Antioxidant Defenses

Perturbations in the ROS elimination pathways appear to be another consequence of chronic oxidative stress. Attention has focused with increasing clarity on the intricate balance between the primary (superoxide dismutase [SOD]) and secondary (catalase [CAT], glutathione peroxidase [GPX], myeloperoxidase [MPO]) steps of the antioxidant pathway, rather than on the absolute levels of the individual enzymes, as the mechanism for maintaining tissue oxidant homeostasis. Alterations in the balance appear to vary according to the particular disease state in question. In a study of the inflamed mucosa from IBD patients, investigators demonstrated that the levels of Cu/Zn-SOD and extracellular SOD were slightly decreased, but the expression of manganese MnSOD was markedly up-regulated.[91] From the early stages of inflammation, the lamina propria in IBD patients is subjected to considerable amounts of H_2O_2. Accumulating phagocytic leukocytes generate high local concentrations of H_2O_2 for prolonged time periods, and they also contain slightly elevated levels of MnSOD. Because H_2O_2 is highly diffusible and stable, excess H_2O_2 may easily reach surrounding cells within the lamina propria or the epithelium. However, the deleterious effects appear to be mitigated by monocytes and macrophages, which contain the H_2O_2-neutralizing enzyme CAT, infiltrating the lamina propria. Balance appears to be maintained in the lamina propria, despite the apparent lack GPX in the lamina propria, and most of the H_2O_2 generated is probably handled by neutrophilic MPO, which, in turn, will down-regulate GPX production. However, MPO reacts with H_2O_2 to form $HOCl^-$, a stable ROS with strong oxidizing properties and multiple proinflammatory effects.[91] High levels of $HOCl^-$-releasing neutrophils in the inflamed lamina propria not only explain the lack of GPX up-regulation with inflammation but also explain how $HOCl^-$-mediated GPX inhibition can create an amplification loop of increasing $HOCl^-$ concentrations in the IBD lamina propria, which might contribute to serious cellular injury and perpetuation of the inflammatory process.[91]

Abnormal Detoxification Pathways

Data from animal models of colitis and human studies of IBD patients suggest that detoxification enzyme depletion may be an important factor in the initiation and progression of ulcerative colitis.[88] Recent studies have highlighted the critical importance of transporters such as ABCB1, multidrug resistance (MDR)1 and ABCC1-3 (MRP1-3) in maintaining the health of IECs by keeping drugs, nutrients, or bacterial compounds in the gut lumen.[92,93] MDR1A knockout mice spontaneously develop colitis upon exposure to normal intestinal flora.[94] MDR1 gene polymorphisms identified in humans have been proposed as susceptibility factors for IBD.[95,96] Using mucosal biopsy specimens from noninflamed areas of the colon and terminal ileum in patients with ulcerative colitis and Crohn's disease, global gene expression profiling was performed to determine alterations in genes associated with detoxification and epithelial membrane integrity. Several dysregulated genes were identified in both disease groups and tissues.[86] A large number of genes were specifically regulated in the ileum of patients with Crohn's disease (934 genes, 67%), and the aberrant genes unique for ulcerative colitis were mainly identified in the colon (64 genes, 23%).[86] A strong down-regulation of several GST genes was noted in ulcerative colitis more than Crohn's disease, which correlated with reduced GST activity due to loss of GST protein levels in nonimmune cells of the mucosa, but not inflammatory cells.[86] Both MDR1 and pregnane x receptor (PXR), a member of the nuclear receptor super-family (which is highly important in regulating xenobiotic metabolism) were strongly down-regulated in the colonic mucosa of ulcerative colitis patients, but not in Crohn's disease.[86]

Immune Regulation

Nuclear factor (NF)-κB is a ubiquitous regulatory factor which plays a prominent role in regulating mucosal inflammation. Many immunological and environmental factors influence the activation status of NF-κB. Protective mechanisms confer a relative resistance to NF-κB activation to prevent inappropriate activation by the normal gut flora.[97] Epithelial cells use this resistance to protect themselves against the background oxidative stress generated by inflammatory cells present in IBD. NF-κB acts as redox sensor in the cell, as ROS can activate NF-κB. Although active NF-κB generates proinflammatory gene products, this is balanced by the simultaneous induction of survival responses, including the production of NO, derived from iNOS and other inhibitors of apoptosis.[97] Epithelial cells seem to be the main cell expressing iNOS in the mucosal inflammation associated with IBD. High levels of NO play a protective role in mucosal inflammation by producing a negative feedback loop that blocks prolonged activation of NF-κB and limits chronic inflammation.[97]

Data from animal models of colitis, as well as human studies of IBD patients, suggest that detoxification enzyme depletion may be important in the initiation and progression of ulcerative colitis and that excess biotransformation may result in colon cancer.[88] Subtle differences in the morphological development of ulcerative-colitis-associated carcinogenesis compared to sporadic colon cancers may well be related to an inflammation-driven carcinogenesis process in ulcerative colitis patients. The available evidence suggests that DNA damage caused by oxidative stress in the characteristic damage-regeneration cycle is at the level of secretion of inflammatory cytokines, which is a major contributor to colorectal cancer (Chapter 17) development in ulcerative colitis patients.

Possible Roles of Antioxidant Therapy in Inflammatory Bowel Disease

Attenuating oxidative stress has been used as a therapeutic strategy for over 50 years, as drugs commonly used for IBD, including sulphasalazine/5-ASA, are potent ROS scavengers. However, these agents also work through a variety of other mechanisms. Specific strategies to address intestinal oxidative stress consist mainly of efforts to inhibit ROS producing enzymes, to directly scavenge ROS, or to augment the inherent capability of existing cellular antioxidant pools.[99]

Therapeutic normalization of Cu/Zn-SOD levels has been successful in various animal models of inflammation, and early uncontrolled trials with bovine SOD demonstrated clinical improvement in patients with IBD;[100] however, delivery difficulties involving its short circulatory half-life, its poor cellular uptake, and its anomalous prooxidant side effect at high doses have hampered generalized clinical use.[100] To circumvent these shortcomings, gene transfer technology has been investigated as a method of delivery. Transgenic mice, bred to over-express human Cu/Zn-SOD, were protected from colitis-associated mortality.[100] Under mild inflammatory conditions, transgenic Cu/Zn-SOD overexpression resulted in a 2- to 3-fold reduction of mucosal MPO activity, which was found to accurately reflect the number of neutrophils, to levels even below those in water control animals.[100] This finding suggests that Cu/Zn-SOD overexpression may assist in the clearance of mucosal neutrophils, thereby ameliorating acute inflammation.

Using antioxidants to block NF-κB activation in disorders complicated by underlying oxidative stress may provide another method for preventing or ameliorating inflammatory conditions. Vitamin A deficiency heightens the intensity of the inflammatory response of peritoneal phagocytes, manifested by increased numbers of circulating leukocytes, enhanced T-cell proliferative responses, and augmented release of NO.[101] Investigators evaluated the effects of vitamin A deficiency on IBD with a trinitro benzesulfonic acid (TNBS) -induced rat model of induced colitis.[101] After inducing vitamin A deficiency in the experimental group, colitis was induced in experimental and control animals. After histological changes were evaluated, DNA-binding of NF-κB in the colons of the colitis and the control groups was compared by electrophoretic mobility shift assay. Vitamin A deficiency led to higher levels of NF-κB binding to DNA in nuclear extracts of both groups of vitamin A deficient rats, compared to colons from noncolitis rats supplemented with vitamin A. Although all animals demonstrated inflammation initially after TNBS exposure, the vitamin A deficient rats demonstrated a markedly worsened histologic picture in the chronic phase, with inflammatory cell infiltrates and enhanced collagen content and fibrosis.[101]

The potent GrTP antioxidant, (-)-epigallocatechin-3-gallate (EGCG), has demonstrated efficacy as an anti-inflammatory agent and has been of major research interest to this group. The initial study has demonstrated the ability of EGCG to block LPS-induced TNF-α gene expression.[102] The anti-inflammatory mechanism was further characterized by exposing the intestinal epithelial cell line IEC-6 to GrTP prior to exposure to TNF-α. GrTPs, especially EGCG, prevented the activation of inhibitor kappa kinase by inhibiting the phosphorylation of IκB.[102] These investigators then showed that GrTP were highly effective at attenuating inflammation in the IL-2 knockout model of IBD (Figure 28-6), and these authors are in the process of initiating clinical trials of GrTPs in IBD.[102]

Conclusion

Although initially believed to be a mere by-product of mucosal inflammation in IBD, oxidative stress has surfaced as an important causative agent of clinical symptoms of IBD as well as an important modulator of the disease process. Most recently, clinical evidence has demonstrated down-regulation of specific detoxification genes in ulcerative colitis (and to a lesser extent, Crohn's disease), which could play an etiological role in the pathogenesis of IBD by increasing the ability of the susceptible individual to xenobiotic stress. Future therapy will likely be directed at mitigating the detrimental effects of free radicals by enhancing preexisting antioxidant pools and inhibiting

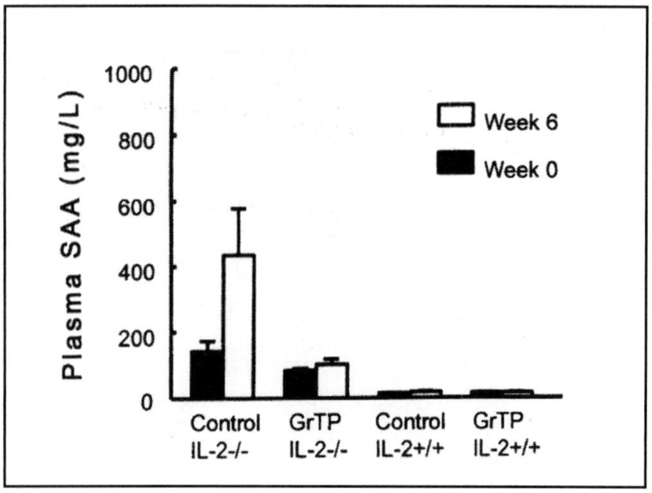

Figure 28-6. Effect of green tea polyphenols (GrTP) on plasma concentrations of serum amyloid A (SAA) in interleukin-2-deficient and IL-2 +/+ mice. Data are means + SEM, n = 14 for GrTP/IL-2 -/- and Control/IL-2-/- and n = 8 for GrTP/IL-2+/+ and Control/IL-2+/+. IL-2-/- (both groups) versus IL-2+/+ (both groups) wk 0, P <.01; GrTP IL-2-/- versus Control IL-2-/- wk 6, P <.01. Reprinted from Varilek GW, Yang F, Lee EY, et al. Green tea polyphenol extract attenuates inflammation in interleukin-2-deficient mice, a model of autoimmunity. *J Nutrition*. 2001;131:2034-2039.

the immunological effects of oxidative stress rather than specific therapy directed at detoxifying the free radicals themselves.

Oxidative Stress in Pancreatic Disease

Similar to liver diseases described above, oxidative stress is proposed to be a significant underlying mechanism for the cell injury in many forms of pancreatic disease. This section will review the role of oxidative stress in acute and chronic pancreatitis.

Acute and Chronic Pancreatitis

Nutrition and pancreatitis are discussed in Chapters 21 (chronic pancreatitis) and 22 (acute pancreatitis).

Acute pancreatitis is an acute inflammatory process of the pancreas coupled with destruction of the gland. The morphology of acute pancreatitis ranges from patchy edema to large areas of necrosis and hemorrhage depending on the severity of the disease.[104] In severe cases, this disease can be life-threatening, as the systemic inflammatory response can lead to multiple organ failure.[105] Gallstones are the leading cause of acute pancreatitis in developed countries, accounting for more than 90% of cases worldwide. Another major cause is alcohol abuse;[106] it is however debated whether acute alcoholic pancreatitis occurs independently from chronic alcoholic pancreatitis. If acute pancreatitis is survived and the bout clears, the prognosis for recovery for the patient is usually quite good.

While also an inflammatory disease, chronic pancreatitis involves a much lower grade of inflammation in comparison to acute pancreatitis, and the inflammatory response tends to occur locally instead of systemically. This disease is characterized by marked tissue destruction, which results in the progressive deterioration of exocrine and endocrine function and leads to multiple associated diseases, such as maldigestion (Chapter 5) and diabetes (Chapter 16).[107,108] The major pathology of chronic pancreatitis is characterized by intra- and interlobular acinar fibrosis as well as fibrotic strictures of pancreatic ducts.[109] Epidemiological evidence suggests that alcohol abuse causally accounts for 70% to 80% of adult chronic pancreatitis in the United States and other industrialized countries,[110,111] and the degree of fibrosis is greater in chronic alcoholic pancreatitis than in nonalcoholic chronic pancreatitis.[109] Importantly, the prevalence of this disease is likely to be underestimated because alcohol abusers often have asymptomatic pancreatic damage.[112]

Oxidative Stress and Antioxidants in Pancreatitis

Regardless of the etiology of injury, oxidative stress is proposed to be pivotal in the progression to parenchymal pancreatic tissue destruction.[113] Indeed, the involvement of free radicals in pancreatic damage has been shown in various forms of acute pancreatitis[114] and alcoholic pancreatitis.[115] Furthermore, humans and animals consuming alcohol also often have a diminished antioxidant status in pancreas[116,117] and in blood.[118] There is also evidence of persistent oxidant stress in patients with chronic pancreatitis[119] as well as increased lipid peroxidation and altered glutathione metabolism.[120] Furthermore, damage mediated by oxidative stress during acute and chronic pancreatitis may contribute to later development of diabetes (Chapter 16) and pancreatic cancer (Chapter 26) in these individuals.[121]

Whether acute or chronic, it is clear that inflammation plays a key role in the progression of pancreatitis. Elevated proinflammatory cytokines have been found in the serum,[122] peripheral blood monocytes[123] and pancreatic tissue[124] of patients with acute and chronic pancreatitis. Given this, the hypothesis that inflammatory cells may be a source of oxidative stress (see above) under these conditions is strongly supported.[114,125] What is less clear is whether oxidative stress contributes to initiation of the disease. However, in the case of alcoholic pancreatitis, there are experimental data supporting the hypothesis that alcohol metabolism in the pancreas may contribute to localized oxidative stress[115,126] analogous to the response of the liver. Another potential mechanism through which alcohol can cause oxidative stress in the pancreas is via hypoxia. It has been shown that ethanol causes pancreatic vasoconstriction and decreases pancreatic blood oxygen tension in the absence of systemic blood pressure changes.[127-130] Later work in an enteral rat model of alcohol-induced pancreatitis demonstrated an increase in hypoxia at the cellular level using the hypoxia marker pimonidazole.[131] While hypoxia can damage cells directly, reoxygenation following hypoxia can, paradoxically, induce more damage by formation of reactive oxygen species, leading to oxidative stress.[132,133] Under these conditions, this early oxidative stress caused by alcohol exposure directly may exacerbate the secondary inflammatory response during pancreatitis.[134] (Nutrition and alcohol abuse are discussed together in Chapter 15.)

Antioxidant Supplementation in Pancreatitis

Regardless of whether oxidative stress plays a causal role in pancreatitis or an exacerbating role in the progression of the disease, antioxidant supplementation is proposed to be a useful therapy. For example, in a prospective trial of 10 patients with chronic and acute recurrent pancreatitis from various etiologies, supplementation with a complex containing vitamin E, vitamin C, and organic selenium resulted in significant pain relief and decreased need for hospital admission during the year of treatment as compared to the year prior to treatment.[135] Furthermore, in a 20-week, double blind, placebo-controlled, crossover trial of supplementation with selenium, beta-carotene, vitamin C, vitamin E, and methionine, most patients reported fewer attacks with significantly less background pain while on treatment.[136] However, large prospective placebo-controlled trials are still needed to support these hypotheses.

Conclusion

Oxidative stress is increasingly recognized as an etiologic factor in many forms of GI diseases. The understanding of the role of ROS has been extended from inducing cell death at high levels of ROS to acting as signaling molecules at much lower levels. In many disease states, there are initial adaptive responses to increased generation of ROS such as induction of antioxidant enzymes (eg, MnSOD). Alcoholic liver disease and nonalcoholic steatohepatitis are examples in which there is altered mitochondrial function with impaired transfer of electrons between mitochondrial respiratory complexes and subsequent leakage of electrons. Initial defense mechanisms compensate for this, but secondary "hits" then cause liver injury. Antioxidant therapy is an attractive and inexpensive intervention in many GI diseases. However, dosing, appropriate combination of agents, and targeting of agents still need to be addressed in individual organ systems. For example, in liver injury it may be beneficial to target antioxidants to the Kupffer cell to down-regulate NFκB. On the other hand, inhibiting NFκB in the hepatocyte may be deleterious as it acts as a survivor factor. Thus, understanding mechanisms of oxidant induced cell injury, cell signaling, and appropriate mechanisms of antioxidant therapy remain areas of active investigation.

References

1. Koppenol WH. The centennial of the Fenton reaction. *Free Radic Biol Med.* 1993;15:645-651.
2. Gerschman R, Gilbert DL, Nye SW, Dwyer P, Fenn WO. Oxygen poisoning and x-irradiation: a mechanism in common. *Science.* 1956;119:623-626.
3. Harman D. Aging: a theory based on free radical and radiation chemistry. *J Gerontol.* 1956;11:298-300.
4. McCord JM, Fridovich I. Superoxide dismutase. An enzymic function of erythrocuprein (hemocuprein). *J Biol Chem.* 1969;244:6049-6055.
5. Sies H. *Oxidative Stress.* London, UK: Academic Press; 1985.
6. Corcoran GB, Mitchell JR, Vaishnav YN, Horning EC. Evidence that acetaminophen and N-hydroxyacetaminophen form a common arylating intermediate, N-acetyl-p-benzoquinoneimine. *Mol Pharmacol.* 1980;18:536-542.
7. Kruidenier L, Verspaget HW. Review article: oxidative stress as a pathogenic factor in inflammatory bowel disease—radicals or ridiculous? *Aliment Pharmacol Ther.* 2002;16:1997-2015.
8. Evans JL, Goldfine ID, Maddux BA, Grodsky GM. Are oxidative stress-activated signaling pathways mediators of insulin resistance and beta-cell dysfunction? *Diabetes.* 2003;52:1-8.
9. Jaeschke H, Gores GJ, Cederbaum AI, Hinson JA, Pessayre D, Lemasters JJ. Mechanisms of hepatotoxicity. *Toxicol Sci.* 2002;65:166-176.
10. Golden MH. The development of concepts of malnutrition. *J Nutr.* 2002;132:2117S-2122S.
11. Toyokuni S. Iron-induced carcinogenesis: the role of redox regulation. *Free Radic Biol Med.* 1996;20:553-566.
12. Sies H. Strategies of antioxidant defense. *Eur J Biochem.* 1993;215:213-219.
13. Arteel GE, Sies H. The biochemistry of selenium and the glutathione system. *Environ Toxicol Pharmacol.* 2001;10:153-158.
14. Allen RG, Tresini M. Oxidative stress and gene regulation. *Free Radic Biol Med.* 2000;28:463-499.
15. Droge W. Free radicals in the physiological control of cell function. *Physiol Rev.* 2002;82:47-95.
16. Forman HJ, Torres M. Redox signaling in macrophages. *Mol Aspects Med.* 2001;22:189-216.
17. Kamata H, Hirata H. Redox regulation of cellular signalling. *Cell Signal.* 1999;11:1-14.
18. Ermak G, Davies KJ. Calcium and oxidative stress: from cell signaling to cell death. *Mol Immunol.* 2002;38:713-721.
19. D'Angio CT, Finkelstein JN. Oxygen regulation of gene expression: a study in opposites. *Mol Genet Metab.* 2000;71:371-380.
20. Hoek JB, Pastorino JG. Ethanol, oxidative stress, and cytokine-induced liver cell injury. *Alcohol.* 2002;27:63-68.
21. Dhakshinamoorthy S, Long DJ, Jaiswal AK. Antioxidant regulation of genes encoding enzymes that detoxify xenobiotics and carcinogens. *Curr Top Cell Regul.* 2000;36:201-216.
22. Zambon A, Waxman K, Daughters K, Eloi L. ATP-MgCl2 added to resuscitation improves survival in an experimental model of hemmorrhagic shock. *Resuscitation.* 1994;28:253-257.
23. Epe B, Ballmaier D, Roussyn I, Briviba K, Sies H. DNA damage by peroxynitrite characterized with DNA repair enzymes. *Nucleic Acids Res.* 1996;24:4105-4110.
24. Arteel G, Marsano L, Mendez C, Bentley F, McClain CJ. Advances in alcoholic liver disease. *Best Pract Res Clin Gastroenterol.* 2003;17:625-647.
25. Arteel GE. Oxidants and antioxidants in alcohol-induced liver disease. *Gastroenterology.* 2003;124(3):778-790.
26. Reinke LA, Lai EK, DuBose CM, McCay PB. Reactive free radical generation in vivo in heart and liver of ethanol-fed rats: correlation with radical formation in vitro. *Proc Natl Acad Sci USA.* 1987;84(24):9223-9227.
27. Meagher EA, Barry OP, Burke A, et al. Alcohol-induced generation of lipid peroxidation products in humans. *J Clin Invest.* 1999;104(6):805-813.
28. Wu D, Cederbaum AI. Ethanol cytotoxicity to a transfected HepG2 cell line expressing human cytochrome P4502E1. *J Biol Chem.* 1996;271(39):23914-23919.
29. Hoek JB, Cahill A, Pastorino JG. Alcohol and mitochondria: a dysfunctional relationship. *Gastroenterology.* 2002;122(7):2049-2063.

30. Morgan K, French SW, Morgan TR. Production of a cytochrome P450 2E1 transgenic mouse and initial evaluation of alcoholic liver damage. *Hepatology.* 2002;36(1):122-134.
31. Kono H, Bradford BU, Yin M, et al. CYP2E1 is not involved in early alcohol-induced liver injury. *Am J Physiol.* 1999;277:G1259-G1267.
32. Adachi M, Ishii H. Role of mitochondria in alcoholic liver injury. *Free Radic Biol Med.* 2002;32(6):487-491.
33. Lluis JM, Colell A, Garcia-Ruiz C, Kaplowitz N, Fernandez-Checa JC. Acetaldehyde impairs mitochondrial glutathione transport in HepG2 cells through endoplasmic reticulum stress. *Gastroenterology.* 2003;124(3):708-724.
34. Colell A, Garcia-Ruiz C, Miranda M, et al. Selective glutathione depletion of mitochondria by ethanol sensitizes hepatocytes to tumor necrosis factor. *Gastroenterology.* 1998;115(6):1541-1551.
35. Kono H, Rusyn I, Yin M, et al. NADPH oxidase-derived free radicals are key oxidants in alcohol-induced liver disease. *J Clin Invest.* 2000;106(7):867-872.
36. Kono H, Rusyn I, Uesugi T, et al. Diphenyleneiodonium sulfate, an NADPH oxidase inhibitor, prevents early alcohol-induced liver injury in the rat. *Am J Physiol Gastrointest Liver Physiol.* 2001;280(5):G1005-G1012.
37. McClain CJ, Barve S, Deaciuc I, Kugelmas M, Hill D. Cytokines in alcoholic liver disease. *Semin Liver Dis.* 1999;19(2):205-219.
38. McClain CJ, Cohen DA. Increased tumor necrosis factor production by monocytes in alcoholic hepatitis. *Hepatology.* 1989;9:349-351.
39. Kugelmas M, Hill DB, Vivian B, Marsano L, McClain CJ. Cytokines and NASH: a pilot study of the effects of lifestyle modification and vitamin E. *Hepatology.* 2003;38:413-419.
40. Hill DB, Marsano L, Cohen D, Allen J, Shedlofsky S, McClain CJ. Increased plasma interleukin-6 concentrations in alcoholic hepatitis. *J Lab Clin Med.* 1992;119(5):547-552.
41. Hill DB, Marsano LS, McClain CJ. Increased plasma interleukin-8 concentrations in alcoholic hepatitis. *Hepatology.* 1993;18(3):576-580.
42. Honchel R, Ray MB, Marsano L, et al. Tumor necrosis factor in alcohol enhanced endotoxin liver injury. *Alcohol Clin Exp Res.* 1992;16(4):665-669.
43. Limuro Y, Gallucci RM, Luster MI, Kono H, Thurman RG. Antibodies to tumor necrosis factor alfa attenuate hepatic necrosis and inflammation caused by chronic exposure to ethanol in the rat. *Hepatology.* 1997;26(6):1530-1537.
44. Kamimura S, Tsukamoto H. Cytokine gene expression by Kupffer cells in experimental alcoholic liver disease. *Hepatology.* 1995;22(4):1304-1309.
45. Nanji AA, Zhao S, Sadrzadeh SM, Waxman DJ. Use of reverse transcription-polymerase chain reaction to evaluate in vivo cytokine gene expression in rats fed ethanol for long periods. *Hepatology.* 1994;19(6):1483-1487.
46. Friedman SL. Liver fibrosis—from bench to bedside. *J Hepatol.* 2003;38(Suppl 1):S38-S53.
47. Lee KS, Buck M, Houglum K, Chojkier M. Activation of hepatic stellate cells by TGF alpha and collagen type I is mediated by oxidative stress through c-myb expression. *J Clin Invest.* 1995;96(5):2461-2468.
48. Zamara E, Novo E, Marra F, et al. 4-Hydroxynonenal as a selective pro-fibrogenic stimulus for activated human hepatic stellate cells. *J Hepatol.* 2004;40(1):60-68.
49. McClain CJ, Hill DB, Song Z, et al. S-Adenosylmethionine, cytokines, and alcoholic liver disease. *Alcohol.* 2002;27(3):185-192.
50. Mato JM, Camara J, Fernandez de Paz J, et al. S-adenosylmethionine in alcoholic liver cirrhosis: a randomized, placebo-controlled, double-blind, multicenter clinical trial. *J Hepatol.* 1999;30(6):1081-1089.
51. Luper S. A review of plants used in the treatment of liver disease: part 1. *Altern Med Rev.* 1998;3(6):410-421.
52. Ferenci P, Dragosics B, Dittrich H, et al. Randomized controlled trial of silymarin treatment in patients with cirrhosis of the liver. *J Hepatol.* 1989;9(1):105-113.
53. Pares A, Planas R, Torres M, et al. Effects of silymarin in alcoholic patients with cirrhosis of the liver: results of a controlled, double-blind, randomized and multicenter trial. *J Hepatol.* 1998;28(4):615-621.
54. Hill DB, Devalaraja R, Joshi-Barve S, Barve S, McClain CJ. Antioxidants attenuate nuclear factor-kappa B activation and tumor necrosis factor-alpha production in alcoholic hepatitis patient monocytes and rat Kupffer cells, in vitro. *Clin Biochem.* 1999;32(7):563-570.
55. de la Maza MP, Petermann M, Bunout D, Hirsch S. Effects of long-term vitamin E supplementation in alcoholic cirrhotics. *J Am Coll Nutr.* 1995;14(2):192-196.
56. Pena LR, Hill DB, McClain CJ. Treatment with glutathione precursor decreases cytokine activity. *JPEN J Parenter Enteral Nutr.* 1999;23(1):1-6.
57. Neuschwander-Tetri BA, Caldwell SH. Nonalcoholic steatohepatitis: summary of an AASLD Single Topic Conference. *Hepatology.* 2003;37(5):1202-19. Review. Erratum in: *Hepatology.* 2003;38(2):536.
58. Sanyal AJ, Campbell-Sargent C, Mirshahi F, et al. Nonalcoholic steatohepatitis: association of insulin resistance and mitochondrial abnormalities. *Gastroenterology.* 2001;120:1183-1192.
59. Sumida Y, Nakashima T, Yoh T, et al. Serum thioredoxin levels as a predictor of steatohepatitis in patients with nonalcoholic fatty liver disease. *J Hepatol.* 2003;38:32-38.
60. Emery MG, Fisher JM, Chien JY, Kharasch ED, Dellinger EP, Kowdley KV, Thummel KE. CYP2E1 activity before and after weight loss in morbidly obese subjects with nonalcoholic fatty liver disease. *Hepatology.* 2003;38:428-435.
61. Sreekumar R, Rosado B, Rasmussen D, Charlton M. Hepatic gene expression in histologically progressive nonalcoholic steatohepatitis. *Hepatology.* 2003;38:244-251.
61. Hui JM, Hodge A, Farrell GC, Kench JG, Kriketos A, George J. Beyond insulin resistance in NASH: TNF-alpha or adiponectin? *Hepatology.* 2004;40(1):46-54.
62. Yang SQ, Lin HZ, Lane MD, Clemens M, Diehl AM. Obesity increases sensitivity to endotoxin liver injury: implications for the pathogenesis of steatohepatitis. *Proc Natl Acad Sci USA.* 1997;94:2557-2562.
63. Chawla RK, Watson WH, Eastin CE, Lee EY, Schmidt J, McClain CJ. S-adenosylmethionine deficiency and TNF-alpha in lipopolysaccharide-induced hepatic injury. *Am J Physiol.* 1998;275: G125-G129.
64. Dixon JB, Bhathal PS, Hughes NR, O'Brien PE. Nonalcoholic fatty liver disease: improvement in liver histological analysis with weight loss. *Hepatology.* 2004;39(6):1647-1654.
65. Lavine JE. Vitamin E treatment of nonalcoholic steatohepatitis in children: a pilot study. *J Pediatr.* 2000;136:734-738.
66. Hasegawa T, Yoneda M, Nakamura K, Makino I, Terano A. Plasma transforming growth factor-beta1 level and efficacy of alpha-tocopherol in patients with non-alcoholic steatohepatitis: a pilot study. *Aliment Pharmacol Ther.* 2001;15:1667-1672.
67. Abdelmalek MF, Angulo P, Jorgensen RA, Sylvestre PB, Lindor KD. Betaine, a promising new agent for patients with nonalcoholic steatohepatitis: results of a pilot study. *Am J Gastroenterol.* 2001;96: 2711-2717.
68. McClain CJ, Mokshagundam SP, Barve SS, Song Z, Hill DB, Chen T, Deaciuc I. Mechanisms of non-alcoholic steatohepatitis. *Alcohol.* 2004;34(1):67-79.
69. Sumida Y, Nakashima T, Yoh T, et al. Serum thioredoxin levels as an indicator of oxidative stress in patients with hepatitis C virus infection. *J Hepatol.* 2000;33(4):616-622.
70. Kitada T, Seki S, Iwai S, Yamada T, Sakaguchi H, Wakasa K. In situ detection of oxidative DNA damage, 8-hydroxydeoxyguanosine, in chronic human liver disease. *J Hepatol.* 2001;35(5):613-618.

71. Valgimigli L, Pedulli GF, Paolini M. Measurement of oxidative stress by EPR radical-probe technique. *Free Radic Biol Med.* 2001;31(6):708-716.
72. Chuang TY, Brashear R, Lewis C. Porpyria cutanea tarda and hepatitis C virus: a case-control study and meta-analysis of the literature. *J Amer Acad Dermatol.* 1999;41:31-36.
73. Lerat H, Honda M, Beard M, et al. Steatosis and liver cancer in transgenic mice expressing the structural and nonstructural proteins of hepatitis C virus. *Gastroenterology.* 2002;122:352-365.
74. Lai M. Hepatitis C virus proteins: direct link to hepatic oxidative stress, steatosis, carcinogenesis and more. *Gastroenterology.* 2002;122:568-569.
75. Okuda M, Li K, Beard M, Showalter L, Scholle F, Lemon S, Weinman S. Mitochondrial injury, oxidative stress, and antioxidant gene expression are induced by hepatitis C virus core protein. *Gastroenterol.* 2002;122:366-375.
76. Gong G, Waris G, Tanveer R, Siddiqui A. Human hepatitis C virus NS5A protein alters intracellular calcium levels, induces oxidative stress, and activates STAT-3 and NF-kappa B. *Proc Natl Acad Sci USA.* 2001;98(17):9599-9604.
77. Pessione F, Ramond M-J, Njapoum C, et al. Cigarette smoking and hepatic lesions in patients with chronic hepatitis C. *Hepatology.* 2001;34:121-125.
78. Morgan TR, Brenner D, Everhart J, et al. Hepatitis C and alcohol: fundamental and translational research directions. *Alcohol Clin Exp Res.* 2003;27(4):726-731.
79. von Herbay A, Stahl W, Niederau C, Sies H. Vitamin E improves the aminotransferase status of patients suffering from viral hepatitis C: a randomized, double-blind, placebo-controlled study. *Free Radic Res.* 1997;27(6):599-605.
80. Jaeschke H, Knight TR, Bajt ML. The role of oxidant stress and reactive nitrogen species in acetaminophen hepatotoxicity. *Toxicol Lett.* 2003;144(3):279-288.
81. McClain CJ, Price S, Barve S, Devalarja R, Shedlofsky S. Acetaminophen hepatotoxicity: an update. *Curr Gastroenterol Rep.* 1999;1:42-49.
82. McClain CJ. Late presentation of acetaminophen hepatotoxicity: an unresolved problem. *Dig Dis Sci.* 1982;27:375-376.
83. Llanos RM, Mercer JF. The molecular basis of copper homeostasis copper-related disorders. *DNA Cell Biol.* 2002;21(4):259-270.
84. Brewer GJ. Zinc acetate for the treatment of Wilson's disease. *Expert Opin Pharmacother.* 2001;2(9):1473-1477.
85. Mizoguchi A, Mizoguchi E, Bhan AK. Immune networks in animal models of inflammatory bowel disease. *Inflammy Bowel Dis.* 2003;9(12):246-259.
86. Langmann T, Moehle C, Maverer R, et al. Loss of detoxification in inflammatory bowel disease: dysregulation of pregnane X receptor target genes. *Gastroenterology.* 2004;127(7):26-40.
87. Groh V, Steinle A, Spies T, et al. Recognition of stress-induced MHC molecules by intestinal epithelial gammadelta T cells. *Science.* 1998;20:219-235.
88. Roediger W, Babidge W. Human colonocyte detoxification. *Gut.* 1997;41:731-734.
89. Koch TR, Yuan LX, Fink JG, et al. Induction of enlarged intestinal lymphoid aggregates during acute glutathione depletion in a murine model. *Dig Dis Sci.* 2000;45(11):2115-2121.
90. Jourd'heuil D, Meddings JB. Oxidative and drug-induced alterations in brush border membrane hemileaflet fluidity, functional consequences for glucose transport. *Biochim Biophys Acta.* 2001;1510(1-2):342-353.
91. Kruidenier L, Kuiper I, Van Duijn W, et al. Imbalanced secondary mucosal antioxidant response in inflammatory bowel disease. *J Pathol.* 2003;201(1):17-27.
92. Ho GT, Moodie FM, Satsangi J. Multidrug resistance 1 gene (P-glycoprotein 170): an important determinant in gastrointestinal disease? *Gut.* 2003;52:759-766.
93. Langmann T, Mauerer R, Zahn A, et al. Real-time reverse transicription-PCR expression profiling of the complete human ATP-binding cassette transporter superfamily in various tissues. *Clin Chem.* 2003;49:230-238.
94. Panwala CM, Jones JC, Viney JL, et al. A novel model of inflammatory bowel disease: mice deficient for the muliple drug resistance gene, mdr1a, spontaneously develop colitis. *J Immunol.* 1998;161:5733-5744.
95. Brant SR, Panhuysen CI, Nicolae D, et al. MDR1 Ala893 polymorphism is associated with inflammatory bowel disease. *Am J Hum Genet.* 2003;73:1282-1292.
96. Schwab M, Schaeffeler E, Marx C, et al. Association between the C3435T MDR1 gene polymorphism and susceptibility for ulcerative colitis. *Gastroenterology.* 2003;124:26-33.
97. Dijkstra G, Moshage H, Jansen PL. Blockade of NF-kappaB activation and donation of nitric oxide: new treatment options in inflammatory bowel disease? *Scand J Gastroenterol.* 2002;236:37-41.
98. Seril DN, Liao J, Yang GY, Yang CS. Oxidative stress and ulcerative colitis-associated carcinogenesis: studies in humans and animal models. *Carcinogenesis.* 2003;24(3):353-362.
99. Kruidenier L, Verspaget HW. Antioxidants and mucosa protectives: realistic therapeutic options in inflammatory bowel disease? *Mediators Inflamm.* 1998;7(3):157-162.
100. Kruidenier L, van Meeteren ME, et al. Attenuated mild colonic inflammation and improved survival from severe DSS-colitis of transgenic Cu/Zn-SOD mice. *Free Radic Biol Med.* 2003;34(6):753-765.
101. Reifen R, Nur T, Ghebermeskel K, et al. Vitamin A deficiency exacerbates inflammation in a rat model of colitis through activation of nuclear factor-kappaB and collagen formation. *J Nutr.* 2002;132(9):2743-2747.
102. Yang F, De Villiers WJ, McClain CJ, Varilek GW. Green tea polyphenols block endotoxin-induced tumor necrosis factor-production and lethality in a murine model. *J Nutr.* 1998;128:2334-2340.
103. Yang F, Oz HS, de Villiers WJ, et al. The green tea polyphenol (-)-epigallocatechin-3-gallate blocks nuclear factor kappa-beta activation by inhibiting IkB kinase activity in the intestinal epithelial cell line IEC-6. *Mol Pharmacol.* 2001;60(3):528-533.
104. Mitchell RM, Byrne MF, Baillie J. Pancreatitis. *Lancet.* 2003;361:1447-1455.
105. Raraty MG, Connor S, Criddle DN, Sutton R, Neoptolemos JP. Acute pancreatitis and organ failure: pathophysiology, natural history, and management strategies. *Curr Gastroenterol Rep.* 2004;6:99-103.
106. Apte MV, Wilson JS. Alcohol-induced pancreatic injury. *Best Pract Res Clin Gastroenterol.* 2003;17:593-612.
107. Ammann RW, Buehler H, Muench R, Freiburghaus AW, Siegenthaler W. Differences in the natural history of idiopathic (nonalcoholic) and alcoholic chronic pancreatitis: a comparative long-term study of 287 patients. *Pancreas.* 1987;2:368-377.
108. Lankisch PG, Lohr-Happe A, Otto J, Creutzfeldt W. Natural course in chronic pancreatitis: pain, exocrine and endocrine pancreatic insufficiency and prognosis of the disease. *Digestion.* 1993;54:148-155.
109. De Angelis C, Valente G, Spaccapietra M, Angonese C, DelFavero G, Naccarato R, Andriulli A. Histological study of alcoholic, nonalcoholic and obstructive chronic pancreatitis. *Pancreas.* 1992;7:193-196.
110. Singh M, Simsek H. Ethanol and the pancreas: current status. *Gastroenterology.* 1990;98:151-162.
111. Sarles H, Bernard JP, Johnson C, Chir M. Pathogenesis and epidemiology of chronic pancreatitis. *Ann Rev Med.* 1989;40:453-468.
112. Renner IG, Savage WT III, Stace NH, Pantoja JL, Schultheis WM, Peters RL. Pancreatitis associated with alcoholic liver disease. A review of 1022 autopsy cases. *Dig Dis Sci.* 1984;29:593-599.
113. McCloy R. Chronic pancreatitis at Manchester, UK. Focus on antioxidant therapy. *Digestion.* 1998;59:36-48.
114. Schulz HU, Niederau C, Klonowski-Stumpe H, Halangk W, Luthen R, Lippert H. Oxidative stress in acute pancreatitis. *Hepatogastroenterology.* 1999;46:2736-2750.
115. Schenker S, Montalvo R. Alcohol and the pancreas. *Recent Dev Alcohol.* 1998;14:41-65.

116. Van Gossum A, Closset P, Noel E, Cremer M, Neve J. Deficiency in antioxidant factors in patients with alcohol-related chronic pancreatitis. *Dig Dis Sci.* 1996;41:1225-1231.
117. Ashakumary L, Vijayammal PL. Additive effect of alcohol and nicotine on lipid peroxidation and antioxidant defence mechanism in rats. *J Appl Toxicol.* 1996;16:305-308.
118. Curran FJ, Sattar N, Talwar D, Baxter JN, Imrie CW. Relationship of carotenoid and vitamins A and E with the acute inflammatory response in acute pancreatitis. *Br J Surg.* 2000;87:301-305.
119. Guyan PM, Uden S, Braganza JM. Heightened free radical activity in pancreatitis. *Free Radic Biol Med.* 1990;8:347-354.
120. Schoenberg MH, Buchler M, Pietrzyk C. Lipid peroxidation and glutathione metabolism in chronic pancreatitis. *Pancreas.* 1995;10:36-43.
121. Farrow B, Evers BM. Inflammation and the development of pancreatic cancer. *Surg Oncol.* 2002;10:153-169.
122. Simovic MO, Bonham MJ, Abu-Zidan FM, Windsor JA. Anti-inflammatory cytokine response and clinical outcome in acute pancreatitis. *Crit Care Med.* 1999;27:2662-2665.
123. McKay CJ, Gallagher G, Brooks B, Imrie CW, Baxter JN. Increased monocyte cytokine production in association with systemic complications in acute pancreatitis. *Br J Surg.* 1996;83: 919-923.
124. Gukovskaya AS, Gukovsky I, Zaninovic V, et al. Pancreatic acinar cells produce, release, and respond to tumor necrosis factor-alpha. Role in regulating cell death and pancreatitis. *J Clin Invest.* 1997;100:1853-1862.
125. Gomez-Cambronero LG, Sabater L, Pereda J, et al. Role of cytokines and oxidative stress in the pathophysiology of acute pancreatitis: therapeutical implications. *Curr Drug Targets Inflamm Allergy.* 2002;1:393-403.
126. Wilson JS, Apte MV. Role of alcohol metabolism in alcoholic pancreatitis. *Pancreas.* 2003;27:311-315.
127. Foitzik T, Fernandez-del Castillo C, Rattner DW, Klar E, Warshaw AL. Alcohol selectively impairs oxygenation of the pancreas. *Arch Surg.* 1995;130:357-361.
128. Foitzik T, Hotz HG, Hot B, Kirchengast M, Buhr HJ. Endothelin-1 mediates the alcohol-induced reduction of pancreatic capillary blood flow. *J Gastrointest Surg.* 1998;2:379-384.
129. Widdison AL, Alvarez C, Schwarz M, Reber HA. The influence of ethanol on pancreatic blood flow in cats with chronic pancreatitis. *Surgery.* 1992;112:202-208.
130. Reber HA, Karanjia ND, Alvarez C, et al. Pancreatic blood flow in cats with chronic pancreatitis. *Gastroenterology.* 1992;103:652-659.
131. McKim SE, Uesugi T, Raleigh JA, McClain CJ, Arteel GE. Chronic intragastric alcohol exposure causes hypoxia and oxidative stress in the rat pancreas. *Arch Biochem Biophys.* 2003;417:34-43.
132. McCord JM. Oxygen-derived free radicals in postischemic tissue injury. *N Engl J Med.* 1985;312:159-163.
133. McCord JM, Fridovich I. The reduction of cytochrome C by milk xanthine oxidase. *J Biol Chem.* 1968;243:5753-5760.
134. Pandol SJ, Gukovsky I, Satoh A, Lugea A, Gukovskaya AS. Animal and in vitro models of alcoholic pancreatitis: role of cholecystokinin. *Pancreas.* 2003;27:297-300.
135. las Heras CG, Garcia dlP, Fernandez MD, Fernandez Forcelledo JL. Use of antioxidants to treat pain in chronic pancreatitis. *Rev Esp Enferm Dig.* 2000;92:375-385.
136. Uden S, Bilton D, Nathan L, Hunt LP, Main C, Braganza JM. Antioxidant therapy for recurrent pancreatitis: placebo-controlled trial. *Aliment Pharmacol Ther.* 1990;4:357-371.

Chapter 29

Perioperative Nutritional Support

Andrew Ukleja, MD

Introduction

The importance of nutritional support in the perioperative period has been well recognized. Malnutrition has been often observed in hospitalized surgical patients. Compromised nutritional status in the perioperative period has an adverse effect on surgical outcome including higher risk of nosocomial infections, poor wound healing, and slow functional recovery. Therefore, identification of patients at risk and optimization of nutritional status perioperatively is very important. Patients with severe malnutrition or rapid deterioration of nutritional status appear to be well-suited candidates for nutritional therapy. However, nutritional support is often instituted to unselected individuals undergoing surgical intervention.

The use of parenteral nutrition (PN) should be limited to patients with dysfunctional gastrointestinal (GI) tract. Enteral nutrition (EN) has been shown to be superior to PN. Despite the extensive literature on this topic, many controversies exist regarding who benefits from nutritional support, when to start nutritional therapy, and which route of support to choose. In this chapter, biologic responses to surgical stress and a nutritional assessment of surgical patients will be addressed with focus on options of perioperative nutritional support and their use in clinical practice.

The Need for Nutritional Support

Malnutrition has been observed in up to 50% of hospitalized patients.[1] The effect of poor nutrition on surgical outcome was first reported in 1936.[2] A higher mortality was observed in surgical malnourished patients with weight loss >20%, compared with well-nourished individuals undergoing ulcer surgery. In addition to preoperative weight loss, low serum albumin has been linked to higher rates of complications in postsurgical patients.[3] Despite compelling evidence that malnutrition affects postoperative morbidity and mortality, perioperative nutrition is often ignored and nutrition therapy is not instituted until occurrence of complications. Therefore, a critical issue in the management of surgical patients is to identify those who may benefit from perioperative nutritional support. A surgical injury induces many changes in body metabolism and can lead to rapid nutritional depletion. Perioperative nutritional support gives the opportunity in selected patients to blunt the effects of surgical stress.

Physiologic Responses to Surgical Trauma

A surgical intervention is a state of stress leading to complex physiologic responses to maintain body homeostasis. These responses are induced by stress and trauma of surgery such as volume loss, tissue damage, pain, and fear. In contrast to accidental injury, surgery results in an "elective" tissue trauma with a controlled injury and predictive responses to a certain degree. The management of surgical patients is designed to attenuate stress responses from tissue injury and organ removal by careful tissue dissection, avoidance of wound contamination, use of vaso-active and pain medications, and close monitoring of cardiovascular responses. Nutritional support and adequate hydration, when needed, are important components of perioperative management.

The stress of surgery creates a catabolic, hypermetabolic state with increased demands for protein and energy.[4] In response to surgical injury, stress hormones—such as corticosteroids, catecholamines, and glucagons—are released.[5] The initial postsurgical period of hypercatabolism is called "adrenergic-corticoid phase." It lasts an average of 1 to 3 days. Because of increased energy and protein requirements, a rapid redistribution of fat, proteins, and glycogen are seen from adipose tissue and skeletal muscle to metabolically active tissues.[6]

Cortisol, released from adrenal cortex, stimulates tissue catabolism and redistributes amino acids from skeletal muscles to the liver to enter gluconeogenesis and synthesis of acute phase proteins. High serum levels of cortisol are seen for 24 to 48 hours following surgery.[7] Glucagon has glycogenolytic and gluconeogenic effects. It induces production of glucose and glucogenic precursors in the liver. Epinephrine and norepinephrine are released from adrenal medulla to help maintain circulatory stability. Norepinephrine also induces metabolic responses by increasing metabolic rate and lipolysis.[8] This hormonal burst can lead to protein-calorie malnutrition and negative nitrogen balance within a few days. Patient's preexisting nutritional status and degree of hypermetabolism will influence the rate of deterioration of the nutritional status.

In response to surgical stress and anesthesia, aldosterone and antidiuretic hormone are secreted to maintain water and electrolyte balance.[9] Excess of these hormones after surgery will impair excretion of water, which leads to water retention and weight gain in some patients. Water can accumulate in surgical wounds and thus affect their healing. Eventually, excess of fluids is eliminated by the kidneys within a few days following surgery.

Cytokines produced at the time of injury stimulate mobilization of amino acids from skeletal muscles to provide nutrients for cellular metabolism and synthesis of acute phase proteins.[10] Acute phase proteins are involved in reduction of the systemic inflammatory responses due to tissue damage, and they help with coagulation and wound healing by inhibiting tissue destruction and protection from infections.[11]

The second phase after surgical injury, called the "adrenergic-corticoid withdrawal phase," lasts 1 to 3 days. The next anabolic phase starts typically within 3 to 6 days from an uncomplicated surgery and is characterized by return of bowel function, improvement of appetite, and resumption of oral intake. A positive nitrogen balance, weight gain, increase in lean body mass, and muscle strength are observed during this period.

At the time of surgical trauma, in a malnourished or a starving patient, progressive depletion of body compartments can occur, leading to adverse clinical outcome. Surgical injury by itself or complicated by hypoxemia, hypotensive shock, sepsis, and protein depletion can lead to impaired intestine permeability and host defense. Patients after surgery are vulnerable because of ileus and intestinal stasis. Intact bowel epithelium and preservation of mucosal perfusion and immune mechanisms allow effective elimination of bacteria and toxins and prevent bacterial translocation.[12] A dysfunction of gut mucosal barrier in malnourished patients or those with complicated course can predispose them to sepsis by allowing entry of bacteria and toxins from the gut to systemic circulation. In this setting, early nutritional support by oral or enteral feeding may help to maintain gut barrier function and prevent bacterial translocation. Any delays in initiation of feeding or nutrition support can result in deterioration of nutritional status and slow recovery time.

Sequelae of Malnutrition in Surgical Patients

Nutritional status is often poorly documented in surgical patients, despite serious nutritional deficits seen in patients undergoing surgical intervention.[13] Nutritional deficiencies result from an underlying disease or an inadequate oral intake. Many patients experience worsening in their nutritional status during their hospital stay as a result of inappropriate cessation of feeding due to withholding because of ongoing diagnostic tests and procedures. Reduced food intake leads to loss of fat and muscle tissue, which is followed by weight loss.[14]

The main concern is that malnourished patients undergoing surgery are at a higher risk for infectious complications, including wound infections, sepsis, and poor wound healing.[15] Malnutrition is associated with impaired function of immune system (reduced production of complement; poor bacterial opsonization; and dysfunctions of neutrophils, macrophages, and lymphocytes), exaggerated stress response, multi-organ failure, and delayed functional recovery.[16] Preoperative hypoalbuminemia has been associated with postoperative organ dysfunction, higher risk of GI bleeding, and nosocomial infections.[17] Increased length of mechanical ventilation, longer intensive care unit stay, and higher rate of hospital death have been reported as results of malnutrition.[18] Deleterious consequences of malnutrition are shown in Table 29-1.

Infection is the major complication observed in the postsurgical period.[19] Infections can initiate severe catabolic responses, which lead to increased proteolysis and lipolysis, accelerated gluconeogenesis, and release of inflammatory mediators. This response may compromise a host of defense mechanisms—especially in undernourished patients, thus increasing the possibility of sepsis, multi-organ system failure, and death.

Nutritional Assessment of Surgical Patient

Nutrition screening is an important part of evaluation prior to surgery. This assessment helps to distinguish patients who need aggressive nutritional support. Both clinical and laboratory data have been used to determine nutritional status. Significant weight loss, protein depletion, low serum albumin, and depressed total lymphocyte count have been associated with increased rate of postoperative complications. Evaluation of nutritional status is best accomplished by taking a good history and physical examination combined with serum levels of visceral proteins. It appears that nutritional deterioration over a short time is a more sensitive indicator in terms of who

TABLE 29-1.

Consequences of Malnutrition in Surgical Patients

Clinical Consequences	Mechanisms
Poor wound healing/suture dehiscence	edema and body fluid ↓ hydroxyl-praline deposition ↓ osmotic pressure
Increased susceptibility to infection (Increased frequency of decubitus ulcers)	immune deficiency cytokine release ↓ lymphocyte migration ↓ neutrophil function, (↓ adherence and chemotaxis)
Bacterial overgrowth of the GI tract	impaired gut mucosal barrier
Prolonged pulmonary intubation	↓ muscle strength and ↑ fatigability

is at risk for surgical complications and who may benefit from nutritional support. Another important issue of nutritional assessment is determination of the patient's level of stress and degree of illness by using the acute physiology and chronic health evaluation (APACHE II) and adjusted trauma index (ATI) scores.[20] Nutritional assessment is discussed in depth in Chapter 1.

The Patient's Medical History

The patient's medical history in relation to nutrition should focus on the presence of GI dysfunction, anorexia, and history of weight loss. Impairment of the GI tract can affect oral intake, nutritional status, route of nutrition delivery, and postoperative recovery. Abdominal bloating or distention, vomiting, and diarrhea can be a limitation to oral or enteral feeding in the perioperative period. A history of weight change is important. Details of recent weight loss prior to admission should be determined. Weight change expressed as a percentage of ideal body weight (IBW) or as a percentage of weight lost from usual body weight (UBW) is a good predictor of nutritional status deterioration. Weight loss exceeding 10% of usual body weight within 3 to 6 months appears to be predictive of significant malnutrition.[21,22]

Other important aspects of the medical history include chronic medical illnesses with nutritional impact such as diabetes mellitus, thyroid disease, inflammatory bowel disease, and liver and renal diseases. Attention should be paid to previous infections and operations, particularly GI surgery. Prolonged hospital stay is often associated with a higher risk of nutritional deficiencies when compared to acute trauma patients who are otherwise well. Good documentation of food intake is important to confirm compliance with nutritional needs. Dietitians play a special role in this matter.

Bedside Physical Examination of the Patient

Physical examination of the patient should focus on findings suggestive of poor nutrition: weight loss, muscle wasting (bitemporal, extremities), leg edema, xerosis, glossitis, and poor dentition. Ecchymoses, pressure ulcers, and surgical wound infections are important signs of nutritional deficiencies. Anthropometric measures—eg, arm muscle circumference, triceps skin-fold thickness, creatinine height index—are helpful to determine fat and body mass, but they have a limited value due to intraobserver variation and poor sensitivity to detect acute changes in nutritional status.[23] Muscle function testing (eg, hand-grip dynamometry) may detect skeletal muscle dysfunction and be a valid indicator of an increased risk for postoperative complications. This test is simple to perform and is inexpensive; however, it seems to be underutilized.[24] Tests evaluating body composition such as dual radiographic absorptiometry or bioelectrical impedance are used mainly in research settings. The evaluation of body composition is discussed in Chapter 2.

Laboratory Tests

Levels of visceral proteins including serum albumin, prealbumin, and transferrin are often used in clinical practice as markers of nutritional status and to monitor response to nutritional support. However, their value is limited after surgery because of their alteration in response to surgical stress such as fluid shifts, increased vascular permeability, and impaired hepatic synthesis. Serum protein status is affected by many factors such as muscle mass, underlying illness, blood loss, wound healing, infections, and GI absorption. Surgery alone decreases serum albumin levels. Low serum albumin levels are also found in patients with hepatic and renal disease. Therefore, low level of serum albumin should not be used solely as a marker of malnutrition.

The close relationship between low protein status and poor wound healing has been observed.[18,24] A serum albumin value of less than 2.5 g/dL generally reflects severity of illness and has been associated with poor outcome.[25] In patients who had undergone pancreas and esophageal surgery, albumin levels <3.25 g/dL were associated with higher rates of complications.[26] Serum transferrin level reflects protein status for 2 to 4 weeks prior to testing. Low transferrin should be considered a reliable indicator of malnutrition only if normal serum iron level is found. Serum prealbumin has shorter half-life of 2 to 3 days, and it reflects protein status for 1 to 2 weeks before the assessment. Its level is influenced by a renal and hepatic disease. In the appropriate setting, total peripheral lymphocyte count <1000/µL is not only an important indicator of malnutrition but is also a predictor of nosocomial infections.[27]

Serum levels of glucose, electrolytes, and BUN/creatinine ratio are helpful in assessment of the overall clinical and volume status. Serum calcium, magnesium, and phosphorous should be measured in the setting of poor oral intake, diarrhea, and malnutrition.[28] Iron level should be measured if microcytic anemia is discovered. Macrocytic anemia should raise suspicion for vitamin B12 or folate deficiency.

How to Determine Nutritional Support Requirements

The accuracy of nutritional support regimen is important. Both underfeeding and overfeeding may have a negative impact on surgical outcome. Negative nitrogen balance and increased mortality have been found in trauma patients who were underfed.[29,30] The Harris-Benedict equation is most often used to calculate caloric requirements. Caloric requirements are best estimated by indirect calorimetry.[31] IBW should be used to determine caloric needs for malnourished patients. Total energy requirement is determined by resting energy requirement adjusted to physical activity level and multiplied by a stress factor depending on type of the injury: postoperative 1 to 1.1; fracture 1.1 to 1.3, infection 1.3 to 1.5, and burn 1.5 to 2.0.[32] Well-nourished patients require, on average, 25 to 30 kcal/kg/day.[33,34] A higher amount of calories is needed by patients in hypermetabolic state (eg, intensive care unit, sepsis).[6,35] Total caloric needs should be calculated by 20% more of IBW for obese patients.

Glucose should constitute 60% to 70% of total energy requirement and should not exceed 6 g/kg/day. Fat should account for 20% to 30% of total calories and not exceed 2.5 g/kg/day. Amino acids should provide 15% to 20% of total calories with daily requirement of 1.2 to 1.5 g/kg/day and will be higher with increased metabolic demands. Protein delivery of more than 2.0 g/kg/day should be avoided except for severe catabolism. Protein intake in severely malnourished patients should be calculated according to the mean between IBW and measured weight and should be 20% higher for obese patients. Overfeeding should always be avoided.[36]

Postoperative Ileus and Enteral Feeding

Gastroparesis and paralytic ileus, commonly seen after surgery, limit the patient's ability to tolerate oral or gastric feedings. Appropriate pain control, avoidance of opioids, intensive mobilization, and limitation of sodium and fluids infusion are helpful to stimulate early return of bowel function. Excess of infused sodium and fluids during surgery has been associated with prolonged ileus.[37] The use of prolonged decompression with nasogastric tube can contribute to insufficient delivery of nutrients.[38] Nasogastric tubes should not be used routinely after abdominal surgery for decompression. Their routine use was associated with a higher rate of pulmonary complications in meta-analysis.[39]

Traditional postoperative care included a period of semi-starvation and nasogastric decompression before return of bowel function. Oral feeding was often delayed because of concern about the dehiscence of the anastomosis and side effects such as nausea, vomiting, and bloating. The peristalsis of small bowel recovers 6 to 8 hours after surgical trauma, and small bowel ability to absorb nutrients is preserved even in the absence of peristalsis and bowel sounds.[40,41] Awaiting the signs of bowel function to return so the patient can resume oral or enteral feeding does not appear to be the case anymore. The use of early feeding regardless of objective signs of bowel function return has been demonstrated to be safe after bowel resection in a few studies.[42-44]

Prolonged Ileus

For patients undergoing complex upper GI surgery with expected prolonged ileus or gastroparesis, elective jejunostomy tube placement intraoperatively should be strongly considered, especially in malnourished patients. Jejunal feeding has been proven to be beneficial in this setting.[45] For patients with inadequate oral intake, anorexia, and predominantly postoperative gastroparesis, the access to the small bowel can be achieved by placement of a nasoenteric tube. Nasoenteric tubes are ideal for short-term perioperative feeding, typically less than 1 month.[46] Percutaneous gastostomy or jejunostomy tube placement should be considered when long-term feeding (>1 month) is anticipated.

Elective Surgery

Most patients undergoing elective surgeries are well nourished. They can withstand a brief perioperative period of starvation without harmful sequelae. Preoperative carbohydrate load has been shown to be superior to fasting in surgical patients in regard to postoperative metabolism, nitrogen losses, and insulin resistance.[47] Well-nourished patients undergoing elective surgery are unlikely to benefit from pre- or postoperative nutritional support because of low likelihood of nutrition-related complications. Patients with adequate nutrition can receive postoperatively a solution of 5% to 10% dextrose for 5 to 7 days after surgery before initiation of oral feeding and without detrimental effects on the outcome.

Oral Supplements

Oral nutrition is always preferred because it is a physiologic way to provide nutrients. Patients with a normal GI tract function should be fed by mouth, and a regular hospital diet provides adequate nutrition. In a step-up approach, during an initial phase, liquids can by supplemented by oral dietary supplements. Among patients who have had general anesthesia, resumption of oral intake is typically possible within a few days. Anorexia is a common factor limiting spontaneous food intake. Therefore, early use of energy-dense foods can be beneficial in patients who have limited oral intake and any degree of malnutrition, allowing them to receive the same amount of calories in smaller, energy-dense meals to meet their caloric needs. Meal supplements with high protein drinks and oral supplements have been found to improve calorie intake after surgery.[43,48] Oral dietary supplements have been shown to be associated with significant benefits in respect to reduction of a patient's morbidity and mortality, less infection complications, and shorter hospital stay.[49,50] Contrary to findings in malnourished patients, the routine pre- and postoperative oral dietary supplements were of no benefit in well-nourished patients undergoing major bowel surgery in randomized controlled trial.[51] The use of high caloric supplements is often limited because of the patient's postoperative anorexia and altered taste sensation as well as poor tolerance for the supplements' taste.

High tolerability (>85%) of early postoperative feedings was demonstrated in a prospective trial of 200 patients after open colon resection.[52] In this trial, a higher intolerance of early oral feeding was found after total colectomy than after partial colon resection, which suggests a possible correlation with the type and extent of bowel resection. In another study of 87 patients, early feeding was tolerated in 90% of participants after open colon resection, which resulted in lower postoperative morbidity and shorter hospital stays.[53] The early oral feeding protocol included clear liquid diet on the evening of postoperative day (POD) 2, followed by a regular diet on POD 3 if clear liquids were tolerated. Early feeding appears to be feasible and safe in all surgical patients.[54,55]

Special Nutritional Considerations in Surgical Patients

Patients who have undergone bowel surgery constitute a unique group of surgical patients. Many of them may have nutritional compromise because of nonfunctional GI tracts prior to surgery. These patients often have a nutritional disadvantage in the early postoperative period because their intestines, the optimal route of nutrients delivery, cannot be used because of ileus and concerns about the anastomosis.[56] Therefore, implementation of oral nutrition is often delayed in the early postoperative period. Resumption of oral intake is dependent on local expertise and often follows standard postoperative care. The early oral feeding should be encouraged based on available data. In mildly malnourished patients, a 5- to 7-day bowel rest is allowed before initiation of PN.[57] Patients with complicated postoperative course such as leak, infection, or sepsis, or who are malnourished at baseline will need early nutritional therapy.

Patients with GI malignancy constitute another challenging group. Cachexia is common in these patients, but the degree of malnutrition varies considerably. Patients are often severely malnourished because of anorexia and bowel dysfunction (eg, nausea, vomiting, constipation, abdominal pain). Early nutritional therapy has been recommended in malnourished patients undergoing surgical intervention.[58] However, perioperative nutritional support has a very limited role in nonmalnourished patients with cancer.[28,59] (Nutrition for patients with GI cancer is discussed in Chapter 26.)

Malnutrition is very common in patients with inflammatory bowel disease (IBD).[60] Patients with Crohn's disease slowly develop progressive nutritional deficits, whereas patients with ulcerative colitis are typically well-nourished, but they develop acute nutritional deficiencies with flare-ups of the disease. These patients are at an increased risk of nutritional deterioration when undergoing surgical procedures. In case of severe malnutrition, surgical intervention should be postponed to correct nutritional deficiencies prior to surgery. Bowel rest and PN may be appropriate in patients with severe diarrhea, obstructive type symptoms, strictures, and enterocutaneous and enteroenteric fistulas. Nutritional support has been studied extensively in the surgical settings in patients with IBD.[61] (See Chapter 18.)

Patients with advanced liver disease deserve special consideration. These patients are often malnourished due to anorexia, inadequate intake, nausea, and ascites.[62] Therefore, perioperative nutritional support has to be considered in many patients, and it has a high priority in management of patients with liver disease. An improvement in survival was found in patients who had better nutrition at the time of liver transplantation.[63] (See Chapter 20.)

Trauma patients typically are well nourished immediately before injury and prior to emergent surgery; however, after surgery, they may be at a high risk for compromise of nutritional status and may require aggressive postoperative nutritional support, depending on complications.

Elderly patients need special attention. They are frequently undernourished, and obtaining good nutritional history is commonly difficult and challenging. Poor functional performance, altered taste, and sluggish bowel function can affect the nutrient delivery and overall recovery after surgery. Aggressive nutritional support may be required in patients at risk. (See Chapter 14.)

Nutritional Interventions

Numerous clinical trials have documented the benefits of nutritional support in selected surgical patients. The main indications for perioperative nutritional support include preexisting nutritional deprivation, anticipated or actual inadequate caloric oral intake, sepsis, and multi-organ system failure. Many trials had been published to evaluate the effects of nutritional interventions on surgical outcomes. It is recognized that the majority of the studies have limitations, such as lack of randomization, uncontrolled and small trials, and use of different noncomparable measures of malnutrition. Two options of nutritional support are available (EN and PN) when it becomes clear that the patient is unable to maintain an adequate oral intake and that undernutrition or malnutrition is found.

Each route of nutritional support has its own risks, and these specific risks must be balanced with the potential benefits. (Indications and contraindications of both EN and PN are discussed in Chapter 34.)

Parenteral Nutrition

The indications for PN in surgical patients became clearer in recent years because of meta-analysis. Many patients prefer intravenous nutrition rather than nasogastric or naso-enteric tube feedings when oral intake is reduced.[64] However, even short-term PN carries a risk of complications, including the most serious: infections. Other PN-related complications include technical (access related), metabolic (hyperglycemia, electrolyte abnormalities), and refeeding syndrome. Complications are discussed in Chapter 38.

PN requires close monitoring, preferably by a nutrition support team. PN is more expensive than EN. Therefore, PN should be considered only if the GI tract does not work.

Preoperative Parenteral Nutrition

The role of preoperative PN is controversial, and its routine use is not recommended. The majority of prospective trials have not shown a clear benefit of preoperative PN. Only two initial studies report benefits.

In the first prospective study, published in two parts, preoperative PN was compared to intravenous fluids and to a regular hospital diet in patients with GI cancer.[59] PN infusion led to two-fold decrease in postoperative complications and four-fold decrease in mortality compared to the control group. The third group of patients who was given higher lipid content in PN (but equal amount of total calories) had infections and mortality rates similar to controls. The results were suggestive of loss of PN benefit, possibly because of the immunosuppressive effect of lipid emulsion.[65] In the second study, 124 patients undergoing resection of hepatocellular carcinoma received PN for 7 days preoperatively, compared to a group who received no nutritional therapy.[58] Patients who received PN had decreased postoperative morbidity from 54% to 34% (controls versus PN group). Improved liver-function tests, less ascites, and weight loss were observed in PN group.

In the largest study, the VA Cooperative study, 395 malnourished patients (99% of them males) undergoing laparotomy or noncardiac thoracotomy were randomly assigned to PN (7 to 15 days preoperatively and 3 days postoperatively) versus either receiving no nutritional support or oral feedings.[66] Patients who received PN had a statistically higher rate of infectious complications (14.1% versus 6.4%) and a nonsignificant reduction in mortality at 30 days (7.3% versus 4.9%). The rates of major complications during the first 30 days after surgery were similar in the two groups, as was the overall 90-day mortality rate. In contrast, severely malnourished patients treated with PN had fewer noninfectious complications than controls (5% versus 42.9%). This study showed favorable effect of PN only in severely malnourished patients and a lack of benefit of PN in borderline malnourished patients.

In a randomized controlled trial of 90 malnourished patients with GI malignancies who received PN (preoperatively for 10 days and postoperatively for 9 days) versus glucose infusion, reductions in complications (mainly noninfectious) and mortality were seen.[67] In a published meta-analysis of 27 randomized trials, including 11 trials of preoperative PN versus oral diet and intravenous dextrose, no difference in mortality was found between patients in both groups.[68] In the majority of studies, PN was provided preoperatively for 5 to 10 days. In another critical review of the literature including 33 trials of perioperative PN, preoperative use of PN was associated with a 10% reduction in complication rates only noted among malnourished patients.[69]

Therefore, PN should not be used indiscriminately, and its use should be limited to those patients in whom enteral administration cannot meet caloric requirements. In general, preoperative PN use should be limited to those patients with severe malnutrition (10% weight loss and serum albumin level <2.5 g/dL) and nonfunctional GI tracts. In that setting, elective surgery should be postponed to correct malnutrition. Preoperative PN for 7 to 10 days in those patients may reduce postoperative morbidity.

Postoperative Parenteral Nutrition

Data on postoperative use of PN has not been favorable. A few studies demonstrated more septic and nonseptic complications in PN group when compared to controls. A statistically higher rate of major complications (45% versus 23%), such as fistulae, abscesses, peritonitis, and anastamotic breakdown, and 3.5-fold increase in mortality have been found in patients undergoing pancreatic resection for malignancy who received PN postoperatively.[70] Infectious complications in PN group were due predominantly to intra-abdominal abscesses, thought to be secondary to bacterial translocation. In the larger study by Sandstrom et al, patients who received PN after emergent or elective major surgery were found to have higher mortality and a higher rate of cardiovascular and central nervous system complications than were control patients receiving glucose solution only.[71]

In a meta-analysis of 9 randomized trials, postoperative PN was associated with a 10% increased risk of complications.[28] In another meta-analysis of 27 randomized controlled trials, including 17 trials of postoperative PN, no difference in complication rates was observed between PN group and controls.[68] Most trials with postoperative PN showed no reduction in complications with even worse outcome in patients receiving postoperative PN alone. Meta-analysis clearly showed a lack of overall effect of PN on mortality. Certain limitations of the trials are recognized, including the amount of calories provided, duration of PN, and lack of adequate glucose control.

A glutamine-supplemented postoperative PN was shown to have positive effect on surgical outcome in GI cancer patients when compared to effects of a standard PN.[72] Synthetic soluble glutamine dipeptide ananyl-GLn, at dose of 0.3 g/kg/day, was added to PN for at least 7 days. Decreased rate of infections, improved nitrogen balance, and shorter hospital stay were observed in the glutamine group. Positive outcome was thought to result from attenuated depletion of muscle protein and nitrogen loss combined with improved immune-cell activation and intestinal permeability.

Overall routine use of PN in postoperative patients should not be recommended. Guidelines suggest that elective surgical patients with preoperative malnutrition or expected inadequate recovery of oral intake within 7 to 10 days should receive PN.[33] If PN is planned to be infused for 5 to 7 days only, perhaps peripheral access can be used for its administration, as long as caloric needs are met. PN use cannot be justified if bowel function is expected to return within 7 days after surgery in nonmalnourished patients because of potential infectious complications. (Complications of PN are discussed in Chapter 38.)

Enteral Nutrition

EN is considered superior to PN in surgical patients. Enteral feeding is more physiologic, stimulating biliary and gastric secretions, and it reduces the risk of metabolic complications. The use of enteral feeding helps maintain the gut integrity and it increases splanchnic blood flow, stimulates the gut immune system, and prevents bacterial translocation. EN has been associated with reduction of septic and nonseptic complications and a lower cost when compared to PN. (Complications of EN are discussed in Chapter 39.) The experience with perioperative EN has been favorable. However, postoperative ileus is often a limiting factor to initiate enteral feeding and to provide adequate nutrition (reach target of >80% daily caloric requirements). This may have a negative effect on the overall surgical outcome.[23,73] Early feeding appears to be critical before the patient develops a hypermetabolic status; otherwise, the beneficial effect of EN can be lost.[74]

Preoperative Enteral Nutrition

The data supporting preoperative enteral feeding appear to be clearer than that supporting PN. However, only a few randomized studies evaluated the preoperative EN. Patients with obstructive jaundice treated with percutaneous transhepatic placement of a biliary drains who received preoperative EN for an average 20 days versus no nutritional support had a significant reduction in perioperative morbidity (17.8% versus 46.8%) and mortality (3.5% versus 12.5%).[75] Decreased rate of infectious complications (10.4% versus 37.2%) and the mortality rate (6% versus 11.7%) were found in another randomized trial of patients given elemental formula through a nasogastric tube for 7 to 10 days before surgery when compared to controls.[76] The EN group had a significant improvement in levels of visceral protein, body weight, and anthropometric measures. A 50% reduction in postoperative complications was observed in patients with head and neck cancer, randomized to nocturnal supplements for 10 to 21 days prior to surgery versus controls receiving regular diet alone.[77] Beneficial effect of preoperative EN, including immune-enhanced formula (IEF), was found in malnourished patients with GI cancer comparing both pre- and postoperative EN with postoperative EN alone.[78] Patients who received both pre- and post EN had a lower rate of infections (18% versus 42%) and a reduction in length of hospital stay. Improvements in quality of life, physical and emotional functioning, and dyspnea were found in 49 severely malnourished patients with neck and head cancer who received IEF in prospective RCT.[79]

In general, postoperative complication rates appear to be substantially lower in the recipients of preoperative EN when compared to controls who received no EN. Seven to 10 days of preoperative EN has become standard care for patients with weight loss of more than 10% of body weight. A longer period of EN may be necessary for patients with a more extreme weight loss.

Postoperative Enteral Nutrition

The beneficial effects of postoperative enteral feeding have been well established. A substantial reduction in sepsis rate (4% versus 26%) was reported in surgical patients with abdominal trauma who received early jejunostomy feeds versus gradual oral intake and intravenous fluids.[80] Reduced requirements for antibiotic coverage and less weight loss were reported in malnourished patients who underwent GI and vascular surgery and then received enteral supplements postoperatively.[81] Other clinical trials have also confirmed a lower rate of infections in patients who were fed enterally.[82,83]

The benefits of postoperative EN were clearly demonstrated in two trials involving orthopedic surgery patients.[84,85] In a large trial, malnourished women with femoral neck fractures who received enteral supplementation via nasogastric tube had shorter rehabilitation stays and an overall decrease in mortality (8% versus 21.7%).[84] Similar results were reported in a smaller randomized trial of elderly women after hip surgery who were given oral supplements and a regular diet versus a regular diet alone.[85] A reduction in complication rate was found from 56% to 13% (controls versus supplement group). In a randomized study of malnourished patients with GI cancer, early postoperative EN significantly reduced the complication rate and hospital stay when compared with PN.[86] In two prospective studies evaluating postoperative nutrition after gastric and esophagus surgery, EN, provided by nasojejunal tube, was compared to PN.[87,88] Fewer infectious complications and lower morbidity were seen in the EN group. Jejunostomy tube placement for EN delivery is important in patients after pancreatic surgery because delayed gastric emptying has been found. In patients undergoing pylorus-preserving Whipple procedure, cyclic EN was found to be more beneficial over continuous EN.[89]

Early EN was shown to be superior to intravenous fluid infusion after liver transplantation in randomized controlled trials by reduction in viral infections (17% to 0%), a 50% reduction of bacterial infections, and an improved nitrogen balance.[90] See Table 29-3 for postoperative enteral-feeding trials.

In hemodynamically unstable patients, jejunal feedings have been associated with the induction or worsening of bowel ischemia. Therefore, enteral feeding should be avoided in septic, hypotensive, and unstable patients.[91] EN is clearly superior to PN in a reduction of morbidity and in cost savings. Because EN is more physiologic, it should be considered as "primary therapy" if the patient's GI tract works. Approach to nutritional support in surgical patients is summarized in Tables 29-2 and 29-3.

TABLE 29-2.

Nutritional Interventions in the Preoperative Period

Nutritional Status (Degree of Malnutrition)	Functional GI Tract	Nutritional Support	Surgery
None or mild		None	Proceed
Moderate	Yes	EN	Proceed
Moderate	No	EN	Proceed
Severe*	Yes	EN (7 to 14 days)	Postpone surgery
Severe	Yes	PN (7 to 14 days)	Postpone surgery

*Severe malnutrition: weight loss >10%, albumin <2.5 g/dl, SGA "C"

TABLE 29-3.

Nutritional Therapy in the Postoperative Period

Nutritional Status (Degree of Malnutrition)	Bowel Function Return (days)	Nutritional Support	Onset of Support (days)
None/mild	Yes	None (gradual oral intake)	
None/mild	No (5 to 7)	PN	5 to 7
None/mild*	No (5 to 7)	PN or EN†	1 to 2
Moderate	Yes	EN	1 to 2
Moderate	No	PN	1 to 2
Severe	Yes	EN	1 to 2
Severe	No	PN	1
Intensive care unit	Yes	IEF	1 to 2

*complicated course: sepsis, leak, infections
†if gut works

Immunonutrition: A New Direction

In addition to the route of nutrient delivery, current focus in surgical nutrition is on formulas with additional benefits: the immunonutrition. IEFs are designed to use specific nutrients to modify the metabolic and immune response to surgery. These diets are aimed to augment the patient's immune system by inhibiting release of interleukin-6 and tumor necrosis factor as well as to improve gut oxygen metabolism and gut barrier function by preventing bacterial translocation.[92] Nutrients being evaluated include arginine, glutamine, nucleotides, and omega-3 fatty acids. Chapter 42 also addresses immunonutrition in its discussion of EN.

Meta-analysis has shown that postoperative immunonutrition may improve the patient's outcome when compared with outcome of those receiving standard feedings.[93] IEFs have been shown to be beneficial in intensive-care–unit trauma patients by decreasing the rate of infectious complication, with no influence on postoperative mortality.[94,95] Interestingly, a subgroup of critically ill patients with ongoing sepsis and infection had a higher mortality rate with a diet rich in arginine.[96] The application of IEFs can help to ameliorate (but not reverse) the catabolic and immunological response to surgical trauma.[97]

In the first study with IEF, malnourished patients undergoing upper GI surgery were randomized to receive standard or IEF diet postoperatively. The group supplemented with IEF had fewer infectious complications and shorter hospital stays but no difference in mortality.[92] In a large randomized study by Senkal et al, 154 patients with upper GI surgery were given IEF or isocaloric formula, starting within 24 hours after surgery with an attempt to reach the target within 5 days.[98] A reduction in infectious complications and in the patients' lengths of hospital stay were found. No difference in complication rate was found in another study of the well-nourished patients undergoing major upper GI surgery that compared IEF given for 5 days to intravenous fluids administered alone.[99] It was thought that no benefit of IEF was demonstrated because well-nourished patients were at low risk for complications. Perioperative supplementation with IEF versus standard formula was evaluated in a randomized controlled trial including 154 patients with upper GI surgery for malignancy.[100] Oral immune-enhanced diet was provided before surgery followed by enteral feedings continued through the postoperative period for at least 6 days. Total complications rate—including rates of pneumonias and wound infections—was significantly reduced in IEF group, especially in the late period (>3 days). IEFs were associated with an overall reduction of postoperative infectious complications and a shorter hospital stay in both well-nourished and malnourished patients. It has been shown that while immunonutrition increases the costs of nutrition in surgical patients, the cost was overcompensated by savings in subsequent postoperative treatment costs in those patients who experienced complications. Similar results with perioperative IEF, given for 7 days prior to surgery, were reported by Braga et al in 206 patients undergoing surgery for stomach, pancreas, and colon cancer.[101] Reduction in infectious complications was found in both the malnourished (14% IEF versus 40% standard diet) and well-nourished (9% versus 20%) group. The beneficial effects of preoperative and early postoperative immunonutrition on immune system (improved phagocytosis, lower C-reactive protein) have been demonstrated in the above studies.

At present, the use of IEF is limited to selected surgical patients because of the higher cost of the formula and limited studies, which involved mostly cancer patients. A key point for success is to start the patient on immunonutrition before surgery (preoperative loading) and continue in the early postoperative period. This can result in improved outcome and reduction of the late postoperative infectious complications.

In conclusion, IEF should be used in high-risk patients prior to surgery for 5 to 7 days and continued for at least 5 days postoperatively to achieve maximum beneficial effect.[102] The cost of the formula may be balanced by potential savings in length of hospital stay and limited antibiotic usage. Further studies are needed to determine which patients benefit from immunonutrition and the optimal duration of its supplementation.

Conclusions

Malnutrition is commonly seen in surgical patients, and it has a negative effect on the surgical outcome. Assessment of the patient's nutritional status should be a standard of preoperative evaluation (Chapter 1). Despite many available studies, the outcome of nutritional therapy in the perioperative period is not consistent and difficult to compare given the broad range of surgical settings and interventions. Early use of the gut after surgery is most beneficial. Among well-nourished patients, resumption of oral intake is usually possible within a few days after surgery, and no supplemental nutrition is required.

Given the lack of clear benefit and documented risks, patients who are not malnourished, or only with mild degree of malnutrition, should not have surgery deferred for provision of nutritional support. On the contrary, severely malnourished patients benefit from delaying elective surgery to provide nutritional support, but they are at a higher risk for infectious complications if PN is given perioperatively. Routine postoperative PN should not be attempted unless bowel rest is anticipated for greater than 7 to 10 days. Careful monitoring of nutritional support is important to optimize its benefits. Patients with severe malnutrition require aggressive nutritional support. Therefore, earlier nutritional intervention is appropriate in malnourished patients at baseline and in those with perioperative complications. Enteral feedings should be considered first if the gut works. EN has proven beneficial in malnourished patients during the pre- and especially postoperative period when considering the patient's gradual resumption of oral diet. Immune-enhancing formulas are desirable and beneficial in selected surgical patients; however, their role in the surgical setting must be clarified. Overall, it is a challenge to distinguish patients who will benefit from nutritional support from those who will not. Additional work is needed to determine whether a more aggressive early nutritional therapy or differently composed formulas may be more effective during the perioperative period.

References

1. Weinsier RL, Hunker EM, Krumdieck CL, Butterworth CE Jr. Hospital malnutrition. A prospective evaluation of general medical patients during the course of hospitalization. *Am J Clin Nutr.* 1979;32:418-426.
2. Studley HO. Percentage of weight loss: a basic indicator of surgical risk in patients with chronic peptic ulcer. *JAMA.* 1936;106:458-460.
3. Gibbs J, Cull W, Henderson W, et al. Preoperative serum albumin level as a predictor of operative mortality and morbidity: results from the National VA Surgical Risk Study. *Arch Surg.* 1999;134:36-42.
4. Souba WW. Homeostasis: bodily changes in trauma and surgery. In: Sabiston D, ed. *Essentials of Surgery.* 2nd ed. Philadelphia, Pa: WB Saunders; 1987:10-23.
5. Hasselgren PO. Catabolic response to stress and injury: implications to regulation. *World J Surg.* 2000;24:1452-1459.
6. Frankenfield DC, Wiles CE, Bagley S, Siegel JH. Relationships between resting and total energy expenditure in injured and septic patients. *Crit Care Med.* 1994;22:1796-1804.
7. Cuthbertson DP. Alterations in metabolism following injury: part I. *Injury.* 1980;11:175-189.
8. Souba WW, Wilmore DW. Diet and nutrition in the care of the patient with surgery, trauma, and sepsis. In: Shils M, Young V, eds. *Modern Nutrition in Health and Disease.* 8th ed. Philadelphia, Pa: Lea & Febiger; 1994: 1202-1240.
9. Cuthbertson DP. The metablolic response to injury and its nutritional implications: retrospect and prospect. *JPEN J Parenter Enteral Nutr.* 1979;3:108-129.
10. Souba WW. Cytokines: key regulators of the nutritional/metabolic response to critical illness. *Curr Prob Surg.* 1994;31:577-652.
11. Fong Y, Lowry SF. Cytokines and the cellular response to injury and infection. In: Wilmore DW, Brennam MF, Harker AH, et al, eds. *Care of the Surgical Patient (Critical Care)*: IV. Trauma. New York, NY: Scientific American Medicine; 1992:1.
12. Braga M, Gianotti L, Constantini E, et al. Impact of enteral nutrition on intestinal bacterial translocation and mortality in burned mice. *Clin Nutr.* 1994;13:256-261.
13. McWhirter JP, Pennington CR. Incidence and recognition of malnutrition in hospital. *Br Med J.* 1994;308:945-948.
14. Elwyn DH, Bryan-Brown CW, Shoemaker WC. Nutritional aspects of body water dislocation in postoperative and depleted patients. *Ann Surg.* 1975;182:76-85.
15. Haydock DA, Hill GL. Impaired wound healing in surgical patients with varying degrees of malnutrition. *JPEN J Parenter Enteral Nutr.* 1986;10:550-554.
16. Mainous MR, Deitch EA. Nutrition and infection. *Surg Clin North Am.* 1994;74:659-676.
17. Rady MY, Ryan T, Starr NJ. Clinical characteristics of preoperative hypoalbuminemia predict outcome of cardiovascular surgery. *JPEN J Parenter Enteral Nutr.* 1997;21:81-90.
18. Reinhardt GF, Myscofski JW, Wilkens DB, et al. Incidence and mortality of hypoalbuminemic patients in hospitalized veterans. *JPEN J Parenter Enteral Nutr.* 1980;4:357-359.
19. Malone DL, Genuit T, Tracy JK, et al. Surgical site infections: reanalysis of risk factors. *J Surg Res.* 2002;103:89-95.
20. Goldhill DR, Sumner A. APACHE II, data accuracy and outcome prediction. *Anaesthesia.* 1998;10:937-943.

21. Warnold I, Lundholm K. Clinical significance of preoperative nutritional status in 215 noncancer patients. *Ann Surg.* 1984;199:299-305.
22. Windsor JA, Hill GL. Weight loss with physiologic impairment—a basic indicator of surgical risk. *Ann Surg.* 1988;207:290-296.
23. Moore FA, Feliciano DV, Andrassy RJ, et al. Early enteral feeding compared with parenteral, reduces postoperative septic complications. *Ann Surg.* 1992;216:172-183.
24. Stack JA, Babineau TJ, Bistran BR. Assessment of nutritional status in clinical practice. *Gastroenterologist.* 1996;4:S8-S15.
25. McClave SA, Snider HL, Spain DA. Preoperative issues in clinical nutrition. *Chest.* 1999;115:64S-70S.
26. Kudsk KA, Tolley EA, DeWitt RC, et al. Preoperative albumin and surgical site identify surgical risk for major postoperative complications. *JPEN J Parenter Enteral Nutr.* 2003;1:1-9.
27. Gorse GJ, Messner RL, Stephens ND. Association of malnutrition with nosocomial infection. *Infect Control Hosp Epidemiol.* 1989;5:194-203.
28. Klein S, Kinney J, Jeejeebhoy K, et al. Nutrition support in clinical practice: review of published data and recommendations for future research directions. Summary of a conference sponsored by the National Institutes of Health, American Society for Parenteral and Enteral Nutrition, and American Society for Clinical Nutrition. *Am J Clin Nutr.* 1997;66:683-706.
29. Ranson JHC, Spencer FC. Prevention, diagnosis, and treatment of pancreatic abscess. *Surgery.* 1977;82:99-106.
30. Bartlett RH, Dechert RE, Mault JR, et al. Measurement of metabolism in multiple organ failure. *Surgery.* 1982;92:771-779.
31. McClave SA, Snider HL. Use of indirect calorimetry in clinical nutrition. *Nutr Clin Pract.* 1992;7:207-221
32. Bozzetti F, Allaria B. Nutritional support in ICU patients: position of scientific societies. *Nestle Nutr Workshop Ser Clin Perform Programme.* 2003;8:279-298.
33. Guidelines for the use of parenteral and enteral nutrition in adult and pediatric patients. *JPEN J Parenter Enteral Nutr.* 2002;26(1):1SA-138SA.
34. Hunter DC, Jaksic T, Lewis D, et al. Resting energy expenditure in the critically ill: estimations versus measurement. *Br J Surg.* 1988;75:875-878.
35. Frankenfield DC, Smith JS, Cooney RN. Accelerated nitrogen loss after traumatic injury is not attenuated by achievement of energy balance. *JPEN J Parenter Enteral Nutr.* 1997;21:324-329.
36. Heyland DK, Novak F, Drover JW, et al. Should immunonutriton become routine in critically ill patients? A systematic review of the evidence. *JAMA.* 2001;286:944-953.
37. Holte K, Sharrock NE, Kehlet H. Pathophysiology and clinical implications of perioperative fluid excess. *Br J Anaesth.* 2002;89:622-632.
38. Donat SM, Slaton JW, Pisters LL, et al. Early nasogastric tube removal combined with metoclopramide after radical cystectomy and urinary diversion. *J Urol.* 1999;162:1599-1602.
39. Cheatham ML, Chapman WC, Hey SP, Sawyers JL. A meta-analysis of selective versus routine nasogastric decompression after elective laparotomy. *Ann Surg.* 1995;221:469-476.
40. Rothnie NG, Kemp Harper RA, Catchpole BN. Early postoperative gastrointestinal motility. *Lancet.* 1963;2:64-67.
41. Woods JH, Erickson LW, Condon RE. Post-operative ileus: a colonic problem. *Surgery.* 1978;84:527-533.
42. Lewis SJ, Egger M, Sylvester PA, Thomas S. Early enteral feeding versus 'nil by mouth' after gastrointestinal surgery: systematic review and meta-analysis of controlled trials. *BMJ.* 2001;323:773-776.
43. Saluja SS, Kaur N, Shrivastava UK. Enteral nutrition in surgical patients. *Surg Today.* 2002;32:672-678.
44. Nygren J, Thorell A, Ljungqvist O. New developments facilitating nutritional intake after gastrointestinal surgery. *Curr Opin Clin Nutr Metab Care.* 2003;6:593-597.
45. Ryan JA, Page CP. Intrajejunal feeding: development and current status. *JPEN J Parenter Enteral Nutr.* 1984;8:187-198.
46. Kirby DF, Delegge MH, Flaming CR. American Gastroenterological Association technical review on tube feeding for enteral nutrition. *Gastroenterology.* 1995;108:1282-1301.
47. Nygren J, Thorell A, Ljungqvist O. Preoperative oral carbohydrate nutrition: an update. *Curr Opin Clin Nutr Metab Care.* 2001;4:255-259.
48. Odlund Olin A, Armyr I, Soop M, et al. Energy-dense meals improve energy intake in elderly residents in a nursing home. *Clin Nutr.* 2003;22:125-131.
49. Rana S, Bray J, Menzies-Gow N. Short term benefits of postoperative oral dietary supplements in surgical patients. *Clin Nutr.* 1992;11:337-344.
50. Keele AM, Bray MJ, Emery PW, et al. Two-phase randomized controlled clinical trial of postoperative oral dietary supplements in surgical patients. *Gut.* 1997;40:393-399.
51. MacFie J, Woodcock NP, Palmer MD, et al. Oral dietary supplements in pre- and postoperative surgical patients: a prospective and randomized clinical trial. *Nutrition.* 2000;16:723-728.
52. DiFronzo LA, Cymerman J, O'Connell TX. Factors affecting early postoperative feeding following elective open colon resection. *Arch Surg.* 1999;134:941-946.
53. DiFronzo LA, Yamin N, Patel K, O'Connell TX. Benefits of early feeding and early hospital discharge in elderly patients undergoing open colon resection. *J Am Coll Surg.* 2003;197:747-752.
54. Petrelli NJ, Cheng C, Driscoll D, et al. Early postoperative oral feeding after colectomy: an analysis of factors that may predict failure. *Ann Surg Oncol.* 2001;8:796-800.
55. Henriksen MG, Hansen HV, Hessov I. Early oral nutrition after elective colorectal surgery: influence of balanced analgesia and enforced mobilization. *Nutrition.* 2002;18:263-267.
56. Souba WW. Nutritional support. *N Engl J Med.* 1997;336:41-48.
57. Bower RH, Talamini MA, Sax HC, et al. Postoperative enteral vs parenteral nutrition. A randomized controlled trial. *Arch Surg.* 1986;121:1040-1045.
58. Fan ST, Lo CM, Lai EC, et al. Perioperative nutritional support in patients undergoing hepatectomy for hepatocellular carcinoma. *N Engl J Med.* 1994;331:1547-1552.
59. Muller JM, Brenner U, Dienst C, Pichlmaier H. Preoperative parenteral feeding in patients with gastrointestinal carcinoma. *Lancet.* 1982;1:68-71.
60. Stokes MA, Hill GL. Total energy expenditure in patients with Crohn's disease: measurement by the combined body scan technique. *JPEN J Parenter Enteral Nutr.* 1993;17:3-7.
61. Rombeau JL, Barot LR, Williamson CE, et al. Preoperative total parenteral nutrition and surgical outcome in patients with inflammatory bowel disease. *Am J Surg.* 1982;143:139-143.
62. Merli M, Nicolini G, Angeloni S, et al. Malnutrition is a risk in cirrhotic patients undergoing surgery. *Nutrition.* 2002;18:978-986.
63. Pikul J, Sharpe MD, Lowndes R, Ghent CN. Degree of preoperative malnutrition is predictive of postoperative morbidity and mortality in liver transplant recipients. *Transplantation.* 1994;57:469-472.
64. Scolapio JS, Picco MF, Tarrosa VB. Enteral versus parenteral nutrition: the patient's preference. *JPEN J Parenter Enteral Nutr.* 2002;26:248-250.
65. Muller JM, Keller HW, Brenner U, et al. Indications and effects of preoperative parenteral nutrition. *World J Surg.* 1986;10:53-63.
66. Perioperative total parenteral nutrition in surgical patients. The Veterans Affairs Total Parenteral Nutrition Cooperative Study Group. *N Engl J Med.* 1991;325:525-530.
67. Bozzetti F, Gavazzi C, Miceli R, et al. Perioperative total parenteral nutrition in malnourished, gastrointestinal cancer patients: a randomized, clinical trial. *JPEN J Parenter Enteral Nutr.* 2000;24:7-14.
68. Heyland DK, Montalvo M, MacDonald S, et al. Total parenteral nutrition in the surgical patient: a meta-analysis. *Can J Surg.* 2001;44:102-111.
69. Torosian MH. Perioperative nutrition support for patients undergoing gastrointestinal surgery: critical analysis and recommendations. *World J Surg.* 1999;23:565-569.

70. Brennan MF, Pisters PW, Posner M, et al. A prospective randomized trial of total parenteral nutrition after major pancreatic resection for malignancy. *Ann Surg.* 1994;220:436-441.
71. Sandstrom R, Drott C, Hyltander A, et al. The effect of postoperative intravenous feeding (TPN) on outcome following major surgery evaluated in a randomized study. *Ann Surg.* 1993; 217:185-195.
72. Di Cosmo L. Glutamine supplemented total parenteral nutrition in major abdominal surgery. *Nutrition.* 2001;17:968-969.
73. Braga M, Gianotti L, Gentilini O, et al. Early postoperative enteral nutrition improves gut oxygenation and reduces cost compared with total parenteral nutrition. *Crit Care Med.* 2001;29:242-248.
74. Cerra FB. How nutrition intervention changes what getting sick means. *JPEN J Parenter Enteral Nutr.* 1990;14:164S-169S.
75. Foschi D, Cavagna G, Callioni F, et al. Hyperalimentation of jaundiced patients on percutaneous transhepatic biliary drainage. *Br J Surg.* 1986;73:716-719.
76. Shukla HS, Rao RR, Banu N, et al. Enteral hyperalimentation in malnourished surgical patients. *Indian J Med Res.* 1984;80:339.
77. Flynn MB, Leightty FF. Preoperative outpatient nutritional support of patients with squamous cancer of the upper aerodigestive tract. *Am J Surg.* 1987;154:359-362.
78. Braga, M, Gianotti, L, Nespoli L, et al. Nutritional approach in malnourished surgical patients: a prospective randomized study. *Arch Surg.* 2002;137:174-180.
79. Van Bokhorst-De Van Der Schueren MA, Langendoen SI, Vondeling H, et al. Perioperative enteral nutrition and quality of life of severly malnourished head and neck cancer patients:a randomized clinical trial. *Clin Nutr.* 2000;19:437-444.
80. Moore FA, Moore EE, Jones TN, et al. TEN versus TPN following major abdominal trauma: reduced septic morbidity. *J Trauma.* 1989;29:916-922.
81. Beattie AH, Prach AT, Baxter JP, Pennington CR. A randomised controlled trial evaluating the use of enteral nutritional supplements postoperatively in malnourished surgical patients. *Gut.* 2000;46:813-818.
82. Beier-Holgersen R, Boesby S. Influence of postoperative enteral nutrition on postsurgical infections. *Gut.* 1996;39:833-835.
83. Braga M, Gianotti L, Vignali A, et al. Artificial nutrition after major abdominal surgery: impact of route of administration and composition of the diet. *Crit Care Med.* 1998;26:24-30.
84. Bastow MD, Rawlings J, Allison SP. Benefits of supplementary tube feeding after fractured neck of femur: a randomised controlled trial. *Br Med J.* 1983;287:1589-1592.
85. Delmi M, Rapin CH, Bengoa JM, et al. Dietary supplementation in elderly patients with fractured neck of the femur. *Lancet.* 1990;335:1013-1016.
86. Bozzetti F, Braga M, Gianotti L. Postoperative enteral versus parenteral nutrition in malnourished patients with gastrointestinal cancer: a randomised multicentre trial. *Lancet.* 2001;358:1487-1492.
87. Baigrie RJ, Devitt PG, Watkins DS. Enteral versus parenteral nutrition after oesophagastric surgery: a prospective randomized comparison. *Aust NZ J Surg.* 1996;66:668-670.
88. Sand J, Luostarinen M, Maitikainen M. Enteral or parenteral feeding after total gastrectomy: a prospective randomized pilot study. *Eur J Surg.* 1997;163:761-766.
89. Van Berge H, Akkermans LM, Van Gulik TM, et al. Prospective, randomized trial on the effect of cyclic versus continuous enteral nutrition on postoperative gastric function after pylorus-preserving pancreatoduodenectomy. *Ann Surg.* 1997;226:677-685.
90. Hasse JM, Blue LS, Leipa GU, et al. Early enteral nutrition support in patients undergoing liver transplantation. *JPEN J Parenter Enteral Nutr.* 1995;19:437-443.
91. Munshi IA, Steingrub JS, Wolpert L. Small bowel necrosis associated with early postoperative jejunal tube feeding in a trauma patient. *J Trauma.* 2000;49:163-165.
92. Daly JM, Lieberman MD, Goldfine L, et al. Enteral nutrition with supplemented arginine, RNA, and omega-3 fatty acids in patients after operation: immunologic, metabolic and clinical outcome. *Surgery.* 1992;112:56-72.
93. Heys SD, Walker LG, Smith I, et al. Enteral nutrition supplementation with key nutrients in patient critically ill and cancer. *Ann Surg.* 1999;229:467-477.
94. Bower RH, Cerra FB, Bershadsky B, et al. Early enteral administration of a formula (Impact) supplemented with arginine, nucleotides, and fish oil in intensive care unit patients: results of a multicenter, prospective, randomized clinical trial. *Crit Care Med.* 1995;23:436-449.
95. Beale RJ, Bryg DJ, Bihari DJ. Immunonutrition in critically ill; a systemic review of clinical outcome. *Crit Care Med.* 1999;27:2799-2805.
96. Bone RC. Sir Issac Newton, sepsis, SIRS and CARS. *Crit Care Med.* 1996;24:1125-1128.
97. Senkal M, Kamen M, Eickhoff U, et al. Preoperative immunonutrition improves the postoperative immune response. *Intensive Care Med.* 1996;22:(S3)353.
98. Senkal M, Mummet A, Eickhoff U, et al. Early postoperative immunonutrition: clinical outcome and cost-comparison analysis in surgical patients. *Crit Care Med.* 1997;25:1489-1496.
99. Heslin MJ, Latkany L, Leung D, et al. A prospective, randomized trial of early enteral feeding after resection of upper gastrointestinal malignancy. *Ann Surg.* 1997;226:567-77.
100. Senkal M, Zumtobel V, Bauer KH, et al. Outcome and cost-effectiveness of perioperative enteral immunonutrition in patients undergoing elective upper gastrointestinal tract surgery. *Arch Surg.* 1999;134:1309-1316.
101. Braga M, Gianotti L, Radaelli G, et al. Perioperative immunonutrition in patients undergoing cancer surgery: results of a randomized double-blind phase 3 trial. *Arch Surg.* 1999;134:428-433.
102. Proceedings from Summit on immune-enhancing enteral therapy. May 25-26, 2000, San Diego, California, USA. *JPEN J Parenter Enteral Nutr.* 2001;25(2):S1-S63.

Section V

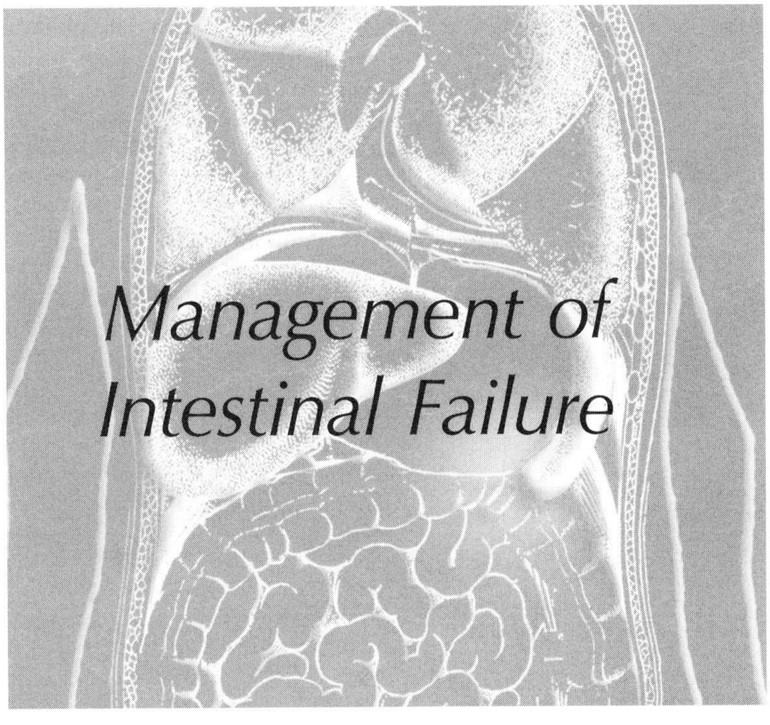

Management of Intestinal Failure

Chapter 30

Dietary Management in Short Bowel Syndrome

Alan L. Buchman, MD, MSPH, and
James S. Scolapio, MD

Definition of Short Bowel Syndrome

Short bowel syndrome is a collection of signs and symptoms occurring after massive surgical intestinal resection and characterized by weight loss and malabsorption of fluids and macro and micronutrients. The normal small intestine is approximately 600 cm in length and the colon is approximately 150 cm. Short bowel syndrome may be a congenital or acquired condition. Infants born with jejunal or ileal atresia constitute the congenital forms. Otherwise, short bowel syndrome results from surgical bowel resection because of multiple resections for recurrent Crohn's disease; massive enterectomy undertaken because of a catastrophic vascular event such as a mesenteric arterial embolism or venous thrombosis; volvulus; trauma; or tumor resection in adults and, in children, gastroschisis, necrotizing enterocolitis (NEC), volvulus, and extensive aganglionosis. Functional short bowel syndrome may also occur in cases of severe malabsorption where the bowel length is often intact. Such conditions may include chronic intestinal pseudo obstruction syndrome, refractory sprue, radiation enteritis, and congenital villous atrophy.

Severe nutrient and fluid malabsorption occurs following extensive small intestinal resection. It should be noted that individuals with less than 100 cm of jejunum remaining generally have a net secretory response to food and, as such, may lose more fluid than they ingest.[1]

Individuals with short bowel syndrome can be grouped into two distinct subgroups: those with intact colon in continuity with their residual small intestine and those without colon in continuity. In those patients whose colon is in continuity, the colon becomes an important digestive organ. Sodium and water are absorbed in the colon[2-4] as is energy from absorbed short chain fatty acids (SCFA) (see discussion under complex carbohydrates and soluble dietary fiber). Energy absorption was assessed in a study of 148 patients with various lengths of residual small and large bowel.[1] Patients with a preserved colon had lower fecal volume and less fecal energy loss than did patients without a colon. Fecal energy excretion values in patients with partial colonic function were not significantly different from those in patients with a full colon. Differences in energy excretion between patients with and without a functional colon were mainly due to differences in carbohydrate excretion, not fat. In patients without a colon, fecal excretion remained stable with lengths of small bowel as short as 150 to 200 cm. Therefore, patients with less than 150 to 200 cm of remaining small intestine without a colon may have significant energy and fluid losses and may require parenteral nutrition (PN) for survival. In contrast, patients with a partial or complete remaining colon in continuity with the small intestine may not have significant fluid and energy loss until less than 50 to 70 cm of the small bowel remains. With shorter lengths, patients may require PN for survival.

Intestinal Adaptation Following Resection

There are exceptions to such length limits as described above. Estimates of the length of the remaining small bowel and health are not always accurate from surgical, endoscopic, or radiographic reports. In addition, the remaining intestine can compensate or adapt with time, resulting in increased surface area and nutrient absorption.[5] The results of this adaptation can be observed clinically in the form of patient weight gain, reduced intestinal fluid losses, and stabilization of micronutrients. These changes usually are clinically obvious approximately 3 months after intestinal resection and may continue for years.

Patients often clinically adapt to the significantly reduced energy absorption associated with short bowel syndrome through hyperphagia and increase their energy intake 1.5 to 2 times their resting energy expenditure.[5] Intestinal absorption also becomes more efficient per unit length. Intestinal hypertrophy occurs following massive enterectomy and as a result the intestine lengthens slightly, but more importantly, villi increase in number, height, and density and thereby absorptive surface area is increased.[6-8] This process may evolve over 1 to 2 years and longer in isolated cases.[2,9,10]

Several factors are important determinants in the functional adaptation process and clinical outcome.[2,11,12] These include the presence or absence of the colon and ileocecal valve, length of residual intestine and colon, the health of the remaining bowel, patient age, and other comorbid conditions. In general, at least 100 cm of residual small intestine in the absence of an intact and functional colon, or 60 cm in the presence of a completely functional colon,[2,9] is necessary to prevent dependence on PN; however, the degree of adaptation and PN-dependence may be highly individualized. Younger individuals have exhibited a greater degree of adaptation than older patients.

Despite the fact that most nutrients are absorbed in the proximal jejunum, the residual ileum adapts and assumes the role of macronutrient absorption. However, jejunal hypertrophy does not replace the loss of the specialized cells of the terminal ileum that absorb vitamin B12/intrinsic factor or bile salts.

Medical Therapy of Short Bowel Syndrome

The goal of medical therapy for short bowel syndrome is that the patient will resume work and a normal lifestyle, or as normal of one as possible. This is undertaken via the use of specific measures that gradually decrease their PN requirement, with eventual elimination as a goal for some individuals. Provision of adequate nutrition, including both macro- and micronutrients with prevention of energy malnutrition and specific nutrient deficiencies, provision of sufficient fluid to prevent dehydration, and prevention/correction acid-base disturbances are the most important aspects of the medical management of the short bowel patient. Given that most carbohydrates, nitrogen, and fat are absorbed within the first 100 cm and up to 150 cm of jejunum dietary intervention has an important role in the medical management of the patient with short bowel syndrome.[13]

Dietary Management

Patients will generally require PN for the first 7 to 10 days following massive enterectomy. (PN and other nutritional support is discussed in Section VI of this text.) Nutritional therapy, even PN, should not be introduced until the patient is hemodynamically stable and fluid management issues are relatively stable. The goal is to provide patients with approximately 25 to 35 kcal/kg/day and 1.0 to 1.5 kg/day of protein. Some debate exists as to whether the patient's actual body weight or ideal body weight should be used in this calculation. For the postoperative patient, standard enteral formula (Chapter 42) are recommended. These should be instituted gradually as tolerated. Once the patient is able to eat, they should be encouraged to eat a regular diet, but modified as described below. There is no value in separating liquids from solids in the diet. Such practices have no effect on macronutrient, electrolyte, or mineral absorption; fecal volume; or fecal weight.[3]

Specific dietary recommendations (Chapter 7) should be based on the presence or absence of a colon. The colon can convert complex carbohydrates by bacterial fermentation to SCFA (acetate, propionate, and butyrate) (Chapter 8), which can provide a source of calories, up to 500 to 1000 kcal/day. In addition, SCFA stimulate colonic sodium and water absorption.

Carbohydrates

The proximal jejunum is rarely resected in patients who require massive enterectomy. Most intestinal disacharidases are present in highest concentration proximally; therefore, a lactose-restricted diet is not recommended for those patients with more distal resections. Marteau et al studied 14 short bowel patients in whom a lactose-free diet was compared to a diet that contained 20 g/day of lactose in no more than 4 g of milk.[14] Lactose absorption, breath hydrogen production, subjective symptoms of flatulence, and diarrhea were similar between diets. These data confirmed the findings of an earlier controlled study, which reported that lactose absorption was enhanced when the lactose was provided in yogurt rather than in milk in 17 short bowel patients.[15] The amount of lactose found in a glass of milk (20 to 25 g) is generally well tolerated, even in patients with an end-jejunostomy.[15] Lactose restriction should be considered in patients with more proximal jejunal resections and in others and only transiently during the immediate postoperative period when hypotension or poor perfusion-induced shock to the intestine may result in transient lactose maldigestion. Otherwise, dietary lactose restriction will result in insufficient dietary calcium intake because most lactose is found in milk-based foodstuff.

Fat

Luminal lipid digestion may be impaired because of impaired bile salt reabsorption related to resected ileum (>100 cm).[16] Bile acids are necessary for adequate nutrient absorption and thus are important for optimizing dietary management. Significant bile acid loss can occur when >100 cm of the terminal ileum is resected or diseased. Unconjugated bile acids such as ursodeoxycholic acid may have a cathartic effect when presented to the colon. Deconjugation to deoxycholic acid (which is responsible for secretions in the small bowel and colon) occurs by the colonic bacterial flora. Therefore, treatment with ox bile supplements has been attempted in three cases to increase the duodenal bile salt concentration to a concentration greater than the level at which micellar solubilization of lipid occurs.[17-19] Unfortunately, this therapy has been associated with significantly increased fecal volume, at least in those patients with intact colon. Cholylsarcosine (Diamalt AG, Munich, Germany) is a conjugated bile acid that is synthesized by conjugation of the amino acid group of sarcosine (N-methylglcine) to the carboxyl group of cholic acid. Because of the additional methyl group of sarcosine, cholylsarcosine appears to be resistant to bacterial deconjugation and dehydroxylation and therefore should be devoid of cathartic effect. A preliminary, open-labeled study of four patients (two with colon in continuity) indicated treatment with the conjugated bile acid cholylsarcosine (6 g/day) was associated with an increase in fat absorption of 17±3 g/day without any effect on stool wet weight, although one of the four patients did experience a significant increase in wet stool output and nausea was experienced by another patient.[20] Commercial conjugated bile acid products are not currently available in the United States. Cholestyramine is not useful in patients with >100 cm of ileal resection and may actually worsen steatorrhea because of its binding of dietary lipid (and fat-soluble vitamins).[21]

Although dietary fat restriction may result in increased fecal fat losses, the percentage of fat absorbed does not differ between high-fat (75% nonprotein calories derived from fat)/low carbohydrate and low-fat/high carbohydrate, isocaloric, and isonitrogenous diets.[22] Fecal weight also did not differ between high- and low-fat diets in this study. However, because fat (9.0 kcal/g) is a more concentrated energy source than is carbohydrate (4.0 kcal/g), fat restriction may deprive the patient of an important energy source. Up to 65% of dietary carbohydrate may be malabsorbed and lost in feces without degradation by colonic bacteria.[23]

Medium chain triglycerides (MCT; C8-C10) do not require solubization with micelles for absorption, are energy dense (8.3 kcal/g), and are absorbed directly into the portal circulation. In addition, MCTs are absorbed by the colon. This may occur because MCTs are water soluble. In a study comparing two high-fat diets (50% of total calories) for 4 days each, 19 patients with short bowel syndrome (mean small bowel length: 143 cm; range: 50 to 250 cm)—10 of whom had colons (mean small bowel length: 203 cm; range: 125 to 300 cm) and 9 of whom were without colons—were randomized in a crossover design.[24] The diets consisted of either long chain triglycerides (LCT) or LCT plus MCT. Energy absorption was significantly increased by the addition of MCT (from 46% to 58%, $P < .05$) in patients with colons but not in those without colons. Fecal volume did not change in patients with a colon, and a trend toward increased output was seen in those without a colon. MCT may exert their positive effects in the colon because of their water-soluble properties, much like SCFA in contrast to the insoluble lipophilic long-chain fatty acids (LCFA). Some, but not all LCT, can be replaced by MCT in the diet. In a short bowel patient eating 10.5 MJ/day (2500 kcal/day), approximately 1.5 to 3 MJ/day (360 to 720 kcal/day; 40 to 80 g) of LCT can be replaced with MCT. However, LCT are still necessary to provide essential fatty acids, primarily linoleic fatty acid, which is not found in LCT. In addition, excessive intake of MCT may result in nausea, vomiting, and ketosis.

The Role of Soluble Fiber, Complex Carbohydrates, and Starch

Soluble nonstarch polysaccharides and some starches are not generally absorbed by the small intestine.[25] Soluble fiber is water soluble and is found primarily in oatmeal, oat bran, psyllium (Metamucil [Procter & Gamble, Cincinnati, Ohio]; Konsyl [Konsyl Pharmaceuticals, Edison, NJ]), barley, artichokes, strawberries, legumes, prunes, grapefruit, and squash—in descending order of concentration. Soluble fiber and starches pass undigested into the colon where colonic bacteria ferment them to hydrogen and methane (hence patient "gas" complaints) but also to SCFA including butyrate, proprionate, and acetate. SCFA are the preferred fuel for the colonocyte.[26] Therefore, the colon becomes an important machine for energy absorption in the patient with short bowel syndrome. Approximately 75 mmol of SCFA are produced from 10 g of unabsorbed carbohydrate.[27]

In one study, eight adult patients with short bowel syndrome (mean length of small bowel: 114 cm; range: 50 to 245 cm), all of whom had a colon, and six patients with end jejunostomies (mean length: 168 cm; range: 100 to 250 cm), who had no colon, were treated for 4 days with an isocaloric, high-carbohydrate:low-fat (60%:20%) diet (HCLF) or a low-carbohydrate:high-fat (20%:60%) diet (LCHF).[28] In patients with a colon, the HCLF diet reduced fecal losses of energy by 500 kcal/day, compared to the LCHF diet, and the absorption of energy increased from 49% to 69%, $P < .001$. Fecal excretion of carbohydrates was low and was not influenced by change in diet, whereas fecal fat was highly dependent on dietary changes. In contrast, patients with end jejunostomies excreted equal amounts of calories on each diet, and the percentage of calories absorbed was not different (HCLF, 55% versus LCHF, 48%; $P = .21$). The excretion of carbohydrate and fat was proportional to the amounts ingested. Both in patients with and in those without a colon, fecal volumes were not significantly affected by either diet. In another study, patients with short bowel syndrome but an intact colon in continuity were able to decrease fecal energy loss by 1.3 to 3.1 MJ/day (310 to 740 kcal/day) when they were fed a diet consisting of 60% carbohydrates.[29] Colonic metabolism of unabsorbed carbohydrate was indicated by decreased fecal carbohydrate losses in the patients with colon in continuity.

It is possible for an intact colon to absorb up to 2.2 to 4.9 MJ (525 to 1170 kcal) daily from dietary fiber.[2,29,30] Colonic energy absorption may also increase somewhat during the postresection adaptation phase, related to increased colonic bacterial carbohydrate fermentation.[30,31] This may be related to increased colonic bacteria in patients with short bowel syndrome as well as an increase in the concentration or activity of various enzymes such as β-galactosidase over time during the adaptation period.

Because SCFA stimulate sodium and water absorption,[32] patients might have decreased fecal fluid and sodium loss, although this has not been observed clinically.[29] It should be noted that not all studies have shown improved energy absorption with HCLF diets. In one study, eight patients with short bowel syndrome (length unknown), = three of whom had a partial colon, were treated with a HCLF and a LCHF diet for 5 days each in a crossover design.[22] There was no difference between diets in effect on stool weights, absorption of fat, total calories, or electrolytes and minerals. There were three patients with a partial colon (transverse colon), but they also exhibited no increase in energy absorption with a HCLF diet. (Dietary fiber is discussed in detail in Chapter 11.)

Proteins/Amino Acids

Dietary protein (Chapter 8) is first digested and then absorbed as di- and tripeptides. Therefore, it was reasoned that dietary protein provided in a predigested form would be more readily absorbed. However, nitrogen absorption is the macronutrient least affected by decreased intestinal absorptive surface. Therefore, the utility of peptide-based diets in such patients is generally without merit.

McIntyre et al compared energy, nitrogen, and fat absorption, as well as stool weight in seven patients with end-jejunostomy and all with <150 cm (range 60 to 150 cm) of remaining small intestine. These patients were fed with either a peptide-based versus an essentially isocaloric and isonitrogenous polymeric formula. Although the study was small, no differences were observed in energy, nitrogen, fat, carbohydrate, electrolyte, mineral, or fluid absorption.[33] Uncontrolled data from Levy et al support these findings.[34] Data from Cosnes, however, in a small study of six patients, all with 90 to 150 cm of residual jejunum and end-jejunostomy, suggested nitrogen absorption may be enhanced by the use of a peptide-based diet.[35] However, energy, other macronutrient, electrolyte, mineral, and fluid absorption were unaffected.[35] Therefore, the clinical affect of the modestly increased nitrogen absorption observed was insignificant. It must be recognized that the above-described studies were all very small, the study populations somewhat heterogeneous, and the various peptide constituents and their respective concentrations in the various formulas differed significantly. There was also variation in the type and amount of fat (LCT versus MCT). Therefore, it is difficult to make definitive comparisons between studies and provide specific clinical recommendations based on these studies.

The amino acid glutamine, together with glucose, is the preferred fuel for the small intestinal enterocyte.[36] Rodent PN models suggested that both parenteral or enteral glutamine supplements could effect more rapid and more significant bowel adaptation following massive enterectomy.[37,38] Therefore, it was thought glutamine supplementation in humans would have a similar effect. Bouteloup et al reported the ingestion of 50 g of glutamine daily led to a slight but statistically significant increase in nitrogen absorption in a group of eight patients who had ileostomies and a mean of 140 cm of resected small intestine. However, it is possible the improved nitrogen balance observed may have been largely related to the increased nitrogen consumption in these patients.[39] Another small study showed no increase in body weight or lean body mass following glutamine supplementation in otherwise well-nourished patients with short bowel syndrome.[40] Scolapio et al showed treatment with oral glutamine (0.45 g/kg/day) had no effect on small intestinal morphology, carbohydrate absorption, fat absorption, or fecal fluid loss.[41] (Studies using a combination of glutamine and growth hormone are discussed in Chapter 33).

Dietary Restriction

Normally, oxalate in the diet binds to dietary calcium and is excreted in the stool. However, in the presence of significant fat malabsorption, dietary calcium preferentially binds to free fatty acids, rendering oxalate free to pass into the colon where it is absorbed; dietary oxalate is only minimally absorbed in the small intestine. Absorption may also be enhanced because of increased colonic permeability caused by injury from malabsorbed bile salts that are also passing into the colon.[42] Once absorbed in the colon, oxalate is filtered by the kidneys, where it binds to calcium, resulting in hyperoxaluria and calcium oxalate nephrocalcinosis and nephrolithiasis.[9] Therefore, dietary oxalate should be restricted in patients with short bowel syndrome who have colon in continuity and hyperoxalouria. Oral calcium supplements may also be of value for the prevention of calcium-oxalate nephrolithiasis.[43] Hyperoxaluria may also develop in patients without colon who are PN-dependent.[44] This is most likely related to metabolism of vitamin C in the PN solution, in the presence of light, to oxalate.[45] It may therefore be beneficial to shield PN (from light) to which vitamin C has been added either as a multivitamin solution or individually, although it remains unclear if dietary oxalate should be restricted in all patients with an end jejunostomy that require PN.

Fluid and Electrolyte Management

Massive enterectomy is associated with transient gastric hypersecretion. Basal acid secretion is significantly increased for several months postoperatively.[46,47] Because the pH of duodenal luminal contents therefore decreases, lipase deconjugation may occur, resulting in decreased fat digestion and enhanced fat malabsorption. Massive small bowel resection is also associated with hypergastrinemia during the initial first 6 months postoperatively.[46] H2 antagonists and proton pump inhibitors are useful in reducing gastric fluid secretion and, therefore, will also reduce fluid losses during this period.[1,48-50] However, absorption of orally dosed medications may be impaired; therefore, either large doses of oral medication or intravenous delivery may be required.

Fluid losses usually require chronic control with antimotility agents such as loperamide hydrochloride or diphenoxylate. Typical doses are 4 to 16 mg/day, although medical malabsorption may occur, necessitating larger doses. If these doses are ineffective, especially in patients with no colon in continuity or those who are left with a minimum of residual jejunum or duodenum, codeine or tincture of opium may be necessary. The usual dose for codeine sulfate is 15 to 60 mg bid to qid. Rarely, patients will require treatment with octreotide. Octreotide may be useful to slow intestinal transit time and increase water and sodium absorption, although its mechanism of action is unknown.[51,52] In one open-labeled study of nine patients with end-jejuonstomies, daily jejunostomy volume decreased from 8.1±1.8 to 4.8±0.7 L/day using a dose of 100 µg SQ, tid 30 minutes before meals.[53] Because use of octreotide does not lead to PN discontinuation, its use should be reserved for patients with high output jejunostomies in whom fluid and electrolyte management is problematic. Octreotide reduces splanchnic protein synthesis and thereby reduces mucosal protein incorporation and villous growth rate; as a result, octreotide may impair postresectional intestinal adaptation.[54] The incidence of cholelithiasis is also increased[55,56] in a group of patients already predisposed to this problem.[57]

Oral rehydration solutions (ORS) are also important in the dietary management of patients with short bowel syndrome primarily because of their effect on fluid and electrolyte absorption. Most of the published success with ORS has been in the context of treating patients with cholera, in which such solutions have substantially reduced mortality. Few data are available in short bowel syndrome. These glucose-polymer-based solutions should be instituted to decrease dehydration and to decrease PN fluid requirements in patients with residual jejunum ending in a jejunostomy. ORS work by the solvent drag mechanism in the jejunum, in which nutrients such as glucose promote the passive absorption of electrolytes and water. To avoid passive secretion of salt and water, solutions should be isotonic with plasma.

As increasing amounts of the small bowel are removed, the volume of the effluent rises. Patients with <100 cm of residual jejunum are at significant risk for dehydration because they secrete more sodium and fluid than consumed orally.[1] Because the jejunum is permeable to sodium and chloride, passively-absorbed solutions with high sodium chloride concentration are readily absorbed. Glucose promotes salt and water absorption by solvent drag.[58] However, sodium and water are not absorbed from hypotonic or isotonic solutions in the jejunum.

Several commercially available ORS formulas are available, although the best, and certainly the least expensive, is that recommended by the World Health Organization.[59] This can be formulated by dissolving the following in 1 L of tap water: sodium chloride (2.5 g), potassium chloride (1.5 g), sodium carbonate (2.5 g), and glucose (table sugar, 20 g). Only the potassium chloride requires a physician prescription. Most, if not all, of the commercially available ORS have substantially less sodium (in the range of 45 to 50 mmol/L). Less sodium chloride may be added, but the optimal sodium concentration should be at least 90 mmol/L, which is the usual concentration of small bowel effluent.[4]

Solutions with lower sodium concentrations lead to increased sodium losses. Standard "sport drinks" have high sugar content and too little sodium. Therefore, patients with short bowel syndrome should be cautioned against consumption of plain water and should be encouraged to drink ORS whenever they are thirsty. Recent evidence has shown that hypotonic (160 mOsmol/kg) ORS leads to decreased intraluminal duodenojejunal fluid flow rate in normal volunteers, although the effect on GI fluid losses or patient hydrational status in short bowel patients has not been evaluated.[60] Rice-based formulas (Ceralyte, 40 g of rice carbohydrate; osmolality, 225 [sodium, 50 mmol/L], 235 [sodium 70], or 260 [sodium 90]) allow more glucose delivery to the small intestine without increasing the osmotic load from free glucose. The addition of glutamine to a standard rehydration formula did not enhance sodium absorption in a study of six patients with end jejunostomies.[61] Several case reports showed successful results (defined as discontinuation of parenteral fluids and electrolytes) of ORS with sodium concentrations between 77 and 116 mmol/L.[62-70] The mean length of jejunum in these studies was 100 cm (range: 25 to 180 cm). Two of the patients (one with 25 cm and one with 30 cm of small intestine) had parts of their colon remaining.

Intake is often limited by palatability. Commercial products with a better taste have been marketed. For patients with residual colon in continuity, ORS may still be of value; however, provided sufficient sodium is present in the diet, the amount of sodium in the ORS may not be as critical because the colon readily absorbs sodium and water against a steep electrochemical gradient.[71] For patients with no remaining jejunum but who have residual ileum, the presence of glucose in the ORS is not critical because ileal water absorption is not affected by the presence of glucose.[72]

In addition to sodium losses, significant quantities of magnesium are lost in jejunal or ileal effluent as well.[73] Given that patients may develop magnesium deficiency (Chapter 3) despite a normal serum concentration, it is prudent to determine 24-hour urine magnesium loss.[74] The median 24-hour urine magnesium in normal volunteers was 127 mg (versus 19 mg for magnesium deficient short bowel patients) in one study.[73] Magnesium deficiency may precipitate calcium deficiency because hypomagnesemia impairs the release of parathyroid hormone.[75] In addition, the majority of patients with short bowel syndrome who remain independent of PN are in negative calcium balance.[76] Therefore, in the absence of PN, oral calcium supplementation is recommended routinely (800 to 1200 mg/day). Unlike calcium supplementation, magnesium replacement is often problematic. Attempts with oral magnesium oxide, or even oral consumption of the injectable form of magnesium, have not generally been successful and have been associated with increased fecal loss because of their cathartic effect.[77] Magnesium gluconate may have the least cathartic effect of commercially available oral magnesium supplements. Although magnesium gluconate is water soluble, magnesium has not generally been a constituent of ORS. Some patients may require periodic parenteral magnesium, despite the absence of a PN or intravenous fluid requirement.

Iron is absorbed in the duodenum, and therefore, in the absence of hemorrhage, is not routinely required as a supplement. Phosphorous deficiency is not well described in short bowel syndrome, and therefore supplementation is rarely, if ever, required. (Mineral deficiencies are discussed at greater length in Chapter 3.)

Vitamins

Micronutrients often require supplementation in short bowel syndrome. Because water-soluble vitamins are absorbed in the proximal jejunum, it is unusual for deficiencies to develop in short bowel patients except in those patients with a proximal jejunostomy or duodenostomy. However, these patients generally require PN in which multivitamins should be routinely provided. Thiamine deficiency has been reported in patients who require PN but generally only in those who have not received supplementation as part of the intravenous multivitamin formulation. This became an important issue during a recent parenteral vitamin shortage.[78] Patients presented with Wernicke's encephalopathy, beriberi, and severe metabolic alkalosis.[79]

If thiamine deficiency is suspected, whole blood thiamine concentration is not helpful; this reflects recent nutritional intake. Erythrocyte transketolase activity should be determined and empiric therapy begun with 100 mg of parenteral thiamine daily. Biotin deficiency has rarely been reported in patients with short bowel syndrome.[80] It is manifested in a scaly dermatitis, alopecia, lethargy, hypotonia, and lactic acidosis. Therapy consists of parenteral biotin supplementation of 0.3 to 1 mg daily, although currently this is not commercially available. Vitamin B12 supplementation is required (300 g/month SQ) in patients who have had a significant portion of their terminal ileum resected (>60 cm).[81] Single-use vials of vitamin B12 contain 1000 mcg; therefore, patients are often given the additional vitamin (without any harmful effects). Folic acid is provided as a constituent of parenteral multivitamins. However, in patients with proximal jejunal resection, folate deficiency may develop.[82] These patients should receive a 1-mg/day supplement.

Fat-soluble vitamin deficiency (A, D, and E) is more common because of the steatorrrhea that occurs in short bowel syndrome and the subsequent decrease in micellar formation and fat digestion.[83] The use of cholestyramine may also result in fat-soluble vitamin deficiency.[84] Night blindness and xerophthalmia have been described in patients with short bowel syndrome.[85] Given that as vitamin A deficiency progresses, corneal ulceration, and permanent visual loss may ensue, short bowel patients who do not receive parenteral multivitamins should have their serum vitamin A concentration monitored. If a low serum vitamin A concentration is detected, therapy is 10,000 to 50,000 IU daily. This may be administered either orally or parenterally. Care should be taken to avoid over supplementation of vitamin A, especially in patients with severe renal insufficiency, as toxicity may result.

Vitamin D deficiency may result in osteomalacia, a defect in bone mineralization. Usually dietary intake is a relatively unimportant source of vitamin D because the majority is endogenously synthesized from 7-dehydrocholesterol via ultraviolet light.[86,87] However, because enterohepatic circulation is disrupted in patients who have undergone significant ileal resections, deficiency may result.[73] Large doses of vitamin D (50,000 to 100,000 IU/day) may be administered orally or by depot injection. In addition, the activated form of vitamin D—1,25-dihydroxyvitamin D (0.25 mg/day)—may be administered. Serum ionized calcium concentration can be monitored. Overzealous supplementation may result in hypercalcemia and extraintestinal soft tissue calcification.

Vitamin E deficiency in patients with short bowel syndrome may manifest in hemolysis[88] and various neurological deficits.[89] Because serum vitamin E concentration reflects serum total lipid concentration, which may be decreased in patients with short bowel syndrome because of massive steatorrhea, a low serum vitamin E concentration alone may not be indicative of a deficient state; the serum vitamin E:total lipid ratio should be calculated.[90,91] Supplementation can be provided orally with 800 to 1200 mg daily; no parenteral form of vitamin E is commercially available.

Most vitamin K is synthesized by colonic bacteria (60%),[92] although dietary intake accounts for about 40% of requirements. Deficiency is therefore uncommon in patients with intact colon. However, vitamin K deficiency is frequent in patients who have no residual colon or who have received recent broad-spectrum antibiotics. The vitamin K requirement is approximately 1 mg daily.[92] (Vitamin deficiencies are discussed at length in Chapter 3.)

Trace Metals

Patients with short bowel syndrome lose a significant amount of zinc and selenium in their feces. A significant amount of zinc is also lost in small bowel effluent (12 mg/L small intestinal fluid and 16 mg/L stool).[93] Zinc deficiency has been associated with growth abnormalities,[94] delayed wound healing,[95] cellular immunity dysfunction.[96] Patients in whom zinc deficiency is suspected should be treated empirically with oral zinc sulfate or zinc gluconate (220 to 440 mg daily) or with parenteral zinc sulfate if the patient requires PN. Serum and leukocyte measurements of zinc concentration, although helpful, may be unreliable.[97]

Selenium deficiency has been associated with cardiomyopathy,[98] peripheral neuropathy, proximal muscle weakness and pain,[99] whitening of the hair, and macrocytosis.[100] Serum selenium is a reliable indicator of selenium status, and if low, oral or parenteral supplementation should be provided (60 to 150 mcg/day).

Chromium is a necessary cofactor for insulin's effects in peripheral tissue.[101] However, current data suggests that there is sufficient chromium available in PN solutions as a contaminant to prevent deficiency from developing. Although there are three reported cases of possible chromium deficiency in patients requiring long-term PN,[102] deficiency has not been reported in short bowel patients who do not require PN; therefore, routine supplementation is not recommended. In addition, routine chromium supplementation may be associated with nephrotoxicity.[103] Copper deficiency is very rare in the patient with short bowel syndrome. Deficiency may result in microcytic anemia, neuropathy, and decreased fertility.[104]

References

1. Nightingale JM, Lennard-Jones JE, Walker ER, Farthing MJ. Jejunal efflux in short bowel syndrome. *Lancet*. 1990;336:765-768.
2. Nightingale JM, Lennard-Jones JE, Gertner DJ, et al. Colonic preservation reduces need for parenteral therapy, increases incidence of renal stones, but does not change high prevalence of gallstones in patients with a short bowel. *Gut*. 1992;33:1493-1497.
3. Woolf GM, Miller C, Kurian R, Jeejeebhoy KN. Nutritional absorption in short bowel syndrome. *Dig Dis Sci*. 1987;32:8-15.
4. Landfoged K, Olgaard K. Fluid and electrolyte absorption and renin-angiotensin-aldosterone axis in patients with severe short-bowel syndrome. *Gastroenterology*. 1979;14:729-735.
5. Crenn P, Morin MC, Joly F, et al. Net digestive absorption and adaptive hyperphagia in adult short bowel patients. *Gut*. 2004;53:1279-1286.
6. Solhaug JH, Tvete S. Adaptive changes in the small intestine following bypass operation for obesity. *Scand J Gastroenterol*. 1978;13:401-408.
7. Dowling RH, Booth CC. Functional compensation after small-bowel resection in man. *Lancet*. 1966;2:146-147.
8. Weinstein LD, Shoemaker CP, Hersh T, Wright HK. Enhanced intestinal absorption after small bowel resection in man. *Arch Surg*. 1969;99:560-561.
9. Messing B, Crenn P, Beau P, et al. Long-term survival and parenteral nutrition dependence in adult patients with short bowel syndrome. *Gastroenterology*. 1999;117:1043-1050.
10. Kurkchubasche AG, Rowe MI, Smith SD. Adaptation in short-bowel syndrome: reassessing old limits. *J Pediatr Surg*. 1071;28:1069-1071.
11. Carbonnel F, Cosnes J, Chevret S, et al. The role of anatomic factors in nutritional autonomy after extensive small bowel resection. *JPEN J Parenter Enteral Nutr*. 1996;20:275-280.
12. Kaufman SS, Loseke CA, Lupo JV, et al. Factors affecting duration of parenteral hyperalimentation in children with short bowel syndrome (abstract). *Gastroenterology*. 1996;110:A809.
13. Borgstrom B, Dahlqvist A, Lundh G, Sjovall J. Studies of intestinal digestion and absorption in the human. *J Clin Invest*. 1957;36:1521-1536.
14. Marteau P, Messing B, Arrigoni E, et al. Do patients with short-bowel syndrome need a lactose-free diet? *Nutrition*. 1997;13:13-16.
15. Arrigoni E, Marteau P, Briet F, et al. Tolerance and absorption of lactose from milk and yogurt during short-bowel syndrome in humans. *Am J Clin Nutr*. 1994;60:926-929.
16. Ohkohchi N, Andoh T, Izumi U, et al. Disorder of bile acid metabolism in children with short bowel syndrome. *J Gastroenterol*. 1997;32:472-479.
17. Little KH, Schiller LR, Bilhartz LE, Fordtran JS. Treatment of severe steatorrhea with ox bile in an ileectomy patient with residual colon. *Dig Dis Sci*. 1992;37:929-933.
18. Fordtran JS, Bunch F, Davis GR. Ox bile treatment of severe steatorrhea in an ileectomy-ileostomy patient. *Gastroenterology*. 1982;82:564-568.
19. Djurdjevic D, Popovic O, Necic D, Hranisavljevic S. Ox bile treatment of severe steatorrhea in a colectomy and ileectomy patient. *Gastroenterology*. 1988;95:1160.
20. Heydorn S, Jeppesen PB, Mortensen PB. Bile acid replacement therapy with cholylsarcosine for short-bowel syndrome. *Scand J Gastroenterol*. 1999;34:818-823.
21. Hofmann AF, Poley R. Role of bile acid malabsorption in pathogenesis of diarrhea and steatorrhea in patients with ileal resection. *Gastroenterology*. 1972;62:918-934.
22. Woolf GM, Miller C, Kurian R, Jeejeebhoy KN. Diet for patients with a short bowel: high fat or high carbohydrate? *Gastroenterology*. 1983;84:823-828.
23. Ameen VZ, Powell GK, Jones LA. Quantitation of fecal carbohydrate excretion in patients with short bowel syndrome. *Gastroenterology*. 1987;92:493-500.
24. Jeppesen PB, Mortensen PB. The influence of a preserved colon on the absorption of medium chain fats in patients with small bowel resection. *Gut*. 1998;478-483.
25. Englyst HN, Trowell H, Southgate DA, Cummings JH. Dietary fiber and resistant starch. *Am J Clin Nutr*. 1987;46:873-874.
26. Bond JH, Currier BE, Buchwald H, Levitt MD. Colonic conservation of malabsorbed carbohydrate. *Gastroenterology*. 1980;78:444-447.
27. Cummings JH, Gibson GR, Macfarlane GT. Quantitative estimates of fermentation in the hind gut of man. *Acta Vet Scand Supp*. 1989;86:76-82.
28. Jeppesen PB, Mortensen PB. The influence of a preserved colon on the absorption of medium chain fat in patients with small bowel resection. *Gut*. 1998;43:478-483.
29. Nordgaard I, Hansen BS, Mortensen PB. Colon as a digestive organ in patients with short bowel. Lancet. 1994;343:373-376.
30. Nordgaard I, Hansen BS, Mortensen PB. Importance of colonic support for energy absorption as small-bowel failure proceeds. *Am J Clin Nutr*. 1996;64:222-231.
31. Ruppin H, Bar-Meir S, Soergel KH, et al. Absorption of short-chain fatty acids by the colon. Gastroenterology. 1980;78:1500-1507.
32. Briet F, Flourie B, Achour L, et al. Bacterial adaptation in patients with short bowel and colon in continuity. Gastroenterology. 1995;109:1446-1453.
33. McIntyre PB, Fitchew M, Lennard-Jones JE. Patients with a high jejunostomy do not need a special diet. *Gastroenterology*. 1986;91:25-33.
34. Levy E, Frileux P, Sandrucci S, et al. Continuous enteral nutrition during the early adaptive stage of the short bowel syndrome. *Br J Surg*. 1988;75:549-553.
35. Cosnes J, Evard D, Beaugerie L, et al. Improvement in protein absorption with a small peptide-base diet in patients with high jejunostomy. *Nutrition*. 1992;8:406-411.
36. Windmueller HG, Spaeth AE. Identification of ketone bodies and glutamine as the major respiratory fuels in vivo for postabsorptive rat small intestine. *J Biol Chem*. 1978;253:69-76.
37. Guarino A, Canani RB, Iafusco M, et al. In vivo and in vitro effects of human growth hormone on rat intestine ion transplort. *Pediatr Res*. 1995;37:576-580.
38. Souba WW, Klimberg VS, Plumley DA, et al. The role of glutamine in maintaining a healthy gut and supporting the metabolic response to injury and infection. *J Surg Res*. 1990;48:383-391.
39. Bouteloup C, Dechelotte P, Hecketsweiler B, et al. Effect of oral glutamine on absorptive function in ileostomized patients. *Clin Nutr*. 1994;13:61S.
40. Dias MC, Faintuch J, Waitzberg DL, et al. Oral diet and glutamine in patients with short bowel syndrome. *JPEN J Parenter Enteral Nutr*. 1999;23:S157.
41. Scolapio JS, McGreevy K, Tennyson GS, Burnett OL. Effect of glutamine in short bowel syndrome. *Clin Nutr*. 2001;20:319-323.
42. Dobbins JW, Binder HJ. Effect of bile salts and fatty acids on the colonic absorption of oxalate. *Gastroenterology*. 1976;70:1096-1100.
43. Barilla DE, Notz C, Kennedy D, Pak CY. Renal oxalate excretion following oral oxalate loads in patients with ileal disease and with renal and absorptive hypercalciurias. Effect of calcium and magnesium. *Am J Med*. 1978;64:579-585.
44. Buchman AL, Moukarzel A, Ament ME. Excessive urinary oxalate excretion occurs in long-term TPN patients both with and without ileostomies. *J Am Coll Nutr*. 1995;14:24-28.
45. Rockwell GF, Campfield T, Nelson BC, Uden PC. Oxalogenesis in parenteral nutrition solution components. *Nutrition*. 1998;14:836-839.
46. Windsor CW, Fejfar J, Woodward DA. Gastric secretion after massive small bowel resection. *Gut*. 1969;10:779-786.
47. Williams NS, Evans P, King RFJ. Gastric acid secretion and gastrin production in the short bowel syndrome. *Gut*. 1985;26:914-919.
48. Jacobsen O, Ladefoged K, Stage JG, Jarnum S. Effects of cimetidine on jejunostomy effluents in patients with severe short bowel syndrome. *Scand J Gastroenterol*. 1986;21:824-828.

49. Nightingale JM, Walker ER, Farthing MJ, Lennard-Jones JE. Effect of omeprazole on intestinal output in the short bowel syndrome. *Aliment Pharmacol Ther.* 1991;5:405-412.
50. Jeppesen PB, Staun M, Tjellesen L, Mortensen PB. Effect of intravenous ranitidine and omeprazole on intestinal absorption of water, sodium, and macronutrients in patients with intestinal resection. *Gut.* 1998;43:763-769.
51. Cooper JC, Williams NS, King RF, Barker MC Effects of a long-acting somatostatin analogue in patients with severe ileostomy diarrhoea. *Br J Surg.* 1986;73:128-131.
52. Ladefoged K, Christensen KC, Hegnhoj J, Jarnum S. Effect of a long-acting somatostatin analogue SMS 201-995 on jejunostomy effluents in patients with severe short bowel syndrome. *Gut.* 1989;30:943-949.
53. O'Keefe SJ, Haymond MW, Bennet WM, et al. Long-acting somatostatin analogue therapy and protein metabolism in patients with jejunostomies. *Gastroenterology.* 1994;107:379-388.
54. Sukhotnik I, Khateeb K, Krausz MM, et al. Sandostatin impairs postresection intestinal adaptation in a rat model of short bowel syndrome. *Dig Dis Sci.* 2002;47:2095-2102.
55. Niv Y, Charash B, Sperber AD, Oren M. Effect of octreotide on gastrostomy, duodenostomy, and cholecystostomy effluents: a physiologic study of fluid and electrolyte balance. *Am J Gastroenterol.* 1997;92:2107-2111.
56. Catnach SM, Anderson JV, Fairclough PD, et al. Effect of octreotide on gall stone prevalence and gall bladder motility in acromegaly. *Gut.* 1993;34:270-273.
57. Roslyn JJ, Pitt HA, Mann LL, et al. Gallbladder disease in patients on long-term parenteral nutrition. *Gastroenterology.* 1983;84:148-154.
58. Fortran JS. Stimulation of active and passive sodium absorption by sugars in the human jejunum. *J Clin Invest.* 1975;55:728-737.
59. World Health Organization. Treatment and prevention of dehydration in diarrhoeal diseases: a guide for use at the primary level. Geneva, Switzerland: WHO; 1976.
60. Pfeiffer A, Schmidt T, Kaess H. The role of osmolality in the absorption of a nutrient solution. *Aliment Pharmacol Ther.* 1998;12:281-286.
61. Beaugerie L, Carbonnel F, Hecketsweiler B et al.: Effects of an isotonic oral rehydration solution, enriched with glutamine, on fluid and sodium absorption in patients with a short-bowel. *Aliment Pharmacol Ther.* 1997;11:741-746.
62. Newton CR, Gonvers JJ, McIntyre PB et al: Effect of different drinks on fluid and electrolyte losses from a jejunostomy. *J R Soc Med.* 1985;78:27-34.
63. Rodriguez-Iturbe B, Herrera J, Garcia R. Relationship between glomerular filtration rate and renal blood flow at different levels of protein-induced hyperfiltration in man. *Clin Sci (Lond).* 1988;74:11-15.
64. Crow M, Meyer GW. "Cholera solution" in short bowel syndrome. *South Med J.* 1978;71:1303-1304.
65. Griffin GE, Fagan EF, Hodgson HJ: Enteral therapy in the management of massive gut resection complicated by chronic fluid and electrolyte depletion. *Dig Dis Sci.* 1982;27:902-908.
66. Laustsen J, Fallingborg J. Enteral glucose-polymer-electrolyte solution in the treatment of chronic fluid and electrolyte depletion in short-bowel syndrome. *Acta Chir Scand.* 1983;149:787-788.
67. MacMahon RA. The use of the World Health Organization's oral rehydration solution in patients on home parenteral nutrition. *JPEN J Parenter Enteral Nutr.* 1984;8:720-721.
68. Ward K, Murray B, Neale G. Treatment of salt losing ileostomy diarrhoea with an oral glucose polymer electrolyte solution. *Ir J Med Sci.* 1984;153:77-78.
69. Camilleri M, Prather CM, Evans MA, Andresen-Reid ML. Balance studies and polymeric glucose solution to optimize therapy after massive intestinal resection. *Mayo Clin Proc.* 1992;67:755-760.
70. Beaugerie L, Cosnes J, Verwaerde F, et al. Isotonic high-sodium oral rehydration solution for increasing sodium absorption in patients with short-bowel syndrome. *Am J Clin Nutr.* 1991;53:769-772.
71. Fordtran JS, Rector FC Jr, Carter NW. The mechanisms of sodium absorption in the human small intestine. *J Clin Invest.* 1968;47:884-900.
72. Davis GR, Santa Ana CA, Morawski SG, Fordtran JC. Permeability characteristics of human jejunum, ileum, proximal colon, and distal colon: results of potential difference measurements and unidirectional fluxes. *Gastroenterology.* 1982;83:844-850.
73. Selby PL, Peacock M, Bambach CP. Hypomagnesaemia after small bowel resection: treatment with 1α-hydroxylated vitamin D metabolites. *Br J Surg.* 1984;71:334-337.
74. Fleming CR, George L, Stoner GL, et al. The importance of urinary magnesium values in patients with gut failure. *Mayo Clin Proc.* 1996;71:21-24.
75. Anast CS, Winnacker JL, Forte LR, Burns TW. Impaired release of parathyroid hormone in magnesium deficiency. *J Clin Endocrinol Metab.* 1976;42:707-717.
76. Hylander E, Ladefoged K, Madsen S. Calcium balance and bone mineral content following small-intestinal resection. *Scand J Gastroenterol.* 1981;16:167-176.
77. Scolapio JS, Tammela L, Stoner G. Injectible magnesium, given orally: attempt at magnesium replacement in short bowel syndrome. *Gastroenterology.* 1999;116:A576.
78. Alloju M, Ehrinpreis MN. Shortage of intravenous multivitamin solution in the United States. *N Engl J Med.* 1997;337:54-55.
79. Schiano TD, Klang MG, Quesada E, et al. Thiamine status in patients receiving long-term home parenteral nutrition. *Am J Gastroenterol.* 1996;91:2555-2559.
80. Mock DM, DeLorimer AA, Liebman WM, et al. Biotin deficiency: an unusual complication of parenteral alimentation. *New Engl J Med.* 1981;304:820-823.
81. Andersson H, Bosaeus I, Brummer RJ, et al. Nutritional and metabolic consequences of extensive bowel resection. *Dig Dis.* 1986;4:193-202.
82. Denburg J, Bensen W, Ali MA, et al. Megaloblastic anemia in patients receiving total parenteral nutrition without folic aid or vitamin B12 supplementation. *Can Med Assoc J.* 1977;117:144-146.
83. Edes TE, Walk BE, Thornton WH Jr, Fritsche KL. Essential fatty acid sufficiency does not preclude fat-soluble-vitamin deficiency in short-bowel syndrome. *Am J Clin Nutr.* 1991;53:499-502.
84. Compston JE, Horton LW. Oral 25-hydroxyvitamin D_3 in treatment of osteomalacia associated with ileal resection and cholestyramine therapy. *Gastroenterology.* 1978;74:900-902.
85. Mokete B, De Cock R. Xerophthalmia and short bowel syndrome. *Br J Gastroenterol.* 1998;82:1340-1341.
86. Stamp TC, Round JM. Seasonal changes in human plasma levels of 25-hydroxyvitamin D. *Nature.* 1974;247:563-565.
87. Haddad JG, Hahn TJ. Natural and synthetic sources of 25-hydroxyvitamin D in man. Nature. 1973;244:515-516.
88. Fritsma GA. Vitamin E and autoxidation. *Am J Med Technol.* 1983;49:453-456.
89. Howard L, Ovesen L, Satya-Murti S, Chu R. Reversible neurological symptoms caused by vitamin E deficiency in a patient with short bowel syndrome. *Am J Clin Nutr.* 1982;36:1243-1249.
90. Meydani M, Cohn JS, Macauley JB, et al. Postprandial changes in the plasma concentration of alpha and gamma tocopherol in human subjects fed a fat-rich meal supplemented with fat-soluble vitamins. *J Nutr.* 1989;119:1252-1258.
91. Thurnham DI, Davies JA, Crump BJ, et al. The use of different lipids to express serum tocopherol: lipid ratios for the measurement of vitamin E status. *Ann Clin Biochem.* 1986;23:514-520.
92. Conly JM, Stein K, Worobetz L, et al. The contribution of vitamin K2 (menaquinones) produced by the intestinal microflora to human nutritional requirements for vitamin K. *Am J Gastroenterol.* 1994;89:915-923.
93. Wolman SL, Anderson GH, Marliss EB, Jeejeebhoy KN. Zinc in total parenteral nutrition: requirements and metabolic effects. *Gastroenterology.* 1979;76:458-467.
94. Prasad AS. Zinc in growth and development and spectrum of human zinc deficiency. *J Am Coll Nutr.* 1988;7:377-384.

95. Golden MH, Golden BE, Jackson AA. Skin breakdown in kwashiorkor responds to zinc. *Lancet.* 1980;1:1256.
96. Golden MH, Golden BE, Harland PS, Jackson AA. Zinc and immunocompetence in protein-energy malnutrition. *Lancet.* 1978;1:1226-1228.
97. Prasad AS. Laboratory diagnosis of zinc deficiency. *J Am Coll Nutr.* 1985;4:591-598.
98. Fleming CR, Lie JT, McCall JT, et al. Selenium deficiency and fatal cardiomyopathy in a patient on home parenteral nutrition. *Gastroenterology.* 1982;83:689-693.
99. Brown M, Cohen HJ, Lyons JM, et al. Proximal muscle weakness and selenium deficiency associated with long-term parenteral nutrition. *Am J Clin Nutr.* 1986;43:549-554.
100. Vinton NE, Dahlstrom KA, Strobel CT, Ament ME. Macrocytosis and pseudoalbinism: manifestations of selenium deficiency. *J Pediatr.* 1987;111:711-717.
101. Roginski EE, Mertz W. Effects of chromium (3+) supplementation on glucose and amino acid metabolism in rats fed a low protein diet. *J Nutr.* 1969;97:525-530.
102. Jeejeebhoy KN, Chu RC, Marliss EB, et al. Chromium deficiency, glucose intolerance, and neuropathy reversed by chromium supplementation, in a patient receiving long-term total parenteral nutrition. *Am J Clin Nutr.* 1977;30:531-538.
103. Moukarzel A, Song MK, Buchman AL, et al. Excessive chromium intake in children receiving total parenteral nutrition. *Lancet.* 1992;339:385-388.
104. Williams DM. Copper deficiency in humans. *Semin Hematol.* 1983;20:118-128.

Chapter 31

Nontransplant Surgery for Short Bowel Syndrome

Kishore Iyer, MBBS, FRCS (Eng), FACS

Introduction

Short bowel syndrome refers to a specific form of intestinal failure resulting from inadequate length of functional small bowel. The syndrome is characterized by a failure to meet the body's needs for calories and macro- and micronutrients via the enteral route. Although the metabolic, nutritional, fluid, and electrolyte consequences of having inadequate functional gut length are predictable, many of the complications related to the syndrome, such as liver disease and frequent life-threatening septic episodes, are related to the provision of total parenteral nutrition (TPN) and the obligatory need for long-term central venous access.

There is considerable disagreement as to what exactly constitutes "short" bowel. The problem is caused by limited data on normal bowel length at different ages in the normal population, difficulties in measuring bowel length, the influence of the site of resection on outcome, and the considerable individual differences in outcomes among patients with apparently similar gut lengths.[1-5] In adult patients, there is general agreement that a residual length of <200 cm of small bowel constitutes short bowel syndrome. The consequences may be considerably ameliorated by presence of the colon, a situation in which a residual length of <60 cm of small bowel may be the length at which short bowel syndrome is apparent. There is even less agreement in attempting to define short bowel syndrome in the pediatric age group. Corresponding critical residual lengths of small bowel may be <100 cm in the absence of any colon or as little as <30 cm of small bowel in the presence of colon. This widespread lack of consensus and widely varying clinical outcomes that appear to be unrelated to gut length (except at the extremes of length) suggest the logic of moving to a more functional term, such as intestinal failure rather than placing undue emphasis on an arbitrary residual gut length.

Historical surgical attempts at improving intestinal function following massive bowel resection were designed to delay intestinal transit and included vagotomy and pyloroplasty, recirculating small bowel loops, antiperistaltic gastric tubes, reversed small bowel segments, and pouch formation.[6] In a series of carefully designed animal studies, Budding and Smith observed that the simplest procedure of creating an ileal reversed segment appeared to produce the best outcome but was still associated with significant complications.[7] They made the landmark observation that "clinical application of corrective surgical procedures in the treatment of massive resection of the small intestine seems justified only when dietary and medical measures fail to keep the patient in satisfactory condition."[7] The experimental success achieved by preileal and prejejunal transposition of the colon in puppies with 90% small intestinal resection has seen only limited clinical application.[8,9] Of these historic attempts, segmental reversal of the small intestine continues to be employed in carefully selected adult patients with short bowel syndrome.[10] Further progress in the surgical management of intestinal failure awaited the momentous development of parenteral nutrition (PN) as a safe and routinely applicable technology.[11-16]

The effects of massive intestinal resection have been studied extensively by many groups.[1,17-22] Collectively, these physiological processes initiate the process of adaptation. Viewed simplistically, adaptation has a structural component that increases available surface area for nutrient absorption and, at the same time, there is a functional increase in various enzymatic and hormonal processes that increase the intestinal capacity for nutrient absorption and digestion. Though a discussion of adaptation is beyond the scope of this chapter, certain observations are noteworthy.[23]

- Over time, the residual intestine dilates and lengthens.
- Residual ileum may be more capable of adaptation than jejunum.
- The adaptive process depends on luminal nutrition, pancreatobiliary secretions, and various gut hormones and mediators.
- The time taken for adaptation is unknown but may be even longer than 2 years.

The medical management of patients with intestinal failure is complex and best undertaken by an experienced multi-disciplinary team that includes gastroenterology, nutrition, and surgical expertise early in the care to ensure optimal outcomes. Such an approach allows graded application of care. Goals of therapy evolve over time from early resuscitation to optimization of PN and enteral nutrition (EN) to prevention of complications of PN in the long term. In this multidisciplinary approach, only a small percentage of patients will require surgical intervention, and an even smaller group of patients will fail all modalities of treatment and become candidates for intestinal transplantation.

Role of the Surgeon in Management of Short Bowel Syndrome

The surgeon with an interest in intestinal failure and nutrition is a key member of the multidisciplinary team caring for the patient with intestinal failure. The role of the surgeon should not be defined purely in terms of technical problem solving. The surgeon should be responsible, ideally in partnership with a gastroenterologist, for the long-term well-being of the patient. The role of the "intestinal failure" surgeon starts from preventing the development of short bowel syndrome and continues with the provision of secure long-term venous access and employing strategies for autologous gut salvage in selected cases.

If all conservative attempts fail to prevent or reverse the occurrence of life-threatening complications of PN, such as the development of liver disease or loss of venous access, the surgeon should play a key role in determining failure and the need for intestinal transplantation. Even in this late stage of the disease, the surgeon, now working with the intestinal transplantation program, can help optimize the care of the patient to allow the best possible outcome from intestinal transplantation.

Principles of Early Surgical Management

Very little data is available on the prevention of short bowel syndrome. A high index of concern for the imminent development of short bowel syndrome, and a conservative approach to potential intestinal catastrophes, may allow prevention of intestinal failure and indeed improve outcomes in some cases.[24-30]

When the risk of development of short bowel syndrome is high, early adoption of a conservative strategy to minimize preventable loss of bowel is mandatory. A successful approach relies on preservation of all bowel of doubtful viability with planned "second-look" laparotomy, as described by Weber and colleagues.[31] The "clip and drop-back" technique, described by Grosfeld and coworkers in the presence of compromised bowel, can be used with excellent results.[28] Also, use of a silastic mesh to close the abdomen in these instances facilitates rapid re-entry into the abdomen while preserving the fascio-aponeurotic layers for subsequent closure. The mesh can also serve to provide additional abdominal domain to reduce the risks of abdominal compartment syndrome secondary to ischemia-reperfusion. In extreme instances, the entire bowel can be exteriorized in a "silo" fashioned from a silastic sheet, allowing edematous bowel to gradually return into the peritoneal cavity, mainly under the influence of gravity.

Irrespective of etiology, once the patient is adequately resuscitated and stabilized, the surgical priority becomes restoration of intestinal continuity. Recruitment of distal unused intestine often facilitates reabsorption and is an important first step towards adaptation. Prevention of disuse mucosal atrophy with restoration of luminal flow and of trophic factors is an important prerequisite for the process. There is growing appreciation of the colon's ability to salvage undigested carbohydrates by bacterial breakdown into short chain fatty acids that can directly enter the portal circulation as energy sources (Chapter 23). This author believes that stomas should be avoided if possible in patients with short bowel syndrome.

Apart from the loss of bowel length inherent in creation (and reversal) of any stoma, clinical experience suggests that patients with difficult-to-manage and poorly placed stomas may be at significant additional risk of catheter-related infections while on long-term PN (Chapter 38). Proximity of the catheter to the stoma site may play a role. Disadvantages and complications of early stoma closure are few but deserve attention. Unreabsorbed bile salts in the colon may stimulate an osmotic diarrhea with severe perineal irritation that requires meticulous skin protection. Nevertheless, barring patients with high end jejunostomies and/or those with no distal bowel other than rectosigmoid, as well as patients with functional disorders such as congenital pseudo-obstruction, closure of any preexisting stomas as an important early step in the overall surgical management.

Definitive Surgical Management

Surgical options in long-term patients with short bowel syndrome fall into four general categories of procedures: 1) to correct slow transit, 2) to improve intestinal motility (dilated bowel), 3) to slow intestinal transit (no bowel dilatation), and 4) to increase mucusal surface area (Table 31-1).

Correcting Slow Transit

Occurrence of slow intestinal transit in patients with short bowel syndrome is uncommon and should prompt

TABLE 31-1.

Four General Categories of Surgical Options in Long-Term Patients With Short Bowel Syndrome

1. Operations to correct slow transit
2. Operations to improve intestinal motility (dilated bowel)
   a. Imbrication
   b. Tapering enteroplasty
   c. Longitudinal intestinal lengthening and tailoring (Bianchi)[32,33]
   d. Transverse intestinal lengthening (Kimura and Georgeson)[34,35]
   e. STEP procedure
3. Operations to slow intestinal transit (no bowel dilatation)
   a. Valves
   b. Reversed segments
   c. Colon interposition
4. Operations to increase mucosal surface area
   a. Creation of neomucosa
   b. Sequential intestinal lengthening

a search for strictures, adhesions, and blind loops that are causing partial obstruction. These are usually left over from the original underlying disease, such as necrotizing enterocolitis or Crohn's disease, and should be treated expeditiously. On rare occasions, prior unsuspected pathology (eg, duodenal webs and missed entero-enteric fistulas) may be the cause, successful treatment of which allows a favorable outcome in patients with short bowel syndrome.

Improving Intestinal Motility

Rapid intestinal transit occurs more frequently in patients with short bowel syndrome. Rapid transit may be a result of inappropriate EN, extremely short length of bowel, or small intestine bacterial overgrowth (SIBO) (Chapter 23). Persistent rapid transit with increased stool losses should prompt investigation to rule out potential structural causes for the rapid transit. These are manifest most often by segmental bowel dilatation. Dilated bowel segments exhibit poor antegrade peristalsis. Such dilated segments may result in significant stasis of intestinal content, leading to SIBO, which, in turn, leads to rapid transit.[36] Hard evidence for bacterial overgrowth and episodic translocation in this setting is lacking. Nevertheless, it is the author's practice to attempt gut decontamination when dealing with rapid intestinal transit in a patient with short bowel syndrome. The demonstration of a dilated segment of bowel in such a patient usually indicates likely failure of medical treatment and the need for surgical intervention. It must be emphasized that the indication for surgery is the failure of medical treatment in a patient with a significantly dilated segment of small bowel; the demonstration of bowel dilatation per se in a patient who is advancing satisfactorily towards enteral autonomy from TPN and is free of complications is in itself not an indication for surgical intervention.

The choice of surgical procedure to tackle the dilated bowel segment in the patient with intestinal failure requires careful judgment. The simplest expedient of resecting the dilated segment is applicable only in the rare instance in which bowel length is demonstrably not an issue with enteral autonomy, having been achieved easily in a patient with adequate remnant bowel length and a very limited segment of dilated bowel. More often, the difficult choice rests between a simpler tapering procedure or a procedure that combines tapering with some potential gain in length.

De Lorimier and Harrison first described an intestinal plication technique that achieved the goal of creating a narrower and, therefore it was hoped, a more streamlined and propulsive loop of bowel without any loss of mucosal surface area.[37] They achieved these twin objectives by simple in-folding of the dilated loop of bowel and suturing adjacent sero-muscular surfaces.[37] Unfortunately, though the operation is effective in the short term, the plication is prone to partial or complete breakdown with recurrence of the dilatation and its attendant complications. Tapering enteroplasty as performed by this author usually consists of removal of a portion of the dilated bowel along the antimesenteric border, leaving behind a segment that is of normal caliber.

Care must be taken to avoid excessive narrowing of the residual bowel with a resultant stricture. If there is any concern, a small enterotomy allows passage of a wide-bore tube (eg, 24 Fr in a neonate), with tapering of the bowel around the tube to ensure a satisfactory remnant lumen. This is usually not necessary, and placement of stay sutures along the antimesenteric border prior to the actual tapering allows visual estimation of the lumen to be left behind. Tapering can be done simply and swiftly with repeated firings of a linear mechanical stapling device incorporating a cutting blade, with additional hand-sewn imbrication of the staple line along the antimesenteric border, if desired.

The Longitudinal Intestinal Lengthening and Tailoring (LILT) procedure, first described by Adrian Bianchi in 1980, is based on the principle that the mesenteric blood supply of the bowel can be separated into two layers, with vessels alternately being allocated to opposite surfaces.[32,33] Development of an avascular window in the mesenteric border of a dilated bowel loop between the two leaves of the mesentery and careful allocation of alternate blood vessels to either side allows division of a dilated loop of bowel longitudinally into two "hemi-loops", each with one-half of the original blood supply. Anastomosis of the two hemi-loops, end-to-end in isoperistaltic fashion in a "lazy-S" configuration, completes the operation. The actual longitudinal division of the bowel may be accomplished in relatively rapid fashion with a mechanical stapling device, dividing the hemi-loops between two double rows of staples, or the division may be carried out by hand using bipolar diathermy with fashioning of the hemi-loops by tedious hand suturing.

The author of this chapter has encountered four patients who developed hemi-loop fistulae between adjacent hemi-loops. Three of the four patients had undergone LILT (stapled technique) at different medical centers as children. The first of these was referred for isolated small bowel transplantation with recurrent life-threatening fungal infections. A dilated loop at the site of his previous LILT was caused by complete breakdown of the adjacent walls of the two hemi-loops, essentially forming a giant recirculating loop. For repair, the fistulae and adjacent staple lines were excised; the mesenteric borders were redefined, preserving the blood supply to the hemi-loops; and a hand-sewn LILT was redone. At over 18 months follow-up, the patient has achieved full enteral autonomy of PN and is free of all infections. This case has led this team to abandon the stapling technique and adopt a traditional free-hand technique in all cases on the basis that it may allow more precise visualization and protection of the mesenteric blood vessels without the additional dissection required to create the space needed for insertion of a stapling device.

Although Bianchi's own follow-up paper indicated that hemi-loop fistulae occurred in two of five study animals, this complication has not been reported until the author's recent inclusion of the above case in a larger report.[38] It is unclear whether reported failures following the Bianchi LILT procedure may, at least partially, be caused by this unrecognized complication. It is also unknown whether adoption of a freehand technique using bipolar diathermy and hand-suturing (as opposed to using a stapling device) will reduce the incidence of this complication. A modification of the Bianchi procedure has been proposed by Chahine and Ricketts, who used a single-wide tapered anastomosis, thus avoiding the need for three smaller anastomosis, as originally proposed by Bianchi.[39]

The results of the Bianchi procedure are somewhat difficult to assess and are largely in the form of individual case series. Formal studies of the physiological effects of this operation are few. In a series of experiments in dogs, Thompson et al demonstrated that LILT attenuated the normal adaptive response to intestinal resection.[40] Animals that had undergone lengthening had diminished body weight, albumin levels, and absorption, compared to those in animals that had undergone only the resection at 4 and 12 weeks of study.[40] Transit time was prolonged after lengthening—these changes appeared related to hypergastrinemia and possibly to decreased enteroglucagon and increased somatostatin levels.[40] The same group reported on their early clinical experience with the procedure in six children: overall outcome was improved in five of six children, with four of the five achieving full enteral autonomy from PN and some improvement being achieved in the 5th.[41] However, Thompson et al reported that one of the six patients died from sepsis related to an anastomotic leak and one of the five survivors had necrosis of one of the hemi-loops.[41] This early report emphasizes the potential morbidity and even mortality from the operation, related as much to the fragility of the patient population as to the procedure.

In one of the few objective studies of the procedure, Weber and Powell documented reduced stool frequency (mean of 8 preoperatively to 3 per day, 6 months after), increased transit time, and normalization of D-xylose and fat absorption after Bianchi LILT procedures in five patients.[42] Four of the five patients attained full enteral autonomy from PN by 6 months after the lengthening procedure. A follow-up report on 16 patients from the same group confirmed their early experience with objective improvements in measured aspects of bowel motility and absorption, as well as achievement of enteral autonomy from PN in 14 of the 16 patients (88%).[43]

Waag et al reported their experience with application of the procedure in 25 children with short bowel syndrome.[44] With a mean follow-up of 6 years, PN was discontinued in 17 of 18 survivors at a mean of 5.1 months after operation.[44] The authors emphasized the frequency of metabolic and septic complications occurring in this group of patients, complications which require constant vigilance and medical and nutritional treatment (Chapter 30) to achieve overall acceptable outcomes in 13 of their 18 survivors. None of the seven deaths in their series were related directly to the procedure: three were due to end-stage liver disease in association with PN, and two were due to sepsis.[44]

Spitz and coworkers reported on the problems leading to failure of the procedure in three children with very short bowel syndrome.[45] In all three cases, the authors concluded that the combination of technical problems and worsening complications of short bowel syndrome may have been reduced considerably by deferring application of the procedure to a time when the infants were bigger and normal adaptation had been completed.[45] Occurrence of hemi-loop entero-enteric fistulae appeared to be the cause of failure in the first patient in the series. We believe loss of early functional improvement following the LILT procedure must be vigorously investigated, particularly to rule out anastomotic narrowing or entero-enteric fistulae between hemi-loops. These may be hitherto under-recognized complications that lead to some of the "failures" following the procedure. Bianchi's own experience with the procedure in 20 children resulted in seven of nine survivors attaining enteral autonomy from PN at a median follow-up of 7 years.[46] In general, survivors had at least 40 cm of small bowel at the time of lengthening and had minimal or no liver disease.[46] A follow-up report (Bianchi, A: personal communication) in over 25 children indicates that the experience is sustained, with perhaps a slightly higher percentage of patients coming off PN in the longer term.

Bianchi's own experience with autologous gut salvage supports the generally accepted notion that the LILT procedure, and indeed other procedures aimed at autologous gut salvage, should not be applied in patients with any degree of PN-associated liver disease other than in its earliest stages. This author recently reported on the extended application of autologous gut salvage procedures in the era of intestinal transplantation.[38] This series included application of the Bianchi LILT procedure in four carefully selected children with advanced liver disease, all of whom had clinical evidence of portal hypertension, significant hyperbilirubinemia, and biopsy evidence of fibrosis in the liver, up to and including cirrhosis. The four participants were part of a series of patients with advanced liver disease who were aggressively treated for PN-associated liver disease with attempts at autologous gut salvage. Four of the 10 children attained full enteral autonomy from PN, and four others had significant (>50%) decrease in PN requirements. Of greatest interest, 9 of the 10 survivors in this cohort exhibited full biochemical and functional liver recovery following the procedure, as did the one patient who died from catheter-related sepsis while being close to full enteral autonomy. Twelve of the 13 children in this report were originally referred for intestinal transplantation, in isolation or combined with the liver. The presence of even advanced degrees of liver dysfunction in very carefully selected children with short bowel syndrome may not be an absolute contraindication to attempts at autologous gut salvage. This conclusion must be viewed against the fact that patients with short bowel syndrome and advanced liver disease may have a very limited window of opportunity for successful combined liver-intestinal transplantation. The needs of such a high-risk group of patients are best served by a multi-disciplinary team with expertise and experience in all aspects of management of intestinal failure and liver disease, while having rapid access to liver-intestinal transplantation.

A small percentage of patients who undergo the Bianchi procedure develop delayed dilatation of the lengthened segment with evidence of dysmotility in the dilated segment. Additionally, some patients have dilatation of only the 2nd and 3rd parts of the duodenum or very proximal jejunum. These patients are not candidates for longitudinal intestinal lengthening, in the former case because the mesentery is now reduced to a single layer and in the latter case for anatomic reasons. For this small cohort of patients, Kimura and Soper reported on a technique of transverse bowel lengthening using an isolated bowel segment.[34,35] The operation relies on developing neovascularization of the dilated segment of bowel by creating a wide myo-enteropexy and anchoring the bowel after denuding it of the sero-muscular layer on its antimesenteric aspect to the undersurface of similarly denuded liver or rectus sheath. At a second stage (about 6 weeks later), if the dilated bowel loop shows evidence of having successfully 'parasitized' itself to its neo-vascular source, the loop can be divided transversely, effectively achieving transverse intestinal lengthening and tapering. Although the isolated bowel loop appears capable of normal function, the actual situations where such novel procedures can be applied are few and far between.[35] According to the author's knowledge, less than a handful of these procedures have been applied worldwide.

Attachment of a loop of bowel to the undersurface of the abdomen also significantly complicates abdominal re-entry, which may be a consideration if a patient is failing all therapies and being considered for intestinal transplantation. With the steadily improving outcomes for intestinal transplantation, the role for such novel procedures with limited available experience and uncertain long-term benefit may be disappearing.

The recently described serial transverse enteroplasty procedure (STEP) has generated considerable interest.[47,48] In principle, lengthening of a loop of bowel is achieved by serial transverse applications of a GIA stapler, from opposite directions, to create a zig-zag channel. The authors reported their initial observations in a group of six pigs in which bowel dilatation was first accomplished by creating a reversed jejunal segment. Bowel lengthening was accomplished using the STEP enteroplasty, and the animals were studied radiologically prior to terminal examination of the bowel at 6 weeks.[47] There appeared to be a significant gain in length of bowel in animals following the procedure, and the zig-zag channel appeared to straighten out at 6 weeks. All lengthened animals gained weight. In their first case report soon after, the authors reported improved bowel function in a 2-year-old patient who had apparent "failure" of a Bianchi procedure performed at the age of 11 months, with significant dilatation of the previously lengthened segment. Bowel length was increased again by application of the novel STEP procedure, from a total of 130 cm to 200 cm. Improvement in bowel function was paralleled by some improvement without normalization of D-xylose absorption.[48]

The remarkable technical simplicity of this novel procedure in comparison to the relative complexity of the Bianchi and other lengthening procedures may explain the considerable interest it has generated including in the lay press (*New York Times*, 2003). Several groups have each performed a small number of STEP procedures. This author's experience suggests the need for caution and further study (Iyer, unpublished observations). Of five patients who have now undergone the STEP procedure in his care, one had some dilatation after a Bianchi procedure approximately 18 years ago; this patient, who was receiving approximately 50% of her caloric intake via PN, experienced no benefit from the procedure, as did one other adult patient with extremely short bowel (45 cm ending in a stoma). The third patient, who had excessive stoma losses with minimally dilated bowel, underwent the STEP and appears to have reduced ostomy losses with modest improvement in PN requirements following the procedure. The fourth patient had rapid worsening of her advanced liver disease following the STEP procedure and died from the complications of end-stage liver disease. The recent patient in this limited series has had very little, if any, improvement in his profound gastrointestinal dysmotility and enteral intolerance after the STEP procedure. This limited early experience suggests the need for further study to better understand the choice of candidates and potential contraindications for what appears to be a technically simple operation.

Slowing Intestinal Transit

The occurrence of refractory rapid intestinal transit in a patient with short bowel syndrome in the absence of bowel dilatation is particularly challenging. Nipple valves, constructed in the manner of an everted ileostomy, at the site of small bowel-colonic anastomosis have been shown to be of benefit in a small series of cases.[23] The biggest drawbacks of the technique are the fact that the optimal length of the valve is unclear: a short valve is ineffective whereas too long of a valve may cause complete intestinal obstruction, particularly if applied in a growing child. Further, constructing an optimal valve may require 8 to 10 cm of bowel in a patient who cannot afford the additional loss of length. Prosthetic valves address these concerns and require only 2 to 3 cm of bowel for their placement; however, placement may be complicated by erosion of the valve into the bowel lumen or obstruction caused by tissue reaction or prosthetic dislodgement.[23]

The potential benefit of reversed intestinal segments in management of short bowel syndrome has been referred to earlier. Panis and coworkers reported on segmental reversal of the small bowel in eight patients at the time of restoration of intestinal continuity 10. The mean length of remnant small bowel at the time of reversal was 46 ± 18 cm and the mean length of the bowel segment used for reversal was 12.7 ± 2.8 cm, with the reversed segment being distal small bowel in all but one patient. Complete mesenteric rotation was avoided by appropriate juxtaposition of the segments to be anastomosed. At a median follow-up of 35 months (range: 2 to 108 months), four patients attained full enteral autonomy from PN, with significant reduction in PN requirements in the remaining patients.[10] Unpredictable bowel growth in children makes the use of reversed segments much less reliable; although reversed loops may initially slow transit, they can cause progressive intestinal obstruction as they grow with the child.

Isoperistaltic colonic interposition to slow intestinal transit has seen only limited clinical application, perhaps because of the risk of eosinophilic colitis causing refractory bleeding.[49] Although the potential value of colonic salvage of undigested carbohydrates, converting them into SCFA, is recognized, it is unclear why a segment of colon taken out of colonic continuity and interposed in the small bowel should be of greater value than in its original anatomical position. This author believes that the procedure does not have any role in the management of short bowel syndrome in the era of intestinal transplantation.

Increasing Mucosal Surface Area

The prospect of creating neomucosa and thus truly expanding mucosal surface area has drawn extensive research over the last decade, but clinically meaningful success remains elusive.[50,51] Georgeson and coworkers have adopted a novel and perhaps more practically relevant approach toward the same goal.[52] In eight children with refractory short bowl syndrome and no signs of intestinal adaptation, dilatation of the small bowel was accomplished by creating a nipple or artificial valve. When the bowel had satisfactorily dilated, intestinal lengthening was carried out in a conventional Bianchi-type procedure. Seven of eight patients achieved a decrease in PN requirement with this sequential approach to intestinal lengthening.[23,52]

Conclusions and Future Direction

Surgical management of short bowel syndrome has evolved considerably over the last four decades, paralleling advances in PN and EN. Improvements in the understanding of the physiology of intestinal failure and adaptation have contributed to the improvement in outcomes. There is a growing realization that indications for surgical intervention in this high-risk patient population are, for the most part, related to failure of nutritional and medical treatment or to onset of complications. A challenge for the future is to better define the position and timing of potentially risky surgical intervention aimed at improving existing gut length or function, weighed against early referral for intestinal transplantation, with the prospects of improved post-transplantation outcomes. Perhaps the best answer is in intestinal transplantation programs working alongside intestinal rehabilitation programs, providing a whole range of expertise: from nutritional and medical intervention to autologous intestinal reconstruction and intestinal transplantation. Patients with intestinal failure will then have specific therapy directed to their disease state rather than having to find different centers offering one or the other but not providing seamless and comprehensive therapy. These comprehensive Intestinal Failure/Rehabilitation Centers may be the practical solution to improved outcomes for the patient with short bowel syndrome, while patients await clinically meaningful advances in creating neomucosa and tissue engineered bowel. Additionally, pre-emptive intestinal transplantation before failure of PN therapy for the patient with intestinal failure may soon become a practical reality based on improving outcomes, analogous to pre-emptive kidney transplantation for the patient with renal failure. Intestinal transplantation may soon become the standard of care for the patient with short bowel syndrome, perhaps even preemptively replacing PN in carefully selected cases.

References

1. Alpers D. How adaptable is the intestine in patients with short-bowel syndrome. *Am J Clin Nutr.* 2002;75:787-788.
2. Nightingale JM, Bartram C, Lennnard-Jones JE. Length of residual bowel after partial resection: correlation between radiographic and surgical measurements. *Gastrointest Radiol.* 1991;16:305-306.
3. Sondheimer JM, Cadnapaphornchai M, Sontag M, Zerbe GO. Predicting the duration of dependence on parenteral nutrition after neonatal intestinal resection. *J Pediatr.* 1998;132:80-84.
4. Messing B, Crenn P, Beau P, Boutron-Ruault MC, Rambaud JC, Matuchansky C. Long-term survival and parenteral nutrition dependence in adult patients with the short bowel syndrome. *Gastroenterology.* 1999;117:1043-1050.
5. Touloukian RJ, Walker-Smith GJ. Normal intestinal length in preterm infants. *J Pediatr Surg.* 1983;18:720-723.
6. Cywes S. The surgical management of massive bowel resection. *J Pediatr Surg.* 1968;3:740-748.
7. Budding J, Smith C. Role of recirculating loops in the management of massive resection of the small intestine. *Surg Gyn Obst.* 1967;125:243-249.
8. Hutcher NE, Salzberg AM. Pre-ileal transposition of colon to prevent the development of short bowel sndrome in puppies with 90 percent small intestinal resection. *Surgery.* 1971;70:189-197.
9. Hutcher NE, Mendez-Picon G, Salzberg AM. Prejejunal transposition of colon to prevent the development of short bowel syndrome in puppies with 90 per cent small intestine resection. *J Pediatr Surg.* 1973;8:771-777.
10. Panis Y, Messing B, Rivet P, et al. Segmental reversal of the small bowel as an alternative to intestinal transplantation in patients with short bowel syndrome. *Ann Surg.* 1997;225:401-407.

11. Wilmore DW, Dudrick SJ. Growth and development of an infant receiving all nutrients exclusively by vein. *JAMA.* 1968;203:860-864.
12. Wilmore DW, Dudrick SJ. Safe long-term venous catheterization. *Arch Surg.* 1969;98:256-258.
13. Wilmore DW, Groff DB, Bishop HC, Dudrick SJ. Total parenteral nutrition in infants with catastrophic gastrointestinal anomalies. *J Pediatr Surg.* 1969;4:181-189.
14. Dudrick SJ, Wilmore DW, Vars HM, Rhoads JE. Long-term parenteral nutrition with growth, development, and positive nitrogen balance. *Surgery.* 1968;64:134-142.
15. Dudrick SJ, Wilmore DW, Vars HM, Rhoads JE. Can intravenous feeding as the sole means of nutrition support growth in the child and restore weight loss in an adult? An affirmative answer. *Ann Surg.* 1969;169:974-984.
16. Dudrick SJ, Groff DB, Wilmore DW. Long term venous catheterization in infants. *Surg Gyn Obst.* 1969;129:805-808.
17. Hanson WR, Osborne JW, Sharp JG. Compensation by the residual intestine after intestinal resection in the rat; I: influence of amount of tissue removed. *Gastroenterology.* 1977;72:692-700.
18. Hanson WR, Osborne JW, Sharp JG. Compensation by the residual intestine after intestinal resection in the rat; II: influence of postoperative time interval. *Gastroenterology.* 1977;72:701-705.
19. Kurkchubasche AG, Rowe MI, Smith SD. Adaptation in short bowel syndrome: reassessing old limits. *J Pediatr Surg.* 1993;28:1069-1071.
20. Wilmore DW, Dudrick SJ, Daly JM, Vars HM. The role of nutrition in the adaptation of the small intestine after massive resection. *Surg Gyn Obst.* 1971;132:673-680.
21. Wilmore DW, Dudrick SJ. Effects of nutrition on intestinal adaptation following massive small bowel resection. *Surg Forum.* 1969;20:398-400.
22. Quigley EM, Thompson JS. The motor repsonse to intestinal resection: motor activity in the canine small intestine following distal resection. *Gastroenterology.* 1993;105:791-798.
23. Georgeson K. Short-bowel syndrome. In: O'Neill Jr J, ed. *Pediatric Surgery.* 5th ed. St Louis, Mo: Mosby-Year Book Inc; 1998:1223-1232.
24. Di Abriola GF, De Angelis P, Dall'oglio L, DiLorenzo M. Strictureplasty: an alternative approach in long segment bowel stenosis Crohn's disease. *J Pediatr Surg.* 2003;38:814-818.
25. Dietz DW, Fazio VW, Laureti S, et al. Strictureplasty in diffuse Crohn's jejunoileitis: safe and durable. *Dis Colon Rectum.* 2002;45:764-770.
26. Kosloske AM, Jewell PF. A technique for preservation of the ileocecal valve in the neonatal short intestine. *J Pediatr Surg.* 1989;24:369-370.
27. Thompson JS, Iyer KR, DiBaise JK, Young RL, Brown CR, Langnas AN. Short bowel syndrome and Crohn's disease. *J Gastrointest Surg.* 2003;7:1069-1072.
28. Vaughan WG, Grosfeld JL, West K, Schere LR III, Villamizar E, Rescorla FJ. Avoidance of stomas and delayed anastomosis for bowel necrosis: the 'clip and drop-back' technique. *J Pediatr Surg.* 1996;31:542-545.
29. Moore T. Management of midgut volvulus with extensive necrosis by "patch, drain and wait". *Ped Surg Int.* 1991;6:313-317.
30. Moore T. Management of nnecrotizing enterocolitis by "patch, drain and wait". *Pediatr Surg Int.* 1989;4:110-113.
31. Weber TR, Lewis JE. The role of second-look laparotomy in necrotizing enterocolitis. *J Pediatr Surg.* 1986;21:323-325.
32. Bianchi A. Intestinal lengthening: an experimental and clinical review. *J R Soc Med.* 1984;77:35-41.
33. Bianchi A. Intestinal loop lengthening—a technique for increasing small intestinal length. *J Pediatr Surg.* 1980;15:145-151.
34. Bianchi A. Longitudinal intestinal lengthening and tailoring: results in 20 children. *J R Soc Med.* 1997;90:429-432.
35. Kimura K, Soper RT. Isolated bowel segment (Model 1): creation by myoenteropexy. *J Pediatr Surg.* 1990;25:512-513.
36. de Lorimier AA, Norman DA, Goodling CA, Preger L. A model for the cinefluoroscopic and manometric study of chronic intestinal obstruction. *J Pediatr Surg.* 1973;8:785-791.
37. de Lorimier AA, Harrison MR. Intestinal plication in the treatment of atresia. *J Pediatr Surg.* 1983;18:734-737.
38. Iyer KR, Horslen S, Torres C, Vanderhoof JA, Langnas AN. Functional liver recovery parallels autologous gut salvage in short bowel syndrom. *J Pediatr Surg.* 2004;39:340-344.
39. Chahine A, Ricketts R. A modification of the Bianchi Intestinal lengthening procedure with a single anastomosis. *J Pediatr Surg.* 1998;33:1292-1293.
40. Thompson JS, Quigley EM, Adrian TE. Effect of intestinal tapering and lengthening on intestinal structure and function. *Am J Surg.* 1995;169:111-119.
41. Thompson JS, Pinch LW, Murray J, Vanderhoof JA, Schultz LR. Experience with intestinal lengthening for the short-bowel syndrome. *J Pediatr Surg.* 1991;26:721-724.
42. Weber TR, Powell MA. Early improvement in intestinal function after isoperistaltic bowel lengthening. *J Pediatr Surg.* 1996;31:61-64.
44. Weber TR. Isoperistaltic bowel lengthening for short bowel syndrome in children. *Am J Surg.* 1999;178:600-604.
45. Waag KL, Hosie S, Wessel L. What do children look like after longitudinal intestinal lengthening? *Eur J Pediatr Surg.* 1998;9:260-262.
46. Huskisson L, Brereton R, Kiely E, Spitz L. Problems with intestinal lengthening. *J Pediatr Surg.* 1993;28:720-722.
46. Kimura K, Soper RT. A new bowel elongation technique for the short bowel syndrome using the isolated bowel segment Iowa models. *J Pediatr Surg.* 1993;28:792-794.
47. Kim HB, Fauza D, Garza J, Oh J-T, Nurko S, Jaksic T. Serial transverse enteroplasty (STEP): a novel bowel lengthening procedure. *J Pediatr Surg.* 2003;38:425-429.
48. Kim HB, Lee PW, Garza J, Duggan C, Fauza D, Jaksic T. Serial transverse enteroplasty for short bowel syndrome: a case report. *J Pediatr Surg.* 2003;38:881-885.
49. Glick PL, de Lorimier AA, Adzick NS, Harrison MR. Colon interposition: an adjuvant operation for short-gut syndrome. *J Pediatr Surg.* 1984;19:719-725.
50. Bianchi A, Lendon M, Ward I. Assessment of surgical techniques for neomucosal growth. *Ped Surg Int.* 1992;7:41-46.
51. Saday C, Mir E. A surgical model to increase the intestinal absorptive surface: intestinal lengthening and growing neomucosa in the same approach. *J Surg Res.* 1996;62:184-191.
52. Georgeson K, Halpin D, Figueroa R, Vincente Y, Hardin W Jr. Sequential intestinal lengthening procedures for refractory short bowel syndrome. *J Pediatr Surg.* 1994;29:316-321.

Chapter 32

INTESTINAL TRANSPLANTATION

Jonathan Fryer, MD

Introduction

Intestinal transplantation is a promising therapeutic alternative to long-term parenteral nutrition (PN) for patients with intestinal failure. The complex interactions between the intestinal graft, the recipient immune system, and the external environment have made successful transplantation a significant challenge. While outcomes with early intestinal transplant efforts were sub-optimal, recent results reveal significant improvements in graft and patient survivals. Ongoing basic research, combined with the increased clinical experience and careful selection of patients, will be necessary to overcome the remaining immunologic and physiologic barriers to long-term success with intestinal transplantation.

Historical Aspects

Intestinal transplantation was first conceptualized by Alexis Carrel at the turn of the century, as one of the many procedures that would become feasible with the development of the vascular anastomosis. In 1959, Lillihei's report on a series of intestinal transplants performed in dogs inspired the first attempt at human intestinal transplantation by Ralph Deterling in 1964. Unfortunately, this effort and several others that followed were unsuccessful because of inadequate immunosuppression. In the early 1980s, when cyclosporine's effectiveness had been established in other organ transplants, interest in intestinal transplantation was renewed. Although the first intestinal transplant using cyclosporine, performed by Cohen in Toronto, was unsuccessful,[1] other centers in France, Germany, and Canada subsequently demonstrated that successful intestinal transplantation was possible, and in the early 1990s, several intestinal transplant programs were established.[2-4] There are now over 60 centers worldwide that together have performed approximately 1000 intestinal transplants.[5]

Functional Changes After Intestinal Transplantation

Short and long-term function of small bowel (SB) grafts has been an important area of investigation. Physiologic changes unrelated to the immune response can influence SB graft function. Sarr et al reported that SB isograft transplantation has little impact on morphology, mucosal disaccharidase activity, and tissue content of regulatory proteins.[6] However, significant changes in the absorption of fluids, electrolytes, and bile salts result from the jejunoileal denervation that accompanies SB transplantation.[7,8] Functional changes can also occur because of ischemia-reperfusion[9] or acute[10] or chronic rejection.[11]

Iwanami et al looked at a D-xylose absorption, cyclosporine absorption, intestinal transit time, in vitro muscle contractility, and mucosal enzyme activity in canine SB allografts. In this study, 50% of allograft recipients survived more than 1 year and maintained comparable weights and SB function to isograft recipients and normal dogs, while the remaining recipients had to be destroyed because of progressive weight loss and malnutrition caused by significantly impaired function. Interestingly, while all allograft recipients had inflammatory changes in the submucosa and muscularis propria, only the latter group had significant mucosal pathology. These results suggest that, while occult inflammation in nonmucosal locations may be ongoing in normally functioning SB allografts, that short-term graft and recipient outcomes may be determined by the ability to control inflammation and injury in the mucosa.[12]

In the human experience, SB absorptive function has been shown to be well preserved in successful SB transplants,[13] although experimental models have shown that defects in fat absorption can exist in the early post-transplant period as intestinal lymphatics are re-established.[14] The malabsorption of immunosuppressive drugs can result in devastating rejection episodes; therefore, a SB allograft's survival depends on its absorptive function. Defects in the SB epithelial cytochrome p450 system and p-glycoprotein[15,16] have been reported and could potentially precipitate a vicious cycle of rejection-related drug malabsorption, which leads to escalating rejection.

The Immunobiology of Intestinal Transplantation

Several factors unique to SB allografts may make success more difficult to achieve with SB transplants than with other organ allografts. The SB's extensive lymphoid tissues may enhance its immunogenicity[17,18] by providing greater potential for early and extensive interaction between donor major histocompatability complex antigens[19-21] and recipient T cells. However, small animal studies have shown that most donor lymphoid cells are replaced by recipient cells within days of the transplant being performed.[22,23] Compared to isografts, this turnover of lymphoid cell populations occurs more rapidly in SB allografts and is associated with a greater increase in tissue chemokine and cytokine levels[22-24] which can augment the rejection response.[25] Conversely, persistence of donor lymphoid cell populations may reflect a donor specific hyporesponsiveness[26-28] or tolerance.

Because of the SB's large population of lymphoid cells, there is greater potential for a bidirectional exchange of cells between the SB graft and the recipient than with most other organ allografts. Whereas a host-to-graft flow of cells is predominant in most organ allografts[22,23] partial or complete repopulation of recipient immune cell populations by donor cells[26-29] has also been demonstrated and may play a role in down-regulating the allograft rejection response.[30-32] Therefore, several strategies have been utilized to manipulate the exchange of donor and recipient cells, including ablation of donor[33-35] or recipient[33,36] lymphoid cell populations by irradiation[33,34,36] or antibody therapy.[35,37-39] Recent clinical efforts have concentrated on the elimination of key recipient immune cell populations prior to transplantation using antilymphocyte antibodies[37,38] followed by use of low-dose post-transplant immunosuppression to encourage tolerogenic immune interactions between donor and recipient cells.[38,40]

The SB's coexistence with microorganisms likely contributes to the high morbidity and mortality seen after SB transplantation. Sepsis and multiorgan failure account for more than 50% of deaths after SB transplantation,[5,41] and a high percentage of the bacterial infections are caused by classic enteric bacteria.[42-44] Translocation of bacteria and bacterial products has been shown to occur in both animal models of SB transplantation[45-51] and in the clinical experience[42,52] and to correlate with septic complications.[53] Bacterial translocation and sepsis occur in association with acute rejection episodes,[50,51] ischemia-reperfusion injury,[42] graft-versus-host disease,[53] and use of immunosuppressive drugs.[47] Other factors that may contribute to bacterial translocation include transplantation of the colon,[42,54] systemic venous drainage of the intestinal graft,[47,55] post-transplant lymphoproliferative disease[43] and bacterial overgrowth.[55,56] Several parameters have been utilized to establish a correlation between early SB barrier dysfunction,[52,57] rejection, and bacterial translocation.[50,51]

In the early phases of SB allograft rejection, prior to the appearance of major histologic changes, there is a significant up-regulation of proinflammatory cytokines.[22,23,58] These proinflammatory cytokines have been shown to alter the epithelial tight junctions[59,60] that normally block paracellular egress of SB luminal antigens and bacterial products that can exacerbate SB mucosal inflammation and augment rejection by a bystander effect.[22] Preliminary data indicate that tight junction proteins and epithelial barrier function are altered in the early phases of SB allograft rejection (Jonathan Fryer, unpublished data, 2005).

Part of the reason for the high incidence of infectious complications seen with intestinal transplants is the high level of immunosuppression used to prevent SB allograft rejection. In general, the maintenance immunosuppression utilized in SB allografts exceeds that for all other solid organ allografts. Several factors may contribute to this practice, including the greater difficulty in detecting rejection in the intestine and the greater potential for lethal consequences if intestinal rejection is missed. Underlying these factors is the basic premise that the intestine is one of the most immunogenic organs used for transplantation. While few experimental studies have actually compared rejection responses between different organ allografts,[61] the cumulative clinical experience supports this premise.[5,33,35,41,62-64]

There are several reasons why the SB may have greater immunogenicity than other organ allografts. Fundamental differences seem to exist in some basic components of the rejection response in SB allografts. There is evidence to suggest that CD8+ cells assume a bigger role in SB allograft rejection than in the rejection of other allografts.[63,64] Co-stimulatory molecule interactions may also differ with SB allografts.[65-70] Blockade of tumor necrosis factor (TNF)-receptor superfamily molecule membrane lymphotoxin,[66] 4-1BB (CD137),[67] has been shown to have co-stimulatory properties that may be unique to SB allograft rejection.[71] The OX-40 (CD134) co-stimulatory pathway also appears to play a unique role in the rejection response to SB allografts.[70]

The SB has a high baseline level of proinflammatory cytokines and chemokines, and these may play a more important in SB allograft rejection than with other allografts. Both TNF and interferon (IFN)-γ induction have been shown to correlate with SB allograft rejection.[22,23,59,60] Interestingly, anti-TNF therapy has not been studied in animal models of SB allograft rejection, although it has been utilized clinically.[25] Veitch et al demonstrated

Table 32-1.

Medicare Criteria for Parenteral Nutrition Failure

1. Impending or overt liver failure
   ↑ bilirubin, ↑ liver enzymes, ↑ spleen, ↑ PT, ↑ INR, ↓ platelets
   varices, stomal bleeding, hepatic fibrosis, cirrhosis
2. Thrombosis of central veins
   ≥2 subclavian, jugular, or femoral veins
3. Frequent central line related sepsis
   ≥2 episodes per year or ≥1 if fungemia, septic shock, or ARDS
4. Frequent severe dehydration

that disruption of the IFNγ-IFNγR interaction inhibits, but does not eliminate, SB allograft rejection.[24] Elimination of donor interferon-inducible protein-10 (IP-10) inhibits the mucosal infiltration of CXCR3+ T cells and also delays but does not eliminate rejection.[23] Other cytokines may inhibit rejection. Zhu et al recently demonstrated that SB allograft recipients who were pretreated with genetically modified interleukin-10–producing dendritic cells rejected SB allografts at a rate that was significantly slower than controls.[71]

The unique properties of the intestinal epithelial cell in SB mucosal inflammation may also contribute to the SB's increased immunogenicity. The intestinal epithelium is the largest epithelial surface in the body and a primary target of the recipient immune response after SB transplantation. Early in SB allograft rejection, or after other mucosal proinflammatory stimuli, there is increased epithelial expression of HLA class-II antigens.[72,73] When activated by endotoxin or proinflammatory cytokines, intestinal epithelial cells produce TNF, thereby creating an autocrine/paracrine positive feedback loop that can lead to escalating inflammation in the SB mucosa. Furthermore, intestinal epithelial cells may function as antigen presenting cells (APCs), potentially initiating the immune response.[74] Due to the ongoing interactions between luminal antigens, epithelial cells, and GALT, the normal SB mucosa is in a constant state of low-grade "physiological" inflammation.[75] with high baseline levels of proinflammatory cytokines including IFN-γ and TNF-α.[76] SB epithelial cells have been shown to be a major source of IP-10 in the SB; therefore, the combination of high baseline levels of proinflammatory cytokines in close proximity to this large source of IP-10 predisposes the SB allograft to a vigorous rejection response.[22,23] In this proinflammatory environment, additional stimuli can trigger significant T-cell infiltration and rejection in an otherwise stable SB allograft.[22]

As rejection is mediated primarily by infiltrating T cells, mechanisms of T-cell trafficking unique to the SB may also contribute to its increased immunogenicity. Recent studies in a mouse model indicate that activated effector/memory T cells are "imprinted" to return to the gut by dendritic cells residing in the intestinal mucosa that induce high levels of α4β7 integrin on the newly activated T cell's surface.[77] Sarnacki et al found that α4β7 blockade did not prolong SB allograft survival but that blockade of another integrin, αLβ2, did.[78] Kellersman et al subsequently found that rejection could be inhibited with monoclonal antibodies to β7 integrins, although it was not inhibited in SB transplants performed using β7 integrin –/– recipients.[79] Although the results in small animal models are somewhat conflicting, the recent clinical availability of monoclonal antibodies to these integrins will likely engender their use in carefully selected clinical scenarios.

The Role of Intestinal Transplantation in Intestinal Failure Management

Prior to the development of PN, most patients with intestinal failure died of malnutrition. With the availability of PN, survival has been made possible for many. However, PN is inconvenient and expensive[80] and can be associated with life-threatening complications (Chapter 38). Patients on long-term PN have significant morbidity and mortality.[81-83] Intestinal transplantation provides a potential alternative to PN for long-term intestinal failure management.

As the early results with intestinal transplantation were suboptimal, thus far it has been used only in situations where PN therapy has failed (Medicare Coverage Policy Decisions: Intestinal and Multivisceral Transplantation, CAG-00036, October 4, 2000). Medicare has defined PN failure as the development of at least one of the following: liver failure, central vein thromboses, frequent or severe central-line–related sepsis, or recurrent dehydration (Table 32-1). Although the Medicare criteria may identify patients who are not thriving on PN, they also define a patient subset that is more likely to have a poor outcome than will other intestinal failure patients. Therefore, comparisons of outcomes in long-term PN patients with intestinal transplant recipients are flawed because candidates for intestinal transplant candidates are, by definition, sicker than other long-term PN patients. Another potential shortcoming of the current Medicare criteria is that they may identify patient subsets that have not received optimal care or that are noncompliant. These patients may not be appropriate for transplantation and some may be at higher risk for failure with any therapy.

As the results with intestinal transplant continue to improve, it would be more valid to compare long-term PN with intestinal transplantation in patient subsets in which the risk of PN failure is high. Patients with less than 50 cm of small intestine, especially those with no colon, are at extremely high risk of developing life-threatening complications, including end-stage liver disease (ESLD), within 5 years.[82,83] Because these patients do poorly with long-term PN, they are appropriate candidates for isolated intestine transplants and would be the most appropriate patient population for comparing the outcomes of long-term PN versus transplantation.

Recurrent or life-threatening central venous catheter-related sepsis is one of the Medicare criteria for PN failure. The Oley registry data indicate that, on average, PN patients were hospitalized for infectious complications approximately once per year.[84] Messing et al found intestinal failure patients on permanent PN have a high mortality rate (>50%, with median follow-up of 64 months), with 31% of deaths attributable to sepsis.[82] In this series, the central venous catheter was clearly identified as the source of sepsis in 50% of septic deaths. It is not always possible to determine whether poor technique and/or compliance are responsible for catheter-related sepsis; therefore, these patients should not automatically be labeled as noncompliant. Bacterial translocation of gastrointestinal (GI) organisms may also contribute to catheter sepsis, despite good catheter technique.[85] Even programs that have reported low infection rates have some individual patients who experience very high rates of infection.[86]

Liver failure (Chapter 20) is another Medicare criterion for PN failure. Liver abnormalities are a recognized complication in long-term PN patients. PN patients who develop ESLD have an extremely high mortality and most die within 2 years.[81] In these circumstances, a combined intestine/liver transplant may be the only option. Although in carefully selected patients, transplanting the liver alone can be successful,[87] transplanting only the intestine in the setting of ESLD is likely to yield poor results. Unfortunately, the stage at which the hepatic pathological process has progressed to the point where an intestine-only transplant is doomed to fail has not been clearly defined. Outcomes data for intestine-only transplant recipients stratified by the stage of their pretransplant liver pathology are needed.

Nontransplant Alternatives for Intestinal Failure Patients

Significant interest exists in developing nonsurgical strategies to eliminate long-term PN dependence. While the shortened small intestine undergoes significant adaptation without intervention, several therapies may augment and/or accelerate this process. Recombinant human growth hormone has recently been approved by the FDA for use in short bowel syndrome. While early clinical studies have produced conflicting results,[88,89] growth hormone appears to augment the short gut's ability to absorb luminal nutrients and therefore reduces PN requirements in short gut patients.[90,91] Animal studies with glucagon-like peptide-2 suggest its potential may exceed that of growth hormone,[92] although only preliminary clinical data are available.[93] Other promising strategies are being evaluated to reduce the complications associated with long-term PN use. Early studies suggest that PN-associated liver disease may be reduced by supplementation of choline.[94]

In some carefully selected patients, surgical procedures other than intestinal transplant can be beneficial to patients with short-gut syndrome.[95] Surgical procedures to reestablish intestinal continuity can benefit short bowel syndrome patients by enhancing conditions for enteral feeding, thereby optimizing nutrient absorption by the residual small intestine. If the colon is in continuity, it enhances absorption of fluid and electrolytes, salvages carbohydrate calories,[96] reduces the risk of ESLD, and prolongs survival in short-gut syndrome patients.[83] Other surgical procedures attempting to lengthen the intestine[97] or decrease intestinal transit time[95] have not been shown to be safe or effective enough for routine use, although they may be helpful in individual situations. These options are discussed in detail in Chapter 31.

Types of Intestinal Transplant Required

Intestinal failure patients who have not developed irreversible liver disease usually require intestine-only transplants. Unfortunately, most patients are not referred for transplant evaluation until they have already developed irreversible liver disease.[5,41,98] In these circumstances, a combined liver-intestine transplant is required. While there is little dispute about the need for intestinal transplantation in these patients, outcomes reveal that most are beyond the point of salvage when referred at this stage, and most do not make it to transplant. The waiting-list mortality in patients requiring combined liver-intestine transplants greatly exceeds that for all other organ transplant recipients, including those for intestine only and liver only.[98,99] Furthermore, outcomes in those patients who do survive to receive a combined transplant are also inferior to all other organ transplant recipients, including those receiving an intestine only.[5,99]

Multivisceral transplants are performed in a small number of intestinal transplant candidates, primarily those with diffuse motility disorders. Generally, these grafts include the stomach, duodenum, and pancreas in addition to the intestine and liver, although numerous variations to this combination also occur. Multivisceral transplants are most commonly performed in patients who have diffuse GI motility disorders (GI motility is discussed in Chapter 23) or in other situations in which replacement of multiple GI organs is indicated. Because the extrinsic denervation associated with graft procurement also results in dysmotility, it is not yet clear in patients with motility disorders whether

TABLE 32-2.

Survival After Intestinal Transplantation*

Survival	Organs	3 months	1 year	3 years
Graft	Intestine only	86.8%	71.8%	43.6%
Graft	Liver-intestine	68.5%	56.1%	39.2%
Patient	Intestine only	88.6%	79.1%	73.1%
Patient	Liver-intestine	73.3%	60.0%	39.2%

*2003 Annual Report of the US Scientific Registry of Transplant Recipients and The Organ Procurement and Transplantation Network. Transplant data 1990-2002. US Department of Health and Human Services, Health Resources and Services Administration, Office of Special Programs, Division of Transplantation, Rockville, MD; United Network of Organ Sharing, Richmond, VA.

the replaced stomach and duodenum of a multivisceral graft has more effective motility post-transplant than the retained, native stomach and duodenum in transplant recipients who do not receive these additional organs. Furthermore, many patients who require combined liver and intestine transplants receive a graft that also includes the pancreas, as this allows preservation of the graft bile duct. Unfortunately, in many reports, it is not always clear if these grafts are included as liver-intestine grafts or as multivisceral grafts. This unfortunately introduces confusion to any interpretation of outcomes in multivisceral transplant recipients.

Outcomes With Intestinal Transplantation

Approximately 1000 transplants have been performed since 1985 in over 60 centers worldwide.[5,41] The total number of intestine transplants performed per year has exceeded 100 only since 2001. Gender distribution has been equal, with 54% of transplants being performed in males and 46% in females. Over 60% of transplants have been performed in patients younger than 18 years of age. The primary diseases responsible for the patients' needs for intestinal transplants are diverse. In children, volvulus, gastroschisis, necrotizing enterocolitis, intestinal atresia, aganglionosis, and pseudo-obstruction account for 75% of intestinal transplant patients. In adults, ischemia, Crohn's, trauma, volvulus, and desmoid tumors account for 63%.[5,41]

The majority of intestinal transplants performed thus far have also required livers. Because the results with liver-intestine transplants are inferior to intestine-only transplants, these data suggest that intestine-transplant candidates are being referred late. This appears to be particularly evident in the pediatric population, in which only 36% of recipients received isolated intestines compared with 52% of the adult recipients. Most pediatric recipients undergo liver-intestine transplants (56%), whereas this is less common with adult recipients (25%). Thus far, multivisceral transplants have been performed less commonly in pediatric (8%) compared with adult (23%) recipients.[4,41]

Intestinal transplant survivors who are beyond 10 years post-transplant are accumulating, with the longest survivor now approaching 15 years post-transplant.[5] The majority of transplants (75.5%) have been performed in the United States,[5] and the US' experience in graft and patient survival are presented in Table 32-2. The disparity between graft and patient survivals for intestine-only transplants reflects the ability to remove the intestine graft, if necessary, when patient survival is threatened. The most common indications for graft removal have been rejection (57%), thrombosis/ischemia or bleeding (20.7%), and sepsis (6.6%). With combined liver-intestine transplants, complete graft removal is uncommon because a replacement graft is required. Therefore, graft survival closely correlates well with patient survival in this subset. The most common causes of death in transplant recipients have been sepsis (46.0%), rejection (11.2%), technical problems (6.2%), and lymphoma (6.2%).[5,41] A factor that likely contributes to the inferior patient survival with combined liver-intestine transplants is the fact that these patients are much sicker patients going into their transplants. This is supported by the much higher waiting list mortality in patients awaiting combined liver-intestine transplants.[98]

Although most intestinal transplants have been performed using deceased donors, living donors have also been utilized. While the small numbers performed preclude robust statistical analysis, recipient outcomes appear no different whether deceased or living donors are used.[5,41] Theoretically, living donors may provide advantages to the recipient by reducing waiting times, facilitating human leukocyte antigen matching, and minimizing ischemic times, although this has yet to be confirmed. Furthermore, long-term postoperative morbidity in living intestine donors needs to evaluated closely to warrant its wider application.

The early post-transplant phase is often difficult with intestine transplant recipients, and close surveillance is necessary to preempt or promptly intervene with potentially disastrous complications, such as rejection and infection. Consequently, hospital stays have been quite long following intestinal transplants and the median stays for intestine-only and combined liver-intestine transplants are 42 and 51 days, respectively. Following discharge, intestine transplant patients have required a median of two readmissions. One common reason for readmission is rejection, and the incidence of rejection is 57% with intestine only grafts and 39% with combined liver-intestine grafts. These results suggest that the liver may protect the intestine graft from rejection. Because of the high incidence of rejection, the difficulty in diagnosing rejection early, and the life-threatening consequences associated with unrecognized rejection, intestine-transplant recipients generally receive more immunosuppression than other transplant recipients. This higher level of immunosuppression with intestinal transplantation likely contributes to the higher incidence of post-transplant lymphoproliferative disorders (PTLDs). Because of the high frequency of Epstein-Barr virus naivety in pediatric recipients, PTLDs are more prevalent in the pediatric intestinal-recipient population, where they are seen in 11.1% of intestine only, 10.4% of liver-intestine, and 18.6% of multivisceral transplants,[5,41] compared with 3.4%, 2.9%, and 6.0%, respectively, in the adult population.

At 6 months post-transplant, over 80% of surviving intestinal transplant recipients are PN-free, which indicates that successful intestinal transplants are effective in eliminating PN dependence. With regard to quality of life, over 80% of successful recipients are functioning at normal levels when evaluated at 6 months post-transplant using the Karnofsky performance score.[5,41]

The overall outcomes with intestinal transplants have improved significantly as the experience has accumulated.[5,41] Several variables clearly influence outcomes, and careful patient selection is clearly important. Graft survival is significantly better in transplants performed in recipients who are outpatients compared with those who are hospitalized at the time transplant (P <0.02). This supports the premise that late referral of sicker patients results in inferior outcomes. Probably as a consequence of this data, patient selection criteria have changed since 2001, with the ratio of outpatients to inpatients undergoing intestinal transplants increasing from approximately 1:1 to 2.5:1. As with other organ transplants, retransplantation is associated with inferior results. Although retransplantation can be successful, graft survival is significantly better in first transplants compared with retransplants (P <0.0001). Finally, immunosuppressive protocols appear to influence graft survival. Induction with some polyclonal (antilymphocyte) or monoclonal (anti-IL2R) antibody preparations followed by maintenance immunosuppression using FK506 has been associated with better outcomes (P <0.003).

Several variables have also been associated with better patient survival. Patient survival is better in recipients who are brought in as outpatients compared with those who are hospitalized (P = 0.0006), as stated earlier. The experience of the center in which the transplant is performed also appears to influence patient survival (P = 0.0118), although this does not appear to be true when the U.S. experience is evaluated independently.[99] Finally, induction with polyclonal (antilymphocyte) or monoclonal (anti-IL2R) antibody preparations combined with FK506 maintenance has been associated with improved patient survival (P <0.02).

In summary, intestinal transplantation is complex, and a better understanding of its unique immunologic and physiologic issues will be necessary to achieve outcomes that are comparable to other organ allografts. In the long-term management of intestinal failure patients, the ultimate role of intestinal transplantation will be determined by its success compared to other available medical and surgical options. Currently, patients are considered for transplant only when life-threatening complications associated with PN failure have already developed. Because many patients who fail PN are too sick to be rescued by transplantation, it will ultimately be more appropriate to consider transplantation in the intestinal failure candidates who are at highest risk for PN failure, so they can be transplanted before they become unsalvageable.

References

1. Cohen Z, Silverman RE, Wassef R, et al. Small intestinal transplantation using cyclosporine. Report of a case. *Transplantation.* 1986;42(6):613-621.
2. Goulet OJ, Revillon Y, Cerf-Bensussan N, et al. Small intestinal transplantation in a child using cyclosporine. *Transplant Proc.* 1988;20(3 [Suppl 3]):288-296.
3. Deltz E, Schroeder P, Gebhardt H, et al. First successful clinical small intestine transplantation. *Tactics and Surgical Technic Chirurg.* 1989;60(4):235-239.
4. Grant D, Wall W, Mimeault R, et al. Successful small-bowel/liver transplantation. *Lancet.* 1990;335(8683):181-184.
5. Sarr MG, Siadati MR, Bailey J, Lucas DL, Roddy DR, Duenes JA. Neural isolation of the jejunoileum. Effect on tissue morphometry, mucosal disaccharidase activity, and tissue peptide content. *J Surg Res.* 1996;61(2):416-424.
6. Herkes SM, Smith CD, Sarr MG. Jejunal responses to absorptive and secretory stimuli in the neurally isolated jejunum in vivo. *Surgery.* 1994;116:576-586.
7. Oishi AJ, Sarr MG. Intestinal transplantation: effects on ileal enteric absorptive physiology. *Surgery.* 1995;117:545-553.
8. Yagmurdur MC, Ozdemir A, Ozenc A, Kiline K. The effects of alpha-tocopherol and verapamil on mucosal functions after gut ischemia/reperfusion. *Turk J Gastroenterol.* 2003;14(1):26-32.
9. Klaus A, Weiss H, Nguyen JH, et al. Histamine-degrading enzymes as cellular markers of acute small bowel allograft rejection. *Transpl Int.* 2003;16(8):474.
10. Pakarinen MP, Kuusanmaki P, Lauronen J, Paavonen T, Halttunen J. Effects of ileum transplantation and chronic rejection on absorption and synthesis of cholesterol in pigs. *Pediatr Surg Int.* 2003;19(9-10):656-661.
11. Iwanami K, Ishikawa T, Nalesnik M, et al. Long-term function and morphology of intestinal autografts and allografts in outbred dogs. *Am J Transplant.* 2003;3(9):1083-1090.
12. Kim J, Fryer J, Craig RM. Absorptive function following small intestinal transplantation. *Dig Dis Sci.* 1998;43(9):1925-1930.
13. Winkelaar GB, Smith LJ, Martin GR, Sigalet DL. Fat absorption after small intestinal transplantation in the rat. *Transplantation.* 1997;64(4):566-571.
14. Kaplan B, Lown K, Craig R, et al. Low bioavailability of cyclosporine microemulsion and tacrolimus in a small bowel transplant recipient: possible relationship to intestinal P-glycoprotein activity. *Transplantation.* 1999;67(2):333-335.
15. Masuda S, Uemoto S, Hashida T, Inomata Y, Tanaka K, Inui K. Effect of intestinal P-glycoprotein on daily tacrolimus trough level in a living-donor small bowel recipient. *Clin Pharmacol Ther.* 2000;68(1):98-103.
16. Frezza EE, Gerunda GE, Fassina A, et al. NK activity during graft-versus-host disease and graft rejection in rats following intestinal semiallogenic and allogenic transplantation with or without mesenteric lymphadenectomy. *Transplantation.* 1994;58(6):698-701.
17. Zhang Z, Zhu L, Quan D, et al. Pattern of liver, kidney, heart, and intestine allograft rejection in different mouse strain combinations. *Transplantation.* 1996;62:1267-1272.
18. Fromont G, Cerf-Bensussan N, Patey N, et al. Small bowel transplantation in children: an immunohistochemical study of intestinal grafts. *Gut.* 1995;37(6):783-790.

19. Cagiannos C, Zhong R, Zang Z, et al. Effect of major histocompatibility complex expression on murine intestinal graft survival. *Transplantation.* 1998;66(10):1369-1374.
20. He G, Hart J, Kim OS, et al. The role of CD8 and CD4 T cells in intestinal allograft rejection: a comparison of monoclonal antibody-treated and knockout mice. *Transplantation.* 1999;67(1):131-137.
21. Zhang Z, Kaptanoglu L, Haddad W, et al. Donor T cell activation initiates small bowel allograft rejection through and IFN-gamma-inducible protein-10-dependent mechanism. *J Immunol.* 2002;168(7):3205-3212.
22. Zhang Z, Kaptanoglu L, Tang Y, et al. IP-10-induced recruitment of CXCR3 host T cells is required for small bowel allograft rejection. *Gastroenterology.* 2004;126(3):809-818.
23. Veitch AM, Higgins LM, Bajaj-Elliot M, Farthing MJG, Macdonald TT. Impaired rejection and mucosal injury of small intestinal allografts lacking the interferon-γ receptor. *Int J Exp Path.* 2003;84:107-113.
24. Pascher A, Radke C, Dignass A, et al. Successful infliximab treatment of steroid and OKT3 refractory acute cellular rejection in two patients after intestinal transplantation. *Transplantation.* 2003;76(3):615-618.
25. Gilroy RK, Coccia PF, Talmadge JE, et al. Donor immune reconstitution after liver-small bowel transplantation for multiple intestinal atresia with immunodeficiency. *Blood.* 2004;103(3):1171-1174.
26. Inoue S, Tahara K, Kaneko T, et al. Long-lasting donor passenger leukocytes after hepatic and intestinal transplantation in rats. *Transpl Immunol.* 2004;12(2):123-131.
27. Loffeler S, Meyer D, Otto C, et al. Different kinetics of donor cell populations after isolated liver and combined liver/small bowel transplantation. *Transpl Int.* 2000;13(Suppl 1):S537-S540.
28. Tryphonopoulos P, Icardi M, Salgar S, et al. Host derived enterocytes in intestinal grafts. *Transplantation.* 2002;74(1):120-138.
29. Starzl TE, Zinkernagel RM. Transplantation tolerance from a historical perspective. *Nat Rev Immunol.* 2002;1:233-239.
30. Starzl TE, Demetris AJ, Murase N, Trucco M, Thomson AW, Rao AS. The lost chord: microchimerism and allograft survival. *Immunol Today.* 1996;17:577-584.
31. Orloff SL, Yin Q, Corless CL, Orloff MS, Rabkin JM, Wagner CR. Tolerance induced by bone marrow chimerism prevents transplant vascular sclerosis in a rat model of small bowel transplant chronic rejection. *Transplantation.* 2000;69(7):1295-1303.
32. Abu-Elmagd K, Reyes J, Todo S, et al. Clinical intestinal transplantation: new perspectives and immunologic considerations. *J Am Coll Surg.* 1998;186:512-525.
33. Murase N, Ye Q, Nalesnik MA, et al. Immunomodulation for intestinal transplantation by allograft irradiation, adjunct donor bone marrow infusion, or both. *Transplantation.* 2000;70:1632-1641.
34. Sudan DL, Kaufman SS, Shaw BW Jr, et al. Isolated intestinal transplantation for intestinal failure. *Am J Gastroenterol.* 2000;95(6):1506-1515.
35. Bakonyi A, Berho M, Ruiz P, et al. Donor and recipient pre-transplant conditioning with non lethal irradiation and antilymphocyte serum improves the grafts survival in a rat small bowel transplant model. *Transplantation.* 2001;72:983-988.
36. Tzakis AG, Kato T, Nishida S, et al. Alemtuzumab (Campath-1H) combined with tacrolimus in intestinal and multivisceral transplantation. *Transplantation.* 2003;75(9):1512-1517.
37. Starzl TE, Murase N, Abu-Elmagd K, et al. Tolerogenic immunosuppression for organ transplantation. *Lancet.* 2003;361(9368):1502-1510.
38. Abu-Elmagd K, Reyes J, Bond G, et al. Clinical intestinal transplantation: a decade of experiences at a single center. *Ann Surg.* 2001;234(3):404-416.
39. Koshiba T, Kitade H, Waer M, et al. Break of tolerance via donor-specific blood transfusion by high doses of steroids: a differential effect after intestinal transplantation and heart transplantation. *Transplant Proc.* 2003;35(8):3153-3155.
40. Grant D. Intestinal transplantation: 1997 Report of the International Registry. *Transplantation.* 1999;67(7):1061-1064.
41. Cicalese L, Sileri P, Green M, Abu-Elmagd K, Kocoshis S, Reyes J. Bacterial translocation in clinical intestinal transplantation. *Transplantation.* 2001;71(10):1414-1417.
42. Sigurdsson L, Reyes J, Kocoshis SA, et al. Bacteremia after intestinal transplantation in children correlate temporarily with rejection or gastrointestinal lymphoproliferative disease. *Transplantation.* 2000;70(2):302.
43. Loinaz C, Kato T, Nishida S, et al. Bacterial infections after intestine and multivisceral transplantation. *Tranplant Proc.* 2003;35(5);1929-1930.
44. Li XC, Zhong R, Quan D, et al. Endotoxin in the peripheral blood during acute intestinal allograft rejection. *Transpl Int.* 1994;7(3):223-226.
45. Cooke KR, Olkiewicz K, Erikson N, Ferrara SL. The role of endotoxin and the innate immune response in the pathophysiology of acute graft versus host disease. *J Endotoxin Res.* 2002;8(6):441-448.
46. Fryer JP, Kim S, Wells CL, et al. Bacterial translocation in a large animal model of small bowel transplantation. Portal vs systemic venous drainage and the effect of tacrolimus immunosuppression. *Arch Surg.* 1996;131(1):77-84.
47. Fryer J, Grant D, Jiang J, et al. Influence of macrophage depletion on bacterial translocation and rejection in small bowel transplantation. *Transplantation.* 1996;62(5):553-559.
48. Gianotti L, Bergamo C, Braga M, et al. In vivo evaluation of timing, degree, and distribution of bacterial translocation following experimental small bowel transplantation. *Transplantation.* 1995;60(9):891-896.
49. Grant D, Hurlbut D, Zhong R, et al. Intestinal permeability and bacterial translocation following small bowel transplantation in the rat. *Transplantation.* 1991;52(2):221-224.
50. Hurlbut D, Zhong R, Wang P, et al. Intestinal permeability and bacterial translocation following orthotopic intestinal transplantation in the rat. *Transplant Proc.* 1990;22(6):2451.
51. Watson CJ, Wraight EP, Neale G, et al. Radionuclide studies in intestinal transplantation. Diagnosis of rejection and assessment of permeability. *Transplantation.* 1996;61(1):155-157.
52. Price BA, Cumberland NS, Clark CL, Pockley AG, Lear PA, Wood RF. The effect of rejection and graft-versus-host disease on small intestinal microflora and bacterial translocation after rat small bowel transplantation. *Transplantation.* 1993;56(5):1072-1076.
53. Todo S, Tzakis A, Reyes J, et al. Small intestinal transplantation in humans with or without the colon. *Transplantation.* 1994;57(6):840.
54. Berney T, Kato T, Nishida S, et al. Portal versus systemic drainage of small bowel allografts: comparative assessment of survival, function, rejection, and bacterial translocation. *J Am Coll Surg.* 2002;195(6):804-848.
55. Deitch EA, Kemper AC, Specian RD, Berg RD. A study of the relationship among survival, gut-origin sepsis, and bacterial translocation in a model of systemic inflammation. *J Trauma.* 1992;32(2):141-147.
56. Grant D, Lamont D, Zhang R, et al. 51Cr-EDTA: a marker of early intestinal rejection in the rat. *J Surg Res.* 1989;46(5):507-514.
57. Quan D, Grant DR, Zhang RZ, et al. Altered gene expression of cytokine, ICAM-1, and class II molecules precedes mouse intestinal allograft rejection. *Transplantation.* 1994;58(7):808-816.
58. Poritz L, Garver KI, Tilberg AF, Koltun WA. Tumor necrosis factor alpha disrupts tight junction assembly. *J Surg Res.* 2004;116:14-18.
59. Ma TY, Iwamoto GK, Hoa NT, et al. TNF-alpha-induced increase in intestinal epithelial tight junction permeability requires NF-kappa B activation. *Am J Physiol Gastrointest Liver Physiol.* 2004;286(3):G367-G376.
61. Fishbein TM, Kaufman SS, Florman SS, et al. Isolated intestinal transplantation: proof of clinical efficacy. *Transplantation.* 2003;76(4):636-640.

62. Newell KA, He G, Hart J, Thistlethwaite JR. Treatment with either anti-CD4 or anti-CD8 monoclonal antibodies blocks alpha beta T cell mediated rejection of intestinal allografts in mice. *Transplantation.* 1997;64:959-965.
63. He G, Hart J, Thisthlethwaite JR Jr, Newell KA. Role of CD8+ and CD4+ T cells in the rejection of murine intestinal allografts. *Transplant Proc.* 1998;30:2592-2593.
64. Newell KA, He G, Guo Z, et al. Cutting edge: blockade of the CD28/B7 co-stimulatory pathway inhibits intestinal allograft rejection mediated by CD4+ but not CD8+ T cells. *J Immunol.* 1999;163:2358-2362.
65. Guo Z, Wang J, Meng L, et al. Cutting edge; membrane lymphotoxin regulates CD8(+) T cell mediated intestinal allograft rejection. *J Immunol.* 2001;167:4796-4800.
66. Wang J, Guo Z, Dong Y, et al. The role of 4-1BB in allograft rejection mediated by CD8+ T cells. *Am J Transplant.* 2003;3:1091-1098.
67. Tian L, Guo W, Yuan Z, et al. Association of the CD134/CD134L co-stimulatory pathway with acute rejection of small bowel allograft. *Transplantation.* 2002;74:133-138.
68. Guo Z, Meng L, Kim O, et al. CD8 T cell-mediated rejection of intestinal allografts is resistant to inhibition of the CD40/CD154 co-stimulatory pathway. *Transplantation.* 2001;71:1351-1354.
69. Trambley J, Bingman AW, Lin A, et al. Asialo GM1(+) CD8(+) T cells play a critical role in costimulation blockade-resistant allograft rejection. *J Clin Invest.* 1999;104:1715-1722.
70. Zhu M, Wei MF, Liu F, Shi HF, Wang G. Interleukin-10 modified dendritic cells induce allo-hyporesponsiveness and prolong small intestine allograft survival. *World J Gastroenterol.* 2003;9(11):2509-2512.
71. Kelly J, Weir DG, Feighery C. Differential expression of HLA-D gene products in the normal and celiac small bowel. *Tissue Antigens.* 1988;31(3):151-160.
72. Sturgess RP, Hooper LB, Spencer J, Hung CH, Nelufer JM, Ciclitira PJ. Effects of interferon-gamma and tumour necrosis factor-alpha on epithelial HLA class-II expression on jejunal mucosal biopsy specimens cultured in vitro. *Scand J Gastroenterol.* 1992;27:907-911.
73. Mayer L. Mucosal immunity and gastrointestinal antigen processing. *J Pediatr Gastroenterol Nutr.* 2000;30 Suppl:S4-S12.
74. Wittig BM, Zeitz M. The gut as an organ of immunology. *Int J Colorectal Dis.* 2003;18(3):181-187.
75. Hurst SD, Cooper CJ, Sitterding SM, et al. The differentiated state of intestinal lamina propria CD4+ T cells results in altered cytokine production, activation threshold, and co-stimulatory requirements. *J Immunol.* 1999;163(11):5937-5945.
76. Mora JR, Bono MR, Manjunath N, et al. Selective imprinting of gut-homing T cells by Peyer's patch dendritic cells. *Nature.* 2003;424:88-93.
77. Sarnacki S, Auber F, Cretolle C, Camby C, Cavazzan-Calvo M, Muller W, Wagner N, Brousse N, Revillon Y, Fischer A, et al. Blockade of the integrin αLβ2 but not of integrins α4 and/or β7 significantly prolongs intestinal allograft survival in mice. *Gut.* 2000;47:97-104.
78. Kellersmann R, Lazarovits A, Grant D, et al. Monoclonal antibody against beta7 integrins, but not beta7 deficiency, attenuates intestinal allograft rejection in mice. *Transplantation.* 2002;74:1327-1334.
79. Richard DM, Deeks JJ, Sheldon TA, Shaffer JL. Home parenteral nutrition: a systematic review. *Health Technology Assessment.* 1997;1(1).
80. Chan S, McCowen KC, Bistrian BR, et al. Incidence, prognosis, and etiology of end-stage liver disease in patients receiving home parenteral nutrition. *Surgery.* 1999;126:28-34.
81. Messing B, Crenn P, Beau P, et al. Long-term survival and parenteral nutrition dependence in adult patients with short bowel syndrome. *Gastroenterology.* 1999;117:1043-1050.
82. Cavicchi M, Beau P, Crenn P, Degott C, Messing B. Prevalence of liver disease and contributing factors in patients receiving home parenteral nutrition for permanent intestinal failure. *Ann Intern Med.* 2000;132:525-532.
83. Howard L, Ament M, Fleming CR, Shike M, Steiger E. Current use and clinical outcome of home parenteral and enteral nutrition therapies in the United States. *Gastroenterology.* 1995;109(2):355-365.
84. Pierro A, Van Saene HKF, Donnell SC, et al. Microbial translocation in neonates and infants receiving long-term parenteral nutrition. *Arch Surg.* 1996;131:176-179.
85. Moukarzel AA, Haddad I, Ament ME, et al. 230 patient years of experience with home long-term parenteral nutrition in childhood: natural history and life of central venous catheters. *J Pediatr Surg.* 1994;29(10):1323-1327.
86. Horslen SP, Kaufman SS, Sudan DL, Fox IJ, Shaw BW, Langnas AN. Isolated liver transplantation in infants with total parenteral nutrition-associated end-stage liver disease. *Transplant Proc.* 2000;32(6):1241.
87. Wilmore DW, Lacey JM, Soultanakis RP, Bosch RL, Byrne TA. Factors predicting a successful outcome after pharmacologic bowel compensation. *Ann Surg.* 1997;226(3):288-292.
88. Scolapio JS, Camilleri M, Fleming CR, et al. Effect of growth hormone, glutamine, and diet on adaptation in short-bowel syndrome: a randomized, controlled study. *Gastroenterology.* 1997;113(4):1074-1081.
89. Seguy D, Vahedi K, Kapel N, Souberbielle JC, Messing B. Low-dose growth hormone in adult home parenteral nutrition-dependent short bowel syndrome patients: a positive study. *Gastroenterology.* 2003;124(2):293-302.
90. Wu GH, Wu ZH, Wu ZG. Effects of bowel rehabilitation and combined trophic therapy on intestinal adaptation in short bowel patients. *World J Gastroenterol.* 2003;9(11):2601-2604.
91. Drucker DJ, DeForest L, Brubaker PL. Intestinal response to growth factors administered alone or in combination with human [Gly2]glucagon-like peptide 2. *Am J Physiol.* 1997;273(6 [Pt 1]): G1252-G1262.
92. Jeppesen PB, Hartmann B, Thulesen J, et al. Glucagon-like peptide 2 improves nutrient absorption and nutritional status in short-bowel patients with no colon. *Gastroenterology.* 2001;120(4):806-815.
93. Buchman AL, Dubin MD, Moukarzel AA, et al. Choline deficiency: a cause for hepatic steatosis during parenteral nutrition that can be reversed with intravenous choline supplementation. *Hepatology.* 1995;22:1399-1403.
94. Thompson JS, Langnas AN. Surgical approaches to improving intestinal function in the short-bowel syndrome. *Arch Surg.* 1999;134(7):706-709.
95. Royall D, Wolever BM, Jeejeebhoy KN. Evidence for colonic conservation of malabsorbed carbohydrate in short bowel syndrome. *Am J Gastroenterol.* 1992;87:751-756.
96. Bueno J, Guitterrez J, Mazariegos GV, et al. Analysis of patients with longitudinal intestinal lengthening procedure referred for intestinal transplantation. *J Pediatr Surg.* 2001;36(1):178-183.
97. Fryer J, Pellar S, Ormond D, Koffron A, Abecassis M. Mortality in candidates waiting for combined liver-intestine transplants exceeds that for other candidates waiting for liver transplants. *Liver Transplantation.* 2003;9(7):748-753.
98. 2003 Annual Report of the US Scientific Registry of Transplant Recipients and The Organ Procurement and Transplantation Network. Transplant data 1990-2002. US Department of Health and Human Services, Health Resources and Services Administration, Office of Special Programs, Division of Transplantation, Rockville, MD; United Network of Organ Sharing, Richmond, Va.

Chapter 33

The Use of Growth Factors in Short Bowel Syndrome

Palle Bekker Jeppesen, MD, PhD

Introduction

Malabsorption of nonessential and essential nutrients, fluids, and electrolytes, if not compensated for by increased intake, will lead to diminished body stores and subclinical and (eventually) clinical deficiencies. By definition, intestinal failure prevails when parenteral support is necessary to maintain nutritional equilibrium. After intestinal resection, adaptation—a progressive recovery from the malabsorptive disorder—may be evident. Research has focused on optimizing remnant intestinal function through dietary or pharmacological interventions. This chapter describes factors responsible for the morphological and functional changes in the adaptive processes and presents results of clinical trials that use either growth hormones or glutamine and glucagon-like peptide (GLP)–2 in short bowel patients.

Short Bowel Syndrome, Intestinal Failure, and Intestinal Adaptation

Short bowel syndrome refers to an aggregation of clinical signs and symptoms, mainly caused by intestinal resection, and the subsequent diarrhea, dehydration, malabsorption of macronutrients, weight loss, malabsorption of vitamins and trace elements, and malnutrition. After a period of intestinal adaptation, the minimal length of small bowel required to maintain nutritional integrity and intestinal autonomy through hyperphagia and to avoid intestinal failure and dependence upon parenteral support has been reported to be 50 to 70 cm of small bowel, if colon is left intact, or 100 to 150 cm, if the resection is associated with a colectomy.[1-4] However, in general, the correlation between remnant intestinal length and absorptive function is poor, and, when considering outcome, the intestinal absorptive function rather than the length is the key determinant. Recent balance studies have demonstrated that intestinal failure may be defined by measurements of wet-weight and energy absorption. Patients who absorb less than 1.4 kg/day of wet weight or less than 84% of their calculated basic energy needs according to the Harris Benedict equations depend on parenteral fluid or energy support, respectively.[5]

The term "intestinal adaptation" may be applied to the progressive recovery from intestinal insufficiency or failure that follows a loss of intestinal length (Chapter 31). Figure 33-1 illustrates a theoretical graphic presentation of intestinal function in relation to time after intestinal resection. A "spontaneous adaptation," or recovery of intestinal function, is generally described, reaching a plateau at a certain time (given as graph "SA" in Figure 33-1). When trying to improve intestinal adaptation, therapies could either reach a higher plateau phase ("hyperadaptation," given as graph "HA" in Figure 33-1) or reduce the time period until the plateau was reached ("accelerated adaptation," presented as "AA", or "accelerated hyper-adaptation," presented as "AHA" in Figure 33-1). The time issue may be relevant in patients who are difficult to maintain on parenteral nutrition (PN) (Chapter 30). However, the maximal increase in the functional absorptive capacity obtained by hyperadaptation, represented by the level of the plateau, is the aim when trying to wean stable patients from parenteral support.

Figure 33-1. Schematic presentation of intestinal adaptation. SA=spontaneous adaptation, AA=accelerated adaptation, HA=hyperadaptation, AHA=accelerated hyperadaptation.

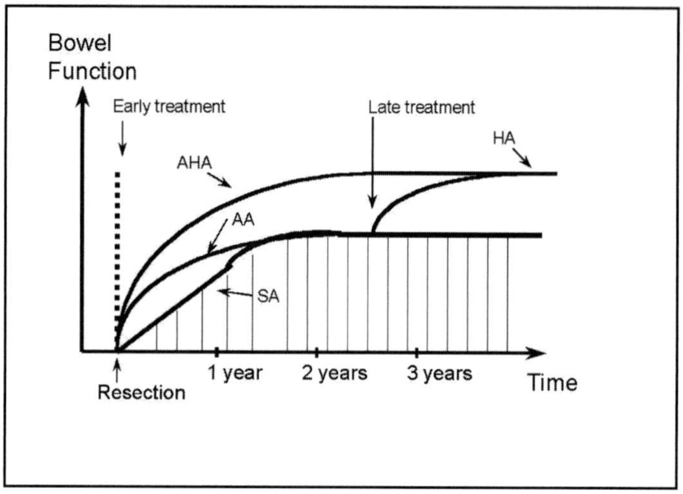

Morphological and Functional Changes During Intestinal Adaptation

Morphological, biochemical, hormonal, and neural systems appear to be involved in intestinal adaptation. Data supporting this are mainly derived from animal studies in which the process of compensatory hyperplasia is extraordinary in some species. It is important to realize that an overall translation of this data to humans cannot be presumed. In the rat, the ileal villi grow to their fully adapted height within about 2 weeks when jejunum is resected.[6] In a human, this process has been demonstrated in patients with jejunoileal bypass operations after which villus heights increased and reached a plateau in 1 year.[7] Most animal and human resection studies describe jejunal changes in short bowels with colon-in-continuity. Thus, conclusions drawn may not hold for patients with a jejunostomy.

Morphological Changes

The process of epithelial turnover is highly dynamic in the intestine. Thus, within 3 to 6 days, the epithelial cells proliferate within the crypts at the base of the villi, mature, differentiate, and move upward toward the tip of a villus, from which they are shed into the bowel lumen.[8] Adaptation is characterized by cellular hyperplasia that increases the crypt depth and villus size.[3-19] The morphological changes are more marked in the mucosal surface area, but changes are also seen in the submucosa or muscularis layers.[14]

The intensity of the adaptive response appears to be proportional to the total length as well as to specific areas of the bowel resected. It is greater in the distal small bowel following proximal resection compared with the proximal bowel after distal resection.[8,14,15] Thus, a significant morphologic adaptive response is seen after proximal resection in the ileum in animal models.[9,11,16,17] Adaptive hyperplasia of colonic mucosa occurs after both jejunal and ileal resection.[18-21] The adaptive response also occurs in the jejunal remnant after ileal resection, but it is less dramatic, more variable, and may partly be related to adaptive changes in food intake.[22] Finally, ileal mucosa may also undergo hyperplasia after colectomy.[23,24]

Functional Changes

Only a few longitudinal studies have been performed in humans with respect to functional changes following intestinal resection. However, it is the clinical experience that short bowel patients with an intact colon show improved absorption with time, whereas patients with jejunostomy do not.[25] Althausen et al described diminished fecal water losses and increased absorption of glucose, galactose, amino acids, and fats during the time after extensive small bowel resection in two patients with preserved colons.[26] The jejunal absorptive capacity of short bowel patients has also been examined by segmental perfusion techniques, and the absorption of glucose, water, and sodium was increased per unit of length compared to that of control subjects.[26,27] Ileostomy adaptation does occur within a period of 6 months; however, this response is lacking in "ileostomists" who have had an ileal resection.[28] Thus, the preservation of the terminal ileum and the colon seems to be of importance in the adaptive response following intestinal resection. The time required to maximum adaptation is not certain. Studies of calcium absorption have suggested that it may continue for more than 2 years,[29] although the main adaptive response seems to take place within a few months.

It seems that the increase in intestinal function with time following intestinal resection may simply be related to the morphologically demonstrated villus hyperplasia, because only minor changes in the activity of specific intestinal disaccharides, hydrolases, enterokinase, and sodium-potassium-ATPase have been demonstrated.[17,30,31] However, functional adaptation may also involve a trend towards normalization of gastric hypersecretion, gastric emptying, and rapid intestinal transit reported in the short bowel syndrome.[32]

Factors Responsible for Morphological and Functional Changes

The signals and precise mechanisms that trigger the hyperplastic adaptive response after small bowel resection are not completely understood. The main factors thought to influence intestinal adaptation are exposure of the remaining mucosa to luminal nutrients and non-nutritive components of the diet, various factors related to the provision of enteral feedings (eg, pancreaticobiliary secretions and enteric hormones), and possibly various growth factors and hormones not secreted from the intestine.

Direct Actions of Luminal Nutrients and Pancreaticobiliary Secretions

It has been suggested that certain preferred substrates directly or through stimulation of bile and pancreatic secretions could have a positive effect on the growth of the epithelial cells.[33-38] Alternatively, the action could be indirect, through the stimulation of the release of enteric hormones with interrelated effects on intestinal secretion, motility, or growth. In animal studies, the significant role of enteral nutrition in the process of bowel adaptation is supported by the finding that the absence of luminal nutrients inhibits the intestinal adaptive hyperplasia, even when the necessary amount of calories is administered via PN.[39-41] In humans, PN, given to normal volunteers, induces a much more muted degree of atrophy in the small intestine, characterized by slightly reduced mucosa thickness, villus height, and cell count; increased permeability to small molecules; and decreased in enterocyte enzyme activities.[42,43] Thus, a difference in the inertia of the adaptive response seems to exist between species.[44]

By infusing single, specific nutrients into the bowel, it is possible to evaluate the adaptive properties in animal models. Similar studies have not been performed in man. It seems that mucosal hyperplasia is stimulated by both metabolized or nonmetabolized substrates, absorbed by both active and diffusion processes.[45-49]

Findings suggest that long chain triglycerides (LCTs) administered intragastrically to rats after resection increase adaptation more efficiently than proteins and polysaccharides.[45] A highly unsaturated fat source was more effective in increasing mucosal weight, DNA content, and bowel protein content after resection than was observed in animals fed diets containing less highly unsaturated fats.[50] Administration of diets containing supplemental linoleic acid exerted a more trophic effect on bowel mucosal protein content after resection than what was observed in animals receiving the minimal requirement of this fatty acid.[51,52] Research also indicates that LCTs are more trophic than medium-chain triglycerides.[45,53]

Short chain triglycerides or short chain fatty acids (SCFAs) have been shown to stimulate intestinal mucosal growth when administered both perorally,[54] intracolonically,[55,56] and intravenously.[57] The absorption of SCFAs stimulates sodium and water absorption with importance for final stool volume.[58,59] The trophic actions of SCFAs during peroral administration have previously been related to the provision of preferred oxidative fuels to the intestinal mucosa: butyrate directly to the colon[55] and via hepatic metabolism of SCFAs to glutamine to the small bowel.[57] However, SCFAs given into the hindgut lumen indirectly stimulated the epithelial cell proliferation of an isolated and denervated jejunal segment of the rat.[60] Thus, the trophic effects in the small intestine might be hormonally mediated through the release of gastrointestinal regulatory peptides. Furthermore, SCFA-supplemented PN has been demonstrated to increase proglucagon abundance,[61] and this abundance together with increased concentrations of proglucagon-derived peptides have been demonstrated to be strongly correlated with cellular proliferation during intestinal adaptation.[62-65]

Clinically, glutamine has been used in promoting intestinal adaptation. Glutamine is an important fuel for rapidly dividing cells, including those of the small intestinal mucosa. It has been suggested to accelerate postresectional hyperplasia and enhance the intestinal glucose and sodium absorption.[66-70] However, Vanderhoof et al were unable to demonstrate a trophic effect of the addition of 5% glutamine to a chow diet following resection in the rat. Glutamine produced less hyperplasia than another amino acid, glycine, which has no specific role in intestinal metabolism.[71,72] Furthermore, Scolapio et al reported that 8 weeks of treatment with oral glutamine and a high-carbohydrate, low-fat diet did not improve intestinal morphology and function in eight short bowel patients.[73]

Enteric Hormones

The search for specific hormones related to the intestinal adaptation occurring after resection has been intensive. The presence of a systemic trophic factor was evidenced by hyperplasia of the intestinal mucosa in an unoperated animal that was in parabiosis with an animal subjected to partial enterectomy.[74] After intestinal resection in rats, mucosal proliferation was observed in ileal fragments transplanted beneath the renal capsule and thus out of continuity with the intestinal lumen.[75] Also, mucosal atrophy of a bypassed intestinal segment, from which nutrients and pancreaticobiliary secretions were absent, was reversed when an animal was fed enterally rather than by PN.[76] Later, it was found that tumors producing enteroglucagon were associated with intestinal mucosal hyperplasia.[77,78]

The term "enteroglucagon" was used to describe the peptide present in the endocrine L-cells mainly found in the distal ileal and colonic mucosa with glucagon-like immunoreactivity demonstrated by antisera raised against the pancreatic hormone glucagons.[79] However, initially the molecular structure of enteroglucagon was unknown, and the serum concentrations were derived by subtracting pancreatic glucagon concentrations from total glucagon-like immunoreactivity. Enteroglucagon was secreted from the terminal ileum and colon in response to malabsorbed food residues and was found in increased concentrations in patients with enterectomy or after jejunoileal bypass.[80,81] In patients with partial ileal resection, enteroglucagon was raised both basally and postprandially.[82] In contrast, patients who underwent colonic resection showed an enteroglucagon profile, which, although not significantly different from that of the control group, had lower enteroglucagon concentrations at each time-point studied.[83] Later, it was found that the peptides responsible for the glucagon-like immunoreactivity initially described was glicentin and oxyntomodulin,[84,85] but the intestinotrophic mediator has been demonstrated to be GLP-2 in rodents.[86-88] Glicentin, oxyntomodulin, GLP-2, and GLP-1 are secreted, through a post-transitional processing of proglucagon, from the L-cells of the distal small intestine[89] and possibly in the colon,[90,91] whereas glucagon, glicentin-related pancreatic peptide, and the major proglucagon fragment are produced by a differential processing of proglucagon in the pancreatic A cells.

It has been speculated that the L-cells, through the secretion of proglucagon-derived peptides, may serve as sensors in the distal intestine, providing feedback information to the upper intestine in order to optimize the nutrient and fluid absorption. Thus, increasing loads of nutrients or fluid into the ileum and colon may stimulate the secretion of glicentin, oxyntomodulin, GLP-1, and GLP-2. Whereas the biological activity of glicentin and oxyntomodulin remains controversial,[92] GLP-1 is a insulinotrophic hormone[93,94] and inhibits gastric secretion and motility by inhibiting central parasympathetic outflow.[95] In addition to mediating increased jejunal absorption through induction of jejunal epithelial proliferation, GLP-2 has been described to decrease gastric emptying,[96] increase intestinal transit time, and inhibit sham-feeding–induced gastric-acid secretion.[97] Therefore, it is likely that a pharmacological replacement tends to restore the physiological feedback, previously described as the ileal brake mechanism (Chapter 23).

Administration of a potent protease-resistant analogue of GLP-2 has been demonstrated to augment the adaptive response to massive intestinal resection in rodents,[98] and postresectional intestinal growth correlates to circulating GLP-2 levels.[99] The postprandial GLP-2 secretion has been measured following a standardized 3.9 MJ test-meal in short bowel patients with[100] and without[101] a preserved colon and compared to gender- and age-matched controls. The median (25% to 75%) fasting GLP-2 value was 72 (69 to 105) pmol/L 23 (19 to 27) pmol/L, P = 0.001, and the meal-stimulated area under the curve 21078 min x pmol/L (14811 to 26610) 11150 min x pmol/L (7151 to 12801), P = 0.01, in the short bowel patients with a preserved colon compared to the control subjects. In the short bowel patients without a preserved colon, the median (25% to 75%) fasting GLP-2 value was 5 (4 to 7) pmol/L 9 (6 to 11) pmol/L, P = 0.07, and the meal-stimulated area under the curve 9272 min x pmol/L (6218 to 10928) 1565 min x pmol/L (1224 to 2662), P = 0.002, compared to the control subjects. Thus, the elevated GLP-2 concentrations in short bowel patients with a preserved colon, as shown in this study,[100] may explain some of the beneficial effects of a preserved colon on intestinal motility and functional adaptation in the ileum-resected short bowel patients. The impaired meal-stimulated GLP-2 response in patients with a jejunostomy has later raised the hypothesis that GLP-2 administration could constitute a new therapeutic strategy; enhancing jejunal adaptation in ileum resected short bowel patients with intestinal failure.

Hormonal Stimulation of Intestinal Adaptation

Two major hormonal candidates—growth hormones and GLP-2—have been suggested in the treatment of patients with short bowel syndrome. Currently, hormonal therapy in short bowel patients should be considered experimental and is only recommended in research settings. The overall aim of any given treatment in short bowel patients is to improve their quality of life. Quality of life may be estimated by the use of standardized questionnaires; however, at present, it is difficult to establish which numerical improvement on the disease-specific inflammatory bowel disease questionnaire or nondisease specific sickness impact profile scales would justify the introduction of a new treatment.

The main focus of research performed in short bowel has been to increase the absolute intestinal absorption. However, in most studies assessing the effects of pharmacological interventions, the dietary intake has been fixated during balance studies. Therefore, in contrast to these "physiological studies", the effect on the dietary intake of these interventions, and thereby on the true absolute absorption, has not been established in vivo in the everyday settings of the patients. For instance, pharmacological agents could (ie, due to an effect on the gastric emptying) induce a sensation of satiety, thereby also reducing the overall dietary intake.

Even in studies in which a true increase in the intestinal absorption has been established, the outcomes may differ in individual patients. It is possible that an improved energy and macronutrient balance in some patients may lead to changes in body weight and composition and, in others, to a change in basal metabolic rate, whereas some may increase their physical activity. Improved fluid and electrolyte balance may allow for increased perspiration and production of urine and sweat. Thus, to get a more precise picture of the individual short bowel patient, each of these parameters ideally should be measured in long-term experiments. Because of the vast requirements and efforts to conduct such experiments, the ability to wean-off patients from parenteral support has been used as a surrogate marker of an effect of given treatments. However, unless the pretreatment need for parenteral support has been verified, such an end-point is invalid. Most home parenteral nutrition (HPN) patients (Chapter 40) can be reduced in parenteral support for shorter or longer periods, and they may even compensate for these changes in the energy, macronutrient, fluid, and electrolyte balances. Despite these difficulties, the search for factors to enhance bowel adaptation and increase the assimilation of macronutrients and absorption of wet weight, thereby decreasing the need for PN, is intensive. Although the evidence-based knowledge is weak, a comparison of the results obtained in short-term clinical trials employing growth hormone and GLP-2 is presented.

Effects of Growth Hormone, Glutamine, and Glucagon-like Peptide 2 in Clinical Studies

Wet-Weight Absorption

Byrne et al were the first to introduce the concept of "bowel rehabilitation" with the introduction of high dose (0.14 mg/kg/day) growth hormone, glutamine, and a high carbohydrate diet in the treatment of short bowel patients.[102,103] In the first study, published by Byrne and Wilmore, the wet-weight absorption increased from 1.7 to 2.4 kg/day, and sodium absorption increased from 74 to 113 mmol/day over 5 weeks of treatment. From the baseline absorptive parameters, the actual need for parenteral fluid and sodium could be questioned in the majority of the patients in that study, according to the borderlines of intestinal failure defined by Jeppesen et al.[5] All eight patients in the Byrne et al study had a colon-in-continuity, and, in addition to dietary changes toward a high-carbohydrate diet, they were also given oral rehydration solutions as a part of the "rehabilitation." Despite claims to the contrary, the effects may, in fact, be related to dietary changes and rehydration solutions, rather than growth hormones and glutamine. Although significant, the effect of growth hormones (0.13 mg/kg/day) and oral glutamine on intestinal sodium and potassium absorption was less than 5 mmol/day in the placebo-controlled, double-blind study by Scolapio et al.[104] In contrast, growth hormone (0.11 mg/kg/day) and glutamine, both orally and parenterally administered, tended to decrease wet-weight absorption and increase fecal excretion of sodium and potassium, which reached significance ($P < 0.05$) in comparison with baseline values from the study of Szkudlarek et al.[105] However, these findings were contrasted by clinical findings of generalized edema, increased body weight, a need for diuretics, and a reduction in parenteral saline during treatment. The patients were probably in the process of excreting water and sodium accumulated during the treatment at the time of the post-treatment balance studies 5 days after termination of treatment. In the lower dose studies from Ellegaard (growth hormone 0.024 mg/kg/day)[106] and Seguy (0.05 mg/kg/day),[107] no significant positive effects on either wet-weight or sodium absorption were seen. It has recently been reported that growth hormones increase extracellular volume by stimulating sodium reabsorption in the distal nephron and preventing pressure natriuresis.[108] Thus, the effects of growth hormones on fluid balance in short bowel patients may be related to effects on the kidneys rather than on the intestine.

In the study with native GLP-2 by Jeppesen et al, eight patients were treated with 400 mcg of GLP-2 twice a day, given subcutaneously for 35 days in an open label study (corresponding to 0.013 ± 0.002 mg/kg/day, a range of 0.011 to 0.017 mg/kg/day).[109] Four patients with a mean residual jejunum of 83 cm received HPN, whereas four patients with a mean ileum resection of 106 cm did not. Their average wet-weight absorption was 1.2 ± 1.7 kg/day at baseline and the wet-weight absorption increased by 420 ± 480 g/day, $P = 0.04$, whereas the effect on sodium absorption did not reach statistical significance (33 ± 49 mmol/day, $P = 0.10$).

Energy Absorption

In studies using growth hormone, there have been conflicting results on intestinal energy and macronutrient absorption. In the study by Byrne et al, the baseline dietary energy intake was 2692 kcal/day, and 1618 kcal/day (~6773 kJ/day, 60%) were absorbed.[102] Thus, according to the borderlines that define intestinal failure suggested by Jeppesen et al,[5] the majority of these patients did not need parenteral energy. After 3 weeks of treatment, the intake and absorption were 2367 and 1759 kcal/day (~7363 kJ/day, 74%), respectively, which was a significant improvement in percentage ($p<0.003$) but only an increase of 141 kcal/day (~590 kJ/day) in absolute amounts. In this study by Byrne and Wilmore, all eight short bowel patients had a colon-in-continuity. As stated, the "rehabilitation" included a high-carbohydrate, low-fat diet, which in itself is know to increase the energy absorption in this segment of short bowel patients. Supporting the hypothesis that diet alone resulted in this effect, intestinal fat absorption did not improve. In the study by Scolapio et al, where only two of eight patients had colon-in-continuity, high-carbohydrate diets were provided in both the placebo and treatment arms.[104] Energy absorption was not measured, but no changes were observed regarding nitrogen or fat absorption. In the studies by Ellegaard et al[106] and Szkudlarek et al,[105] no changes were found in intestinal energy or in fat or nitrogen absorption. In the study by Seguy et al, growth hormone (0.05 mg/kg/day, 9 of 12 patients with colon-in-continuity) and an unrestricted hyperphagic diet increased intestinal absorption of nitrogen by 14% ± 6% ($P < 0.040$), carbohydrates by 10% ± 4% ($P <0.040$), and energy by 15% ± 5% ($P <0.002$), which in absolute terms was 427 kcal/day (~1787 kJ/day).[107] Fat absorption was unaffected by the treatment.

In the study with native GLP-2, the absolute energy absorption tended to increase by 441 ± 634 kJ/day ([105 ± 151 kcal/day] $P = 0.09$). Treatment with GLP-2 increased the energy absorption by 3.5% ± 4.0%—from 49.9% ± 20.3% to 53.4% ± 18.1% ($P = 0.04$)—which was equivalent to an increase of 13.1% ± 22.3% in percentage of the absorption at baseline (49.9%). Absorption of carbohydrates improved by 0.35 ± 0.44 MJ/day ($P = 0.06$), which was borderline significant, whereas the relative absorption showed an insignificant increasing trend of 4.4 ± 7.5% ($P = 0.14$) from 69.7% ± 22.0% to 74.1% ± 15.9%. Excretion of protein (nitrogen) decreased 0.14 ± 0.13 MJ/day ($P = 0.02$), but the effect on the absolute absorption did not reach statistical significance ($P = 0.16$). This was in contrast to the improvement in the relative absorption of protein which increased by 4.7% ± 5.4% from 47.4% ± 29.3% to 52.1 ± 28.4% ($P = 0.04$). The effect of GLP-2 on fat absorption was not significant. The improvement in the absolute amount of energy absorbed was obtained despite an insignificant decrease in intake of 0.17 MJ/day, which means that the reduction in the energy malabsorbed (equal to the stomal excretion) was proportionally larger: 0.62 MJ/day.

Body Weight, Composition, and Urine Creatinine Excretion

In the growth-hormone study by Byrne et al, a weight gain of 5.4 ± 1.2 kg was described in the eight patients after 21 days of treatment.[102] Occurrence of edema were not reported, but increases in body weight are difficult to explain considering the magnitude of the effect of approximately 12.4 MJ (590 kJ/day) on the energy balance over the 21 days of treatment. In the study by Byrne et al, neither body composition nor urine creatinine excretion was measured. In the 8-week growth-hormone (0.024 mg/kg/day) study by Ellegaard et al, an increase in lean body mass of 2.5 kg and a decrease in fat mass of 0.1 kg were found.[106] Total body potassium increased 4.7%, equivalent to 1.1 ± 0.4 kg of body cell mass, which was parallel to the 5.6% increase in lean body mass measured by dual energy x-ray absorptiometry (DEXA) (Chapter

2). Ellegaard et al concluded that the increase in lean body mass was derived from both increased body cell mass and extracellular water. Using DEXA measurements, Scolapio et al found an increase in lean body mass of 3.96 ± 0.5 kg and a decrease in the percent of body fat of 2.51±0.4%, which corresponded to approximately 1.0 kg compared to placebo.[110] Scolapio et al concluded that the increased body weight during treatment with high doses of growth hormone was mainly caused by the increase in extracellular water and the presence of peripheral edema, which was encountered in all eight patients treated. In the study by Szkudlarek et al, a weight gain of 1.0 ± 0.3 kg (P <0.050) was measured daily for 5 days after 4 weeks of treatment. DEXA evaluation indicated that lean body mass increased 2.9 kg (P <0.001) and fat mass decreased 2.4 kg (P <0.001) compared with baseline, whereas the changes were not significant in comparison to placebo. No changes were seen in urinary creatinine excretion.[111] The most likely explanation of the rather modest weight gain and increase in lean body mass in the study of Szkudlarek et al could be the timing of measurements. The patients had been off growth hormone and glutamine for 5 days, when the DEXA-scan measurements were performed. At this time, generalized edemas, which occurred in all eight patients, were on the decline. In the other studies, lean body mass was measured while patients were still receiving treatment. In the study by Seguy et al, body weight increased 2.0 kg (P <0.003), and the lean body mass, measured by bioimpedance (Chapter 2), increased 2.2 kg (P <0.006).[107] No adverse events to the growth-hormone treatment were encountered.

In the 35-day study with native GLP-2 treatment, the overall increase in energy absorption of 15 MJ translated into a significant increase in body weight of 1.2 ± 1.0 kg (P = 0.010).[109] Lean body mass improved with 2.9 ± 1.9 kg (P = 0.004), and fat mass decreased by 1.8 ± 1.3 kg (P = 0.007). The study demonstrated positive findings on urine creatinine excretion (0.7 ± 0.7 mmol/day, P = 0.02), which suggests an increase in muscle mass in relation to GLP-2 treatment.

Conclusion

In recent years, increased attention has been addressed to the pharmacological enhancement of bowel adaptation aimed at weaning patients with intestinal failure from parenteral support. In these patients, apart from posing a threat of causing line sepsis, thrombosis, and liver damage, the complex technology of HPN significantly impairs quality of life.[112] Although the initial trials employing growth hormone and glutamine were positive, the subsequent controlled trials have been disappointing. However, in the low-dose study of Seguy et al, an impressive effect of 427 kcal/day (~1787 kJ/day) on intestinal energy absorption was seen.

Also, in a recent study, only published in abstract form, Byrne et al demonstrated the ability of weaning short bowel patients from parenteral support over 4 weeks of growth-hormone treatment. The weekly requirements of the parenteral volume were reduced by 3.9 L/week (~557 mL/day) and parenteral energy by 3084 kcal/week (441 kcal/day = 1844 kJ/day) employing growth hormone (0.1 mg/kg/day), glutamine supplementation, and a high carbohydrate diet. However, the weaning of the short bowel patients from parenteral support led to a significant weight loss of 5.2 kg, when the patients were evaluated at 18 weeks. Thus, when nutritional balance studies are not performed, such results are hard to interpret.

The presence and severity of adverse events is a concern when considering long-term pharmacological growth-hormone treatment to promote hyperadaptation in short bowel patients. Thus, the myalgia, arthralgia, gynecomastia, carpal tunnel syndrome, nightmares, and insomnia reported in most growth-hormone studies in short bowel patients may jeopardize the positive effects on quality of life, which should be the ultimate goal of such treatment.

Hopes have been directed towards GLP-2 because the physiologic effects of GLP-2 appear rather specific for the gut, which is concordant with the localization of the GLP-2 receptor. The peptide has intestinotrophic, antisecretory, and transit-modulating effects in the short bowel patients and the adverse events, even in supraphysiological doses, seem limited. So far, the effects of GLP-2 are not clinically dramatic, but in the first human trial, the dose of GLP-2 and the duration of therapy were chosen arbitrarily. The optimal duration and concentration requirements for GLP-2 to induce beneficial effects on intestinal secretion, motility, morphology, and (most important) absorption are not known. However, GLP-2 analogs with a more slowly degradation has been developed,[113] and preliminary results are positive, almost doubling the effects seen in the study employing native GLP-2. Optimal dosage and administration of this new treatment to short bowel patients may eventually result in long-term improvements in nutritional status and independence of PN in a larger fraction of short bowel patients.

References

1. Carbonnel F, Cosnes J, Chevret S, et al. The role of anatomic factors in nutritional autonomy after extensive small bowel resection. *JPEN J Parenter Enteral Nutr.* 1996;20(4):275-280.
2. Nightingale JM, Lennard Jones JE, Walker ER, Farthing MJ. Jejunal efflux in short bowel syndrome. *Lancet.* 1990;336(8718):765-768.
3. Nightingale JM, Lennard Jones JE, et al. Colonic preservation reduces need for parenteral therapy, increases incidence of renal stones, but does not change high prevalence of gall stones in patients with a short bowel. *Gut.* 1992;33(11):1493-1497.
4. Messing B, Crenn P, Beau P, et al. Long-term survival and parenteral nutrition dependence in adult patients with the short bowel syndrome. *Gastroenterology.* 1999;117:1043-1050.
5. Jeppesen PB, Mortensen PB. Intestinal failure defined by measurements of intestinal energy and wet weight absorption. *Gut.* 2000;46(5):701-706.
6. Forrester JM. The number of villi in rat's jejunum and ileum: effect of normal growth, partial enterectomy, and tube feeding. *J Anat.* 1972;111(2):283-291.
7. Friedman HI, Chandler JG, Peck CC, Nemeth TJ, Odum SK. Alterations in intestinal structure, fat absorption and body weight after intestinal bypass for morbid obesity. *Surg Gynecol Obstet.* 1978;146(5):757-767.
8. Eastwood GL. Gastrointestinal epithelial renewal. *Gastroenterology.* 1977;72(5[Pt 1]):962-975.

9. Dowling RH, Booth CC. Structural and functional changes following small intestinal resection in the rat. *Clin Sci.* 1967;32(1):139-149.
10. Obertop H, Nundy S, Malamud D, Malt RA. Onset of cell proliferation in the shortened gut. Rapid hyperplasia after jejunal resection. *Gastroenterology.* 1977;72(2):267-270.
11. Nygaard K. Resection of the small intestine in rats. 3. Morphological changes in the intestinal tract. *Acta Chir Scand.* 1967;133(3):233-248.
12. Booth CC, Evans KT, Menzies T, Street DF. Intestinal hypertrophy following partial resection of the small bowel in the rat. *Br J Surg.* 1958;46;403-410.
13. Porus RL. Epithelial hyperplasia following massive small bowel resection in man. *Gastroenterology.* 1965;48(6):753-757.
14. Hanson WR, Osborne JW, Sharp JG. Compensation by the residual intestine after intestinal resection in the rat. I. Influence of amount of tissue removed. *Gastroenterology.* 1977;72(4[Pt 1]):692-700.
15. Hanson WR, Osborne JW, Sharp JG. Compensation by the residual intestine after intestinal resection in the rat. II. Influence of postoperative time interval. *Gastroenterology.* 1977;72(4[Pt 1]):701-705.
16. Tilson MD, Wright HK. Adaptation of functioning and bypassed segments of ileum during compensatory hypertrophy of the gut. *Surgery.* 1970;67(4):687-693.
17. Weser E, Hernandez MH. Studies of small bowel adaptation after intestinal resection in the rat. *Gastroenterology.* 1971;60(1):69-75.
18. Tilson MD, Michaud JT, Livstone EM. Early proliferative activity in the left colon of the rat after partial small-bowel resection. *Surg Forum.* 1976;27(62):445-446.
19. Williamson RC, Bauer FL, Ross JS, Malt RA. Proximal enterectomy stimulates distal hyperplasia more than bypass or pancreaticobiliary diversion. *Gastroenterology.* 1978;74(1):16-23.
20. Nundy S, Malamud D, Obertop H, Sczerban J, Malt RA. Onset of cell proliferation in the shortened gut. Colonic hyperplasia after ileal resection. *Gastroenterology.* 1977;72(2):263-266.
21. Solhaug JH, Tvete S. Adaptative changes in the small intestine following bypass operation for obesity. A radiological and histological study. *Scand J Gastroenterol.* 1978;13(4):401-408.
22. Young EA, Weser E. Nutritional adaptation after small bowel resection in rats. *J Nutr.* 1974;104(8):994-1001.
23. Wright HK, Poskitt T, Cleveland JC, Herskovic T. The effect of total colectomy on morphology and absorptive capacity of ileum in the rat. *J Surg Res.* 1969;9(5):301-304.
24. Woo ZH, Nygaard K. Small-bowel adaptation after colectomy in rats. *Scand J Gastroenterol.* 1978;13(8):903-910.
25. Nightingale JM, Lennard-Jones JE. The short bowel syndrome: what's new and old? *Dig Dis.* 1993;11(1):12-31.
26. Dowling RH, Booth CC. Functional compensation after small-bowel resection in man. Demonstration by direct measurement. *Lancet.* 1966;2(7455):146-147.
27. Weinstein LD, Shoemaker CP, Hersh T, Wright HK. Enhanced intestinal absorption after small bowel resection in man. *Arch Surg.* 1969;99(5):560-562.
28. Hill GL, Mair WS, Goligher JC. Impairment of "ileostomy adaptation" in patients after ileal resection. *Gut.* 1974;15(12):982-987.
29. Gouttebel MC, Saint Aubert B, et al. Intestinal adaptation in patients with short bowel syndrome. Measurement by calcium absorption. *Dig Dis Sci.* 1989;34(5):709-715.
30. McCarthy DM, Kim YS. Changes in sucrase, enterokinase, and peptide hydrolase after intestinal resection. The association of cellular hyperplasia and adaptation. *J Clin Invest.* 1973;52(4):942-951.
31. Tilson MD, Wright HK. An adaptive change in ileal Na-K-ATPase activity after jejunectomy or jejunal transposition. *Surgery.* 1971;70(3):421-424.
32. Remington M, Malagelada JR, Zinsmeister A, Fleming CR. Abnormalities in gastrointestinal motor activity in patients with short bowels: effect of a synthetic opiate. *Gastroenterology.* 1983;85(3):629-636.
33. Williamson RC. Intestinal adaptation (second of two parts). Mechanisms of control. *N Engl J Med.* 1978;298(26):1444-1450.
34. Weser E, Heller R, Tawil T. Stimulation of mucosal growth in the rat ileum by bile and pancreatic secretions after jejunal resection. *Gastroenterology.* 1977;73(3):524-529.
35. Altmann GG. Influence of bile and pancreatic secretions on the size of the intestinal villi in the rat. *Am J Anat.* 1971;132(2):167-177.
36. Miazza BM, Levan H, Veja S, Dowling RH. Effect of pancreatico-bilary diversion (PBD) on jejunal and ileal structure and function in the rat. In: Robinson JW, Dowling RH, Riecken EO, eds. *Mechanisms of Intestinal Adaptation.* Lancaster: MTP Press Limited; 1982:467-476.
37. Weser E, Drummond A, Tawil T. Effect of diverting bile and pancreatic secretions into the ileum on small bowel mucosa in rats fed a liquid formula diet. *JPEN J Parenter Enteral Nutr.* 1982;6(1):39-42.
38. Gelinas MD, Morin CL. Effects of bile and pancreatic secretions on intestinal mucosa after proximal small bowel resection in rats. *Can J Physiol Pharmacol.* 1980;58(9):1117-1123.
39. Ford WD, Boelhouwer RU, King WW, de Vries JE, Ross JS, Malt RA. Total parenteral nutrition inhibits intestinal adaptive hyperplasia in young rats: reversal by feeding. *Surgery.* 1984;96(3):527-534.
40. Feldman EJ, Dowling RH, McNaughton J, Peters TJ. Effects of oral versus intravenous nutrition on intestinal adaptation after small bowel resection in the dog. *Gastroenterology.* 1976;70(5 PT.1):712-719.
41. Levine GM, Deren JJ, Yezdimir E. Small-bowel resection. Oral intake is the stimulus for hyperplasia. Am J Dig Dis 1976; 21(7):542-546.
42. Buchman AL, Moukarzel AA, Bhuta S, et al. Parenteral nutrition is associated with intestinal morphologic and functional changes in humans. *JPEN J Parenter Enteral Nutr.* 1995;19(6):453-460.
43. Guedon C, Schmitz J, Lerebours E, et al. Decreased brush border hydrolase activities without gross morphologic changes in human intestinal mucosa after prolonged total parenteral nutrition of adults. *Gastroenterology.* 1986;90(2):373-378.
44. Hughes CA, Dowling RH. Speed of onset of adaptive mucosal hypoplasia and hypofunction in the intestine of parenterally fed rats. *Clin Sci.* 1980;59(5):317-327.
45. Morin CL, Grey VL, Garafalo C. Influence of lipids on intestinal adaptation after resection. In: Robinson JW, Dowling RH, Riecken EO, eds. *Mechanisms of Intestinal Adaptation.* Lancaster: MTP Press Limited; 1982:175-185.
46. Spector MH, Levine GM, Deren JJ. Direct and indirect effects of dextrose and amino acids on gut mass. Gastroenterology 1977; 72(4 Pt 1):706-710.
47. Spector MH, Traylor J, Young EA, Weser E. Stimulation of mucosal growth by gastric and ileal infusion of single amino acids in parenterally nourished rats. *Digestion.* 1981;21(1):33-40.
48. Weser E, Vandeventer A, Tawil T. Stimulation of small bowel mucosal growth by midgut infusion of different sugars in rats maintained by total parenteral nutrition. *J Pediatr Gastroenterol Nutr.* 1982;1(3):411-416.
49. Weser E, Vandeventer A, Tawil T. Non-hormonal regulation of intestinal adaptation. *Scand J Gastroenterol.* 1982;17(Suppl 74):105-113.
50. Vanderhoof JA, Park JH, Herrington MK, Adrian TE. Effects of dietary menhaden oil on mucosal adaptation after small bowel resection in rats. *Gastroenterology.* 1994;106(1):94-99.
51. Park JH, Grandjean CJ, Hart MH, Baylor JM, Vanderhoof JA. Effects of dietary linoleic acid on mucosal adaptation after small bowel resection. *Digestion.* 1989;44(2):57-65.
52. Hart MH, Grandjean CJ, Park JH, Erdman SH, Vanderhoof JA. Essential fatty acid deficiency and postresection mucosal adaptation in the rat. *Gastroenterology.* 1988;94(3):682-687.

53. Vanderhoof JA, Grandjean CJ, Kaufman SS, Burkley KT, Antonson DL. Effect of high percentage medium-chain triglyceride diet on mucosal adaptation following massive bowel resection in rats. *JPEN J Parenter Enteral Nutr.* 1984;8(6):685-689.
54. Kripke SA, De Paula JA, Berman JM, Fox AD, Rombeau JL, Settle RG. Experimental short-bowel syndrome: effect of an elemental diet supplemented with short-chain triglycerides. *Am J Clin Nutr.* 1991;53(4):954-962.
55. Kripke SA, Fox AD, Berman JM, Settle RG, Rombeau JL. Stimulation of intestinal mucosal growth with intracolonic infusion of short-chain fatty acids. *JPEN J Parenter Enteral Nutr.* 1989;13(2):109-116.
56. Frankel WL, Zhang W, Singh A, et al. Mediation of the trophic effects of short-chain fatty acids on the rat jejunum and colon. *Gastroenterology.* 1994;106:375-380.
57. Windmueller HG, Spaeth AE. Identification of ketone bodies and glutamine as the major respiratory fuels in vivo for postabsorptive rat small intestine. *J Biol Chem.* 1978;253(1):69-76.
58. Ruppin H, Bar Meir S, Soergel KH, Wood CM, Schmitt MG, Jr. Absorption of short-chain fatty acids by the colon. *Gastroenterology.* 1980;78(6):1500-1507.
59. Roediger WE, Moore A. Effect of short-chain fatty acid on sodium absorption in isolated human colon perfused through the vascular bed. *Dig Dis Sci.* 1981;26(2):100-106.
60. Sakata T. Stimulatory effect of short-chain fatty acids on epithelial cell proliferation of isolated and denervated jejunal segment of the rat. *Scand J Gastroenterol.* 1989;24(7):886-890.
61. Tappenden KA, Drozdowski LA, Thomson AB, McBurney MI. Short-chain fatty acid-supplemented total parenteral nutrition alters intestinal structure, glucose transporter 2 (GLUT2) mRNA and protein, and proglucagon mRNA abundance in normal rats. *Am J Clin Nutr.* 1998;68(1):118-125.
62. Bloom SR, Polak JM. The hormonal pattern of intestinal adaptation. A major role for enteroglucagon. *Scand J Gastroenterol Suppl.* 1982;14:93-103.
63. Sagor GR, Ghatei MA, Al Mukhtar MY, Wright NA, Bloom SR. Evidence for a humoral mechanism after small intestinal resection. Exclusion of gastrin but not enteroglucagon. *Gastroenterology.* 1983;84(5[Pt 1]):902-906.
64. Roundtree DB, Ulshen MH, Selub S, et al. Nutrient-independent increases in proglucagon and ornithine decarboxylase messenger RNAs after jejunoileal resection. *Gastroenterology.* 1992;103(2):462-468.
65. Taylor RG, Verity K, Fuller PJ. Ileal glucagon gene expression: ontogeny and response to massive small bowel resection. *Gastroenterology.* 1990;99(3):724-729.
66. Souba WW, Smith RJ, Wilmore DW. Glutamine metabolism by the intestinal tract. *JPEN J Parenter Enteral Nutr.* 1985;9(5):608-617.
67. Tamada H, Nezu R, Matsuo Y, Imamura I, Takagi Y, Okada A. Alanyl glutamine-enriched total parenteral nutrition restores intestinal adaptation after either proximal or distal massive resection in rats. *JPEN J Parenter Enteral Nutr.* 1993;17(3):236-242.
68. Rhoads JM, Keku EO, Quinn J, Woosely J, Lecce JG. L-glutamine stimulates jejunal sodium and chloride absorption in pig rotavirus enteritis. *Gastroenterology.* 1991;100(3):683-691.
69. Gardemann A, Watanabe Y, Grosse V, Hesse S, Jungermann K. Increases in intestinal glucose absorption and hepatic glucose uptake elicited by luminal but not vascular glutamine in the jointly perfused small intestine and liver of the rat. *Biochem J.* 1992;283(Pt 3):759-765.
70. O'Dwyer ST, Smith RJ, Hwang TL, Wilmore DW. Maintenance of small bowel mucosa with glutamine-enriched parenteral nutrition. *JPEN J Parenter Enteral Nutr.* 1989;13(6):579-585.
71. Vanderhoof JA, Blackwood DJ, Mohammadpour H, Park JH. Effects of oral supplementation of glutamine on small intestinal mucosal mass following resection. *J Am Coll Nutr.* 1992;11(2):223-227.
72. Michail S, Mohammadpour H, Park JH, Vanderhoof JA. Effect of glutamine-supplemented elemental diet on mucosal adaptation following bowel resection in rats. *J Pediatr Gastroenterol Nutr.* 1995;21(4):394-398.
73. Scolapio JS, McGreevy K, Tennyson GS, Burnett OL. Effect of glutamine on intestinal function in short-bowel. *Clin Nutr.* 2001;20:319-323.
74. Loran MR, Carbone JV. The humoral effect of intestinal resection on cellular proliferation and maturation in parabiotic rats. In: Sullivan MF, ed. *Gastrointestinal Radiation Injury.* Amsterdam: Excerpta Medica Foundation; 1968:127-139.
75. Tilson MD, Livstone EM. Radioautography of heterotopic autografts of ileal mucosa in rats after partial enterectomy. *Surg Forum.* 1975;26:393-394.
76. Dworkin LD, Levine GM, Farber NJ, Spector MH. Small intestinal mass of the rat is partially determined by indirect effects of intraluminal nutrition. *Gastroenterology.* 1976;71(4):626-630.
77. Gleeson MH, Bloom SR, Polak JM, Henry K, Dowling RH. Endocrine tumour in kidney affecting small bowel structure, motility, and absorptive function. *Gut.* 1971;12(10):773-782.
78. Stevens FM, Flanagan RW, O'Gorman D, Buchanan KD. Glucagonoma syndrome demonstrating giant duodenal villi. *Gut.* 1984;25(7):784-791.
79. Unger RH, Eisentraut AM, Sims K, McCall MS, Madison LL. Site of origin of glucagon in dogs and humans. *South Soc Clin Res.* 1961;9:53.
80. Andrews NJ, Irving MH. Human gut hormone profiles in patients with short bowel syndrome. Dig Dis Sci 1992; 37(5):729-732.
81. Holst JJ, Sorensen TI, Andersen AN, et al. Plasma enteroglucagon after jejunoileal bypass with 3:1 or 1:3 jejunoileal ratio. *Scand J Gastroenterol.* 1979;14(2):205-207.
82. Bloom SR. Hormonal changes after jejuno-ileal bypass and their physiological significance. In: Maxwell JD, Gazet JC, Pilkington TR, eds. *Surgical Management of Obesity.* London, UK: Academic Press; 1980:115-123.
83. Bloom SR, Besterman HS, Adrian TE, et al. Gut hormone profile following resection of large and small bowel. *Gastroenterology.* 1979;76(5):1001.
84. Holst JJ. Evidence that glicentin contains the entire sequence of glucagon. *Biochem J.* 1980;187(2):337-343.
85. Thim L, Moody AJ. The primary structure of porcine glicentin (proglucagon). *Regul Pept.* 1981;2(2):139-150.
86. Drucker DJ, Erlich P, Asa SL, Brubaker PL. Induction of intestinal epithelial proliferation by glucagon-like peptide 2. *Proc Natl Acad Sci USA.* 1996;93(15):7911-7916.
87. Tsai CH, Hill M, Drucker DJ. Biological determinants of intestinotrophic properties of GLP-2 in vivo. *Am J Physiol.* 1997;272(3[Pt 1]):G662-G668.
88. Tsai CH, Hill M, Asa SL, Brubaker PL, Drucker DJ. Intestinal growth-promoting properties of glucagon-like peptide- 2 in mice. *Am J Physiol.* 1997;273(1[Pt 1]):E77-E84.
89. Orskov C, Holst JJ, Knuhtsen S, et al. Glucagon-like peptides GLP-1 and GLP-2, predicted products of the glucagon gene, are secreted separately from pig small intestine but not pancreas. *Endocrinology.* 1986;119(4):1467-1475.
90. Varndell IM, Bishop AE, Sikri KL, Uttenthal LO, Bloom SR, Polak JM. Localization of glucagon-like peptide (GLP) immunoreactants in human gut and pancreas using light and electron microscopic immunocytochemistry. *J Histochem Cytochem.* 1985;33(10):1080-1086.
91. Larsson LI, Holst J, Hakanson R, Sundler F. Distribution and properties of glucagon immunoreactivity in the digestive tract of various mammals: an immunohistochemical and immunochemical study. *Histochemistry.* 1975;44(4):281-290.
92. Holst JJ. Enteroglucagon. *Annu Rev Physiol.* 1997;59:257-271.
93. Holst JJ, Orskov C, Nielsen OV, Schwartz TW. Truncated glucagon-like peptide I, an insulin-releasing hormone from the distal gut. *FEBS Lett.* 1987;211(2):169-174.
94. Mojsov S, Weir GC, Habener JF. Insulinotropin: glucagon-like peptide I (7-37) co-encoded in the glucagon gene is a potent stimulator of insulin release in the perfused rat pancreas. *J Clin Invest.* 1987;79(2):616-619.
95. Holst JJ. Glucagonlike peptide 1: a newly discovered gastrointestinal hormone. *Gastroenterology.* 1994;107(6):1848-1855.

96. Wojdemann M, Wettergren A, Hartmann B, Holst JJ. Glucagon-like peptide-2 inhibits centrally induced antral motility in pigs. *Scand J Gastroenterol.* 1998;33(8):828-832.
97. Wojdemann M, Wettergren A, Hartmann B, Hilsted L, Holst JJ. Inhibition of sham feeding-stimulated human gastric acid secretion by glucagon-like peptide-2. *J Clin Endocrinol Metab.* 1999;84(7):2513-2517.
98. Scott RB, Kirk D, MacNaughton WK, Meddings JB. GLP-2 augments the adaptive response to massive intestinal resection in rat. *Am J Physiol.* 1998;275(5[Pt 1]):G911-G921.
99. Thulesen J, Hartmann B, Kissow H, et al. Intestinal growth adaptation and glucagon-like peptide 2 in rats with ileal--jejunal transposition or small bowel resection. *Dig Dis Sci.* 2001;46(2):379-388.
100. Jeppesen PB, Hartmann B, Thulesen J, et al. Elevated plasma glucagon-like peptide 1 and 2 concentrations in ileum resected short bowel patients with a preserved colon. *Gut.* 2000;47(3):370-376.
101. Jeppesen PB, Hartmann B, Hansen BS, et al. Impaired meal stimulated glucagon-like peptide 2 response in ileal resected short bowel patients with intestinal failure. *Gut.* 1999;45(4):559-563.
102. Byrne TA, Morrissey TB, Nattakom TV, Ziegler TR, Wilmore DW. Growth hormone, glutamine, and a modified diet enhance nutrient absorption in patients with severe short bowel syndrome. *JPEN J Parenter Enteral Nutr.* 1995;19(4):296-302.
103. Byrne TA, Persinger RL, Young LS, Ziegler TR, Wilmore DW. A new treatment for patients with short-bowel syndrome. Growth hormone, glutamine, and a modified diet. *Ann Surg.* 1995;222(3):243-254.
104. Scolapio JS, Camilleri M, Fleming CR, et al. Effect of growth hormone, glutamine, and diet on adaptation in short-bowel syndrome: A randomized, controlled study. *Gastroenterology.* 1997;113(4):1074-1081.
105. Szkudlarek J, Jeppesen PB, Mortensen PB. Effect of high dose growth hormone with glutamine and no change in diet on intestinal absorption in short bowel patients: a randomised, double blind, crossover, placebo controlled study. *Gut.* 2000;47(2):199-205.
106. Ellegaard L, Bosaeus I, Nordgren S, Bengtsson BA. Low-dose recombinant human growth hormone increases body weight and lean body mass in patients with short bowel syndrome. *Ann Surg.* 1997;225(1):88-96.
107. Seguy D, Vahedi K, Kapel N, Souberbielle JC, Messing B. Low-dose growth hormone in adult home parenteral nutrition-dependent short bowel syndrome patients: a positive study. *Gastroenterology.* 2003;124(2):293-302.
108. Johannsson G, Sverrisdottir YB, Ellegard L, Lundberg PA, Herlitz H. GH increases extracellular volume by stimulating sodium reabsorption in the distal nephron and preventing pressure natriuresis. *J Clin Endocrinol Metab.* 2002;87(4):1743-1749.
109. Jeppesen PB, Hartmann B, Thulesen J, et al. Glucagon-like peptide 2 improves nutrient absorption and nutritional status in short-bowel patients with no colon. *Gastroenterology.* 2001;120(4):806-815.
110. Scolapio JS. Effect of growth hormone, glutamine, and diet on body composition in short bowel syndrome: a randomized, controlled study. *JPEN J Parenter Enteral Nutr.* 1999:23(6);309-313.
111. Jeppesen PB, Szkudlarek J, Hoy CE, Mortensen PB. Effect of high-dose growth hormone and glutamine on body composition, urine creatinine excretion, fatty acid absorption, and essential fatty acids status in short bowel patients: a randomized, double-blind, crossover, placebo-controlled study. *Scand J Gastroenterol.* 2001;36(1):48-54.
112. Jeppesen PB, Langholz E, Mortensen PB. Quality of life in patients receiving home parenteral nutrition. *Gut.* 1999;44(6):844-852.
113. Drucker DJ, Shi Q, Crivici A, et al. Regulation of the biological activity of glucagon-like peptide 2 in vivo by dipeptidyl peptidase IV. *Nat Biotechnol.* 1997;15(7):673-677.

Section VI

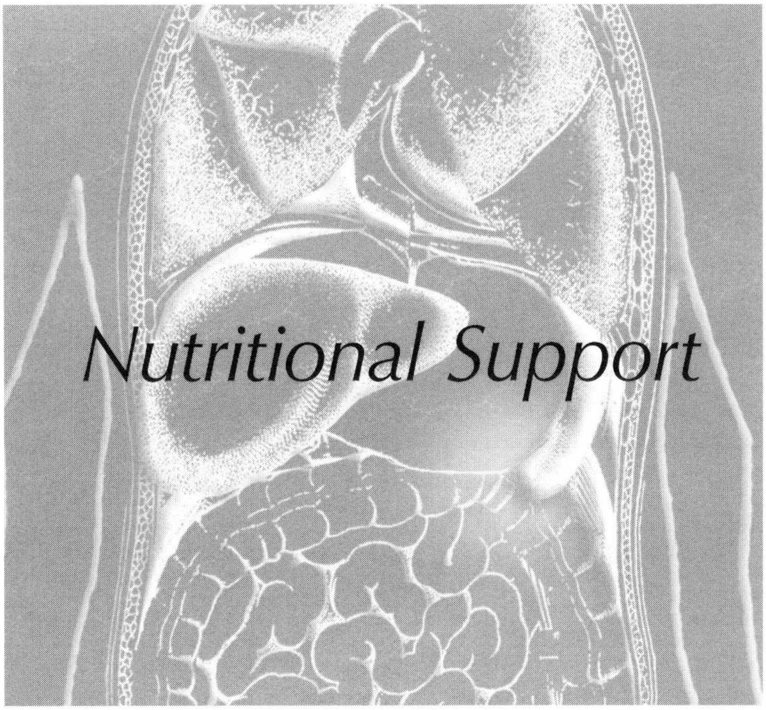

Nutritional Support

Chapter 34

Indications and Contraindications to Enteral and Parenteral Nutrition

Ronald L. Koretz, MD

Introduction

Indication: a symptom or particular circumstance that indicates the advisability or necessity of (as a special medical treatment or procedure).
—Webster's Third New International Dictionary

Over the past several decades, the cost of healthcare in the United States has increased rapidly. Americans are currently spending in excess of $1 trillion (or as a former President of the United States put it, "a million million dollars") annually, which translates into about 15% of the Gross Domestic Product (GDP). Furthermore, it has been projected that the growth in such spending will continue, and the expense of healthcare may be as high as $16 trillion (32% of the GDP) in 2030.[1]

Obviously, this level of growth is not sustainable, and some force will intervene to curtail it. There are several options for controlling expenditures. The simplest is to decide how much one wants to cut on a percentage basis and then make that percentage cut across the board. Oregon attempted to control its Medicaid expenditures by stratifying its healthcare needs and drawing a line when the money ran out; everything above the line was funded and everything below it (including organ transplantation) was not. Currently, special interest groups (via marketing techniques) appear to be directing most of our expenditures.

The most rational method would be to use evidence to determine resource allocation. Interventions best supported by evidence would get the most resources; those with evidence of inefficacy or net harm would get none. This chapter focuses on evidence that is available to assess the efficacy of the therapeutic intervention of nutrition support. Four different types of nutrition support are discussed: parenteral nutrition (PN), protein sparing therapy (PST), enteral nutrition (EN), and volitional nutritional support (VNS). These are defined in Table 34-1.

Not all sources of evidence are equal; the major distinguishing characteristic in the reliability of evidence is the effort that was made to reduce the influence of bias. The randomized controlled trial eliminates many of the confounding factors that arise when control groups are identified and is thus afforded more credibility in the evidence hierarchy.[2] However, randomized controlled trials can still have problems. These include Type I or Type II errors, inability to extrapolate data from a study population, inappropriate data analysis (eg, not using intent to treat), lack of blinding, use of surrogate end points, or defects in the randomization process.[3]

An even higher level of evidence is the "systematic review". For therapeutic interventions, this usually consists of an evaluation of randomized controlled trials, often with a statistical combination of the data (meta-analysis).[4] A systematic review should not be confused with the more commonly available narrative review. In the latter, an expert summarizes what he or she believes to be important; obviously, preexistent beliefs can lead to biased interpretations.[5]

In a systematic review, a question is formulated, a strategy is designed to find all of the relevant and high-quality data regarding that question, and those data are employed to answer the question. The methodology that is to be used to perform each of these steps is defined before the searching, data abstraction, and analysis is even begun. The data drive the conclusions.

For purposes of defining "indication" or "contraindication", this chapter employs data from

TABLE 34-1.

Definitions for Different Types of Nutrition Support

Type of Nutrition Support	Definition
Parenteral Nutrition	The intravenous (central or peripheral venous catheter) provision of nitrogen (as amino acids or protein hydrolysate) and >10 kcal/kg/day of non-nitrogenous calories
Protein Sparing Therapy	The intravenous provision of nitrogen (as amino acids or protein hydrolysate) and <10 kcal/kg/day of non-nitrogenous calories
Enteral Nutrition	The nonvolitional infusion of a putative complete (including essential micronutrients if given in caloric sufficiency) nutrient liquid formulation through a tube placed in the upper GI tract*
Volitional Nutritional Support	A liquid formulation containing at least a nonprotein source of calories (carbohydrate and/or fat) and nitrogen (as intact protein, digested protein, and/or amino acids) that is taken orally by the patient, with specific instructions regarding its consumption on a scheduled basis†

*It will have been the intent of the investigator to provide a source of nitrogen (intact protein, protein hydrolysate, and/or free amino acids) and >10 kcal/kg/day of non-nitrogenous calories.

†This formulation may be provided as a supplement to the ad-lib intake of standard food; these formulations differ from supplemental "snacks" prepared from real food (eg, milk shakes, sandwiches, etc.) (Note: VNS requires the patient to consume the nutrient solution him- or herself rather than having medical personnel infuse the liquid; as such, it is being referred to as "volitional" and is considered separately from EN.)

randomized controlled trials whenever possible. The chapter also, in general, takes a Food and Drug Administration (FDA) position with regard to formulating conclusions. Before it allows any pharmaceutical product to be released, the FDA has to receive efficacy data from randomized controlled trials. This is a more restrictive point of view than that employed in many "evidence-based guidelines". In these latter exercises, when no data are available, recommendations are based on the opinions of experts. (By definition, "expert opinion" does not require data; it is the lowest level of evidence.)

The numbers of randomized controlled trials that specifically compared some form of nutrition support to no therapy, or that compared EN to PN, in various disease states are displayed in Table 34-2. My colleagues and I used these randomized controlled trials as the basis for two systematic reviews. The first considered the parenteral infusion of nutrients (PN and PST).[6] The second evaluated EN and VNS.[7]

Meta-analyses were conducted as part of these systematic reviews for a number of the disease states.[6,7] The estimated effect calculated by meta-analysis can be expressed in several ways; these are summarized in Table 34-3. In these systematic reviews[6,7] the estimated effect was usually presented as absolute risk difference. A statistically significant difference in these computations is traditionally defined as a 95% confidence interval that does not cross the line of equivalence (0.0 for absolute risk difference and 1.0 for both relative risk and odds ratio).

Nutrition support is a therapeutic intervention and is not just eating. Nutritional interventions are procedures that produce adverse side effects and utilize healthcare resources. Weighed against these costs would be the putative better outcome. From a patient's perspective, a favorable outcome is a reduction in the likelihood of mortality or morbidity of an underlying disease, or at least a reduction in the duration of hospitalization (or the cost of the care).

With these as the outcomes of interest, this chapter considers the role of nutrition support in specific disease states.

Nutrition Support in Specific Disease States

PERIOPERATIVE NUTRITION SUPPORT

Summary of the Data

The estimated effects of the various types of perioperative nutrition support are summarized in Table 35-4. None of the nutritional interventions had any effect on mortality. The estimated effect of PN tended to be (slightly) beneficial with regard to postoperative complication rates, but these estimates did not achieve statistical significance. In one subgroup analysis, preoperative PN did appear to reduce the subsequent rate of major postoperative complications in patients undergoing surgery for cancer of the stomach or esophagus by 18%. (In other words, for every 5.5 of these patients who were given preoperative PN, one did not have a major postoperative complication.) PST had no effect on any postoperative morbidity.

TABLE 34-2.

Number of Randomized Controlled Trials of Nutrition Support

	Comparing no nutrition therapy to				*Comparing*
Disease State	**PN**	**PST**	**EN**	**VNS**	**EN to PN**
Perioperative	41	20	11	9	19
Liver disease:					
Alcoholic hepatitis	2	5	1	2[1]	–
CLD	–	–	2	3	1
Liver transplant	1	–	2	1	1
Acute pancreatitis	2	1[2]	1[3]	N/A	5
IBD	2	–	–	1	6[4]
Critical illness	1[5]	–	2	N/A	11
Oncology	2[6]	–	2	4	–
LBW infants	5	1	–	N/A	2
Pulmonary:					
COPD	1	–	–	8	–
Cystic fibrosis	1	–	1	–	–
AIDS	1	–	–	3	1[6]
Geriatrics	N/A	N/A	1	11	–
Hip fracture	–	–	3	6	–
Stroke	–	–	–	1	–

N/A = Not applicable; CLD = Chronic liver disease; IBD = Inflammatory bowel disease; LBW = Low birth weight; COPD = Chronic obstructive pulmonary disease; AIDS = Acquired immunodeficiency syndrome; PN = parenteral nutrition; PST = protein sparing therapy; EN = enteral nutrition; VNS = volitional nutritional support

[1] One of these implemented EN if patient unable to consume sufficient nutrient formulation voluntarily

[2] Second arm of one of the PN randomized controlled trials

[3] No clinical data except organ failure score

[4] Two of these randomized controlled trials compared VNS to PN

[5] Second arm of one of the EN randomized controlled trials

[6] VNS compared to PN

EN tended to reduce the incidence of infections, but the estimated effect only became significant in trials that were of low methodologic quality. When EN was compared to PN, the former usually produced better outcomes.

VNS had an "across-the-board" beneficial effect. These patients had to consume the supplements and probably were less ill than were those in the EN trials. The methodologic quality of these VNS trials was, for the most part, low.

Specialized enteral formulations containing putative immunonutrients (φ-3 fatty acids, arginine, ribonucleic acid, and/or glutamine) are becoming popular (Chapter 42). When standard formulas were compared to these specialized ones in surgical patients, the specialized ones resulted in fewer infections.[8]

None of the nonvolitional forms of nutrition support (PN, PST, and EN) had an effect on the duration of hospitalization. While VNS appears to have resulted in shorter hospital stays, four other randomized controlled trials that could not be included in the meta-analysis (insufficient statistical information) failed to find any such decreases.

There were virtually no data assessing costs.

Implications of the Data

While nutrition support was not shown to reduce postoperative complications with statistical certainty, trends in that direction were often present. However, even if a true beneficial effect does exist, it is not dramatic, and a small benefit must be weighed against the cost. For example, if a week of preoperative PN reduces the total complication rate by 5%, 20 patients would need to be treated for 7 days each to prevent one adverse event. The therapy would only be economically justifiable if these complications were very expensive.[9]

Almost all of the randomized controlled trials specifically excluded severely malnourished patients. One of these trials contained a subgroup analysis that suggested that severely malnourished patients benefited from PN.[10] While the differences did not achieve statistical significance, the rates of major postoperative complications were 20% to 25% in severely malnourished given PN and 40% to 50% in the nutritionally comparable controls. This information is inadequate to establish the presence or absence of efficacy of nutrition support in the severely malnourished surgical patient.

Even though PST improves nitrogen balance[11-21] it does not affect mortality or morbidity when it is provided postoperatively. This dissociation between nutritional and clinical outcomes, observed in other trials of nutrition support,[22] emphasizes the importance of focusing on clinical outcomes rather than surrogate nutritional markers.

We know that low quality trials usually overestimate the treatment effect.[23] Thus, the effect of VNS may not be as great as it appears. Nonetheless, this form of

TABLE 34-3.

Methods of Expressing the Estimated Treatment Effect Calculated in Meta-analysis

Method of Expression	Definition
Absolute risk difference[1]	The arithmetical difference between the rate of the outcome in the treated group and the rate of that outcome in the control group
Relative risk ratio[1]	The incidence of the outcome in the treated group divided by the incidence of the outcome in the control group[2]
Odds ratio[1]	The odds of a particular outcome occurring in the intervention group divided by the odds of it occurring in the control group[3]
Weighted mean difference[4]	The difference between the average value of the outcome in the treated group and that value in the control group

[1] Used for dichotomous (outcome present or absent, a form of categorical data) data.
[2] For example, a risk ratio of 0.75 means that the event occurred only three-quarters as often in the treated group as in the control group.
[3] The odds ratio is not easy to grasp intuitively; when the rates of the event are small in each group, the odds ratio approximates the risk ratio.
[4] Used for continuous (non-categorical) data.

nutrition therapy may have the most cost-effective therapeutic potential.

LIVER DISEASE

Summary of the Data

In addition to the randomized controlled trials noted for alcoholic hepatitis, one randomized controlled trial tested the combination of VNS and an anabolic steroid.[24] Another randomized controlled trial compared EN to steroid therapy.[25]

Survival was not improved by PN, PST, EN, or VNS.[6,7] When 4 weeks of inpatient EN was compared to steroid therapy in 71 patients with alcoholic hepatitis,[25] there was no difference in hospital mortality (31% versus 25%). During the longer-term outpatient follow-up, significantly more patients in the steroid group expired (8% versus 37%). Most of the late deaths in the steroid group were from infections, and the steroid therapy may have masked these conditions earlier. Thus, in the absence of a true control group, we cannot know if EN prevented late deaths or if steroids predisposed the patients to a mortal outcome.

Five randomized controlled trials, including one that combined VNS with anabolic steroids,[24] did not find that a variety of nutrition support regimens had any effect on the complication rates in alcoholic hepatitis. Intravenous nutrition support was associated with a faster decline in serum bilirubin.

The role of nutrition support was assessed in other forms of chronic liver disease. Although the data were limited, no effect was observed on survival, infectious or other liver-related complications, or on duration of hospitalization. EN and PN appeared to be equivalent.

The utility of nutrition support in patients undergoing liver transplantation was also studied. The data were limited, but none of these treatments had any apparent effect on mortality, morbidity, duration of hospitalization, or rejection rates.

Branched-chain amino acids (BCAAs) compete with aromatic amino acids for transport into the central nervous system; because aromatic amino acids may be precursors of compounds that produce hepatic encephalopathy, BCAAs might be a useful (pharmacologic) treatment. Although these amino acids did appear to provide a modest benefit in one meta-analysis, the effect disappeared if the analysis was limited to the trials of higher quality.[26]

Implications of the Data

There is no apparent effect of nutrition support in patients with a variety of liver diseases. Although intravenous infusions may produce a faster resolution of hyperbilirubinemia, the clinical relevance of such an improvement is undefined.

BCAA-enriched solutions (alone or as part of a nutrition support regimen) may be beneficial in treating hepatic encephalopathy. This is a pharmacologic rather than nutritional effect, and the expense of BCAAs is higher than that of other available therapies.[9]

ACUTE PANCREATITIS

Summary of the Data

Two randomized controlled trials evaluated the role of PN in patients with relatively mild acute pancreatitis; one included a second treatment arm (PST).[6] Five randomized controlled trials compared PN to EN7; each of these trials employed a predigested formulation that was delivered directly into the jejunum. At least three of these trials assessed patients with relatively severe pancreatitis and one enrolled patients with relatively mild disease. One randomized controlled trial compared EN to no treatment but provided no clinical data except for an organ failure score.[27] One other compared intragastric to intrajejunal EN.[28]

TABLE 34-4.

Meta-analyses of Perioperative Trials*

Outcome	Absolute Risk Difference[1]	Confidence Intervals	Number of Studies (Patients) Included
Parenteral Nutrition:			
Mortality	0%	-2%, +2%	37 (2164)
Total complications	-6%	-13%, +1%	32 (2062)
Infectious complications	-2%	-8%, +3%	29 (1612)
Major complications	-3%[2]	-9%, +3%	22 (1648)
Wound complications	-2%	-6%, +2%	29 (1800)
Intra-abdominal complications	0%[3]	-5%, +4%	21 (1375)
Postoperative pneumonia	-2%	-4%, +2%	23 (1684)
Duration hospitalization	+0.2 days[4]	-0.72 days, +1.04 days	10 (246)
Protein Sparing Therapy:			
Mortality	+1%	-2%, +3%	13 (1033)
Total complication rate	-3%	-7%, +1%	16 (1182)
Infectious complication rate	+2%	-1%, +5%	16 (1109)
Major complications	-1%	-6%, +4%	6 (773)
Wound complications	0%	-4%, +3%	11 (1005)
Intra-abdominal complications	+1%	-3%, +5%	10 (950)
Postoperative pneumonia	+1%	-2%, +3%	10 (957)
Enteral Nutrition:			
Mortality	-1%	-4%, +3%	8 (604)
Total complications	-15%	-37%, +10%	8 (536)
Infectious complications	-12%	-27%, +2%[5]	7 (506)
Major complications	+1%	-6%, +8%	7 (506)
Wound complications	-7%	-16%, +1%	8 (648)
Intra-abdominal/thoracic complications	-5%	-11%, +1%	8 (566)
Postoperative pneumonia	-3%	-9%, +3%	5 (448)
Enteral Nutrition versus Parenteral Nutrition:[6]			
Mortality	-1%	-3%, +1%	16 (1391)
Total complication rate	-5%	-12%, +1%	14 (1308)
Infectious complication rate	-10%	-14%, -5%	15 (1306)
Major complications	-6%	-10%, -1%	9 (941)
Wound complications	-3%	-6%, +1%	8 (841)
Intra-abdominal/thoracic complications	-4%	-8%, 0%	9 (944)
Postoperative pneumonia	-4%	-8%, 0%	8 (888)
Duration hospitalization	-1.76 days[4]	-2.74 days, -0.77 days	4 (639)
Volitional Nutrition Support:			
Mortality	0%	-2%, +2%	7 (640)
Total complication rate	-13%	-23%, -3%	9 (789)
Infectious complication rate	-10%	-18%, -1%	8 (637)
Major complications	-14%	-22%, -6%	5 (416)
Wound complications	-11%	-22%, 0%	6 (477)
Intra-abdominal/thoracic complications	-10%	-18%, -2%	4 (376)
Postoperative pneumonia	-3%	-7%, +1%	5 (451)
Duration hospitalization	-2.38 days[4]	-4.03 days, -0.73 days	4 (365)

* Data from references 6 and 7.

[1] Difference between the outcome in the treated group and the control group; a negative number represents a benefit for the treated group

[2] In trials that only included patients with upper GI cancers who were undergoing surgery, absolute risk difference = -18% (-31%, -6%)

[3] Actual estimate is -0.3%, so estimated risk differences for each of the complication rates in the parenteral nutrition meta-analysis were negative

[4] Weighted mean difference (difference between average duration of hospitalization in the treated and the control group)

[5] Confidence interval did not overlap 0 when only trials of low quality considered

[6] Enteral nutrition considered to be the experimental arm and parenteral nutrition considered to be the control arm

None of these trials found any differences in mortality. Compared with standard therapy, PN resulted in more complications and a longer hospitalization in one trial.[6] Intravenous nutrient infusions did not appear to have any effect on the development of pseudocysts or phlegmons.

Compared to those given EN, the recipients of PN appeared to have more problems (infections, hyperglycemia, and structural [pseudocysts, phlegmons, and/or abscesses]).[7] No statistically significant differences in durations of hospitalization were observed.

Powell et al randomized 27 patients who were believed to have a poor prognosis to either intrajejunal EN or no nutritional therapy.[27] The assessed outcomes were mostly inflammatory markers and measures of gut permeability. No differences were seen in an organ failure score. Intragastric and intrajejunal infusions were comparable.[28]

Implications of the Data

It would appear that EN is safer and more effective than is PN in patients with pancreatitis. The difficulty that exists in interpreting this information is the scarcity of data about the absolute value of either modality compared to doing nothing. In one randomized controlled trial, the recipients of PN had a worse outcome than did untreated controls. The single trial comparing EN to no nutrition treatment was not powered to see clinical differences, and very little clinical information was even provided.[27] At this time, we have no probative data to support a policy of providing nutrition support to patients with pancreatitis; in fact, there is some concern about the harmfulness of PN.

Inflammatory Bowel Disease

Summary of the Data

None of the trials found any effect of nutrition support on mortality, but deaths are rare anyway. PN did not improve the remission rate in patients with colitis. In one 6-month outpatient trial of VNS, gastrointestinal (GI) side effects limited the ability of the patients to consume the formula.[7] No significant differences were observed. PN was comparable to EN.[7]

Pediatricians may use nutrition support to maintain the growth of children with inflammatory bowel disease. There are no randomized controlled trials to assess this practice.

Implications of the Data

PN was not helpful in treating Crohn's or ulcerative colitis. PN is equivalent to EN in treating patients with active Crohn's disease of the small intestine. By inference, PN is inferior to standard therapy because three separate meta-analyses have concluded that clinical remission in Crohn's disease is achieved more frequently with corticosteroids than with EN.[29-31]

The data for using nutrition support in inflammatory bowel disease all suggest that there is no reason to believe that these patients derive benefit from being kept in a fasting state.[6,7,32] We have no information from randomized controlled trials to guide a decision regarding the use of nutrition support in affected children to maintain growth.

Critical Illness

Summary of the Data

Only a few trials compared nutrition support to no treatment. Neither PN nor EN significantly affected mortality.[6,7] One randomized controlled trial compared immediate to delayed EN;[33] no patients died. No differences were appreciated with regard to survival when EN was compared to PN.[7]

Another systematic review of nutrition support in the intensive care unit considered the question of early versus later intervention with nutrition support and concluded that those receiving such treatment within 1 to 2 days of admission tended to have better survival (relative risk 0.52, 95% confidence interval 0.25, 1.08).[34] However, the analysis is limited by the study designs of a number of the included randomized controlled trials; some of the control groups received PN (an intervention that may cause excess infections[6]), one of the trials may not have been randomized,[7] and one other included patients who were not necessarily in an intensive care unit.[7]

PN did not reduce the rate of infections in one trial.[6] Infectious complications tended to be more frequent in the control groups of both EN trials. The use of immunonutrient formulations (compared to standard ones) may result in fewer infections.[8] Burn patients who had EN initiated at the time of admission tended to have fewer episodes of sepsis (3/10 versus 7/10, $P > 0.10$).[34] Those who had the EN continued during surgery had fewer wound infections (2/40 versus 9/40, $P < 0.05$).[35] The systematic review of randomized controlled trials in the intensive care unit described a trend for the EN patients to have fewer infectious complications (relative risk 0.66, 95% CI 0.36, 1.22).[34] Infectious complications occur more frequently in those given PN (compared to EN).[34]

Although there were only a small number of randomized controlled trials available, nutrition support did not appear to affect either the length of time mechanical ventilation was required or the duration of stay in the intensive care unit or hospital.[6,7]

Implications of the Data

Although we have only a limited number of randomized controlled trials that compared PN or EN to no treatment, there is no compelling evidence that supports either intervention in the critically ill. Nonetheless, many intensivists have accepted the dictum that such treatment is important and have focused on comparing different forms of nutritional interventions (be it EN versus PN or standard versus immunonutrient formulations).

The trial that most supports EN has an inherent flaw.[36] Control patients who were not eating by day 5 were given PN, an intervention that may actually create infections.[6] (This problem confounds the interpretation of all of the randomized controlled trials comparing EN to PN.)

Limited data may appear to suggest that EN is beneficial in burn patients.[33,35] In addition to the usual caveats that apply to small studies, both trials have another possible flaw, namely lack of randomization. In one, it is stated that the patients "were randomly assigned by a case-control method;"[33] in the other, patients were "randomly assigned" to the treatment group and "matched" to patients who had infusions withheld for surgery.[35]

Oncologic Applications (Cancer Chemotherapy or Radiation Therapy)

Summary of the Data

The data for nutrition support has been particularly disappointing with regard to its utility in patients receiving oncotherapy. In general, PN, EN, and VNS did not have any effect on mortality.[6,7] In one randomized controlled trial of bone marrow transplant patients, the group that received in-hospital PN had better long-term (beginning several months later) survival.[37] Patients with end-stage malignancies receiving no specific cancer therapy lived significantly longer if they received PN (46 versus 7 days), although the clinical relevance of this observation is unclear.[38]

PN increased the complication rates;[6] the absolute risk differences were 40% (total complications) and 16% (infectious complications). There were far fewer EN or VNS trials; no effects (good or bad) were observed.[7] The tumor response rates were also adversely affected by PN.[6] (It may be that exogenous nutrients stimulate tumor growth.[6]) No differences in tumor response were seen in one EN and two VNS trials.[7]

Appetite stimulants (eg, megesterol, corticosteroids, or cyproheptadine) could be viewed as a variant of VNS. Such treatment does improve appetite and usually produces weight gain.[7] The treatment may also create a better sense of well-being.[7] However, this did not translate into improved survival or decreased morbidity from the malignant disease.[7]

Implications of the Data

PN did not alter survival in patients receiving radiation or chemotherapy. The data cannot exclude the possibility that PN will favorably affect long-term survival in patients undergoing bone marrow transplantation. In all other aspects, the use of PN in cancer patients receiving chemotherapy, radiation therapy, or bone marrow transplantation was clearly associated with net harm, namely increases in total and infectious complication rates and an impaired tumor response to chemotherapy.

There was no apparent positive or negative effect from the enteral provision of nutrients (either through a tube or by drinking), but the data are limited. No trials assessed EN or VNS in hematologic malignancies.

Pediatrics

Summary of the Data

The only pediatric condition for which nutrition support was evaluated with randomized controlled trials was low birth weight infants. There is no evidence that PN or PST (or, by inference EN) alters survival or complication rates.[6,7]

Pediatricians often fear that EN induces necrotizing enterocolitis in very premature infants. The hypothesis that small amounts of enteral nutrient delivery would facilitate an ultimate transition to full enteral feeding (so-called "trophic feeding") was addressed in a systematic review.[39] There was no increased or decreased risk of necrotizing enterocolitis from this intervention. The recipients of the minimal feedings had an overall reduction in the time to full feeding (2.7 days) and a 15.6-day reduction in the length of hospitalization.

Additional nutrients should promote more rapid weight gain (and a subsequent earlier discharge) in neonates who are only hospitalized because of low birth weight. However, more rapid weight gain did not translate into an earlier discharge in the PN trials.[6]

Nutrition support is often advocated for children with a variety of underlying conditions who are failing to grow normally. Although anecdotal reports suggest that this is useful, no randomized controlled trials were identified other than the material discussed below in the section on cystic fibrosis.

Implications of the Data

No benefits from PN (and from EN, at least by inference from two randomized controlled trials comparing it to PN) were observed in low birth weight infants. Although this nutritional intervention may increase the rate of weight gain, there is no evidence that this translated into any meaningful clinical outcome, including an earlier hospital discharge. It is generally believed that such neonates require early nutrition support because of: 1) a lack of intrinsic energy stores, and 2) nutrient requirements for growth and development. We have no direct data assessing how long such babies can endure starvation.

One meta-analysis showed what appeared to be a positive effect from the trophic feeding.[40] However, those reviewers noted the methodologic problems in the randomized controlled trials, including lack of blinding, inadequate provision of the details about the randomization process, dropouts, and generally small trials (possible publication bias). The largest trial did not show a benefit, reinforcing the concern about publication bias. The conclusion of the review was that it was unclear if this intervention was helpful.

Pulmonary (Including Cystic Fibrosis)

Summary of the Data

Neither PN nor EN appeared to influence mortality or morbidity.[6,7] A trial of PN in cystic fibrosis assessed the utility of 4 months of PN delivered at home.[40] The average number of days spent in the hospital was not significantly different between the two groups.

Most of the data that were provided in the VNS trials dealt with intermediate outcomes in patients with chronic obstructive pulmonary disease. For the most part, no improvements were described with regard to exercise capacity, handgrip strength, pulmonary function, respiratory muscle strength, or quality of life.[7] A systematic review concluded that there is no evidence that nutrition interventions are of benefit in this condition.[41]

Another systematic review assessed techniques for achieving weight gain in patients with cystic fibrosis.[42] Although only one of the included trials was a randomized controlled trial, the authors concluded that almost any type of intervention would achieve the desired end (increased weight), be it behavioral therapy, VNS, EN, or PN. Pulmonary function stabilized or seemed to improve in some of the reports. (This same observation was made with megestrol.[43]) However, as these reviewers pointed out, it is unknown if weight gain translates into any meaningful improvements in the underlying disease. Three other systematic reviews also commented on the lack of good outcome data regarding the use of EN, supplements, or fish oil in cystic fibrosis.[44-46]

Implications of the Data

There are only limited data available assessing the role of nutrition support in lung disease. No benefit has been identified.

Acquired Immunodeficiency Disease

Summary of the Data

The single PN trial in patients with acquired immunodeficiency disease (AIDS) evaluated the utility of 2 months of home PN. No difference in survival was reported in the initial report; three patients in each group died.[47] (Subsequently, the investigators reported that survival was improved in the recipients of PN, but these data were not analyzed in accordance with the initial treatment assignment.[48]) No mortality difference was seen in the single randomized controlled trial of VNS that provided this information.[49]

Although the recipients of PN had improved anthropometric measurements and weight gain and subjectively felt better, no difference in the incidence of AIDS-related complications was observed.[47] Similarly, the VNS trials did not find that this intervention resulted in any differences in infectious complications, CD4 counts, grip strength, or overall quality of life.[7]

Kotler et al compared VNS to PN in 23 malabsorbing outpatients.[50] (Only 16 of them completed the 8-week trial.) No differences were seen with regard to CD4 counts or overall quality of life; the VNS group had better physical functioning. PN was more expensive.

Appetite stimulants produce weight gain and senses of well-being.[51-53] However, no meaningful change in performance status or the course of the underlying AIDS occurred.

Implications of the Data

Nutrition support improves body weight and subjective feelings of well-being. However, there is no evidence that it alters the natural history of AIDS.

Renal Failure

Summary of the Data

No randomized controlled trials have compared nutrition support to no such treatment in patients with acute or chronic renal failure.[54] The provision of amino acids and calories during (intradialytic)[55-58] or after (intravenous)[59] hemodialysis in patients with chronic renal failure has been assessed. None of these trials reported clinical outcomes, and a systematic review of these techniques concluded that the evidence was weak and a clear recommendation could not be made.[60]

Five randomized controlled trials evaluated the use of essential amino acid-based PN during acute renal failure. The control groups all received either isocaloric amounts of dextrose (no amino acids).[61-63] or standard PN.[64,65] Although a meta-analysis concluded that the essential amino acid-based PN improved recovery from the acute episode of organ dysfunction but not rates of overall survival,[66] the trial designs make any interpretation difficult. Why give oliguric control patients large amounts of dextrose and no insulin or insulin secretogogue (essential amino acids)?

Implications of the Data

There is no evidence that nutrition support is of value in acute or chronic renal failure.

Cardiac Disease

Summary of the Data

One randomized controlled trial compared the use of a high-calorie VNS formulation to a "placebo" (a 1:10 dilution of the VNS formulation) in patients with congestive heart failure.[67] Only intermediate or surrogate outcomes were reported. No differences were seen.

Summary and Implications

No randomized controlled trials have directly addressed the utility of nutrition support in heart disease.

Geriatrics

Summary of the Trials

Ten trials of VNS in the geriatric population are available.[7] Nine of them, enrolling 1276 patients, were combined in a meta-analysis estimating the effect of VNS on mortality.[7] Two large randomized controlled trials accounted for about two-thirds of the patients;[68,69] no difference in survival was demonstrated. No difference in septic complications was seen in one of the two large trials.[69]

Another published meta-analysis, less restrictive in its definition of supplements and employing a less conservative statistical approach, found that oral supplements were associated with reduced mortality and shortened hospital stay.[70]

In some studies, individual measures of functional status appeared to have been improved by the VNS. However, different measures improved in different studies, and measures that did improve in one trial did not necessarily improve in another. Quality of life scores, assessed in two trials, were not changed by the VNS.

Three randomized controlled trials (two of VNS and one of EN) assessed the ability of nutrition support to prevent pressure ulcers;[7] no effect was found. An additional small randomized controlled trial compared "nutritional support" (ranging from VNS to EN to PN) to standard care in patients who already had developed pressure ulcers.[71] No differences in healing were observed.

None of the nine randomized controlled trials demonstrated an effect of nutrition support on the survival of patients with hip fractures.[7] Neither VNS nor EN had any effect on the total complication rate. Similarly, VNS had no significant effect on infectious complications. No consistent effect on the duration of hospitalization, quality of life, or functional status was observed, although a subgroup analysis of one of the EN trials suggested that the rehabilitation time in the very thin patients may have been shortened.

One randomized controlled trial failed to identify any benefit of VNS in patients with strokes.[7]

Implications of the Data

The randomized controlled trials were small and of poor quality; most of the data failed to show any benefit. There is a modicum of evidence for using VNS in geriatric patients in general or for using EN in very thin ones with hip fractures. Another systematic review of hip fractures (that included quasirandomized and unpublished trials as well as other types of supplements) concluded that the evidence was very weak, but noted that such supplements may reduce the long-term complications and number of days spent in rehabilitation wards.[72]

Pregnancy

Summary of the Data

One systematic review assessed various attempts to increase energy and/or protein intake in pregnant women;[73] no benefits could be attributed to these nutritional interventions.

Implications of the Data

Although pregnant women should certainly eat adequately, there is no evidence to suggest that VNS will provide any further benefit.

Allergic Disorders

Summary of the Data

In theory, if natural foodstuffs, proteins in particular, can act as allergens, there might be value in consuming predigested diets. One randomized controlled trial in adults with asthma compared the ingestion of a protein hydrolysate-containing diet to one containing intact protein.[74] The asthmatic adults who consumed the protein hydrolysate-containing diet were more likely to improve (9/21 versus 1/16, $P < 0.05$). A similarly designed trial in infants with colic suggested that the low-allergen diet appeared to lessen the magnitude of the discomfort.[75]

In another pediatric trial, children with atopic dermatitis were randomized to antigen-restricted diets along with whey or casein hydrolysate supplements or to their usual diet.[76] The hydrolyzed protein diet did appear to improve the dermatitis, but the dropout rates in both groups were very high. Because some of those dropouts occurred because of worsening disease, it is difficult to interpret the data.

Two randomized controlled trials randomized infants believed to be at risk of allergic disorders (because of positive family histories) to either an intact protein formula or one containing protein hydrolysates for 4 months; they were then followed for 4 to 5 years.[77,78] The subsequent incidences of asthma and/or eczema were lower in the group that consumed the hydrolysates.

One randomized controlled trial randomized 20 adult patients with rheumatoid arthritis to either a low-fat, amino-acid based synthetic diet or to a "standard" one.[79] Joint tenderness significantly improved only in the group consuming the experimental diet; the erythrocyte sedimentation rate and platelet count significantly improved only in the control group.

Implications of the Data

Formulations containing digested protein seem to provide benefit in some allergic disorders. However, the randomized controlled trials were not blinded and the outcome assessment could have been influenced by observer bias.

Primary Starvation

Summary of the Data

Any organism that is deprived of nutrients for a long enough period will eventually develop morbidity and, ultimately, die. With regard to nutrition support, we need to know how long that period is before "primary starvation" contributes its own adverse outcomes to patients with underlying conditions.

The randomized controlled trials that compared some form of nutrition support to no nutrition support usually were conducted for at least a week. In fact, when the meta-analyses were confined only to those studies, the conclusions did not differ.[6,7] In an effort to assess this factor more closely, one of our systematic reviews undertook an analysis of the surgical trials in which PN was used or withheld for periods in excess of 7 days (">7", 7 to 10, 8, 9.4 [mean], 10, 12, 13, and 18 days respectively). Even then, PN had no effect on any of the clinical outcomes.

Experiences with famines and fasts indicate that even healthy people will get into trouble eventually, albeit only after a matter of weeks.[80] We do not know if patients with underlying illnesses get into trouble faster because of some degree of depleted reserves and/or increased needs, or if they can endure longer periods because of metabolic adaptations. Given the fact that nutrition support for 1 to 2 weeks does not seem to provide any benefit, it does appear to be reasonable to conclude that, whatever the period of time is before primary starvation becomes an important clinical issue, that period is measured in weeks (plural), not days (at least in those who are not severely malnourished at the outset).

For patients whose GI tract is permanently damaged, the parenteral infusion of nutrients (home PN) is life-saving. We do not need randomized controlled trials to test this proposition. Controls are required if an outcome is unpredictable for any given patient. If that outcome is absolutely predictable, the fact that an intervention changes it is proof of efficacy.

Much of the home PN in the United States is provided to cancer patients.[81] There is a dramatic difference in survival between patients with benign disease (especially Crohn's disease) and those with malignancy.[82] The respective 1-year survival rates are >90% and 15% to 30%.

There is limited information about quality of life and functional assessment of patients receiving home PN. In general, these parameters are better in younger individuals with benign disease who have been on the therapy for longer periods of time.[82] These patients still do not perceive their lives as being normal, but rather being comparable to those of dialysis patients.[82]

Home PN is associated with important medical complications. These include catheter complications, (sepsis, occlusion, or central vein thrombosis), liver disease, metabolic bone disease, and psychiatric problems (especially depression). The cost is about $100,000/year.[81,82]

There is another group of patients for whom long-term nutrition support is an issue. These are patients who have intact GI tracts but who, for a variety of reasons cannot or will not eat; this group is typified by patients with strokes who have swallowing disorders or by individuals with advanced dementia. EN, particularly with percutaneous gastrostomy tubes, has become very popular for such individuals. For patients with strokes who otherwise have some reasonable amount of functional capacity, the issue is analogous to using PN for inadequate bowel syndrome. (Because the patients cannot swallow, fatal starvation must occur unless nutrients are supplied artificially.)

In patients with end stage dementia, the use of such nutrient infusions is controversial. Families may request the therapy, viewing it as "eating". Sometimes such tubes are placed to facilitate hospital discharge and nursing home placement. No randomized controlled trials are available, and the short-term (1 to 6 months) mortality in such intubated patients is high.[83-86] Palliation may not even be accomplished.[87] These patients are immobile and do not communicate needs to defecate; the nutrient infusions could actually cause more harm than good (incontinence and/or decubiti).

Implications of the Data

For nonseverely malnourished patients who are expected to resume oral food intake, the period of time before nutrient deprivation will be an issue is a matter of weeks, not days. We have no such insight into the time that is dangerous for the severely malnourished patient. Patients with irreversible GI tract failure will succumb to starvation unless parenteral nutrients are provided. The use of home PN in this scenario is analogous to providing hemodialysis to patients with end-stage renal disease. Patients with intact GI tracts, but underlying disorders that do not allow the normal assimilation of food, are candidates for long-term EN. However, such therapy should only be offered when it is clear that the benefits outweigh the medical risks and costs.

Potential Limitations of the Data

It is widely accepted that protein-energy malnutrition is accompanied by adverse clinical consequences. It would seem to be intuitively obvious that the correction of that state of malnutrition should improve clinical outcome. Thus, the data from the randomized controlled trials have been disappointing. Why haven't these randomized controlled trials demonstrated a more impressive benefit? The simplest answer is that nutrition support is not an effective therapeutic intervention. After all, there is no reason to believe that the association between poor nutritional status and poor outcome is causative. This chapter has already documented examples in which the nutritional parameters improved but the clinical ones did not. Even if malnutrition were partly responsible for the poor outcome, the side effects of the nutrition support might equal the benefits it provided. In such a case, no net effect would result.

The investigators may be using the wrong nutritional formulations. A number of the randomized controlled trials were conducted at a time when the standard was to provide large amounts of calories. The resultant metabolic abnormalities, especially hyperglycemia, may have been responsible for infections and other complications. Current regimens employ fewer calories.

The randomized controlled trials may not have included (and have not identified) the patients who will benefit. We certainly lack data regarding the effect of nutrition support in the severely malnourished.

There may be other randomized controlled trials that were not identified. Computer searches of MEDLINE can miss pertinent studies.[88] For that reason, a number of methods were used to find trials.[6,7] Unpublished studies always create a problem, but publication bias usually favors the trials that show beneficial effects.[88]

As noted at the outset, even randomized controlled trials have pitfalls. Type I errors are not likely to be an issue, because this review found few positive effects. Although both a large number of randomized controlled trials and meta-analysis reduce the likelihood of type II errors, we cannot exclude the possibility that favorable trends actually represent true differences (especially in the clinical conditions with only limited amounts of data).

Inappropriate data analysis (such as not using intent to treat), lack of blinding, defective randomization allocation, and other lacks of methodologic rigor can impact on the size of the observed treatment effect. The degree of rigor is referred to as the "quality" of the trial and, as previously noted, low quality is associated with an overestimation of that effect. Most of the randomized controlled trials were of relatively poor quality, which suggests that the true effects of nutrition support may be even less beneficial than the data indicated.

TABLE 34-5.

Indications and Contraindications for Nutrition Support[1]

Disease State	*PN*	*PST*	*EN*	*VNS*
Perioperative	No[2]	No	No	Possible benefit[3]
Liver disease:				
Alcoholic hepatitis	No[4]	No[4]	No[4]	No[4]
CLD	Unknown	Unknown	No	No
Liver transplant	No	Unknown	No	No
Acute pancreatitis	No[5]	No	No[6]	N/A
IBD[7]	No	Unknown	No	No
Critical illness	No	Unknown	No[8]	N/A
Oncology	No[9]	Unknown	No[10]	No[10]
Pediatrics:				
LBW infants	No	No	Possible benefit of trophic feeding[3]	N/A
Other conditions[7]	Unknown	Unknown	Unknown	Unknown
Pulmonary	No	Unknown	No[6]	No
AIDS	No	Unknown	Unknown	No
Renal failure	Unknown	Unknown	Unknown	Unknown
Cardiac disease	N/A	N/A	Unknown	Unknown
Geriatrics	N/A	N/A	No[6]	Possible benefit[3,11]
Hip fracture	Unknown	Unknown	Possible less rehabilitation time[3]	Possible benefit[3]
Stroke	N/A	N/A	Unknown	No[6]
Pregnancy	N/A	N/A	Unknown	No
Allergic disorders	N/A	N/A	N/A	Possible benefit[12]

No = Data from >1 randomized controlled trial unable to demonstrate benefit
Unknown = No data from randomized controlled trials available
N/A (not applicable) = This type of nutrition support inappropriate for this disease state
[1] Virtually no data from randomized controlled trials for effect of nutrition support in severely malnourished
[2] Subgroup analysis indicated potential utility for preoperative PN in patients with upper GI (esophagus/stomach) cancer
[3] Randomized controlled trials that suggested the presence of a benefit were of low quality
[4] Branched chain amino acid solutions may improve hepatic encephalopathy (pharmacologic effect)
[5] Increased morbidity in patients with mild pancreatitis
[6] Data only available from single randomized controlled trial
[7] No data from randomized controlled trials regarding effect of nutrition support on growth retardation in children
[8] Trends for EN to reduce infection rates, but differences not statistically significant
[9] Excess morbidity and poorer tumor response with chemotherapy or radiation therapy; one randomized trial suggested improved long-term survival with PN in patients undergoing bone marrow transplantation
[10] Unknown for hematologic malignancies
[11] In those at risk of malnutrition (discordant results in different meta-analyses)
[12] Use of preformulated nutrient solutions containing digested protein

Indications and Contraindications for Nutrition Support

The term "nutrition support" may conjure up an image of a patient sitting at the dinner table enjoying a meal with the rest of his or her family. However, nutrition support is not eating. It requires the placement of a tube in some channel (intestine or vein) or, at the very least, the consumption of a liquid that has been prescribed by a healthcare worker. It is a therapeutic intervention and must be assessed as one.

Very little evidence supports the use of this therapy, despite the existence of a large number of randomized controlled trials. At this time, there are only a few disease states for which healthcare providers can advocate its implementation. The data-based recommendations are summarized in Table 34-5.

The "indications" for nutrition support are the following:

1. Preoperative PN appears to reduce the incidence of major postoperative complications in patients scheduled to undergo attempted curative surgery for cancer of the esophagus or stomach. (Even here, it should be pointed out that this conclusion is based on a subgroup analysis of data that, overall, failed to show an effect.)
2. Perioperative VNS was associated with a positive effect, but this conclusion rests on data from low quality randomized controlled trials.
3. PN may improve long-term survival in patients undergoing bone marrow transplantation.
4. VNS may be effective in geriatric populations who are malnourished or at risk of becoming so. This conclusion rests on a relatively liberal interpretation of low quality studies.
5. Both EN and VNS may be of benefit as adjunctive therapy in patients (especially malnourished ones) with hip fractures.
6. BCAAs may be helpful in the management of hepatic encephalopathy, but this is an expensive pharmacologic (non-nutritional) effect.
7. Trophic feeding may be helpful in low birth weight infants, although this conclusion also rests on data from low quality studies.
8. While it may be correct to provide nutrition support to children who are failing to grow normally because of an underlying disease, we have no data from randomized controlled trials to justify this practice.
9. Diets containing hydrolyzed protein may be useful in some allergic disorders.
10. Home PN has never been assessed in randomized controlled trials, but that is not necessary; the intervention is indicated in patients in whom the GI tract will be inoperative for months (or even permanently) if the benefit to be gained justifies the resource expenditure that has to be made.
11. Similarly, patients who cannot access an intact GI tract (eg, functioning stroke victims with swallowing disorders) are candidates for home (or long-term institutional) intestinal tube infusions, with the same proviso that the benefits have to outweigh the risks. (The benefits may not outweigh the risks in patients with end-stage dementia.)

There are no data available to assess the role of nutrition support in the severely malnourished. No recommendation can be made.

There are conditions in which nutrition support produces net harm. This is particularly the case for PN in patients who are receiving chemotherapy or radiation therapy for cancer. PN also appears to be problematic in patients with mild pancreatitis. (PN may even predispose all patients to getting infections without necessarily providing any compensatory benefit.) For the remainder of the disease states that have been considered, there is either no randomized controlled trial available to assess the situation or at least one randomized controlled trial that has failed to show benefit.

While nutrition support has been advocated for decades, the evidence belies this enthusiasm. Given our limitations, this is one area where it would appear that resource utilization can be safely curtailed.

Take nothing on its looks. Take everything on evidence. There is no better rule.
— Charles Dickens (in *Great Expectations*)

References

1. Burner ST, Waldo DR, McKusick DR. National health expenditures projections through 2030. *Health Care Financ Rev.* 1992;14(1):1-29.
2. Younossi Z, Guyatt G. Evidence-based medicine: a method for solving clinical problems in hepatology. *Hepatology.* 1999;30:829-832.
3. Moher D, Schulz KF, Altman DG. The CONSORT statement: revised recommendations for improving the quality of reports of parallel-group randomised trials. *Lancet.* 2001;357:1191-1194.
4. Cook DJ, Mulrow CD, Haynes RB. Systematic reviews: synthesis of best evidence for clinical decisions. *Ann Intern Med.* 1997;126:376-380.
5. Mulrow CD. The medical review article: state of the science. *Ann Intern Med.* 1987;106:485-488.
6. Koretz RL, Lipman TO, Klein S. AGA technical review on parenteral nutrition. *Gastroenterology.* 2001;121:970-1001.
7. Koretz RL, Avenell A, Lipman TO, et al. Enteral nutrition. Gastroenterology, in submission.
8. Heyland DK, Novak F, Drover JW, Jain M, Su X, Suchner U. Should immunonutrition become routine in critically ill patients? A systematic review of the evidence. *JAMA.* 2001;286:944-953.
9. Ofman J, Koretz RL. Clinical economics review: nutritional support. *Aliment Pharmacol Ther.* 1997; 11:453-471.
10. Veterans Affairs Total Parenteral Nutrition Cooperative Study Group. Perioperative total parenteral nutrition in surgical patients. *N Engl J Med.* 1991;325:525-532.
11. Hansell DT, Davies JWL, Shenkin A, et al. The effects of an anabolic steroid and peripherally administered intravenous nutrition in the early postoperative period. *JPEN J Parenter Enteral Nutr.* 1989;13:349-358.
12. Hwang T-L, Mou S-C, Chen M-F. The importance of a source of sufficient protein in postoperative hypocaloric partial parenteral nutrition support. *JPEN J Parenter Enteral Nutr.* 1993;17:254-256.
13. Abbott WC, Bistrian BR, Blackburn GL. The effect of dextrose and amino acids on respiratory function and energy expenditure in morbidly obese patients following gastric bypass surgery. *J Surg Res.* 1986;41:225-235.
14. Culebras-Fernandez JM, de la Hoz Riesco M, Villares Garcia C, et al. Improvement of the nutritional condition with hypocaloric peripheral parenteral nutrition (HPPN) in the immediate postoperative period of elective abdominal surgery. *Infusionsther Klin Ernahr.* 1987;14:202-208.
15. Doglietto GB, Gallitelli L, Pacelli F, et al. Protein-sparing therapy after major abdominal surgery. Lack of clinical effects. *Ann Surg.* 1996;223:357-362.
16. Figueras J, Puig P, Rafecas A, et al. Postoperative hypocaloric parenteral nutrition. *Acta Chir Scand.* 1988;154:435-438.
17. Freund H, Hoover HC, Atamian S, Fischer JE. Infusion of the branched chain amino acids in postoperative patients. *Ann Surg.* 1979;190:18-23.

18. Hensle TW. Protein-sparing therapy in cystectomy patients. *J Urol.* 1978;119:355-358.
19. Hogbin BM, Smith AM, Craven AH. An evaluation of peripheral essential amino acid infusion following major surgery. *JPEN J Parenter Enteral Nutr.* 1984;8:511-514.
20. Jimenez Jimenez FJ, Ortiz Leyba C, Jimenez Jimenez LM, Garcia Valdecasas MS, Garnacho Montero J. Study of hypocaloric peripheral parenteral nutrition in postoperative patients (European project). *Clin Nutr.* 1995;14:88-96.
21. Lopez-Hellin J, Lopez-Lara M, Mercader S, et al. Early curbing of protein hypercatabolism in postoperative patients by nutritional support with glucose plus amino acids, but not with glucose alone. *Clin Nutr.* 1997;16:67-73.
22. Koretz RL. Is nutritional support worthwhile? In: Heatley RV, Green JH, Losowsky MS, eds. *Consensus in Clinical Nutrition.* Cambridge: Cambridge University Press; 1994:158-191.
23. Moher D, Pham B, Jones A, et al. Does quality of reports of randomised trials affect estimates of intervention efficacy reported in meta-analyses? *Lancet.* 1998;362:609-613.
24. Mendenhall CL, Moritz TE, Roselle GA, et al. A study of oral nutritional support with oxandrolone in malnourished patients with alcoholic hepatitis: results of a Department of Veterans Affairs cooperative study. *Hepatology.* 1993;17:564-576.
25. Cabre E, Rodriguez-Iglesias P, Caballeria J, et al. Short- and long-term outcome of severe alcohol-induced hepatitis treated with steroids or enteral nutrition: a multicenter randomized trial. *Hepatology.* 2000;32:36-42.
26. Als-Nielsen B, Koretz RL, Kjaergaard LL, Gluud C. Branched chain amino acids for hepatic encephalopathy (Cochrane Review). In: The Cochrane Library, Issue 2. Oxford: Update Software; 2003.
27. Powell JJ, Murchison JT, Fearon KCH, Ross JA, Siriwardena AK. Randomized controlled trial of the effect of early enteral nutrition on markers of the inflammatory response in predicted severe acute pancreatitis. *Br J Surg.* 2000;87:1375-1381.
28. Eatock FC, Chong P, Menezes N, et al. A randomized study of early nasogastric versus nasojejunal feeding in severe acute pancreatitis. *Am J Gastroenterol.* 2005;100:432-439.
29. Griffiths AM, Ohlsson A, Sherman PM, Sutherland LR. Meta-analysis of enteral nutrition as a primary treatment of active Crohn's disease. *Gastroenterology.* 1995;108:1056-1067.
30. Fernandez-Banares F, Cabre E, Esteve-Comas M, Gassull MA. How effective is enteral nutrition in inducing clinical remission in active Crohn's disease? A meta-analysis of the randomized clinical trials. *JPEN J Parenter Enteral Nutr.* 1995;19:356-364.
31. Messori A, Trallori G, D'Albasio G, et al. Defined-formula diets versus steroids in the treatment of active Crohn's disease. A meta-analysis. *Scand J Gastroenterol.* 1996;31:267-272.
32. Lochs H, Meryn S, Marosi L, Ferenci P, Hortnagl H. Has total bowel rest a beneficial effect in the treatment of Crohn's disease? *Clin Nutr.* 1983;2:61-64.
33. Chiarelli A, Enzi G, Casadei A, Baggio B, Valerio A, Mazzoleni F. Very early nutrition supplementation in burned patients. *Am J Clin Nutr.* 1990;51:1035-1039.
34. Heyland DK, Dhaliwal R, Drover JW, Gramlich L, Dodek P, and the Canadian Critical Care Clinical Practice Guidelines Committee. Canadian clinical practice guidelines for nutrition support in mechanically ventilated, critically ill adult patients. *JPEN J Parenter Enteral Nutr.* 2003;27:355-373.
35. Jenkins ME, Gottschlich MM, Warden GD. Enteral feeding during operative procedures in thermal injuries. *J Burn Care Rehabil.* 1994;15:199-205.
36. Moore EE, Jones TN. Benefits of immediate jejunostomy feeding after major abdominal trauma: a prospective, randomized study. *J Trauma.* 1986;26:874-881.
37. Weisdorf SA, Lysne J, Wind D, et al. Positive effect of prophylactic total parenteral nutrition on long-term outcome of bone marrow transplantation. *Transplantation.* 1987;43:833-838
38. Solassol C, Joyeaux H, Dubois JB. Total parenteral nutrition (TPN) with complete nutritive mixtures: an artificial gut in cancer patients. *Nutr Cancer.* 1979;1:13-18.
39. Tyson JE, Kennedy KA. Minimal enteral nutrition for promoting feeding tolerance and preventing morbidity in parenterally fed infants (Cochrane Review). In: The Cochrane Library, Issue 4. Oxford: Update Software; 2002.
40. Kirvela O, Stern RC, Askanazi J, et al. Long-term parenteral nutrition in cystic fibrosis. *Nutrition.* 1993;9:119-126.
41. Ferreira IM, Brooks D, Lacasse Y, Goldstein RS, White J. Nutritional supplementation for stable chronic obstructive pulmonary disease (Cochrane Review). In: The Cochrane Library, Issue 1. Oxford, Update Software; 2003.
42. Jelalian E, Stark LJ, Reynolds L, Seifer R. Nutrition intervention for weight gain in cystic fibrosis: a meta-analysis. *J Pediatr.* 1998;132:486-492.
43. Eubanks V, Koppersmith N, Wooldridge, et al. Effects of megestrol acetate on weight gain, body composition, and pulmonary function in patients with cystic fibrosis. *J Pediatr.* 2002;140:439-444.
44. Conway SP, Morton A, Wolfe MA. Enteral tube feeding for cystic fibrosis (Cochrane Review). In: The Cochrane Library, Issue 4. Oxford: Update Software; 2002.
45. Beckles Willson N, Elliott TM, Everard ML. Omega-3 fatty acids (from fish oils) for cystic fibrosis (Cochrane Review). In: The Cochrane Library, Issue 4. Oxford: Update Software; 2003.
46. Smyth R, Walters S. Oral calorie supplements for cystic fibrosis (Cochrane Review). In: The Cochrane Library, Issue 1. Oxford, Update Software; 2003.
47. Melchior JC, Chastang C, Gelas P, et al. Efficacy of 2-month total parenteral nutrition in AIDS patients: a controlled randomized prospective trial. *AIDS.* 1996;10:379-384.
48. Melchior J-C, Gelas P, Carbonnet F, et al. Improved survival by home total parenteral nutrition in AIDS patients: follow-up of a controlled randomized prospective trial. *AIDS.* 1998;12:336-337.
49. Keithley JK, Swanson B, Zeller JM, et al. Comparison of standard and immune-enhancing oral formulas in asymptomatic HIV-infected persons: a multicenter randomized controlled clinical trial. *JPEN J Parenter Enteral Nutr.* 2002;26:6-14.
50. Kotler DP, Fogleman L, Tierney AR. Comparison of total parenteral nutrition and an oral, semielemental diet on body composition, physical function, and nutrition-related costs in patients with malabsorption due to acquired immunodeficiency syndrome. *JPEN J Parenter Enteral Nutr.* 1998;22:120-126.
51. Van Roenn JH, Armstrong D, Kotler DP, et al. Megestrol acetate in patients with AIDS-related cachexia. *Ann Intern Med.* 1994;121:393-399.
52. Oster MH, Enders SR, Samuels SJ, et al. Megestrol acetate in patients with AIDS and cachexia. *Ann Intern Med.* 1994;121:400-408.
53. Beal JE, Olson R, Laubenstein L, et al. Dronabinol as a treatment for anorexia associated with weight loss in patients with AIDS. *J Pain Symptom Manage.* 1995;10:89-97.
54. Zarazaga A, Garcia-de-Lorenzo L, Garcia-Luna PP, et al. Nutritional support in chronic renal failure: systematic review. *Clin Nutr.* 2001;20:291-299.
55. Cano N, Labastie-Coeyrehourq J, Lacombe P, et al. Perdialytic parenteral nutrition with lipids and amino acids in malnourished hemodialysis patients. *Am J Clin Nutr.* 1990;52:726-730.
56. Wolfson M, Jones MR, Kopple JD. Amino acid losses during hemodialysis with infusion of amino acids and glucose. *Kidney Int.* 1982;21:500-506.
57. McCann L, Feldman C, Hornberger J, et al. Effect of intradialytic parenteral nutrition on delivered Kt/V. Am J Kidney Dis 1999;33:1131-1135.
58. Jones M, Hagen T, Boyle CA, et al. Treatment of malnutrition with 1.1% amino acid peritoneal dialysis solution: results of a multicenter outpatient study. *Am J Kidney Dis.* 1998;32:761-769.
59. Guarnieri G, Faccini L, Lipartiti T, et al. Simple methods for nutritional assessment in hemodialyzed patients. *Am J Clin Nutr.* 1980;33:1598-1607.
60. Foulks CJ. An evidence-based evaluation of intradialytic parenteral nutrition. *Am J Kidney Dis.* 1999;33:186-192.

61. Abel R, Beck CH, Abbott WM, et al. Improved survival from acute renal failure after treatment with intravenous essential l-amino acids and glucose. *N Engl J Med.* 1973;288:695-699
62. Leonard CD, Luke RG, Siegel RR. Parenteral essential amino acids in acute renal failure. *Urology.* 1975;6:154-157.
63. Feinstein EI, Blumenkrantz MJ, Healy M, et al. Clinical and metabolic responses to parenteral nutrition in acute renal failure. *Medicine.* 1981;60:124-137.
64. Feinstein EI, Kopple JD, Silberman H, Massry SG. Total parenteral nutrition with high or low nitrogen intakes in patients with acute renal failure. *Kidney Int.* 1983;26(Suppl 16):S319-S323.
65. Mirtallo JM, Schneider PJ, Mavko K, Ruberg RL, Fabri PJ. A comparison of essential and general amino acid infusions in the nutritional support of patients with compromised renal function. *JPEN J Parenter Enteral Nutr.* 1982;6:109-113.
66. Naylor CD, Detsky AS, O'Rourke K, Fonberg E. Does treatment with essential amino acids and hypertonic glucose improve survival in acute renal failure? A meta-analysis. *Renal Failure.* 1987-8;10:141-152.
67. Broqvist M, Arnqvist H, Dahlstrom U, et al. Nutritional assessment and muscle energy metabolism in severe chronic congestive heart failure: effects of long-term dietary supplementation. *Eur Heart J.* 1994;15:1641-1650.
68. Larsson J, Unosson M, Ek AC, et al. Effect of dietary supplementation on nutritional status and clinical outcome in 501 geriatric patients: a randomized study. *Clin Nutr.* 1990;9:179-184.
69. Norregaard O, Tottrup A, Saaek A, Hessov I. Effects of oral nutritional supplements to adults with chronic obstructive pulmonary disease. *Clin Resp Physiol.* 1987;23(Suppl 12):388S.
70. Milne AC, Potter J, Avenell A. Protein and energy supplementation in elderly people at risk from malnutrition (Cochrane Review). In: The Cochrane Library, Issue 1. Oxford, Update Software; 2003.
71. Myers SA, Takiguchi S, Slavish S, Rose CL. Consistent wound care and nutritional support in treatment. *Decubitus.* 1990; 3:16-28.
72. Avenell A, Handoll HHG. Nutritional supplementation for hip fracture aftercare in the elderly (Cochrane Review). In: The Cochrane Library, Issue 4. Oxford: Update Software; 2002.
73. Kramer M. Effects of energy and protein intakes on pregnancy outcome: an overview of the research evidence from controlled clinical trials. *Am J Clin Nutr.* 1993;58:627-635.
74. Hoj L, Osterballe O, Bundgaard A, Weeke B, Weiss M. A double-blind controlled trial of elemental diet in severe, perennial asthma. *Allergy.* 1981;36:257-262.
75. Hill DJ, Hudson IL, Sheffield LJ, et al. A low allergen diet is a significant intervention in infantile colic: results of a community-based study. *J Allergy Clin Immunol.* 1995;96:886-892.
76. Mabin DC, Sykes AE, David TJ. Controlled trial of a few foods diet in severe atopic dermatitis. *Arch Dis Child.* 1995;73:202-207.
77. Mallet E, Henocq A. Long-term prevention of allergic diseases by using protein hydrolysate formula in at-risk infants. *J Pediatr.* 1992;121:S95-S100.
78. Chandra RK. Five-year follow-up of high-risk infants with family history of allergy who were exclusively breast-fed or fed partial whey hydrolysate, soy, and conventional cow's milk formulas. *J Ped Gastroenterol Nutr.* 1997;24:380-388.
79. Haugen MA, Kjeldsen-Kragh J, Forre O. A pilot study of the effect of an elemental diet in the management of rheumatoid arthritis. *Clin Exp Rheumatol.* 1994;12:275-279.
80. Frommel D, Gautier M, Questiaux E, Schwarzenberg L. Voluntary total fasting: a challenge for the medical community. *Lancet.* 1984;1:1451-1452.
81. Howard L, Ament M, Fleming CR, Shike M, Steiger E. Current use and clinical outcome of home parenteral and enteral nutrition therapies in the United States. *Gastroenterology.* 1995;109:355-365.
82. Richards DM, Deeks JJ, Sheldon TA, Shaffer JL. Home parenteral nutrition: a systematic review. *Health Technol Assess.* 1997;1(1):1-59.
83. Sanders DS, Carter MJ, D'Silva J, et al. Survival analysis in percutaneous endoscopic gastrostomy feeding: a worse outcome in patients with dementia. *Am J Gastroenterol.* 2000; 95:1472-1475.
84. Sanders DS, Carter MJ, D'Silva J, et al. Percutaneous endoscopic gastrostomy: a prospective audit of the impact of guidelines in two district general hospitals in the United Kingdom. *Am J Gastroenterol.* 2002;97:2239-2245.
85. Murphy LM, Lipman TO. Percutaneous endoscopic gastrostomy does not prolong survival in patients with dementia. *Arch Intern Med.* 2003;163:1351-1353.
86. Meier DE, Ahronheim JC, Morris J, Baskin-Lyons S, Morrison RS. High short-term mortality in hospitalized patients with advanced dementia: lack of benefit of tube feeding. *Arch Intern Med.* 2001;161:594-599.
87. Finucane TE, Christmas C, Travis K. Tube feeding in patients with advanced dementia: a review of the evidence. *JAMA.* 1999;282:1365-1370.
88. Dickersin K, Min Y-I, Meinert CL. Factors influencing publication of research results. *JAMA.* 1992;267:374-378.

Chapter 35

Vascular Access for the Patient Receiving Parenteral Nutrition

Sandeep Gupta, MD; Ezra Steiger, MD; and Mark Sands, MD

Introduction

The development of parenteral nutrition (PN) in the 1960s enhanced the clinician's ability to treat many severe gastrointestinal disorders that interfered with oral or enteral nutrient intake. Effective administration of PN, whether given to the patient in the hospital or at home, is dependent on obtaining and maintaining safe, prolonged vascular access. Complications associated with vascular-access–device insertion and maintenance can be serious and even life threatening. The early diagnosis and treatment of complications will help to prevent disastrous outcomes.[1] The use of PN in the hospital or home setting necessitates different vascular-access devices and techniques of placement. The complications associated with their continued use usually present in the same way and are often similarly treated.

Vascular Access for the Hospitalized Patient

Device Selection

Choosing a suitable catheter type for an individual patient requires the evaluation of many factors. The caloric needs of the patient are the most important preliminary consideration that guides the choice of catheter type. The next most important factor is the length of time that vascular access is needed. Additionally, available facilities, equipment, and physician services at individual hospitals will all ultimately factor in to the decision of which catheter type is appropriate for a given patient.

PN solutions are either glucose based or lipid based. The glucose-based solutions use dextrose as the main calorie source and are markedly hypertonic; they must be delivered by a central venous device with the distal end of the device in the superior vena cava near its junction with the right atrium. This position allows for the rapid dilution of the hypertonic fluid with less likelihood of vein-wall irritation leading to phlebitis and thrombosis.[2] The infusion of PN into central veins is referred to as central parenteral nutrition (CPN). Lipid-based PN solutions use isotonic lipid solutions as the major kilocalorie source, are less hyperosmolar (osmolarity <900 mOsm), and can be safely given through short, intravenous cannulas placed in the hand or forearm. Lipid-based PN is commonly referred to as peripheral parenteral nutrition (PPN) because it is given via peripheral veins.

Peripheral Catheters

There are many types of peripheral catheters; however, they are relatively similar and do not offer a distinct advantage over each other. Two types of peripheral venous-access devices include angio-catheters and midline catheters. The traditional angio-catheter can be kept in a forearm vein for up to 4 days, and peripheral formulas can be infused through it. The cost is about $15.[3] The midline catheter is introduced in an antecubital vein and is 7 to 8 inches in length. It is advanced into the cephalic or basilic vein. These catheters have an insertion and device cost of $95 to $165 and $33, respectively.[4]

The advantages of peripheral access include low cost and complication rates. In contrast to central catheters, these catheters create no risk of perforation of the great vessels, the pleural space, or the heart. The most common complication of peripheral access is thrombophlebitis, which presents with pain as its first symptom. In addition, catheter sepsis can occur but is relatively infrequent. Both of these complications can be treated

TABLE 35-1.

Calculating the Osmolarity of Parenteral Nutrition Solutions

Total grams of amino acids per liter of solution	x 10
+ Total grams of dextrose per liter of solution	x 5
+ Total grams of lipid per liter of solution (using 30% lipid)	x 0.67
+ Toal mEq of sodium, potassium, calcium and magnesium per liter of solution	x 2
= Total milliosmoles per liter of solution	

by catheter removal and antibiotic therapy. A large controlled trial on the effect of differing dressing regimens for peripheral catheters showed no difference in catheter-site colonization or phlebitis when comparing transparent dressings with simple gauze. Additionally, the transparent dressings could be left on the peripheral catheters without changing them for the life of the catheter.[5]

Peripheral catheters are restricted to short-term use. They are useful in situations in which PN supplementation is needed for short periods of time (ie, perioperatively [1 to 2 weeks]).

The major limitation of peripheral veins is the type of solutions that can be infused through them. Peripheral formulas should be used for low to moderate nutritional deficiencies. Peripheral access is limited to a 3-in-1 solution containing protein, carbohydrate, and large amounts of lipid in a base solution. Osmolarity cannot exceed 900 mOsm/L because the formula can be caustic to peripheral veins including the common femoral vein. Osmolarity of a PN solution can be calculated by knowing its dextrose, amino acid, lipid, and electrolyte contents (Table 35-1).

Both types of peripheral catheters are inexpensive, easy to place, and useful for short-term nutritional supplementation. Central venous catheters placed through the femoral vein should be treated as peripheral catheters because the tip lies in the iliac vein or very proximal inferior vena cava (Figure 35-1). Central PN solutions should be avoided, and the less hyperosmolar PPN solutions should be infused through these catheters.

Central Venous Catheter

The central venous catheter is the vascular-access device most commonly used for CPN in the hospital setting. Although infection is more likely to occur in multi-lumen catheters compared to single lumen catheters,[6] their utility in managing patients who require multiple intravenous therapies makes these catheters more practical to use in the hospital setting. They are placed percutaneously via the subclavian or jugular veins using the Seldinger technique and are not tunneled. Two central principles are observed to avoid complications when placing any intravenous line with this technique: always have control of the guide wire and never advance against resistance.

Catheters placed by the percutaneous subclavian approached are reported to have a lower rate of infection[7] compared to catheters placed via the jugular vein. The decreased incidence of infections is probably related to the ease of maintaining the sterile occlusive dressing over the exit site on the chest wall more readily than that on the neck. Femoral vein catheterization should be avoided because of the high rate of infection,[8,9] thrombosis,[10] and difficulty in maintaining cleanliness around the catheter exit site in the groin. Educational videos demonstrating safe central venous catheter placement techniques were developed by the Food and Drug Administration and are very useful for resident training, even though some of the equipment and supplies have changed over the years.[11]

Peripherally Inserted Central Catheters

A central access catheter can also be inserted by cannulating the basilic or cephalic vein at the antecubital space or upper arm and advancing a long catheter through the peripheral access vein into the superior vena cava. These catheters, called peripherally inserted central catheters (PICC), have been available since the 1970s and have been increasingly popular because of the ease of placement and comparatively lower cost than other available long-term catheters. Available in both single- and double-lumen configurations, they are typically used for weeks or months. This catheter can usually be placed at the bedside by a nurse at a cost of about $400.[3] When there is difficulty in identifying a suitable cephalic, basilic, or median antecubital vein for cannulation, ultrasound at the bedside or by a radiologist in interventional radiology is very useful. Central formulas, including both 2-in-1 and 3-in-1 solutions, can be infused through this catheter. The risks are usually similar to peripheral angio-catheters, limited to local thrombophlebitis and catheter sepsis. However, as with any centrally located catheter, the risks of major venous thrombosis, malposition, and cardiac arrhythmias are possible. There is almost no risk of pneumothorax, vascular perforation, or hemothorax.[4]

The contraindications to placement are previous venous surgery on that extremity, major venous thrombosis, local infection, lymphedema, ipsilateral axillary node dissection, or a history of extremity trauma. Once the catheter is placed, a chest x-ray should be checked to confirm the catheter tip location, ideally at the junction of the superior vena cava and right atrium, and the catheter may then be used immediately. With its low cost and low complication rate and its ability to infuse high tonicity parenteral solutions, this catheter can be used in and out of the hospital for PN as well as antibiotics. The exit site position in the

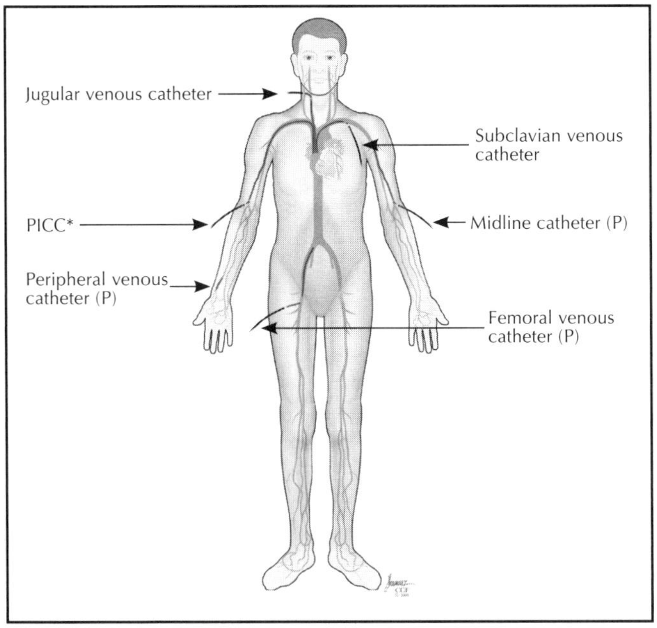

Figure 35-1. Vascular access devices used to deliver parenteral nutrition fluids to hospitalized patients. (P) denotes devices used for peripheral parenteral nutrition (PPN) only. *PICC = peripherally inserted central catheter.

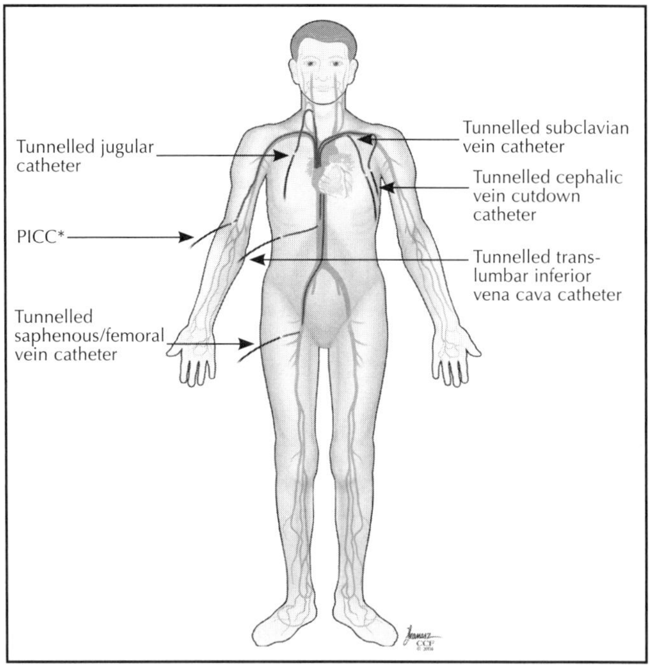

Figure 35-2. Vascular access devices used to deliver parenteral nutrition fluids to patients at home or alternate site settings. Subcutaneous ports can also be inserted at the exit sites instead of the external catheter segments. *PICC = peripherally inserted central catheter.

antecubital space makes it necessary for the patient to care for the catheter with only one hand, which can be a disadvantage for some patients.

Although complications associated with their insertion are less than those with percutaneous subclavian catheterization, the incidence of phlebitis, thrombosis, and catheter dysfunction is usually higher[12,13] than with other central lines.

Vascular Access for the Home Patient

Device Selection

Patients discharged to outpatient settings require devices that are readily maintained with limited danger of accidental removal. Tunneled cuffed catheters (Broviac, or Hickman, Bard Access Systems, Salt Lake City, Utah) or subcutaneous ports are most commonly used. Placement of these devices takes place in the interventional radiology suite or in the operating room, and charges range from \$3500 to \$4200.[3] In some patients who require outpatient access for relatively short periods of time (several weeks to 2 months), PICC may be more appropriate and, if inserted at the bedside, costs \$400.[3] Tunneled catheters can be placed percutaneously through the internal jugular vein or subclavian vein in the operating room or the interventional radiology suite, or by cutdown via the internal or external jugular vein or cephalic vein in the operating room (Figure 35-2). The catheter is tunneled subcutaneously from the previously marked exit site on the chest wall to the cutdown or percutaneous site. Excess catheter length is excised so that the tip of the catheter lies at the junction of the superior vena cava and right atrium. The Dacron velour cuff is positioned 2 to 4 cm proximal to the exit site in the subcutaneous tunnel to allow tissue ingrowth that stabilizes the catheter and theoretically prevents ascending catheter tract infection. Until tissue ingrowth secures the catheter, an exit site suture around the catheter is left in place for at least 4 weeks. The patient or caregiver can readily access the catheter hub at the external portion of the catheter. Some activities are limited with the external tunneled catheter to keep the exit site clean and dry.

The subcutaneous port is inserted using similar techniques and venous routes as tunneled catheters; however, it lies entirely in a subcutaneous pocket, usually on the anterior chest wall. It must be accessed via a percutaneously placed noncoring needle for infusions. When PN infusion is not needed, the access needle can be removed allowing for full activity without regard to keeping a dressing clean and dry. Most patients who have subcutaneous ports, however, leave the cannulating needle in place for 2 to 7 days at a time if they require daily infusions.

Morbidity of Central Venous Catheters

Complications of Central Line Insertion

Most complications of central venous catheters can be separated into short and long term. Short-term complications include pneumothoraces, which occur in 1% to 4% of patients receiving central venous catheters.[14] This is defined as a lung parenchymal injury during venipuncture allowing inspired air to leak between the visceral and parietal pleura. The visceral pleural can act as a one-way valve, causing progressive accumulation of air, which results in a tension pneumothorax. This can compress the adjacent lung and vena cava and shift the mediastinum to the contralateral side, which requires immediate needle decompression in the second intercostals space in the midclavicular line followed by tube thoracostomy. Nontension pneumothoraces can be treated without tube decompression if it is <30% of the pleural space and fails to progress over serial x-rays over a 24-hour period and if the patient remains clinically stable.[15-17]

Vascular perforation can occur as an immediate complication at the time of insertion of the catheter. A local wound hematoma can occur in more coagulopathic patients. This can be managed with manual compression of the vascular exit site and correction of an underlying coagulopathy. Perforation of central vascular structures is relatively infrequent. The hypothetical mechanism of injury is the failure of the relatively inflexible dilator to negotiate the turns of the subclavian veins into the brachiocephalic vein or superior vena cava. A mediastinal hematoma or hemothorax can develop from this. If a vascular perforation exists, the removal of the catheter could make a relatively controlled hemorrhage uncontrollable. If the patient is hemodynamically unstable, a tube thoracostomy should be placed to drain a hemothorax and Advanced Cardiac Life Support algorithm protocol should be initiated. Pericardial tamponade can also occur with a mortality approaching 90%.[18] This is a result of perforation of central vein or cardiac wall into the pericardial space, which results in rapid deterioration of blood pressure and oxygen saturation. Beck's triad of hypotension, muffled heart sounds, and distended neck veins ensues. High clinical suspicion is extremely important when this procedure results in such catastrophic outcomes, and urgent cardiothoracic surgery consultation is necessary. Inadvertent perforation of the carotid artery during jugular vein cannulation is best managed with surgical consultation prior to removal of the misplaced cannula.[1]

The use of ultrasound to mark the position of the subclavian vein in an attempt to reduce complications has not been of proven benefit in a randomized prospective study;[19] however, it was shown to be of value when real-time ultrasound guidance was used in a group of patients who would otherwise be difficult-access cases.[20] The incidence of insertion complications increases with multiple attempts and in very thin patients.[19] A postinsertion–attempt chest x-ray is mandatory prior to catheter use to ascertain proper position of any centrally directed catheter and to rule out the occurrence of a pneumothorax.

Catheter pinch-off occurs when a medially placed percutaneous subclavian catheter becomes occluded between the clavicle and first rib. Typically, flow through the catheter is temporarily restored by raising the patient's arm or rolling the shoulder on the same side that the catheter is on.[21] A chest x-ray will show indentation of the catheter at the junction of the clavicle and first rib. The catheter can be severed by the scissors-like motion of the clavicle against the first rib; these catheters should be removed and a new catheter placed more laterally. Less common complications associated with catheter insertion include air embolus and right atrial and major venous perforations.[22]

Catheter Infections

Catheter-related infections can be subdivided into local and systemic types. Local types include exit-site, tunnel, and port-pocket infections. Purulent exit-site infections of nontunneled catheters are best treated by removal of the temporary central catheter. Tunneled cuffed catheter purulent exit site infections may be treated with antibiotics and wound care as long as the Dacron velour cuff and tunnel are not involved. However, if the clinical situation deteriorates from sepsis or if a port becomes exposed, the device must be removed. Both tunnel infection and port pocket infections usually require device removal to eradicate the infection.

Catheter-related blood-stream infection (CRBSI) is a frequent complication of prolonged central venous access in the hospital or home setting. CRBSI is estimated to affect more than 200,000 patients per year in the United States[23,24] and the Communicable Disease Center (CDC) estimates that the attributable cost per infection is $34,508 to $56,000.[25] CRBSI occurs when a patient develops bacteriemia with positive blood cultures and has clinical or microbiologic evidence that the catheter is the source of infection. Most often, the patient in the hospital presents with fever without a readily apparent source of infection. Shaking chills and fever associated with infusion of the parenteral nutrition solution occurs frequently in the home patient but can also occur in the hospital setting. The catheter exit site is usually benign appearing, even with noncuffed catheters.[26]

The etiology of CRBSI is thought to be from one of three sources: 1) contamination from the catheter exit site, which is more likely to occur with the temporary catheter than with the tunneled catheter; 2) contamination of the hub, a more likely cause of catheter sepsis in the home patient but one that can also occur in the hospitalized patient; and 3) hematogenous seeding from a distant site—such as an intra-abdominal abscess—that colonizes the catheter.[24] The possibility of hematogenous seeding necessitates the use of prophylactic antibiotics whenever a patient with a vascular access device in place undergoes oral surgery, teeth cleaning, or surgery involving a contaminated part of the body. Antibiotics should be given parenterally if malabsorption is significant.

Diagnosing Catheter Infections

Diagnosing CRBSI without removing the catheter can be done by one of three techniques:[27] 1) paired quantitative blood cultures from the vascular access device and from a peripheral vein showing greater growth from the blood drawn through the catheter; 2) time to positivity showing growth from blood drawn through the catheter at least 2 hours before growth in the blood drawn by the peripheral vein; and 3) endoluminal brush cultures, where the brush passed through a catheter can sample the biofilm on the endoluminal surface and is considered positive if more than 100 colony-forming units per milliliter grow. CRBSI usually presents with the patient experiencing a persistent fever in the hospital setting. In the home setting, the sudden appearance of fever and chills in the patient upon the

TABLE 35-2.

Recommendations for Placement of Intravascular Catheters

- Educate healthcare workers regarding proper indications, procedures for insertion and maintenance, and appropriate infection control measures
- Do not routinely culture catheter tips
- Observe proper hand hygiene procedures even if sterile gloves are worn
- Maintain aseptic technique for the insertion and care of intravascular catheters
- Sterile gloves should be worn when inserting arterial or central catheters
- Do not routinely use cutdown procedures to insert catheters
- Disinfect clean skin with an appropriate antiseptic before catheter insertion
- Do not apply organic solvents to the skin before inserting catheters
- Sterile gauze or sterile transparent semi-permeable dressing can be used to cover the catheter exit site
- Do not use topical antibiotic ointments or creams on insertion site
- Select catheter, insertion technique, and site that has the lowest incidence of complications for the anticipated intravenous therapy
- Promptly remove any catheter that is no longer needed

Adapted from CDC MMWR Recommendations and Reports. *Guidelines for the Prevention of Intravascular Catheter Related Infections.* Aug. 9, 2002.

start of the PN solution is almost always diagnostic of a catheter infection. If the patient presents with severe sepsis and hypotension, even with no other apparent source, the catheter should be removed and cultured immediately after blood cultures are obtained through the catheter and a peripheral vein. The most common organisms infecting catheters include *Staphylococcus epidermidis*, *Staphylococcus aureus*, and *Candida* species. The initial antibiotic therapy should include vancomycin to cover the gram-positive organisms. Immunocompromised patients should also receive gram-negative coverage because of their susceptibility to a wide variety of organisms.

Many catheter infections can be treated with antibiotic therapy alone; however, certain organisms, such as *Candida* and *Staphylococcus aureus* are very difficult to eradicate and most often require removal of the indwelling catheter. In addition, the persistence of positive blood cultures or the patient's failure to improve clinically are other reasons that mandate prompt removal of the indwelling intravenous line. Home parenteral nutrition patients with suspected catheter or port sepsis should be admitted to the hospital with appropriate cultures taken, and the suspected device should be used only for antibiotic administration as well as that of 5% dextrose and electrolyte solutions. If the catheter or port is removed, a new device may be placed when post device removal blood cultures are negative. Complicating endocarditis, osteomyelitis, and endophthalmitis may be the cause of persistently positive blood cultures after device removal. Consultation with an infectious disease specialist is very helpful in the management of the patient with suspected vascular access infection.

Prevention of Catheter Infection

Judicious use of central venous catheters will limit unnecessary complications (Table 35-2). The routine changing of catheters has not been shown to decrease catheter infection rate in several studies.[28] In addition, prevention of catheter infection has been studied in a randomized prospective double-blind study on preoperative vancomycin versus placebo. There was no benefit for the treatment group.[29] The use of antibiotic flushes have met with limited success and in some cases led to growth of resistant organisms. A prospective study of catheter-related infections in patients receiving PN in the hospital showed a decline in the rate of infection from 33% to 4% with the hiring of a nurse to assume the responsibility for the catheter care.[30] The only significant predictive variable influencing the risk of infectious outcome is the patient diagnosis. Younger male patients with hematological malignancies are at the greatest risk for infectious complications.[31,32]

Additionally, there is some evidence to suggest that certain catheter materials may reduce infectious complications. In a retrospective study, the use of chlorhexidine-silver-sulfadiazine–impregnated central venous catheters in intensive care unit patients at high risk for catheter-related infections reduced the incidence of CRBSI and provided significant savings.[33] Similar results were found in a randomized prospective study.[34] Minocycline and ethylene diamine tetra-acetate (EDTA) solutions have been shown to be effective against microorganisms embedded in biofilm on catheter surfaces in in-vitro and ex-vivo experiments[35] and may, in the future, be effective flush solutions to reduce the incidence of catheter infections. Evidence-based recommendations for the prevention of catheter-related infections were recently published[25] as guidelines for practitioners who insert catheters and for persons involved in infection surveillance and control in hospitals. These guidelines are very helpful in diagnosing, managing, and preventing catheter-related infections in the patient receiving PN in the hospital or at home.

CATHETER OCCLUSION

Sudden cessation of fluid flow through the catheter can be caused by mechanical or thrombotic complications. Common mechanical problems include occluded intravenous tubing by clamps or kinked intravenous tubing, acute angulation of the catheter, or catheter pinch off by compression of the clavicle over the first rib. Physical exam or a chest x-ray can readily diagnose these mechanical problems.

Thrombotic occlusion of the catheter usually occurs more slowly: over hours or days. There is a gradual decrease in flow rate and difficulty aspirating blood from the catheter. Fibrin sheath at the tip of the catheter allows flushing but not withdrawal of blood because of a one-way valve effect. A thrombus within the lumen of the catheter or at the tip of the catheter is usually the cause. Change in the patient's position, repeated flushing, or instillation of tissue plasminogen activator[36,37] will usually restore catheter function. Precipitate occlusion of the catheter can be caused by calcium phosphate precipitates, lipid emulsion, or drug precipitates. Hydrochloric acid, 70% alcohol, and sodium hydroxide have been suggested for clearing catheters of these obstructions.[38] An amount of fluid equal to the internal volume of the catheter is left in place for 30 to 90 minutes before aspirating. The dwell time can be increased as long as 12 hours if the catheter patency cannot be readily restored after the first instillation.

Catheter-Associated Thromboses

Thrombosis is associated with central venous catheters in 0% to 50% of patients.[39-43] Symptoms include ipsilateral arm swelling, edema, and dull achy pain. Subcutaneous collateral venous branches may become engorged from diversion of occluded blood. The rate of pulmonary embolus can be as high as 15%[44] and these patients need standard anticoagulation. Risk factors for vascular thrombosis include those with hypercoagulability, underlying malignancy, and an immunocompromised host. Diagnostic investigation includes a venous duplex of the affected subclavian and internal jugular vein. Secondary changes in the venous system of both axillary and jugular veins can be used to diagnose its occlusion. If the duplex ultrasound does not show a thrombus and the clinical suspicion is high, contrast venography remains the gold standard for diagnosis.

Treatment for thrombosis includes heparinisation with a partial thromboplastin time of 55 to 70 seconds while coumadin therapy is initiated to keep the International Normalized Ratio between 2.0 and 3.0 for a minimum of 3 months. Central catheter removal is more controversial. The long-term venous access dependence of the patient needs to be considered before deciding on its removal. In chronic PN patients, given their life-long need for venous access, the catheter may be kept in if it remains functional. If the central access device must continue to be used long term, therapeutic anticoagulation should be maintained indefinitely. The principle of the prevention of catheter thrombosis centers on the catheter tip placement, technique, and biomaterial of catheter. Studies testing low-dose warfarin for prophylaxis against thrombosis are few; however, findings show efficacy in patients with cancer.[43] If thrombolytic or anticoagulant therapy is begun early, the lysis of the clot or its stabilization can help to prevent long-term sequellae.[45]

When a suspected septic thrombus occurs, thrombolytic agents should not be used and a course of antibiotic or antifungal agents should be given for at least 4 to 6 weeks as the patient is converted from heparin to coumadin. The vascular access device is best left in place until the thrombus stabilizes.

The Role of the Interventional Radiologist in Difficult Vascular Access

The use of image guidance to facilitate vascular access procedures has resulted in significant reductions in procedure length, the number of failed access attempts, and the number and severity of procedurally related complications.[46-48] An additional benefit has been the improved ability to establish vascular access in the sub-group of patients with limited remaining usable sites. In these patients, image guidance by ultrasound, fluoroscopy, or computed tomography (CT) permits consideration of non-traditional access routes, including the inferior vena cava and hepatic veins.

Prior to 1990, the establishment of suitable access in cases of upper body venous occlusion was a frequent topic of discussion in radiologic and surgical publications. Direct surgical placement of catheters in the superior vena cava, right atrium, or azygous vein was the usual alternative. In 1989 and 1990, reports of successful direct catheter placement to the inferior vena cava for the purpose of long-term access were published in the surgical literature.[49,50]

Shortly thereafter, Denny et al[51] reported the successful placement and use of the translumbar route in the fluoroscopy suite with interventional catheter and guide wire techniques in six patients. In this report, there were no instances of catheter migration or inferior vena cava thrombosis. The procedure followed for translumbar placement is somewhat analogous to that of translumbar aortography: the patient is placed in a prone position, and working from a point over the right iliac crest with a cephalo-medial oblique angulation, a 21-gauge needle is advanced to enter the inferior vena cava caudal to the level of renal veins at the L2 to L3 level. Contrast injection under fluoroscopy confirms intravascular location, and subsequent catheter and guide-wire exchanges permit the introduction of a peel-away sheath through which the access device can be introduced. Venography, ultrasound, or CT may be utilized to facilitate inferior vena cava access in patients with difficult anatomy.

Lund et al[52] reported on the placement of 46 catheters in 40 patients with devices ranging from 9.6 to 14.4 Fr in size. There were no procedural complications, and CT scans performed on 31 patients within 1 to 10 weeks of placement revealed no evidence of retroperitoneal hemorrhage. Inferior vena cava thrombus formation occurred in eight patients, with two thrombi-causing caval occlusions. All were successfully lysed with urokinase. Ten catheter malpositions were noted. Five catheters were replaced, four were repositioned with interventional techniques, and one spontaneously resumed its original position.

Transhepatic access to the inferior vena cava can be used in those instances where the more caudal inferior vena cava is unsuitable for access. In 1989, Crummy et al reported the first[53] of several reports detailing few complications and good long-term results.[54,55] The procedure is performed similarly to percutaneous transhepatic biliary drainage, with a 21-gauge needle used to access a branch of the right or middle hepatic vein. Ultrasound is useful in avoiding inadvertent portal vein traversal. Catheter length must be chosen to allow adequate position within the inferior vena cava such that diaphragmatic movement does not result in catheter tip malposition/displacement.

Imaging guidance coupled with interventional radiologic techniques permit the use of still other unusual vascular access sites. Very small caliber steerable guidewires and catheters permit the establishment of access via collateral veins to larger central veins. In other situations, combined radiologic and surgical procedures may be feasible, enabling access to vascular structures not otherwise achievable.[56]

The assistance of the interventional radiology service is often sought for difficult access patients. However, image-guided placement of vascular access devices has evolved to become the method of choice in many institutions as a result of safety, economic, and practical considerations.

Conclusion

The provision of PN to patients requires the skills of a multidisciplinary team. Obtaining and maintaining safe vascular access requires the cooperative expertise of interventional radiologists, surgeons, nurses, and experienced physicians. Complications associated with vascular access insertion are minimized when skilled and knowledgeable clinicians are involved.

The patient going home with a long-term vascular access device should be educated regarding its proper care and maintenance. Potential complications of prolonged vascular access can be managed successfully if diagnosed early. Obtaining safe reliable vascular access for a patient needing PN should almost always be possible when a team of skilled clinicians cares for the patient.

References

1. Shah PM, Babu SC, Goyal A, Mateo RB, Madden RE. Arterial misplacement of large-caliber cannulas during jugular vein catheterization: case for surgical management. *J Am Coll Surg.* 2004;198:939-944.
2. Cadman A, Lawrance JAL, Fitzsimmons L, Spencer-Shaw A, Swindell R. To clot or not to clot? That is the question in central venous catheters. *Clin Radiol.* 2004;59:349-355.
3. Horattas MC, Trupiano J, Hopkins S, Pasiini D, Martina C, Murty A. Changing concepts in long-term central venous access: catheter selection and cost savings. *Am J Infect Control.* 2001;29(1):32-40.
4. Ryder MA. Peripheral access options. *Surg Oncology Clin N Am.* 1995;4:395-427.
5. Maki DG, Ringer M. Evaluation of dressing regimens for prevention of infection with peripheral intravenous catheters: gauze, transparent polyurethane dressing, and an iodophor-transparent dressing. *JAMA.* 1987;258:2396-2403.
6. Dezfulian C, Lavelle J, Nallamothu BK, Kaufman SR, Saint S. Rates of infection for single-lumen versus multilumen central venous catheters: a meta-analysis. *Crit Care Med.* 2003;31(9):2385-2390.
7. Kemp L, Burge J, Choban P, Harden J, Mirtallo J, Flancbaum L. The effect of catheter type and site on infection rates in total parenteral nutrition patients. *JPEN J Parenter Enternal Nutr.* 1994;18:71-74.
8. Harden JL, Kemp L, Mirtallo J. Femoral catheters increase risk of infection in total parenteral nutrition patients. *Nutr Clin Pract.* 1995;10:60-66.
9. Goetz AM, Wagener MM, Miller JM, Muder RR. Risk of infection due to central venous catheters: effect of site of placement and catheter type. *Infect Control Hosp Epidemiol.* 1998;19:842-845.
10. Trottier SJ, Veremakis C, O'Brien J, Auer AI. Femoral deep vein thrombosis associated with central venous catheterization: results from a prospective randomized trial. *Crit Care Med.* 1995;23:52-59.
11. Scott W. Central venous catheter complications: a three-part video series [videotape]. DHHS/FDA/CVC-WG-Production; 1994.
12. Cardella JF, Cardella K, Bacci N, Fox PS, Post JH. Cumulative experience with 1,273 peripherally inserted central catheters at a single institution. *J Vasc Interv Radiol.* 1996;7:5-13.
13. Duerksen DR, Papineau N, Siemens J, Yaffe C. Peripherally inserted central catheter for parenteral nutrition: a comparison with centrally inserted catheters. *JPEN J Parenter Enternal Nutr.* 1999;23:85-89.
14. Norton JA, Bollinger RR, Chang AE, et al. Surgery: basic science and clinical evidence. *Vascular Access for Cancer.* 2001;88(6):1803.
15. Broadwater JR, Henderson MA, Bell JL, et al. Outpatient percutaneous central venous access in cancer patients. *Am J Surg.* 1990;160:676-680.
16. Morton JE, Jan-Mohamed RM, Barker HF, Milligan DW. Percutaneous insertion of subclavian Hickman catheters. *Bone Marrow Transplant.* 1991;7:739-741.
17. Ray S, Stacey R, Imrie M, Filshie J. A review of 560 Hickman catheter insertions. *Anaesthesia.* 1996;51:981-985.
18. Collier PE, Ryan JJ, Diamond DL. Cardiac tamponade from central venous catheters. Report of a case and review of the English literature. *Angiology.* 1984;35:595-600.
19. Mansfield PF, Hohn DC, Fornage BD, Gregurich MA, Ota DM. Complications and failures of subclavian-vein catheterization. *N Engl J Med.* 1994;331:1735-1738.
20. Fry WR, Clagett GC, O'Rouke PT. Ultrasound-Guided Central Venous Access. *Arch Surg.* 1999;134(7):738-741.
21. Andris DA, Krzywda EA, Schulte W, Ausman R, Quebbeman EJ. Pinch-off syndrome: a rare etiology for central venous catheter occlusion. *JPEN J Parenter Enternal Nutr.* 1994;18:531-533.
22. Feliciano DV, Mattox KL, Graham JM, Beall AC Jr, Jordan GL Jr. Major complications of percutaneous subclavian vein catheters. *Am J Surg.* 1979;138:869-874.
23. Maki DG. Infections caused by intravascular devices used for infusion therapy. In: Bistro AI, Waldvogel FA, eds. *Infections Associated With Indwelling Medical Devices.* 2nd ed. Washington, DC: ASM Press; 1994:155-205.
24. Raad LL. Intravascular catheter-related infections. *Lancet.* 1998; 351:893-898.
25. CDC MMWR Recommendations and Reports. Aug. 9, 2002. Guidelines for the Prevention of Intravascular Catheter Related Infections.
26. Safdar N, Maki DG. Inflammation at the insertion site is not predictive of catheter-related blood stream infection with short-term, non-cuffed central venous catheters. *Crit Care Med.* 2002;30:2632-2635.
27. Raad II, Hanna HA. Intravascular catheter-related infections: new horizons and recent advances. *Arch Int Med.* 2002;162(8):871-878.
28. Cook D, Randolph A, Kernerman P, et al. Central venous catheter replacement strategies: a systematic review of the literature. *Crit Care Med.* 1997;25:1417-1424.
29. Ranson MR, Oppenheim BA, Jackson A, Kamthan AG, Scarffe JH. Double-blind placebo controlled study of vancomycin prophylaxis for central venous catheter insertion in cancer patients. *J Hosp Infect.* 1990;15:95-102.

30. Keohane PP, Jones BJ, Attrill H, et al. Effect of catheter tunneling and a nutrition nurse on catheter sepsis during parenteral nutrition: a controlled trial. *Lancet.* 1983;2:1388-1390.
31. Whitman ED. A neural network to predict prospectively the risk of central venous access device infection. *Surg Forum.* 1996;KL VII:630-632.
32. Schwarz RE, Groeger JS, Coit DG. Subcutaneously implanted central venous access devices in cancer patients: a prospective analysis. *Cancer.* 1997;79:1635-1640.
33. Veenstra DL, Saint S, Sullivan SD. Cost-effectiveness of antiseptic-impregnated central venous catheters for the prevention of catheter-related bloodstream infection. *JAMA.* 1999;11:554-560.
34. Collin G. Decreasing catheter colonization through the use of an antiseptic impregnated catheter: a continuous quality improvement project. *Chest.* 1999;115(6):1632-1640.
35. Raad I, Chatzinikolaou I, Chaiban G, et al. In vitro and ex vivo activities of minocycline and EDTA against microorganisms embedded in biofilm on catheter surfaces. *Antimicrob Agents Chemother.* 2003;47:3580-3585.
36. Timoney JP, Malkin MG, Leone DM, et al. Safe and cost effective use of alteplase for the clearance of occluded central venous access devices. *J Clin Oncol.* 2002;20(7):1918-1922.
37. Deitcher SR, Fesen MR, Kiproff PM, et al. Safety and efficacy of alteplase for restoring function in occluded central venous catheters: results of the cardiovascular thrombolytic to open occluded lines trial. *J Clin Oncol.* 2001;20:317-324.
38. Grant J. Recognition, prevention, and treatment of home total parenteral nutrition central venous access complications. *JPEN J Parenter Enternal Nutr.* 2002;26:S21-S28.
39. Haire WD, Lieberman RP, Edney J, et al. Hickman catheter-induced thoracic vein thrombosis. Frequency and long-term sequelae in patients receiving high-dose chemotherapy and marrow transplantation. *Cancer.* 1990;66:900-908.
40. Haire WD, Lieberman RP, Lund GV, Edney JA, Kessinger A, Armitage JO. Thrombotic complications of silicone rubber catheters during autologous marrow and peripheral stem cell transplantation: prospective comparison of Hickman and Groshong catheters. *Bone Marrow Transplant.* 1991;7:57-59.
41. Anderson AJ, Krasnow SH, Boyer MW, et al. Thrombosis: the major Hickman catheter complication in patients with solid tumor. *Chest.* 1989;95:71-75.
42. Horne MK III, May DJ, Alexander HR, et al. Venographic surveillance of tunneled venous access devices in adult oncology patients. *Ann Surg Oncol.* 1995;2:174-178.
43. Bern MM, Lokich JJ, Wallach SR, et al. Very low doses of warfarin can prevent thrombosis in central venous catheters. *Ann Intern Med.* 1990;112:423-428.
44. Monreal M, Raventos A, Lerma R, et al. Pulmonary embolism in patients with upper extremity DVT associated to venous central lines—a prospective study. *Thromb Haemo.* 1994;72(4):548-550.
45. Joffe HV, Goldhaber SZ. Upper-extremity deep vein thrombosis. *Circulation.* 2002;106(14):1874-1880.
46. Mauro MA. Interventional Radiologic Placement of Central Venous Catheters. *Hospital Physician.* 1996;55-59.
47. Mauro M, Jaques P. Radiologic placement of long-term central venous catheters: a review. *J Vasc Intervent Radiol.* 1993;4(1):127-137.
48. Lund GB, Trerotola SO, Scheel PF Jr, et al. Outcome of tunneled hemodialysis catheters placed by radiologists. *Radiology.* 1996;198(2):467-472.
49. Boddie AW Jr. Translumbar catheterization of the inferior vena cava for long term angioaccess. *Surg Gynecol Obstet.* 1989;168:55-57.
50. Voeller GR, Frederick RC, Luther RW. Direct transcaval placement of both a Greenfield filter and a Hickman catheter. *Surgery.* 1990;107:110-112.
51. Denny DF Jr, Greenwood LH, Morse SS, Lee GK, Baquero J. Inferior vena cava: translumbar catheterization for central venous access. *Radiology.* 1989;174:1013-1014.
52. Lund GB, Lieberman R, Haire W, Martin V, Kessinger A, Armitage J. Translumbar inferior vena cava catheters for long-term venous access. *Radiology.* 1990;174:31-35.
53. Crummy AB, Carlson P, McDermott JC, Andrews D. Percutaneous transhepatic placement of a Hickman catheter. *AJR Am J Roentgenol.* 1989;153:1317-1318.
54. Azizkhan RG, Taylor LA, Jaques PF, Mauro MA, Lacey SR. Percutaneous translumbar and transhepatic inferior vena caval catheters for prolonged venous access in children. *J Pediatric Surg.* 1992;27:165-169.
55. Kaufman JA, Greenfield AJ, Fitzpatrick GF. Transhepatic cannulation of the inferior vena cava. *J Vasc Interv Radiol.* 1991;2:331-334.
56. Meranze SG, McLean GK, Stein EJ, Jordan HA. Catheter placement in the azygous system: an unusual approach to venous access. *AJR Am J Roentgenol.* 1985;144:1075-1076.

Chapter 36

Parenteral Nutrition Formulas

David F. Driscoll, PhD

Introduction

The safe and successful application of parenteral nutrition (PN) therapy is contingent upon prescribing reasonable amounts of nutrients in a final volume commensurate with the patient's clinical condition. A variety of patient scenarios may dramatically alter the amounts necessary to meet metabolic demands, as the clinical condition may preclude this objective. For example, if nutrition support is indicated to support the protein synthetic response to injury (ie, during acute metabolic stress), then the amounts of energy prescribed are often hypocaloric, with greater emphasis on protein (at least 1 g/kg/day), fluid, electrolyte, and acid-base homeostasis. Once corrected, the prescribing pattern shifts towards achieving eucaloric nutrition support. Alternatively, if nutritional rehabilitation is the goal of PN therapy, a eucaloric and rarely a hypercaloric supply of macro- and micronutrients are often indicated. At other times, issues—such as the availability of venous access sites—may also affect the amount and types of nutrients prescribed. In every case, such patient conditions guide the contents of the final PN formulation, which might affect the stability, compatibility, and ultimately the safety of the infusion.

Patients' Needs for Parenteral Nutrition Formulas

The types of PN formulas prescribed can vary for a given patient condition. Thus, the historical approach of "one size fits all" (ie, the classic 1000 mL of 8.5% amino acids plus 1000 mL of 50% dextrose plus additives with a variable infusion rate) has since been rejected by today's standards, and many have adopted an individualized approach to PN therapy, particularly during critical illness.[1] The critical care period represents the most sensitive time during hospitalization, when even subtle changes in metabolic homeostasis may assume major clinical significance. Thus, the need for a patient-specific approach to PN therapy is most necessary during this time to avoid introducing iatrogenic complications. In less critical patient care scenarios, the PN approach can be less stringent but, nonetheless, would be optimized in accordance with meeting the patient's protein, calorie, and fluid needs while addressing the metabolic issues coincident with comorbid disease(s). The mere fact the patient needs PN therapy in the first place points to the significance of such active disease(s).

The safe approach to meeting the nutritional needs via PN therapy is based on establishing the correct amounts of nutrients for the individual patient's weight. Table 36-1 outlines the general PN requirements for adults. Using this baseline, the amounts of fluid and nutrients are adjusted according to the metabolic fluctuations commonly associated with acute metabolic stress (changes in intravascular volume, electrolyte and acid-base imbalance, ventilatory defects, etc). This review is intended to outline the various strategies for optimizing PN therapy in a variety of clinical conditions in adults.

Protein and Energy Requirements

There are specific amounts of protein and calories that should be supplied to the patient incapable of oral alimentation. Depending on the patient's clinical condition, if not judiciously provided, even seemingly

TABLE 36-1.

General Parenteral Nutrition Requirements for Adults

Nutrient	Amounts
Protein (amino acids)	1.5 g/kg/day
Energy (70% to 80% dextrose, 20% to 30% lipids)	25 kcal/kg/day
Volume	25 mL/kg/day
Sodium	60 to 100 mEq/day
Potassium	40 to 80 mEq/day
Calcium	10 mEq/day
Magnesium	10 mEq/day
Chloride/Acetate	as per acid-base status
Trace Minerals-5	3 mL/day
Multivitamins	10 mL/day

"basal" amounts of nutrients can produce harm. More is not better, nor will it improve nitrogen balance; but, of course, there has to be a baseline amount of nutrients that achieves a eucaloric state. Although these amounts will be enumerated below, they should serve as a foundation or goal quantities to maintain lean body mass; yet such goals at this stage of nutrition support may not be achievable until the acute metabolic stress subsides. Hence, the early efforts of PN therapy in the critical care period will be hypocaloric, whereas the approach during nutritional rehabilitation (ie, restoration of lean body mass) will be hypercaloric. Ultimately, however, once the approach to acute period (usually days) or to the chronic rehabilitation period (usually months) is sufficiently addressed, the nutrition support regimen will revert to the baseline or eucaloric state. Application of these strategies will be discussed later in this chapter.

PROTEIN (AMINO ACIDS)

The basal amount of protein necessary to meet the needs of adults is approximately 0.8 g/kg/day. During metabolic stress, the rate of endogenous nitrogen breakdown (catabolism) increases, anabolism decreases, and utilization of exogenous sources of protein are less efficient. To compensate for these heightened protein requirements, the amounts needed approximately double to 1.5 g/kg/day during this time. Higher amounts of protein may have small, incremental improvements in nitrogen balance, but these effects appear to reach a plateau at intakes of up to 2 g/kg/day; for above this, most of the additional amounts of protein administered are converted to urea.[2,3] A possible exception to these upper limits of protein intake may be in patients with severe burn injury or head trauma, but for most metabolically stressed patients it is prudent to provide 1.5 g/kg/day.

In general, the use of conventional amino acids is indicated. For patients with nitrogen accumulation disorders of either renal or hepatic origin, specialized amino acid formulations may be considered. The primary benefit associated with improved utilization of protein is largely derived from higher amounts of the branched-chain amino acids (BCAAs)—ie, leucine, isoleucine, and valine—whereas the importance of using formulations that emphasize essential amino acids (in renal failure) or reductions in the concentration of aromatic amino acids (in hepatic failure) are no longer routinely recommended.[4] For example, attempts to meet the protein needs with the essential amino acids formulation in an acutely ill patient have caused hyperammonemic encephalopathy[5] and neither the renal nor hepatic formulations contain the proper ratio of amino acids necessary to achieve nitrogen balance. In the conventional amino acid formulation, the BCAAs comprise between 18% and 25% of the total amino acids, whereas those formulations that are "BCAA-enriched" contain between 45% and 50%. The selection of BCAA-enriched amino acid formulations engenders significant increases in costs (approximately three-fold more per gram), and their use is generally based on the ability of the patient to "tolerate" conventional amino acids. Tolerance is predicated on adverse outcomes; therefore, if a significant medical risk exists, the decision should be weighted accordingly.

For example, if a patient's blood urea nitrogen (BUN) is approaching 100 mg% or higher, and dialysis is not readily available, and continued feeding of conventional protein may increase the risk of uremic-associated bleeding, BCAA-enriched formulas might provide a reasonable option to slow the rate of rise in BUN. This would often be employed as a temporizing maneuver until effective dialysis begins. Similarly, if a patient has severe encephalopathy and enteral feeding is being contemplated, using a BCAA-enriched formula may lessen the nitrogen burden and reduce the risk of aspiration pneumonia from impairments of the swallowing and/or gag reflex. In either event, if the risk of continued feeding with conventional protein heightens the medical risks to the patient, BCAA-enriched formulations may be used for a short time. The ultimate goal is to provide a full complement of amino acids to support the protein synthetic response to injury and facilitate nutritional rehabilitation.

ENERGY (GLUCOSE AND LIPIDS)

The basal amount of calories (including those from protein) provided to the adult patient lies between 25 and 30 kcal/kg/day.[6] During metabolic stress, it is often mistakenly believed that higher amounts of calories are necessary to combat "hypermetabolism" from severe metabolic stress. In fact, it was commonplace to calculate the basal needs and then multiply the total caloric intake by various "stress" factors, so that the greater the patient's stress, the more calories were indicated.[7] Unfortunately, during acute illness, which is accompanied by numerous metabolic derangements, administration of excess nutrients may be harmful. In fact, during the critical care period, energy is deliberately prescribed in hypocaloric quantities until the stress response remits to more stable levels.[8]

Glucose

Glucose is an essential energy source required for certain vital organs and tissues of the body including, for example, the brain, red blood cells, and renal medulla. During metabolic stress, it is a rapid source of energy to meet the acute needs of the patient; however, readily available body stores are limited to approximately 400 to 700 g of glucose stored as glycogen. The liver is the principal reservoir for mobilizable glycogen and can be depleted in less than 24 hours of severe metabolic stress.[9] In the absence of exogenous glucose supply during injury, muscle proteolysis occurs to release gluconeogenic amino acids for heightened glucose production by the liver. The amount of energy supplied as glucose is often in the range of 70% to 80% of the total calories. During acute illness, it is prudent to start glucose infusions gradually at rates that approximate basal requirements and gradually advance to levels that meet up to 80% of energy needs but not to exceed its optimal glucose oxidation rate. Basal needs are approximately 2 mg/kg/minute with optimal glucose oxidation rates of up to double the basal amounts or approximately 4 mg/kg/minute. In most clinical scenarios that include lipids as a daily caloric source in recommended quantities, overfeeding with glucose and its attendant complications (hyperglycemia and infection, hepatic steatosis, respiratory dysfunction) are rare.

Lipids

Typically, lipids are derived from neutral triglycerides, such as soybean oil, which is highly polyunsaturated and rich in the 18-carbon, omega-6 and omega-3 long chain triglyceride (LCT), essential fatty acids, and linoleic and linolenic acids. Historically, the first successful LCT injectable lipid emulsion was made from 100% soybean oil (ie, Intralipid) and has remained the major lipid source found in these formulations. Other long chain fatty acids (LCFA), ranging from 16 to 22 carbons in length, have been used. For example, there are LCTs derived from marine sources such as menhaden oil that is rich in omega-3 LCFA (eicosapentanoic and docosahexanoic acids), which are also highly polyunsaturated (5 and 6 double bonds, respectively) with hydrocarbon chains as long as 22 carbons in length. Finally, olive oil—which is an 18-carbon, monounsaturated, omega-9 LCFA) has also been used. The omega-3, 6, and 9 nomenclature is used to indicate the position of the first double bond in the hydrocarbon chain. For example, an omega-9 fatty acid (ie, olive oil) has 1 double bond occurring at the number 9-carbon atom from the methyl end of the triglyceride structure.

Alternatively, common medium chain triglyceride (MCT) sources, whose hydrocarbon chain length varies from 8 to 10 hydrocarbons and that are fully saturated (ie, no double bonds), include oils from tropical plants such as coconut and palm kernel. They are a readily metabolized source of energy and exist in various "mixtures" with soybean oil in amounts ranging from 40% to 75% of a given formulation. Reducing the soybean oil content limits the metabolic problems associated with rapid infusion rates[10,11] but supplies ample amounts of the essential fatty acids, which are not present in MCTs. Thus, these alternative injectable lipid emulsion mixtures may be safer metabolic alternatives. Unfortunately, at the present time, only LCT-based injectable lipid emulsions are available in the United States made from either 100% soybean oil or as a 50:50 physical mixture (by weight) with safflower oil.

Lipids are an important energy source provided on a daily basis in amounts that typically represent about 20% to 30% of total energy needs. Higher amounts may be provided but have not been associated with significant clinical benefits above 30% of total calories.[12] Ideally, lipids are administered continuously over 24 hours and mixed in a single PN bag, known as an all-in-one or total nutrient admixture (TNA). Alternatively, they can be given separate from the PN admixture, but this method of intravenous delivery is associated with metabolic complications (hypertriglyceridemia, immune dysfunction, etc) related to their infusion rate and can be worsened by infectious risks associated with protracted infusion times.[13] The Centers for Disease Control (CDC) has determined that the administration of a single lipid infusion container for periods greater than 12 hours increases infectious morbidity. Limiting the infusion rate of omega-6 LCTs, such as soybean oil-in-water emulsions, to no greater than 0.1 g/kg/ hour reduces the risk of metabolic complications,[14] but when the LCT is given as an intermittent infusion, it is difficult to provide the entire dose of lipids over 12 hours when using common commercially available products. For example, unless the patient weighs in excess of 80 kg, a 500 mL container of a 20% emulsion should not be administered.[15] Thus, smaller sizes (such as 200 or 250 mL) of 20% soybean oil-in-water emulsion are preferable and safer for most adult patients. Table 36-2 lists the various commercially available lipid emulsions.

Volume

The volume needs of unstressed adults necessary to maintain fluid homeostasis are empirically based on achieving a euvolemic state where inputs essentially equals outputs. Fluid intake is assessed at between 20 to 40 mL/kg/day.[16] In general, the basal amount of fluid that should be prescribed for adults via PN therapy is approximately 25 mL/kg/day, bearing in mind the patient will receive fluids from other sources. In the stable clinical setting, these may include various intravenous medications, hydration solutions, spontaneous oral intake, hydrated mechanical ventilation (if present) that, when combined, will provide ample fluid intake. If his or her renal function is adequate, the patient will maintain normal fluid balance.

During acute metabolic stress, however, these intakes often require significant modification. For example, postoperative patients may be acutely volume-overloaded following major thoracoabdominal surgery, with fluid restrictions imposed by the primary care team that results in severely limiting the volume allotted for the delivery of

TABLE 36-2.

Various Commercially Available Lipid Emulsions (Not Inclusive)

Product	*Company*	*Lipid Composition**	*Concentration*	*Size† (ml)*
Liposyn II	Abbott (USA)	Soybean/safflower 50:50	10%, 20%	100, 200, 500
Liposyn III		Soybean oil 100%	10%, 20%, 30%	100, 200, 500
Intralipid	Fresenius/Kabi	Soybean oil 100%	10%, 20%, 30%	50, 100, 250, 500
Structolipid	(Sweden)	Soybean/MCT 36:64	20%	500
Lipofundin N	B. Braun (Germany)	Soybean Oil 100%	10%, 20%	100, 250, 500
Lipofundin MCT/LCT		Soybean/MCT	10%, 20%	100, 250, 500
Lipoplus		MCT/soybean/fish oil 50:40:10	10%, 20%	100, 250, 500
Lipovenous	Fresnius (Germany)	Soybean oil 100%	10%, 20%, 30%	100, 250, 500
Lipovenous MCT		Soybean/MCT 50:50	10%, 20%	250, 500
Omegaven		Fish oil 100%	10%	50, 100
Clinoleic	Baxter (France)	Olive oil/soybean 80:20	20%	100, 250, 500
Colip	Baxter (USA)	MCT/soybean oil 75:25	20%	500

*Proportion by weight

Adapted from Driscoll DF, Adolph M, Bistrian BR. Lipid emulsions in parenteral nutrition. In: Rombeau JL, Rolandelli RH, eds. *Clinical Nutrition. Parenteral Nutrition.* 3rd edition. Philadelphia, Pa; WB Saunders, 2001:37.

nutrition support.[17] Often, the volume for PN may be no more than 1000 mL/day, and in many patients the fluid intakes fall to 10 to 15 mL/kg. Although a calorically dense formulation could be made in such a volume using highly concentrated macronutrient products (ie, 15% amino acids, 70% dextrose, and 30% lipid emulsion), there is no clinical evidence supporting the achievement of a eucaloric feeding state from the outset of nutrition support; however, there is evidence it may do harm, particularly with respect to the glycemic control.[18] Consequently, it makes little sense to attempt full PN therapy with volumes less than 700 to 750 mL. Moreover, PN formulas in volumes less than 700 mL are so highly concentrated that the risk of incompatibilities is greatly increased[19,20] and that may ultimately compromise the safety of the formulation.

In contrast, other patients, such as those with inflammatory bowel disease, may require supraphysiologic amounts of volume to maintain fluid homeostasis. This is especially true in patients with ostomies and those with severe short bowel syndrome in whom fluid requirements may double the normal intakes, particularly in the first 3 to 6 months following small bowel resection. Antisecretory agents may be used to reduce the fluid (and electrolyte) losses. Meeting the patient's fluid needs can be accomplished via the PN admixture using a dilute formula, but extremely dilute formulas that result in nearly isotonic concentrations of nutrients (analogous to a peripheral vein PN admixture) may pose significant compatibility problems (eg, with calcium and phosphate solubility).[21] In this circumstance, it is more prudent to provide a baseline volume via the PN admixture and supplement with the additional volume of fluid via separate infusions of simple intravenous solutions, such as lactated ringers or other suitable alternatives.

Electrolytes, Vitamins, Minerals, and Drugs

ELECTROLYTES

The electrolyte needs of patients receiving PN therapy must be met by specific additions to the PN admixture and must meet the official requirements of the United States Pharmacopeia (USP). The amounts prescribed should be based on normal end-organ function; however, as with the macronutrients and fluids described above, the clinician must work from established baseline requirements, recognizing that, under various patient scenarios, significant modifications will be necessary. Of the multiple parenteral electrolytes required to maintain homeostasis, there are three—calcium, magnesium, and phosphorus—that should be routinely prescribed in set quantities, unless the patient's condition dictates otherwise.

In adults, the amount of elemental calcium required via PN should be equal to 200 mg/day (10 mEq or 5 mmol daily) and should be provided as the organic salt, calcium gluconate injection, USP 10%. Although there are other parenteral salt forms of calcium (such as chloride and acetate), they should not be used in PN admixtures as they pose major compatibility problems. Elemental magnesium should be administered at 120 mg/day (10 mEq or 5 mmol per day) and should be provided as the inorganic salt, magnesium sulfate injection, USP 50%. For elemental phosphorus, the only FDA-approved forms include the sodium or potassium salts as inorganic monobasic and dibasic phosphate mixtures, such as sodium phosphates injection, USP, or potassium phosphates injection. The amount necessary to meet daily needs is 1000 mg (30 mmol) of elemental phosphorus. (The use of mEq units to express the amount of elemental phosphorus is not used because these salts exist as two different species—mono- and dibasic forms—with a pH range spanning between 0.8 and 1 unit. This latter point—ie, the variable pH range of these products—precludes the use of the mEq unit as it requires the valence of the phosphate species. Thus, because there are two species and the pH is not fixed, mEq units are not used for phosphate supplements.[21])

Other electrolyte requirements (ie, sodium, potassium, chloride, and acetate) are not as specific as those presented previously. Rather, these supplements are largely dictated by the clinical status of the patient and, therefore, can be highly variable. In general, assuming the patient has a normal end-organ function, sodium is often prescribed in amounts between 60 and 100 mEq (1380 to 2300 mg or 60 to 100 mmol); potassium between 40 and 80 mEq (1560 to 3120 mg or 40 to 80 mmol); and chloride salts of these are typically prescribed unless the patient is academic. In that case, equivalent forms as acetate are used. Under no circumstances is the use of bicarbonate salts (eg, sodium bicarbonate) justified in any PN admixture, as the risk of precipitation is too great with, for example, calcium ions. Acetate salts provide equal alkalinizing power without the risk of clinically significant incompatibilities.

Vitamins

Parenteral multivitamins have undergone recent and significant formulation changes in accordance with the Food and Drug Administration (FDA) directive, Docket Number 79N to 0113.[22] Specifically, the FDA has mandated that the standard parenteral multivitamin product be reformulated by increasing the daily amounts of: ascorbic acid (from 100 to 200 mg); folic acid (from 0.4 to 0.6 mg); thiamine (from 3 to 6 mg); and pyridoxine (from 4 to 6 mg). In addition, the FDA required the inclusion of phylloquinone or vitamin K1 (to 0.15 mg), which was not previously included. (At this time, all are compliant with the FDA mandate.)

The change in composition is noteworthy in that this is the first change in the formulation since it was first proposed by the American Medical Association (AMA) in 1975. Of these changes, the addition of vitamin K1 appears to be most significant and is of particular concern in patients receiving long-term, home parenteral nutrition (HPN) therapy. Many of these patients receive mini-dose warfarin therapy to reduce the incidence of central vein thrombosis from the placement of permanent infusion catheters. As the mechanism of action for warfarin is to interfere with vitamin-K–dependent clotting factors (II, VII, IX, and X), the routine provision of vitamin in this population is new and untested. The daily supply of 0.15 mg of phylloquinone may adversely alter the efficacy of mini-dose warfarin prophylaxis and increase the incidence of thrombosis of the large central veins of the upper venous system, requiring the placement of catheters into less successful, and more risky, venous access site (eg, left atrial appendage, femoral vein). The clinical issue is heightened further considering that the efficacy of low-dose warfarin is not measured by routine laboratory tests, such as the international normalized ratio; warfarin is empirically dosed in the range of 1 to 2 mg/day.[23,24] Typically, if prolongation of the prothrombin time occurs, the dose is scaled back accordingly. In the case of mini-dose warfarin, however, its effects have been shown to be linked to increases in the generation of plasma under-γ-carboxylated prothrombin (PIVKA-II) proteins.[25]

All PN admixtures should contain parenteral multivitamins. The national parenteral vitamin shortages in 1988 and again in 1996 were associated with significant clinical morbidity and mortality when PN was provided without them.[26,27] Of greatest importance, the three deaths attributed to refractory lactic acidosis in association with acute thiamine deficiency, and the pivotal role hypertonic dextrose (a major PN additive) played in these unfortunate circumstances, starkly points out the clinical significance of parenteral multivitamins.[26] A common characteristic of each of these patients was their heightened sensitivity to acute vitamin deficiencies because of either pre-existing malnutrition and/or comorbid conditions (case 1: HPN for short bowel syndrome for 3 years; case 2: abdominal gunshot wounds; and case 3: ulcerative colitis) that made them exquisitely sensitive to water-soluble vitamin deficiencies.

Trace Minerals

Trace mineral supplements are important additives in PN therapy. Although maybe not as critical in the acute care setting over brief periods (5 to 7 days) of PN administration in most patients, they are vitally important in patients receiving long-term HPN therapy. It should also be stated that, for patients with pre-existing malnutrition and/or gastrointestinal (GI) disease, as with the vitamin cases described above, routine supplementation of trace minerals should be supplied each day in the PN admixture. Typically, a trace mineral cocktail providing 12 mcg of chromium, 1.2 mg of copper, 0.3 mg of manganese, 60 mcg of selenium, and 3 mg of zinc is indicated.

Drugs

Finally, certain drugs may be added to the PN admixture that may reduce the volume load in susceptible patients. In so doing, the volume allocated to the patient from the addition of drugs is a fraction of the amount normally provided via the conventional intermittent delivery of medications in small individual infusion bags, such as 50 mL of 5% dextrose in water or 0.9% sodium chloride. The use of pharmacological agents for control of gastric acidity, small bowel secretions, and peptic ulcer disease are commonly added to PN admixtures, such as the histamine-2 receptor antagonists. For example, instead of receiving the drug every 6 to 12 hours in 50 mL diluents (total volume: 100 to 200 mL/day), only the drug is added (total volume 1 to 8 mL), which results in up to a 99% net reduction of volume for a single drug. Such maneuvers are of greatest clinical value in the severely volume-overloaded, critically ill patients.

The selection of what type of drugs may be added is contingent upon at least three main factors: 1) the dose must be effective via continuous infusion; 2) drug stability (and/or compatibility) must be ascertained by stability-indicating assays in accordance with the USP specifications for at least 24 hours; and 3) the drug dose must be stable for 24 hours.[28] The first point deals with the pharmacokinetics of the drug and specifically addresses whether such dosing results in optimizing the therapeutic response. This is true for many drugs but may not be appropriate for others, such as for certain antimicrobial agents. The second point addresses the efficacy of the drug as well but from a potential safety perspective. On one hand, if the drug is unstable and therefore rendered pharmacologically inactive, the ensuing therapeutic failure may be clinically significant, such as in the case, for example, of stress ulcer prophylaxis. A therapeutic failure in this case could result in a life-threatening GI bleed. As well, once the drug degrades to an inactive product, it is possible that the degradation product may form insoluble co-precipitates with other components in the PN admixture. For example, dosing of supraphysiologic doses of ascorbic acid for its putative antioxidant effects may result in high amounts of oxalic acid that can react with free calcium ions, forming the insoluble calcium oxalate product.[29] Finally, the third point speaks to a safety issue as well, as drug doses that change in accordance with the patients clinical status are not appropriate additions to the PN admixture, and the infusion rate is constant and should not be altered. An example of this would be for heparin: although an appropriate PN additive when used as prophylaxis against central venous thrombosis, it should never be added for full therapeutic anticoagulation when the dose may change multiple times over 24 hours in accordance with bleeding times.

Parenteral Nutrition Formulations

There are a number of approaches that might be taken in prescribing a given PN formulation. Typical sterile components that are used in compounding these formulations are shown in Table 36-3. As discussed previously, the initial approach during acute metabolic stress often results in prescribing a formulation that is hypocaloric; examples of these regimens in a fluid-restricted patient are provided for a range of adult weights (40 to 80 kg) in Table 36-4. Once the stress response remits and fluid restrictions are lifted, a eucaloric regimen may be considered; examples of these formulations appear in Table 36-5. A similar approach to repleting the malnourished patient may also be necessary, with calories given at levels above needs, and the amounts depend upon the individual goal weight assessed for a given patient. Ultimately, once that weight is achieved over several months, a eucaloric regimen is reinstituted for long-term nutrition support and weight maintenance.

Continuous Versus Cycled Parenteral Nutrition Infusions

As a general rule, all hospitalized and acutely ill patients should receive PN therapy via a continuous infusion over 24 hours whenever possible. A metabolically unstable patient may not tolerate cycled infusions and, in certain conditions, they may be harmful. This is particularly true in patients with end-organ dysfunction. In no case, however, should any PN bag infuse for a period exceeding 24 hours, as such a practice is flawed on both clinical and pharmaceutical grounds. For example, PN admixture infusions of the same bag for periods exceeding 24 hours fosters less attention on the metabolic aspects of patient care, may increase infectious risks, allows greater degradation of many PN admixture components, and consequently can lead to physicochemical incompatibilities that result in therapeutic failures or worse, precipitation, and possibly pulmonary embolism.

Exceptions to this rule would be in patients with limited venous access and receiving life-saving multiple-drug therapy that may not be compatible as a co-infusion into the same intravenous line with the PN admixture. In this case, if possible, the PN infusion can be scheduled around the pharmacotherapy as long as there is a reasonable time allotted for the infusion of PN. Generally, this would be at least 8 hours, and the admixture will likely be hypocaloric. Movement towards a more eucaloric regimen will be dictated by the clinical status of the patient and additional time for infusion. Alternatively, hospitalized patients who are metabolically stable and will receive HPN are often cycled prior to discharge. This is done to assess patient tolerance to an idealized infusion rate (usually between 8 to 12 hours), generally occurring over 3 to 4 days, and to familiarize the patient with infusion procedures. Often, the 24-hour infusion is cycled at a rate starting between 16 and 18 hours and the time of infusion is reduced each day until the goal rate is achieved. It should be noted here that, if such patients are receiving drug therapy, the doses in the PN admixture should be scaled back accordingly, with supplemental doses provided during the "off-cycle" period. For example, for the ostomy patient receiving H2–receptor antagonist therapy (ie, 200 mg of ranitidine to control GI losses during the 24-hour continuous infusion) and now is cycled over 12 hours, only 100 mg should be included in the PN admixtures, with one or two doses administered separately during the off-cycle. Otherwise, if no supplemental drug dose(s) is given outside the PN for 12 hours, ostomy losses may greatly increase, which leads to dehydration and possible readmission to the hospital. This proportionalized approach should be applied for any drug in a cycled PN infusion.[28]

TABLE 36-3.

Common Sterile Components and Concentrations of Nutrients Used in Compounding Total Parenteral Nutrition Admixtures

Additive	*Concentration(s)*
Conventional crystalline amino acids	10% to 15%
BCAA	7%
Dextrose	50% to 70%
Lipid emulsion	20%
Sodium chloride	4 mEq/mL
Sodium acetate	2 mEq/mL
Sodium phosphates	4 mEq of sodium + 3 mmol phosphate/mL
Potassium chloride	2 mEq/mL
Potassium acetate	2 mEq/mL
Calcium gluconate	0.465 mEq/mL
Magnesium sulfate	4.05 mEq/mL
Trace minerals—5 (per 3 mL)	
Chromium	12 μg
Copper	1.2 mg
Manganese	0.3 mg
Selenium	60 μg
Zinc	3 mg
Parenteral multivitamins (per 10 mL)	
Retinol*	1 mg
Ergocalciferol*	5 μg
α-tocopherol*	10 mg
Phylloquinone*	150 μg
Ascorbic acid†	200 mg
Folic acid†	600 μg
Niacin†	40 mg
Riboflavin†	3.6 mg
Thiamine†	6 mg
Pyridoxine†	6 mg
Cyanocobalamin†	5 μg
Pantothenic acid†	15 mg
Biotin†	60 μg

* fat-soluble vitamins
† water-soluble vitamins
BCAA = branched-chain amino acid

Parenteral Nutrition Stability and Compatibility

The stability of PN admixtures is complex, given the number of components present in a typical formulation. For example, there are 15 to 20 crystalline amino acids, dextrose, 10 to 12 electrolyte salts, 12 to 13 vitamins, 5 to 7 trace minerals, and possibly lipid emulsion and drugs. Combined, there are 50 or more individual chemical entities that compose a PN admixture. Degradation processes most commonly encountered include those involving oxidation, hydrolysis, and emulsion breakdown.

One of the most significant examples of instability that may be encountered in PN admixtures includes destabilization of lipid emulsion when included in a formulation, forming a 3-in-1 or total nutrient admixture (TNA). There are many benefits associated with TNA therapy compared to the separate administration of lipid emulsions, such as reduced infectious risk, related to both the formulation and elimination of separate administration sets and/or peripheral catheters; improved metabolic utilization of lipid emulsions when given over 24 hours versus 12 hours or less; and cost effectiveness. However, if the composition of the TNA formulation is pushed beyond the limits imposed by the manufacturer—whether it results from excess cations (sodium, potassium, and especially calcium and magnesium), excessively long beyond-use date assignments by the compounding pharmacist, or poor storage conditions—the emulsified submicron droplets can coalesce, forming large fat globules in excess of 1 μm. When these globules reach a dimension of 5 μm or more, they are capable of obstructing the vessels of the microvasculature and, if infused in sufficient quantities, can lead

TABLE 36-4.

Hypocaloric 1000 mL Total Parenteral Nutrition Regimens as a Single Versus Mixed-Fuel System in Intensive Care Unit Patients

		Single Fuel		*Mixed Fuel*		
Weight (kg)	Total kcal/day*	Amino acids†	Glucose‡	Amino acids	Glucose	Lipids§
40	600	40 g/266 mL(4%)	128 g/183 mL(12.8%)‖	40 g/266 mL(4%)	75 g/107 mL(7.5%)	20 g/100 mL(2%)‖
50	750	50 g/333 mL(5%)‖	160 g/228 mL(16%)‖	50 g/333 mL(5%)‖	96 g/137 mL(9.6%)‖	24 g/120 mL(2.4%)‖
60	900	60 g/400 mL(6%)‖	192 g/275 mL(19.2%)‖	60 g/400 mL(6%)‖	115 g/164 mL(11.5%)‖	29 g/145 mL(2.9%)‖
70	1050	70 g/466 mL(7%)‖	224 g/320 mL(22.4%)‖	70 g/466 mL(7%)‖	135 g/192 mL(13.5%)‖	34 g/170 mL(3.4%)‖
80	1200	80 g/533 mL(8%)‖	256 g/366 mL(25.6%)‖	80 g/533 mL(8%)‖	154 g/220 mL(15.4%)‖	39 g/195 mL(3.9%)‖

* Calories from the hypocaloric regimen consists of 1 g/kg/day of protein and 15 kcal/kg/day total or approximately 50%-60% of needs. Hypocaloric regimens that are intended as permissive underfeeding are often intended for patients whose present weight is within 10% of ideal body weight.
† Assumes a stock bottle of 15% amino acids at 4.1 kcal/g
‡ Assumes a stock bottle of 70% hydrated dextrose at 3.4 kcal/g
§ Assumes a stock bottle of 20% lipid emulsion at 9 kcal/g and providing approximately 20% of total calories
‖ Final concentration of nutrient in 1000 mL of TPN fluid

Adapted from Driscoll DF. Formulation of parenteral and enteral admixtures. In: Pichard C, Kudsk KA, eds. *Update in Intensive Care and Emergency Medicine. From Nutrition Support to Pharmacologic Nutrition in the ICU.* Berlin, Germany: Springer-Verlag; 2000:141.

TABLE 36-5.

Eucaloric, Euvolemic Total Parenteral Nutrition Regimens as a Single- Versus Mixed-Fuel System in Intensive Care Unit Patients

		Single Fuel		*Mixed Fuel*		
Weight (kg)	Total kcal/day*	Amino acids†	Glucose‡	Amino acids	Glucose	Lipids§
40	1000	60 g/400 mL	222 g/317 mL	60 g/400 mL	166 g/237 mL	21 g/105 mL
50	1250	75 g/500 mL	277 g/396 mL	75 g/500 mL	208 g/297 mL	26 g/130 mL
60	1500	90 g/600 mL	333 g/476 mL	90 g/600 mL	250 g/357 mL	31 g/155 mL
70	1750	105 g/700 mL	388 g/554 mL	105 g/700 mL	290 g/414 mL	37 g/185 mL
80	2000	120 g/800 mL	444 g/634 mL	120 g/800 mL	333 g/476 mL	42 g/210 mL

* Calories from the eucaloric and euvolemic regimen consists of 1.5 g/kg/day of protein, 25 kcal/kg/day and 25 mL/kg/day. Eucaloric and euvolemic regimens are in conformance with the ASPEN Guidelines for safe TPN formulations and intended for patients whose present weight is within 10% of ideal body weight.
† Assumes a stock bottle of 15% amino acids at 4.1 kcal/g
‡ Assumes a stock bottle of 70% hydrated dextrose at 3.4 kcal/g
§ Assumes a stock bottle of 20% lipid emulsion at 9 kcal/g and providing approximately 25% of total calories

Adapted from Driscoll DF. Formulation of parenteral and enteral admixtures. In: Pichard C, Kudsk KA, eds. *Update in Intensive Care and Emergency Medicine. From Nutrition Support to Pharmacologic Nutrition in the ICU.* Berlin, Germany: Springer-Verlag; 2000:141.

to fat embolism. Thus, strict adherence to the lipid manufacturer's guidelines regarding safe ranges of amino acids, dextrose, lipids, and electrolytes must be observed.

With respect to storage and beyond-use date assignments, the issues differ between the hospital and home care setting. In the hospital, TNA admixtures are commonly compounded on a daily basis with the aid of an automated compounding device, which has a specific mixing sequence. After compounding, the pharmacist generally assigns a 30-hour beyond-use date to the formulation. Such dating allows for the transport of the admixture to the patient care units, and leaves sufficient time for the PN formulation to be infused over 24 hours. Hence, the 30-hour assignment is reasonable from clinical, pharmaceutical, and logistical perspectives. In the home care setting, the PN formulations are often prepared in amounts ranging from 7 to 10 day supplies, which are refrigerated until the time of use. If a TNA admixture is prescribed, the safest means of preparing and storing this formulation is via the use of multi-chamber bags. Commonly, dual-chamber bags are used, where the lipid emulsion resides in a compartment separate from the other ingredients (ie, amino acids, dextrose, electrolytes, vitamins, and minerals). The patient is instructed to remove the dual-chamber PN bag from the refrigerator and mix the contents prior to infusion. In this way, the beyond-use date of the TNA is commensurate with cycled infusion: ie, the period of time when the emulsion is mixed with the other admixture components is often less than 12 hours compared to the 30-hour beyond-use dates typically assigned for hospital-prepared formulations. It is this author's opinion that this the safest way to provide TNA therapy in the home, compared to 7 to 10 day beyond-use assignments that would be applied in the absence of using dual-chamber bags. Finally, it should be noted that polyvinyl chloride bags or administration set tubing constructed with the plasticizer diethylhexylphthalate (DEHP) should never be used with TNA formulations because of the leaching of DEHP and possible disruption of emulsion stability;[30] only DEHP-free products, such as those made from ethyl vinyl acetate, should be used.

The compatibility of PN admixtures containing multiple additives is equally complex. The biggest concern is the interaction of two or more components forming an insoluble co-precipitate. In fact, the formation of crystalline precipitates is likely more dangerous than coalesced large fat globules, given their rigid structure compared to the flexible and deformable surfaces of similarly sized fat globules.[31] Consider the scenario where a 10-µm crystalline precipitate or a 10-µm fat globule approaches a 5-µm capillary. The normal physiological response to the initial occlusion would be an increase in pulmonary artery pressure. In the case of the rigid crystalline precipitate, the arterial pressure would continue to increase, whereas with the fat globule, the increasing pressure causes the flexible lipid surfaces to deform and pass through the vessel. Hence, the occlusion is complete in the former circumstance and incomplete in the latter. In other words, one could conclude that the LD50 for the same concentration of similarly sized species for rigid crystals would be a fraction of the LD50 for fat globules.

Evidence to support the lethality of rigid crystalline precipitates was demonstrated in the 1994 FDA Safety Alert, in which two patients died and at least two others nearly died as a result of an incompatible combination of calcium and phosphate in PN admixtures.[32] In fact, calcium and phosphate additives present one of the most significant incompatibilities encountered in PN therapy and has been associated with significant morbidity and mortality. As a general rule, meeting the recommended dietary allowances for calcium and phosphate in PN admixtures should be reserved for high osmolality PN formulations (ie, final concentration of amino acid are ≥4% and dextrose ≥10%) intended for central venous delivery and should never be attempted in low osmolality formulations intended for peripheral vein administration, where the incompatibility is most prevalent.[21]

Conclusion

PN formulas are complex mixtures and should be reserved for those patients with significant temporary or even permanent dysfunction of the GI tract. The correct dosing of nutrients is vital to the success of PN therapy, and, in the acute care setting, achieving a eucaloric state should not be the goal from the outset, but rather, be initiated in a gradual manner (ie, hypocaloric) so as to avoid nutrition-related complications (eg, hyperglycemia and infection). Achievement of a eucaloric state (~25 kcal/kg/day) may take several days to accomplish and generally occurs as the patient's stress response remits. In no circumstance should nitrogen balance be the driving force during this time, but rather the goal should be directed at reducing the degree of net negative nitrogen balance. In most cases, nitrogen balance is reached after discharge from the hospital during the recuperative phase in the home setting.

In patients receiving long-term nutrition support at home, the initial PN therapy is often designed to replete the losses in lean body mass endured during the acute and/or chronic phases of malnutrition. In this setting, where the metabolic stress is minimal or nonexistent, providing calories in excess of energy expenditure (~35 kcal/kg/day) to restore body cell mass may be indicated for several months. Once the desired weight is achieved, the amounts of nutrients prescribed are reduced at levels that maintain a desired body weight.

Delivery of PN in the acute care setting is most safely accomplished when infused continuously over 24 hours. Cycling of PN admixtures to infusion periods of 12 hours or less should be reserved principally for administration to HPN patients and, under limited conditions, in the acute care setting. The stability and compatibility of PN formulations must be ascertained throughout the beyond-use date assignment and supported by data from the manufacturer of nutritional products, as well as information appropriately gleaned from the literature. Both stability and compatibility are generally compromised when low osmolality PN admixtures are designed for administration via the small peripheral veins. Hence, the composition of such formulations should be simple and not intended to meet the full needs of the patient, and they should be viewed as a temporary infusion until either central venous access is available or the patient demonstrates tolerance of food via normal consumption of protein and calories by the GI tract.

References

1. Shikora SA, Martindale RG, Schwaitzberg SD. Preface. In: Shikora SA, Martindale RG, Schwaitzberg SD, eds. *Nutritional Considerations in the Intensive Care Unit*. Dubuque, IA: Kendall/Hunt Publishing Company; 2002:xi.
2. Shaw JH, Wildbore M, Wolfe RR. Whole body protein kinetics in severly septic patients: the response to glucose infusion in total parenteral nutrition. *Ann Surg.* 1987;205:288-294.
3. Shaw JH, Wolfe RR. Whole-body protein kinetics in patients with early and advanced gastrointestinal cancer: the response to glucose infusion in total parenteral nutrition. *Surgery.* 1988;103:148-155.
4. Driscoll DF, Bistrian BR. Parenteral nutrition (macronutrient fuels). In: Shikora SA, Martindale RG, Schwaitzberg SD, eds. *Nutritional Considerations in the Intensive Care Unit*. Dubuque, IA: Kendall/Hunt Publishing Company; 2002:39-49.
5. Lamiell JJ, Ducey JP, Freese-Kepczyk BJ, et al. Essential amino acid-induced hyperammonemic encephalopathy and hypophosphatemia. *Crit Care Med.* 1990;18:451-452.
6. Bistrian BR. Update on total parenteral nutrition. *Am J Clin Nutr.* 2001;74:153-154.
7. Sherman MS. Parenteral nutrition and cardiopulmonary disease. In: Rombeau JL, Rolandelli R, eds. *Clinical Nutrition. Parenteral Nutrition*. Philadelphia, Pa: WB Saunders Company; 2001:335-352.
8. Driscoll DF, Bistrian BR. Parenteral and enteral nutrition in the intensive care unit. In: Irwin RS, Rippe JM, eds. *Intensive Care Medicine*. Philadelphia, Pa: Lippincott Williams & Wilkins; 2003:2057-2069.
9. Wolfe RR. Carbohydrate metabolism in the critically ill patient. *Crit Care Clin.* 1987;3:11-24.
10. Hwang TL, Huang SL, Chen MF. Effects of intravenous fat emulsion on respiratory failure. *Chest.* 1990;97:934-938.
11. Mathru M, Dries DJ, Zecca A, et al. Effect of fast vs slow intralipid infusion on gas exchange, pulmonary hemodynamics, and prostaglandin metabolism. *Chest.* 1991;99:426-429.
12. Delafosse B, Viale JP, Tissot S, et al. Effects of glucose-to-lipid ratio and type of lipid on substrate oxidation rate in patients. *Am J Physiol.* 1994;267:E775-E780.
13. Sacks GS, Driscoll DF. Does lipid hang time make a difference? Time is of the essence. *Nutr Clin Prac.* 2002;17:284-290.
14. Klein S, Miles JM. Metabolic effects of long-chain and medium-chain triglyceride emulsions in humans. *JPEN J Parenter Enternal Nutr.* 1994;18:396-397.
15. Driscoll DF. Intravenous lipid emulsions: 2001. *Nutr Clin Prac.* 2001;16:215-218.
16. National Advisory Group on Standards and Practice Guidelines for Parenteral Nutrition. Safe practices for parenteral nutrition formulations. *JPEN J Parenter Enternal Nutr.* 1998;22:49-66.
17. Lowell JA, Schifferdecker C, Driscoll DF, Benotti PN, Bistrian BR. Postoperative fluid overload: not a benign problem. *Crit Care Med.* 1990;18:728-733.
18. McCowen KC, Malhotra A, Bistrian BR. Stress-induced hyperglycemia. *Crit Care Clin.* 2001;74:107-124.
19. Driscoll DF. Drug-induced metabolic disorders and parenteral nutrition in the intensive care unit: a pharmaceutical and metabolic perspective. *DICP, Ann Pharmacother.* 1989;23:363-371.
20. Driscoll DF. Formulation of enteral and parenteral mixtures. In: Pichard C, Kudsk KA, eds. *Update in Intensive Care Medicine*. Brussels, Belgium: Springer-Verlag; 2000:138-150.
21. Driscoll DF. Compounding TPN admixtures: then and now. *JPEN.* 2003;27:433-438.
22. Department of Health and Human Services. Food and Drug Administration. Parenteral multivitamin products; Drugs for human use; Drug efficacy Study Implementation; Amendment. Federal Register 2000;65:21200-21201.
23. Bern MM, Bothe A Jr, Bistrian BR et al. Prophylaxis against central vein thrombosis with low-dose warfarin. *Surgery.* 1986;99:216-221.
24. Bern MM, Lokich JJ, Wallach SR et al. Very low doses of warfarin can prevent thrombosis in central venous catheters. *Ann Intern Med.* 1990;112:423-428.
25. Bach AU, Anderson SA, Foley AL, et al. Assessment of vitamin K status in human subjects administered "minidose" warfarin. *Am J Clin Nutr.* 1996;64:894-902.
26. Centers for Disease Control (CDC). Deaths associated with thiamine-deficient total parenteral nutrition. *MMWR Morb Mortal Wkly Rep.* 1989;38:43-46.
27. Centers for Disease Control (CDC). Lactic acidosis traced to thiamine deficiency related to nationwide shortage of multivitamins for total parenteral nutrition. *MMWR Morb Mortal Wkly Rep.* 1997;46:523-528.
28. Driscoll DF, Baptista RJ, Mitrano FP, et al. Parenteral nutrient admixtures as drug vehicles: theory and practice in the critical care setting. *DICP.* 1991;25:276-283.
29. Gupta VD. Stability of vitamins in total parenteral nutrition solutions. *Am J Health Sys Pharma* 1986;43:2132.
30. Driscoll DF, Bhargava HN, Li L, et al. Physicochemical stability of total nutrient admixtures. *Am J Hosp Pharm.* 1995;52:623-634.
31. Driscoll DF. Physicochemical assessment of total nutrient admixture stability and safety: Quantifying the risk. *Nutrition.* 1997;12:166-167.
32. Lumpkin MM. Safety alert: hazards of precipitation associated with parenetral nutrition. *Am J Hosp Pharm.* 1994;51:1247-1248.

Chapter 37

Pediatric Parenteral Nutrition

Adib Moukarzel, MD, FAAP, FACN, CNSP

Introduction

Venous nutrition in pediatrics was first described nearly 50 years ago when, in 1944, Helfrick and Abelson reported the successful intravenous delivery of a complete diet to a 5-month-old male with severe marasmus.[1] The regimen included alternate peripheral vein infusions of a mixture of 50% glucose and 10% casein hydrolysate and a 10% olive oil-lecithin emulsion, providing 130 kcal/kg/day. After 5 days, the authors report, "The fat fads of the check had returned, the ribs were less prominent, and the general nutritional status was much improved." Since then, parenteral nutrition (PN) has become a well-accepted medical practice in neonates, infants, and children. When oral feeding is impossible for prolonged periods of time, total intravenous alimentation may provide sufficient fluid, dextrose, amino acids, lipid emulsion, minerals, vitamins, and trace metals not only to maintain the weight and the nutritional status (as in adults), but also to sustain growth in the pediatric patient.

This technique has been lifesaving for infants who have had intractable diarrhea syndromes or extensive resection of bowel, and PN is crucial to allow low birthweight infants to achieve high survival rate. Infusions may be administered through an indwelling central vein catheter, an umbilical vein catheter, or a peripheral vein. Despite its usage for the last 40 years, metabolic, mechanical, and infectious complications still occur.

This chapter reviews PN in pediatrics and focuses on what is pertinent to children.

Indications and Contraindications

PN is generally limited to patients who have been refractory to all other forms of treatment [eg, enteral nutrition (EN)] or for whom other forms of treatment (eg, surgery) are inadvisable. The most common indications and conditions for PN are listed in Table 37-1. Some patients require complete PN, whereas others receive supplemental or intermittent support. PN for oncology patients is often indicated for mucositis in graft-versus-host disease and in children with anorexia or vomiting that is associated with chemo- or radiation therapy. PN is utilized with patients with acquired immunodeficiency syndrome who have intractable diarrhea or pancreatitis. PN can also be indicated as a nutritional supplement, before organ transplantation.[2]

Another frequent indication for PN is low birthweight and premature delivery of newborns. Premature infants, especially those with respiratory distress syndrome who are incapable of full oral feeds, often receive PN because of their extremely limited substrate reserve, very rapid growth rate, and perceived susceptibility to irreversible brain damage secondary to malnutrition. In addition, during the newborn period and first months of life, PN is used in infants with intractable diarrhea and those undergoing gastrointestinal (GI) surgery.

In fact, any child who cannot receive adequate nutrition via the GI tract for more than a few days should receive PN. Some patients may not be able to receive full nutrition enterally; they then need supplemental PN.

TABLE 37-1.

Common Indications for Parenteral Nutrition in Children and Newborns

Short Bowel Syndrome
- Secondary to jejuno-ileal atresia
- Secondary to necrotizing enterocolitis
- Secondary to midgut volvulus with strangulation
- Associated with gastroschisis
- Congenital short bowel
- Secondary to Crohn's disease

Intestinal Motility Disorders
- Chronic intestinal pseudo-obstructive syndromes (neuropathic, myopathic, unknown)
- Secondary to chemotherapy and radiation therapy

Intractable Diarrhea
- Failure of enteral nutrition
    - Refractory sprue
    - Autoimmune mucosal disease
    - Crohn's disease
    - Intestinal lymphangiectasia
    - Hypoplastic villous syndrome
    - Secretory tumors
    - Unknown etiology

Inflammatory Bowel Disease

Ascites
- Intractable chylous ascites

Other
- Cystic fibrosis
- Pre orthotopic liver transplantation
- Respiratory failure

Cancer-related
- After bone marrow transplantation- graft-versus-host disease
- Radiation damage to intestine with obstruction and/or diarrhea
- Diarrhea, anorexia, vomiting secondary to chemotherapy

Acquired immunodeficiency syndrome
- Refractory diarrhea
- Pancreatitis

Hypermetabolic conditions
- Sepsis
- Burns
- Major trauma
- Malignancy

Other conditions
- Liver disease
- Congenital heart disease
- Inborn errors of metabolism
- Chronic renal disease

Newborn receiving PN in the neonatal unit
- Surgical diagnosis:
    - Gastroschisis
    - Small bowel atresia
    - Tracheoesophageal fistula
    - Obstruction
    - Omphalocele
    - Imperforate anus and fistula
    - Large bowel atresia
    - Diaphragmatic hernia
    - Malrotation
    - Multiple anomalies
    - Other
- Medical diagnosis:
    - Necrotizing enterocolitis
    - Premature ± Respiratory distress syndrome
    - Sepsis
    - Malabsorption
    - Other

PN may also be used in the malnourished child to supplement enteral feeds.

Contraindications for PN include a functional, available GI tract, or other extenuating circumstances precluding vascular access and the use of PN. Whenever enteral feeding is possible, it should be utilized. Patients with anorexia nervosa are not candidates for PN.

Children who have some intestinal function should be encouraged to feed as much as possible. Even small amounts of liquid should be given by mouth, as soon as possible, to ensure maximal stimulation of the GI tract for its adaptation and diminish bacterial translocation. This also applies to infants who have minimal chance of surviving without PN. They should receive at least 5% of their daily caloric requirements orally (either liquid or pureed food). Failure to initiate oral feeding in infants can later result in sucking or swallowing problems. Infants can really "unlearn" how to suck and swallow. In addition, failure to offer supplemental foods by 6 months may result in the child's difficulty in accepting solid foods later and can delay the timely appearance of other developmental milestones, such as neuromuscular control of head and neck, chewing, and swallowing ability.[3]

Route of Administration

PN can be administered through peripheral veins (peripheral PN) using standard peripheral intravenous catheters and solutions with an osmolarity of 300 to 900 mOsm/L. When solutions of higher osmolarity are used, larger veins (central veins) with a high blood flow must be used to avoid sclerosis and inflammation of the wall of the vein (central PN).

The decision to choose central or peripheral venous nutrition is based on four basic issues: 1) extent of caloric need and enteric functional status, 2) volume tolerance, 3) anticipated duration of intravenous therapy, and 4) venous access. The first step, therefore, is to establish the child's caloric need including the demands of growth, even in the face of acute disease. The nutritional status is determined by anthropometric analysis, documentation of nutrient deficiency, and the impact of the disease. Enteric function is assessed for degree of maldigestion or malabsorption. In peripheral PN solution, because of the need of lower osmolarity, there is a restriction of a lower concentration (10% in children to 12.5% in newborns) of dextrose. This contrasts with a possible higher concentration of dextrose up to 35% in central venous solutions. Therefore, central venous PN allows for greater caloric delivery from dextrose than the peripheral route. Volume intolerance from chronic cardiopulmonary or renal disease is the most common rate-limiting factor in peripheral intravenous nutrition. In patients who are fluid restricted, central PN may be the only way to provide adequate calories. Generally, if the patient is expected to need total PN for less than 2 weeks, a peripheral catheter may suffice. It is often difficult to maintain peripheral access sites for longer than 2 weeks while delivering adequate calories.

Peripheral venous nutrition offers the advantages of rapid initiation with no requirement for the risk that is entailed in acquiring central vein access. Other advantages include reduced rates of line sepsis and major vein thrombosis. There are no significant differences in total cost, pharmacy expense, or nursing time required for care of the line. The disadvantage of peripheral venous nutrition is the reduced volume and concentration of caloric delivery that can be achieved when contrasted to central venous nutrition. The major complication of peripheral venous nutrition is phlebitis of the peripheral vein, which correlates with duration of vein use and osmolarity of the infusate. If the osmolality exceeds 600 mOsm/L (10% glucose solution with electrolytes), phlebitis will develop in up to 70% of patients. The frequency of phlebitis can be reduced by combining lipid emulsion with the solution of dextrose and protein, which lowers the final osmolality of the admixture. Although controversial and unproven, low-dose heparin in the infusate also is used frequently. Kamala et al[4] performed a double-blind trial of heparin (1 IU/mL) added to the PN admixtures in 66 infants who were fed via peripherally inserted central catheters (PICC). There were no significant differences in outcome between the two groups; however, a modest numerical advantage to the heparin group in terms of blocked catheters was offset by the more general concerns in respect to heparin toxicity (especially thrombocytopenia). Briefly, peripheral PN is usually used for patients with normal nutritional status, short anticipated period of no or inadequate enteral feedings, and normal nutritional and fluid status.

Patients who require PN for a long period, have abnormal nutritional status, have increased requirements, or require concentrated PN should receive a centrally placed venous catheter. This may be a tunneled catheter, a PICC line, or an implantable catheter system.

The central vein tunneled catheters are made of a flexible material, such as silicone elastomer or polyurethane. The cuffed, tunneled central venous catheters, such as Hickman or Broviac catheters, have been commonly used. These may be placed by either a cut-down or a percutaneous method in a central vein under sterile technique. These catheters provide stability and decrease the risk of infection by subcutaneously tunneling the catheter to a distant exit site. After the catheter is placed, a separate incision is made on the patient's chest or abdomen so the distal end of the catheter can be directed through a subcutaneous tunnel between the two incisions. The catheter is trimmed to an appropriate estimated length so it will terminate in the superior or inferior vena cava.

These catheters differ from the traditional ones: 1) Teflon reinforces the neck to reduce the risk of cracking and breaking, and 2) the distal end of the catheter has a Luer lock connector to enable a better fit of the intravenous tubing end or to allow it to be screw-capped when not in use. These catheters also have a Dacron cuff attached to the mid-portion. This material stimulates the formation of dense fibrous adhesions, which anchor the catheter securely and create a barrier for ascending bacteria. It takes approximately 2 weeks for this type of adhesion to develop. It is best for the catheter tip to float in the superior vena cava instead of the right atrium.[5,6] Cardiac arrhythmias can occur if the catheter is in the atrium.

The size of the Broviac catheter used depends on the size of the child and the major vein as well as the purpose for which the central catheter will be used. A Hickman catheter is a larger version of the Broviac catheter and may be used in a child of school age.[7,8] It has greater internal and external diameters and is typically used for nutrition, administration of blood products, taking blood samples, and giving chemotherapy. The physician should be aware that there is an infant Broviac catheter as well as a standard Broviac catheter.[9]

Dual and triple lumen catheters are used in pediatric patients, specifically oncologic and transplantation patients. These catheters require considerably more care and have greater incidence of infection than do single lumen catheters.[10]

Certain catheters and cuffs are coated or impregnated with antimicrobial or antiseptic agents, such as chlorhexidine and silver sulfadiazine,[11] minocycline and rifampin,[12] platinum and silver, or silver cuffs. These catheters can decrease the risk for infection and potentially decrease hospital costs associated with treating infections, despite the additional acquisition cost of an antimicrobial- or antiseptic-impregnated catheter.[13] All of the studies involving antimicrobial- or antiseptic-impregnated catheters have been conducted using triple lumen, non-cuffed catheters in adult patients whose catheters remained in place <30 days. Although all of the studies have been conducted in adults, these catheters have been approved by Food and Drug Administration (FDA) for use in patients weighing >3 kg. Currently, no antiseptic- or antimicrobial-impregnated catheters are available for use in patients who weigh <3 kg.

PICC are becoming increasingly popular as an alternative for patients needing intermediate to long-term access.[14]

Finck et al[15] recently investigated whether percutaneous subclavian central venous catheterization, using the Seldinger technique, is safe and successful in children younger than 1 year of age, as in some units an open surgical cut-down approach has been preferred. The investigators retrospectively considered 84 infants who had required central venous access, identified from their medical procedure index covering a 1-year period. The 84 children had together received 110 central venous lines. The success rate was 79% in those under 6 months of age, and 96% in those aged 6 to 12 months. Remarkably, no complications were recorded. This retrospective audit supports the safety and success of percutaneous central line insertion, even in small children.

A totally implantable venous access system was developed in the 1980s for the treatment of cancer patients with chemotherapy. This device (Infuse-A-Port; Intermedics Infusaid Corporation, Norwood, Mass) consists of a silicone rubber catheter connected to a subcutaneously placed, molded-plastic injection port or reservoir. Venous access is gained through the subclavian vein into the superior vena cava, using the silicone rubber catheter.[16] The catheter is attached to the reservoir, which is implanted subcutaneously and sutured to muscular fascia for stability. Entry into the venous system is achieved with the use of a specially deflected, pointed Huber needle, which prevents coring of the self-sealing subcutaneous reservoir. Similar implantable systems have also been reported and used for the administration of drugs, blood products, and PN. Complications in using the implanted catheter systems can be categorized into five groups: venous thrombosis, catheter migration, infection, extravasation, and withdrawal occlusion.[17]

These catheters are considered "central" if the tip of the catheter is at the junction of the superior vena cava and the right atrium. It is important to document the position of the line by radiologic methods (x-ray) so that malposition of the line can be avoided.

Umbilical venous catheters may also be used for the administration of PN. In the case of lines placed in the lower extremities (femoral lines), every attempt is made to have the tip of the catheter in the inferior vena cava above the level of the diaphragm. PN can also be delivered via peritoneal or hemodialysis catheters.

Occasional use has been made of arteriovenous fistulas or shunts for vascular access in PN.[18-20] When a shunt is used, a small "T" is placed in the shunt and access is achieved through the "T," infusing the solution through the catheter while blood flow is maintained. When an arteriovenous fistula is used, a small bore needle is percutaneously placed into the access, similar to what is done in dialysis. The PN solutions are infused either continuously or cyclically. Use of an arteriovenous fistula or shunt may be associated with an increased incidence of thrombosis of the vascular access. This risk, along with fear of bleeding from the access due to arterial pressure, has limited its use for PN. The rate of infection of an arteriovenous fistula is lower than that of a catheter.

Nutrient Requirements

Fluid

Fluid and electrolyte deficits should be corrected before PN is initiated whenever possible. After this, maintenance fluid needs and extra-physiologic losses should be met and verified daily by monitoring the patient's weight and intake and output records. Extraneous fluid loss (eg, through nasogastric solution, fistula, ostomy drainage, diarrhea, and emesis) should be replaced with a separate intravenous solution in amounts equal to measured losses. The solution should contain similar electrolytes content as the fluid. Using PN solution to replace extraneous fluid and electrolyte losses should be avoided because daily fluctuations cause frequent PN-solution–order changes, increasing wastage, labor, and cost. Maintenance-fluid needs are usually met with PN and fat emulsion, whereas replacement solutions should be tailored to specific losses. Daily maintenance fluid requirements for children[21,22] are outlined in Table 37-2.

Multiple factors determine the fluid requirements of infants and children. These include the hydration status, size, age, environmental factors, and underlying disease. Factors that increase fluid requirements include radiant warmers, conventional single-walled incubators, and phototherapy. Those that decrease fluid requirements include heat shields, thermal blankets, and double-walled incubators.

Should the patient need fluid restriction, he or she can still intake the same amount of calories with reduced daily volume of PN solution and increased dextrose concentration. The maximal possible dextrose concentration is 35%. The amino acid concentration may also be increased to

TABLE 37-2.

Fluid Recommendations (Maintenance Requirements) for Parenteral Nutrition

Initial Volume For Patients Free of Cardiovascular or Renal Disease	
<10 kg	100 mL/kg
11 to 20 kg	1000 cc + 50 mL/kg for each kg >10 kg
>20 kg	1500 cc + 20 mL/kg for each kg >20 kg

Volume may be increased by:
10 mL/kg/day in infants until the desired caloric intake is achieved (to a maximum of 200 mL/kg/day, if tolerated)
>10 kg: by 10% of initial volume per day until desired caloric intake is achieved (to a maximum of 4000 mL/m²/day, if tolerated)

TABLE 37-3.

Suggested Guidelines for Fluid Intakes in Newborns (mL/kg/day)*

Birthweight (g)	Day 1 to 2	Day 3	Days 15 to 30
751 to 1,000	105	140	150
1,001 to 1,250	100	130	140
1,251 to 1,500	90	120	130
1,501 to 2,000	80	110	130
> 2,000 (term infant)	70	80	90 to 100

*In clinical practice, 150 to 180 ml/kg of fluid are often administered

maintain adequate protein intake. A higher proportion of calories may also be supplied using fat emulsion 20% (at 2 kcal/mL) or even 30%.

Premature newborns have unique fluid requirements[23] (Table 37-3). In these neonates, fluid therapy is designed to avoid variations in serum osmolality, dehydration, and overhydration and to provide stable electrolyte, glucose levels, and acid-base balance. Excess fluid intake (>150 mL/kg/day) in very-low-birthweight (VLBW) infants[24] may be associated with patent ductus arteriosus,[25] bronchopulmonary dysplasia,[26] necrotizing enterocolitis,[27] and intraventricular hemorrhage.[28,29]

Energy Requirements and Resting Energy Expenditure

Energy requirements vary widely with age and gender during infancy, childhood, and adolescence (Table 37-4). Based on data from several thousand children over 1 year of age, the World Health Organization (WHO) recommendations provide an estimated resting energy expenditure (REE), which may then be multiplied by a factor to adjust for catch-up growth, activity, and medical status to provide an estimate of total daily caloric needs[30] (Tables 37-5 and 37-6). In obese patients (>120% ideal body weight), the Schofield height/weight equation more accurately predicts energy needs[31] (Table 37-7).

In addition, there are many different recommendations and equations to estimate the caloric needs of children.[32-39] These estimates have numerous limitations. They are a statistical average, which does not necessarily apply to the child who is about to receive the PN or accurately reflect the individual patient's needs.[32] Furthermore, because of genetic differences and differences in other factors affecting energy expenditure, there may be significant inter-individual variations in energy expenditure in children and even among normal newborns where energy requirements do not fall within narrow margins.[40,41] White et al have shown that in the pediatric intensive care unit there is a day-to-day variation in energy expenditure of patients: as high as 21 ± 16% (mean ± SD).[42] In many studies, estimates of REE are measured on healthy nonhospitalized children, often on enteral feeding and not receiving PN. Few studies estimate REE of children receiving PN with different medical conditions; they show that an equation based on lean body mass or 24-hour urinary creatinine excretion could be a more accurate estimate of REE than conventional methods based on weight or height, and the equation may be applicable to diverse nutritional states.[38,39] Another inaccuracy is that children generally require less parenteral than enteral calories because a portion of the enterally supplied calories is lost in the stool and expanded in the process of digestion and absorption. This is especially true in the immature infant.[43]

It should be pointed out that the parenteral requirements for various nutrients depend on the goal to be achieved. The requirements for normal growth, for example, are considerably greater than those for preserving existing body composition. Theoretically, if protein intake is adequate, an energy intake approximating the REE is sufficient for maintenance (prevention of weight loss), whereas an energy intake in excess of REE is necessary to achieve weight gain. The total energy intake necessary to produce a specific rate of weight gain will be greater in

TABLE 37-4.

Recommended Energy and Protein Intakes

Age (year) (kcal/kg)	Energy* (mean) kcal/day	Energy* (mean) (g/kg) (g/day)	Protein
Preterm	100 to 120		2.5 to 3.5 g/kg
Infants and children			
0 to 0.5	115	300	2.2 g/kg
0.5 to 1	105	600	2.0 g/kg
1 to 3	100	1300	1.8 g/kg
4 to 6	85	1700	1.5 g/kg
7 to 10	85	2400	1.2 g/kg
Adolescents			
Boys			
11 to 14		2800	45 g/day
15 to 18		3000	56 g/day
Girls			
11 to 14		2400	46 g/day
15 to 18		2100	46 g/day

*Best assessed by estimation of resting energy expenditure REE (indirect calorimetry)

TABLE 37-5.

Estimated Resting Energy Expenditure for Children (in kcal)

Gender	1 to 3 yr	3 to 10 yr	10 to 18 yr	18 to 30 yr
Male	60.9W – 54	22.7W + 495	17.5W + 651	15.3W + 679
Female	61.0W – 51	22.5W + 499	12.2W + 746	14.7W + 496

W = weight in Kg,
Adapted from World Health Organization (WHO), Geneva: Energy and protein requirements, Technical Report Series. 1985;724:71.[30]

TABLE 37-6.

Disease Activity/Stress Factors*

1.3	Well-nourished child at rest with mild to moderate stress (minor surgery)
1.5	Normal active child with mild to moderate stress Inactive child with severe stress (trauma, cancer, extensive surgery) Malnourished child requiring catch-up growth with minimal activity
1.7	Active child requiring catch-up growth Active child with severe stress

*Multiply REE times disease activity/stress factor for estimated daily energy requirements.
Adapted from World Health Organization (WHO), Geneva: Energy and protein requirements, Technical Report Series. 1985;724:71.[30]

Table 37-7.

Predicting Resting Energy Expenditure: Schofield Height/Weight Equations (kcal/day)

Age	*0 to 3 Years*	*3 to 10 Years*	*10 to 18 Years*
Female	16.252W + 1023.2H – 413.5	16.969W + 161.8H + 371.2	8.265W + 465H + 200
Male	0.167W + 1517.4H – 617.6	19.59W + 130.3H + 414.9	16.25W + 137.2H – 515.5

W = weight in kg; H = height in cm

infants with higher REE.[44] For example, the REE of infants with bronchopulmonary dysplasia is 10% to 30% greater than that of infants without it.[45] Hence, for the same rate of weight gain, infants with bronchopulmonary dysplasia require a greater energy intake than those without this condition. The same is true for children receiving PN for Henoch Schönlein purpura and with other chronic or acute conditions.[44]

Traditionally, it is accepted that the energy intake of the surgical patient would be higher than that of a "nonstressed" patient. However, recently, this concept has been challenged, as the increased energy expenditure associated with surgery in newborns and children is short-lived and lasts only 24 hours after the procedure.[41] For example, although newborns have a 20% increase in REE after major surgery, this elevation returns to baseline within 12 to 24 hours.[45] Nonventilated surgical neonates (gastroschisis, atresia, or volvulus) who remain critically ill and require PN also do not appear to require increased energy intakes.[40] Preterm infants (25 weeks gestation) and children who have not undergone surgery behave similarly.[31,41,46,47] Taken together, these data support the idea that in most cases there is little need to provide postoperative or critically ill infants and children with much more than their REE, which in most cases will be an amount similar to their basal metabolic rate.

By estimating energy requirements from body weight, age, or other formulas, one should be capable of directing a regimen that would meet the calories a patient needs and avoid overfeeding. However, a child weighing 10 kg for instance, will need an amount of calories based on his or her metabolic status and degree of malnutrition (ie, his or her body composition) rather than body weight or age. Therefore, exactly measuring the energy requirements in an individual patient is ideal. This can be accomplished through measurement of oxygen consumption and carbon dioxide production, and determination of REE by indirect calorimetry when the patient becomes "stable."[48] The indirect calorimetry is crucial for the patient with increased needs, in critically ill patients, and for those not responding to nutritional therapy.

Measuring energy expenditure during the first 24 hours after surgery will overestimate the energy requirements for the entire postoperative period, potentially resulting in excess energy intake (overfeeding) with its potential consequences. These include hepatic dysfunction, hyperglycemia, elevations in blood urea nitrogen, cholesterol, and triglyceride, delayed weaning from ventilators, fluid overload, hyperosmolar states, and increased secretion of norepinephrine and urinary catecholamines.[49] Diet-induced thermogenesis from overfeeding and lipogenesis becomes a metabolic stress.[50] PN administration itself increases metabolic rate.[51] The more malnourished the patients, the greater the stimulatory effect of PN on metabolic rate.[52]

In clinical practice, indirect calorimetry may not be practical because of the expensive equipment and the expertise required. If indirect calorimetry technology in the nonintubated child not receiving supplemental oxygen is well standardized, measurements in the newborn infant and the intubated patient receiving supplemental oxygen are technically difficult. A patient in the intensive care setting who has a Swan-Ganz catheter to measure cardiac output can also have his or her REE calculated according to cardiac output.[53]

In summary, one should be flexible regarding the "appropriate" energy intake and monitor the child for weight gain (fluid versus tissue) and evidence of overfeeding. Stable nonstressed infants should gain weight without excess fluid. If they do not, and regardless of the estimated caloric requirements, there is a need to increase nutrients (and calories) until appropriate weight is gained but without inducing overfeeding. Here is an indication for indirect calorimetry.

Administration of PN, which provides all nutritional requirements, should be avoided in the first couple of days of a patient's critical illness, as it will further increase the metabolic rate[52] and do little to stem the protein catabolic response to the illness. An exception is the preterm infant. PN is required after birth (first day of life as opposed to the first few days of life) because of the premature infant's limited nutritional stores.[54] This may induce fewer infections during hospitalization, and infants are more likely to reach 10th percentile for weight or height at the time of discharge.[55]

Amino Acids (Protein)

Protein hydrolysate solutions were the first to be used in PN solutions. They induced hyperammonemia, poor utilization of nitrogen, decreased amounts of arginine, high amount of glycine, hyperchloremic metabolic acidosis, and non-negligible amount of aluminum and parenteral-associated osteopenia.[56] These formulations are currently replaced by synthetic crystalline amino acid solutions. Most of the first marketed formulations of amino acid were designed according to the requirements of normal, orally fed adult subjects and not for growing infants and children.[57] Use of these solutions in neonate and small infants leads to high plasma concentrations of methionine, glycine, and phenylalanine (a cause for concern regarding safety), and to low plasma concentrations of the branched-chain amino acids (BCAA) tyrosine, and cysteine.[57-59]

The design and production of amino acids solutions—such as TrophAmine (McGaw, Irvine, Calif)—specifically designed to meet the needs of neonates resolved these problems.[58,59] These "neonatal" amino acid solutions have been used in neonates to promote growth and to normalize plasma amino acid levels within the range recommended by Wu and others.[60] TrophAmine differs from adult formulations in that it contains 1) taurine (considered essential in neonates because of their delayed maturation of cystathionase and cysteine sulfinic acid decarboxylase); 2) glutamic and aspartic acids (found in high concentrations in human milk); 3) less phenylalanine, methionine, and glycine; 4) more tyrosine and histidine (due to limited synthetic ability); and 5) high concentration of BCAA. TrophAmine may be used in newborn infants including preterm infants until at least 6 months of age and probably beyond 24 months of age.[61] Unlike adult-type amino acid solutions, use of this product is associated with a decrease in PN-related cholestasis, probably in part because of the solution's taurine content, which results in "normal" plasma levels of taurine.[62] Because, these solutions contain higher concentration of BCAA, they may be used in patients with chronic liver disease and cholestasis, replacing in children specialized solutions, such as HepatAmine. TrophAmine has a lower pH than do standard amino acid solutions and allows larger amounts of calcium and phosphorus to be added to the PN solution without precipitation.[63]

Since the introduction of TrophAmine, other neonatal formulations have been studied. Among them are American-made solutions Aminosyn-PF (Abbott Laboratories),[64] Neopham (modeled after the amino acid pattern in human breast milk),[65] and pediatric formula IV proposed by Imura and others66 and European formulations Primene (Clintec) and Vaminolac (Pharmacia). The development of amino acid solutions specific to the needs of neonates may ultimately allow adequate growth with lower protein and calorie intakes than previous amino acid solutions. There are reports of positive nitrogen balance (>200 mg/kg/day) and weight gain (>10 g/kg/day) with low doses of TrophAmine (2 g/kg/day) and calories (50 kcal/kg/d) in preterm infants receiving PN.[57] In the past, these results were achievable only with higher calorie and standard protein intakes.

Novamine 15% is a highly concentrated formulation of regular, crystalline amino acids that allows the final PN solution to contain higher maximum amino acids concentrations than do the standard regular formulation. It may be used for patients over 6 months of age.

HepatAmine is a specialized formulation that is high in BCAA and low in methionine and aromatic amino acids. It has been designed for patients with altered serum amino acid profiles who develop hepatic encephalopathy or liver failure. Although data evaluating these formulations are encouraging,[67] no data have shown a change in mortality. Furthermore, data comparing these formulations with standard amino acids are lacking. The neonatal amino acid solutions have concentrations of essential amino acids including BCAA, which are fairly close to those in the specialized amino acids solutions. The benefit of specialized amino acid solutions for patients with renal disease also is not clear.[68,69]

Other Sources of Nitrogen

Glutamine is the most abundant amino acid in the body.[70] However, it is unstable in water and is absent from the currently available amino acid solutions. The nutritional requirement for this non-essential amino acid during catabolic illness differs greatly from that during health.[70] Glutamine exported from the muscle serves as an ammonia donor, supports rapidly proliferating tissue such as fibroblasts or lymphocytes, and is a primary fuel source for enterocytes and colonocytes.[71] Glutamine supplemented PN preserves gut structure and improves gut immune function in animal models.[72] The use of glutamine containing dipeptides is proposed because of the instability of glutamine. In adult humans, there are data showing that glutamine supplemented PN improves the nitrogen balance,[73] has clinical and metabolic efficacy after bone marrow transplantation,[74-76] and prevents intestinal atrophy and increased permeability in critically ill patients.[77] However, convincing definitive data are still lacking in children.

Another source of nitrogen is represented by ornithine ketoglutarate. This salt is a precursor of glutamine and may have an effect on the secretion of anabolic hormones (insulin, growth hormones) and the synthesis of metabolites such as polyamines, arginine, and ketoacids.[78] It has been successful in inducing a better nitrogen balance in malnourished, traumatized, burned, and surgical patients.[79-81] In prepubertal children on PN, it is reported that daily parenteral administration of 15 g of ornithine ketoglutarate reverses growth retardation and increased insulin-like growth factor I plasma levels.[82] A more specific approach to protein metabolism might be achieved in the future.

Guidelines for amino acid requirements in PN are shown in Table 37-4. They vary from 2.5 to 3.5 g/kg/day for preterm infants to 0.75 g/kg/day for adolescents.[57-59] (Composition of commonly used amino acid solutions are shown in Table 37-2.) Similar to energy requirements, amino acid requirements vary from individual to individual under normal circumstances.

To promote efficient net protein utilization and not use protein as an energy source, the calorie-to-nitrogen ratio—150 to 200 nonprotein calories per 1 gram of nitrogen—are recommended. One gram of protein contains 0.16 grams of nitrogen; therefore, 24 to 32 non-nitrogen calories must be supplied per gram of protein to yield a desirable calorie-to-nitrogen ratio of 150 to 200:1.

Although it has been stated in the literature that the amino acid intake should be gradually increased over the first few days of PN administration (to maintain adequate calorie-to-nitrogen ratio), this practice is not justified. Moreover, a recent review of the literature on the use of early amino acid introduction found no metabolic abnormalities (elevated blood urea nitrogen (BUN), serum pH, ammonia, serum aminogram) associated with this practice, even in preterm infants if neonatal amino acid formulations are used.83 It is, therefore, safe to give most newborn patients their entire daily protein requirements of neonatal-type formulations on the first day of PN. Gradually increasing the amino acid concentration or volume only postpones the time at which the infant receives adequate intake. In addition, in situations where fluid intake is significantly restricted, energy intake should be sacrificed at the expense of maintaining a greater amino acid intake, particularly when more than REE can be provided (making transiently the calorie-to-nitrogen ratio low, despite the traditional recommendations).

Another reason for amino acid requirements to be a priority in prescribing PN is that immunodeficiency associated with malnutrition is largely related to protein malnutrition as opposed to energy malnutrition. Practically, neonates start at 1.5 to 2.5 g/kg/day of amino acids and increase to the desired goal. Older infants and children start at the goal dose.[84] The only exceptions are critically ill neonates, infants, and children; patients with hepatic and renal insufficiency not on dialysis; and patients with disorders of protein metabolism.

Monitoring Protein Intake

The BUN is the easiest and readily available tool to monitor the protein intake. If renal function and hydration are normal, a low BUN (<5 mg/dL) reflects inadequate amino acid intake and conversely, a high BUN (>20 mg/dL) suggests that the amino acid intake may be too great. For many children, a BUN between 10 and 15 mg/dL is a good target and reflects an amino acid intake that is adequate for protein anabolism. Serum prealbumin (transthyretin) and transferrin are often used as short-term (1 to 2 day) measures of the response to amino acid intake. In addition, serum pH, ammonia, serum aminogram may be monitored.

The intake of energy and amino acids in combination result in the greatest protein gain. Amino acid intake is the main determinant of protein gain. That is, there is a much larger gain in protein accretion with increases in amino acid intake (neonatal type formulations) than with increases in energy intake.

Lipids

Fat is included in PN to prevent essential fatty acid (EFA) deficiency and promote normal development of the nervous system.[85] In addition, fat emulsion provides the most concentrated calories (20% fat emulsion supplies 2.0 kcal/mL, whereas 5% dextrose solution provides 10 times fewer calories, ie, 0.2 kcal/mL). To infuse fat intravenously, it has to be emulsified (with phospholipids) and the resulting emulsion needs to become isotonic. Note that the amount of phospholipids is the same in 10%, 20%, or 30% fat emulsions. The 20% emulsion is used most often. The 10% is infrequently used; the 30% emulsion can only be used in a total nutrient admixture and cannot be infused alone into a peripheral vein.

Patients who cannot tolerate large glucose or fluid loads can receive sufficient calories if fat emulsion is added to the glucose-and-amino–acid regimen. In addition, continuous administration of fat emulsion (which is isotonic) with the PN regimen prolongs the viability of peripheral intravenous lines in infants who may have limited venous access.[86]

Rate of Intralipid Infusion and Monitoring

Infusion of fat is discussed in Chapter 36, and guidelines are similar to those for adult patients. Slower infusion rates are required for small-for-gestational-age infants. Infusion rates of 0.12 g/kg/hour or less resulted in less elevation of plasma lipid levels than did rates of 0.17 g/kg/hour or more.[87]

Intravenous fat emulsions with high concentrations of phospholipids (ie, 10% emulsions) should be avoided as they carry a higher risk of producing high serum levels of triglycerides, cholesterol, and phospholipids than do other emulsions (ie, 20% and 30% emulsions).[89-91] Phospholipid is believed to inhibit lipoprotein lipase. Four g/kg/day of 20% of intravenous fat emulsions caused less increase of plasma lipids than 2 g/kg/d of 10% of intravenous fat emulsion.[87]

A number of other factors decrease the rate of clearance of intravenous fat emulsions. In preterm infants and malnourished patients, there is a slower rate of clearance resulting from lower levels of lipoprotein lipase. This is due to the decreased capillary mass where the lipoprotein lipase resides.[90] Another factor that alters the clearance of intravenous fat emulsion and induces hypertriglyceridemia is the concurrent administration of steroids or other lipolytic drugs.[91] Additionally, drugs such as propofol and amphotericin B contain lipid and should be taken into account in nutritional calculations.

Another factor that may alter the tolerance to intravenous fat emulsion and induces hypertriglyceridemia is the patient medical condition. This includes patients who have organ dysfunction (such as liver or renal disease) or who are metabolically stressed (sepsis, trauma). In these settings, the high levels of catecholamines, cortisol, and cytokines promote the lipolysis of lipid.[92-94] Of note, children with sepsis and liver disease[95,96] and infants with cyanotic heart disease (ventricular septal defects or transposition of the great vessels) can tolerate and utilize intravenous fat emulsions.[97]

Monitoring Fat Infusion

Serum triglyceride and cholesterol levels should be measured before PN is initiated and after any increase in dose of lipids, to be sure the patient can tolerate the new dosage. The serum triglyceride levels may be either a through level (fasting level for 6 to 8 hours after stopping the fat infusion) or a peak level (measured 4 hours after starting an intravenous fat infusion or 4 hours after any increase in infusion rate), as it is at this time that hypertriglyceridemia is most likely to occur.[98-99] A sudden increase in the triglyceride level may be indicative of sepsis. Patients on long-term PN who infuse lipids on a regular basis should have triglyceride and cholesterol determinations quarterly.

Ideally, the triglyceride level should be "normal." The problem resides on the little data of the physiologic level of triglyceride in breast-fed normal full-term or premature newborns. Some authors define a high level any level above 100 mg/dL,[101] while others accept 200 mg/dL and even 400 mg/dL. Of note, some common methods

TABLE 37-8.

Dosing for Intravenous Lipid Emulsions in g/kg/day

Starting Age	*Daily Dose*	*Dose Increase*	*Maximum Dose*
Preterm	0.5 to 1.0	1.0	3.5 to 4
Full-term (0 to 6 mo)	1.0 to 1.5	1.0 to 1.5	3.5 to 4
Older infant (6 to 12 mo)	1.0 to 1.5	1.0 to 1.5	3 to 4
Children (1 to 10 yr)	1.0	1.0 to 1.5	3 to 4
Adolescents (11 to 18 yr)	1.0	1.0	2 to 3

of measuring triglycerides measure the free glycerol released from the triglyceride molecule.[102] Given that intravenous fat emulsions contain free glycerol in addition to triglycerides, the serum triglyceride level measured by evaluating glycerol will be an overestimation of the true serum triglyceride level. Unfortunately, there are no data defining the level at which one should be concerned.

Postprandially, the serum triglyceride of normal adults may approach 500 mg/dL.[103] Even values above 1500 mg/dL do not appear to have harmful effects.[103] The American Gastroenterological Association Technical Review on Parenteral Nutrition states that intravenous fat emulsion should not be administered to patients whose serum triglyceride levels exceed 400 mg/dL.[54] No data are provided to support this statement but we agree that serum triglyceride levels <400 mg/dL are unlikely to cause clinically relevant problems.

A normal plasma triglyceride level does not mean that exogenous triglycerides are adequately used (oxidation) or stored (in the adipose tissue). Indeed part of the exogenous lipid may be cleared by other mechanisms, especially capture by the reticuloendothelial system (which may lead to fat overload syndrome).

Essential Fatty Acid Deficiency

A key role for intravenous fat emulsion is the prevention of EFA deficiency. EFAs are required for brain and somatic growth, wound healing, skin integrity, and immune function. EFA deficiency causes a generalized, scaly dermatitis composed of thickened, erythematous, desquamating plaques. Additional manifestations of EFA deficiency include poor hair growth or alopecia, thrombocytopenia, failure to thrive or reduced growth rate, increased susceptibility to infections, and impaired wound healing.[104,105] Microscopically, the horny layer of the skin is cracked, the barrier function of the skin is disturbed, and transepidermal water loss is increased.

Biochemical evidence of EFA deficiency has been observed in the serum of fasted newborn infants as early as 2 days after initiating fat-free PN.[85,105] Linoleic (18:2 n-6) and arachidonic (20:4 n-6) acids are deficient, and an abnormal metabolite—5,8,11-eicosatriaenoic acid (20:3 n-9)—is present in the plasma. An EFA deficiency can be assessed by determination of the ratio of 5,8-11-eicosatetraenoic to arachidonic acid (triene-to-tetraene ratio). A ratio >0.4 generally is assumed an early indicator of EFA deficiency. Recently, it has been suggested that measurement of n-6 and n-3 long-chain polyunsaturated fatty acids is more reliable than the more commonly used triene-to-tetraene ratio.[106]

Topical application of sunflower seed oil that contains linoleic acid has been reported to ameliorate the clinical and biochemical skin manifestations.[107] However, this finding could not be duplicated in subsequent studies.[108] Interestingly, 15 mL twice a day of corn oil, sunflower oil, or safflower oil enterally provides as much linoleic acid as 150 mL of 10% of intravenous fat emulsions at less than 5% of the cost. Many PN patients not on complete bowel rest tolerate such a regimen.[109]

Given that intravenous fat emulsions contain approximately 50% EFAs by weight, 0.5 to 1 g/kg/day of intravenous fat emulsion (2% to 4% of total calories as fat emulsion (ie, 1% to 2% linoleic acid) is usually recommended to prevent EFA deficiency in patients receiving total PN.85,112 However, there appears to be a fair amount of inter-individual variation in EFA requirements based on age, disease, and nutritional status.[85,111-115] For instance, in patients receiving no intravenous fat emulsion, some studies suggest that fatty acid deficiency develops faster when total energy intake is low than when total energy intake is high.[116,117] Therefore, there is debate as to the appropriate amount of intravenous fat emulsion required to prevent EFA deficiency. In adolescents and adults, the recommendation of 1.5 g/kg (approximately 500 mL of 20% intravenous fat emulsion) twice weekly seems more than adequate for some investigators or too low for others.[111-114] In infants (including preterms) who are most susceptible, a minimum of 0.5 g/kg/day should be used.

Amount of Intravenous Fat Emulsions

Care must be taken to keep the percentage of total calories from fat in the range of 30% to 40% of total nonnitrogen calories. It should not exceed 60% of total calories, which constitute a ketogenic diet. Suggested dosing for intravenous fat emulsions is shown in Table 37-8.

Other Types of Intravenous Fat Emulsions

Conventional intravenous fat emulsions contain long chain triglycerides (LCT) and are usually made of soybean and safflower oils. Concerns have been raised about providing children and infants with soybean or safflower oil emulsions. Conventional and new intravenous fat emulsions are discussed in Chapter 36. Newly developed emulsions (with medium chain triglycerides—MCT) have been shown to improve nitrogen balance in adults and children,[118-121] but this effect remains controversial. MCT emulsions have also been used in patients receiving PN for long term with beneficial effect in reducing cholestasis.[121]

Structured lipids (medium chain fatty acids and long chain fatty acids [LCFA] attached to the same glycerol molecule) have been synthesized. They are different from physical mixtures of MCT and LCT. Such structured emulsions have been shown to improve nitrogen retention and muscle protein in adults;[122] however, there is no available study in pediatric patients. Fish oil-based emulsions provide a high amount of long chain polyunsaturated fatty acid. These fatty acids are essential for brain development and have potentially beneficial anti-inflammatory effects.[123-125] Olive oil-based emulsions, which provide higher levels of monounsaturated fatty acids, may lower the incidence of cardiovascular morbidity,[126] as well as preserve EFA and fatty acid elongation, decrease total cholesterol, and improve antioxidant activity against lipid peroxidation.[127] These emulsions may be valuable alternative for PN of preterm infants who are often exposed to oxidative stress, while their antioxidative defense is weak.[128] Supplementation with alpha-tocopherol (vitamin E) at a dose of 0.6 mg/g of unsaturated fatty acids has also been recommended.

Carnitine

Carnitine, a quaternary amino acid, plays an important role in the oxidation of LCFA.[129] Both breast milk and infant formulas contain carnitine. Solutions currently used for intravenous alimentation contain no carnitine, but they do contain all the precursors for its endogenous production.[130] Nonsupplemented parenterally fed infants have low tissue and plasma carnitine levels.[129-132] The clinical significance of this is uncertain.[133] Normalization of serum carnitine levels occurs in infants receiving long-term PN and supplemental oral L-carnitine (50 µmol/kg/day = 8.1 mg/kg/day)[134] or intravenous L-carnitine.[135,136]

Carnitine deficiency may be an etiological factor in the limited ability of premature babies to utilize parenteral lipid. In vitro studies suggest that fatty acid oxidation is impaired when the tissue carnitine levels fall below 10% of normal. Therefore, relative carnitine deficiency may impair fatty acid oxidation, thus reducing the available energy and impairing growth.[129,130]

The VLBW infants requiring PN develop low carnitine levels and impaired ketogenesis that appeared to improve with parenteral carnitine. In 1,001- to 1,500-g VLBW infants on PN supplemented with L-carnitine (50 µmol/kg/day), increased carnitine levels and improved tolerance to intravenous fat emulsions were noted.[136] Other studies of carnitine supplementation have failed to demonstrate significant improvement in clinical outcome.[136,137] In the absence of specific recommendations, a supplementation of 2 to 10 mg/kg/day intravenous L-carnitine has been suggested.[138] Higher doses of carnitine seem to have pharmacologic effects, leading to increased protein and fat oxidation with associated energy loss. Supplementation with 48 mg L-carnitine/kg/day increased the metabolic rate, decreased fat and protein accretion, and prolonged the time to regain birthweight in preterm infants receiving PN with lipids.[139] A recent Cochrane Database Review found no evidence to support the routine supplementation of parenterally fed neonates with carnitine.[129] However, the studies available did not assess the use of carnitine in long-term PN. It is possible that, in this setting, the effects of carnitine deficiency may be too subtle to be easily identified but are still metabolically relevant, given the central role of carnitine in metabolism.[130] (This author does not routinely supplement PN solutions with carnitine.)

Precautions, Side Effects, and Contraindications to the Use of Fat Emulsions

Despite the need to correct any EFA deficiency and the advantage of fat emulsions, there may be several classic contraindications, including the initial phase of sepsis, thrombocytopenia, disseminated intravascular coagulation, respiratory distress syndrome, and metabolic acidosis. When clearance of the intravenous fat is altered, there is a risk of developing hypertriglyceridemia. This may lead to reticuloendothelial system overload, and the so-called "fat overload syndrome."

Fat overload syndromes occur when patients receive excessive quantities of lipids, usually more than 3 g/kg. In the acute syndrome, clinical and biological expression mimics septic syndrome; however, it is related to macrophage activation by capture of exogenous fat particles. Common features include high fever, hepatosplenomegaly, jaundice, respiratory distress, bleeding, thrombopenia, disseminated intra-vascular coagulation, metabolic acidosis, hypoalbuminemia, and hypertriglyceridemia.[140-142] Decrease in platelet count associated with an increase in transaminases, and a further increase in plasma bilirubin, should lead to strong suspicion of lipid toxicity.[143] Bone marrow aspirate, liver biopsy, and temporary suspension or decrease in lipid infusion should be discussed. Lipid infusion should be stopped until normalization of bilirubin and platelet count. In addition to removing or decreasing the lipids, treatment of fat overload syndrome consists of giving supportive care as indicated. Occasionally, parenteral steroids are used.

Possible deleterious effects of fat emulsions on pulmonary function, immune status, platelets, liver and pancreas, and kernicterus are briefly discussed below.

Fat and Pulmonary Function

Pulmonary vascular lipid deposition are more common in preterm infants who received intravenous fat emulsion and are correlated with the duration of lipid therapy, although some infants who never received intravenous fat emulsion also demonstrated lipid deposition.[144]

Intravenous fat emulsions may alter pulmonary function (decreased diffusion capacity, oxygenation, intrapulmonary shunting). These effects were believed to be related to the serum triglyceride level.[145-147] However, serum triglyceride values above 1500 mg/dL do not appear to decrease the carbon monoxide diffusing capacity in healthy adults.[103] It appears more likely that these changes in pediatric patients are because of the conversion of polyunsaturated fatty acids in the emulsions to prostaglandins, which then can cause vasodilatation or vasoconstriction.[147,148] In addition, peroxides, sometimes found in the fat emulsion,[149] promote increased prostaglandin levels.[150] The adverse effects appear to depend on the dose and rate of administration, presence of peroxides, and clinical state of the lungs.[145-147,149,150]

The review of the available data in preterm infants suggests that administration of intravenous fat emulsion at normal rates does not affect oxygenation.[87] Studies showing some adverse effects have usually used inappropriately rapid rates of infusion.[151-153] Observed decreases in transcutaneous pCO_2 may be related to decline in subcutaneous perfusion by local vasoconstriction and not systemic oxygenation.[150,154] In addition, there appears to be no adverse impact on the development of chronic lung disease and possibly a beneficial effect.[87,155]

Fat, Infection, and Immune Status

There is a controversy regarding the effect of intravenous fat emulsions on immune function.[156-159] Some studies show a beneficial effect, some no effect, and some an adverse effect.[156]

A study in adult and pediatric bone-marrow–transplant patients found no increase in the risk of bacteremia or fungemia in patients receiving intravenous fat emulsions.[160] In contrast, a retrospective study of preterm infants identified fat emulsion as a potentially contributing factor to the development of coagulase negative staphylococcal infection. However, in this study, there was no temporal relationship between lipid administration and infection.[161] Many of the effects of intravenous fat emulsions on immune function appear to be related to the generation of leukotrienes and other polyunsaturates from the emulsions. There also is evidence the LCFAs may alter cellular function by changing membrane fluidity.[158] Newer intravenous fat emulsions not yet available in the United States using olive oil or structured lipids may obviate some of these immune-related concerns.[162]

In conclusion, studies on pediatric patients and tissues have not revealed evidence suggesting an impairment of immune function by intravenous fat emulsions.[163-169]

Fat and Platelets

In rare cases, intravenous fat emulsion has been associated with thrombocytopenia. However, prospective and retrospective studies suggest that under normal circumstances they do not induce thrombocytopenia.[142,170] Of note, EFA deficiency itself is a cause of hematologic abnormalities.[171]

Liver and Pancreatic Disease

Liver or pancreatic diseases are not in themselves contraindications to the use of intravenous fat emulsion.

Fat Emulsion and Kernicterus in Neonates

Fat emulsion increases the risk of kernicterus in neonates with jaundice because hydrolysis of lipids increases plasma levels of free fatty acids, which compete with bilirubin for albumin-binding sites, therefore displacing non-conjugated bilirubin from albumin. The American Academy of Pediatrics (AAP) recommends that infants with bilirubin levels of 8 to 10 mg/dL, assuming an albumin concentration of 2.5 to 3.0 g/dL, should receive the amount of fat emulsion required to prevent EFA deficiency (0.5 g/kg/day of fat emulsions).[172]

Carbohydrates

Historically, galactose, sorbitol, fructose, glucose, glycerol, and ethanol all have been used as sources of carbohydrate in infants. The small amount of glycerol present in lipid emulsions contributes to carbohydrate calories. The other carbohydrate sources have no advantage over glucose and can produce serious side effects. D-glucose for intravenous use is currently the unique carbohydrate used during PN. It is provided in the monohydrate form, reducing its caloric yield to 3.4 kcal/g, rather than the 4 kcal/g of enteral glucose. Glucose provides most of the osmolality in the PN solution; glucose concentrations in peripheral PN should be limited to 10% in children and 12.5% in newborn. There is no limit to glucose concentration in solutions to be infused in central veins. The carbohydrate load is initiated in a stepwise fashion to allow an appropriate response of endogenous insulin. The consequences of acute intolerance to glucose are serum hyperosmolarity, hyperglycemia, glucosuria, and osmotic diuresis, which can be avoided by careful monitoring. Hypoglycemia is usually related to the sudden cessation of the PN solution. A newly occurring hyperglycemia or a glucosuria in a previously stable patient receiving PN may be the first sign of a metabolic stress or sepsis.

Optimal Glucose Intake

Few data are available for establishing the optimal (minimum and maximal) glucose intake for children receiving PN and thus avoiding under- or overfeeding from glucose. Estimates of glucose utilization by the brain vary with age and are shown in Table 37-9.[173] These estimates reflect the minimum amount of exogenous glucose that must be provided to prevent hypoglycemia under most circumstances, even if gluconeogenesis may provide a significant amount of this glucose endogenously (even in preterm infants).[174,175] In addition, this amount of exogenous glucose is sufficient to minimize nitrogen loss.[173]

If there is a minimum amount of glucose that must be provided to prevent hypoglycemia, there is also a maximum that may lead to deleterious effects including the production of excessive CO_2 and hepatic steatosis. The rate of parenteral glucose should not exceed the maximal rate of glucose oxidation. This maximal rate varies considerably from infant to infant according to age and clinical status. On average, it does not exceed 6 to 7 mg/kg/minute (9.5 g/kg/day) in preterm 1000- to 2000-g infants.[176] In term surgical infants, or stable short-term or long-term PN (1- to 50-month-old) children, the maximal rate of glucose oxidation is approximately 12.5 mg/kg/minute (18 g/kg/day).[177-179] Stable adult patients on long-term PN have a maximal rate much lower than children and infants.[52,54] Clinical status can modify glucose oxidative capacity significantly. Stressed children decrease their maximal rate of glucose oxidation. For instance, in critically burned children, it is 5 mg/kg/minute (7.2 g/kg/day).[180] Therefore, glucose intake has to be adapted to age, clinical situations (prematurity, severe malnutrition, sepsis, critical illnesses), use of drugs (somatostatin, steroids, tacrolimus), expected weight gain for normal or catch-up growth, oral or enteral intake, and individual variations. Table 37-10 shows recommended initial glucose intake in stable infants and children and a stepwise increase until reaching the goal (in the absence of glucosuria or hyperglycemia).

TABLE 37-9.

Estimates of Glucose Consumption by the Brain

	Utilization	
Age	**(mg. Kg^{-1} .min^{-1})**	**(g. Kg^{-1}. d^{-1})**
Newborn	8.0	11.5
1 year	7.0	10.1
5 years	4.7	6.8
Adolescent	1.9	2.7
Adult	1.0	1.4

TABLE 37-10.

Suggestive Range of Parenteral Glucose Intake for Stable Infants and Children*

Glucose (g/kg/day)	Day 1	Day 2	Day 3	Day 4 and 5
Infant <10 kg	8	12	14	16 to 18
Child <15 kg	6	8	10	12 to 14
15 to 20 kg	4	6	8	10 to 12
20 to 30 kg	4	6	8	<12
> 30 kg	3	5	7	<10

*Rate of advancement may be limited by glucose tolerance (hyperglycemia, glucosuria).

Consequences of Excessive Glucose Administration

When glucose is administered in excess of the amount that can be directly oxidized for energy production and glycogen production, the excess is directed to fat synthesis (lipogenesis)[52,178-180] and promotes fat deposition, which may be a nutritional goal in specific clinical situations (eg, preterm infants). This conversion of glucose to fat is inefficient and probably accounts, in part, for the increase in energy expenditure seen with high rates of glucose infusion.[52] In addition, lipogenesis from glucose results in a large increase CO_2 production relative to O_2 consumption (ie, high respiratory quotient). The greater the proportion of glucose in the PN energy mix, the larger the increase in CO_2 production and minute ventilation.[178,179,181-185] Malnourished patients are least and hypermetabolic individuals are most susceptible. A more important factor with an impact on CO_2 production is total energy intake. There is a linear relationship between energy intake and CO_2 production and increased minute ventilation.[186,187] The greater the total energy intake, the greater the effect will be. Under normal circumstances, the increased CO_2 production is handled easily by increasing the respiratory rate and/or depth. Problems potentially arise in patients with respiratory compromise. In selected patient groups, giving glucose in amounts above the maximal oxidative rate may be appropriate (eg, preterm infants who need to deposit fat). However, the greater the amount of glucose, the greater the risk of adverse consequences.

Excessive glucose administration can affect liver function and induce steatosis, although its contribution to the development of cholestasis in humans is unclear.[188,189] Hepatic steatosis results when export of the very low density lipoprotein (VLDL) triglycerides does not keep pace with the increased de novo synthesis of the VLDL triglycerides, primarily because of stimulation of the secretion of preformed fatty acids by high carbohydrate and prolonged hyperinsulinemia.[184,190] Recent data suggest that the increase in infectious complications related to PN may be partially explained as overfeeding with glucose.[191] Hyperglycemia is a known risk factor for infection.[192,193]

Recently, hyperglycemia was associated with an increased risk of infection in children with burns.[194] Whether this effect is related to overfeeding with glucose (without hyperglycemia) or to hyperglycemia per se requires further investigations.[195] Finally, in critically ill patients, glucose intakes above the maximal glucose oxidation rate are unlikely to enhance energy balance or even reduce protein catabolism.[173]

Glucose as the sole calorie source leads to greater water retention than it does when combined with lipids.[196]

In summary, a balanced PN solution, including carbohydrate and fat (as non-nitrogen calories) may avoid 1) fatty infiltration of the liver, 2) water retention, 3) worsening respiratory compromise in acutely ill ventilator-dependent patients, and 4) may decrease the risk of PN-related infections. Insulin should not be routinely added to the solution because of unpredictable responses in infants. In newborns, there have been numerous studies showing that continuous insulin administration helps control plasma glucose concentration, achieve increased caloric intake, and promote nitrogen retention and growth. However, there is need for more data on its safety and long-term consequences as a growth-promoting agent.[197-201] For instance, suppression of muscle proteolysis by insulin may not be desirable, as the glutamine released from the muscle is an important substrate for intestinal epithelial cells and the immune system. In addition, it is not known whether increased glucose utilization deprives the brain of this important substrate and whether increased glucose taken up by the cells will be efficiently oxidized or converted to fat.

In practice, 6 g/kg/day (4 to 5 mg/kg/minute) of intravenous glucose are started on the first day in VLBW infants (<1500 g). If this is tolerated, it may be increased progressively to 12 to 18 g/kg/day. If it is not tolerated, progression of glucose will be stopped and insulin perfusion will be considered according to clinical and nutritional status with an initial dose of 0.05 IU/kg/hour.[200] Recently, it has been proposed that high amino acid intake—2 to 3 g/kg/day from the first day—in addition to preventing catabolism and promoting anabolism may have several other beneficial effects, including decreased frequency and severity of neonatal hyperglycemia by stimulating endogenous insulin secretion and stimulating growth by enhancing the secretion of insulin and insulin-like growth factors.[202] In older children and adolescents, insulin may be required to improve caloric intake in the face of hyperglycemia. It is not recommended to add insulin to the bag but rather to deliver the insulin as a separate infusion that can be titrated according to serum glucose.

Electrolytes, Minerals, and Trace Elements

Most electrolyte needs can be adequately met by standard PN solution. Abnormalities due to supraphysiologic fluid losses should be treated with equal volumes of an IV fluid apart from the PN solutions. This is far less costly, makes better physiologic sense, and facilitates care. Deficiencies due to other causes should be first treated with IV piggyback infusions. Table 37-11 shows the range of recommended daily intake of electrolytes and minerals for PN solutions in children and infants.[203,204]

The failure to provide adequate calcium and phosphorus is critical in the development of nutrition-related bone disorders.[56,205-207]

Continuous infusion of calcium in PN solutions is preferable to bolus administration. Calcium and phosphorus should not be given independently, as administrating one without the other leads to renal wasting of the infused mineral.[208] The use of alternate PN infusions of calcium and phosphorus to increase the delivery of these minerals while avoiding calcium-phosphorus precipitation in the solutions results in lower calcium and phosphorus retention (42% to 63%),[208-210] compared to the rates attained when these minerals are infused simultaneously (83% to 97%).[208,211,213] In addition, hypercalcemia and hypophosphatemia may occur during high calcium infusion, whereas hyperphosphatemia and hypocalcemia may occur during high phosphorus infusion.[208]

There are no documented major complications associated with the currently recommended higher calcium and phosphorus intake for premature infants receiving PN. Higher parenteral intake of these two nutrients, similar to the recommended intake of 12.5 to 15 mmol/L (500 to 600 mg/L) of calcium and 13 to 14.5 mmol/L (400 to 450 mg/L) of phosphorus[214] delivered at 120-150 mL/kg/day (see Table 38-11), are reported to result in stable normal serum concentrations of calcium, phosphorus, parathyroid hormone, calcitonin, vitamin D metabolites (25-hydroxy vitamin D and 1,25-dihydroxy vitamin D), and normal renal tubular reabsorption of phosphate.[205,215] Additional data supporting the use of these levels of calcium and phosphorus content of PN solutions include several balance studies demonstrating a mean fractional retention of 88% to 94% for calcium and 83% to 97% for phosphorus in clinically stable infants receiving 1.45 to 1.9 mmol/kg/day (58 to 76 mg/kg/day) calcium and 1.23 to 1.74 mmol/kg/day (38 to 54 mg/kg/day) phosphorus from PN.[211-213] With these solution 60% to 70% of the in utero accretion of these two nutrients can be achieved.

Calcium and Phosphorus Solubility

Precipitation of calcium and phosphate in PN solutions has been a continual problem. It is particularly prevalent in solutions for neonates because their calcium and phosphate needs are high, yet fluid requirements are restricted and amino acid concentrations are low.[63,230] To minimize the risk of precipitation, recommendations for calcium and phosphorus intake are based on concentration per liter of solution rather than in amount per kilogram. Of note, calcium and phosphorus requirements in some preterm infants may exceed the solubility of these two elements in the PN solutions. This typically occurs during fluid restriction when the ideal amount of calcium and phosphorus cannot be provided. Factors that enhance precipitate formation include high calcium and phosphate concentrations, decreased amino acid concentration, increased environmental temperature, higher pH amino acid mixture and of the PN solution, and prolonged hanging time.[217-221] Increasing the amount of amino acid, adding cysteine, and lowering the pH of the solution allows higher amounts of calcium and phosphorus to be added to the PN solution without precipitation. Maximal calcium and phosphorus concentrations in PN solutions in neonatal solutions with or without cysteine have been published[63,222] and Tables 37-12 and 37-13 give general guidelines. Because of the individual nature of formulations and mixing techniques, these tables should not be used in lieu of the pharmacist verification for incompatibilities. For instance, administration of intravenous fat emulsions into the same catheter may reduce solubility by 10% to 20%. Addition of acetate without the addition of cysteine also may reduce solubility by 5% to 10%.[221]

Calcium gluconate is traditionally used instead of calcium chloride in parenteral fluids because it is far less likely than calcium chloride to react with phosphate. Calcium glycerophosphate has been shown to be more soluble than calcium gluconate plus phosphate.[223] Therefore, administering sufficient amounts of calcium and phosphorus in PN solutions is no longer a problem in countries where organic phosphate preparation is available. However, limited information exists on the use of alternate sources of inorganic[212,224] and organic salts[225-228] of calcium and phosphorus in PN solutions and on bone mineralization[229] in infants receiving what appears to be adequate calcium and phosphorus.

The titratable acidity of the PN solution offers a protective effect on calcium phosphate compatibility. The higher the concentration of amino acids, the lower the pH and

Table 37-11.

Daily Intravenous Electrolyte Requirements in Patients With Adequate Renal Function

	Adolescents	*Children*	*Infants*	*Preterm Infants****	
	mMol/24 Hr	mMol/kg/24 hr	mMol/kg/24 hr	mMol/kg/24 hr	mMol/L**
Sodium	60-150	2-4	2-4	2-3	
Potassium	70-180	2-4	2-3	2-3	
Chloride	60-150	2-4	2-4	2-3	
Calcium*	5-20	0.25-1.6	0.25-2.0	1.5-2.25	12.5-15.0
Phosphate	15-30	0.5 – 2.0	1-1.5	1.5-2.25	12.5-15.0
Magnesium	4-16	0.125-0.25	0.125-0.25	0.18-0.30	1.5-2.0

*The product obtained by multiplying the total number of mEq of calcium per liter by the total number of mEq of phosphate per liter must not exceed 200 to prevent precipitation of the calcium phosphate complex. Must include calcium and phosphate content of base solutions. Increased concentration of administration on the basis of fluid restriction may result in precipitation.

Based on an intake of 120-150 mL/kg/day. **Note: For Ca, Mg, and P, concentration-based (mmol/L), as per kg per day, recommendations should be used since alterations of fluid volumes by clinical circumstances (such as restriction) could inadvertently result in high mineral concentrations and precipitation of minerals. Ca and P could be adjusted accordingly to biochemical measurements within the range of 1:1 to 1,3:1 molar ratio or 1.3:1 by weight

***Newborn infants may not need sodium or chloride the first day of life. They may need potassium beyond the second day of life. Premature infants may require increased levels of sodium (4-7.5 mEq/kg) due to their inability to effectively reabsorb sodium

Conversion:

Ca 1 mmol = 2 mEq = 40 mg = 430.5 mg calcium gluconate (1 ml of a 10% solution provides 9.3 mg calcium element)
Mg 1 mmol = 2 mEq = 24 mg = 120.3 mg magnesium sulfate
P 1 mmol = 31 mg

Table 37-12.

Highest Compatible Concentration for Calcium and Phosphate in TrophAmine (storage 37°C for 24 hours)

1% TrophAmine 10% Dextrose		*2% TrophAmine 20% Dextrose*		*2% TrophAmine 20% Dextrose Cysteine**	
Phosphate (mmol/L)	Calcium (mEq/L)	Phosphate (mmol/L)	Calcium (mEq/L)	Phosphate (mmol/L)	Calcium (mEq/L)
25	5	50	5	70	14
20	5	40	6	55	15
15	9	30	6	45	18
12	10	25	7	31	25
10	15	20	9	21	30
9	40	15	10	18	40
7	50	13	15		
		11	20		
		9	35		
		9	60		

*50 mg cysteine HCl per gram protein.

TABLE 37-13.

Maximal Calcium and Phosphorus Concentrations in Parenteral Nutrition Solutions*

g/dL (%) Amino acids	Without Cysteine Calcium mEq/L	Without Cysteine Phosphorus mMol/L	With Cysteine Calcium mEq/L	With Cysteine Phosphorus mMol/L
1.0	50	12	50	23
	2	50	2	50
1.5	50	11	50	18
	5	50	12	50
2.0	50	12	50	25
	7	50	12	50
2.5	50	22	50	38
	6	50	28	50

*Presumes the base amino acid solution has a pH of <5.5.
(40 mg/g of amino acids)

the greater amount of calcium and phosphorus that can be admixed to the solution without precipitation.[217,218] Of note, the titratable acidity and pH of the commercially available amino acid solutions varies. In this regard, the pediatric amino acid mixtures (TrophAmine and Aminosyn), which have acidic pH to allow for the addition of adequate amounts of calcium and phosphorus, are of particular benefit.[211,220-222] Other additives normally used in clinical practice, such as magnesium, can influence the calcium phosphate reaction.[217] As the pH rises, the more soluble monobasic phosphate salt is converted to dibasic phosphate salt, which is available to bind calcium and precipitate. Acidification of the solution by adding cysteine hydrochloride can improve solubility. However, cysteine and other sulfate-containing amino acids have detrimental effects on calcium balance during PN.[229,230] Admixture of alkaline drugs, such as aminophylline, in a PN solution may result in calcium phosphate precipitation in solutions containing low amounts of amino acids.[231] The pH of the solution may also be increased by the addition of lipid emulsion.[218] However, pH changes in the solution because aminophylline or lipid emulsion are less appreciable as the amino acid concentration increases from 1% to 2%.[218,231] Of concern, the addition of sodium bicarbonate to acidic PN solutions has the potential for causing carbon dioxide formation, with loss of the bicarbonate ion and formation of insoluble calcium and magnesium carbonates.[232] As a result, most clinicians use acetate salts, which serve as precursors to bicarbonate. At room temperature, conventional dextrose-amino acid mixtures (eg, 25% dextrose and 4% to 5% amino acids) rarely pose an incompatibility problem if calcium gluconate concentrations are 5 mmol/L or less and phosphate concentrations are 30 mmol/L or less.[219] However, insoluble complexes may precipitate when the PN solution is warmed, as in infusing the solution into the patient.

VITAMINS

In 1979, the Nutrition Advisory Group of the Department of Food and Nutrition, American Medical Association (AMA) proposed adult and pediatric guidelines for parenteral multivitamins.[233] Since then, there has not been a recent significant evaluation or reformulation of parenteral vitamin products for premature infants, infants, or children (younger than 11 years of age).[233-235] The currently used intravenous pediatric multivitamin (MVI) preparations were designed to meet the needs of preterm and term infants and children.[236,237] Table 38-14 lists the vitamin requirements and composition of commonly available preparations. The specific recommendation from a 1988 review is to use one vial of MVI-pediatric per day for term-infants and children and 40% of a vial/kg/day for preterm infants.[236] Pediatric MVI should be used in children up to 10 to 11 years of age. Above that age, the adult formulation meets the needs of the older child more adequately. The adult formulations are not recommended for use in low-birthweight infants <1500 g because of concerns about the toxicity of the propylene glycol and polysorbate additives.[238,239] The adult formulation MVI 12 (AAIPharma) lacks vitamin K; however, it may be supplemented. In April 2000, the FDA amended the adult multivitamin formulation to bring it into accordance with the 1988 recommendations of the AMA FDA Public Workshop Committee.[240] Currently, InFuvite (Sabex, Inc, Boucherville, Canada) has the same formulation as MVI 12 (AAIPharma) except for additional 150 µg of vitamin K per vial. One potential problem with the introduction of vitamin K into the new adult formulation is its possible interference with anticoagulants, such as warfarin. Additionally, intravenous fat emulsions contain vitamin K in varying amounts (approximately 13 to 70 µg/dL) that can make titrating anticoagulant therapy even more problematic.[241,242]

A recent Cochrane review suggests that an increased vitamin A intake (via the intramuscular route) is beneficial in the preterm infant.[243] Whether dosing of vitamin A in PN will provide a similar benefit is unclear. Regardless, the current recommendation for vitamin A seems to be too low when administered in the glucose/amino acid solution[59,244-246] and therefore prudence suggests checking its level in pediatric patients receiving PN.

Vitamin deficiency has not been apparent in most individuals reported on PN. It is exceedingly uncommon and should not occur if the infants and children are provided with the appropriate supplementation.[247,248] The multiple

TABLE 37-14.

Daily Intravenous Vitamin Requirements, Recommendations, and Products

	Preterm (per kg)	*Term & Children >1 y*	*MVI PED*	*MVI 12* (5 ml)*
Vitamin A (retinol) (IU)	700 to 1500	2300	2300	3300
Vitamin D (IU)	40 to 160	400	400	200
Vitamin E (tocopherol) (IU)	3.5	7	7	10
Vitamin C (mg)	15 to 25	80	80	100
Folate (ug)	56	140	140	400
Niacin (mg)	4.0 to 6.8	17	17	40
Riboflavin (mg)	0.15 to 0.2	1.4	1.4	3.6
Thiamine (mg)	0.2 to 0.35	1.2	1.2	3
Vitamin B6 (mg)	0.15 to 0.2	1	1	4
Vitamin B12 (ug)	0.3	1	1	5
Pantothenic acid (mg)	1 to 2	5	5	15
Biotin (ug)	8	20	20	60
Vitamin K (mg)	0.3	0.2	0.2	__**

*Patient receiving MVI 12 (AAIPharma) should recieve 0.2 mg/day of vitamin K
**InFuvite (Sabex, Inc, Boucherville, Canada) has the same formulation as MVI 12 except for additional 0.150 mg vitamin K) per vial
Vitamin E: 1 mg = 1 IU; Vitamin A: 500 µg = 1643IU

vitamin preparations should be added to the PN solutions just before administration to minimize losses while the solution is hanging.

TRACE MINERALS

Ten trace minerals are nutritionally essential for humans: zinc, copper, selenium, molybdenum, chromium, manganese, iodine, iron, fluoride, and cobalt. When the patient is not receiving them enterally, they need to be provided by the PN. Trace mineral requirements and metabolism have been reviewed elsewhere.[236,249-251] Guidelines for intravenous administration of trace elements to pediatric patients are summarized in Table 37-15. The intake should be adjusted in cases of catabolic stress, such as infection or intestinal losses. Zinc, copper, and selenium need to be added to the PN, even for short-term PN. Deficiencies of trace minerals are discussed in Chapter 3.

Zinc has the widest range of functions of all the trace minerals and is particularly important in wound healing and immune function. Patients with GI losses due to diarrhea, ileostomies, or even nasogastric suction are at risk for zinc deficiency because of the high zinc content of GI fluids.[253] Zinc deficiency in parenterally fed patients should no longer occur, because zinc is routinely added to PN solutions. However, it is important to recognize that more than normal zinc supplementation is required in patients who have massive diarrhea and malabsorption, as these increase the zinc losses.[254,255] No studies have been done in pediatric patients with regard to the amount of additional zinc replacement that is required for these losses. From adult studies, we know that approximately 17 mg of zinc are lost per kilogram of stool or ileostomy output and 12 mg/kg of small bowel fluid lost via fistulas or stomas. Serum zinc levels, although not entirely reliable, are easily obtained and zinc intake can be titrated appropriately, Copper is essential in humans. Several cuproenzymes play critical metabolic roles, and their activities are generally depressed by copper deprivation. Acquired copper deficiency in infants was first described in 1964.[256] The cases had recurrent episodes of diarrhea and malnutrition. They were treated with cow milk, which is low in copper. During the early years of PN, it was thought that frequent plasma or blood transfusions provided the necessary trace minerals. Report of copper (and zinc) deficiencies in these infants demonstrated the inadequacy of this approach. The same syndrome occurs in pediatric patients receiving PN unsupplemented with copper. Experimentally, copper deficiency results in low lysyl oxidase activity and consequent failure of elastin and collagen cross-linking, resulting in vascular rupture and osteoporosis. Nowadays, with the current supplementation, copper deficiency is highly uncommon and rarely reported.[257,258] Copper should not be given to patient with cholestasis. The importance of selenium as an antioxidant is well known.[259,260] Selenium deficiency in pediatric patients receiving PN may be recognized both clinically and by certain suggestive laboratory tests. Erythrocyte macrocytosis, loss of pigmentation in the hair and skin, and muscle weakness are characteristic of the condition. Elevated transaminases and creatinine levels may also be found.[261] Intravenous supplementation with 2 µg/kg/day of selenium can totally reverse the signs and symptoms of selenium deficiency including the secondary myopathy within a period of 6 weeks.[262] Selenium should always be included as one of the trace metals necessary in patients with chronic diarrhea and large ostomy output. A recent report suggests that the current recommended intake of selenium for preterm infants may be low.[263] Furthermore, selenium renal homeostasis is impaired in patients receiving long-term PN.[264] It is prudent to check serum selenium levels and glutathione peroxidase activity.[253,260,263,265]

Molybdenum deficiency symptoms (tachycardia, tachypnea, vomiting, and central scotomas, with rapid progres-

TABLE 37-15.

Recommended Intravenous Intakes of Trace Elements

Element	Infants (μg/kg/day) Preterm	Term	Children (μg/kg/days) (maximum μg/day)
Zinc	400.00	250 <3 mo 100 >3 mo	50 to 200 (5000)
Copper*	20	20	20 (300)
Selenium +	2	2	2 (30)
Molybdenum (see text) +	0.25	0.25	0.25 (5)
Manganese*	1	1	1 (50)
Iodine (see text)	1	1	1 (1)
Chromium (see text) +	0.0 to -0.2	0.2	0.14 to 0.2
Iron >2 month (see text)	0.2 mg/kg	0.1 mg/kg	0.1 mg/kg

* Omit in patients with obstructive jaundice.
\+ Omit in patients with renal dysfunction.

sion to coma) have been reported in an adult on long-term PN but have not been studied in pediatric patients.[266,267]

Chromium, manganese, iodine, and fluoride are important; however, very often they are not added to PN solutions. Moukarzel and others[268] evaluated the chromium status of children on long-term PN receiving the standard recommendations. Elevated serum chromium levels and lower glomerular filtration rates (GFR) were noted.[269] The GFR were significantly inversely correlated with serum chromium concentration. After 1 year of PN without supplemental chromium, the mean serum chromium levels had fallen but were still higher than in controls. No change occurred in the GFR. Unplanned chromium contamination of the PN solutions still provided 0.05 μg/kg of chromium, which is one-fourth of the current recommendation. These data are consistent with other studies and imply that the addition of chromium to PN at recommended levels in combination with chromium contamination in the PN fluids raises serum chromium levels above that desired.[270-274] In 1990, this author discontinued chromium supplementation in all PN patients.[268,275]

Manganese often contaminates PN solution components in amounts sufficient for daily requirements.[249,252,257] Manganese intoxication causes Parkinsonian-like symptoms with muscular weakness, stiffness, tremors, ataxia, abnormal gait, asthenia, and difficulty with speech.[276] Manganese is a contributor to the development and the severity of PN-associated cholestasis and is excreted in bile.[277,278] Therefore, it is suggested that patients with any liver disease should not receive manganese in their PN.[249,252,276,278,279] Recent data suggests that manganese should not be given to individuals on PN for <30 days and that levels have to be monitored in patients receiving PN with manganese for >30 days.[252,279] This author uses whole blood manganese, red blood cell manganese, or manganese superoxide dismutase as measures of tissue deposition[276] as these correlate with MRI-documented manganese deposition.[279]

Iodine is not added to PN solutions because patients usually receive enough iodine from unavoidable contamination of PN.280 Typically, the iodine is provided in the water of PN plus as natural contaminants in many of the salts that are added to the solutions. Furthermore, if iodine antiseptic solutions are used to clean the site at which the catheter enters the body, this iodine may be absorbed through the skin and contribute to the normal iodine levels.[253,280]

Intravenous iron needs to be provided in pediatric patients who are unable to absorb it through the enteral route. Because iron is absorbed proximally in the duodenum and jejunum, a trial of an oral iron preparation should always be given first. Parenteral iron can be infused as an intermittent intravenous infusion or as a diluted total dose infusion. After a test dose, dilute forms of iron dextran have been added to PN solutions without any serious consequences. This author has seen no consequences with providing 0.5 to 1 mg of an iron dextran preparation daily despite the report of risk of anaphylaxis.[281] Despite its widespread use, total dose infusion is not approved by the FDA.[282-285] Two new iron products free of dextran have recently been approved in 1999 and 2000 for use in the United States: sodium ferric gluconate complex in sucrose (Ferrlecit; Watson, Inc., Morristown, NJ) and iron sucrose (Venofer; Luitpold Pharmaceuticals, Inc, Shirley, NY). Both products have been used extensively in Europe. These products appear to be safe and effective in children[286] and have fewer side effects than those of iron dextran, although, like iron dextran, they can cause hypotension.[287,288] To document that sufficient iron is being provided, serum iron, total iron binding capacity, and percent saturation should be followed. This should prevent secondary hemochromatosis.

There is a variety of other trace metals, but it is not clear whether they should be supplemented. These include fluoride[56,253] and cobalt (part of the cobalamin, vitamin B12). There is no question that other trace metals should be added to the PN solutions,[275,289] but a strong documentation is lacking.

Although PN solutions may be contaminated with small amounts of aluminum, they are not nearly as contaminated as they were in earlier years of PN.[290] In the past, the major source of aluminum contamination was casein hydrolysate; aluminum contributed to the impairment of bone matrix formation and mineralization.[291] With the use of crystalline amino acids, sterile water, and dextrose, the contamination of the solutions is relatively low. The calcium salts contribute up to 80% of the total aluminum load in the PN solutions.[56] Other substances commonly administered intravenously, including phosphorus salts and albumin, have high levels of aluminum. Premature infants may accumulate aluminum and show evidence of toxicity.[292] Studies haves documented development delay in premature infants receiving PN contaminated with 45 µg/kg/day.[293] The FDA has proposed labeling requirements concerning aluminum contents on PN additives, establishing an upper limit permitted in PN additives.[294] Aluminum intake should be determined in children at high risk for toxicity: preterm infants, patients receiving long-term PN, and patients with impaired renal function.

Formulating a Regimen, Monitoring, Advancing Parenteral Nutrition, and Transition to Enteral Nutrition or to Home Parenteral Nutrition

A complete laboratory assessment of the pediatric patient's electrolytes, acid-base status, calcium, phosphorus, magnesium, BUN, creatinine, and triglyceride levels should be performed. An assessment of the patient's nutritional status should be made to determine the child's caloric needs based on age, severity of illness, activity level, and degree of catch-up growth required. Next, the route of administration should be decided. If it is anticipated that the patient will need concentrated PN solution for more than 7 to 14 days, a central venous catheter should be placed.[295] Once, the patient's nutritional requirements and fluid needs are assessed, a PN solution is prescribed.

This initiation phase of PN lasts for 3 to 5 days in pediatric patients and up to 7 days in neonates <1.5 kg.[296] This phase is a time of gradual increase in glucose, fat, and amino acids and is determined by the patient's tolerance. The total daily protein requirement can begin on the first day unless hepatic or renal insufficiency is present, in which case the amount of protein given is titrated based on clinical parameters.

It is customary to start the intravenous lipid dose at 1.0 to 1.5 g/kg/day; if triglyceride levels remain low (see above for the acceptable level), lipids can be increased (see Table 37-8). It is usual to start the patient on 3 to 8 g/kg/day of glucose and increase this by 1 to 2 g/kg/day every day if there is no hyperglycemia or glucosuria until the goal of the PN regimen is reached (see Table 37-10). Initially, the monitoring of weight gain or loss, electrolytes, and fluid balance needs to be performed daily to assess the adequacy and appropriateness of the regimen, and adjustments must be made when necessary. A suggested monitoring is shown in Table 37-16.

An important psychosocial component of the pathway involves incorporating age or developmentally appropriate touch therapy.[296] Infants or children who are unable to eat should not miss the other benefits of feeding time, including holding, cuddling, and communicating. Nonnutritive sucking provides comfort and stimulates normal sucking and swallowing activities.[3] The family of the child will require emotional support and explanations of the various treatments (eg, oro-motor therapy to deal with avoiding feeding aversion) that are required for their child and information about what is developmentally appropriate. A handout is helpful for parents to review in non-technical language what PN is, how it is supplied, and what parents can do to help their child during PN therapy.

The maintenance phase begins when the targeted glucose, fat, and amino acid doses have been achieved. Table 37-17 indicates the typical ingredients of a PN solution. If long-term PN is anticipated, the infusion time is decreased. Schedules for chronic PN infusions vary from 24 hours a day to an 8-hour infusion. The majority of patients receive their PN at home over 10 to 12 hours while they sleep at night and then are disconnected from the PN source. Infusion times vary with the patient's individual PN formula, volume, nutrition needs, metabolic response, and personal preference. Cyclic PN is described below and has some advantages.[297]

The transition phase occurs when the pediatric patient progresses to oral or enteral feedings. There is a decrease in the frequency of laboratory monitoring during these two phases. Calorie counts may be necessary to assess patient's progress as he or she attempts to change modes of feeding. Most parents are concerned about when and what their child eats. Occupational therapists (who are experts in oro-motor therapy) should become involved with children having potential or actual feeding aversion. The discontinuation phase occurs when patients are able to absorb approximately 70% of their caloric needs via the GI tract. Some patients may be discharged from the hospital for PN at home.[204]

Monitoring laboratory work for each phase is shown in Table 37-16. Monitoring the weight at baseline, daily, and then every month is important, as are monitoring the pediatric patient's height or length, head circumference, and arm anthropometrics at baseline and monthly.

PN solutions are ordered daily on a preprinted sheet. A dosing protocol approved by the medical staff allows the pharmacist to adjust PN constituents within recommended limits on concentration and formulation stability.

Parenteral Nutrition Admixtures

Total nutrient admixtures (TNA), also called Three-in-One solutions, or All-in-One solutions, make use of the fact that under certain conditions the glucose amino acid solution may be mixed with intravenous fat emulsion and administered to the patient in one bag.[298] Their major advantages are easier administration (only one infusion pump is required), decreased cost and nursing time, decreased pharmacist preparation time, increased compliance of administering fat emulsion in the home patient population, and reduced risk of bacterial growth in intravenous fat emulsion even after 24 hours.[299]

TABLE 37-16.

Parenteral Nutrition Monitoring Schedule

Laboratory Studies	*Initial Period*	*Later Period*
Glucosuria	Daily	Daily
Glycemia	*	Weekly
BUN	3 times/week	Weekly
Hematocrit	Weekly	Weekly
Complete blood count	Baseline	As indicated
Reticulocyte count	Baseline	As indicated
Serum electrolytes and CO_2	3 times/week	Weekly
Triglycerides	4 hrs after an Increase In dose	Weekly
Cholesterol	Weekly	Weekly
Minerals (Ca, Mg, P)	3 times/week	Weekly
Total protein, albumin, prealbumin, transferrin	Weekly	Weekly
Liver function tests (ALT, GGTP, ALPH)	Weekly	Weekly
Iron studies (TIBC, ferritin, % saturation)	Baseline	Monthly
Vitamins (A, E, 25-OH D, PT/PTT)	Baseline	3 months
Trace elements (Se, Zn, Cu, Mn)	Baseline	3 months
Clinical observation (temperature, activity...)	Daily	Daily
Culture	As indicated	As indicated

*Blood glucose should be monitored closely during a period of glucosuria and for 2 to 3 days after cessation of PN to determine the degree of hypoglycemia. Frequent fingertip venous blood glucose constitutes adequate screening.

ALT = alanine transferase, GGTP = gamma-glutamyltranspeptidase, ALP = alkaline phosphatase, TIBC = total binding iron capacity, PT = prothrombin time, PTT = partial thromboplastin time.

TABLE 37-17.

Typical Infant/Child Total Parenteral Nutrition With Vitamin Ingredients

	*Final Concentrations**	
	Infants	*Children*
Neonatal amino acids	2%	
Balanced amino acids		3.5 to 4.25
Dextrose**	10% to 25%	10% to 25%
Sodium	30 mEq/L	35 mEq/L
Potassium	25 mEq/L	30 mEq/L
Calcium	10 mEq/L	5 mEq/L
Magnesium	10 mEq/L	10 mEq/L
Phosphate	7.5 mmol/L	10 mmol/L
Chloride	30 mEq/L	35 mEq/L
Acetate	27 mEq/L	64 mEq/L
Zinc	2 mg/L	2 mg/L
Copper	1 mg/L	1 mg/L
Selenium	20 μg/L	20 μg/L

*One vial (5 ml) of pediatric MVI is added per day for infants less than 11 years, and one vial of adult MVI is added daily for children older than 11 years.
**Higher concentrations may be used if there is reason to restrict fluid volume. D30 and D35 may be used.

Recently, a bag has been developed that allows the solution to be made with the three components (amino acids, glucose, fat) stored in separate compartments separated by inner seals (Kabiven Multichamber Parenteral Nutrition Packaging System, Fresenius Kabi, Uppsala, Sweden). The bag and components can be stored up to 24 months with the seals between the chambers intact. Seals are opened just before use. The egg yolk phospholipids in the fat emulsion act as the emulsifier and make the solution stable. Other factors affecting solution stability include amino acid, dextrose, calcium, magnesium and iron concentrations, order of addition of PN components, and pH.

The disadvantage of TNA solutions is that the PN components can precipitate and, because TNAs are cloudy, any precipitate needs to be 50 μm or larger to be seen with the naked eye. Particulate matter (mobile, undissolved substances that are unintentionally present in products) can be life threatening, and deaths have been reported presumably because of precipitation of calcium and phosphorus in admixtures.[300,301] The use of appropriate (1.2 or 5 μm) in-line filters can help decrease this complication.

A number of questions remain about PN admixtures for adults as well as pediatric patients. These include the appropriate dosing of some vitamins, the true risks related to particulate matter and fat droplet size, and drug compatibilities. For example, there is less loss of fat-soluble vitamins such as vitamin A than in traditional (two-in-one) PN because the intravenous fat emulsion is protective.[247] Some drugs are compatible with PN admixtures but not with traditional PN and vice versa.[302] PN admixtures should be used in stable patients only.

Cycling Parenteral Nutrition

"Cycling" PN refers to the administration of fluid intermittently with regular breaks from infusion.[297] Initially, a patient is established on a 24-hour infusion. Once the maximal concentration of dextrose solution and the maximal amount of fat to be used are reached, the number of hours of support is decreased by 1 to 2 hours per day. The rate of administration is increased, but the volume administered remains constant. Gradually, over a period of 7 days, the number of hours of infusion is decreased to 10 to 14 hours per day.

The younger the infant, the more hours the infusion is allowed to run.[204] The hyperinsulinemic response prevents hyperglycemia even at a rate of glucose infusion as high as 1.4 g/kg/hour. In school-age children, most infusions are given during a 10-hour infusion period so the patient has a maximal amount of time to be free of attachment to an infusion system. At the end of the infusion, the rate of administration is reduced twice by 50% over a period of 30 minutes. Occasionally, patients may require the infusion rate to be reduced by 25% every 15 minutes over 1 hour to reduce the risk of hypoglycemia.

At completion of the PN infusion, the catheter is flushed with 3 mL of 100 units/mL heparin and then capped with a sterile male Luer lock cap. In infants and small children, the heparin dose is adjusted to 50 units/kg body weight and then diluted with saline to a final volume of 3 mL to prevent over heparinization. At the initiation of the infusion, a similar gradual increase of the rate is needed to avoid hyperglycemia.[295]

In addition to adequacy for home parenteral nutrition and physical and psychological benefit, potential advantages of cyclic PN include improvement in protein synthesis, prevention of liver disease, and achievement of insulin glucagon balance.[303-305] Cycling PN is well tolerated and may be used from 3 to 6 months of age. Guidelines for cycling in infants >6 months of age has been described.[306] Details are provided in Table 37-18.

Complications of Parenteral Nutrition

Complications of PN are fewer when PN protocols are administered by a team with substantial experience and familiar with the techniques. The three types of complications that can occur are infectious, technical, and metabolic (Table 37-19). A detailed review of the complications of PN is presented in Chapter 38; however, pediatric-specific details are included below.

Infectious and Technical Problems

Despite the widespread use of PN, infectious complications are the most frequent PN-related problem; these complications result in increased morbidity, mortality, and healthcare costs. Sepsis rates vary and depend on the definition, methodology, and institution. PN infections are always caused by some known or unsuspected break in technique.

With each fever, a careful examination and a history of the pediatric patient is taken to determine if there is a known cause for the fever. If there is no recognizable source, the most likely possibility is either a catheter infection or a viral infection. The patient has both central line and peripheral blood cultures conducted for aerobes, anaerobes, and fungi. A complete blood count with differential, urinalysis, and chest x-ray are also done. Other tests depend on the clinical findings and suspicions of the examining physician.[307]

If a specific source of infection is identified, the patient should be treated appropriately. Because most patients receiving PN cannot effectively absorb oral antibiotics, the drugs are usually given intravenously.[308] If no obvious source of infection is found, intravenous antibiotic coverage may be started to treat the suspected infection in the central catheter. Vancomycin is usually the initial therapy of choice in suspected catheter infection.[307] Typically, gentamicin is added to the initial regime, pending final culture report and sensitivities. Catheter infections in PN patients are usually treated with intravenous antibiotics for 4 weeks. Removal of tunneled catheters or implantable catheter systems is avoided when there is a long-term need for vascular access for PN.

Intravenous antibiotics are most effective in cases of gram-positive bacteria, but success in gram negative is possible. The most common cause of infection is gram-positive bacteria (including oxacillin resistant coagulase negative staphylococci), followed by gram-negative bacteria, fungi, and mycobacteria. Standards for catheter removal, discussed in Chapter 38, are consistent for adult and pediatric patients.

TABLE 37-18.

Guidelines for Cycling From Use of Cyclic Parenteral Nutrition in Infants Less Than 6 Months of Age

Criteria for Initiating

- Need for continued PN support longer than 2 weeks
- Stable metabolic and hemodynamic status
- Consistent weight gain and growth
- Central venous access

Procedure/Monitoring

Taper off by decreasing the hourly rate by one half for 30 to 60 min, then decrease the hourly rate by one fourth for 30 min
- Inject a heparin solution of 10 U/mL into central lines (heparin-lock)
- Taper on by starting with one half the hourly rate for 30 to 60 min
  - For example: Initial rate; 15mL/hx24 h
  - Taper off: 7mL/hx30min, 3mL/hx30min, then discontinue
  - 2 h off
  - Taper on: 8mL/hx30min
  - New hourly infusion rate: 17mL/h x 20.5 h
  - Taper off: 8mL/h x 30min, 4mL/h x 30 min, then discontinue 4 h off
  - Taper on: 9mL/h x 30min
  - New hourly infusion rate: 19mL/h x 18.5 h

Cycle off PN at the time of line changes/new PN hanging or as convenient for parental (caregiver) schedule
Check capillary glucose concentration 30 to 60 min after capping line and halfway through time off PN until on stable schedule
Check urine dip sticks every void initially, then once per shift when on stable schedule

Criteria for Advancing Hours off PN

Begin with 1 to 2 h off depending on age, amount of enteral feedings, and medications
Increase by 1 to 2 h off every day or as tolerated
If capillary glucose concentration or urine dip stick is abnormal, then do not advance time off
If abnormal glucose or urine parameters continue at a certain amount of time off, then return to previous schedule or change taper-off schedule.
Limit to 4 to 6 h off for those without enteral feedings

TABLE 37-19.

Complications of Parenteral Nutrition

Infectious

Infections: Systemic or local (tunnel infection)
Sepsis

Metabolic

Electrolyte, mineral, and acid base abnormalities:
- Hypo-/Hypernatremia
- Hypo-/Hyperkalemia
- Hypo-/Hypercalcemia
- Hypo-/Hyperphosphatemia
- Hypo-/Hypermagnesemia
- Acidosis/Alkalosis

Hydration-related
- Dehydrated/fluid overload

Carbohydrate-related complications
- Hypo-/Hyperglycemia
- Overfeeding

Protein-related complications
- Hyperammonemia
- Uremia

Lipid-related complications:
- Hypertriglyceridemia
- Hypercholesterolemia
- Essential fatty acid deficiency
- Fat overload syndrome

Refeeding syndrome
Liver disease
- Metabolic bone disease

Renal disease (decreased glomerular filtration rate)
Altered visual function

In the stable children receiving long-term PN at home, the typical catheter remains in place for more than 700 days.[307] Recent data clearly confirm that critically ill children are at increased risk for bloodstream infections, especially those associated with intravascular device placement. According to the Centers for Disease Control and Prevention (CDC), between 1995 and 2000, the mean associated bloodstream infection rate for patients in pediatric intensive care units was 7.7/1000 catheter days.[309] The rate of bloodstream infections was higher among children whose birthweight was <1000 g and those who had umbilical catheters.[327] Other risk factors include the presence of multiple venous catheters or arterial catheters,[310] the number of central catheter days, and interventions such as central venous catheter placement, arterial catheter placement, and PN administration.[312]

New guidelines[313] for the prevention of intravascular catheter-related infections have been developed recently by the AAP, CDC, and other organizations to replace the 1996 guidelines for prevention of intravascular device-related infections published.[314] In this new set of recommendations, there are special considerations intended to prevent these infections in children. These guidelines emphasized: 1) educating and training healthcare providers who insert and maintain catheters; 2) using maximal sterile barrier precautions during central venous catheter insertion; 3) using a 2% chlorhexidine preparation for skin antisepsis; 4) avoiding routine replacement of central venous catheters as a strategy to prevent infection; and 5) using antiseptic- and antibiotic-impregnated short-term central venous catheters if the rate of infection is high despite adherence to other strategies (ie, education and training, maximal sterile barrier precautions, and 2% chlorhexidine for skin antisepsis). In addition, the document provides recommendations related to specific types of catheters, including peripheral venous catheters, central venous catheters, peripheral arterial catheters, pressure monitoring devices, and umbilical catheters.

Catheter occlusion may be caused by a clot or thrombus, fat deposition, calcium-phosphorus precipitation, or drug precipitation (Table 37-20). There are different protocols to deal with each type of occlusion. Infusion 70% ethanol for fat deposition, 0.1 N hydrochloric acid for calcium-phosphorus precipitation, and 0.1 N HCl or 0.1 N NaOH for medication precipitates.[315] Urokinase was widely used to treat catheter thrombosis before its removal from the market because of its significant contamination with infectious agent. Currently, Alteplase (t-PA) is used instead; it is effective and well tolerated.[317] Prophylactic warfarin therapy in adults may be of some benefit.[318,319]

Metabolic Problems

Electrolyte and mineral abnormalities, acid-base disorders, glucose disturbances, and fluid imbalances should be prevented by careful monitoring. It is important to keep PN infusion rate constant and perform cyclic PN while carefully monitoring the glucose homeostasis. Iatrogenic hypermagnesemia in two premature infants receiving PN has been reported.[320] In both cases, the clinical consequences mimicked profound septic shock, but cultures were negative and plasma magnesium levels were in excess of 20 mmol/L. The problem arose through malfunction of an automated PN mixing device. Its catastrophic consequences send an important message to all who regularly treat hypomagnesemia, because there has been a perception that apart from transient symptoms from vasodilatation, the infusion of magnesium is a reliably safe intervention. Overfeeding from an excessive amount of glucose or calories is best prevented by measuring the energy expenditure, as stated above. Protein-related complications are avoided by: 1) choosing the correct quantity and quality of amino acid (amino acid formulation), 2) making sure to give the protein by the enteral rather than the parenteral route when possible, and 3) monitoring BUN and, when indicated, ammonemia (see Table 37-16).

Lipid and Platelets

The complications related to the intravenous fat emulsions have been discussed previously in this chapter. These include hypertriglyceridemia, hypercholesterolemia, EFA deficiency, and fat overload syndromes. Additional information has been reviewed.[157,162]

Refeeding Syndrome

The refeeding syndrome is a potentially lethal condition associated with metabolic, cardiopulmonary, and neurologic complications (hypophosphatemia, hypokalemia, hypoglycemia, hypomagnesemia, hypocalcemia, and sometimes thiamine deficiency) seen in severely malnourished patients undergoing renutrition orally, enterally, or parenterally.[321] During starvation, the catabolism of fat and muscle occurs, resulting in loss of lean body mass, minerals, and water with preservation of serum levels.[322] During the reinstitution of nutrition, especially with a carbohydrate-rich regimen, insulin is released, causing increased intracellular uptake of glucose, phosphorus, and other nutrients. A severe hypophosphatemia may occur, which results in cardiac decompensation, neurologic dysfunction, and red cell and white cell dysfunction.[323]

At-risk patients include those with anorexia nervosa, kwashiorkor, marasmus, morbid obesity with massive weight loss, prolonged fasting, and chronic malnutrition. In at-risk patients—pediatric and adult—the most important measure in the prevention of refeeding syndrome is the adequate provision of phosphorus, magnesium, and potassium. Twice the recommended dose of phosphorus is a reasonable starting point.[324] Usually the risk for clinically significant declines in these minerals lasts for 7 to 10 days after the patient becomes anabolic. During this period, it is important to follow serum phosphorus, potassium, and magnesium closely (every other day or more often) as well as weight change, fluid, and electrolyte balance, cardiovascular condition, caloric intake, and the patient's clinical condition. Caloric intake should be slowly increased only if serum levels of these nutrients are normal. After this time, supplementation can gradually be reduced.[325]

The refeeding syndrome is discussed in detail in Chapter 45.

Cholelithiasis, Cholecystitis, and Chronic Liver Disease

The chance of developing gallbladder sludge because of PN is almost 100% after patients have been receiving PN for 6 full weeks. Any patient who receives PN for more then 30 days and develops abdominal pain should

TABLE 37-20.
Mechanical Complications of Central Venous Access Device

Complications following the placement of the catheter:
Air embolism
Pneumothorax
Hemothorax
Hydrothorax
Perforation of an organ
Malposition: arrhythmias, cardiac tamponade, brachial nerve injury
Extravasation
Thrombosis at vascular access
Early diagnosis and treatment essential
Echocardiography for early detection
Prophylactic warfarin therapy in adults may be of benefit
Crack, breakage, or aneurysm of catheter
Broken catheter requiring repair (use special repair kit)
Catheter occlusion or slow infusion by blood clot
Clear blockage with urokinase or Alteplase (t-PA)
Drug precipitate occlusion
Clear blockage with HCl

be evaluated for cholecystitis. It is possible that stimulating the gallbladder by more frequent feeding would reduce the incidence of biliary sludge and stones.[295] This is discussed in greater detail in Chapter 38.

The pathogeny of liver disease in PN is not well known.[326] Many factors contribute to the PN-associated cholestasis,[327] and these are presented in Chapter 38.[327] A preliminary study in adults suggested that steatosis could be reversed with intravenous choline supplementation.[329] These results encourage similar studies in children and infants, especially that choline pharmacokinetics during choline infusion in humans receiving PN are known[330] and that plasma choline levels in normal newborns, infants, toddlers, and in VLBW neonates requiring PN have been published.[331] The incidence of PN-induced liver disease occurs less frequently because of a change in most protocols in initiating enteral nutrition sooner (even as little as 1 to 5 mL per feed in the preterm neonate) and because of the use of a balanced amino acid solution specifically designed for infants, which reduces the toxicity occurring with pediatric use of adult formulations.[204,332] Despite that, amino acids still contribute to the development of PN-associated cholestasis.[333-335] It has been shown that in the VLBW infant, provision of protein enterally while other nutrients (primarily carbohydrate) are provided intravenously can lessen the severity or reduce the risk of PN-associated cholestasis.[333] In infants and children at risk for cholestasis, consideration as much as possible of enteral rather than parenteral administration of protein is helpful.[336] In addition, the stimulation of the entero-biliary axis by ingestion of LCT or breast milk or by injection of cholecystokinin analogs may reduce the cholestasis.[337] The reduction of intraluminal bacterial overgrowth caused by intestinal stasis by giving metronidazole or performing tapering enteroplasty (in short bowel syndrome) has been found to limit or reverse liver disease.[338] The treatment with 10 to 20 mg/kg/day of ursodeoxycholic acid or taurodeoxycholic acid could decrease liver injury.[339,340] Suggestions to adjust PN to limit liver injury are shown in Table 37-21.

Monitoring patients for evidence of early cholestasis can be done by measuring the alkaline phosphatase, gamma glutamyl transferase activities (GGT), 5′-nucleotidase, ALT, and serum direct bilirubin. When cholestasis occurs, infection, drug toxicity, or biliary obstruction should be investigated.[341] The association of thrombocytopenia with cholestasis may suggest fat overload syndrome. Baseline and repeat ultrasound examinations of gallbladder for sludge may be appropriate for long-term PN in the pediatric patient.

Bone Disease

Osteopenia is a characteristic of patients who receive long-term PN and is multifactorial[206] (Table 37-22). It is usually not associated with clinical symptoms. Chapter 38 discusses this complication in detail. In addition to aluminum toxicity,[342,343] inadequate provision of calcium and phosphorus,[214,229,344-347] hypercalciuria,[205,209,213,216,222,249,259,343] excess vitamin D or disorder in its metabolites,[348,349] and deficiency in zinc[350] or copper,[351] a number of factors have been considered that may contribute to the decreased mineralization. Deficiencies in manganese, fluoride,[352] boron,[353] and silicone[354] have been hypothesized as potential factors. Serum silicone levels in children receiving long-term PN were 50% lower than those in non-PN controls.[354] Furthermore, the significant correlation between silicone intake and degree of demineralization in these children suggests an involvement of silicone in the pathogenesis of the bone disease.[354] In addition, other potential agents have been hypothesized including chronic use of heparin, excess vitamin A, and deficiency of vitamin C, and toxins such as cadmium and strontium.[56,206]

TABLE 37-21.

Suggestions in Ordering PN to Limit Liver Injury

Using the new pediatric and neonatal-adapted amino acid solutions, which provide appropriate amount of amino acid and taurine.
Limiting glucose intake to reduce hepatic steatosis.
Using appropriate amount (and type if available) of IV fat emulsions, which provide EFA, reduce glucose load and limit per oxidation.
Decreasing or stopping lipid supply as soon as thrombopenia, hyperbilirubinemia appear.
Performing cyclic PN, which helps to reduce hyperinsulinism and steatosis
Adapting iron intake and decreasing aluminum content of PN solutions.

Prevention of this bone disease include providing adequate amount of calcium, phosphorus, magnesium, zinc, copper, nitrogen, and vitamin D; decreasing aluminum intake; decreasing supplies of amino acid, especially sulfur containing amino acid;[56,229,346] and monitoring urinary calcium, which should not exceed 5 mg/kg/day. The monitoring should include alkaline phosphatase, calciuria, and measurement of bone mineral content (DEXA scan or other methods). DEXA and other body mass composition procedures are discussed in Chapter 2.

Renal Disease

Glomerular filtration rate may be reduced in children receiving long-term PN.[355] No nephrocalcinosis or tubular dysfunction was identified in the group of patients that this author studied.[356] The decrease in glomerular filtration rate was not related to the underlying disease, infectious episodes, nephrotoxic drugs used, or the excessive urinary oxalate excretion that may occur in long-term PN patients (with or without ileostomy).[357] Although high amino acid intake has been implicated, the cause remains uncertain, but there is a correlation between the duration of PN and the decrease in glomerular filtration rate.

Visual Function

Visual function may be altered in children receiving long-term PN.[358-361] Despite normal visual acuity, one-half of the children had at least one and usually two abnormalities in their electroretinogram. Although deficiency of vitamins A and E, zinc, selenium, linolenic acid, and taurine[359-361] have each been implicated as causes of retinal dysfunction, the etiology and progression of the visual alteration is unknown.

Conclusions

Both the size and age of the pediatric patient are important in determining the appropriate quantities of nutrients administered in PN. There is a minimal amount of calories and a maximum amount. There is a minimum amount of glucose that must be provided to prevent hypoglycemia and a maximum that results in the production of excessive CO_2 and/or hepatic steatosis; and there is a minimum requirement (both dose and frequency) for intravenous fat emulsion to prevent EFA deficiency but a maximum beyond which intravenous fat may have deleterious effects. Amino acids must be provided in adequate amounts to prevent hypoproteinemia; however, there are adverse consequences of giving an excess. In addition, the recommendations of electrolytes, mineral, vitamins, and trace minerals needs to be tailored to the child's conditions.

Theoretically, PN should be possible to provide nutritional support for patients of all ages. One of its goals is to have the same nutritional efficacy as that of normal oral feeding or in-utero nutrition. With astute monitoring and ongoing nutritional assessments, complete nutritional support may be carried out without serious complications in most cases. Future objectives should include studying the efficacy of new substrates (eg, amino acid, lipids, growth factors), minimizing the consequences of the intestinal morphologic and functional changes induced by the PN,[362-364] and improving the anabolism in quickly growing children, especially during illnesses during the phase of immaturity.

PN should be reserved for infants and children who are unable to satisfy adequate nutritional intake for the correction of malnutrition or normal growth through the enteral route. A multidisciplinary nutrition team minimizes inappropriate prescription and allows for the minimal complications.

Table 37-22.

Pathogenesis of Parenteral Nutrition-Related Bone Disease

Nutrients	
Deficiency:	copper, calcium, phosphorus hypercalciuria
Excess:	vitamin D
Toxins:	
aluminum	
Potential agents*	
Nutrients:	vitamin A↑, vitamin C↓, zinc↓↑, manganese↓, silicone↓↑, fluoride↑↓, boron↓
Toxins:	cadmium, strontium
Drugs:	furosemide, heparin, acetate

*Down or up arrows indicate deficiency or excess, respectively.

References

1. Helfrick FW, Abelson NM. Intravenous feeding of a complete diet in a child: a report of a case. *J Pediatr.* 1944;25:400-403.
2. Moukarzel A, Najm I, Vargas J, McDiarmid SV, Busuttil R, Ament, ME. Effect of nutritional status on outcome of orthotopic liver transplantation in pediatric patients. *Transplant Proc.* 1990;22:1560-3.
3. Underwood BA, Hofvander F. Appropriate timing for complementary feeding of the breast-fed infant: a review. *Acta Paediatr Scand Suppl.* 1982;294:1–32.
4. Kamala F, Boo NY, Cheah FC, et al. Randomized controlled trial of heparin for prevention of blockage of peripherally inserted central catheters in neonates. *Acta Paediatr.* 2002;91:1350-1356.
5. Pithie A, Soutar JS, Pennington CR. Catheter tip positions in central vein thrombosis. *JPEN J Parenter Enter Nutr.* 1988;12:613-614.
6. Moukarzel A, Azancot A, Brun P, Vitoux C, Cezard JP, Navarro J. M-Mode and two-dimensional echocardiography in the routine follow-up of central venous catheters in children receiving total parenteral nutrition. *JPEN J Parenter Enter Nutr.* 1991;15:551-555.
7. Broviac JW, Cole JJ, Scribner BH. A silicone rubber atrial catheter for prolonged parenteral alimentation. *Surg Gynecol Obstet.* 1973;136:602-606.
8. Hickman RO, Buckner CD, Clift R, et al. A modified right atrial catheter for access to the venous system in marrow transplant recipients. *Surg Gynecol Obstet.* 1979;148:871-5.
9. Maksimak M, Ament ME, Fonkalsrud EW. Comparison of the pediatric silastic catheter with a standard no. 3 French silastic catheter for central venous alimentation. *J Pediatr Gastroenterol Nutr.* 1982;1:227-31.
10. McCarthy MC, Shives JK, Robinson RJ, et al. Prospective evaluation of single and triple lumen catheters in total parenteral nutrition. *JPEN J Parenter Enter Nutr.* 1987;11:259-262.
11. Bassetti S, Hu J, D'Agostino RB Jr, Sherertz RJ. Prolonged antimicrobial activity of a catheter containing chlorhexidine-silver sulfadiazine extends protection against catheter infections in vivo. *Antimicrob Agents Chemother.* 2001;45:1535–1538.
12. Raad II, Darouiche R, Dupuis J, et al. Central venous catheters coated with minocycline and rifampin for the prevention of catheter-related colonization and bloodstream infections: a randomized, double-blind trial. The Texas Medical Center Catheter Study Group. *Ann Intern Med.* 1997;127:267–274.
13. Veenstra DL, Saint S, Saha S, Lumley T, Sullivan SD. Efficacy of antiseptic-impregnated central venous catheters in preventing catheter-related bloodstream infection: a meta-analysis. *JAMA.* 1999;281: 261–267.
14. Loughran SC, Borzatta M. Peripherally inserted central catheters: a report of 2506 catheter days. *JPEN J Parenter Enteral Nutr.* 1995;19:133–136.
15. Finck C, Smith S, Jackson R, et al. Percutaneous subclavian central venous catheterization in children younger than one year of age. *Am Surg.* 2002;68:401-404.
16. Ecoff L, Barone RM, Simons RM. Implantable infusion port (Port-A-Cath). *J Natl Intraven Ther Assoc.* 1983;6:406-8.
17. Lokich JJ, Bothe A, Benotti P, Moore C. Complications and management of implanted venous access catheters. *J Clin Oncol.* 1985;3:710-7.
18. Ricour C, Revillon Y, Bougle D, et al. Nutrition parenterale par fistule arterio-veineuse. *Arch Fr Pediatr.* 1983;40:457-460.
19. Shils ME, Wright WL, Turnbull A. et al. Long-term parenteral nutrition through an external arteriovenous shunt. *N Engl J Med.* 1970;283:341-44.
20. Heizer WD, Orringer EP. Parenteral nutrition at home for 5 years via arteriovenous fistulae. Supplemental intravenous feedings for a patient with severe short bowel syndrome. *Gastroenterology.* 1977;72:527-532.
21. Adamkin DH. Total parenteral nutrition in hyaline membrane disease. In: Lebenthal E, ed. *Total Parenteral Nutrition: Indications, Utilization, Complications, Pathophysiologic Considerations.* New York, NY: Raven Press; 1986.
22. Pittard WB, Levkoff AH. Parenteral nutrition for the neonate. In: Tsang RC, Nichols BL, eds. *Nutrition During Infancy.* Philadelphia, PA: Hanley and Belfus; 1988.
23. Nash MA. The management of fluid and electrolyte disorders in the neonate. *Clin Perinatol.* 1981;8:251.
24. Ekblad H, Kero P, Takala J, Korvenranta H, Valimaki I. Water, sodium and acid-base balance in premature infants: therapeutical aspects. *Acta Paediatr Scand.* 1987;76:47–53.
25. Bell EF, Warburton D, Stonestreet BS, et al. Effect of fluid administration on the development of symptomatic patent ductus arteriosus and congestive heart failure in premature infants. *N Engl J Med.* 1980;302:598-604.
26. Brown ER, Stark A, Sosenko I, et al. Bronchopulmonary dysplasia: possible relationship to pulmonary edema. *J Pediatr.* 1978;92:982-4.

27. Goldman HI. Feeding and necrotizing enterocolitis. *Am J Dis Child.* 1980;134:553.
28. Goldberg RN, Chung D, Goldman SL, et al. The association of rapid volume expansion and intraventricular hemorrhage in the preterm infant. *J Pediatr.* 1980;96:1060-3.
29. Kerner JA. Fluid requirements. In: Kerner JA, ed. *Manual of Pediatric Parenteral Nutrition.* New York, NY: John Wiley and Sons; 1983.
30. World Health Organization (WHO). Geneva: Energy and protein requirements, Technical Report Series. 1985;724:71.
31. Schofield WN. Predicting basal metabolic rate, new standards and review of previous work. *Hum Nutr Clin Nutr.* 1985;39 (Suppl 1):5-41.
32. Kaplan AS, Zemel BS, Neiswender KM, et al. Resting energy expenditure in clinical pediatrics: measured versus prediction equations. *J Pediatr.* 1995;127:200–205.
33. Koen FM, Joosten KFM, Verhoeven JJ, Hazelzet JA. Energy expenditure and substrate utilization in mechanically ventilated children. *Nutrition.* 1999;15:444-48.
34. Duro D, Rising R, Cole C, Valois S, Cedillo M, Lifshitz F. New equations for calculating the components of energy expenditure in infants. *J Pediatr.* 2002;140:534-9.
35. Pierro A, Jones MO, Hammond P, Donnell SC, Lloyd DA. A new equation to predict the resting energy expenditure of surgical infants. *J Pediatr Surg.* 1994;29:1103-8.
36. White MS, Shepherd RW, McEniery JA. Energy expenditure in 100 ventilated, critically ill children: improving the accuracy of predictive equations. *Crit Care Med.* 2000;28:2307-2312.
37. Dietz WH, Bandini LG, Schoeller DA. Estimates of metabolic rate in obese and nonobese adolescents. *J Pediatr.* 1991;118:146-49.
38. Salas J, Moukarzel A, Goulet O, Putet G, Ricour C. Estimating resting energy expenditure by simple lean body mass indicators in children on total parenteral nutrition. *Am J Clin Nutr.* 1990;51:958-962.
39. Moukarzel A, Salas J, Goulet O, Ricour C. Estimate of specific energy expenditure of the different body tissues in children receiving total parenteral nutrition. *J Leban Med.* 2003;51:206-210.
40. Jaksic T, Shew SB, Keshen TH, Dzakovic A, Jahoor F. Do critically ill surgical neonates have increased energy expenditure? *J Pediatr Surg.* 2001;36:63-7.
41. Lloyd DA. Energy requirements of surgical newborn infants receiving parenteral nutrition. *Nutrition.* 1998;14:101-04.
42. White MS, Shepherd RW, McEniery JA. Energy expenditure measurements in ventilated critically ill children: within- and between-day variability. *JPEN J Parenter Enteral Nutr.* 1999;23:300-4.
43. Reichman B, Chessex P, Putet G, et al. Diet, fat accretion, and growth in premature infants. *N Engl J Med.* 1981;305:1495-1500.
44. Moukarzel A, Colomb V, Gorski AM, Goulet O, Ricour C. Hypermetabolic children on total parenteral nutrition, maintenance activity cost and energy for repleting tissue deficit. *Clin Nutr.* 1987;6:1.
45. Weinstein MR, Oh W. Oxygen consumption in infants with bronchopulmonary dysplasia. *J Pediatr.* 1981;99:958-961.
45. Pierro A, Jones MO, Donnell SC. Total parenteral nutrition in surgical infants. *Biochem Soc Trans.* 1998;26:131-6.
46. Garza JJ, Shew SB, Keshen TH, Dzakovic A, Jahoor F, Jaksic T. Energy expenditure in ill premature neonates. *J Pediatr Surg.* 2002;37:289-93.
47. Coss-Bu JA, Klish WJ, Walding D, Stein F, Smith EO, Jefferson LS. Energy metabolism, nitrogen balance, and substrate utilization in critically ill children 1-3. *Am J Clin Nutr.* 2001;74:664-69.
48. Pencharz PB, Azcue MP. Measuring resting energy expenditure in clinical practice. *J Pediatr.* 1995;127:269-271.
49. Mullen JL. Indirect calorimetry in critical care. *Proc Nutr Soc.* 1991;50:239-244.
50. Mann S, Westenskow DR, Houtchens BA. Measured and predicted caloric expenditure in the acutely ill. *Crit Care Med.* 1985;13:173-7.
51. Fernandez Mondejar E, Duro Lombardo M, Perez de la Cruz AJ, Merida Morales A, Torres Ruiz JM, Ferron Orihuela JA. Variations in oxygen consumption and carbon dioxide production during parenteral nutrition. *Intensive Care Med.* 1982;8:169-72.
52. Elwyn DH, Askanazi J, Kinney JM, Gump FE. Kinetics of energy substrates. *Acta Chir Scand Suppl.* 1981;507:209-19.
53. Liggett SB, St John RE, Lefrak SS. Determination of resting energy expenditure utilizing the thermodilution pulmonary artery catheter. *Chest.* 1987;91:562-566.
54. Koretz RL, Lipman TO, Klein S. AGA technical review on parenteral nutrition. *Gastroenterology.* 2001;121:970-1001.
55. Wilson DC, Cairns P, Halliday HL, Reid M, McClure G, Dodge JA. Randomized controlled trial of an aggressive nutritional regimen in sick very low birthweight infants. *Arch Dis Child Fetal Neonatal Ed.* 1997;77:F4-11.
56. Moukarzel A. Metabolic bone disease in total parenteral nutrition. In: Lifshitz F, ed. *Pediatric Endocrinology.* 2nd ed. New York, NY: Marcel Dekker, Inc.; 1995: 535-546.
57. Heird WC. Amino acids in pediatric and neonatal nutrition. *Curr Opin Clin Nutr Metab Care.* 1998;1:73-8.
58. Brunton JA, Ball RO, Pencharz PB. Current total parenteral nutrition solutions for the neonate are inadequate. *Curr Opin Clin Nutr Metab Care.* 2000;3:299-304.
59. National Advisory Group on Standards and Practice Guidelines for Parenteral Nutrition. Safe practices for parenteral nutrition formulations. *JPEN J Parenter Enteral Nutr.* 1998;22:49-66.
60. Wu PY, Edwards NB, Storm MC. Plasma amino acid pattern in normal term breast-fed infants. *J Pediatr.* 1986;109:347.
61. Heird WC, Hay W, Helms RA, et al. Pediatric parenteral amino acid mixture in low birth weight infants. *Pediatrics.* 1988;81:41-50.
62. Cooper A, Betts JM, Pereira GR. Taurine deficiency in the severe hepatic dysfunction complicating total parenteral nutrition. *J Pediatr Surg.* 1984;19:462.
63. Fitzgerald KA, MacKay MW. Calcium and phosphate solubility in neonatal parenteral nutrient solutions containing TrophAmine. *Am J Hosp Pharm.* 1986;43:88.
64. Adamkin DH, McClead RE, Desai NS, et al. Comparison of two neonatal intravenous amino acid formulations in preterm infants: a multicenter study. *J Perinatol.* 1991;11:375-82.
65. Coran AG, Drongowski RA. Studies on the toxicity and efficacy of a new amino acid solution in pediatric parenteral nutrition. *JPEN J Parenter Enter Nutr.* 1987;11:368.
66. Imura K, Okada A, Fukui Y, et al. Clinical studies on a newly devised amino acid solution for neonates. *JPEN J Parenter Enteral Nutr.* 1988;12:496-504.
67. Chin SE, Shepherd RW, Thomas BJ, et al. Nutritional support in children with end-stage liver disease: a randomized crossover trial of a branched-chain amino acid supplement. *Am J Clin Nutr.* 1992;56:158-63.
68. Heyman MB. General and specialized parenteral amino acid formulations for nutrition support. *J Am Diet Assoc.* 1990;90:401-8.
69. Koretz RL. Does nutritional intervention in protein-energy malnutrition improve morbidity or mortality? *J Ren Nutr.* 1999;9:119-21.
70. Neu J, Demarco V, Li N. Glutamine: clinical applications and mechanisms of action. *Curr Opin Clin Nutr Metab Care.* 2002;5:69-75.
71. Hankard R, Goulet O, Ricour C, et al. Glutamine metabolism in children with short bowel syndrome: a stable isotope study. *Pediatr Res.* 1994;36:202-206.
72. Calder PC. Glutamine and the immune system. *Clin Nutr.* 1994;13:2-8.
73. Tremel H, Kienle B, Weilemann LS, et al. Glutamine dipeptide supplemented parenteral nutrition maintains intestinal function in the critically ill. *Gastroenterology.* 1994;107:1595-1601.
74. Schloerb PR, Amare M. Total parenteral nutrition with glutamine in bone marrow transplantation and other clinical applications. *JPEN J Parenter Enteral Nutr.* 1993;17:407-413.

75. Ziegler TR, Young LS, Benfell K, et al. Clinical and metabolic efficacy of glutamine supplemented parenteral nutrition after bone marrow transplantation. *Ann Intern Med.* 1992;116:821-828.
76. Furst P, Stehle P. The potential use of parenteral dipeptides in clinical nutrition. *Nutr Clin Pract.* 1993;8:106-114.
77. Jiang ZM, Cao JD, Zhu XG, et al. The impact of glutamine dipeptide on nitrogen balance, intestinal permeability and clinical outcome of post operative patients. *JPEN J Parenter Enteral Nutr.* 1999;23:S62-S66.
78. Hammarqvist F, Wernerman J, Von Der Decken A, Vinnars E. Alpha ketoglutarate preserves protein synthesis and free glutamine in skeletal muscle after surgery. *Surgery.* 1991; 109:28-31.
79. Wernerman J, Hammarqvist F, Ali MR, Vinnars E. Glutamine and ornithine Ketoglutarate but not branched chain amino acids reduce the loss of muscle glutamine after surgical trauma. *Metabolism.* 1989; 38:63-66.
80. Cynober LA. The use of alpha-ketoglutarate salts in clinical nutrition and metabolic care. *Curr Opin Clin Nutr Metab Care.* 1999;2:33-37.
81. Dumas F, De Baudt JP, Colomb V, et al. Enteral ornithine alpha-ketoglutarate enhances intestinal adaptation to massive resection in rats. *Metabolism.* 1998;46:1366-1371.
82. Moukarzel A, Goulet O, Salas J, Marti-Henneberg C, Buchman A, Cynober L, Rappaport R, Ricour C. Growth retardation in children receiving long-term total parenteral nutrition: Effects of ornithine alpha-Ketoglutarate. *Am J Clin Nutr.* 1994;60:408-413.
83. Brown MR, Thunberg BJ, Golub L, Maniscalco WM, Cox C, Shapiro DL. Decreased cholestasis with enteral instead of intravenous protein in the very low-birth-weight infant. *J Pediatr Gastroenterol Nutr.* 1989;9:21-7.
84. Thurreen PJ. Early aggressive nutrition in the neonate. *Pediatr Rev.* 1999;20:e45-e55.
85. Gutcher GR, Farrell PM. Intravenous infusion of lipid for the prevention of essential fatty acid deficiency in premature infants. *Am J Clin Nutr.* 1991;54:1024-8.
86. Phelps SJ, Cochran EB. Effect of continuous administration of fat emulsion on the infiltration of intravenous lines in infants receiving peripheral parenteral nutrition solutions. *JPEN J Parenter Enteral Nutr.* 1989;13:628.
87. Putet G. Lipid metabolism of the micropremie. *Clin Perinatol.* 2000;27:57-69.
88. Haumont D, Deckelbaum RJ, Richelle M, et al. Plasma lipid and plasma lipoprotein concentrations in low birth weight infants given parenteral nutrition with twenty or ten percent lipid emulsion. *J Pediatr.* 1989;115:787-93.
89. Haumont D, Richelle M, Deckelbaum RJ, Coussaert E, Carpentier YA. Effect of liposomal content of lipid emulsions on plasma lipid concentrations in low birth weight infants receiving parenteral nutrition. *J Pediatr.* 1992;121:759-63.
90. Rossner S, Eklund B, Freyschuss U, Hallberg D, Kaijser L, Olsson A. Elimination of parenterally administered fat. Studies on removal sites for intralipid in normo-and hyperlipidaemic subjects. *Acta Chir Scand Suppl.* 1976;466:56-7.
91. Amin SB, Sinkin RA, McDermott MP, Kendig JW. Lipid intolerance in neonates receiving dexamethasone for bronchopulmonary dysplasia. *Arch Pediatr Adolesc Med.* 1999;153:795-800.
92. Hasselgren PO. Catabolic response to stress and injury: implications for regulation. *World J Surg.* 2000;24:1452-9.
93. Plank LD, Hill GL. Sequential metabolic changes following induction of systemic inflammatory response in patients with severe sepsis or major blunt trauma. *World J Surg.* 2000;24:630-8.
94. Dahn MS, Kirkpatrick JR, Blasier R. Alterations in the metabolism of exogenous lipid associated with sepsis. *JPEN J Parenter Enteral Nutr.* 1984;8:169-73.
95. Druml W, Fischer M, Ratheiser K. Use of intravenous lipids in critically ill patients with sepsis without and with hepatic failure. *JPEN J Parenter Enteral Nutr.* 1998;22:217-23.
96. Nordenstrom J, Carpentier YA, Askanazi J, et al. Metabolic utilization of intravenous fat emulsion during total parenteral nutrition. *Ann Surg.* 1982;196:221-31.
97. Lundell KH, Sabel KG, Eriksson BO. Plasma metabolites after a lipid load in infants with congenital heart disease. *Acta Paediatr.* 1999;88:718-23.
98. Zaidan H, Dhanireddy R, Hamosh M, Pramanik AK, Chowdhry P, Hamosh P. Effect of continuous heparin administration on Intralipid clearing in very low-birth-weight infants. *J Pediatr.* 1982;101:599-602.
99. Griffin EA, Bryan MH, Angel A. Variations in intralipid tolerance in newborn infants. *Pediatr Res.* 1983;17:478-81.
100. Benderly A, Rosenthal E, Levi J, Brook G. Effect of heparin on lipoprotein profile during parenteral fat infusions. *JPEN J Parenter Enteral Nutr.* 1983;7:37-9.
101. Forget PP, Fernandes J, Begemann PH. Utilization of fat emulsion during total parenteral nutrition in children. *Acta Paediatr Scand.* 1975;64:377-84.
102. D'Harlingue A, Hopper AO, Stevenson DK, Shahin SM, Kerner JA Jr. Limited value of nephelometry in monitoring the administration of intravenous fat in neonates. *JPEN J Parenter Enteral Nutr.* 1983;7:55-8.
103. Newball HH, Friedewald WT, Roberts B, Levy RI, Lenfant CJ. Effect of elevated triglycerides on the diffusing capacity of man. *Am Rev Respir Dis.* 1975;112:83-8.
104. Wheeler N. Parenteral nutrition. In: Kelts DG, Jones RD, eds. *Manual of Pediatric Nutrition.* Boston: Little, Brown & Co.; 1984.
105. Friedman Z, Danon A, Stahlman MT, et al. Rapid onset of essential fatty acid deficiency in the newborn. *Pediatrics.* 1976; 58:640-9.
106. Foote KD, MacKinnon MJ, Innis SM. Effect of early introduction of formula vs fat-free parenteral nutrition on essential fatty acid status of preterm infants. *Am J Clin Nutr.* 1991;54:93-7.
107. Friedman Z, Shochat SJ, Maisels MJ, et al. Correction of essential fatty acid deficiency in newborn infants by cutaneous application of sunflower-seed oil. *Pediatrics.* 1976; 58:650-4.
108. O'Neill JA, Caldwell MD, Meng HC. Essential fatty acid deficiency in surgical patients. *Ann Surg.* 1977;185:536.
109. Pelham LD. Rational use of intravenous fat emulsions. *Am J Hosp Pharm.* 1981;38:44.
110. Friedman Z. Essential fatty acids revisited. Am J Dis Child 1980;134:397-408.
111. Mascioli EA, Lopes SM, Champagne C, Driscoll DF. Essential fatty acid deficiency and home total parenteral nutrition patients. *Nutrition.* 1996;12:245-9.
112. Jeppesen PB, Hoy CE, Mortensen PB. Differences in essential fatty acid requirements by enteral and parenteral routes of administration in patients with fat malabsorption. *Am J Clin Nutr.* 1999;70:78-84.
113. Jeejeebhoy KN, Langer B, Tsallas G, Chu RC, Kuksis A, Anderson GH. Total parenteral nutrition at home: studies in patients surviving 4 months to 5 years. *Gastroenterology.* 1976;71:943-53.
114. Barr LH, Dunn GD, Brennan MF. Essential fatty acid deficiency during total parenteral nutrition. *Ann Surg.* 1981;193:304-11.
115. Wolfram G, Eckart J, Walther B, Zollner N. Factors influencing essential fatty acid requirement in total parenteral nutrition (TPN). *JPEN J Parenter Enteral Nutr.* 1978;2:634-9.
116. Anderson TL, Muttart CR, Bieber MA, Nicholson JF, Heird WC. A controlled trial of glucose versus glucose and amino acids in premature infants. *J Pediatr.* 1979;94:947-51.
117. Nube M, Bos LP, vd Boomgaard DM, Hekkens WT. Energy intake and the appearance of 5,8,11-eicosatrienoic acid in serum lipids during parenteral nutrition without fat. *JPEN J Parenter Enteral Nutr.* 1982;6:134-9.
118. Dennison AR, Ball M, Hands LJ, et al. Total parenteral nutrition using conventional and medium-chain triglycerides: effects on liver functions test, complement, and nitrogen balance. *JPEN J Parenter Enteral Nutr.* 1988;12:15-19.
119. Hyltander A, Sandstrom R, Lundhold K. Metabolic effects of structured triglycerides in humans. *Nutr Clin Prac.* 1995;10:91–97.
120. Beaufrere B, Chassard D, Broussolle C, et al. Effects of D-beta-hydroxybutyrate and long- and medium-chain triglycerides on leucine metabolism in humans. *Am J Physiol.* 1992;262:E268-E274.

121. Goulet O, De Potter S, Postaire M, et al. Long-term total parenteral nutrition in children: utilization of medium chain triglycerides. *Nutrition.* 1992;8:33-37.
122. Chambrier C, Guiraud M, Gibault JP, et al. Medium- and long-chain triacylglycerols in postoperative patients: structured lipids versus a physical mixture. *Nutrition.* 1999;15:274-277.
123. Waitzberg DL, Lotierzo PH, Logullo AF, et al. Parenteral lipid emulsions and phagocytic systems. *Br J Nutr.* 2002;87:S49-S57.
124. Mayer K, Gokorsch S, Fegbeutel C, et al. Parenteral nutrition with fish oil modulates cytokine response in patients with sepsis. *Am J Respir Crit Care Med.* 2003;167:1321-1328.
125. Bell SJ, Mascioli EA, Bistrian BR, et al. Alternative lipid sources for enteral and parenteral nutrition: long- and medium-chain triglycerides, structured triglycerides, and fish oils. *J Am Diet Assoc.* 1991;91:74-78.
126. Louheranta AM, Porkkala-Sarataho EK, Nyssonen MK, et al. Linoleic acid intake and susceptibility of very-low-density and low-density lipoproteins to oxidation in men. *Am J Clin Nutr.* 1996;63:698-703.
127. Goulet O, de Potter S, Antebi H, et al. Long-term efficacy and safety of a new olive oil-based intravenous fat emulsion in pediatric patients: a double-blind randomized study. *Am J Clin Nutr.* 1999;70:338-345.
128. Gobel Y, Koletzko B, Bohles HJ, et al. Parenteral fat emulsions based on olive and soybean oils: a randomized clinical trial in preterm infants. *J Pediatr Gastroenterol Nutr.* 2003;37:161-67.
129. Cairns PA, Stalker DJ. Carnitine supplementation of parenterally fed neonates (Cochrane Review). In: The Cochrane Library, Issue 2, 2004.
130. Borum PR. Should carnitine be added to parenteral nutrition solutions? *Nutr Clin Prac.* 2000;15:153-4.
131. Dahlstrom KA, Ament ME, Moukarzel A, Vinton NE, Cederblad G. Low blood and plasma carnitine levels in children receiving long term parenteral nutrition. *J Pediatr Gastroenterol Nutr.* 1990;11:375-379.
132. Moukarzel AA, Dahlstrom KA, Buchman AL, Ament ME. Carnitine status of children receiving long term total parenteral nutrition: A longitudinal prospective study. *J Pediatr.* 1992;120:759-762.
133. Buchman AL, Moukarzel A, Ament M. Low plasma carnitine levels are not secondary to vitamin B6 deficiency in long term TPN patients. *J Clin Nutr Gastroenterology.* 1993;8:31-33.
134. Helms RA, Whitington PF, Mauer EC, et al. Enhanced lipid utilization in infants receiving oral L-Carnitine during long-term parenteral nutrition. *J Pediatr.* 1986;108:984-8.
135. Bowyer BA, Fleming CR, Haymond MW, Miles JM. L-Carnitine: effect of intravenous administration on fuel homeostasis in normal subjects and home-parenteral-nutrition patients with low plasma carnitine concentrations. *Am J Clin Nutr.* 1989;49:618-23.
136. Stahl GE, Spear ML, Hamosh M. Intravenous administration of lipid emulsions to premature infants. *Clin Perinatol.* 1986;13:133.
137. Innis SM. Fat. In: Tsang RC, Lucas A, Uauy R, Zlotkin S, eds. *Nutritional Needs of the Preterm Infant.* Baltimore, MD: Williams & Wilkins; 1993.
138. Penn D, Ludwigs B, Schmidt-Sommerfeld E, Pascu F. Effect of nutrition on tissue carnitine concentrations in infants of different gestational ages. *Biol Neonate.* 1985;47:130-135.
139. Sulkers EJ Lafeber HN, Degenhart HJ, et al. Effects of high carnitine supplementation on substrate utilization in low-birth-weight infants receiving total parenteral nutrition. *Am J Clin Nutr.* 1990;52:889.
140. Wesson DE, Rich RH, Zlotkin SH, Pencharz PB. Fat overload syndrome causing respiratory insufficiency. *J Pediatr Surg.* 1984;19:777-778.
141. Heyman MB, Storch S, Ament ME. The fat overload syndrome. *Am J Dis Child.* 1981;135:628-30.
142. Dahlstrom KA, Goulet OJ, Roberts RL, Ricour C, Ament ME. Lipid tolerance in children receiving long-term parenteral nutrition: a biochemical and immunologic study. *J Pediatr.* 1988;113:985-90.
143. Colomb V, Jobert-Giraud A, Lacaille F, et al. Role of lipid emulsions in cholestasis associated with long-term parenteral nutrition in children. *JPEN J Parenter Enteral Nutr.* 2000;24:345-350.
144. Shulman RJ, Langston C, Schanler RJ. Pulmonary vascular lipid deposition after administration of intravenous fat to infants. *Pediatrics.* 1987;79:99-102.
145. Skeie B, Askanazi J, Rothkopf MM. Intravenous fat emulsions and lung function: a review. *Crit Care Med.* 1988:16:183-94.
146. Hageman JR, Hunt CE. Fat emulsions and lung function. *Clin Chest Med.* 1986;7:69-77.
147. Hwang TL, Huang SL, Chen MF. Effects of intravenous fat emulsion on respiratory failure. *Chest.* 1990;97:934-8.
148. Adamkin DH, Gelke KN, Andrews BF. Fat emulsions and hypertriglyceridemia. *JPEN J Parenter Enteral Nutr.* 1984;8:563-7.
149. Helbock HJ, Motchnik PA, Ames BN. Toxic hydroperoxides in intravenous lipid emulsions used in preterm infants. *Pediatrics.* 1993;91:83-7.
150. Lavoie JC, Chessex P. The increase in vasomotor tone induced by a parenteral lipid emulsion is linked to an inhibition of prostacyclin production. *Free Radic Biol Med.* 1994;16:795-9.
151. Periera GR, Fox WW, Stanley CA, Baker L, Schwartz JG. Decreased oxygenation and hyperlipemia during intravenous fat infusions in premature infants. *Pediatrics.* 1980;66:26-30.
152. Marks KH, Turner MJ, Rothberg AD. Effect of Intralipid infusion on transcutaneous oxygen and carbon dioxide tension in sick neonates. *S Afr Med J.* 1987;72:389-91.
153. Sun SC, Ventura C, Verasestakul S. Effect of Intralipid-induced lipaemia on the arterial oxygen tension in preterm infants. *Resuscitation.* 1978;6:265-70.
154. Lundman P, Eriksson M, Schenck-Gustafsson K. Transient triglyceridemia decreases vascular reactivity in young, healthy men without risk factors for coronary heart disease. *Circulation.* 1997;96:3266-68.
155. Alwaidh MH, Bowden L, Shaw B, Ryan SW. Randomized trial of effect of delayed intravenous lipid administration on chronic lung disease in preterm neonates. *J Pediatr Gastroenterol Nutr.* 1996;22:303-6.
156. Shulman RJ. The effect of Intralipid on the cytotoxicity of leukocytes for herpes simplex virus-infected cells: a clinical concern? *J Infect Dis.* 1983;148:181-2.
157. Adolph M. Lipid emulsions in parenteral nutrition. *Ann Nutr Metab.* 1999:43:1-13.
158. Guillou PJ. The effects of lipids on some aspects of the cellular immune response. *Proc Nutr Soc.* 1993;52:91-100.
159. Pomposelli JJ, Bistrian BR. Is total parenteral nutrition immunosuppressive? *New Horiz.* 1994:2:224-9.
160. Lenssen P, Bruemmer BA, Bowden RA, Gooley T, Aker SN, Mattson D. Intravenous lipid dose and incidence of bacteremia and fungemia in patients undergoing bone marrow transplantation. *Am J Clin Nutr.* 1998;67:927-33.
161. Avila-Figueroa C, Goldmann DA, Richardson DK, Gray JE, Ferrari A, Freeman J. Intravenous lipid emulsions are the major determinant of coagulase-negative staphylococcal bacteremia in very low birth weight newborns. *Pediatr infect Dis J.* 1998;17:10-7.
162. Carpentier YA. Dupont IE. Advances in intravenous lipid emulsions. *World J Surg.* 2000;24:1493-7.
163. Wheeler JG, Boyle RJ, Abramson JS. Intralipid infusion in neonates: effects on polymorphonuclear leukocyte function. *J Pediatr Gastroenterol Nutr.* 1985:4:453-6.
164. Usmani SS, Harper RG, Usmani SF. Effect of a lipid emulsion (Intralipid) on polymorphonuclear leukocyte functions in the neonate. *J Pediatr.* 1988:113:132-6.
165. Sirota L, Straussberg R, Notti I, Bessler H. Effect of lipid emulsion on IL-2 production by mononuclear cells of newborn infants and adults. *Acta Paediatr.* 1997:86:410-3.
166. Usmani SS, Harper RG, Sia CG, Suntharalingam K, Robeson WR. In vitro effect of Intralipid on polymorphonuclear leukocyte function in the neonate. *J Pediatr.* 1986:109:710-2.

167. English D, Roloff JS, Lukens JN, Parker P, Greene HL, Ghishan FK. Intravenous lipid emulsions and human neutrophil function. *J Pediatr.* 1981:99:913-6.
168. Puri P, Reen DJ, Browne O, Guiney EJ. Immune status of the neonate maintained on total parenteral nutrition. *Arch Dis Child.* 1981:56:283-6.
169. Strunk RC, Murrow BW, Thilo E, Kunke KS, Johnson EG. Normal macrophage function in infants receiving Intralipid by low-dose intermittent administration. *J Pediatr.* 1985;106:640-5.
170. Spear ML, Spear M, Cohen AR, Pereira GR. Effect of fat infusions on platelet concentration in premature infants. *JPEN J Parenter Enteral Nutr.* 1990;14:165-8.
171. Bistrian BR, Bothe A Jr, Blackburn GL, DeFriez Al. Low plasma cortisol and hematologic abnormalities associated with essential fatty acid deficiency in man. *JPEN J Parenter Enteral Nutr.* 1981;5:141-4.
172. American Academy of Pediatrics Committee on Nutrition. Use of intravenous fat emulsions in pediatric patients. *Pediatrics.* 1981;68:738-743.
173. Kalhan SC, Kilic I. Carbohydrate as nutrient in the infant and child: range of acceptable intake. *Europ J Clin Nutr.* 1999;53:S94-S100.
174. Denne SC, Karn CA, Wang J, Liechty EA. Effect of intravenous glucose and lipid on proteolysis and glucose production in normal newborns. *Am J Physiol.* 1995;269:E361-7.
175. Sunehag AL, Haymond MW, Schanler RJ, Reeds PJ, Bier DM. Gluconeogenesis in very low birth weight infants receiving total parenteral nutrition. *Diabetes.* 1999;48:791-800.
176. Lafeber HN, Sulkers EJ, Chapman TE, Sauer PJ. Glucose production and oxidation in preterm infants during total parenteral nutrition. *Pediatr Res.* 1990;28:153-7.
177. Jones MO, Pierro A, Hammond P, Nunn A, Lloyd DA. Glucose utilization in the surgical newborn infant receiving total parenteral nutrition. *J Pediatr Surg.* 1993;128:1121-5.
178. Nose O, Tipton JR, Ament ME. Effect of the energy source on changes in energy expenditure, respiratory quotient, and nitrogen balance during total parenteral nutrition in children. *Pediatr Res.* 1987;21:538-41.
179. Bresson JL, Narcy P, Putet G, Ricour C. Energy substrate utilization in infants receiving total parenteral nutrition with different glucose to fat ratios. *Pediatr Res.* 1989;25:645-8.
180. Sheridan RL, Yu YM, Prelack K. Young VR, Burke JF, Tompkins RG. Maximal parenteral glucose oxidation in hypermetabolic young children: a stable isotope study. *JPEN J Parent Enteral Nutr.* 1998;22:212-6.
181. Schears GJ, Deutschman CS. Common nutritional issues, in pediatric and adult critical care medicine. *Crit Care Clinic.* 1997;13:669-90.
182. Cerra FB, Benitez MR, Blackburn GL, et al. Applied nutrition in ICU patients. *Chest.* 1997;111:769-78.
183. Chan S, McCowen KC, Blackburn GL. Nutrition management in the ICU. *Chest.* 1999;115:145-48.
184. Klein CJ, Stanek GS, Wiles CE III. Overfeeding macronutrients to critically ill adults: metabolic complications. *J Am Diet Assoc.* 1998;98:795-806.
185. Shikora SA, Benotti PN. Nutritional support of the mechanically ventilated patient. *Respir Care Clin N Am.* 1997;3:69-90.
186. Talpers SS, Romberger DJ, Bunce SB, Pingleton SK. Nutritionally associated increased carbon dioxide production. Excess total calories vs high proportion of carbohydrate calories. *Chest.* 1992;102:551-5.
187. Rodriguez JL, Askanazi J, Weissman C, Hensle TW, Rosenbaum SH, Kinney JM. Ventilatory and metabolic effects of glucose infusions. *Chest.* 1985;88:512-8.
188. Burke JF, Wolfe RR, Mullany CJ, Mathews DE, Bier DM. Glucose requirements following burn injury. Parameters of optimal glucose infusion and possible hepatic and respiratory abnormalities following excessive glucose intake. *Ann Surg.* 1979;190:274-85.
189. Tulikoura I, Huikuri K. Morphological fatty changes and function of the liver, serum free fatty acids, and triglycerides during parenteral nutrition. *Scand J Gastroenterol.* 1982;17:177-85.
190. Aarsland A, Chinkes D, Wolfe RR. Contributions of de novo synthesis of fatty acids to total VLDL-triglyceride secretion during prolonged hyperglycemia/hyperinsulinemia in normal man. *J Clin Invest.* 1996;98:2008-17.
191. Bistrian BR. Hyperglycemia and infection: which is the chicken and which is the egg? *JPEN J Parenter Enteral Nutr.* 2001;25:180-1.
192. Engelich G, Wright DG, Hartshorn KL. Acquired disorders of phagocyte function complicating medical and surgical illnesses. *Clin Infect Dis.* 2001;33:2040-8.
193. Khaodhiar L, McCowen K, Bistrian B. Perioperative hyperglycemia, infection or risk? *Curr Opin Clin Nutr Metab Care.* 1999;2:79-82.
194. Gore DC, Chinkes D, Heggers J. Association of hyperglycemia with increased mortality after severe burn injury. *J Trauma.* 2001;51:540-44.
195. McCowen KC, Friel C, Sternberg J, et al. Hypocaloric total parenteral nutrition: effectiveness in prevention of hyperglycemia and infectious complications-a randomized clinical trial. *Crit Care Med.* 2000;28:3606-11.
196. Macfie J, Smith RC, Hill GL. Glucose or fat as a non-protein energy source? A controlled clinical trial in gastroenterological patients requiring intravenous nutrition. *Gastroenterology.* 1981;80:103.
197. Vaucher YE, Walson PD, Morrow G. Continuous insulin infusion in hyperglycemic, very low birth weight infants. *J Pediatr Gastroenterol Nutr.* 1982;1:211.
198. Ostertag SG, Jovanovic L, Lewis B, et al. Insulin pump therapy in the very low birth weight infant. *Pediatrics.* 1986; 78:625-30.
199. Binder ND, Raschko PK, Benda GI, et al. Insulin infusion with parenteral nutrition in extremely low birth weight infants with hyperglycemia. *J Pediatr.* 1989;114:273-80.
200. Kanarek KS, Santeiro ML, Malone JI: Continuous infusion of insulin in hyperglycemic low-birth-weight infants receiving parenteral nutrition with and without lipid emulsion. *JPEN J Parenter Enter Nutr.* 1991:15:417.
201. Collins JW, Hoppe M, Brown K, et al. A controlled trial of insulin infusion and parenteral nutrition in extremely low birth weight infants with glucose intolerance. *J Pediatr.* 1991;118:921-7.
202. Thureen PJ, Melara D, Fennessey V, et al. Effect of low versus high intravenous amino acid intake on very low birth weight infants in the early neonatal period. *Pediatr Res.* 2003;53:24-32.
203. Koo WWK, Tsang RC. Mineral requirements of low-birth-weight infants. *J Am Coll Nutr.* 1991;10:474-486.
204. Moukarzel AA, Ament ME. Home parenteral nutrition in infants and children. In: Rombeau JL, Caldwell MD, eds. *Clinical Nutrition: Parenteral Nutrition* (Clinical Nutrition, Vol 2). Philadelphia: WB Saunders; 1993: 791-813.
205. Koo WW, Tsang RC, Succop P, et al. Minimal vitamin D and high calcium and phosphorus needs of preterm infants receiving parenteral nutrition. *J Pediatr Gastroenterol Nutr.* 1989;8:225-233.
206. Koo WW. Parenteral nutrition-related bone disease. *JPEN J Parenter Enteral Nutr.* 1992;16:386-394.
207. Hylander E, Ladefoged K, Madsen S. Calcium balance and bone mineral content following small intestine resection. *Scand J Gastroenterol.* 1981;16:167-170.
208. Kimura S, Nose O, Seino Y. Effects of alternate and simultaneous administrations of calcium and phosphorous on calcium metabolism in children receiving total parenteral nutrition. *JPEN J Parenter Enteral Nutr.* 1986;10:513-16.
209. Chessex P, Pineault M, Zebiche H, Ayotte RA. Calciuria in parenterally fed preterm infants: role of phosphorus intake. *J Pediatr.* 1985;107:794-796.
210. Hoehn GJ, Carey DE, Rowe JC, et al. Alternate day infusion of calcium and phosphate in low birth weight infants: wasting of the infused mineral. *J Pediatr Gastroenterol Nutr.* 1987;6:752-757.
211. Pelegano JF, Rowe JC, Carey DE, et al. Simultaneous infusion of calcium and phosphorus in parenteral nutrition for premature infants: use of physiologic calcium/phosphorus ratio. *J Pediatr.* 1989;114:115-119.

212. Chessex P, Pineault M, Brisson G, et al. Role of the source of phosphate salt in improving the mineral balance of parenterally fed low birth weight infants. *J Pediatr.* 1990;116:765-772.
213. Pelegano JF, Rowe JC, Carey DE, et al. Effect on calcium/phosphorus ratio on mineral retention in parenterally fed premature infants. *J Pediatr Gastroenterol Nutr.* 1991;12:351-355.
214. Klein L, Ament ME, Slatopolsky E, Coburn JW. Urinary mineral excretion during long-term total parenteral nutrition. In: Urban & Schwarzenberg, eds. *Metabolic Bone Disease in Total Parenteral Nutrition.* Baltimore, MD: Munish; 1985: 101-128.
215. Koo WW, Tsang RC, Steichen JJ, et al. Parenteral nutrition for infants: effect of high versus low calcium and phosphorus content. *J Pediatr Gastroenterol Nutr.* 1987;6:96-104.
216. Knight P, Heer D, Abdenour G. Ca X P and Ca/P in the parenteral feeding of preterm infants. *JPEN J Parenter Enteral Nutr.* 1983;7:110-114.
217. Niemiec PW Vanderveen TW. Compatibility considerations in parenteral nutrient solutions. *Am J Hosp Pharm.* 1984;41:893-911.
218. Eggert LD, Rusho WJ, MacKay MW, et al. Calcium and phosphorus compatibility in parenteral nutrition admixtures. *Am J Hosp Pharm.* 1982;39:49-53.
219. Poole RL, Rupp CA, Kerner JA. Calcium and phosphorus in neonatal parenteral nutrition solutions. *JPEN J Parenter Enteral Nutr.* 1983;7:358-360.
220. Koo WW. Calcium, phosphorus and vitamin D requirements of infants receiving parenteral nutrition. *J Pediatr.* 1988;8:263-268.
221. Dunham B, Marcuard S, Khazanie PG, Meade GT, Nichols K. The solubility of calcium and phosphorus neonatal in total parenteral nutrition solutions. *JPEN J Parenter Enteral Nutr.* 1991;5:608-611.
222. Lenz GT, Mikrut BA. Calcium and phosphate solubility in neonatal parenteral nutrient solutions containing Aminosyn-PF or TrophAmine. *Am J Hosp Pharm.* 1988;45:2367-2371.
223. Hanning RM, Mitchell MK, Atkinson SA. In vitro solubility of calcium glycerophosphate versus conventional mineral salts in pediatric parenteral nutrition solutions. *J Pediatr Gastroenterol Nutr.* 1989;9:67-71.
224. MacMahon P, Mayne PD, Blair M, et al. Calcium and phosphorus solubility in neonatal intravenous feeding solutions. *Arch Dis Child.* 1990;65:352-353.
225. Hanning RM, Atkinson SA, Whyte RK. Efficacy of calcium glycerophosphate vs conventional mineral salts for total parenteral nutrition in low-birth weight infants: a randomized clinical trial. *Am J Clin Nutr.* 1991;54:903-908.
226. Draper HH, Yuen DE, Whyte RK. Calcium glycerophosphate as a source of calcium and phosphorus in parenteral nutrition solutions. *JPEN J Parenter Enteral Nutr.* 1991;15:176-180.
227. Raupp R, von Kries R, Pfahl HG, Manz F. Glyceroglucose-phosphate in parenteral nutrition of premature infants: a comparative in vitro evaluation of calcium and phosphorus compatibility. *JPEN J Parenter Enteral Nutr.* 1991;15:469-473.
228. Prinzivalli M, Ceccarelli S. Sodium D-fructose-1,6-diphosphonate vs. sodium monohydrogen phosphate in total parenteral nutrition: a comparative in vitro assessment of calcium phosphate compatibility. *JPEN J Parenter Enteral Nutr.* 1999;23:326-332.
229. Cole DE, Zlotkin SH. Increased sulfate as an etiological factor in the hypercalciuria associated with total parenteral nutrition. *Am J Clin Nutr.* 1983;37:108-113.
230. Schmidt GL, Baumgartner TG, Fischlishweiger W, et al. Cost containment using cysteine HCl acidification to increase calcium/phosphate solubility in hyperalimentation. *JPEN J Parenter Enteral Nutr.* 1986;10:203-207.
231. Kirkpatrick AE, Holcombe BJ, Sawyer WT. Effect of retrograde aminophylline administration on calcium and phosphate solubility in neonatal total parenteral nutrient solutions. *Am J Hosp Pharm.* 1989;46:2496-2500.
232. Henann NE, Jacks TT. Compatibility and availability of sodium bicarbonate in total parenteral nutrient solutions. *Am J Hosp Pharm.* 1985;42:2718-2720.
233. American Medical Association, Department of Foods and Nutrition. Multivitamin preparations for parenteral use: a statement by the Nutrition Advisory Group 1975. *JPEN J Parenter Enteral Nutr.* 1979;3:258.
234. Greene HL, Moore ME, Phillips B. Evaluation of a pediatric multiple vitamin preparation for total parenteral nutrition. II. Blood levels of vitamins A, D, and E. *Pediatrics.* 1986;77:539-47.
235. Moore MC, Greene HL, Phillips B, et al. Evaluation of a pediatric multiple vitamin preparation for total parenteral nutrition in infants and children. I. Blood levels of water-soluble vitamins. *Pediatrics.* 1986:77:530-8.
236. Greene HL, Hambidge KM, Schanler R, Tsang RC. Guidelines for the use of vitamins, trace elements, calcium, magnesium, and phosphorus in infants and children receiving total parenteral nutrition: report of the Subcommittee on Pediatric Parenteral Nutrient Requirements from the Committee on Clinical Practice Issues of the American Society for Clinical Nutrition. *Am J Clin Nutr.* 1988;48:1324-42.
237. American Medical Association Department of Foods and Nutrition. Multivitamin preparations for parenteral use. A statement by the Nutrition Advisory Group. *JPEN J Parenter Enteral Nutr.* 1979:3:258-62.
238. Alade SL, Brown RE, Paquet A Jr. Polysorbate 80 and E-Ferol toxicity. *Pediatrics.* 1986;77:593-7.
239. MacDonald MG, Getson PR, Glasgow AM, Miller MK, Boeckx RL, Johnson EL. Propylene glycol: increased incidence of seizures in low birth weight infants. *Pediatrics.* 1987;79:622-5.
240. Department of Health and Human Services Food and Drug Administration. Parenteral multivitamin products; Drugs for Human Use; Drug efficacy study implementation; Amendment. Federal Register. 2000;56:21200-21201.
241. Drittij-Reijnders MJ, Sels JP, Rouflart M, Thijssen HH. Vitamin K status and parenteral nutrition; the effect of Intralipid on plasma vitamin Kl levels. *Eur J Clin Nutr.* 1994;48:525-7.
242. Lennon C, Davidson KW, Sadowski JA, Mason JB. The vitamin K content of intravenous lipid emulsions. *JPEN J Parenter Enteral Nutr.* 1993;17:142-4.
243. Darlow BA, Graham PJ. Vitamin A supplementation for preventing morbidity and mortality in very low birthweight infants. Cochrane Database Syst Rev. 2000;(2):CD00050l.
244. Pediatric Parenteral Multivitamin Products; Drug Efficacy Study Implementation; Announcement of Marketing Conditions. Federal Register. 2000;65:4253-4256.
245. Porcelli PJ, Greene HL, Adcock EW. Retinol (vitamin A) and riboflavin (vitamin B2) administration and metabolism in very low birth weight infants. *Semin Perinatol.* 1992;16:170-80.
246. Greene HL, Phillips BL, Franck L, et al. Persistently low blood retinol levels during and after parenteral feeding of very low birth weight infants: examination of losses into intravenous administration sets and a method of prevention by addition to a lipid emulsion. *Pediatrics.* 1987;79:894-900.
247. Smith JL, Canham JE, Kirkland WD, Wells PA. Effect of Intralipid, amino acids, container, temperature, and duration of storage on vitamin stability in total parenteral nutrition admixtures. *JPEN J Parenter Enteral Nutr.* 1988;12:478-83.
248. Smith JL, Canham JE, Wells PA. Effect of phototherapy light, sodium bisulfite, and pH on vitamin stability in total parenteral nutrition admixtures. *JPEN J Parenter Enteral Nutr.* 1988;12:394-402.
249. Hardy G, Reilly C. Technical aspects of trace element supplementation. *Curr Opin Clin Nutr Metab Care.* 1999:2:277-85.
250. Van Gossum A, Neve J. Trace element deficiency and toxicity. *Curr Opin Clin Nutr Metab Care.* 1998;1:499-507.
251. Allwood MC. Aluminium in parenteral nutrition admixtures: an unnecessary risk? *Nutrition.* 1999;15:958-9.
252. Klein GL. Aluminum in parenteral solutions revisited-again. *Am J Clin Nutr.* 1995;61:449-56.
253. Moukarzel AA, Ament ME. Trace elements in parenteral nutrition. In: Lifshitz F, ed. *Childhood Nutrition.* Boca Raton, FL: CRC Press, Inc.; 1995: 159-182.

254. Guidelines for essential trace element preparations for parenteral use. A statement by an expert panel. AMA Department of Foods and Nutrition. *JAMA*. 1979;241:2051-4.
255. Wolman SL, Anderson GH, Marliss EB, Jeejeebhoy KN. Zinc in total parenteral nutrition: requirements and metabolic effects. *Gastroenterology*. 1979;79:458-467.
256. Cordano A, Baertl JM, Graham GG. Copper deficiency in infancy. *Pediatrics*. 1964; 34:324.
257. Shulman RJ. Zinc and copper balance studies in infants receiving total parenteral nutrition. *Am J Clin Nutr*. 1989;49:879-83.
258. Dahlstrom KA, Ament ME, Medhin MG, Meurling S. Serum trace elements in children receiving long-term parenteral nutrition. *J Pediatr*. 1986;109:625-30.
275. Observations on effect of sodium selenite in prevention of Keshan disease. *Chin Med J*. 1979;92:471.
260. Yusuf SW, Rehman Q, Casscells W. Cardiomyopathy in association with selenium deficiency: a case report. *JPEN J Parenter Enteral Nutr*. 2002:26:63-6.
261. Vinton NE, Dahlstrom KA, Strobel CT, Ament ME. Macrocytosis and pseudoalbinism: manifestations of selenium deficiency. *J Pediatr*. 1987;111:711-717.
262. Kelly DA, Coe AW, Shenkin A, Lake BD, Walker-Smith JA. Symptomatic selenium deficiency in a child on home parenteral nutrition. *J Pediatr Gastroenterol Nutr*. 1988;7:783-786.
263. Klinger G, Shamir R, Singer P, Diamond EM, Josefsberg Z, Sirota L. Parenteial selenium supplementation in extremely low birth weight infants: inadequate dosage but no correlation with hypothyroidism. *J Perinatol*. 1999:19:568-72.
264. Buchman AL, Moukarzel A, Ament ME. Selenium renal homeostasis is impaired in patients receiving long term parenteral nutrition. *JPEN J Parenter Enteral Nutr*. 1994;18:231-233.
265. Hatanaka N, Nakaden H, Yamamoto Y, Matsuo S, Fujikawa T, Matsusue S. Selenium kinetics and changes in glutathione peroxidase activities in patients receiving long-term parenteral nutrition and effects of supplementation with selenite. *Nutrition*. 2000;16:22-6.
266. Abumrad NN, Schneider AJ, Steel D, Rogers LS. Amino acid intolerance during prolonged total parenteral nutrition reversed by molybdate therapy. *Am J Clin Nutr*. 1981;34:2551-9.
267. Abumrad NN. Molybdenum: is it an essential trace metal? *Bull N Y Acad Med*. 1984;60:163.
268. Moukarzel AA, Song MK, Buchman AL, et al. Excessive chromium intake in children receiving total parenteral nutrition. *Lancet*. 1992;339:385-388.
269. Moukarzel AA, Ament ME, Buchman AL, Dahlstrom KA, Vargas J. Renal function of children receiving long term parenteral nutrition. *J Pediatr*. 1991;119:864-868.
270. Buchman AL, Moukarzel AA, Ament ME. The role of chromium and cadmium toxicity in TPN-induced nephropathy. *J Clin Nutr Gastroenterol*. 1992;7:39-41.
271. Pluhator-Murton MM, Fedorak RN, Audette RJ, Marriage BJ, Yatscoff RW, Gramlich LM. Trace element contamination of total parenteral nutrition. 1. Contribution of component solutions. *JPEN J Parenter Enteral Nutr*. 1999;23:222-7.
272. Bougle D, Bureau F, Deschrevel G, et al. Chromium and parenteral nutrition in children. *J Pediatr Gastroenterol Nutr*. 1993;17:72-4.
273. Hak EB, Storm MC, Helms RA. Chromium and zinc contamination of parenteral nutrient solution components commonly used in infants and children. *Am J Health Syst Pharm*. 1998;55:150-4.
274. Mouser JF, Hak EB, Helms RA, Christensen ML, Storm MC. Chromium and zinc concentrations in pediatric patients receiving long-term parenteral nutrition. *Am J Health Syst Pharm*. 1999;56:1950-6.
275. Moukarzel AA, Ament ME. Home parenteral nutrition. *Home Infusion News*. 1993;2:3-7.
276. Dickerson RN. Manganese intoxication and parenteral nutrition. *Nutrition*. 2001;17:689-693.
277. Masumoto K, Suita S, Taguchi T, et al. Manganese intoxication during intermittent parenteral nutrition: report of two cases. *JPEN J Parenter Enteral Nutr*. 2001;25:95-9.
278. Fok TF, Chui KK, Cheung R, Ng PC, Cheung KL, Hjelm M. Manganese intake and cholestatic jaundice in neonates receiving parenteral nutrition: a randomized controlled study. *Acta Paediatr*. 2001;90:1009-15.
279. Fitzgerald K, Mikalunas V, Rubin H, McCarthey R, Vanagunas A, Craig RM. Hypermanganesemia in patients receiving total parenteral nutrition. *JPEN J Parenter Enteral Nutr*. 1999;23:333-6.
280. Moukarzel AA, Buchman AL, Salas JS, et al. Iodine supplementation in children receiving long-term parenteral nutrition. *J Pediatr*. 1992;121:252-254.
281. Wan KK, Tsallas G. Dilute iron dextran formulation for addition to parenteral nutrient solutions. *Am J Hosp Pharm*. 1980;37:206-210.
282. Reed MD, Bertino JS Jr, Halpin TC Jr. Use of intravenous iron dextran injection in children receiving total parenteral nutrition. *Am J Dis Child*. 1981;135:829-31.
283. Halpin TC Jr, Bertino JS, Rothstein FC, Kurczynski EM, Reed MD. Iron-deficiency anemia in childhood inflammatory bowel disease: treatment with intravenous iron-dextran. *JPEN J Parenter Enteral Nutr*. 1982;6:9-11.
284. Surico G, Muggeo P, Muggeo V, et al. Parenteral iron supplementation for the treatment of iron deficiency anemia in children. *Ann Hematol*. 2002;81:154-7.
285. Mamula P, Piccoli DA, Peck SN, Markowitz JE, Baldassano RN. Total dose intravenous infusion of iron dextran for iron-deficiency anemia in children with inflammatory bowel disease. *J Pediatr Gastroenterol Nutr*. 2002;34:286-90.
286. Pollak A, Hayde M, Hayn M, et al. Effect of intravenous iron supplementation on erythropoiesis in erythropoietin-treated premature infants. *Pediatrics*. 2001;107:78-85.
287. Charytan C, Levin N, Al-Saloum M, Hafeez T, Gagnon S, Van Wyck DB. Efficacy and safety of iron sucrose for iron deficiency in patients with dialysis-associated anemia: North American clinical trial. *Am J Kidney Dis*. 2001;37:300-7.
288. Michael B, Coyne DW, Fishbane S, et al. Sodium ferric gluconate complex in hemodialysis patients: adverse reactions compared to placebo and iron dextran. *Kidney Int*. 2002;61:1830-9.
289. Nielsen FH. New essential trace elements for the life sciences. *Biol Trace Element Res*. 1990;26-27:599-611.
290. Moukarzel A, Ament ME, Vargas J, et al. Non aluminum dependent osteopathy in children on long term parenteral nutrition. *Am J Clin Nutr*. 1990;51:520.
291. Koo WW, Kaplan LA. Aluminum and bone disorders: with specific reference to contamination of infant nutrients. *J Am Coll Nutr*. 1988;7:199-214.
292. American Academy of Pediatrics, Committee on Nutrition. Aluminum toxicity in infants and children. *Pediatrics*. 1996;97:413-416.
293. Bishop NJ, Morley R, Day JP, Lucas A. Aluminum neurotoxicity in preterm infants receiving intravenous-feeding solutions. *N Engl J Med*. 1997;336:1557-61.
294. Klein GL, Leichtner AM, Heyman MB. Aluminum in large and small volume parenterals used in total parenteral nutrition: response to the Food and Drug Administration notice of proposed rule by the North American Society for Pediatric Gastroenterology and Nutrition. *J Pediatr Gastroenterol Nutr*. 1998;27:457-460.
295. Moukarzel AA, Ament ME. Home parenteral nutrition. In: Lifshitz F, ed. *Childhood Nutrition*. Boca Raton, FL: CRC Press, Inc., 1995:183-196.
296. Fisher AA, Poole RL, Machie R, et al. Clinical pathway for pediatric parenteral nutrition. *Nutr Clin Pract*. 1997;12:76-80.
297. MacFie J. Cyclic parenteral nutrition. *Nutrition*. 1997;13:46-55.
298. Driscoll DF. Total nutrient admixture: theory and practice. *Nutr Clin Pract*. 1885;10:114-119.

299. Didier ME, Fischer S, Maki DG. Total nutrient admixtures appear safer than lipid emulsion alone as regards microbial contamination: growth properties of microbial pathogens at room temperature. *JPEN J Parenter Enteral Nutr.* 1998;22:291-6.
300. Driscoll DF. Stability and compatibility assessment techniques for total parenteral nutrition admixures: setting the bar according to pharmacopeial standards. *Curr Opin Clin Nutr Metab Care.* 2005;8:297-303.
301. McKinnon BT. FDA safety alert: hazards of precipitation associated with parenteral nutrition. *Nutr Clin Pract.* 1996;11:59-65.
302. Trissel LA, Gilbert DL, Martinez JF, Baker MB, Walter WV, Mirtallo JM. Compatibility of medications with 3-in-l parenteral nutrition admixtures. *JPEN J Parenter Enteral Nutr.* 1999;23:67-74.
303. Friel C, Bistrian B. Cycled total parenteral nutrition: is it more effective? *Am J Clin Nutr.* 1997;65:1078-9.
304. Tukehara H, Hino M, Kameoka K. A new method of total parenteral nutrition for surgical neonates: it is possible that cyclic TPN prevents intrahepatic cholestasis. *Tokushima J Exp Med.* 1990;37:97-102.
305. Hwang TL, Lue MC, Chen LL. Early use of cyclic TPN prevents further deterioration of liver functions for the TPN patients with impaired liver function. *Hepatogastroenterology.* 2000;47:1347-50.
306. Collier S, Crouch J, Hendricks K, Caballero B. Use of cyclic parenteral nutrition in infants less than 6 months of age. *Nutr Clin Pract.* 1994;9:65-68.
307. Moukarzel AA, Haddad I, Ament ME, et al. 230 patient years of experience with home long-term parenteral nutrition in childhood: natural history and life of central venous catheters. *J Pediatr Surg.* 1994;29:1323-1327.
308. Buchman AL, Moukarzel A, Goodson B, et al. Catheter related infections associated with home parenteral nutrition and predictive factors for the need for catheter removal in their treatment. *JPEN J Parenter Enteral Nutr.* 1994;18:297-302.
309. National Nosocomial Infections Surveillance (NNIS) System report, data summary from January 1992–June 2001, issued August 2001. *Am J Infect Control.* 2001;6:404-421.
310. O'Grady NP, Alexander M, Dellinger EP, et al. Guidelines for the prevention of intravascular catheter-related infections. Centers for Disease Control and Prevention. *MMWR Recomm Rep.* 2002;51:1-29.
311. Yogaraj JS, Elward AM, Fraser VJ. Rate, risk factors, and outcomes of nosocomial primary bloodstream infection in pediatric intensive care unit patients. *Pediatrics.* 2002;110:481-485.
312. Grohskopf LA, Sinkowitz-Cochran RL, Garrett DO, et al. A national point-prevalence survey of pediatric intensive care unit-acquired infections in the United States. *J Pediatr.* 2002;140:432-8.
313. O'Grady NP, Alexander M, Dellinger EP, et al. Guidelines for the Prevention of Intravascular Catheter-Related Infections. *Pediatrics.* 2002;110:e51.
314. Pearson ML. Guideline for prevention of intravascular device-related infections. Part I. Intravascular device-related infections: an overview. The Hospital Infection Control Practices Advisory Committee. *Am J Infect Control.* 1996;24:262-277.
315. Garcia MG, Poole RL, Rubin GD, Kerner JA Jr. Successful use of repeated ethanol injections to clear a central venous catheter occlusion after Urokinase failure. *J Pediatr Pharm Pract.* 1999;4:152-156.
316. http://www.pediatrics.org/cgi/content/full/110/5/e51. Accessed May 30, 2005.
317. Haire WD, Herbst SL. Use of Alteplase (t-PA) for the management of thrombotic catheter dysfunction: guidelines from a consensus of the National Association of Vascular Access Networks (NAVAN). *Nutr Clin Pract.* 2000;15:265-275.
318. Bern MM, Lokich JJ, Wallach SR, et al. Very low doses of warfarin can prevent thrombosis in central venous catheters. A randomized prospective trial. *Ann Intern Med.* 1990;112:423-8.
319. Bern MM, Bothe A, Bistrian B, et al. Prophylaxis against central vein thrombosis with low-dose warfarin. *Surgery.* 1986;99:216-21.
320. Ali A, Walentik C, Mantych GJ, et al. Iatrogenic acute hypermagnesemia after total parenteral nutrition infusion mimicking septic shock syndrome: two case reports. *Pediatrics.* 2003;112:e70-e72.
321. Weinsier RL, Krumdieck CL. Death resulting from overzealous total parenteral nutrition: the refeeding syndrome revisited. *Am J Clin Nutr.* 1981;34:393-399.
322. Crook MA, Hally V, Panteli JV. The importance of the refeeding syndrome. *Nutrition.* 2001;17:632-7.
323. Brooks MJ, Melnik G. The refeeding syndrome: an approach to understanding its complications and preventing its occurrence. *Pharmacotherapy.* 1995;15:713-26.
324. Shulman RJ, Philips S. Parenteral nutrition in infants and children. *J Pediatr Gastroenterol Nutr.* 2003;36:587-607.
325. Solomon SM, Kirby DF. The refeeding syndrome: a review. *JPEN J Parenter Enteral Nutr.* 1990;14:90-97.
326. Quigley EM, Marsh MN, Shaffer JL, Markin RS. Hepatobiliary complications of total parenteral nutrition. *Gastroenterology.* 1993;104:286-301.
327. Teitelbaum DH. Parenteral nutrition-associated cholestasis. *Curr Opin Pediatr.* 1997;9:270-5.
328. Buchman AL, Moukarzel A, Jenden DJ, Roche M, Rice K, Ament ME. Hepatic transferase abnormalities are associated with low plasma free choline in patients receiving long term parenteral nutrition. *Clin Nutr.* 1993;12:33-37.
329. Buchman AL, Dubin MD, Moukarzel AA, et al. Choline deficiency: a cause of hepatic steatosis during parenteral nutrition that can be reversed with intravenous choline supplementation. *Hepatology.* 1995;22:1399-1403.
330. Buchman AL, Jenden DJ, Moukarzel A, et al. Choline pharmacokinetics during intermittent intravenous choline infusion in human subjects. *Clin Pharmacol Therapeutics.* 1994;55:277-283.
331. Buchman AL, Sohel M, Moukarzel A, et al. Plasma choline in normal newborns, infants, toddlers, and in very-low-birth-weight neonates requiring total parenteral nutrition. *Nutrition.* 2001;17:18-21.
332. Sokol RJ. Total parenteral nutrition-related liver disease. *Acta Paed Sin.* 1997;38:418-28.
333. Brown MR, Thunberg BJ, Golub L, Maniscalco WM. Decreased cholestasis with enteral instead of intravenous protein in the very low-birth-weight infant. *J Pediatr Gastroenterol Nutr.* 1989;9:21-7.
334. Moss RL, Amii LA. New approaches to understanding the etiology and treatment of total parenteral nutrition-associated cholestasis. *Semin Pediatr Surg.* 1999;8:140-7.
335. Senger H, Boehm G, Beyreiss K, Braun W, Raiha N. Evidence for amino acid induced cholestasis in very-low-birth-weight infants with increasing enteral protein intake. *Acta Paediatr Scand.* 1986;75:724-8.
336. Kaufman SS. Prevention of parenteral nutrition-associated liver disease in children. *Pediatr Transplant.* 2002;6:37-42.
337. Ling PR, Sheikh M, Boyce P, et al. Cholecystokinin (CCK) secretion in patients with severe short bowel syndrome (SSBS). *Dig Dis Sci.* 2001;46:859-864.
338. Capron JP, Gineston JL. Herve MA. Metronidazole in prevention of cholestasis associated with total parenteral nutrition. *Lancet.* 1983;1:446-447.
339. Spagnuolo MI, Iorio R, Vegnente A, Guarino A. Ursodeoxycholic acid for the treatment of cholestasis in children on long term total parenteral nutrition: a pilot study. *Gastroenterology.* 1996;111:716-719.
340. Heudi JE, Weichmann DA, Creutzinger V, et al. Tauroursodeoxycholic acid (TUDCA) in the prevention of total parenteral nutrition-associated liver disease. *J Pediatr.* 2002;141;237-242.
341. Colomb V, Jobert-Giraud A, Maier-Redelsperger M, et al. Hematologic disorders following prolonged use of intravenous fat in children. *JPEN J Parenter Enteral Nutr.* 1986;10:284-288.
342. Anderson C, Danylchuk KD. The effect of chronic excess zinc administration on the Haversian bone remodelling system and its possible relationship to "Itai Itai" disease. *Environ Res.* 1979;20:351-357.

343. Moukarzel A, Ament ME, Vargas J, et al. Parenteral nutrition bone disease in children. *Clin Res.* 1990;38:190A.
344. Goodman WG, Lemann J, Lennon EJ, et al. Production, excretion and net balance of fixed acid in patients with renal acidosis. *J Clin Invest.* 1966;44:495-497.
345. Kim Y, Linkswiler HM. Effect of level of protein intake on calcium metabolism and on parathyroid and renal function in the adult human male. *J Nutr.* 1979;109:1399-1404.
346. Buchman AL, Moukarzel A. Metabolic bone disease associated with total parenteral nutrition. *Clin Nutr.* 2000;19:217-231.
347. Karton MA, Rettmer R, Lipkin EW, et al. D-Lactate and metabolic bone disease in patients receiving long-term parenteral nutrition. *JPEN J Parenter Enteral Nutr.* 1989;13:132-135.
348. Hurley DL, McMahon M. Long-term parenteral nutrition and metabolic bone disease. *Endocrinol Metab Clin North Am.* 1990;19:113-131.
349. Shike M, Sturtridge WC, Tam CS, et al. A possible role of vitamin D in the genesis of parenteral nutrition induced metabolic bone disease. *Ann Intern Med.* 1981;95:560-568.
350. Koo WW, Succop P, Hambidge KM. Serum alkaline phosphatase and serum zinc concentrations in preterm infants with rickets and fractures. *Am J Dis Child.* 1989;143:1342-1345.
351. Koo WW, Succop P, Hambidge KM. Sequential serum copper and ceruloplasmin concentrations in preterm infants with rickets and fractures. *Clin Chem.* 1991;37:556-559.
352. Moukarzel AA, Ament ME, Vargas J, McDiarmid S, Reyen L, Guss W. Is fluoride deficiency related to the bone disease of parenteral nutrition? (abstract). *Clin Nutr.* 1990;9:65.
353. Moukarzel A, Song MK, Vargas J, et al. Boron deficiency is not an etiological factor in the osteopenia of parenteral nutrition bone disease in children (abstract). *JPEN J Parenter Enteral Nutr.* 1992;16:31S.
354. Moukarzel A, Song MK, Haddad I, et al. Is silicon deficiency involved in the pathogenesis of metabolic bone disease of children receiving parenteral nutrition? (abstract). *JPEN J Parenter Enteral Nutr.* 1992;16-3S.
355. Moukarzel A, Ament M, Buchman A. Renal function of children receiving long term parenteral nutrition. *J Pediatr.* 1991;119:864-8.
356. Buchman AL, Moukarzel A, Ament ME, et al. Serious renal impairment is associated with long term parenteral nutrition. *JPEN J Parenter Enteral Nutr.* 1993;17:438-444.
357. Buchman AL, Moukarzel A, Ament ME. Excessive urinary oxalate excretion occurs in long-term TPN patients both with and without ileostomies. *J Am Coll Nutr.* 1995;14:24-28.
358. Vinton NE, Heckenlively JR, Laidlaw SA, et al. Visual function in patients undergoing long term total parenteral nutrition. *Am J Clin Nutr.* 1990;52:895-902.
359. Geggel HS, Ament ME, Heckenlively JR, Martin DA, Kopple JD. Nutritional requirement for taurine in patients receiving long-term parenteral nutrition. *New Engl J Med.* 1985;312:142-6.
360. Vinton NE, Laidlaw SA, Ament ME, Kopple JD. Taurine concentrations in plasma and blood cells of patients undergoing long term TPN. *Am J Clin Nutr.* 1986;44:398-404.
361. Vinton NE, Laidlaw SA, Ament ME, Kopple JD. Taurine concentrations in plasma, blood cells and urine of children undergoing long term TPN. *Pediatr Res.* 1987;21:399-403.
362. Buchman AL, Moukarzel AA, Eckhert C, Bhuta S, Mestecky J, Hollader D. The effects of total parenteral nutrition on intestinal morphology and function in man. *Transplantation Proc.* 1994;26:1457.
363. Buchman AL, Mestecky J, Moukarzel AA, Ament ME. Intestinal immune function is unaffected by parenteral nutrition in man. *J Am Coll Nutr.* 1995;14:656-661.
364. Buchman AL, Moukarzel AA, Bhuta S, et al. Parenteral nutrition is associated with intestinal morphologic and functional changes in humans. *JPEN J Parenter Enteral Nutr.* 1995;19:453-460.

Chapter 38

Complications of Long-Term Parenteral Nutrition

Alan L. Buchman, MD, MSPH

Survival

Most patients who require home parenteral nutrition (HPN) die from causes related to their underlying disease rather than as a complication of the parenteral nutrition (PN).[1,2] Survival is 87% at 1 year for patients that have benign gastrointestinal (GI) disorders (91%, 70%, and 62% survival at 1, 3, and 5 years[2]) although survival for patients with nonbenign (including malignancies and radiation enteritis) GI disorders is only 10% to 50% at 1 year.1 Survival is >90% for younger patients with Crohn's disease. PN-related complications with rehospitalization accounted for 5% of deaths in the USA (11% in France[2]).[1] PN-related complications occur approximately once a year except for patients with acquired immunodeficiency syndrome (AIDS), malignancy or hyperemesis gravidarum, where the incidence of PN-related complications is 3 to 4 times per year.[1] The death rate in patients who require HPN is unrelated to the length of residual bowel but is associated with the existence of either intestinal obstruction or pseudo-obstruction.[2] Several potentially serious complications may be encountered that may have significant impact on patient survival and morbidity. Complications related to PN are listed in Table 38-1.

Catheter-Related Complications

Catheter-Related Infections

The most commonly encountered catheter-related complication is infection. There are three types of catheter-related infections (Figure 38-1): 1) catheter sepsis, the most common[4]; 2) exit-site or cuff infection (erythema or purulence at the catheter skin exit site caused by an infection in the subcutaneous cuff that anchors the catheter); and 3) tunnel infections (erythema and tenderness over the subcutaneous catheter tract), the least common.

Catheter Sepsis

The diagnosis of early catheter sepsis often requires a high index of suspicion. The patients with catheter-related sepsis may present with fever or shortness of breath only during PN infusion or flushing of their catheter, prior to development of rigors, hypotension, and other systemic manifestations of sepsis. The patient must be trained to recognize these symptoms and, if present, to notify his or her physician immediately.

The algorithm in Figure 38-2 addresses the diagnosis and treatment of catheter-related infection. Blood cultures should be obtained from both the catheter and a peripheral vein. A blood smear should be examined for the presence of budding yeast[6] and blood fungal cultures obtained. It is important that sufficient blood be obtained for culture (10 to 20 mL).[5] Contaminated PN solutions are extremely rare in the United States, although, if that is suspected, an aliquot should be obtained from the patient's PN bag for culture. In general, therapy should be initiated in the hospital, although patients may be discharged home to complete their antimicrobial course as soon as they are stable. Sometimes, if the patient lives close to a medical facility and is otherwise stable, cultures can be obtained by home nurses and empiric antibiotics initiated at home. This is best done in patients who are familiar with the administration of home intravenous antibiotics.

Table 38-1.

Complications of Home Parenteral Nutrition

Infections	Metabolic Bone Disease
Catheter sepsis	Osteoporosis
	Osteomalacia
Exit-Site Infections	
Tunnel infections	Hepatic Dysfunction
	Hepatic steatosis
Catheter Occlusion	Cholestasis
Catheter thrombosis	Phospholipidosis
Pulmonary embolism	Hepatic failure
Superior/inferior venal cava syndrome	
Nonthrombotic occlusion (lipid or protein)	Biliary Disease
	Acalculous cholecystitis
Gastrointestinal	Gallstones
Gastroparesis	Calculous cholecystitis
Intestinal villus hypoplasia	
Renal	
Decreased glomerular filtration rate	
Tubular dysfunction	

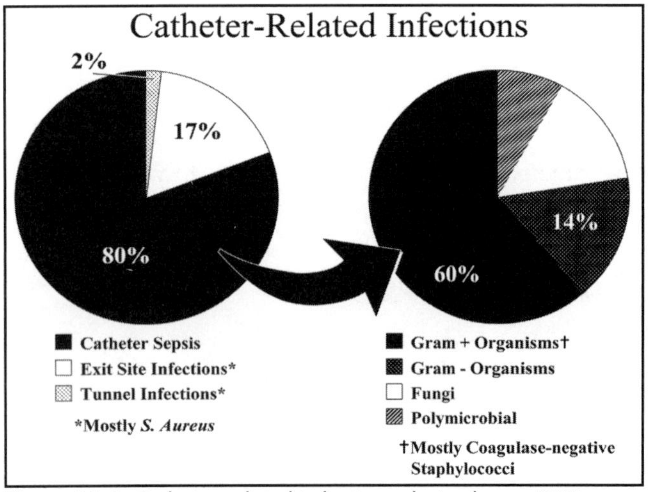

Figure 38-1. Catheter-related infections during home TPN. (Adapted from Buchman AL. Complications of long-term home total parenteral nutrition: their identification, prevention and treatment. *Dig Dis Sci.* 2001;46:1-18.)[3]

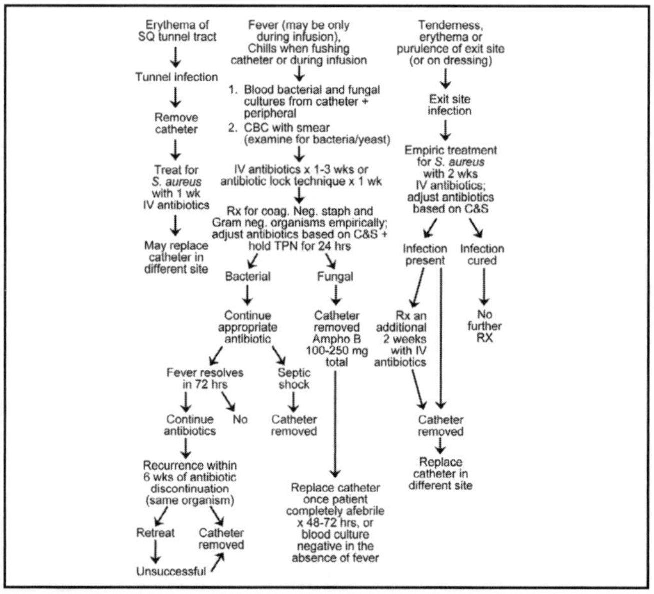

Figure 38-2. Suggested algorithm for the diagnosis and treatment of catheter-related infections. (Adapted from Buchman AL, Scolapio J, Fryer J. AGA technical review on short bowel syndrome and intestinal transplantation. *Gastroenterology.* 2003;124:1111-1134.)[5]

A single bacterial count of >100 cfu/mL from the catheter or a colony count ratio of 4:1 (central versus peripheral blood) is a reliable identifier of catheter sepsis.[8,9] However, the diagnosis must often be made on a clinical basis when other potential infection sources have been excluded, especially if blood cannot be obtained from the catheter and one is considering an attempt at catheter salvage. A large variety of organisms may cause catheter infections (see Figure 38-1). Most are gram-positive bacteria, although infection with gram-negative bacteria or fungi are frequent. Most exit-site and tunnel infections are caused by *Staphaloccocus* species.

Treatment of Catheter Sepsis

PN should be withheld for 24 hours (longer if the patient is unstable) to effect catheter sterilization and to prevent further bloodstream seeding. Intravenous fluids may be infused via a peripheral intravenous line. Aggressive initial antimicrobial therapy with broad spectrum antibiotics (such as vancomycin) and an aminoglycoside (such as gentamicin) may be useful in keeping the mortality rate low.[4] Therapy can be adjusted once blood culture results are available.[4,10-13] A convenient antimicrobial therapy regimen should be selected that can be administered once or twice daily (eg, before and after the PN infusion) to avoid excessive catheter manipulations, which are inconvenient and potentially invite the risk of yet another infection. The provider should select antimicrobial agents that are compatible with PN, although vigorous catheter flushing can be done before and after the medications are infused. It is recommended to continue antibiotic treatment for 4 weeks if the catheter remains in situ, although the supporting data are largely anecdotal.[4] Others have used a median of 7 days of intravenous antibiotic therapy and have reported a <10% recurrence.[14] Scaring may occur to the central vein with catheter removal and insertion and may ultimately lead to venous occlusion. Therefore, given that long-term HPN patients require life-long venous access, every attempt should be made to treat infections with the catheter in situ. However, catheter salvage should be attempted only for bacterial infections.

A major issue in the treatment of PN-related infections is catheter removal (see Figure 38-2). Most episodes of catheter sepsis can be treated successfully without catheter removal.[4,10-12,15] The catheter should always be removed with fungemia,[4,11,12,16] septic shock, or failure to defervesce and otherwise improve within 48 to 72 hours from the start of antibiotic therapy. Increased mortality may occur in patients for whom catheter removal is delayed when fungemia is present.[16,17] Catheter replacement may be undertaken once the patient has been completely afebrile for 48 to 72 hours. Catheter removal should be followed by 1 week of appropriate intravenous antibiotics, although there is little data on optimal treatment duration. Fungal infections generally require a total dose of 100 to 250 mg of Amphotericin B in addition to catheter removal.[4] There has been little experience with fluconazole and other antifungal treatment in this setting.[18]

The antibiotic lock technique, in which a highly concentrated antibiotic solution is instilled into the catheter in a volume sufficient only to fill the catheter, twice daily (eg, before and after PN infusion) for 1 to 2 weeks, has been described more recently for treatment of patients with uncomplicated catheter sepsis.[19-21] Success rates have been reported >90%, although treatment of fungemia has not generally been effective.[20] Amikacin (1.5 mg/mL), gentamicin (5 mg/mL), minocycline (0.2 mg/mL), and vancomycin (1.0 to 5.0 mg/mL) have been used. The antibiotic lock technique is much less expensive than the delivery of systemic antibiotics, appears to be more successful (although the currently available data are rather limited), and is more convenient for the patient.

Prevention of Catheter Sepsis

The risk of infection appears similar with either tunneled (Hickman/Broviac/Groshong-type) external catheters or an implanted reservoir catheter,[22,23] although two large, retrospective studies have suggested infection risk is increased in patients with implanted catheters.[24,25] However, infection risk is significantly greater when either multi-lumen catheters or nontunneled catheters (other than percutaneously-inserted central catheter or PICC) are used for PN delivery.[26-29] A tunneled catheter is inserted through the skin and "tunneled" subcutaneously for several centimeters until it is directed into the central vein. This helps inhibit bacteria and fungal translocation via the catheter into the bloodstream by providing a more difficult route for skin flora.

The infection risk may be greater when a needle-less catheter system is used,[30] although that probably relates to a hub design that permits infusion solution or blood to remain in the injection cap where it may become contaminated, either by skin flora or during the catheter preparation for use.

The infection rate is greater in children, most likely because of a child's inability to effect good catheter care and greater chance for contamination of the exit site.[4] (PN for pediatric patients is discussed in Chapter 37.) Infection rates are also significantly greater in patients with AIDS.[4,31] This might be related to immunosuppression, although patients who have undergone recent chemotherapy or bone-marrow transplant patients who use a similar catheter-care protocol as that of patients with AIDS do not appear to have such an increased infection risk.[4,31] There is no data on the incidence of central venous catheter infection in patients with AIDS in the era of antiretroviral therapy.

Prophylactic antibiotic infusion prior to invasive procedures on the basis of an indwelling catheter does not prevent subsequent catheter infection and is, therefore, not recommended.[32]

Catheter Care

Catheter care technique is arguably the most important determinant of the risk of catheter infection.[4,29,32] Contamination of the catheter skin exit site[33] and catheter hub 32 to 34 are the primary sources for infections. Proper cleaning of these sites is essential. Evidence suggests that the nurse or patient's hand may contaminate both the exit site and catheter hub during catheter manipulations, including connecting or disconnecting PN.[37] Even a single inoculum may be sufficient to result in catheter sepsis for virulent organisms such as *Pseudomonas aeruginosa*.[38] Endoluminal bacterial seeding begins with hub contamination at the junction between the catheter and infusion line.[39] Luer locks themselves have no antibacterial properties and require strict aseptic manipulation. Improvement in catheter hub care results in significantly decreased infection risk.[36] This includes avoidance of three-way stopcocks because of the risk of hub contamination.[40,41]

Exit-Site and Tunnel Infections

Most exit-site and tunnel infections are caused by skin flora, most notably *Staphylococcus* species.[4] Purulent drainage from the exit site should be cultured and initial therapy provided with intravenous vancomycin until culture results are available.[4,45] Neither exit-site or tunnel infections are systemic infections, and they are rarely associated with fever or leukocytosis. However, delayed treatment may lead to more serious sequelae. Duration of therapy has been recommended for 2 weeks, although the data are largely anecdotal.[4] Most exit-site infections can be treated successfully without catheter removal;[4,10-12,15] however, antibiotic penetration of the subcutaneous tunnel is suboptimal. Therefore, catheter removal is required for tunnel infections.

Prevention of Exit-Site and Tunnel Infections

As with the prevention of catheter sepsis, exit-site care is the most reliable determinant of infection risk. Newly designed hubs and connection devices, not currently

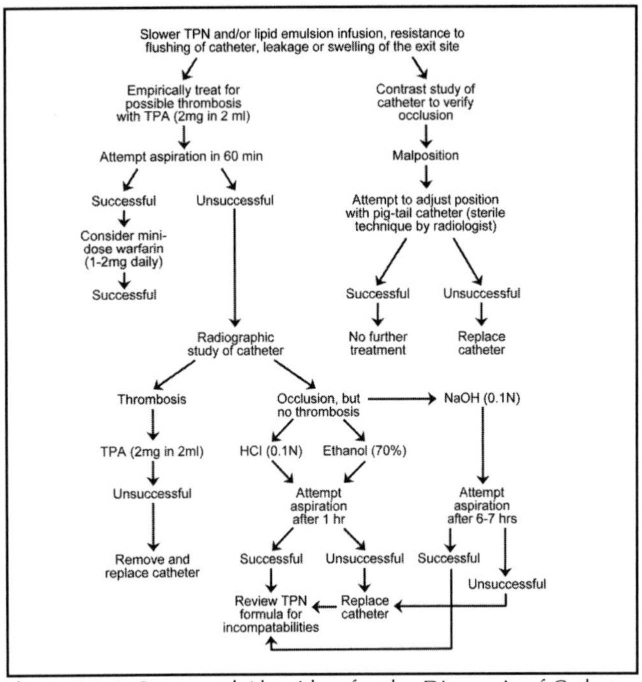

Figure 38-3. Suggested Algorithm for the Diagnosis of Catheter-Related Occlusion (thrombotic and nonthrombotic). (Adapted from Buchman AL, Scolapio J, Fryer J. AGA technical review on short bowel syndrome and intestinal transplantation. *Gastroenterology.* 2003;124:1111-1134.)[5]

available in the USA, have been associated with a lower incidence of infection,[43-45] although an antibiotic-impregnated catheter cuff was not.[46] Regardless of how good the equipment or the technique are, catheter-related infection is most easily avoided if the catheter is not used for anything other than PN.[47] In the rare absence of a peripheral vein for medication delivery, the catheter must be prepared aseptically each time, prior to medication injection.

Catheter Dressings and Dressing Changes

Less frequent dressing changes and the use of gauze rather than transparent polyurethane dressings have been associated with a lower risk for catheter infection.[48-53] Increased bacterial colonization was noted under the transparent dressings, which may result in part from moisture accumulation under such dressings. These data are from inpatient populations. There have been no studies on the optimal frequency for dressing changes in HPN patients who have tunneled or peripherally inserted catheters. Similarly, no studies have compared gauze to transparent dressings in HPN patients. It is unclear if the results from inpatient studies can be generalized to this patient group.

Catheter Occlusions

Occlusions are the second most common catheter-related problem. These may occur because of thrombus, precipitate formation, or mechanical problems (Figure 38-3).

Thrombosis

Thrombosis generally results from disruption of the intimal surface of the vein followed by development of a fibrin sheath around the catheter.[54,55] Although catheter thrombosis is relatively uncommon, if unrecognized and untreated, it may lead to the need for catheter removal and long-term loss of a venous access site. Over time (>10 years in some cases), thrombosed veins may recanalize. The incidence of catheter thrombosis is greater in some patients, such as those with a history of mesenteric venous thrombosis, and the incidence of subclinical catheter thrombosis may be much greater.[56-58] However, it is unknown whether blood clots found on routine, scheduled catheter checks result in development of clinically significant thromboses.

Superior vena cava (SVC) or inferior vena cava (IVC) syndrome is a rare (incidence of 0.02 to 0.04/catheter year)[59-61] but serious sequela of catheter thrombosis. One study showed that 68% of patients with SVC or IVC syndrome had at least a single prior catheter thrombosis, and nearly 40% of patients who developed catheter thrombosis subsequently developed SVC/IVC syndrome.[59] Intracardiac thrombosis has also been reported and is related to catheter tip position in the right atrium.[61,62] Pulmonary embolism is a rare complication of catheter thrombosis.[62-65]

Very low dose warfarin (1 to 2 mg daily) does not alter the prothrombin time or a partial thromboplastin time but may prevent catheter thrombosis.[66,67] This may be related to incomplete but critical inhibition of vitamin K-dependent factors.[68-70] Patients who develop catheter thrombosis despite low-dose warfarin should be fully anticoagulated as long as they require HPN.[70,71] Anticoagulation may require increased warfarin for patients who receive more lipid emulsion because vitamin K is intrinsically contained in lipid emulsions.[72] Vitamin K-containing multivitamins should not be administered to patients who require warfarin anticoagulation. Long-term heparin use is not recommended because of the risk of osteoporosis,[73] although low-molecular weight heparin may have less detrimental effects on bone than will unfractionated heparin.[74] Intravenous heparin is incompatible with lipid emulsion (3-in-1 emulsions),[75] although catheter flushing with heparin 100 U/mL (0.6 to 3 mL, depending on the catheter volume) is recommended.[76,77] There is limited data on the use of low-molecular weight heparin in HPN patients.

Catheter thrombosis may be treated using urokinase (5000 U/mL, 2 mL for tunneled catheters and 1 mL for ports)[78,79] or tissue plasminogen activator (TPA, 2 mg/ml, 2 ml for tunneled catheters and 1 mL for ports) (see Figure 39-3).[80,81] If medical treatment is unsuccessful, removal and replacement of the catheter in another site are necessary. Thrombosed veins may recanalize over several years, and it may be possible to reuse a former site for catheter placement.

Nonthrombotic Occlusion

Up to 50% of nonthrombotic occlusions may be related to mechanical problems with the catheter. These include catheter migration from the SVC or IVC into a smaller vessel, damage to the catheter,[55,79,82] medication-PN incompatibilities leading to precipitation within the catheter,[83-87] and lipid deposition within the catheter.[88,89] Hydrochloric acid dissolves some mineral and medication precipitates that form because of low calcium/phosphate solubility in PN solutions. This occurs most frequently when medications that have a low pKa are used in the

PN solutions.[83-87] Sodium hydroxide (0.1 N) may also dissolve some mineral precipitates, although it may require up to 6 to 7 hours after instillation into the catheter before any attempt at aspiration can be made.[87] Ethanol may be used to dissolve waxy lipid deposits around the catheter (see Figure 38-3).[86,88]

It is often difficult to determine whether a catheter occlusion is thrombotic or nonthrombotic in origin, although lipid-based precipitates generally have a more gradual onset than thrombosis. Lipid occlusions also generally occur in association with the use of 3-in-1 emulsions and not when lipids are infused separately from the dextrose/amino acid components of PN.[89,90]

Renal Complications

PN-associated nephropathy is the most recent systemic complication of long-term PN described.[91-93] Creatinine clearance declines by approximately 3.5% per year in adults.[91] The etiology of this decline is unknown, but age, nephrotoxic drug use, and previous bloodstream infections are all contributing factors.[91] Tubular function is also impaired in adults,[91] although not necessarily in children.[92] Short-term PN leads to dramatically increased creatinine clearance, probably because of glomerular hyperfiltration, and nephromegaly may result.[94,95] Glomerular sclerosis could result over the long term.

No correlation has been found between the decline in renal function and intravenous amino acid intake in either adults or children.[91,92] Excessive chromium infusion (primarily in the form of contaminates in the PN solutions) is associated with decreased renal function in children[96] but not in adults.[91,97] Chromium deposited to a significant degree in a rodent PN model and was associated with renal tubular abnormalities.[98] Cadmium and other heavy metal contaminants in PN do not appear to play a role.[97]

Hyperoxaluria occurs in adult HPN patients and probably children as well.[99,100] Despite increasing the risk for nephrolithiasis, there is no correlation with renal dysfunction.[99] The hyperoxaluria may be related to endogenous production from vitamin C contained in PN solutions.[100] PN solution acidity may contribute as well.[91]

Gastrointestinal Complications

Gastroparesis

Studies in normal volunteers have demonstrated that intravenous infusion of long-chain-triglyceride–based emulsions will delay gastric emptying, although it is unclear whether this results in clinically significant sequelae such as early satiety.[101] The etiology for this finding is unknown. Hyperglycemia may also cause gastroparesis as well as decreased gastric and pancreatic secretions.[102,103]

Intestinal Hypoplasia

Although intestinal villus hypoplasia (not atrophy) has been well described in rodent models of PN, it has not been observed to a similar degree in humans.[104-108] Slight, but statistically significant decreases in jejunal villus height have been observed in some, although not all studies;[104-107] these changes were not clinically significant. Crypt depth remains unchanged.[104-106] Similarly, no decrease in intestinal villus height was observed in obese volunteers who were starved for 2 weeks[107,109] or in the excluded jejunal or ileal segments of patients who had either jejunal or ileal bypasses 3.5 to 6 years previous.[110] Virtually all HPN patients eat something; many have hyperphagia. Therefore, the intestinal changes related to the lack of luminal nutrients would be unlikely to occur in HPN patients.

Intestinal permeability to macromolecules increases in volunteers who receive PN and no oral food intake, although this observation was unrelated to changes in intestinal morphology.[104,108] The etiology or clinical significance of the increase in intestinal permeability remains unknown. Some patients develop intercellular edema, although both the relationship with increased intestinal permeability and clinical significance are speculative. There is little data to support any functional impairment of the GI tract during PN. Although Guedon et al observed a decrease in duodenal disaccharidase concentrations after 2 to 3 weeks of PN,[105] no functional deficit has been observed.[104] Contrary to animal studies, PN is not associated with intestinal immune dysfunction.[111,112]

Metabolic Bone Disease

PN-associated metabolic bone disease was first described by Shike et al and Klein et al separately in 1980.[113,114] Many factors may be involved, including lifestyle and the underlying diseases (Table 38-2). Its prevalence is unknown but may be as great as 40% to 100%.[115]A relationship with body mass index and age at HPN onset has been shown.[116] Patients may be asymptomatic or may manifest bone and back pain or fractures (usually vertebral). The disease may manifest in osteomalacia with excessive organic bone matrix, in osteoporosis with decreased bone mass where bone formation is exceeded by bone resorption but bone mineralization and osteoid content remain normal, or in a combination of both osteomalacia and osteoporosis. Low trabecular bone density (lumbar spine), measured either by quantitative computed tomography or dual-energy absorptiometry, signifies increased fracture risk. Bone biopsy following double tetracycline labeling (to determine if bone formation is decreased and if osteoid is increased) may also be useful in the diagnosis if osteomalacia is suspected.

Metabolic bone disease associated with PN was originally characterized by transient hypercalciuria, high normal plasma 25 hydroxyvitamin D3 [$25(OH_2)D_3$], hypercalcemia, either normal or low serum parathyroid hormone (PTH) concentration (although Klein et al reported normal to elevated PTH[114]), and negative calcium balance with normal serum phosphorus with increased osteoid and decreased mineralization evident on bone biopsy.[117] Decreased serum 1,25 dihydroxyvitamin D3 [$1,25(OH_2)D_3$] concentration has also occasionally been reported.[117]

(Metabolic bone disease in patients with GI disease is discussed in detail in Chapter 13 of this text. Methods for assessing body composition, including measurement for bone density, are discussed in Chapter 2.)

Table 38-2.

Parenteral Nutrition Associated Metabolic Bone Disease

Nutrient Deficiencies	
Minerals:	copper, calcium, fluoride, phosphorous, silicon
Vitamins:	D, K
Hormones:	androgens, estrogen, hyperparathyroidism, hypoparathyroidism
Toxicities	
Metals:	aluminum, strontium
Vitamins:	A, D
Medications:	acetate, corticosteroids, cyclosporine, diuretics, heparin, tacrolimus, theophylline, warfarin, excessive amino acid infusion
Other:	acidosis, underlying disease, sedentary lifestyle, cigarette smoking

Potential Etiologies

Hypercalciuria may reflect the cycled nature of HPN, increased bone resorption, excessive amino acid infusion, vitamin A toxicity, or hyperinsulinemia.[118-120] Increasing the phosphorous concentration in the PN may reduce the hypercalciuria,[121] although care must be provided to avoid calcium precipitation. Most current adult PN solutions contain a standard phosphate concentration of 10 to 15 mmol/L (usually 30 to 45 mmol/day), which is less than is recommended based on balance studies[122] and that concentration used by Wood et al to treat hypercalciuria.[121]

Chronic acidosis has also been associated with both hypercalciuria and metabolic bone disease,[123-126] although one of the treatments for chronic acidosis (acetate) itself has been associated with osteoblast proliferation inhibition in vitro.[127] However, other studies have shown that treatment of chronic acidosis with acetate (replacement of 160 mmol Cl with 160 mmol Ac) leads to decreased hypercalciuria.[128]

Aluminum toxicity—manifested by elevated plasma, urine, and bone aluminum concentrations and by low turnover bone disease—was once found to be a significant contributor to the development of PN-associated osteomalacia.[129,130] Reduced bone formation and reduced serum 1,25(OH_2)D_3 concentration is characteristic of aluminum bone toxicity.[129-131] Casein protein hydrolysate was once the source of amino acids for the PN solutions, but significant aluminum contamination was present. By mid 1981, these solutions were discontinued and crystalline-free amino-acid–based formulas were substituted. Studies showed that this substitution resulted in increased bone formation.[131,132] Reduction in the degree of aluminum contamination was also associated with increased serum 1,25(OH_2)D_3.[131]

Although aluminum contamination has been reduced significantly, other PN components—including sodium phosphate, calcium gluconate, and multivitamins—still contain rather large concentrations of aluminum, although their contribution to the overall PN solution is fairly small.[133] Unfortunately, low bone formation characterized by low bone mineral content continues to be a problem in some, but not all, HPN patients, despite the lack of significant aluminum exposure.[132,134-137] In addition, there remain a few patients who have received HPN since the time prior to introduction of the crystalline-free amino-acid solutions.

Other potential causes of metabolic bone disease in patients requiring HPN include their underlying disorder[135,138] (eg, dehydration, primary hyperparathyroidism, hypoparathyroidism, which are often related to magnesium deficiency from chronic diarrheal losses, vitamin D malabsorption, cytokine activity in active Crohn's disease, or connective tissue disease) and medication-induced osteopenia from corticosteroids, methotrexate, cyclosporine, or tacrolimus, which may be used in the therapy of the underlying disorder. Plasma fluoride concentration correlates significantly with bone mineral density in children who require long-term HPN, although there are no studies with fluoride supplementation that have been undertaken in HPN patients.[139]

Shike suggested that the vitamin D in the multivitamin preparations used in PN may have a toxic effect on bone.[113,140] Hypercalciuria decreased in three patients who had vitamin D withdrawn from their PN solutions, and osteomalacia improved in one of the patients who had follow-up bone biopsies.[113] However, the patients may have had secondary hyperparathyroidism prior to beginning PN, a disease in which bone mineralization is impaired but osteoid formation is increased.[140] In a subsequent study, Shike et al found significant aluminum contamination was present in these patients' PN (based on the likelihood at least some patients received casein hydrolysate during their early days of PN), although only 3 of 12 had positive aluminum bone staining.[140] Bone biopsies of these patients showed reduced osteoid and total bone volume (consistent with decreased bone matrix formation and normal mineralization) with normal resorption activity, although osteoid and mineralization were reportedly normal in patients with positive aluminum staining. This contrasts with the previously described studies in which osteoid was increased and mineralization decreased in association with low serum vitamin D and PTH concentrations. In the Shike study, serum 25(OH_2)D_3 and 1,25(OH_2)D_3, calcium and PTH concentrations were all within the normal ranges, although the serum aluminum concentration was elevated.[140] In addition, a decrease in the osteoid area with a concurrent increase in bone mineralization was described in patients who were switched from casein-based amino acids to crystalline amino acids.[131]

Others have found a significant correlation between serum 1,25(OH_2)D_3 and biochemical measures of bone formation in patients who did not receive significant aluminum, suggesting that increased serum 1,25(OH_2)D_3 may stimulate bone formation, rather than depress it.[142] However, long-term (4.5 years) vitamin D withdrawal in patients with depressed serum PTH and 1,25(OH_2)D_3 only has been associated with a significant increase in lumbar bone mineral density and normalization of both PTH and 1,25(OH_2)D_3.[143] PN-associated bone disease and the role of vitamin D remain poorly understood.

Potential Therapies

There is little data on the treatment of PN-associated metabolic bone disease. Two small studies have suggested intermittent intravenous biphosphonate therapy may increase bone metabolism disease in some patients.[144,145]

There is no data on the use of additional vitamin D supplementation, calcitonin, PTH, or even a home-based, low-impact exercise program for the treatment of PN-associated metabolic bone disease. Given the heterogeneous nature of this disease, it is unlikely that any of these potential therapies will be useful for all patients with PN-associated metabolic bone disease. However, intravenous biphosphonates should probably be administered to patients with osteopenia and who have no evidence of osteomalacia. Oral calcium supplements (1000 to 1500 mg daily) may be useful. Serum 25(OH_2)D_3 concentration should be measured at least yearly, and serum PTH and testosterone concentrations should be determined if clinically appropriate. Long-term heparin therapy should be avoided, although long-term use of warfarin, because of its vitamin K antagonistic effects, may also be problematic. Any underlying inflammatory diseases should receive optimal therapy. Finally, regular exercise and smoking cessation should be encouraged. For a more in depth review of PN-associated metabolic bone disease, the reader is referred to Buchman and Moukarzel's review.[146]

Hepatic Disease

Liver Test Abnormalities and Morphologic Changes

PN-associated liver disease was first described in 1971.[147] Different centers have reported the development of end-stage liver disease in 15% to 40% in their adult HPN patient population; the prevalence is greater in neonates.[148-150] The association between hepatic aminotransferase abnormalities and PN has been well documented, and three distinctive morphologic abnormalities in the liver have been described. It is important to realize, however, that liver test abnormalities are nonspecific and insensitive indicators for specific hepatic morphologic lesions,[151] and therefore non-PN or intestinal failure-related causes of hepatic abnormalities should be sought out. Serum hepatic aminotransferase concentrations often become elevated within 4 to 7 weeks of PN initiation and may remain elevated as long as PN is continued.[152,153] In adult patients, serum bilirubin elevation is unusual,[154] but it is more common in infants. The increase in serum alkaline phosphatase may be related in part to metabolic bone disease and not liver disease alone.[114] Alkaline phosphatase isoenzyme concentrations can be determined. Liver function during PN has not been evaluated in humans. Morphologic abnormalities in adults include steatosis (macro- and microvesicular, Figure 38-4) and cholestasis (Figure 38-5), either of which may progress to fibrosis (Figure 38-6) and cirrhosis, and phospholipidosis. PN-associated liver disease in adults usually manifests as hepatic steatosis or steatohepatitis,[151,155-157] although this may be progressive with subsequent development of cirrhosis and hepatic failure.[158-164] Frank cholestasis, manifested morphologically in ballooning of hepatocytes, Kupffer cell hyperplasia, and bile duct plugging, is uncommon in adults, although the incidence appears to be increasing. Patients with the shortest residual intestine[2,159] and those patients who are infused moderate and larger doses of lipid emulsion (>1.0 g/kg/day)[148,149,158] appear particularly at risk.

Possible Etiologies

This observation that patients with the shortest residual intestine are at greatest risk for development of significant hepatic abnormalities[2,159] suggests the likelihood of either severe malabsorption or the level of PN dependence as the most likely causes for PN-associated liver disease. Carbohydrate overfeeding (primarily with dextrose) was once a common cause of benign hepatic steatosis (although severe steatosis with hepatomegaly may be painful) in an era of overfeeding when patients were routinely provided with 50 to 60 kcal/kg/day.[164,165] This is much less likely when patients receive 25 to 40 kcal/kg/day of energy.

Because the widespread use of lipid emulsions became popular in the early 1980s, essential fatty acid deficiency in patients with intestinal failure who require PN has become uncommon. However, such patients must receive a minimum of 2% to 4% of their calories as linoleic fatty acid (eg, 4% to 8% of daily calories as lipid emulsion) to prevent essential fatty acid deficiency.[166,168] A plasma triene:tetrene ratio >0.4171 or a low plasma linoleic fatty acid concentration is indicative of biochemical fatty acid deficiency and can develop as early as 2 weeks following withdrawal of lipids.[164] Clinical signs may include skin rash, neuropathy, hepatosplenomegaly, and thrombocytopenia.

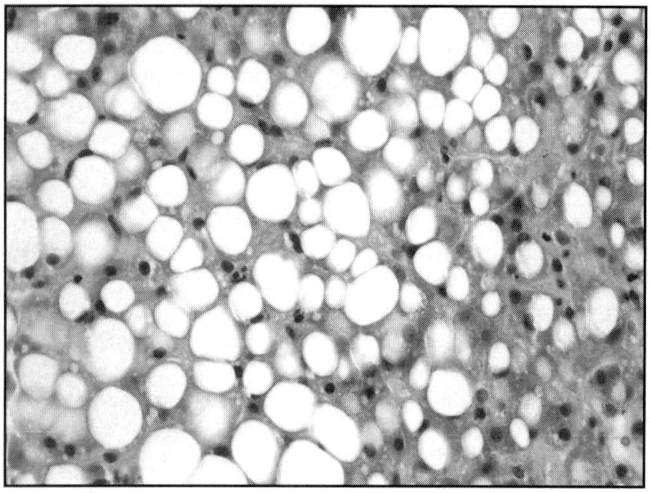

Figure 38-4. Macro- and microsteatosis of the liver associated with PN. (Courtesy of Dr. Sambasiva Rao of Northwestern University Medical School, Chicago, IL.)

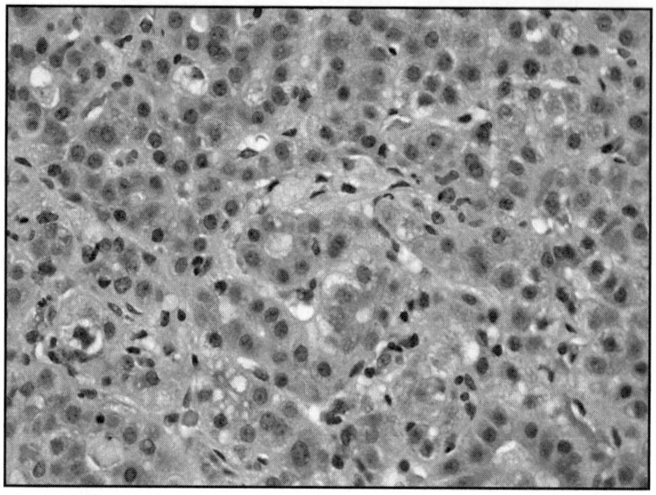

Figure 38-5. Cholestasis associated with PN. (Courtesy of Dr. Sambasiva Rao of Northwestern University Medical School, Chicago, IL.)

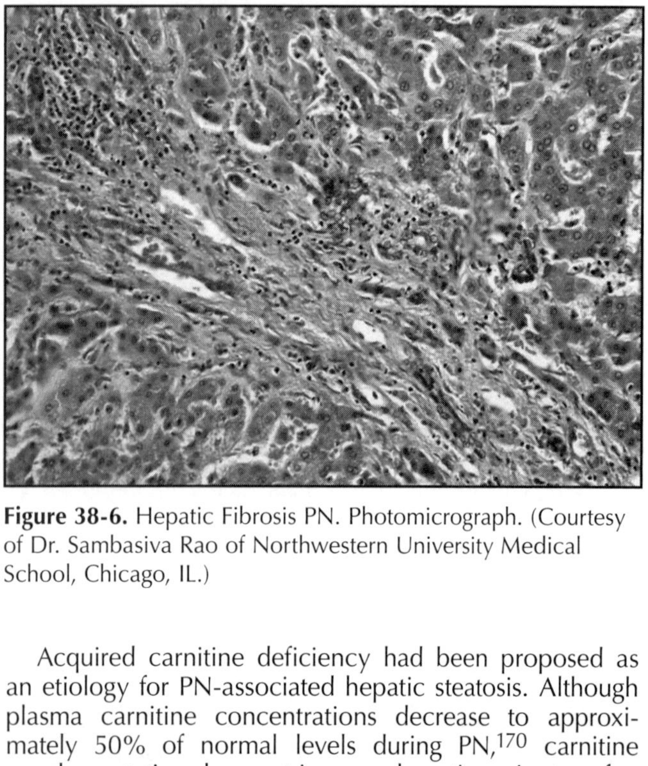

Figure 38-6. Hepatic Fibrosis PN. Photomicrograph. (Courtesy of Dr. Sambasiva Rao of Northwestern University Medical School, Chicago, IL.)

Acquired carnitine deficiency had been proposed as an etiology for PN-associated hepatic steatosis. Although plasma carnitine concentrations decrease to approximately 50% of normal levels during PN,[170] carnitine supplementation does not improve hepatic aminotransferase abnormalities, the degree of hepatic steatosis, or lipid utilization in PN-requiring patients.[171,172] Despite these data, carnitine supplementation is routinely provided to patients in some institutions. Carnitine can be synthesized from the amino acids lysine and methionine contained in the PN solutions.

Low plasma free choline concentration has been observed in most patients who require PN.[157,173-177] Significant correlations exists between both hepatic aminotransferase concentrations and degree of hepatic steatosis as well as with the plasma free choline concentration.[157,173-177] Choline is required for very low density lipoprotein (VLDL) synthesis. When VLDL synthesis is insufficient, defective triglyceride transport from the liver becomes impaired.[178,179] Hepatocellular carcinoma, possibly related to choline deficiency, has also been reported.[180,183] Massive lecithin (13% choline) doses led to a significant increase in plasma free choline concentration and a corresponding, but incomplete, decrease in hepatic steatosis in a study of HPN patients with hepatic steatosis.[157]

Whether or not manganese toxicity occurs and contributes to cholestasis is unclear.[183,184] Manganese is excreted via the biliary system, and elevated serum manganese concentration may simply reflect underlying hepatic abnormalities. It has been proposed that plant sterols contained in lipid emulsion may lead to phytosterolemia when large doses of lipid emulsion are infused (>1.4 g/kg/day) in children, although the serum concentration of phytosterols did not necessarily correspond to the amount of lipid emulsion infused.[185] In three of the five patients with severe hepatic dysfunction, total serum bilirubin and aspartate aminotransferase concentrations decreased in parallel with a decrease in the plasma phytosterol concentration, which followed a decrease in the volume of lipid infused. Further study is warranted. Phospholipidosis has also been rarely described following prolonged infusion of lipid emulsion.[186]

Potential Therapies

In a preliminary study, intravenous choline supplementation restored plasma-free choline concentrations to normal and ameliorated hepatic steatosis.[173] A double-blinded, placebo-controlled trial of choline-supplemented PN confirmed the findings of the previous open-label study and showed significant improvements in hepatic aminotransferase abnormalities.[177] It appears choline may be an essential nutrient for PN-dependent patients, although it is currently undergoing further testing and is not commercially available.

There are few treatment options for PN-associated cholestasis. Copper and manganese are excreted via the biliary system and therefore should not be provided to patients who have significant cholestasis or hepatic dysfunction. Phenobarbital and antibiotics such as gentamicin are useless.[187,188] Some studies have shown ursodeoxycholic acid (UCDA) at a dose of 10 to 45 mg/kg/day to significantly improve cholestasis in preterm infants whereas others have shown less impressive results.[189,190] Data in adults are limited to a study of 10 patients who had generally limited improvement when treated with UCDA (6 to 15 mg/kg/day).[191,192] Cholecystokinin (0.04 ug/kg bid) injections were associated with numerically, but not significantly lower, serum direct bilirubin concentration in neonates who required PN.[193] This has not been studied in adults. Tauroursodeoxycholic acid was not useful for the prevention of PN-associated liver disease in a study of 22 infants.[194] Similarly, two randomized trials of taurine-supplemented versus standard neonatal PN showed the former failed to prevent PN-associated liver disease.[195,196] One retrospective study suggested hepatic aminotransferase abnormalities were less severe in patients who received metronidazole.[197] Combined liver-small intestinal transplantation may be the only potentially viable option for a patient with PN-associated hepatic failure. However, in patients with early fibrosis but no evidence of cirrhosis, isolated intestinal transplantation may be useful for the prevention of further liver abnormalities, although fibrosis remains unchanged.[198]

Biliary Disease

HPN patients are at risk for both acalculous and calculous cholecystitis.[199] Acalculous cholecystitis occurs because of decreased food-mediated cholecystokinin (CCK) release, which results in decreased gallbladder.[200,201] Narcotic use, bile stasis, and increased bile lithogenecity may decrease gallbladder contraction.[200-202] Massive gallbladder dilation may develop; percutaneous cholecystostomy is required for drainage. The gallbladder dysmotility and abnormal emptying during PN may result in false positive iminodiacetic (IDA) hepatic scintigraphy,[203-205] although the use of an intravenous morphine bolus injection may improve scan specificity.[204] Patients should be encouraged to eat on a daily basis—to ensure adequate gallbladder emptying and to help prevent development of cholecystitis—even if they are completely PN-dependent because of severe malabsorption.

Biliary sludge develops in 50% of patients following 4 to 6 weeks of PN and in virtually 100% of patients after 6 weeks of PN.[205,206] Some of these patients will ultimately develop gallstones. However, sludge resolves in virtually all patients after 4 weeks of enteral/oral refeeding.[205] Gallbladder stasis may be the most important risk factor for the development of gallstones, which is similar to acalculous cholecystitis.[207,208] However, most gallstones found in patients who receive long-term PN are calcium-bilirubinate in composition, rather than cholesterol.[209-211] This suggests the possibility that a chronic infectious process involving the biliary tree may play a role in the stone formation, although the exact etiology for pigmented stones is uncertain.[212]

CCK injections have been used to induce gallbladder contraction and reduce the prevalence of biliary sludge.[213-215] However, this treatment is not universally successful and has been associated with cholecystitis, nausea, and flushing in some patients.[214-216] Rapid, high-dose intravenous amino-acid infusions (0.3 to 2.1 g/minutes versus 0.12 to 0.14 g/minutes for cyclic HPN patients) have also been used to stimulate gallbladder contraction.[217,218] However, this approach is clinically impractical, and lower amino acid infusion rates do not generally stimulate gallbladder contraction.[218] Relatively rapid infusion of lipid emulsion (10% emulsion for 100 mL/hour for 3 hours) also stimulates gallbladder contraction and may be useful preventative therapy.[219,220] This may be mediated via CCK release,[221] although presumably the effect would be centrally mediated. Intravenous chenodeoxycholate infusion has shown promise in the prairie dog model for the prevention of calcium bilrubinate gallstones, although it has not been studied in humans.[222] The prevention of calculous cholecystitis still remains suboptimal in HPN patients, which has led some to recommend prophylactic cholecystectomy in patients. The best and least expensive means to prevent cholecystitis in HPN patients is to simply encourage patients to eat.

Conclusion

Patients who require long-term PN have impressive survival when compared with small bowel transplantation. However, both survival and morbidity are significantly affected by potentially serious complications related to the use of long-term PN. These complications may result from nutrient deficiencies, nutrient excesses, and/or mechanical problems associated with the delivery system. Infectious complications, the most common, are often related to insufficient patient or caregiver education, which results in suboptimal catheter care. The etiology and prognosis of other complications (such as metabolic bone disease, nephropathy, and hepatobiliary disease) are more obscure and are, therefore, challenging to manage appropriately.

References

1. Howard L, Ament M, Fleming CR, Shike M, Steiger E. Current use and clinical outcome of home parenteral and enteral nutrition therapies in the United States. *Gastroenterology.* 1995;109:355-365.
2. Messing B, Lemann M, Landais P, et al. Prognosis of patients with nonmalignant chronic intestinal failure receiving long-term home parenteral nutrition. *Gastroenterology.* 1995;108:1005-1010.
3. Buchman AL. Complications of long-term home total parenteral nutrition: their identification, prevention and treatment. *Dig Dis Sci.* 2001;46:1-18.
4. Buchman AL, Moukarzel A, Goodson B, et al. Catheter-related infections associated with home parenteral nutrition and predictive factors for the need for catheter removal in their treatment. *JPEN J Parenter Enteral Nutr.* 1994;18:297-302.
5. Buchman AL, Scolapio J, Fryer J. AGA technical review on short bowel syndrome and intestinal transplantation. *Gastroenterology.* 2003;124:1111-1134.
6. Buchman AL, Lee S, Miller J, Valdecantos A. Candida fungemia diagnosed from peripheral blood smear. *JAMA.* 1988;260:2926.
7. Mermel LA, Maki DG. Detection of bacteremia in adults: consequences of culturing an inadequate volume of blood. *Ann Intern Med.* 1993;119:270-272.
8. Mosca R, Curtas S, Forbes B, Meguid MM. The benefits of isolator cultures in the management of suspected catheter sepsis. *Surgery.* 1987;102:718-723.

9. Capdevila JA, Planes AM, Palomar M, et al. Value of differential quantitative blood cultures in the diagnosis of catheter-related sepsis. *Eur J Microbiol Infect Dis.* 1992;11:403-407.
10. Johnson PR, Decker MD, Edwards KM, Schaffner W, Wright PF. Frequency of broviac catheter infections in pediatric oncology patients. *J Infect Dis.* 1986;154:570-578.
11. Widmer AF. Management of catheter-related bacteremia and fungemia in patients on total parenteral nutrition. *Nutrition.* 1997;13:18S-25S.
12. Wang EE, Prober CG, Ford-Jones L, Gold R. The management of central intravenous catheter infections. *Pediatr Infect Dis.* 1984;3:110-113.
13. Prince A, Heller B, Levy J, Heird WC. Management of fever in patients with central vein catheters. *Pediatr Infect Dis.* 1986;5:20-24.
14. Rannem T, Ladefoged K, Tvede M, Lorentzen JE, Jarnum S. Catheter-related septicaemia in patients receiving home parenteral nutrition. *Scand J Gastroenterol.* 1986;21:455-460.
15. King DR, Komer M, Hoffman J, et al. Broviac catheter sepsis: the natural history of an iatrogenic infection. *J Pediatr Surg.* 1985;20:728-733.
16. Lecciones JA, Lee JW, Navarro EE, et al. Vascular catheter-associated fungemia in patients with cancer: analysis of 155 episodes. *Clin Infect Dis.* 1992;14:875-883.
17. Dato VM, Dajani AS. Candidemia in children with central venous catheters: role of catheter removal and amphotericin B therapy. *Pediatr Infect Dis J.* 1990;9:309-314.
18. Rex JH, Bennett JE, Sugar AM, et al. Intravenous catheter exchange and duration of Candidemia. *Clin Infect Dis.* 1995;21:994-996.
19. Messing B, Peitra-Cohen S, Debure A, Beliah M, Bernier JJ. Antibiotic-lock technique: a new approach to optimal therapy for catheter-related sepsis in home-parenteral nutrition patients. *JPEN J Parenter Enteral Nutr.* 1988;12:185-189.
20. Benoit JL, Carandang G, Sitrin M, Arnow PM. Intraluminal antibiotic treatment of central venous catheter infections in patients receiving parenteral nutrition at home. *Clin Infect Dis.* 1995;21:1286-1288.
21. Krzywda EA, Andris DA, Edmiston CE Jr, Quebbeman EJ. Treatment of Hickman catheter sepsis using antibiotic lock technique. *Infect Control Hosp Epidemiol.* 1996;16:596-598.
22. Howard L, Claunch C, McDowell R, Timchalk M. Five years of experience in patients receiving home nutrition support with the implanted reservoir: a comparison with the external catheter. *JPEN J Parenter Enteral Nutr.* 1989;13:478-483.
23. Wurzel CL, Halom K, Feldman JG, Rubin LG. Infection rates of Broviac-Hickman catheters and implantable venous devices. *Am J Dis Child.* 1988;142:536-540.
24. Santarpia L, Pasanisi F, Alfonsi L, et al. Prevention and treatment of implanted central venous catheter (CVC)-related sepsis: a report after six years of home parenteral nutrition (HPN). *Clin Nutr.* 2002;21:207-211.
25. Bozzetti F, Mariani L, Bertinet DB, et al. Central venous catheter complications in 447 patients on home parenteral nutrition: an analysis of over 100,000 catheter days. *Clin Nutr.* 2002;21:475-485.
26. Savage AP, Picard M, Hopkins CC, Malt RA. Complications and survival of multilumen central venous catheters used for total parenteral nutrition. *Br J Surg.* 1993;80:1287-1290.
27. McCarthy MC, Shives JK, Robinson RJ, Broadie TA. Prospective evaluation of triple and single lumen catheters in total parenteral nutrition. *JPEN J Parenter Enteral Nutr.* 1987;11:259-262.
28. Yeung C, May J, Hughes R. Infection rate for single v triple lumen subclavian catheters. *Infect Control Hosp Epidemiol.* 1988;9:154-158.
29. Keohane PP, Jones BJ, Attrill H, et al. Effect of catheter tunneling and a nutrition nurse on catheter sepsis during parenteral nutrition. *Lancet.* 1983;2:1388-1390.
30. Danzig LE, Short LJ, Collins K, et al. Bloodstream infections associated with a needleless intravenous infusion system in patients receiving home infusion therapy. *JAMA.* 1995;273:1862-1864.
31. Raviglione MC, Battan R, Pablos-Mendez A, et al. Infections associated with Hickman catheters in patients with acquired immunodeficiency syndrome. *Am J Med.* 1989;86:780-786.
32. O'Keefe SJ, Burnes JU, Thompson RL. Recurrent sepsis in home parenteral nutrition patients: an analysis of risk factors. *JPEN J Parenter Enteral Nutr.* 1994;18:256-263.
33. Maki DG, Band JD. A comparative study of polyantibiotic and iodophor ointments in prevention of vascular catheter-related infections. *Am J Med.* 1981;70:739-744.
34. Sitges-Serra A, Linares J, Garau J. Catheter sepsis: the clue is the hub. *Surgery.* 1985;97:355-357.
35. Salzman MB, Rubin LG. Relevance of the catheter hub as a portal for microorganisms causing catheter-related bloodstream infections. *Nutrition.* 1997;13:15S-17S.
36. Stotter AT, Ward H, Waterfield AH, Hilton J, Sim AJ. Junctional care: the key to prevention of catheter sepsis in intravenous feeding. *JPEN J Parenter Enteral Nutr.* 1987;11:159-162.
37. De Cicco M, Panarello G, Chiaradia V, et al. Source and route of microbial colonization of parenteral nutrition catheters. *Lancet.* 1989;2:1258-1261.
38. Segura M, Alia C, Valverde J, et al. Assessment of a new hub design and the semiquantitative catheter culture methods using an in vivo experimental model of catheter sepsis. *J Clin Microbiol.* 1990;28:2551-2554.
39. Sitges-Serra A, Puig P, Linares J, et al. Hub colonization as the initial step in an outbreak of catheter-related sepsis due to coagulase-negative staphylococci during parenteral nutrition. *JPEN J Parenter Enteral Nutr.* 1984;8:668-672.
40. Brismar B, Jordahl L, Nystrom B, Pettersson N. Bacterial contamination of intravenous line side ports of different designs. *Clin Nutr.* 1987;6:31-33.
41. Snydman DR, Murray SA, Kornfeld SJ, Majka JA, Ellis CA. Total parenteral nutrition-related infections. *Am J Med.* 1982;73:695-699.
42. Goulet O, Larchet M, Gaillard JL, et al. Catheter related sepsis during long-term parenteral nutrition in paediatric gastroenterology patients: a study of 185 consecutive central venous catheters. *Clin Nutr.* 1990;9:73-78.
43. Segura M, Alvarez-Lerma F, Tellado JM, et al. A clinical trial on the prevention of catheter-related sepsis using a new hub model. *Ann Surg.* 1996;223:363-369.
44. Inoue Y, Nezu R, Matsuda H, et al. Experimental study of hub contamination: effect of a new connection device: the I system. *JPEN J Parenter Enteral Nutr.* 1992;16:178-180.
45. Halpin DP, O'Byrne P, McEntee G, Hennessy TP, Stephens RB. Effect of a betadine connection shield on central venous catheter sepsis. *Nutrition.* 1991;7:33-34.
46. Burnes J, Kelly D, O'Keefe S, Devine R. Evaluation of a subcutaneous antimicrobial cuff in the reduction of catheter related infection in patients receiving home parenteral nutrition. *JPEN J Parenter Enteral Nutr.* 1998; 22:S15.
47. Dimick JB, Swoboda S, Talamini MA, Pelz RK, Hendrix CW, Lipsett PA. Risk of colonization of central venous catheters: catheters for total parenteral nutrition vs other catheters. *Am J Crit Care.* 2003;12:328-335.
48. Stebbins J, O'Neill M, Steiger E. The effect of decreased catheter care on primary sepsis rate in central venous catheters (CVC) used in parenteral nutrition. *JPEN J Parenter Enteral Nutr.* 1989;13:16S.
49. Powell C, Regan C, Fabri PJ, Ruberg RL. Evaluation of Opsite catheter dressings for parenteral nutrition: a prospective, randomized trial. *JPEN J Parenter Enteral Nutr.* 1982;6:43-46.
50. Andersen PT, Herlevsen P, Schaumburg H. A comparative study of "op-site" and "nobecutan gauze" dressings for central venous line care. *J Hosp Infect.* 1986;7:161-168.
51. Conly JM, Grieves K, Peters B. A prospective, randomized study comparing transparent and dry gauze dressings for central venous catheters. *J Infect Dis.* 1989;159:310-319.
52. Hoffmann KK, Weber DJ, Samsa GP, Rutala WA. Transparent polyurethane film as an intravenous catheter dressing. *JAMA.* 1992;267:2072-2076.

53. Powell CR, Traetow MJ, Fabri PJ, et al. Op-site dressing study: a prospective randomized study evaluating povidone iodine ointment and extension set changes with 7-day Op-site dressings applied to total parenteral nutrition subclavian sites. *JPEN J Parenter Enteral Nutr.* 1985;9:443-446.
54. Hoshal VL Jr, Ause RG, Hoskins PA. Fibrin sleeve formation on indwelling subclavian central venous catheters. *Arch Surg.* 1971;102:353-358.
55. Cassidy FP, Zajko AB, Bron KM, et al. Noninfectious complications of long-term central venous catheters: radiologic evaluation and management. AJR *Am J Roentgenol.* 1987;149:671-675.
56. Burt ME, Dunnick NR, Drudy AG, Maher MM, Brennan MF. Prospective evaluation of subclavian vein thrombosis during total parenteral nutrition by contrast venography. *Clin Res.* 1981;20:264A.
57. Bozzetti F, Scarpa D, Terno G, et al. Subclavian venous thrombosis due to indwelling catheters: a prospective study on 52 patients. *JPEN J Parenter Enteral Nutr.* 1983;7:560-562.
58. Fabri PJ, Mirtalo JM, Ruberg RL, et al. Incidence and prevention of thrombosis of the subclavian vein during total parenteral nutrition. *Surg Gyne Obstet.* 1982;155:238-240.
59. Buchman AL, Misra S, Moukarzel A, Ament ME. Catheter thrombosis and superior/inferior vena cava syndrome are rare complications of long term parenteral nutrition. *Clin Nutr.* 1994;13:356-360.
60. Beers TR, Burnes J, Fleming CR. Superior vena caval obstruction in patients with gut failure receiving home parenteral nutrition. *JPEN J Parenter Enteral Nutr.* 1990;14:474-479.
61. Schmidt-Sommerfeld E, Snyder G, Rossi TM, Lebenthal E. Catheter-related complications in 35 children and adolescents with gastrointestinal disease on home parenteral nutrition. *JPEN J Parenter Enteral Nutr.* 1990;14:148-151.
62. McCulloch I, Pennington CR. Intracardiac thrombus complicating prolonged parenteral nutrition in an adult. *JPEN J Parenter Enteral Nutr.* 1989;13:557-559.
63. Dollery CM, Sullivan ID, Bauraind O, Bull C, Milla PJ. Thrombosis and embolism in long-term central venous access for parenteral nutrition. *Lancet.* 1994;344:1043-1045.
64. Mailloux RJ, DeLegge MH, Kirby DF. Pulmonary embolism as a complication of long-term total parenteral nutrition. *JPEN J Parenter Enteral Nutr.* 1993;17:578-582.
65. Leiby JM, Purcell H, DeMaria JJ, Kraut EH, Sagone AL, Metz EN. Pulmonary embolism a result of Hickman catheter-related thrombosis. *Am J Med.* 1989;86:228-231.
66. Bern MM, Bothe A Jr, Bistrian BR, et al. Prophylaxis against central vein thrombosis with low-dose warfarin. *Surgery.* 1986;99:216-221.
67. Bern MM, Lokich JJ, Wallach SR, et al. Very low doses of warfarin can prevent thrombosis in central venous catheters. *Ann Intern Med.* 1990;112:423-428.
68. Wessler T, Gittel SN, Bank H, Martinowitz U, Stephenson RC. An assay of the antithrombotic action of warfarin: its correlation with the inhibition of stasis thrombosis in rabbits. *Thromb Haemost.* 1978;40:486-496.
69. Bertina RM, Westhoek-Kuipers ME, Alderkamp GH. The inhibitor of prothrombin conversion in plasma of patients on oral anticoagulant treatment. *Thromb Haemost.* 1981;45:237-241.
70. Gitel SN, Wessler S. Dose-dependent antithrombotic effect of warfarin in rabbits. *Blood.* 1983;61:435-438.
71. Veerabagu MP, Tuttle-Newhall J, Maliakkal R, Champagne C, Mascioli EA. Warfarin and reduced central venous thrombosis in home total parenteral nutrition patients. *Nutrition.* 1995;11:142-144.
72. Lutomski DM, Palascak JE, Bower RH. Warfarin resistance associated with intravenous lipid administration. *JPEN J Parenter Enteral Nutr.* 1987;11:316-318.
73. Griffith GC, Nichols G Jr, Asher JD, Flanagan B. Heparin osteoporosis. *JAMA.* 1965;193:85-88.
74. Pettila V, Leinonen P, Markkola A, Hiilesmaa V, Kaaja R. Postpartum bone mineral density in women treated for thromboprophylaxis with unfractionated heparin or LMW heparin. *Thromb Haemost.* 2002;87:182-186.
75. Johnson OL, Washington C, Davis SS, Schaupp K. The destabilization of parenteral feeding emulsions by heparin. *Int J Pharm.* 1989;53:237-240.
76. Buchman AL. *Handbook of Nutritional Support.* Philadelphia, Pa: Williams and Wilkins; 1997:946-947.
77. Moreno JM, Valero MA, Gomis P, Leon-Sanz M. Central venous catheter occlusion in home parenteral nutrition patients. *Clin Nutr.* 1998;17:35-36.
78. Glynn MFX, Langer B, Jeejeebhoy KN. Therapy for thrombotic occlusion of long-term intravenous alimentation catheters. *JPEN J Parenter Enteral Nutr.* 1980;4:387-390.
79. Stephens LC, Haire WD, Kotulak GD. Are clinical signs accurate indicators of the cause of central venous catheter occlusion? *JPEN J Parenter Enteral Nutr.* 1995;19:75-79.
80. Atkinson JB, Bagnall HA, Gomperts E. Investigational use of tissue plasminogen activator (t-PA) for occluded central venous catheters. *JPEN J Parenter Enteral Nutr.* 1990;14:310-311.
81. Semba CP, Deitcher SR, Li X, Resnansky L, Tu T, McClusky ER. Treatment of occluded central venous catheters with alteplase: results in 1,064 patients. *J Vasc Interv Radiol.* 2002;13:1199-1205.
82. Johnson RL, Lieberman RP, Kaplan PA, Haire WD. Silicone rubber catheter venography using standard angiographic techniques. *Cardiovasc Interventional Radiol.* 1988;11:45-49.
83. Breaux CW Jr, Duke D, Georgeson KE, Mestre JR. Calcium phosphate crystal occlusion of central venous catheters used for total parenteral nutrition in infants and children: prevention and treatment. *J Pediatr Surg.* 1987;22:829-832.
84. Shulman RJ, Reed T, Pitre D, Laine L. Use of hydrochloric acid to clear obstructed central venous catheters. *JPEN J Parenter Enteral Nutr.* 1988;12:509-510.
85. Pennington CR, Pithie AD. Ethanol lock in the management of catheter occlusion. *JPEN J Parenter Enteral Nutr.* 1987;11:507-508.
86. Werlin SL, Lausten T, Jessen S, et al. Treatment of central venous catheter occlusions with ethanol and hydrochloric acid. *JPEN J Parenter Enteral Nutr.* 1995;19:416-418.
87. Sando K, Fujii M, Tanaka K, et al. Lock method using sodium hydroxide solution to clear occluded central venous access devices. *Clin Nutr.* 1997;16:185-188.
88. Johnston DA, Walker K, Richards J, Pennington CR. Ethanol flush for the prevention of catheter occulsion. *Clin Nutr.* 1992;11:97-100.
89. Beau P, Matuchansky C. Lipid delivery and catheter obstruction during cyclic total parenteral nutrition. *Lancet.* 1987;2:1095-1096.
90. Messing B, Beiiah M, Girard-Pipau F, Leeve D, Bernier JJ. Technical hazards of using nutritive mixes in bags for cyclical intravenous nutrition: comparison with standard intravenous nutrition in 48 gastroenterological patients. *Gut.* 1982;23:297-303.
91. Buchman AL, Moukarzel A, Ament ME, et al. Serious renal impairment is associated with long-term parenteral nutrition. *JPEN J Parenter Enteral Nutr.* 1993;17:438-444.
92. Moukarzel AA, Ament ME, Buchman AL, Dahlstrom KA, Vargas J. Renal function of children receiving long-term parenteral nutrition. *J Pediatr.* 1991;119:864-868.
93. Boncompain-Gerard M, Robert D, Fouque D, Hadj-Aissa A. Renal function and urinary excretion of electrolytes in patients receiving cyclic parenteral nutrition. *JPEN J Parenter Enteral Nutr.* 2000;24:234-239.
94. Graf H, Stummven HK, Luger A, Prager R. Effect of amino acid infusion on glomerular filtration rate. *N Engl J Med.* 1983;308:159-160.
95. Cochran ST, Pagani JJ, Barbaric ZL. Nephromegaly in hyperalimentation. *Radiology.* 1979;130:603-606.
96. Moukarzel A, Song MK, Buchman AL, et al. Excessive chromium intake in children receiving total parenteral nutrition. *Lancet.* 1992;339:385-388.
97. Buchman AL, Moukarzel A, Ament ME. The role of chromium and cadmium toxicity in TPN-induced nephropathy. *J Clin Nutr Gastroenterol.* 1992;7:39-41.
98. Buchman AL, Neely M, Grossie VB Jr, et al. Organ heavy-metal accumulation during parenteral nutrition is associated with pathologic abnormalities in rats. *Nutrition.* 2001;17:600-606.

99. Buchman AL, Moukarzel AA, Ament ME. Excessive urinary oxalate excretion occurs in long-term TPN patients both with and without ileostomies. *J Am Coll Nutr.* 1995;14:24-28.
100. Rockwell G, Nelson B, Campfield T, et al. Oxalogenesis in neonatal nutrition solutions. *JPEN J Parenter Enteral Nutr.* 1997;21:S8.
101. Casaubon PR, Dahlstrom KA, Vargas J, et al. Intravenous fat emulsion (intralipid) delays gastric emptying, but does not cause gastroesophageal reflux in healthy volunteers. *JPEN J Parenter Enteral Nutr.* 1989;13:246-248.
102. MacGregor IL, Wiley ZD, Lavigne ME, Way LW. Slowed rate of gastric emptying of solid food in man by high caloric parenteral nutrition. *Am J Surg.* 1979;138:652-654.
103. Kotler DP, Levine GM. Reversible gastric and pancreatic hyposecretion after long-term total parenteral nutrition. *N Engl J Med.* 1979;300:241-242.
104. Buchman AL, Moukarzel AA, Bhuta S, et al. Parenteral nutrition is associated with intestinal morphologic and functional changes in humans. *JPEN J Parenter Enteral Nutr.* 1995;19:453-460.
105. Guedon C, Schmitz J, Lerebours E, et al. Decreased brush border hydrolase activities without gross morphologic changes in human intestinal mucosa after prolonged total parenteral nutrition in adults. *Gastroenterology.* 1986;90:373-378.
106. Van der Hulst RRJ, van Kreel BK, von Meyenfeldt MF, et al. Glutamine and the preservation of gut integrity. *Lancet.* 1993;341:1363-1365.
107. Sedman PC, MacFie J, Palmer MD, Mitchell CJ, Sagar PM. Preoperative total parenteral nutrition is not associated with mucosal atrophy or bacterial translocation in humans. *Br J Surg.* 1995;82:1663-1667.
108. Knudsen KB, Bradley EM, Lecocq FR, Bellamy HM, Welsh JD. Effect of fasting and refeeding on the histology and disaccharidase activity of the human intestine. *Gastroenterology.* 1968;55:46-51.
109. Adibi SA, Allen ER. Impaired jejunal absorption rates of essential amino acids induced by either dietary, caloric or protein deprivation in man. *Gastroenterology.* 1970;59:404-413.
110. Tompkins RK, Waisman J, Watt CMH, Corlin R, Keith R. Absence of mucosal atrophy in human small intestine after prolonged isolation. *Gastroenterology.* 1977;73:1406-1409.
111. Buchman AL, Mestecky J, Moukarzel AA, Ament ME. Intestinal immune function is unaffected by parenteral nutrition in man. *J Am Coll Nutr.* 1995;14:656-661.
112. van der Hulst RRJ, von Meyenfeldt MF, Tiebosch A, Buurman WA, Soeters PB. Glutamine and intestinal immune cells in humans. *JPEN J Parenter Enteral Nutr.* 1997;21:310-315.
113. Shike M, Harrison JE, Sturtridge WC, et al. Metabolic bone disease in patients receiving long-term total parenteral nutrition. *Ann Intern Med.* 1980;92:343-350.
114. Klein GL, Ament ME, Targoff CM, et al. Bone disease associated with total parenteral nutrition. *Lancet.* 1980;2:1041-1044.
115. Hurley DL, McMahon M. Long-term parenteral nutrition and metabolic bone disease. *Endocrinol Metab Clin North Am.* 1990;19:113-131.
116. Pironi L, Labate AM, Pertkiewicz J, et al. Prevalence of bone disease in patients on home parenteral nutrition. *Clin Nutr.* 2002;21:289-296.
117. Klein GL, Horst RL, Norman AW, Ament ME, Slatopolsky E, Coburn JW. Reduced serum levels of 1,25-dihydroxyvitamin D during long-term total parenteral nutrition. *Ann Intern Med.* 1981;94:638-643.
118. Bengoa JM, Sitrin MD, Wood RJ, Rosenberg IH. Amino acid-induced hypercalciuria in patients on total parenteral nutrition. *Am J Clin Nutr.* 1983;38:264-269.
119. Wood RJ, Bengoa JM, Sitrin MD, Rosenberg IH. Calciuretic effect of cyclic versus continuous total parenteral nutrition. *Am J Clin Nutr.* 1985;41:614-619.
120. DeFronzo RA, Cooke CR, Andres R, Faloona GR, Davis PJ. The effect of insulin on renal handling of sodium, potassium, calcium, and phosphate in man. *J Clin Invest.* 1975;55:845-855.
121. Wood RJ, Sitrin MD, Cusson GJ, Rosenberg IH. Reduction of total parenteral nutrition-induced urinary calcium loss by increasing the phosphorus in the total parenteral nutrition prescription. *JPEN J Parenter Enteral Nutr.* 1986;10:188-190.
122. Rudman D, Millikan WJ, Richardson TJ, Bixler TJ II, Stackhouse J, McGarrity WC. Elemental balances during intravenous hyperalimentation of underweight adult subjects. *J Clin Invest.* 1974;55:94-104.
123. Karton MA, Rettmer R, Lipkin EW, Ott SM, Chait A. D-lactate and metabolic bone disease in patients receiving long-term parenteral nutrition. *JPEN J Parenter Enteral Nutr.* 1989;13:132-135.
124. Lemann J Jr, Litzow JR, Lennon EJ. The effects of chronic acid loads in normal man: further evidence for the participation of bone mineral in the defense against chronic metabolic acidosis. *J Clin Invest.* 1966;45:1608-1614.
125. Lemann J Jr, Litzow JR, Lennon EJ. Studies of the mechanism by which chronic metabolic acidosis augments urinary calcium excretion in man. *J Clin Invest.* 1967;46:1318-1328.
126. Cunningham J, Fraher LJ, Clemens TL, Revell PA, Papapoulos SE. Chronic acidosis with metabolic bone disease. *Am J Med.* 1982;73:199-204.
127. Saitta JC, Lipkin EW, Howard GA. Acetate inhibition of chick bone cell proliferation and bone growth in vitro. *J Bone Miner Res.* 1989;4:379-386.
128. Berkelhammer CH, Wood RJ, Sitrin MD. Acetate and hypercalciuria during total parenteral nutrition. *Am J Clin Nutr.* 1988;48:1482-1489.
129. Klein GL, Alfrey AC, Miller NL, et al. Aluminum loading during total parenteral nutrition. *Am J Clin Nutr.* 1982;35:1425-1429.
130. Ott SM, Maloney NA, Klein GL, et al. Aluminum is associated with low bone formation in patients receiving chronic parenteral nutrition. *Ann Intern Med.* 1983;98:910-914.
131. Vargas JH, Klein GL, Ament ME, et al. Metabolic bone disease of parenteral nutrition: course after changing from casein to amino acids in parenteral solutions with reduced aluminum content. *Am J Clin Nutr.* 1988;48:1070-1078.
132. Lipkin EW, Ott SM, Klein GL. Heterogeneity of bone histology in parenteral nutrition patients. *Am J Clin Nutr.* 1987;46:673-680.
133. Koo WW, Kaplan LA, Horn J, Tsang RC, Steichen JJ. Aluminum in parenteral nutrition solution: sources and possible alternatives. *JPEN J Parenter Enteral Nutr.* 1986;10:591-595.
134. Heyman MB, Klein GL, Wong A, et al. Aluminum does not accumulate in teenagers and adults on prolonged parenteral nutrition containing free amino acids. *JPEN J Parenter Enteral Nutr.* 1986;10:86-87.
135. Saitta JC, Ott SM, Sherrard DJ, Walden CE, Lipkin EW. Metabolic bone disease in adults receiving long-term parenteral nutrition: longitudinal study with regional densitometry and bone biopsy. *JPEN J Parenter Enteral Nutr.* 1993;17:214-219.
136. Moukarzel A, Ament ME, Vargas J, et al. Non aluminum dependent osteopathy in children on long term parenteral nutrition. *Am J Clin Nutr.* 1990;51:520S.
137. Pironi L, Zolezzi C, Ruggeri E, Paganelli F, Pizzoferrato A, Miglioli M. Bone turnover in short-term and long-term home parenteral nutrition for benign disease. *Nutrition.* 2000;16:272-277.
138. Staun M, Tjellesen L, Thale M, Rannem T, Schaadt O, Jarnum S. Bone mineral content in patients on home parenteral nutrition. *Clin Nutr.* 1994;13:351-355.
139. Moukarzel AA, Buchman AL, Vargas J, Baron HI, Ament ME. Is fluoride deficiency related to the bone disease of parenteral nutrition? *Gastroenterology.* 1992;102:A568.
140. Shike M, Shils ME, Heller A, et al. Bone disease in prolonged parenteral nutrition: osteopenia without mineralization defect. *Am J Clin Nutr.* 1986;44:89-98.
141. Podenphant J, Johansen JS, Thomsen K, Riis BJ, Leth A, Christiansen C. Bone turnover in spinal osteoporosis. *J Bone Miner Res.* 1987;2:497-503.
142. Lipkin EW, Ott SM, Klein GL, Deftos LJ. Serum markers of bone formation in parenteral nutrition patients. *Calcif Tissue Int.* 1990;47:75-81.

143. Verhage AH, Cheong WK, Allard JP, Jeejeebhoy KN. Increase in lumbar spine bone mineral content in patients on long-term parenteral nutrition without vitamin D supplementation. *JPEN J Parenter Enteral Nutr.* 1995;19:431-436.
144. Haderslev KV, Tjellesen L, Sorensen HA, Staun M. Effect of cyclic intravenous clodronate therapy on bone mineral density and markers of bone turnover in patients receiving home parenteral nutrition. *Am J Clin Nutr.* 2002;76:482-488.
145. Nishikawa RA, Siepler SE, Siepler JK, Diamantidis T, Okamoto R. Intravenous pamidronate improves bone mineral density in home parenteral nutrition patients. *Clin Nutr.* 2003;22:S88.
146. Buchman AL, Moukarzel A. Metabolic bone disease associated with total parenteral nutrition. *Clin Nutr.* 2000;19:217-231.
147. Penden VH, Witzleben CL, Skelton MA. Total parenteral nutrition. *J Pediatr.* 1971;78:180-181.
148. Cavicchi M, Beau P, Crenn P, Degott C, Messing B. Prevalence of liver disease and contributing factors in patients receiving home parenteral nutrition for permanent intestinal failure. *Ann Intern Med.* 2000;132:525-532.
149. Chan S, McCowen KC, Bistrian BR, et al. Incidence, prognosis, and etiology of end-stage liver disease in patients receiving home parenteral nutrition. *Surgery.* 1999;126:28-34.
150. Sondheimer JM, Asturias E, Cadnapaphornchai M. Infection and cholestasis in neonates with intestinal resection and long-term parenteral nutrition. *J Pediatr Gastroenterol Nutr.* 1998;27:131-137.
151. Sax HC, Talamini MA, Brackett K, Fischer JE. Hepatic steatosis in parenteral nutrition: failure of fatty infiltration to correlate with abnormal serum hepatic enzyme levels. *Surgery.* 1986;100:697-704.
152. Grant JP, Cox CE, Kleinman LM, et al. Serum hepatic enzyme and bilirubin elevations during parenteral nutrition. *Surg Gynecol Obstet.* 1977;145:573-580.
153. Robertson JFR, Garden OJ, Shenkin A. Intravenous nutrition and hepatic dysfunction. *JPEN J Parenter Enteral Nutr.* 1986;10:172-176.
154. Host WR, Serlin O, Rush BF Jr. Hyperalimentation in cirrhotic patients. *Am J Surg.* 1972;123:57-62.
155. Baker AL, Rosenberg IH. Hepatic complications of total parenteral nutrition. *Am J Med.* 1987;82:489-497.
156. Sheldon GF, Peterson SR, Sander R. Hepatic dysfunction during hyperalimentation. *Arch Surg.* 1978;113:504-508.
157. Buchman AL, Dubin M, Jenden D, et al. Lecithin increases plasma free choline and decreases hepatic steatosis in long-term total parenteral nutrition patients. *Gastroenterology.* 1992;102:1363-1370.
158. Chambier C, Lemann M, Vahedi K, et al. Chronic cholestasis in patients supported by prolonged parenteral nutrition. *JPEN J Parenter Enteral Nutr.* 1998;22:S16.
159. Stanko RT, Nathan G, Mendelow H, Adibi SA. Development of hepatic cholestasis and fibrosis in patients with massive loss of intestine supported by prolonged parenteral nutrition. *Gastroenterology.* 1987;92:197-202.
160.. Craig RM, Neumann T, Jeejeebhoy KN, Yokoo H. Severe hepatocellular reaction resembling alcoholic hepatitis with cirrhosis after massive small bowel resection and prolonged total parenteral nutrition. *Gastroenterology.* 1980;79:131-137.
160. Jobert A, Colomb V, Goulet O, Fournet JC, Lacaille F, Corriol O, Ricour C. Cholestasis associated with parenteral nutrition in children: role of lipid emulsions. *Clin Nutr.* 1997;16:S51.
161. Rabeneck L, Freeman H, Owen D. Death due to TPN-related liver failure. *Gastroenterology.* 1984;86:1215.
162. Bowyer BA, Fleming CR, Ludwig J, Petz J, McGill DB. Does long-term home parenteral nutrition in adult patients cause chronic liver disease? *JPEN J Parenter Enteral Nutr.* 1985;9:11-17.
163. Powell EE, Cooksley WG, Hanson R, Searle J, Halliday JW, Powell LW. The natural history of nonalcoholic steatohepatitis: a follow-up study of forty-two patients for up to 21 years. *Hepatology.* 1990;11:74-80.
164. Lowry SF, Brennan MF. Abnormal liver function during parenteral nutrition: relation to infusion excess. *J Surg Res.* 1979;26:300-307.
165. Meguid MM, Akahoshi MP, Jeffers S, Hayashi RJ, Hammond WG. Amelioration of metabolic complications of conventional total parenteral nutrition. *Arch Surg.* 1984;119:1294-1298.
166. Langer B, McHattie JD, Zohrab WJ, Jeejeebhoy KN. Prolonged survival after complete bowel resection using intravenous alimentation at home. *J Surg Res.* 1973;15:226-233.
167. McDonald ATJ, Philips MJ, Jeejeebhoy KN. Reversal of fatty liver by Intralipid in patients on total parenteral nutrition. *Gastroenterology.* 1973;64:885.
168. Reif S, Tano M, Oliverio R, Young C, Rossi T. Total parenteral nutrition-induced steatosis: reversal by parenteral lipid infusion. *JPEN J Parenter Enteral Nutr.* 1991;15:102-104.
169. Holman RT. The ratio of the trienoic:tetraenoic acids in tissue lipids as a measure of essential fatty acid requirement. *J Nutr.* 1960;70:405-410.
170. Moukarzel AA, Dahlstrom KA, Buchman AL, Ament ME. Carnitine status of children receiving long-term total parenteral nutrition: A longitudinal prospective study. *J Pediatr.* 1992;120:759-762.
171. Bowyer BA, Miles JM, Haymond MW, Fleming CR. L-carnitine therapy in home parenteral nutrition patients with abnormal liver tests and low plasma carnitine concentrations. *Gastroenterology.* 1988;94:434-438.
172. Lave T, Lutz O, Frey A, Ehret C, Bach AC. Carnitine supplementation and fat emulsion clearance and utilization. *Infusiontherapie.* 1988;15:152-157.
173. Buchman AL, Dubin MD, Moukarzel AA, et al. Choline deficiency: a cause of hepatic steatosis during parenteral nutrition that can be reversed with intravenous choline supplementation. *Hepatology.* 1995;22:1399-1403.
174. Chawla RK, Wolf DC, Kutner MH, Bonkovsky HL. Choline may be an essential nutrient in malnourished patients with cirrhosis. *Gastroenterology.* 1989;97:1514-1520.
175. Burt ME, Hanin I, Brennan MF. Choline deficiency associated with parenteral nutrition. *Lancet.* 1980;2:638-639.
176. Buchman AL, Moukarzel A, Jenden DJ, et al. Hepatic transaminase abnormalities are associated with low plasma free choline in patients receiving long term parenteral nutrition. *Clin Nutr.* 1993;12:33-37.
177. Buchman AL, Ament ME, Sohel M, et al. Choline deficiency causes reversible hepatic abnormalities in patients during parenteral nutrition: proof of a human choline requirement; a placebo-controlled trial. *JPEN J Parenter Enteral Nutr.* 2001;25:260-268.
178. Yao Z, Vance DE. The active synthesis of phosphatidylcholine is required for very low density lipoprotein secretion from rat hepatocytes. *J Biol Chem.* 1988;263:2998-3004.
179. Lombardi B, Ugazio G, Raick AN. Choline-deficiency-fatty liver: relation of plasma phospholipids to liver triglycerides. *Am J Physiol.* 1968;210:31-36.
180. Vileisis RA, Sorensen K, Gonzalez-Crussi F, Hunt CE. Liver malignancy after parenteral nutrition. *J Pediatr.* 1982;100:88-90.
181. Ghoshal AK, Farber E. The induction of liver cancer by dietary deficiency of choline and methionine without added carcinogens. *Carcinogenesis.* 1984;5:1367-1370.
182. Yokoyama S, Sells MA, Reddy TV, Lombardi B. Hepatocarcinogenic and promoting action of a choline-devoid diet in the rat. *Cancer Res.* 1985;45:2834-2842.
183. Fell JM, Reynolds AP, Meadows N, et al. Manganese toxicity in children receiving long-term parenteral nutrition. *Lancet.* 1996;347:1218-1221.
184. Beath SV, Gopalan S, Booth IW. Manganese toxicity and parenteral nutrition. *Lancet.* 1996;347:1773-1774.
185. Clayton PT, Bowron A, Mills KA, Massoud A, Casteels M, Milla PJ. Phytosterolemia in children with parenteral nutrition-associated liver disease. *Gastroenterology.* 1993;105:1806-1813.
186. Degott C, Messing B, Moreau D, et al. Liver phospholipidosis induced by parenteral nutrition: histologic, histochemical, and ultrasound investigation. *Gastroenterology.* 1988;95:183-191.

187. Gleghorn EE, Merritt RJ, Subramanian N, Ramos A. Phenobarbital does not prevent total parenteral nutrition-induced cholestasis in noninfected neonates. *JPEN J Parenter Enteral Nutr.* 1986;10:282-283.
188. Spurr SG, Grylack LJ, Mehta NR. Hyperalimentation-associated neonatal cholestasis: effect of oral gentamicin. *JPEN J Parenter Enteral Nutr.* 1989;13:633-636.
189. Cocjin J, Vanderhal A, Sehgal S, Rosenthal P. Ursodeoxycholic acid therapy for total parenteral nutrition-associated cholestasis in the neonate. *Gastroenterology.* 1993;104:A615.
190. Spagnuolo MI, Iorio R, Vegnente A, Guarino A. Ursodeoxycholic acid for treatment of cholestasis in children on long-term total parenteral nutrition: a pilot study. *Gastroenterology.* 1996;111:716-719.
191. Lindor KD, Burnes J. Ursodeoxycholic acid for the treatment of home parenteral nutrition-associated cholestasis. *Gastroenterology.* 1991;101:250-253.
192. Beau P, Labat-Labourdette J, Ingrand P, Beauchant M. Is ursodeoxycholic acid an effective therapy for total parenteral nutrition-related liver disease? *J Hepatol.* 1994;20:240-244.
193. Teitelbaum DH, Han-Markey T, Drongowski RA, et al. Use of cholecystokinin to prevent the development of parenteral nutrition-associated cholestasis. *JPEN J Parenter Enteral Nutr.* 1997;21:100-103.
194. Heubi JE, Wiechmann DA, Creutzinger V, Setchell KD, Squires R Jr, Couser R, Rhodes P. Tauroursodeoxycholic acid (TUDCA) in the prevention of total parenteral nutrition-associated liver disease. *J Pediatr.* 2002;141:237-242.
195. Snyder J, Love K, Bratton B, Elkayam O, Fields S, Heyman MB. TPN cholestasis in neonates: results of randomized, double-blind study of amino acid composition. *Gastroenterology.* 2003;124:A30.
196. Cooke RJ, Whitington PF, Kelts D. Effects of taurine supplementation on hepatic function during short-term parenteral nutrition in the premature infant. *J Pediatr Gastroenterol.* 1984;3:234-238.
197. Lambert JR, Thomas SM. Metronidazole prevention of serum liver enzyme abnormalities during total parenteral nutrition. *JPEN J Parenter Enteral Nutr.* 1985;9:501-503.
198. Hasegewa T, Sasaki T, Kimura T, et al. Effects of isolated small bowel transplantation on liver dysfunction caused by intestinal failure and long-term total parenteral nutrition. *Pediatr Transplant.* 2002;6:235-239.
199. Roslyn JJ, Pitt HA, Mann LL, Ament ME, DenBesten L. Gallbladder disease in patients on long-term parenteral nutrition. *Gastroenterology.* 1983;84:148-154.
200. Flati G, Flati D, Jonsson PE, et al. Role of cholesterol and calcium bilrubinate crystals in acute postoperative acalculous cholecystitis. *Ital J Surg Sci.* 1984;14:333-336.
201. Deitch EA, Engel JM. Acute acalculous cholecystitis. Ultrasonic diagnosis. *Am J Surg.* 1981;142:290-292.
202. Warner BW, Hamilton FN, Silberstein EB, et al. The value of hepatobiliary scans in fasted patients receiving total parenteral nutrition. *Surgery.* 1987;102:595-601.
203. Shuman WP, Gibbs P, Rudd TG, Mack LA. PIPIDA scintigraphy for cholecystitis: false positives in alcoholism and total parenteral nutrition. *AJR Am J Roentgenol.* 1982;138:1-5.
204. Flancbaum L, Alden SM. Morphine cholescintigraphy. *Surg Gynecol Obstet.* 1990;171:227-232.
205. Messing B, Bories C, Kunstlinger F, Bernier JJ. Does total parenteral nutrition induce gallbladder sludge formation and lithiasis? *Gastroenterology.* 1983;84:1012-1019.
206. Messing B, Aprahamian M, Rautureau M, Baries C, Bisalli A, Stock-Damge S. Gallstone formation during total parenteral nutrition: a prospective study in man. *Gastroenterology.* 1984;86:1183.
207. Roslyn JJ, Denbesten L, Pitt HA, Kuchenbecker S, Polarek JW. Effect of cholecystokinin on gallbladder stasis and cholesterol gallstone formation. *J Surg Res.* 1981;30:200-204.
208. Mashako MN, Cezard JP, Boige N, et al. The effect of artificial feeding on cholestasis, gallbladder sludge and lithiasis in infants: correlation with plasma cholecystokinin levels. *Clin Nutr.* 1991;10:320-327.
209. Allen B, Bernhoft R, Blanckaert N, et al. Sludge is calcium bilirubinate associated with bile stasis. *Am J Surg.* 1981;141:51-56.
210. Pitt HA, Berquist WE, Mann LL, Porter-Fink V, Fonkalsrud EW, Ament ME, DenBesten L. Parenteral nutrition induces calcium bilirubinate gallstones. *Gastroenterology.* 1983;84:1274.
211. O'Brien CB, Berman JM, Fleming CR, Malet PF, Soloway RD. Total parenteral nutrition gallstones contain more calcium bilirubinate than sickle cell gallstones. *Gastroenterology.* 1986;90:1752.
212. Stewart L, Smith AL, Pellegrini CA, Matson RW, Way LW. Pigment gallstones form as a composite of bacterial microcolonies and pigment solids. *Ann Surg.* 1987;206:242-250.
213. Doty JE, Pitt HA, Porter-Fink V, Denbesten L. Cholecystokinin prophylaxis of parenteral nutrition-induced gallbladder disease. *Ann Surg.* 1985;201:76-80.
214. Sitzmann JV, Pitt HA, Steinborn PA, Pasha ZR, Sanders RC. Cholecystokinin prevents parenteral nutrition induced biliary sludge in humans. *Surg Gynecol Obstet.* 1990;170:25-31.
215. Apelgren KN, Willard DA, Vargish T. TPN alters gallbladder responsitivity to cholecystokinin. *JPEN J Parenter Enteral Nutr.* 1988;12:11S.
216. Dawes LG, Muldoon JP, Greiner MA, Bertolotti M. Cholecystokinin increases bile acid synthesis with total parenteral nutrition but does not prevent stone formation. *J Surg Res.* 1997;67:84-89.
217. de Boer SY, Masclee AAM, Lam WF, Jansen JBMJ, Lamers CBHW. Intravenous amino acids stimulate gallbladder contraction. *Gastroenterology.* 1993;104:A358.
218. Kalfarentzos F, Vagenas C, Michail A, et al. Gallbladder contraction after administration of intravenous amino acids and long-chain triacylglycerols in humans. *Nutrition.* 1991;7:347-349.
219. Doty JE, Pitt HA, Porter-Fink V, Denbesten L. The effect of intravenous fat and total parenteral nutrition on biliary physiology. *JPEN J Parenter Enteral Nutr.* 1984;8:263-268.
220. Priori P, Pezzilli R, Panuccio D, Nardi R, Gullo L. Stimulation of gallbladder emptying by intravenous lipids. *JPEN J Parenter Enteral Nutr.* 1997;21:350-352.
221. Guedon C, Ducrotte P, Chayvialle JA, Lerebours E, Denis P, Colin R. Effects of intravenous and intraduodenal fat on jejunal motility and on plasma cholecystokinin in man. *Dig Dis Sci.* 1988;33:558-564.
222. Broughton G, Fitzgibbons RJ Jr, Geiss RW, Adrian TE, Anthone G. IV chenodeoxycholate prevents calcium bilirubinate gallstones during total parenteral nutrition in the prairie dog. *JPEN. J Parenter Enteral Nutr* 1996;20:187-193.

Chapter 39

Complications of Enteral Nutrition

Eduard Cabré, MD, and
Miguel A. Gassull, MD, PhD

Introduction

In the last 30 years, significant advances in the design of both enteral access devices and chemically defined formula diets have resulted in a widespread use of enteral feeding in clinical practice. A major reason for preferring enteral feeding is its greater safety as compared to parenteral nutrition (PN). In fact, in pioneer studies, the morbidity rate of artificial nutrition in a district hospital was higher with PN[1] than enteral nutrition (EN),[2] especially for metabolic and septic complications. Even in recent meta-analytic studies, a lower complication rate (mainly infectious) is confirmed with EN than with PN.[3]

However, patients on enteral feeding may develop both mechanical and gastrointestinal (GI) side effects related to nutritional support. With properly administered support, these complications are rarely life threatening (eg, pulmonary aspiration); however, they often contribute to diminish the nutritional intake and hence the effectiveness of enteral feeding.[4] The incidence of complications can be reduced either by optimizing the enteral delivery technique and nursing care or by properly selecting the formula diet. These aspects are especially relevant for gastroenterological and critically ill patients.

Complications Related With the Enteral Access

Despite the widespread use of soft fine-bore nasogastric or nasoenteral tubes for enteral feeding, the risks of mechanical complications due to the obsolete wide-bore tubes must be emphasized. Nasopharyngeal discomfort, esophagitis, esophageal erosions, and ulcers (with the late development of strictures) are the most common problems with these tubes. Most of these complications do not occur with fine-bore feeding tubes,[5] but some potentially hazardous side-effects may complicate the tube's use.

Tube Malposition

The most serious complication associated with fine-bore tubes is their inadvertent passage into the tracheobronchial tree and the subsequent infusion of the enteral diet into the airway. Fortunately, this is very rare, usually occurring in unconscious or severely ill patients and in those with depressed cough or swallowing reflexes.[6,7] Although pneumonia is the most frequent consequence of infusion of the enteral diet into the airway, this occurrence may also result in pleural effusion and empyema, pneumomediastinum, bronchopleural fistula, pneumonitis, and sometimes fatal pneumothorax or hydropneumothorax.[8-15]

Prevention of tube misplacement includes tube insertion by well-trained personnel and careful checking of its proper position into the stomach, either by aspirating gastric contents or by auscultation of the epigastrium during air insufflation. However, auscultatory confirmation of tube placement may be misleading.[6] Gastric aspiration through small-diameter tubes may be difficult except for those with a specially designed outflow port.[5,16] Routine x-ray confirmation is probably unnecessary in alert patients; however, it must be carried out in obtunded, noncooperative patients or whenever any difficulty in tube insertion arises. In some cases, tube insertion under fluoroscopic control may also be indicated.

Nasopharyngeal Discomfort

Nasopharyngeal subjective distress during tube insertion is minimal with fine-bore tubes compared with discomfort during insertion of the traditional wide-bore ones. Some patients complain of residual nasopharyngeal discomfort due to scarce salivation, breathing through the mouth, or feeling of foreign body caused by the tube. The patient can overcome this by washing the mouth or gargling. In one study, silicone rubber tubes appeared to be less distressing than those made of polyurethane.[17] However, in most cases, nasopharyngeal discomfort is the result of "psychological intolerance" to tube feeding, which involves deprivation of tasting, chewing, and swallowing.[18]

Tube Obstruction

Occlusion of fine-bore feeding tubes may occur in as many as 10% of patients and is a common cause of tube replacement, which increases the cost of enteral feeding. Although some claim that viscous enteral formulas containing whole protein facilitate tube clogging, inadequate nursing care is the most frequent cause of tube blockade. Although different techniques for clearing obstructed tubes—eg, passing an endoscopic cytology brush[19] or a pancreatic enzyme solution[20]—have been described, the best policy is to prevent tube obstruction by irrigation with 10 to 20 mL of water every 6 to 8 hours or whenever the infusion is stopped.[21] The use of wires to unblock feeding tubes does not seem advisable because of the risk of perforation. Using bullet-tipped polyurethane feeding tubes diminishes the risk of clogging.[16]

Tube Removal

Inadvertent tube removal is an event occurring in >50% of patients. It occurs most often in stuporous or agitated subjects but is also frequent in conscious cooperative individuals.[4] There is no evidence that the use of a weighted tube or its transpyloric passage would reduce the risk of removal. Proper tube attachment and accurate nursing care are needed to prevent this problem.[4]

Gastrostomy and Jejunostomy-Related Complications

Although complications of surgical gastrostomy and jejunostomy will be not covered in this chapter, problems related to more specific nutrition accesses—eg, percutaneous endoscopic gastrostomy (PEG) and needle-catheter jejunostomy (NCJ)—deserve mention.

In the last years, PEG has replaced surgical gastrostomy as routine enteral access for patients in whom long-term enteral feeding is envisaged.[22-24] PEG is cheaper and less time consuming than is surgical gastrostomy.[25] Both retrospective and prospective studies showed no differences in major morbidity, but a higher rate of minor complications for PEG than for surgical gastrostomy has been described.[25-27]

In an early large series of 314 patients,[28] major complications occurred in 9 patients (3%), with 3 deaths (1%) attributable to the procedure. Fatalities were not related to PEG insertion but to the endoscopy itself (gastric aspiration, laryngospasm). The remaining major complications included gastric perforation, bleeding, and hematoma. Minor morbidity occurred in 39 cases (13%), consisting of infection at the tube site in 18 of them.[28] Similar results have been reported in more recent studies.[29,30] After discharge, PEG-related minor morbidity account for readmission in about 25% of patients.[31] Although antibiotic prophylaxis failed to reduce the infectious complications related to PEG in a randomized controlled trial,[32] many other trials have shown that prophylactic antibiotics reduce both local and systemic infections associated to this procedure.[33-36] Therefore, administration of a prophylactic antibiotics (eg, a cephalosporin) is a recommended prior to PEG placement.[37] Pneumoperitoneum may occur but its clinical relevance is low.[38] Stomal leakage and tube migration have also been described, and cologastric fistula has occasionally been reported in pediatric patients.[4]

NCJ is a safe procedure for postoperative enteral feeding.[39-43] Catheter obstruction and dislodgement with intraperitoneal leakage of enteral diet are the most frequent complication associated with this technique. Nevertheless, its frequency is not greater than 1% in the largest series.[44] Catheter dislodgement with intraperitoneal leakage requires re-laparotomy and is associated with a high mortality rate.[45] It may be prevented by suturing the jejunal loop to the abdominal wall. Although this maneuver can theoretically increase the risk of developing volvulus or intestinal obstruction, such complications have not been reported.

Intestinal perforation and pneumatosis intestinalis secondary to NCJ have also been described.[46,47] A case of late jejunal variceal bleeding after NCJ in a cirrhotic patient has been reported, and the authors suggest that portal hypertension may be a contraindication for NCJ.[48] However, NCJ was placed when an esophageal transection and splenectomy were performed, and no jejunal varices were observed during the surgical procedure. Because esophageal transection plus splenectomy favors the development of collateral veins in areas other than the esophagus, it cannot be concluded that NCJ is contraindicated in unoperated patients with portal hypertension or in those undergoing a portal-systemic derivative procedure.

Intestinal ischemia and necrosis without obstruction have been occasionally described in patients fed through NCJ.[49,50] The pathogenesis of such a complication is unclear as, in most cases, other risk factors for mesenteric low flow were present.

Problems Related to Diet Infusion

Inadvertent intravenous administration of an enteral formula diet is a very rare but devastating complication of EN. Sepsis, microembolization, hypersensitivity reactions to various components of the diet, and the development of multi-organ failure have been reported as causes of poor outcome in these patients.[51] In addition to this exceptional and unfortunate complication, food regurgitation, bronchopulmonary aspiration, and diarrhea are the most common problems arising in patients receiving an otherwise well-selected enteral diet.

Gastroesophageal Reflux, Regurgitation, and Bronchopulmonary Aspiration

A potentially fatal complication in patients on continuous tube feeding is regurgitation and aspiration of enteral formula into the airway.[52] The incidence of pulmonary aspiration may be as high as 50%, but it is probably clinically significant in only a few patients. Subjects with swallowing disturbances and mechanically ventilated intensive care patients are particularly at risk for developing this complication.[7,53]

Regurgitation may occur in patients with well-placed nasogastric tubes or PEG and less often in those with nasoduodenal or nasojejunal infusion of the diet.[54,55] Regurgitation and bronchial aspiration may be favored by several conditions: eg, decreased level of consciousness, supine position, and different drugs that may delay gastric emptying.[56] Monitoring gastric residuals has been advocated as a measure to prevent reflux and aspiration, particularly in critically ill patients. However, this policy has been questioned by some authors,[57] and a systematic review of the literature on this topic supports this latter view.[58] Although some studies have shown that gastroesophageal reflux is less frequent in patients with fine-bore than wide-bore nasoenteral tubes,[59] there is no complete agreement on this issue.[56] In patients with incompetent lower esophageal sphincter or hiatal hernia, even fine-bore feeding tubes may facilitate reflux of gastric contents into the esophagus.

Raising the head of the bed is mandatory in all tube-fed patients to prevent bronchial aspiration. Although some physicians avoid the use of high-osmolality energy-dense formulas, there is no evidence that osmolality would influence gastric emptying of diets administered by continuous infusion.[4] Using pump-assisted infusion of the diet contributes to minimize the risk of aspiration, particularly in bedridden patients.[60,61] To prevent acid reflux, H2 blockers or proton-pump inhibitors should be administered to patients with a history of peptic disease, gastric hypersecretion, or gastroesophageal reflux. Otherwise, these drugs should not be routinely administered. Some prokinetic drugs (eg, metoclopramide, cisapride, erythromycin) have been evaluated, although their effects on clinical outcomes are not well established.[62]

Variceal Bleeding

Bleeding from esophageal varices may be a complication of wide-bore nasogastric tubes. However, there is no evidence that fine-bore feeding tubes are able to cause variceal bleeding in cirrhotic patients on EN.[63-66] In a controlled study, the incidence of variceal bleeding was similar in tube-fed cirrhotic patients and those receiving an oral diet.[63]

Diarrhea

Diarrhea is the most common complication of EN. It is reported to occur in 2.3% to 68% of enterally fed patients.[23] Differences in the clinical definition of diarrhea may account, at least in part, for this wide-range incidence of diarrhea associated with enteral feeding.[67] Diagnosing diarrhea in enterally fed patients requires both an accurate interview of the patient and close nursing control on the frequency, volume, and consistency of the stools, especially in patients with underlying GI disease.[68] Many patients on residue-free EN pass 1 to 3 scanty loose or watery stools every 24 to 72 hours without disturbance. This cannot be considered diarrhea. Likewise, only significant worsening of previous bowel habits should be considered diarrhea attributable to enteral feeding. With such a restrictive criterion, the incidence of diarrhea do not exceed 10% even in patients with intestinal diseases.[4]

Multiple etiologies for EN-associated diarrhea are postulated and can be considered a multifactorial process. Causes include: 1) inadequate choice of formula diet in patients with intestinal dysfunction, 2) excessive infusion rate (particularly in patients with extensive bowel disease), 3) high diet osmolality, 4) concurrent administration of drugs (eg, antibiotics, laxatives, prokinetics), 5) intestinal bacterial overgrowth, and 6) bacterial contamination of the formula-diet.[4]

Infusing the enteral diet at an excessive rate is a major mechanism for diarrhea associated to enteral feeding. Proper contact between nutrients and the intestinal absorptive surface is a sine qua non for good digestive tolerance and effectiveness of EN. In patients with intestinal diseases and those with bowel dysfunction (eg, postoperative, critically ill, or severely malnourished patients), this implies the administration of the diet at a slow continuous rate, which can only be achieved with the aid of a peristaltic pump.[60,69] Thus, pump-assisted enteral feeding is mandatory in these cases as well as in those with normal intestinal function undergoing jejunal feeding.[22]

The administration of a hyperconcentrated formula diet has been traditionally considered to produce a high osmolar load into the duodenum and to be an important cause of EN-induced diarrhea. However, this mechanism seems to be particularly operative for sip or bolus feeding but not for continuously infused diets. Moreover, the pylorus regulates the duodenal load of intragastrically infused diets. In a controlled clinical trial, the incidence of diarrhea in patients with normal or near-normal GI function who were receiving polymeric enteral tube feeding was not influenced by the osmolality of the diet.[70] Diets with an osmolality higher that 700 mosmol/L can be well tolerated provided they are slowly infused with the aid of a peristaltic pump.[64,71] This implies that the infusion rate rather than the osmolality of the diet is a major determinant of the development of diarrhea in tube-fed patients. In the light of these data, some authors have recommended against the use of progressive starter regimens when feeding patients with normal GI function[72] or even in those with some digestive diseases.[73] However, some physicians use starter regimens in patients with severe diseases of the small bowel and those fed intrajejunally.

Simultaneous administration of drugs may cause of diarrhea in patients who are receiving EN. The drugs that can cause this include lactulose, lactitol or other osmotic laxatives, magnesium hydroxide-containing antacids, prokinetic drugs, sedatives, analgesics, and anticholinergics, which may impair intestinal motility and lead to intestinal bacterial overgrowth. Some authors have described a stronger-than-expected association between the administration of oral and parenteral antibiotics and the development of diarrhea in enterally fed patients compared with orally fed patients receiving antibiotics.[70,74] It has been hypothesized that the detrimental effect of antibiotics on fermentative capabilities of colonic bacteria would decrease the local production of short-chain fatty acids (SCFA), which would adversely affect colonic sodium and water handling. However, this hypothesis seems little plausible when fiber-free enteral diets are used. Antibiotic-associated diarrhea in enterally fed patients can result from the overgrowth of *Clostridium difficile*, other bacteria, and *Candida spp.*[75,76]

The existence of intestinal bacterial overgrowth may be a significant and often unrecognized cause of diarrhea in enteral feeding. Small-intestinal bacterial overgrowth may develop not only because of structural abnormalities of the bowel (ie, strictures, diverticula, and blind loops) but also because of motility disturbances of the intestine, as occur in many patients on enteral feeding.[77] Bacterial overgrowth may produce diarrhea as a consequence of bacterial deconjugation of bile acids, impairment of brush-border enzyme activities, or direct damage of the intestinal mucosa. To prevent diarrhea secondary to bacterial overgrowth, metronidazole (250 mg tid) should be administered orally to patients with some of the factors for developing intestinal bacterial colonization. Moreover, metronidazole therapy should be attempted in tube-fed patients with unexplained diarrhea. With this policy, many cases of digestive intolerance to enteral feeding can be overcome without discontinuing the diet.[4]

Several microorganisms (eg, enteric gram-negative bacilli, *Staphylococci, Streptococci*, and fungi) have been isolated from enteral feedings.[78,79] Bacterial contamination of the enteral formula has been reported to significantly relate to the presence of diarrhea in tube-fed patients,[80] but other studies failed to demonstrate such an association.[81] Nevertheless, gastroenteritis caused by the presence of enterotoxin-producing bacteria in contaminated diets is a real hazard, especially in neonates, children, and critically ill cachectic patients.[79,82,83] Likewise, septicemia has been reported to occur in association with the administration of contaminated enteral formulas,[84,85] and the development of long-lasting bouts of nosocomial bacteriemia in contaminated enteral feeding has been documented.[86]

Despite the potential risks, the overall clinical significance of bacterial contamination of enteral diets is minimal,[87] although it has been suggested that contaminated formulas can lose part of their nutritional value. Thus, efforts must be made to prevent this source of potentially serious complications of enteral feeding.

Use of commercial diets rather than homemade ones markedly reduces the risk of contamination. Aseptic manipulation of formula diets further diminishes their contamination rate. Ready-to-use diets are less prone to become contaminated than are those requiring manipulation.[82,88] Furthermore, the use of large-volume containers and changing the delivery set daily are advisable.[89]

Ascending contamination of enteral reservoirs may occur, especially in jejunostomy-fed patients[85] or those with decreased gastric acidity. Thus, treatment with antisecretory drugs (H2 blockers or proton-pump inhibitors) can theoretically increase the risk of microbial contamination of enteral diets. However, in the authors' experience, no case of clinically significant bacterial contamination of the diet has been observed in patients on this therapy.

The possibility that dietary fiber could prevent diarrhea associated to enteral feeding was suggested by study assessing the effect of pectin on the bowel habit of 13 healthy volunteers receiving EN.[90] The administration of a fiber-free enteral formula to these subjects resulted in a significant increase in the frequency of liquid stools as compared to those resulting from the intake of a conventional oral diet (60% versus 0%). After 7 days on fiber-free enteral feeding, the subjects were randomized to receive the same fiber-free enteral solution with or without 1% pectin added. Those subjects kept on the fiber-free diet persisted with a 72% rate of liquid stools, whereas this returned to 0% in those subjects fed the pectin-enriched diet, indicating that dietary fiber could prevent the EN-induced diarrhea.

These promising results were unfortunately not confirmed in some early randomized controlled trials in intensive care unit patients using soy polysaccharide as added fiber.[74,91,92] It has to be taken into account, however, that soy polysaccharide is a scarcely fermentable fiber source, and SCFA resulting from bacterial metabolism of dietary fiber and other unabsorbed carbohydrates seem to be responsible for the antidiarrheal effect of fiber. In fact, SCFA are the principal luminal anions in the colon. The magnitude of the daily colonic load and absorption of SCFA is comparable with that of colonic sodium. Like other weak electrolytes, SCFA may be either protonated or ionized. Protonated (un-ionized) SCFA can readily diffuse across membranes, but at normal colonic luminal pH most SCFA are ionized. SCFA absorption in the proximal colon is linked to the activity of Na+ to H+ exchanger system, suggesting that H+ secretion may create a low pH microclimate at the apical surface that promotes diffusion of the protonated SCFA into the cell. The large concentration gradient for SCFA across the colonic epithelium (>50 mM) may be important in stimulating sodium (and, hence, water) absorption by this mechanism.

The results of randomized controlled trials supplementing EN with fermentable fiber support the view that fermentability is a sine qua non for preventing diarrhea with dietary fiber. In a large randomized controlled trial assessing the effect of partially hydrolyzed guar gum (PHGG) in acute medical and surgical patients requiring enteral feeding for more than 5 days, the incidence of diarrhea was only 12% with PHGG-enriched enteral formula, as compared to 30% with fiber-free diet ($p < 0.05$).[93] A more recent trial in 25 critically ill patients confirmed the beneficial effect of PHGG in improving EN-related diarrhea.[94] The role of other fermentable fibres (eg, pectin) for this purpose has been scarcely explored without conclusive results.[95] (The role of dietary fiber is discussed in Chapter 11.)

Other Gastrointestinal Complaints

Nausea and vomiting have been reported to occur in 10% to 22% of enterally fed patients.[70,96] As mentioned, the role of diet osmolality in delaying gastric emptying when enteral feeding is continuously infused appears to be negligible. In fact, no differences in the incidence of nausea and vomiting have been found between either polymeric and oligomeric diets or polymeric diets with different osmolality.[70,96,97] Excessive infusion rate, nasogastric tube dislodgment, and psychogenic factors are more plausible causes for nausea and vomiting in tube-fed patients.

Abdominal bloating and cramps may occur in patients on EN, but the pathogenesis of these occurrences is poorly understood. In patients with intestinal bacterial overgrowth, bloating may be caused by the fermentation of carbohydrates by the intestinal bacteria, which may yield variable amounts of hydrogen, methane, and carbon dioxide. In these patients, oral administration of metronidazole may contribute to improve their symptoms. Increased bloating has been reported in patients fed diets supplemented with highly fermentable fiber sources.[93]

Constipation may be a complication in patients on long-term EN, although its incidence is not known. Low-residue diets have been implicated as the main cause of constipation in these cases; therefore, efforts have been made to increase the bulk-forming capabilities of enteral diets by adding fiber to them. The bulking effect of fiber mostly depends on its ability to generate residue, to retain water, and to increase peristalsis and is maximal for non-fermentable fibers (ie, lignin, cellulose, etc). However, non-fermentable fibers may also increase the stool weight by increasing the bacterial mass (biomass). It has been estimated that regular intake of 20 g/day of guar gum can increase the stool weight by 20%, and this effect can be even greater with pectin. The maintenance of a regular bowel habit has been on of the aims of adding fiber to EN, particularly for those patients requiring long-term enteral feeding. Adding lignin or cellulose to the tube-feeding formulas is not possible. Thus, other non-fermentable (mainly soy polysaccharide) and even fermentable fibers have been assayed for this purpose.

A number of published studies explored the effect of adding fiber to enteral formulas on the stool characteristics of healthy volunteers.[98-103] All of them compared the effects of different fiber supplements with fiber-free enteral formulas and with self-selected oral diets using a crossover random design. Although most studies showed an acceleration of intestinal transit using soy polysaccharide or mixed fibers, the effect on stool weight was much less conclusive. This may be due, at least in part, to the fact that the period of administration of the diets was very short (ranging from 4 to 18 days). The amount of fiber supplement may be another factor. In this sense, it is noteworthy that similar effects on bowel habit can be obtained with a lower amount of a mixture of fibers (including carboxymethylcellulose) as compared to soy polysaccharide alone.[104]

More inconclusive are the results of the four short-term randomized double-blind crossover studies that were performed in patients requiring enteral feeding.[105-108] Only one of the studies[108] reported an increase in the daily stool weight and frequency using a mixture of soy polysaccharide and oat fiber. Again, the short study period (7 to 28 days) may partly account for the lack of positive results.

In this sense, the results of a small pilot series of patients requiring very long-term enteral tube feeding[109] are particularly illustrative. Eleven profoundly mentally handicapped patients were studied while they were on enteral tube feeding for 1 year. The study period was divided into four stages: 1) patients received a fiber-free enteral diet for 60 days; 2) then, patients received formula with 20 g/L soy polysaccharide for a further 60 days; 3) this regime was maintained for the next 6 months; and 4) during the last two 30-day periods, the amount of supplemented fiber was increased to 30 g/L. Feces were collected during the last 5 days of each nutritional period daily for stool weight measurement. Daily fecal weight significantly increased with the fiber-supplemented formula as compared to those weighed during the baseline period when patients were on a fiber-free diet.[109] These results should be confirmed in large controlled trials in patients requiring long-term enteral feeding.

Complications Related to Inappropriate Choice of Diet

Several complications developing in tube-fed patients relate to the fact that the enteral diet chosen does not fit well with the pathophysiological changes induced by the underlying disease. This occurs mainly in patients with GI or liver disease, respiratory failure, carbohydrate intolerance, and severe malnutrition.

Gastrointestinal Disease

As mentioned, the administration of an inadequate enteral diet to a patient with GI disease may cause diarrhea. An extreme example of this would be the intestinal failure resulting from either massive intestinal resection or extensive bowel disease (short bowel syndrome). However, many of the following comments regarding short bowel syndrome may also apply to less severe forms of bowel disease.

Glucose polysaccharides (eg, maltodextrins or polycose) are as well absorbed as is glucose in the first 100 cm of jejunum, even in the absence of pancreatic exocrine secretions. In addition, intestinal disaccharidase (ie, lactase) deficiency is a frequent event in patients with GI disease. Therefore, there is no reason for including mono- or disaccharides, which would unnecessarily increase osmolality, in enteral diets for patients with intestinal failure.[110]

The belief that low-fat diets may be of benefit in intestinal insufficiency has been questioned by controlled trials.[111] In addition, long-chain fatty acids play a major role in promoting intestinal adaptation. However, the quality of lipids in the diet must be adapted to the individual digestive and absorptive capacities of the patient. In diseases in which absorption of long-chain triglycerides is severely impaired (eg, exocrine pancreatic insufficiency, bile salt deficiency, and intestinal lymphangiectasia), part, but not all, of the lipid amount should be supplied as medium-chain triglycerides.

Whole-protein–based polymeric diets are as well tolerated as are peptide-based elemental diets in stable chronic intestinal failure. However, polymeric diets may be poorly absorbed in the early stages after intestinal resection or in patients with severe pancreatic insufficiency. In these cases, diets containing a peptide-based nitrogen source may be useful.[110]

Other changes in enteral diets have been suggested to prevent diarrhea in intestinal failure. First, supplementing sodium to the diet to reach a sodium concentration between 80 and 90 mM has been recommended because intraluminal sodium concentrations below this level result in net intraluminal sodium and water secretion.[112] Second, the addition of fermentable fiber, such as pectin, to the diet has been suggested to improve diarrhea in both healthy subjects[90] and short bowel patients.[113] Early studies claimed for a beneficial effect of adding glutamine and growth hormone to the nutritional regimen of short bowel patients,[114,115] but recent controlled trials have not confirmed this view.[116,117]

Liver Disease

Sodium and water retention and hepatic encephalopathy are major complications of chronic liver disease that may be worsened by standard EN.

Enteral formulas for cirrhotic patients must be low in sodium, and water intake must be restricted.[118] Because this is difficult to achieve with standard diets providing 1 kcal/mL, energy dense (1.3- to 1.5-kcal/mL) formulas should be used in these patients. These diets do not cause diarrhea when administered slowly with the aid of a peristaltic pump.[64,71]

There is agreement that most cirrhotic patients can receive a standard protein supply without risk of developing hepatic encephalopathy.[118] However, protein-intolerant patients who easily develop encephalopathy with standard dietary protein would benefit from branched-chain amino acids (BCAA).[119,120] BCAA have been claimed to be useful to improve liver function in cirrhotic patients,[121] but this view is not widely agreed upon.[122]

Respiratory Disease

A high-carbohydrate load increases carbon dioxide production, oxygen consumption, and ventilatory requirements. It is not clear whether this phenomenon is clinically important in chronic obstructive pulmonary disease without acute respiratory failure. However, it is harmful in critically ill hypercapnic patients. Because the complete oxidation of fat produces less carbon dioxide than do isocaloric amounts of carbohydrates, formula diets in which some of the carbohydrate calories are replaced with fat calories should be used in these patients.[123]

Severe Malnutrition—Refeeding Syndrome

Protein-energy malnutrition has important consequences on the morphology and function of the GI tract and pancreas. Severely malnourished patients may show intestinal villous atrophy and malabsorption, as well as impairment in immune gut response and mucosal barrier function. Therefore, most of the above-mentioned maneuvers to avoid diarrhea in intestinal failure may also apply to patients with severe protein-energy malnutrition.

The potential adverse effects of therapeutic refeeding in severely malnourished patients (either acute or chronic) and those undergoing prolonged starvation were already recognized before the advent of artificial nutrition and have been noted in both parenterally and enterally fed patients, both children and adults.[124-126]

A major pathogenic mechanism for refeeding syndrome is the intracellular shift of some minerals to meet the needs for feeding-stimulated anabolic protein synthesis. This may result in severe hypophosphatemia, hypokalemia, and hypomagnesaemia. Thiamine deficiency, often occurring in malnourished alcoholics, has also been ascribed to refeeding syndrome,[124] although this issue is still controversial. Similarly, the combination of hypertonic dehydration, hypernatremia, and prerenal azotemia, occurring in as many as 5% to 10% of patients receiving hyperosmolar enteral diets, can also be considered part of this syndrome.[124] The clinical consequences of refeeding syndrome include cardiorespiratory, GI, neuromuscular, renal, and hematological disturbances, which can result in a patient's death.[125,127] Prevention of refeeding syndrome requires: 1) recognition of those patients at risk; 2) administration of small amounts of nutrients, instead of attempting hyperalimentation, in the early phases of refeeding; and 3) close monitoring of the electrolyte status, including phosphorus, potassium, and magnesium, over the first week of refeeding.[124,126]

Other Complications

Carbohydrate Intolerance

Hyperglycemia may constitute a problem in diabetic and other critically ill or severely malnourished patients on EN. Hyperglycemia may be deleterious, as it may result in osmotic diuresis, dehydration, hypotension, hyperosmolar nonketotic coma, and ketoacidosis. High total carbohydrate content and the presence of variable amounts of disaccharides in some enteral formulas may partly account for glucose intolerance associated with enteral feeding. Likewise, insulin resistance is a common event in critically ill patients.

Two recent trials investigated the metabolic effects of disease-specific enteral formulas in critically ill patients with diabetes mellitus or stress hyperglycemia[128] and with type 1 diabetics,[129] respectively. Both trials showed a better control of glycaemia in patients receiving the diabetes-adapted diet as compared to the standard formula.[128,129] In both studies, the diabetes-adapted diet included the following modifications, as compared to the standard control formula: 1) supplements of fiber, mostly containing partially hydrolyzed guar gum; 2) partial replacement of maltodextrin by fructose and starch; and 3) increased amounts of lipids as monounsaturated fat. The second of the trials listed above[129] included a third therapeutic arm of patients receiving a similar formula in which only the fiber supplement was added. Interestingly, the glycaemic response of these patients did not differ from that of patients receiving the standard control formula,[129] a result that suggests that the contribution of added fiber is not much relevant to the effects of disease-specific diets for diabetics. This is not surprising if one keeps in mind that viscosity is a sine qua non for the decrease in glycaemic response associated to dietary fiber,[130] and this property is lost with hydrolysis.

LIVER DYSFUNCTION

Abnormal liver-function tests—including increased serum alkaline phosphatase, glutamyl transpeptidase, and aminotransferase activities—were reported early in enterally fed patients. However, the clinical significance of these complications is much less with enteral than with parenteral feeding.

Experimental studies have demonstrated that animals fed intragastrically show a lower incidence of fatty liver than those fed intravenously.[131] Moreover, liver dysfunction secondary to PN clearly improves or even disappears when oral feeding is allowed along with intravenous feeding.[132] In controlled trials, the appearance of liver-function–test derangement in patients with inflammatory bowel disease was similar in individuals on EN and those receiving an oral hospital diet,[133] but significantly lower in enterally than in parenterally fed patients,[134] In addition, in some patients on PN, this had to be discontinued because of the severity of liver dysfunction, whereas it did not occur in any case with enteral feeding.[134]

Conclusion

EN is a safe procedure for feeding most patients who require artificial nutritional support, including those with diseases of the GI tract. Although tube-feeding–related complications are scarce and often mild, they may sometimes be severe and even fatal. In any case, they always contribute to diminish the effectiveness of EN.

The technique of administration must be accurate to prevent life-threatening complications: eg, tube misplacement with intrapulmonary infusion of the diet and bronchoaspiration. Both inadequate technique and inappropriate choice of diet account for diarrhea and other forms of digestive intolerance, which are probably the most frequent and troublesome complications of EN. Finally, metabolic complications, most of them included in the concept of refeeding syndrome, are rare but can be severe.

The judicious use of the various available devices for enteral access and formula diets allows minimization of the morbidity rate of EN. On the other hand, the limitations of the technique must be considered. In this sense, enteral feeding aims to provide adequate nutrition to the patient while maintaining or improving the trophism of his or her bowel. In some circumstances (eg, acute intestinal failure), only the second objective can be met, and the simultaneous use of both EN and PN is mandatory. Administering full-strength enteral feeding alone in these cases may be a source of complications and disappointing results.

References

1. Jones KW, Seltzer MH, Slocum BA, et al. Parenteral nutrition complications in a voluntary hospital. *JPEN J Parenter Enternal Nutr.* 1984;8:385-390.
2. Cataldi-Betcher EL, Seltzer MH, Slocum BA, Jones KW. Complications occurring during enteral nutrition support: a prospective study. *JPEN J Parenter Enternal Nutr.* 1983;7:546-552.
3. Braunschweig CL, Levy P, Sheean PM, Wang X. Enteral compared with parenteral nutrition: a meta-analysis. *Am J Clin Nutr.* 2001;74:534-542.
4. Cabré E, Gassull MA. Complications of enteral feeding. *Nutrition.* 1993;9:1-9.
5. Silk DBA, Rees RGP, Keohane PP, Attrill H. Clinical efficacy and design changes of "fine bore" nasogastric feeding tubes: A seven-year experience involving 809 intubations in 403 patients. *JPEN J Parenter Enternal Nutr.* 1987;11:378-383.
6. Woodall BH, Winfield DF, Bisset GS. Inadvertent tracheobronchial placement of feeding tubes. *Radiology.* 1987;165:727-729.
7. Sitzmann JV. Nutritional support of the dysphagic patient: Methods, risks, and complications of therapy. *JPEN J Parenter Enternal Nutr.* 1990;14:60-63.
8. Torrington KC, Bowman MA. Fatal hydrothorax and empyema complicating a malpositioned nasogastric tube. *Chest.* 1981;79:240-242.
9. Culpepper JA, Veremakis C, Guntupalli KK, Sladen A. Malpositioned nasogastric tube causing pneumothorax and bronchopleural fistula. *Chest.* 1982;81:389.
10. Balogh GJ, Adler SJ, Van der Woude J, et al. Pneumothorax as a complication of feeding tube placement. *Am J Roentgeol.* 1983;141:1275-1277.
11. Aronchick JM, Epstein DM, Gefter WB, Miller WT. Pneumothorax as a complication placement of a nasoenteric tube. *JAMA.* 1984; 52:3287-3288.
12. Hand RW, Kempster M, Levy JH, Rogol PR, Spirn P. Inadvertent transbronchial insertion of narrow-bore feeding tubes into the pleural space. *JAMA.* 1984;251:2396-2397.
13. Dorsey JS, Cogordan J. Nasotracheal intubation and pulmonary parenchymal perforation. An unusual complication of naso-enteral feeding with small-diameter feeding tubes. *Chest.* 1985;87:131-132.
14. Lipman TO, Kessler T, Arabian A. Nasopulmonary intubation with feeding tubes: case reports and review of the literature. *JPEN J Parenter Enternal Nutr.* 1985;9:618-620.
15. Yavascaoglu B, Acar H, Iscimen R, Gurbet A, Uysal H, Kutlay O. Fatal hydrothorax due to misplacement of a nasoenteric feeding tube. *J Int Med Res.* 2001;29:437-440.
16. Rees RGP, Attrill H, Quinn D, Silk DBA. Improved design of nasogastric feeding tubes. *Clin Nutr.* 1986;5:203-207.
17. Herrmann ME, Liehr RM, Tanhoefner H, Emde C, Riecken EO. Subjective distress during continuous enteral alimentation: superiority of silicone rubber to polyurethane. *JPEN J Parenter Enternal Nutr.* 1989;13:281-285.
18. Bayer LM, Bauers CM, Knapp SR. Psychosocial aspects of nutritional support. *Nurs Clin North Am.* 1983;18:119-128.
19. Caos A, Gogel HK. A simple method for clearing enteral feeding tubes. *Gastrointest Endosc.* 1986;32:55.
20. Marcuard SP, Stegall KL. Unclogging feeding tubes with pancreatic enzyme. *JPEN J Parenter Enternal Nutr.* 1990;14:198-200.
21. Krupp KB, Heximer B. Going with the flow. How to prevent feeding tubes from clogging. *Nursing.* 1998;28:54-55.
22. American Gastroenterological Association Medical Position Statement: Guidelines for the use of enteral nutrition. *Gastroenterology.* 1995;108:1280-1281.

23. Kirby DF, DeLegge MH, Fleming CR. American Gastroenterological Association technical review on tube feeding for enteral nutrition. *Gastroenterology.* 1995;108:1282-1301.
24. Payne James JJ. Enteral nutrition: tubes and techniques of delivery. In: Payne-James J, Grimble G, Silk DBA, eds. *Artificial Nutrition Support in Clinical Practice.* London: Edward Arnold, 1995:197-213.
25. Jones M, Santanello SA, Falcone RE. Percutaneous endoscopic vs surgical gastrostomy. *JPEN J Parenter Enternal Nutr.* 1990;14:533-534.
26. Stiegmann GV, Goff JS, Silas D, Pearlman N, Sun J, Norton L. Endoscopic versus operative gastrostomy: Final results of a prospectiva randomized trial. *Gastrointest Endosc.* 1990;36:1-5.
27. Scott JS, De la Torre RA, Unger SW. Comparison of operative versus percutaneous endoscopic gastrostomy tube placement in the elderly. *Am Surg.* 1991;57:338-340.
28. Larson DE, Burton DD, Schroeder KW, DiMagno EP. Percutaneous endoscopic gastrostomy. Indications, success, complications, and mortality in 314 consecutive patients. *Gastroenterology.* 1987;93:48-52.
29. DeLegge MH, Duckworth PF, McHenry L, et al. Percutaneous endoscopic gastrojejunostomy: A dual center safety and efficacy trial. *JPEN J Parenter Enternal Nutr.* 1995;19:239-243.
30. Schurink CA, Tuynman H, Scholten P, et al. Percutaneous endoscopic gastrostomy: complications and suggestions to avoid them. *Eur J Gastroenterol Hepatol.* 2001;13:819-823.
31. Sanders DS, Carter MJ, D'Silva J, et al. Percutaneous endoscopic gastrostomy: a prospective analysis of hospital support required and complications following discharge to the community. *Eur J Clin Nutr.* 2001;55:610-614.
32. Jonas SK, Neimark S, Panwalker AP. Effect of antibiotic prophylaxis in percutaneous endoscopic gastrostomy. *Am J Gastroenterol.* 1985; 80:438-441
33. Dormann AJ, Wigginghaus B, Risius H, et al. A single dose of ceftriaxone administered 30 minutes before percutaneous endoscopic gastrostomy significantly reduces local and systemic infective complications. *Am J Gastroenterol.* 1999;94:3220-3224.
34. Dormann AJ, Wigginghaus B, Risius H, et al. Antibiotic prophylaxis in percutaneous endoscopic gastrostomy (PEG): results from a prospective randomized multicenter trial. *Z Gastroenterol.* 2000;38:229-234.
35. Panigrahi H, Shreeve DR, Tan WC, Prudham R, Kaufman R. Role of antibiotic prophylaxis for wound infection in percutaneous endoscopic gastrostomy (PEG): result of a prospective double-blind randomized trial. *J Hosp Infect.* 2002;50:312-315.
36. Ahmad I, Mouncher A, Abdoolah A, et al. Antibiotic prophylaxis for percutaneous endoscopic gastrostomy: a prospective, randomised, double-blind trial. *Aliment Pharmacol Ther.* 2003;18:209-215.
37. Rey JR, Axon A, Budzynska A, Kruse A, Nowak A. Guidelines of the European Society of Gastrointestinal Endoscopy (E.S.G.E.): antibiotic prophylaxis for gastrointestinal endoscopy. *Endoscopy.* 1998;30:318-324.
38. Dulabon GR, Abrams JE, Rutherford EJ. The incidence and significance of free air after percutaneous endoscopic gastrostomy. *Am Surg.* 2002;68:590-593.
39. Eddy VA, Snell JE, Morris JA. Analysis of complications and long-term outcome of trauma patients with needle catheter jejunostomy. *Am Surg.* 1996;62:40-44.
40. De Gottardi A, Krahenbuhl L, Farhadi J, et al. Clinical experience of feeding through a needle catheter jejunostomy after major abdominal operations. *Eur J Surg.* 1999;165:1055-1060.
41. Biffi R, Lotti M, Cenciarelli S, et al. Complications and long-term outcome of 80 oncology patients undergoing needle catheter jenunostomy placement for early postopertative enteral feeding. *Clin Nutr.* 2000;19:277-279.
42. Chin KF, Townsend S, Wong W, Miller GV. A prospective cohort study of feeding needle catheter jejunostomy in an upper gastrointestinal surgical unit. *Clin Nutr.* 2004;23:691-696.
43. Weimann A, Braunert M, Müller T, Bley T, Wiedemann B. Feasibility and safety of needle catheter jejunostomy for enteral nutrition in surgically treated severe acute pancreatitis. *JPEN J Parenter Enternal Nutr.* 2004;28:324-327.
44. Myers JG, Page CP, Stewart RM, et al. Complications of needle catheter jejunostomy in 2022 consecutive applications. *Am J Surg.* 1995;170:547-551.
45. Han-Geurts IJ, Verhoef C, Tilanus HW. Relaparotomy following complications of feeding jejunostomy in esophageal surgery. *Dig Surg.* 2004;21:192-196.
46. Smith CD, Sarr MG. Clinically significant pneumatosis intestinalis with postoperative enteral feedings by needle catheter jejunostomy: an unusual complication. *JPEN J Parenter Enternal Nutr.* 1991;15:328-331.
47. Wolthuis AM, Vanrijkel JP, Aelvoet C, De Weer F. Needle catheter jejunostomy complicated by pneumatosis intestinalis: a case report. *Acta Chir Belg.* 2003;103:631-632.
48. Edington H, Zajko A, Reilly JJ. Jejunal variceal hemorrhage: an unusual complication of needle catheter jejunostomy. *JPEN J Parenter Enternal Nutr.* 1983;7:489-491.
49. Smith-Choban P, Max MH. Feeding jejunostomy: a small bowel stress test? *Am J Surg.* 1988;155:112-117.
50. Munshi IA, Steingrub JS, Wolpert L. Small bowel necrosis associated with early postoperative jejunal tube feeding in a trauma patient. *J Trauma.* 2000;49:163-165.
51. Ulicny KS, Korelitz JL. Multiorgan failure from the inadvertent intravenous administration of enteral feeding. *JPEN J Parenter Enternal Nutr.* 1989;13:658-660.
52. Kazi N, Mobarhan S. Enteral feeding associated gastroesophageal reflux and aspiration pneumonia: a review. *Nutr Rev.* 1996; 54:324-328.
53. Jacobs S, Chang RWS, Lee B, Bartlett FW. Continuous enteral feeding: A major cause of pneumonia among ventilated intensive care unit patients. *JPEN J Parenter Enternal Nutr.* 1990;14:353-356.
54. Heyland DK, Drover JW, MacDonald S, Novak F, Lam M. Effect of postpyloric feeding on gastroesophageal regurgitation and pulmonary microaspiration: results of a randomized controlled trial. *Crit Care Med.* 2001;29:1495-1501.
55. Heyland DK, Drover JW, Dhaliwal R, Greenwood J. Optimizing the benefits and minimizing the risks of enteral nutrition in the critically ill: role of small bowel feeding. *JPEN J Parenter Enternal Nutr.* 2002;26(Suppl):S51-S57.
56. Metheny NA. Risk factors for aspiration. *JPEN J Parenter Enternal Nutr.* 2002;26(Suppl):S26-S33.
57. Lin HC, Van Citters GW. Stopping enteral feeding for arbitrary gastric residual volume may not be physiologically sound: Results of a computer simulation model. *JPEN.* 1997;21:286-289.
58. McClave SA, Snider HL. Clinical use of gastric residual volumes as a monitor for patients on enteral tube feeding. *JPEN J Parenter Enternal Nutr.* 2002;26(Suppl):43-S50.
59. Ibáñez J, Peñafiel A, Marsé P, Jordá R, Raurich JM, Mata F. Incidence of gastroesophageal reflux and aspiration in mechanically ventilated patients using small-bore nasogastric tubes. *JPEN J Parenter Enternal Nutr.* 2000;24:103-106.
60. Shang E, Geiger N, Sturm JW, Post S. Pump-assisted versus gravity-controlled enteral nutrition in long-term percutaneous endoscopic gastrostomy patients: a prospective controlled trial. *JPEN J Parenter Enternal Nutr.* 2003;27:216-219.
61. Shang E, Geiger N, Sturm JW, Post S. Pump-assisted enteral nutrition can prevent aspiration in bedridden percutaneous endoscopic gastrostomy patients. *JPEN J Parenter Enternal Nutr.* 2004;28:180-183.
62. Davies AR, Bellomo R. Establishment of enteral nutrition: prokinetic agents and small bowel feeding tubes. *Curr Opin Crit Care.* 2004;10:156-161.

63. Keohane PP, Attrill H, Grimble G, Spiller R, Frost P, Silk DBA. Enteral nutrition in malnourished patients with hepatic cirrhosis and acute hepatic encephalopathy. *JPEN J Parenter Enternal Nutr.* 1983;7:346-350.
64. Cabré E, González-Huix F, Abad A, et al. Effect of total enteral nutrition on the short-term outcome of severely malnourished cirrhotics: a randomized controlled trial. *Gastroenterology.* 1990;98:715-720.
65. De Lédinghen V, Beau P, Mannant PR, et al. Early feeding or enteral nutrition in patients with cirrhosis after bleeding from esophageal varices? A randomized controlled study. *Dig Dis Sci.* 1997;42:536-541.
66. Cabré E, Rodríguez-Iglesias P, Caballería J, et al. Short- and long-term outcome of severe alcohol-induced hepatitis treated with steroids or enteral nutrition. A multicenter randomized trial. *Hepatology.* 2000;32:36-42.
67. Bliss DZ, Guenter PA, Settle RG. Defining and reporting diarrhea in tube feed patients—what a mess! *Am J Clin Nutr.* 1992;55:753-759.
68. Guenter PA, Sweed MR. A valid and reliable tool to quantify stool output in tube-fed patients. *JPEN J Parenter Enternal Nutr.* 1998;22:147-151.
69. Jones BJM, Payne S, Silk DBA. Indications for pump-assisted enteral feeding. *Lancet.* 1980;1:1057-1058.
70. Keohane PP, Attrill H, Love M, Frost P, Silk DBA. Relation between osmolality of diet and gastrointestinal side effects in enteral nutrition. *Br Med J.* 1984;288:678-680.
71. Smith J, Horowitz J, Henderson JM, Heymsfield SB. Enteral hyperalimentation in undernourished patients with cirrhosis and ascites. *Am J Clin Nutr.* 1982;35:56-72.
72. Bowling TE, Silk DBA. Diarrhea and enteral nutrition. In: Rombeau JL, Rolandelli RH, eds. *Clinical Nutrition: Enteral and Tube Feeding.* Philadelphia: W.B. Saunders Co.; 1997:540-553.
73. Rees RGP, Keohane PP, Grimble G, Frost P, Attrill H, Silk DBA. Elemental diet administered nasogastrically without starter regimens to patients with inflammatory bowel disease. *JPEN J Parenter Enternal Nutr.* 1986;10:258-262.
74. Guenter PA, Settle RG, Perlmutter S, et al. Tube feeding-related diarrhea in acutely ill patients. *JPEN J Parenter Enternal Nutr.* 1991;15:277-280.
75. Broom J, Jones K. Causes and prevention of diarrhoea in patients receiving enteral nutritional support. *J Hum Nutr.* 1981;35:123-127.
76. Gupta TP, Ehrinpreis MN. Candida-associated diarrhea in hospitalized patients. *Gastroenterology.* 1990;98:780-785.
77. Greeg CR, Toskes PP. Enteric bacterial flora and small bowel bacterial overgrowth syndrome. In: Feldman M, Friedman LS, Sleisenger MH, eds. *Sleisenger & Fordtran's Gastrointestinal and Liver Disease* (7th ed.). Philadelphia: W.B. Saunders Co.; 2002:1783-1793.
78. Mickschl DB, Davidson LS, Fluomoy DJ, Parker DE. Contamination of enteral feedings and diarrhea in patients in intensive care units. *Heart Lung.* 1990;19:362-370.
79. Anderton A. Bacterial contamination of enteral feeds and feeding systems. *Clin Nutr.* 1993;12(Suppl):S16-S32.
80. Anderson KR, Norris DJ, Godfrey LB, Avent CK, Butterworth CE. Bacterial contamination of tube-feeding formulas. *JPEN J Parenter Enternal Nutr.* 1984;8:673-678.
81. Belknap DC, Davidson J, Flournoy DJ. Microorganisms and diarrhea in enterally fed intensive care unit patients. *JPEN J Parenter Enternal Nutr.* 1990;14:622-628.
82. Freedland CP, Roller RD, Wolfe BM, Flynn NM. Microbial contamination of continuous drip feedings. *JPEN J Parenter Enternal Nutr.* 1989;13:18-22.
83. Marion ND, Rupp ME. Infection control issues of enteral feeding systems. *Curr Opin Clin Nutr Metabol Care.* 2000;3:363-366.
84. Casewell MW, Cooper JE, Webster M. Enteral feeds contaminated with Enterobacter cloacae as a cause of septicaemia. *Br Med J.* 1981;282:973.
85. Baldwin BA, Zagoren AJ, Rose N. Bacterial contamination of continuously infused enteral alimentation with needle catheter jenunostomy. Clinical implications. *JPEN J Parenter Enternal Nutr.* 1984;8:30-33.
86. Levy J, Van Laethem Y, Verhaegen G, et al. Contamined enteral nutrition solutions as a cause of nosocomial bloodstream infection: A study using plasmid fingerprinting. *JPEN J Parenter Enternal Nutr.* 1989;13:228-234.
87. Oie S, Kamiya A, Hironga K, Koshira A. Microbial contamination of enteral feeding solutions and its prevention. *Am J Infect Control.* 1992;20:202-205.
88. Dentinger B, Faucher KJ, Ostrom SM, Schmidl MK. Controlling bacterial contamination of an enteral formula through the use of a unique closed system. *Nutrition.* 1995;11:747-750.
89. Rees RGP, Ryan J, Attrill H, Silk DBA. Clinical evaluation of two-liter prepacked enteral diet delivery system: a controlled trial. *JPEN J Parenter Enternal Nutr.* 1988;12:274-277.
90. Zimmaro DM, Rolandelli RH, Koruda MJ, et al. Isotonic tube feeding formula induces liquid stool in normal subjects: reversal by pectin. *JPEN J Parenter Enternal Nutr.* 1989;13:117-123.
91. Frankenfield DC, Beyer PL. Soy-polysaccharide fiber: effect on diarrhea in tube-fed, head-injured patients. *Am J Clin Nutr.* 1989;50:533-538.
92. Dobb GJ, Towler SC. Diarrhoea during enteral feeding in the critically ill: a comparison of feeds with and without fibre. *Intensive Care Med.* 1990; 16:252-255.
93. Homann HH, Kemen M, Fuessenich C, Senkal M, Zumtobel V. Reduction in diarrhea incidence by soluble fiber in patients receiving total or supplemental enteral nutrition. *JPEN J Parenter Enternal Nutr.* 1994;18:486-490.
94. Spapen H, Diltoer M, Van Malderen C, et al. Soluble fiber reduces the incidence of diarrhea in septic patients receiving total enteral nutrition: a prospective, double-blind, randomized, and controlled trial. *Clin Nutr.* 2001;20:301-305.
95. Schultz AA, Ashby-Hughes B, Taylor R, Gillis DE, Wilkins M. Effects of pectin on diarrhea in critically ill tube-fed patients receiving antibiotics. *Am J Crit Care.* 2000;9:403-411.
96. Jones BJM, Lees R, Andrews J, Frost P, Silk DBA. Comparison of and elemental and polymeric enteral diet in patients with normal gastrointestinal function. *Gut.* 1983;24:78-84.
97. Viall C, Porcelli K, Terán JC, Varma RN, Steffee WP. A double-blind clinical trial comparing gastrointestinal side effects of two enteral feeding formulas. *JPEN J Parenter Enternal Nutr.* 1990;14:265-269.
98. Slavin JL, Nelson NL, McNamara EA, Cashmere K. Bowel function of healthy men consuming liquid diets with and without dietary fiber. *JPEN J Parenter Enternal Nutr.* 1985;9:317-321.
99. Lampe JW, Effertz ME, Larson JL, Slavin JL. Gastrointestinal effects of modified guar gum and soy polysaccharide as part of an enteral formula diet. *JPEN J Parenter Enternal Nutr.* 1992;16:538-544.
100. Kapadia SA, Raimundo AH, Silk DBA. The effect of a fibre free and fibre supplemented polymeric enteral diet on normal human bowel function. *Clin Nutr.* 1993;12:272-276.
101. Meier R, Beglinger C, Schnieder H, Rowedder A, Gyr K. Effect of a liquid diet with and without soluble fiber supplementation on intestinal transit and cholecystokinin release in volunteers. *JPEN J Parenter Enternal Nutr.* 1993;17:231-235.
102. Kapadia SA, Raimundo AH, Grimble GK, Aimer P, Silk DBA. Influence of three different fiber-supplemented enteral diets on bowel function and short-chain fatty acid production. *JPEN J Parenter Enternal Nutr.* 1995;19:63-68.
103. Silk DBA, Walters ER, Duncan HD, Green CJ. The effect of a polymeric enteral formula supplemented with a mixture of six fibres on normal human bowel function and colonic motility. *Clin Nutr.* 2001;20:49-58.
104. Sunvold GD, Titgemeyer EC, Bourquin LD, Fahey GC, Garleb KA. Alteration of the fiber and lipid components of a defined-formula diet: Effects on stool characteristics, nutrient digestibility, mineral balance, and energy metabolism in humans. *Am J Clin Nutr.* 1995;62:1252-1260.

105. Patil DH, Grimble G, Keohane PP, Attrill H, Love M, Silk DBA. Do fibre containing enteral diets have advantages over existing low residue diets? *Clin Nutr.* 1985;4:67-71.
106. Heymsfield SB, Roongspisuthipong C, Evert M, Casper K, Heller P, Akrabawi SS. Fiber supplementation of enteral formulas: effects on the bioavailability of major nutrients and gastrointestinal tolerance. *JPEN J Parenter Enteral Nutr.* 1988;12:265-273.
107. Shankardass K, Chuchmach S, Chelswick K, et al. Bowel function of long-term tube-fed patients consuming formulae with and without dietary fiber. *JPEN J Parenter Enteral Nutr.* 1990;14:508-512.
108. Zarling EJ, Edison T, Berger S, Leya J, DeMeo M. Effect of dietary oat and soy fiber on bowel function and clinical tolerance in a tube feeding dependent population. *J Am Coll Nutr.* 1994;13:565-568.
109. Liebl BH, Fischer MH, Van Calcar SC, Marlett JA. Dietary fiber and long-term large bowel response in enterally nourished nonambulatory profoundly retarded youth. *JPEN J Parenter Enteral Nutr.* 1990;14:371-375.
110. Scolapio JS, Fleming CR. Short bowel syndrome. *Gastroenterol Clin North Am.* 1998;27:467-479.
111. Jeejeebhoy KN. Therapy of the short-gut syndrome. *Lancet.* 1983;1:1427-1429.
112. Spiller RC, Jones BJM, Silk DBA. Jejunal water and electrolyte absorption from two proprietary enteral feeds in man: importance of sodium content. *Gut.* 1987;28:681-687.
113. Koruda MJ, Rolandelli RH, Settle RG, Saul SH, Rombeau JL. The effect of a pectin-supplemented elemental diet on intestinal adaptation to massive small bowel resection. *JPEN J Parenter Enteral Nutr.* 1986;10:343-350.
114. Byrne TA, Morrissey TB, Nattakom TV, Ziegler TR, Wilmore DW. Growth hormone, glutamine, and a modified diet enhance nutrient absorption in patients with severe short bowel syndrome. *JPEN.* 1995;19:296-302.
115. Wilmore DW. Growth factors and nutrients in the short bowel syndrome. *JPEN J Parenter Enteral Nutr.* 1999;23(Suppl):S117-S120.
116. Li L, Irving M. The effectiveness of growth hormone, glutamine and a low-fat diet containing high-carbohydrate on the enhancement of the function of remnant intestine among patients with short bowel syndrome: a review of published trials. *Clin Nutr.* 2001;20:199-204.
117. Scolapio JS, Mcgreevy K, Tennyson GS, Burnett OL. Effect of glutamine in short-bowel syndrome. *Clin Nutr.* 2001;20:319-323.
118. Plauth M, Merli M, Kondrup J, Weimann A, Ferenci P, Müller MJ. ESPEN guidelines for nutrition in liver disease and transplantation. *Clin Nutr.* 1997;16:43-55.
119. Horst D, Grace ND, Conn HO, et al. Comparison of dietary protein with an oral, branched chain-enriched amino acid supplement in chronic portal-systemic encephalopathy: A randomized controlled trial. *Hepatology.* 1984;4:279-287.
120. Marchesini G, Dioguardi FS, Bianchi G, et al. Long-term oral branched-chain amino acid treatment in chronic hepatic encephalopathy. A randomized double-blind case in-controlled trial. *J Hepatol.* 1990;11:92-101.
121. Marchesini G, Bianchi G, Merli M, et al. Nutritional supplementation with branched-chain amino acids in advanced cirrhosis: a double-blind, randomized trial. *Gastroenterology.* 2003;124:1792-1801.
122. Charlton M. Branched-chain amino acid-enriched supplements as therapy for liver disease: Rasputin lives. *Gastroenterology.* 2003;124:1980-1982.
123. Radrizzani D, Iapichino G. Nutrition and lung function in the critically ill patient. *Clin Nutr.* 1998;17:7-10.
124. Solomon SM, Kirby DF. The refeeding syndrome: A review. *JPEN J Parenter Enteral Nutr.* 1990;14:90-97.
125. Crook MA, Hally V, Panteli JV. The importance of the refeeding syndrome. *Nutrition.* 2001;17:632-637.
126. Afzal NA, Addai S, Fagbemi A, et al. Refeeding syndrome with enteral nutrition in children: a case report, literature review and clinical guidelines. *Clin Nutr.* 2002;21:515-520.
127. Weinsier RL, Krumdieck CL. Death resulting from overzealous total parenteral nutrition: The refeeding syndrome revisited. *Am J Clin Nutr.* 1980;34:393-399.
128. Mesejo A, Acosta JA, Ortega C, et al. Comparison of a high-protein disease-specific enteral formula with a high-protein enteral formula in hyperglycemic critically ill patients. *Clin Nutr.* 2003;22:295-305.
129. Crespillo MC, Olveira G, Ruiz de Adana MS, et al. Metabolic effects of an enteral nutrition formula for diabetes: comparison with standard formulas in patients with type 1 diabetes. *Clin Nutr.* 2003;22:483-487.
130. Jenkins DJA, Wolever TMS, Leeds AR, et al. Dietary fibres, fibre analogues, and glucose tolerance: importance of viscosity. *Br Med J.* 1978;1:1392-1394.
131. King WWK, Boelhouwer RU, Kingsnorth AN, et al. Nutritional efficacy and hepatic changes during intragastric, intravenous, and prehepatic feeding in rats. *JPEN.* 1983;7:443-446.
132. Pallarés R, Sitges Serra A, Fuentes J, et al. Factores etiopatogénicos posiblemente implicados en la disfunción hepática asociada a nutrición parenteral: Estudio prospectivo de 104 pacientes adultos. *Med Clin* (Barc). 1984;83:832-836.
133. Dolz C, Xiol X, Abad A, et al. Changes in liver function tests in patients with inflammatory bowel disease on enteral nutrition. *JPEN J Parenter Enteral Nutr.* 1989;13:401-405.
134. Abad A, González-Huix F, Esteve M, et al. Liver function tests abnormalities in patients with inflammatory bowel disease receiving artifical nutrition: a prospective randomized study of total enteral nutrition vs total parenteral nutrition. *JPEN J Parenter Enteral Nutr.* 1990;14:618-621.

Chapter 40

Home Parenteral Nutrition in Infants, Children, and Adults

David Ziring, MD, and Marvin Ament, MD

Introduction

For the past 30 years, the delivery of parenteral nutrition (PN) in the home has allowed patients the ability to thrive and maintain an active lifestyle without the need for hospitalization. Despite incremental changes in delivery systems, the basic formula of home PN has remained unchanged since the early 1970s. With growing confidence in its safety, practitioners have utilized home PN in an expanding population of patients.

Moving home PN beyond the realm of intestinal failure, physicians have used home PN in a number of patients who would not traditionally be treated with PN. These include patients with ulcerative colitis, improving nutritional status as a bridge to surgery, growing adolescents with inflammatory bowel disease (IBD) to maximize caloric intake during a potential time of maximal growth velocity, and patients awaiting orthotopic liver transplantation.

Medicine continues to progress in decreasing the incidence of catheter-related sepsis, although PN-related cholestasis remains a significant problem. However, home PN has remained the only life sustaining therapy for many patients prior to the advent of successful small bowel transplantation.

More than 3,000 patients in the United States receive home PN at any one time, particularly in immature and premature infants, of which 10% to 20% are children less than 18 years old.[1] Most of these pediatric patients are able to attend school, and the adults can work during the day and are able to participate in sporting activities including running and swimming. Many adults are trained to care for their catheters and to administer their own PN, and adolescents too have gained independence by performing these skills themselves.

History

The delivery of PN for children at home was pioneered by Drs. Scribner, Broviac, and Ament in 1971, while treating two pediatric patients. One child was a 9-year-old girl who had diffuse mast cell disease in which her gastrointestinal (GI) mucosa was flat, causing a significant malabsorptive and secretory diarrhea. The other child was a 3-year-old boy with end-stage acrodermatitis enteropathica. Both patients survived for several years on PN but died of complications from their illnesses.

Indications

Home PN has primarily been used in patients with intestinal failure. Intestinal failure is defined as the inability to maintain adequate nutrition and hydration with enteral feedings. This group encompasses a wide variety of disease entities, but consists most often of a few diagnoses, including short bowel syndrome, patients with motility disorders, severe mucosal injury, congenital malabsorptive syndromes, trauma and vascular accidents, radiation enteritis, and Crohn's disease (Table 40-1).

Home PN is not something that should be used for patients needing only limited nutrition support. To justify the time and expense in training the patient and his or her family members, as well as the risk inherent to having an indwelling central venous catheter, the patient should require at least 30 days of support at home. Home PN is increasingly used for several months, as a relatively short-term nutritional adjunct. For patients with more complex disorders, home PN is administered for years, allowing the gut time to grow and adapt to

TABLE 40-1.

Common Indications for Home Total Parenteral Nutrition

Indication
Short Bowel Syndrome
Secondary to jejunoileal atresia
Secondary to necrotizing enterocolitis
Secondary to midgut volvulus with strangulation
Associated with gastroschisis
Congenital short bowel
Secondary to Crohn's disease
Intestinal Motility Disorders
Chronic intestinal pseudo-obstructive syndromes (neuropathic, myopathic, unknown)
Secondary to chemotherapy and radiation injury
Intractable Diarrhea
Failure of enteral nutrition
Refractory sprue
Autoimmune mucosal disease
Crohn's disease
Intestinal lymphangiectasia
Hypoplastic villous syndrome
Microvillus inclusion disease
Autoimmune or post-infectious enteropathy
Collagenous enteropathy
Secretory tumors, etiology unknown
Ascites
Intractable chylous ascites
Other
Cystic fibrosis
Pre-orthotopic liver transplantation, small bowel transplantation
Cancer Related
After bone marrow transplantation
Graft-versus-host disease
Radiation damage to intestine with obstruction and/or diarrhea
Diarrhea, anorexia, vomiting secondary to chemotherapy
Acquired Immunodeficiency Syndrome

enteral feedings. In fact, there are some patients who have required a lifetime of home PN because of their chronic, irreversible intestinal failure. There are cases in which patients have been on home PN for as long as 30 years without developing significant complications.

Short Bowel Syndrome

The majority of patients with short bowel syndrome are children who either are born with congenital short bowel syndrome or who have had significant GI surgical resections in the neonatal period secondary to jejunoileal atresia or gastroschisis or who have suffered from necrotizing enterocolitis. These patients have often been maintained on PN for several months while in the neonatal intensive care unit, while their parents were trained prior to hospital discharge to care for the central catheter and to administer PN.

Patients with short bowel syndrome often receive home PN while simultaneously on enteral feedings. The enteral feeds not only provide trophic nutrients for intestinal adaptation but also provide a measure of protection against the development of PN-associated cholestasis.

Motility Disorders

Patients with intestinal neuropathies or myopathies resulting in chronic intestinal pseudo-obstruction often encounter long periods of time when they are intolerant to enteral feedings and require the fluids and calories that home PN provides. By coordinating with the GI clinical nurse specialists and PN pharmacy, families are able to coordinate a schedule of short-term home PN infusions needed when patients become symptomatic. Home PN allows them to maintain adequate hydration and caloric intake during times of enteral feeding intolerance.

Severe Mucosal Injury

The authors of this chapter have diagnosed several children with a significant enteropathy after they have presumably contracted viral enteritides. Nearly the entire mucosal surface of their small intestine has lost villous structure, leaving them not only with little absorptive capacity but with a profound secretory diarrhea as well. During hospitalization, PN was a vital treatment. After discharge from the hospital, these children have been maintained on home PN, with replacement intravenous fluids and occasionally intermittent albumin infusions for as long as 1 year after contracting their original illnesses. Patients with autoimmune enteropathies with circulating anti-intestinal antibodies have suffered from a similar clinical syndrome and have also benefited from long-term home PN. Some of these patients have been able to gradually discontinue home PN after successful immunosuppressive therapy.

Congenital Malabsorptive Syndromes

Traditionally, patients with congenital malabsorption syndromes, including microvillus inclusion disease, have had very poor prognoses. With the recent advent of small bowel transplantation, these children have had a second chance at a successful outcome. They have benefited from years of home PN, time that they have spent growing and thriving. Despite occasional episodes of line sepsis or thromboses, they were able to enjoy a normal nutritional status through their late teens, enabling them to become excellent candidates for intestinal transplantation.

Trauma and Vascular Accidents

Occasionally, procoagulant conditions have led to vascular catastrophes, such as when a mesenteric arterial thrombosis causes near total gut ischemia and resulting necrosis and the need for sub-total enterectomy. The same condition has occasionally occurred in patients who have been the victims of trauma who suffered from crush injuries or gunshot wounds to the abdomen. These patients also benefit from home PN and have been maintained on nightly PN, usually requiring replacement fluids to account for gastric fluids that comprise non-physiologic end-duodenostomy losses.

Intractable Chylous Ascites/Chylothorax

Patients who suffer the complications of thoracic duct or other lymphatic injury or obstruction from surgery or neoplasm resulting in chylothorax or chylous ascites are often difficult to manage with special diet alone. Despite receiving the majority of their enteral fats as medium chain triglycerides (absorbed directly into the venous channels), they continue to leak large amounts of triglyceride-rich fluid into the chest or abdominal cavity. Home PN has been successfully used as an adjunct therapy in these patients while the injured lymphatics heal or during chemotherapy as a malignancy regresses. Once treated, home PN may be discontinued without recurrence of the fluid accumulation.

Inflammatory Bowel Disease

Home PN has been used successfully for many years to allow for "bowel rest" so patients with severe, often steroid-dependent IBD can attain quiescence of active disease. There is a significant population of children who have delayed the decision for a surgical cure for their ulcerative colitis and who have become malnourished in the interim, while becoming poor surgical candidates with poor wound-healing capability. These patients often benefit from short-term home PN as their nutritional status improves, making them better candidates for colectomy. IBD causes depletion of protein stores, not only because of inadequate oral intake during times of illness but also because profoundly inflamed intestine causes net excretion of protein in stool. Home PN provides a source of anabolic protein as well as non-protein calories used for short-term energy needs and long-term storage of calories.

Contraindications

There are no absolute contraindications to receiving home PN. Patients or their caregivers understand the risks, must demonstrate that they are capable of maintaining good care of the central catheter and performing the daily clean and aseptic techniques required in delivering the PN, and must keep in contact with the treating physicians.

Formulations

Despite some promising trials using supplements of branched chain amino acids[2] and omega 3 fatty acids[3-5] in severely ill patients, PN formulations have changed little in the last 30 years. PN provides maintenance fluid needs, a carbohydrate source, and an anabolic supply of protein and fatty acids in a carefully balanced formulation. Physicians with expertise in nutritional therapy are skilled and knowledgeable in prescribing PN and in monitoring patients during initiation and maintenance of their home PN regimen. They must work closely in collaboration with the primary care physician. PN is usually initiated in a hospital setting, allowing practitioners to initiate treatment in a controlled environment to monitor parameters such as serum electrolytes, triglycerides, and blood glucose values. They are able to "compress" the length of time of PN administration prior to patient discharge from the hospital. Patients are also able to spend considerable time with the clinical nurse specialists, who train the patients to care for the line and use the intravenous pump in preparation for discharge home.

Formulations are prepared in sterile conditions using laminar flow hoods with double filtration systems.[6] These nutritional products should be routinely cultured and tested for pyrogens to insure their safety prior to dispensing. Intralipids should be discarded after 24 hours of use to reduce the risk of bacterial contamination.[7]

PN is typically delivered to the patient in a "3-in-1" bag in which the dextrose, amino acids, and intravenous lipid emulsions are mixed together in a multi-liter polyethylene bag. Prior to initiating the PN infusion, the patient adds an appropriate multivitamin formulation to the bag.

In-line filters have pore sizes of 1.2-5 μm, to prohibit particulates (or air) in emulsions from reaching the pulmonary arterial bed.[8] In 1994, the US Food and Drug Administration recommended that in-line filters be used when delivering PN from "all-in-one" formulations.[9] Over the past 30 years, in-line filters have caused some problems, as noted by the author's home PN program, because of the filters' high frequency of breaking and cracking. These filters also have not been proven to reduce the incidence of sepsis in home PN.[10,11] Interestingly, however, is the fact that the clogging of these filters in other programs has led to an evolution by pharmacists in preparing "stable" admixtures of PN solutions. PN formulations can be judged unstable not only because of precipitating minerals but also because of contaminating trace elements and vitamin additives that degrade when exposed to light. The stability of these formulations is judged by ever-increasingly complex systems, including (most recently) acoustic attenuation spectroscopy, which has been used to evaluate emulsion droplet size.[8]

Home PN companies typically deliver PN solutions to patients either once or twice weekly, when they must be promptly refrigerated. Prudent discharge planning necessitates a social worker or nurse visit the home to make sure that the family has the requisite refrigerated storage space for PN and that the environment is clean and conducive to home PN administration.

It is strongly recommended that the home PN patient receive his or her PN through a reputable home care company that has considerable experience in the care of such patients; many do not but welcome the care of such a patient because of the financial remuneration. It is also strongly recommended, because of the complexities involved with home PN, that patients requiring this specialized therapy be referred to a center with a physician experienced in the care of such patients. Because the patient at home should be stable, minimal changes in the PN prescription should be required. If frequent laboratory monitoring and changes in the PN formulation are necessary, the patient is probably not ready for discharge.

Delivery

The vast majority of patients on home PN are on a cycled, intermittent infusion. The time of their PN delivery has been "compressed" in the hospital, prior to their discharge, to provide their infusion overnight so they may lead an active lifestyle during the day. Usually, infusion pumps are programmed to taper the infusion slowly over the last hour prior to discontinuation in order to prevent hypoglycemia.

Patients who have end-duodenostomies because of catastrophic gut loss caused by ischemia or trauma may require hydration that may total more than 4 L/day; because of these large volumes, they must receive their infusions over a 24-hour period. Several of these patients are still able to continue their active lifestyles because of the use of portable infusion pumps. These pumps weigh only a few pounds and can be placed in a backpack-type bag that holds the PN and tubing. Typically, patients are able to travel easily with this apparatus to their place of employment or to school.

Catheters

The Broviac and Hickman catheters have remained the mainstay of PN delivery since the late 1970s. These catheters are durable, easily repaired, and secured subcutaneously with a Dacron cuff in a process that typically takes 7 to 14 days after surgical placement. The Broviac and Hickman catheters end in a Luer lock, which makes their use convenient in the home setting. These locks are infused with a heparin solution to prevent thrombosis and then capped following use. Other means of central access include the implanted Port-a-Cath system (Pharmacia Laboratories [Pfizer Inc], New York, NY) and the Infuse-a-port system (Intermedics Infusaid Corporation, Norwood, MA).

Catheters are typically implanted in the infraclavicular subclavian vein, exiting the anterior chest wall. Placing the catheter in this location has the advantages of allowing the patient ease of mobility and maintenance of the sterile site. Femoral venous placement is also an option but may be more difficult to keep sterile, especially in infants wearing diapers. These femoral venous catheters are placed either below the renal veins or immediately inferior to the diaphragm. As sites are eventually lost to thrombosis, other locations must be found for placement, including an azygous vein or superior vena cava placement via thoracotomy.

Catheter and Site Care

Proper technique in caring for the central venous catheter and the surrounding skin are essential for avoiding the complication of catheter-related sepsis. In fact, several studies have found that better-educated patients who receive care in highly experienced PN centers have significantly fewer episodes of sepsis than do patients in less-experienced settings.[12]

Several approaches are in use. It is believed that the iodine released during skin and catheter care in a sustained fashion from the povidone-iodine solution exerts an antibacterial effect.[13] Chlorhexidine 0.5% in 75% isopropyl alcohol has been increasingly used on insertion sites to disinfect the skin. In fact, a recent prospective study showed that combining these agents when disinfecting the skin with a solution of propanol/chlorhexidine followed by povidone-iodine was superior in the preventing microbial colonization of the central venous catheter (CVC) compared to either of the regimens alone.[14] The authors advocate the routine use of 70% alcohol swabs followed by application of a povidone-iodine scrub. These solutions should be applied with a circular motion, applying friction to the skin progressing from the insertion site to peripheral, adjacent sites. The efficacy of ointments used at the insertion site of CVCs has been less clear, although recent authors have suggested the efficacy of Polysporin[15] with hemodialysis catheter sites and other centrally placed, uncuffed percutaneous catheters.[16]

Dressing Changes

A recent meta-analysis of 23 studies found that there was no difference in catheter-related infection rates between using gauze and tape and three types of transparent films.[17] A novel study comparing CVC sepsis rates of adult cancer patients randomized to use standard CVC site dressings or to use a no-dressing strategy found no difference in sepsis rates but earlier rates of infection in the dressing group, hypothesized secondary to a potential reservoir of infectious organisms on the skin.[18] A more frequent rate (ie, daily) of dressing changes is thought to prevent infection more than a less frequent rate.[19,20] One study found a 3.5% rate of positive skin cultures in 530 patient days using daily dressing changes.[21]

Fluid Requirements in Home Parenteral Nutrition

Water is the most abundant component of the human body. The percentage of body weight of water is greatest in the premature infant (80%), intermediate in weight in the term infant (70%), and least in the adult (60%). Water is found in two major compartments of the body: intracellular water and extracellular water. The extracellular compartment may be further subdivided into three subcompartments: interstitial lymph fluid space, plasma space, and transcellular fluid space. As body fat increases at or after birth and as women mature, a greater proportion of the body is made of fat instead of water.

The fluid requirement of infants, children, and adults may be determined by three methods: 1) volume/weight, 2) volume/surface area, and 3) volume/kcal. The preferred method for calculation is based on volume/weight. Other fluid requirements will depend on other factors, such as if the patient has ostomy outputs that need to be replaced. The volume of replacement fluids can be estimated on the basis of what is lost or, preferably, can be based on the known measured losses. The replacement fluids may be given concurrent with the PN solution or after the PN solution has been infused. Often these fluids may be replaced quite rapidly (over a period of 1 to 2 hours). In rare cases, patients may need to replace ostomy losses during the middle of the day because the volume they lose is so large. Some patients whose ostomy outputs equal the total basic fluid requirements should be considered for somatostatin injection therapy, which may reduce ostomy output by 30% to 40%.

The rate at which fluids are given intravenously in home PN patients depends on what each patient can safely tolerate. Patients who have cardiac, pulmonary, renal, or neurologic diseases may require restricted volumes and should be carefully monitored.

When a patient is started in a PN program in the hospital, many factors have to be considered in establishing the ultimate routine that will be used at home. Daily body weight, fluid intake (parenteral and enteral), and fluid output (urine, diarrhea, nasogastric suction, gastrostomy, jejunostomy) need to be measured daily in the hospital to determine what type and volume of fluids need to be replaced.

Serum electrolytes need to be monitored at least daily for the first 3 days when initiating a PN regime and then every other day for the remainder of the week. Subsequently, as the patient stabilizes, weekly electrolyte measurement may be sufficient. After the patient is established on a home PN routine, electrolyte determinations may be as frequent as twice a week to as infrequent as every 3 months.

Nutrient Requirements in Home Parenteral Nutrition

Electrolytes

Minerals present in ionic form in the body are categorized as electrolytes. The plasma portion of the extracellular space has a significant concentration of sodium, chloride, and bicarbonate with small amounts of potassium, calcium, magnesium, phosphate, sulfate, organic acid, and protein. Interstitial fluid is similar to plasma in electrolyte composition but lacks significant amounts of protein. Conversely, the intracellular space contains potassium and magnesium as the major cationic components with phosphates and sulfates as the anions in smaller concentrations.

A number of formulas may be used to correct water and electrolyte imbalances. These formulas are especially useful when correcting for free-water deficits in hypernatremic dehydration and symptomatic electrolyte disturbances.

Sodium is the major cation of extracellular fluid and functions principally in the control of water distribution, fluid, and electrolytes and contribution to the osmotic pressure of body fluids. It is important along with chloride and bicarbonate in the regulation of acid-base balance. Osmoreceptors in the supraoptic and paraventricular nuclei of the hypothalamus have an important role in regulating sodium balance and extracellular fluid.

If plasma sodium concentration increases, vasopressin or antidiuretic hormone (ADH) is released in response from the neurohypophysis to restore normal sodium concentration levels. ADH acts at the renal level to reduce excretion of solute-free water and increases water reabsorption, which leads to urinary concentration. When ADH response is deficient, urinary dilution occurs.

Regulation of plasma osmolality is precise. An increase of 1% leads to stimulation of thirst and ADH release. The major stimuli of ADH release are physical injury, emotional stress, hypoxia, liver disease, adrenal insufficiency, cardiac failure, and volume depletion.

Chloride

Chloride is the major extracellular anion and is handled in close association with sodium. It is essential to normal growth and development. Hyperchloremia with intravenous infusions may occur as a result of excessive flush of lines with sodium chloride and use of some chloride containing medications.

Potassium

Potassium is the major cation of intracellular fluid and is essential for maintenance of acid-base balance and isotonicity. The intracellular concentration of potassium is 150 mEq/L, and the extracellular concentration is 3 to 5 mEq/L. Total body potassium and lean body mass are closely correlated. In females, total body potassium is lower than in their male counterparts. Ninety percent of total body potassium is available for exchange with the serum even though most is found in the intracellular space.

During PN administration, hypokalemia may occur as potassium leaves the intravascular compartment and enters the intracellular space as positive nitrogen balance occurs.

In hypokalemia the decreased extracellular potassium results in an increase in electronegativity across the cell membrane and hyperpolarization of the cell. Attainment of threshold potential is more difficult and may result in muscle weakness and paralytic ileus. In severe hyperkalemia, the converse may occur with profound muscle weakness and diastolic arrest of the heart.

Bicarbonate

There is no specific requirement for bicarbonate. Acetate, gluconate, lactate, and citrate are organic ions that are hydrogen ion acceptors and that produce bicarbonate during their metabolism. Acetate is most commonly used in PN solutions to prevent acidosis. When metabolized, acetate produces hydroxyl radicals, which increases the base excess if there is no disease that interferes with normal acetate metabolism (such as select inborn errors of metabolism).

Carbohydrates

Monohydrous glucose is the only form of carbohydrate used in PN in the United States and its major energy source, containing 3.4 kcal/g. Glucose should make up 60% to 75% of the nonprotein energy calories in the PN solution with the remainder supplied by lipid. The glucose infusion rate is the rate at which it is delivered to the body. To prevent hyperosmolarity and hyperinsulinemia glucose infusion rates should be increased gradually in a careful, stepwise manner.

In premature infants, a PN glucose concentration of 2.5% to 5% is usually tolerated as the initial concentration, whereas 7.5% in term infants and 10% in older children and adults are recommended. The advancement in the concentration of glucose should range from 2.5% to 5.0% per day as tolerated until the goal of 60% to 75% of the total nonprotein calories is reached.

Premature infants and term infants may tolerate glucose infusion rates of between 8 and 14 mg/kg/minute. Blood glucose determination should be done every 2 to 8 hours for 24 hours when changing glucose infusion rates to maintain a glucose level in a range of 80 to 140 mg/L.

At the present time, there are no acceptable alternative carbohydrate choices for PN because of their potential hepatotoxicity and/or need for insulin similar to glucose.

Lipids in Home Parenteral Nutrition

Intravenous lipid emulsions consist of three basic components: an aqueous component, a lipid phase, and an emulsifying or a stabilizing system. The lipid phase provides essential fatty acids and the majority of calories. The lipid emulsions contain glycerin in the aqueous phase to make the emulsions isotonic. Egg phosphatide stabilizes the fat particles in the emulsion preventing separation of the lipid and aqueous phases. Lipid emulsions contribute 1.8 kcal/ml for 20% solutions and 0.9 kcal/ml for 10% emulsions. Glyceril provides and additional 0.2 kcal/ml for both concentrations.

Lipids are provided in a home PN regime for two purposes: 1) a source of linoleic acid to prevent essential fatty acid deficiency, and 2) to provide additional energy calories.

Neonates who are put on home PN support have a minimum requirement of 0.6 to 0.8 g/kg/day to get their essential fatty acid requirement. However, older infants, children, and adults may receive anywhere from 0.5 to 1.0 g/kg/day to prevent essential fatty acid deficiency and up to 2.0 g/kg/day to provide concentrated calories.

Lipids are a more effective source of energy than are an equicaloric quantity of glucose alone. Resting energy expenditures are greater in those individuals receiving carbohydrate dominant PN solutions because of the generation of excessive carbon dioxide and increased need for oxygen.

Plasma triglycerides remain stable when lipid is infused as long as the rate of lipid infusion is less than or equal to the rate of hydrolysis. Most individuals can tolerate a rate of infusion of 0.1 to 0.15 g/kg/hour, which is sufficient for an infusion program of 12 hours. Some individuals can tolerate a greater lipid infusion rate. Patients on a home PN infusion program should have their triglyceride level checked at least 4 hours after the lipid infusion has stopped on days 1, 3, 7, and 14 to determine if the clearance is maintained and an accumulation of lipids is not occurring.

If triglyceride levels are monitored and remain in the normal range, a low probability exists for the patient to become hepatotoxic from the lipid administration.

Parenteral Proteins

Twenty amino acids must be present in the required amounts for protein synthesis to occur. The amino acid that limits protein synthesis is the one in the lowest quantity in relation to the need for that amino acid. Amino acids present in quantities above their need for protein synthesis are oxidized as an energy source. Amino acid solutions are formulated to provide an amino acid profile that maximizes protein synthesis and minimizes the degradation of amino acids.

There are many different amino acids preparations available commercially. Some are devised specifically for pediatric use. The pediatric solutions were based on a presumed biological ideal: breast milk, a reference plasma amino acid profile such as cord blood or the breast-fed term infant. Adult amino acid profiles in solutions are based on reference ideal proteins such as egg proteins.

Pediatric PN solutions have a higher ration of essential amino acids to total amino acids than do adult formulations because of childrens' need for growth and brain development.

Calcium, Magnesium, and Phosphorus

Calcium, magnesium, and phosphorus have to be supplied to patients in the proper quantities for normal metabolic processes critical to daily metabolism and to provide for bone growth and remodeling. We know that even if we provide these minerals parenterally in quantities normally required enterally, patients still may have osteopenia. Trace elements are a family of elements found in the human body at concentrations less than 0.01%. Those present in the lowest concentrations are the ultratrace elements. The most abundant trace metal is iron, with zinc being second. Despite their low concentration, many of the trace metals are essential in nutrition. Some elements found in the body in small amounts are not yet recognized as having a role in maintaining health. Examples of this type of trace element are arsenic, vanadium, boron, nickel, lithium, and strontium. Some of the trace metals may require replacement at more than maintenance levels.

Because zinc and selenium may be lost in large amounts in ostomy fluids and in patients with chronic diarrhea, replacement may need to be doubled.

Copper is excreted mainly in the bile. Cholestatic conditions and biliary obstruction lead to progressive copper accumulation.

Manganese is a contaminant in many of the salts used in PN solutions. We have not found any of our patients to have low manganese levels; therefore, it is not deliberately added.

Iodine is an essential trace element; however, it is ubiquitous and does not need to be added to the PN solutions. Patients who have been monitored after years of PN usually have normal iodine levels, despite the absence of iodine in their PN solutions.

Molybdenum is a cofactor for a number of redox enzymes including sulfite oxidase and xanthine oxidase. Circulating molybdenum levels are used as an index of molybdenum status, and this element is not routinely added to PN solutions.

Complications of Home Parenteral Nutrition

Patients receiving PN can experience similar complications, whether they receive nutrition at home or in the hospital. These complications are discussed in Chapter 38 of this text. Metabolic bone disease, which can result because of long-term PN, is discussed in detail in Chapter 13, and Chapter 3 discusses micronutrient deficiencies.

Mortality

The number one cause of death related to home PN is sepsis. Death due to sepsis often results from a delay in seeking care or in initiating treatment, including early use of broad-spectrum antibiotics. Liver failure is an infrequent cause of death related to PN.

Cost

Home PN is a relatively expensive therapy, but it is cost effective when one compares it to an inpatient stay for PN infusion. The direct and indirect costs related to home PN (cost of the solution, supplies needed for administration and site care, and support staff time) approaches $100,000 per year.

Outpatient Care

At outpatient visits, pertinent laboratory tests are reviewed and patients are evaluated, weighed, and measured. Pertinent laboratory tests include complete blood count, electrolytes, calcium, magnesium, total protein, albumin, and prealbumin. The physician performs a careful physical exam to assess for any overt nutritional deficiencies. The frequency of outpatient visits changes over time as the regimen and the patient's condition becomes more stable. The patient's first visit should occur within 1 week from discharge from the hospital. Visits may then be spaced out initially to every 2 weeks for 1 month, then monthly for the first year, and then as infrequently as every 2 to 3 months for the second year.

Team-Centered Care

Taking care of patients on home PN requires the coordination of a team of specialists including the physicians, nutritionists, clinical nurse specialists, and social workers. These team members often have a weekly clinic in which they are able to see patients on home PN to chart their progress. A team-centered approach provides a "medical home" for these patients and is most likely to result in a successful outcome.

Each team member has an important role to play. The clinical nurse specialist may review important teaching points about line care, can draw blood from the line for testing using sterile technique, and can repair a broken line. Patients are able to review concerns about their home environment or financial difficulties with the social worker. Nutritionists are able to provide their input regarding the success of the PN in achieving optimal health, growth, and development.

Discontinuing Home Parenteral Nutrition

The decision of when to discontinue PN varies with the individual. Patients who are transitioned to enteral feedings and are able to maintain their weight with normal nutritional parameters electrolyte values and to meet fluid requirements are transitioned slowly off of PN. Initially, they are given PN for fewer days during the week, then with fewer calories per infusion, until they are given a trial period without PN. If they are able to maintain good nutrition without the aid of PN for a period of several weeks, consideration can be given to removal of the CVC.

References

1. Ament ME. Home total parenteral nutrition. In: *Pediatric Gastrointestinal Disease*, vol. 2. Walker WA, Durie PR, Hamilton JR, Walker-Smith JA, Watkins JB, eds. Philadelphia, PA: B.C. Decker Inc; 1991: 1676-1688.
2. Wang XY, Li N, Gu J, Li WQ, Li JS. The effects of the formula of amino acids enriched BCAA on nutritional support in traumatic patients. *World J Gastroenterol.* 2003;9(3):599-602.
3. Mayer K, Gokorsch S, Fegbeutel C, Hattar K, Rosseau S, Walmrath D, Seeger W, Grimminger F. Parenteral nutrition with fish oil modulates cytokine response in patients with sepsis. *Am J Respir Crit Care Med.* 2003;167(10):1321-1328.
4. Mayer K, Fegbeutel C, Hattar K, Sibelius U, Kramer HJ, Heuer KU, Temmesfeld-Wollbruck B, Gokorsch S, Grimminger F, Seeger W. Omega-3 vs. omega-6 lipid emulsions exert differential influence on neutrophils in septic shock patients: impact on plasma fatty acids and lipid mediator generation. *Intensive Care Med.* 2003;29(9):1472-1481.
5. Mayer K, Meyer S, Reinholz-Muhly M, et al. Short-time infusion of fish oil-based lipid emulsions, approved for parenteral nutrition, reduces monocyte proinflammatory cytokine generation and adhesive interaction with endothelium in humans. *J Immunol.* 2003;171(9):4837-4843.
6. Brier KL, Latiolais CJ, Schneider PJ, Moore TD, Buesching WJ, Wentworth BC. Effect of laminar air-flow and clean-room dress on contamination rates of intravenous admixtures. *Am J Hospital Pharm.* 1981;38:1144-1147.
7. Crocker KS, Noga R, Filibeck DJ, Krey SH, Markovic M, Steffee WP. Microbial growth comparisons of five commercial parenteral lipid emulsions. *JPEN.* 1984;8:391-395.
8. Ball PA. Methods of assessing stability of parenteral nutrition regimens. *Curr Opin Clin Nutr Metab Care.* 2001;4(5):345-349.
9. Lumpkin MM. Safety alert: hazards of precipitation associated with parenteral nutrition. *Am J Hosp Pharm.* 1994;51:1427-1428.
10. O'Grady NP, Alexander M, Dellinger EP, et al. Guidelines for the prevention of intravascular catheter-related infections. *Infect Control Hosp Epidemiol.* 2002;23(12):759-769.
11. Fennessy PA, Antonis P, Anderson J. What is the efficacy of in-line filters in reducing microbiological contamination of intravenous fluids. 1999. Unpublished Work.
12. Moukarzel AA, Haddad I, Ament ME, Buchman AL, Reyen L, Maggioni A, Baron HI, Vargas J. 230 patient years of experience with home long-term parenteral nutrition in childhood: natural history and life of central venous catheters. *J Pediatr Surg.* 1994;29:1323-1327.
13. Lokich JJ, Bothe A Jr., Benotti P, Moore C. Complications and management of implanted venous access catheters. *J Clin Oncol.* 1985;3:710-717.
14. Langgartner J, Linde HJ, Lehn N, Reng M, Scholmerich J, T. Gluck. Combined skin disinfection with chlorhexidine/propanol and aqueous povidone-iodine reduces bacterial colonisation of central venous catheters. *Intensive Care Med.* 2004;15.
15. Lok CE, Stanley KE, Hux JE, Richardson R, Tobe SW, Conly J. Hemodialysis infection prevention with polysporin ointment. *J Am Soc Nephrol.* 2003;14(1):169-179.
16. Safdar N, Kluger DM, Maki DG. A review of risk factors for catheter-related bloodstream infection caused by percutaneously inserted, noncuffed central venous catheters: implications for preventive strategies. *Medicine* (Baltimore). 2002;81(6):466-479.
17. Gillies D, O'Riordan E, Carr D, O'Brien I, Frost J, Gunning R. Central venous catheter dressings: a systematic review. *J Adv Nurs.* 2003;44(6):623-632.
18. Olson K, Rennie RP, Hanson J, et al. Evaluation of a no-dressing intervention for tunneled central venous catheter exit sites. *J Infus Nurs.* 2004;27(1):37-44.
19. Curchoe RM, Powers J, El-Daher N. Weekly transparent dressing changes linked to increased bacteremia rates. *Infect Control Hosp Epidemiol.* 2002;23:730-732.
20. Engervall P, Ringertz S, Hagman E, Skogman K, Bjorkholm M. Change of central venous catheter dressings twice a week is superior to once a week in patients with haematological malignancies. *J Hosp Infect.* 1995;29:275-286.
21. Jarrard MM, Olson CM, Freeman JB. Daily dressing change effects on skin flora beneath subclavian catheter dressings during total parenteral nutrition. *JPEN.* 1980;4:391-392.
22. Journeycake JM, Buchanan GR. Thrombotic complications of central venous catheters in children. *Curr Opin Hematol.* 2003;10(5):369-374.
23. Buchman AL, Moukarzel A, Goodson B, et al. Catheter-related infections associated with home parenteral nutrition and predictive factors for the need for catheter removal in their treatment. *JPEN.* 1994;18:297-302.
24. Begala JE, Maher K, Cherry JD. Risk of infection associated with the use of Broviac and Hickman catheters. *Am J Infect Control.* 1982;10:17-23.
25. Graham DR, Keldermans MM, Klemm LW, Semenza NJ, Shafer ML. Infectious complications among patients receiving home intravenous therapy with peripheral, central, or peripherally placed central venous catheters. *Am J Med.* 1991;91:95S-100S.
26. Buchman AL, Guss W, Ament ME. Staphylococcus aureus Hickman catheter infections. *Am J Med.* 1991;91:103-104.
27. Wurzel CL, Halom K, Feldman JG, Rubin LG. Infection rates of Broviac-Hickman catheters and implantable venous devices. *Am J Dis Child.* 1988;142:536-540.
28. Lipkin EW, Ott SM, Klein GL. Heterogeneity of bone histology in parenteral nutrition patients. *Am J Clin Nutr.* 1987;46:673-680.
29. Cohen-Solal M, Baudoin C, Joly F, Vahedi K, D'Aoust L, De Vernejoul MC, Messing B. Osteoporosis in patients on long-term home parenteral nutrition: a longitudinal study. *J Bone Miner Res.* 2003;18(11):1989-1994.
30. Lawson PT, Lovaglio J, Lipkin EW. Osteopenia in rats supported by intravenous nutrition. *Am J Clin Nutr.* 1995;61:346-352.
31. Nishikawa RA, Siepler SE, Siepler JK, Diamantidis T, Okamoto R. Intravenous pamidronate improves bone mineral density in home parenteral nutrition patients. *Clin Nutr.* 2003;22(S1):S88.
32. Clayton PT, Whitfield P, Iyer K. The role of phytosterols in the pathogenesis of liver complications of pediatric parenteral nutrition. *Nutrition.* 1998;14:158-164.
33. Carter BA, Prendergast DR, von Furstenberg R, Karpen SJ. Soy lipid-derived stigmasterol suppresses bile acid-activated bile salt export pump (BSEP, ABCB11) gene expression-role in parenteral nutrition associated cholestasis (PNAC), AASLD 2004.
34. Iyer KR, Spitz L, Clayton P. BAPS prize lecture—new insight into mechanisms of parenteral nutrition-associated cholestasis: role of plant sterols. *J Pediatr Surg.* 1998;33:1-6.
35. Pitt HA, King W III, Mann LL, Roslyn JJ, Berquist WE, Ament ME, DenBesten L. Increased risk of cholelithiasis with prolonged total parenteral nutrition. *Am J Surg.* 1983;145:106-112.
36. Roslyn JJ, Berquist WE, Pitt HA, Mann LL, Kangarloo H, DenBesten L, Ament ME. Increased risk of gallstones in children receiving total parenteral nutrition. *Pediatrics.* 1983;71:784-789.
37. Dawes LG, Greiner M, Joehl RJ. Altered gallbladder bile acidification with long-term total parenteral nutrition. *J Surg Res.* 1999;81:21-26.
38. Li J, Stahlgren LH. Glutamine prevents the biliary lithogenic effect of total parenteral nutrition in rats. *J Surg Res.* 1995;58:491-495.
39. Broughton G, Fitzgibbons RJ Jr., Geiss RW, Adrian TE, Anthone G. IV chenodeoxycholate prevents calcium bilirubinate gallstones during total parenteral nutrition in the prairie dog. *JPEN.* 1996;20:187-193.

Chapter 41

Administration Routes for Enteral Nutrition

Mark H. DeLegge, MD, FACG

Introduction

Nutritional support of the hospitalized patient is important in improving patient outcome. The past 40 years have shown tremendous improvement in medicine's ability to deliver nutrition to at risk patients. The use of parenteral nutrition (PN) was introduced in the 1960s and has continued to be an important tool for the nutrition support of patients with gastrointestinal (GI) impairment. Advances in the development of specialized enteral nutrition (EN) feeding solutions has created interest in the development of disease-specific nutrition management.[1]

The use of EN is preferred to PN because EN is less costly than PN and has the advantages of reduced infectious and metabolic complications.[2] In addition, EN maintains gut integrity and is fundamental in supporting gut immunity, an important defense system for the at risk patient.

In a patient who can eat and drink, the provision of EN support is focused on the use of nutritional supplements, dietary counseling, and appetite stimulation. However, in those patients who will not eat or cannot eat secondary to some dysfunction of the GI tract, an enteral route, or feeding tube, to provide feedings is necessary. Thus, obtaining enteral access becomes the foundation of any attempt at providing EN. The science of enteral access and nutrition support in general has evolved dramatically in recent years.

The radiologist, gastroenterologist, or surgeon usually places the enteral access devices. This can be done at the patient's bedside, fluroscopically, endoscopically, or in the operating room, depending on the specific device used and the expertise available. Medicare trends from 1997 to 2000 have shown a significant increase in enteral access procedures in the United States. Interestingly, the greatest increase in enteral access procedures was among radiologists, closely followed by gastroenterologists. The percentage of surgeons performing enteral access procedures has decreased.[4]

Nasoenteric Tube Access

Nasoenteric access placement techniques—for the bedside, endoscopic, fluoroscopic, and surgical placement—each have indications, benefits, and risks. The final position of an enteral access tube is either the stomach, for gastric feedings, or the jejunum, for small bowel feedings. A patient who is intolerant of gastric feedings, such as a patient with gastroparesis or a patient who has had their stomach surgically removed, will receive small bowel feedings. Nasoenteric tubes have associated early complications (Table 41-1).

The use of small bowel feedings to prevent tube feeding aspiration events is a much more complicated and contentious issue. Some studies have shown a decrease in aspiration episodes in patients who are fed into the small bowel compared with the stomach.[5,6] A recent, prospective trial by Neumann et al directly compared the use of gastric feedings versus small bowel feedings in the intensive care unit. There was no difference in aspiration episodes between gastric or small bowel feedings. However, it took longer to initiate small bowel feedings because of the difficulty in obtaining adequate tube position.[7] A recent consensus conference, after review of the literature, documented that small bowel feeding is recommended for the prevention of aspiration pneu-

Table 41-1.

Complications of Nasogastric or Nasojejunal Tube Placement

Nasal mucosal ulceration
Otitis media
Pharyngitis
Pneumothorax
Sinsusitis
Tracheoesophageal fistula
Tube migration
Aspiration pneumonia
Tube obstruction

monia in critically ill patients.[8] This debate certainly will continue as further aspiration studies are performed.

For those patients who have known gastroparesis, who are intolerant to gastric feedings, or who have had a witnessed tube feeding aspiration event with gastric feedings, small bowel access and feedings should be initiated. The cost-effectiveness of obtaining nasojejunal (NJ) access has been well documented. Nicholas et al described their experience with the use of early NJ tube placement in the critically ill surgical patient. In a large group of patients, the findings demonstrated a significant reduction in the daily census of patients on PN and a 71% reduction in overall PN use.[9]

Bedside nasoenteric tube placement is the most common enteral access technique used in the hospital and in long-term care environments. Either a nasogastric (NG) or NJ tube may be placed. The decision of which tube to use is based on concerns with the patient's tube feeding tolerance and aspiration risk. There are many techniques available for passing bedside NG tubes. Typically, an 8 to 12 Fr NG tube is passed into the stomach after the tube has been lubricated, the head is flexed, and the patient ingests sips of water to assist in passing the tube into the stomach.[10] Many centers promote bedside auscultation for confirmation of an adequate position of the NG tube before use. However, this can be misleading, as inappropriate tube locations (eg, in the lung, in the pleural cavity after perforation, or coiled in the esophagus) may be misinterpreted as being in proper position by bedside auscultatory techniques. For this reason, every patient should have a radiograph to confirm proper position of a NG tube before initiating feedings.[11]

It is not unusual for a physician to have a patient who is comatose and therefore unable to assist with the passage of an NG tube. In these instances, the tube can again be passed at the bedside after tube lubrication and head flexion. The patient is monitored for coughing and wheezing that is consistent with a bronchial placement. Auscultation of the abdominal cavity and a radiograph can confirm proper tube location.

A number of techniques have been promoted for bedside placement of an NJ tube. Thurlow et al promoted the use of a stylet filled tube and a corkscrew motion.[12] Zaloga confirmed the reliability of this technique with a greater than 90% success rate in tube passage.[13] In a separate technique by Ugo et al, the patient is placed into the right lateral decubitus position and the nasoenteric tube is tracked into proper position in the small bowel by auscultation. This technique resulted in an 83% successful bedside NJ tube placement.[14] Lord et al promoted the use of unweighted feeding tubes for these bedside passages, as their success rate for spontaneous small bowel placement was far greater than that documented for weighted tubes (92% versus 56%).[15] In this study, metoclopramide was used as a promotility agent in an attempt to promote passage of the tube from the stomach into the small bowel. More recently, there have been published reports of successful NJ tube placement with a "self-propelled" NJ tube. These tubes have a spiral tip at the distal end. It is believed that the stomach can propel this type of tip through the pylorus easier as compared to a standard straight distal tip. Berger reported on the use of the "self-propelled" feeding tube in 105 critically ill patients.[16] The success rate of post pyloric passage of the NJ tube was 50%. The concurrent use of narcotics decreased the likelihood of successful tube placement.

Good success with NJ tube placement requires practice and familiarity with a standard technique. The "corkscrew" method of NJ tube placement has a proven published efficacy and should be used as the reference technique for those learning bedside NJ tube placement.

There is some concern of inadvertent passage of nasoenteric tubes into the lung or pleural space.[17] This is especially true in comatose patients who cannot assist in their blind, bedside nasoenteric tube passage and who may not cough with a bronchial insertion of a nasoenteric tube. Raff and colleagues report on a technique to avoid intrapulmonary placement of nasoenteric tubes in high-risk patients. They suggest measuring the tube's length before insertion from the earlobe to the xiphoid process. Once the tube is passed to this length, an anterior-posterior radiograph is obtained to determine that the tube is in the esophagus before passing it further into the small intestine.[18]

There have been many attempts to position a tube beyond the pylorus with the use of pharmacologic agents. The results have been mixed. Seifert et al and Kittinger et al reported no benefit of the use of metoclopramide in assisting NJ tube placement.[19,20] In contrast, Whatley et al and Kalafarentzos et al noted a benefit of the use of metoclopramide, with NJ tube placements with a success rate of up to 90%.[21,22] However, controversy exists as to whether a promotility agent assists in successful NJ tube passage. In a literature review, Silva et al noted that

TABLE 41-2.

Endoscopic Methods of Nasoenteric Tube Placement

Methods	Technique
Drag-and-pull	Suture on end of a tube pulled with forceps into position
Over-the-guidewire	Tube pushed into position over a guidewire
Through-the-scope	Tube pushed through biopsy channel of endoscope into small bowel
Nasal endoscopy	Tube passed over guidewire placed through a nasal endoscope

metoclopramide, given intravenously or intramuscularly, was effective in promoting successful nasoenteric tube placement into the small bowel.[23] Griffith et al confirmed the utility of another promotility agent, erythromycin, for promoting successful NJ tube placement at the bedside in critically ill patients.[24] The use of promotility agents given prior to blind, bedside NJ tube passage is gaining popularity.

Failure to blindly pass an NJ tube at the bedside requires the use of fluoroscopic or endoscopic methods of passage. The preference of either technique is center dependent. In those centers with available C-arm fluoroscopy and modified fluoroscopy beds, fluoroscopic passage of NJ tubes can be done at the patient's bedside. Success of fluoroscopic guidance of NJ tube passage can approach 100%.[25] However, in those institutions without bedside fluoroscopic capabilities, transport of patients to the radiology suite, especially critically ill patients, can be time consuming, expensive, and hazardous.[26] In these instances, bedside endoscopic passage of NJ tubes is preferred.

Endoscopic placement of NJ feeding tubes can be done at the bedside with conscious sedation. Table 41-2 lists the techniques for bedside, endoscopic nasoenteric tube passage. The drag-and-pull method is the method with the most history. In this technique, a suture or other material is attached to the end of a NJ tube. This suture is used to drag the NJ tube into position in the small intestine by the use of a grasping forceps. Difficulty usually occurs in releasing the suture from the grasping forceps, which can result in inadvertent displacement of the NJ tube back into the stomach. A second common technique, the over-the-guidewire technique, requires the initial placement of a guidewire into the small intestine. The patient is endoscoped into the distal duodenum or proximal jejunum, and a guidewire is passed through the biopsy channel beyond the tip of the endoscope and well into the proximal jejunum. The endoscope is removed and the guidewire is left in place. A feeding tube is subsequently passed blindly or with fluoroscopic assistance into position in the small intestine. Patrick et al reported a 94% success rate using this technique.[27] More recently, Kulling et al described the use of an ultrathin endoscope to perform nasal endoscopy. A guidewire is placed into the small bowel and the ultrathin endoscope removed. An NJ tube is passed over the guidewire into position.[28] This avoids the need to do an oral-nasal transfer of the feeding tube. Other methods of endoscopic NJ placement are used more infrequently (see Table 41-2).

The decision to use a jejunal (J) tube also should warrant some very specific instructions regarding its care. The lumen of these tubes is much smaller than that of a gastric tube and therefore is prone to clogging. J-tubes should never be checked for residual content, as they are a poor indicator of residual content of the small bowel. In addition, checking residuals through these small-bore tubes increases their probability of clogging. These tubes should be flushed after every tube feeding and medication instillation. Only liquid medications or completely dissolved medications should be placed through a J-tube to reduce the chances of tube occlusion. Care should be taken to stop tube feedings during infusion of medication such as theophylline or potassium chloride—products that are known to coagulate tube feedings or obstruct the J-tube. Collier et al has shown that the use of a fiber-containing formula is quite safe, even through a 5 Fr needle catheter jejunostomy.[29] However, the use of supplemental protein powder in tube feedings or an immune enhancing formula may promote obstruction of smaller (<8 Fr) J-tubes.

Nasoenteric tube placement is the most common method of enteral access. However, nasoenteric tubes may fail early, secondary to either tube occlusion or tube dislodgment and interrupt tube feeding and medication regimens. Therefore, nasoenteric tubes should be used in patients who require either gastric or jejunal access for <1 month. More recently, a procedure for clipping the tip of the NJ tube onto the small bowel mucosa has been described using an endoscopic clipping device. This practice was able to add a few days to the projected longevity of NJ tubes by presumably reducing the risk for NJ tube migration.[30] Patients who have experienced repeated early failure of nasoenteric tubes should receive more permanent enteral access, such as a percutaneous endoscopic gastrostomy or a surgical jejunostomy.

Percutaneous Endoscopic Enteral Access

If a patient will require enteral access for >1 month, endoscopic percutaneous procedures are preferred. These procedures include percutaneous endoscopic gastrostomy (PEG), percutaneous endoscopic gastrojejunostomy (PEG/J), and direct percutaneous endoscopic jejunostomy (DPEJ). All of these procedures require the use of conscious sedation and can be performed in the endoscopy

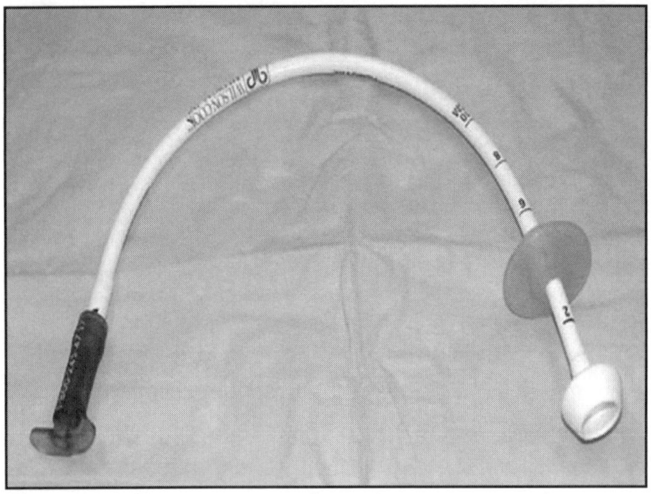

Figure 41-1. Percutaneous endoscopic gastrostomy tube.

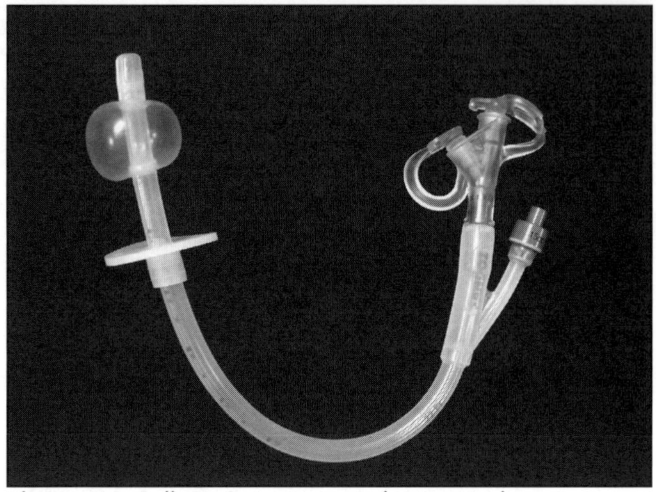

Figure 41-2. Balloon gastrostomy replacement tube.

suite, in the operating room, or at the bedside. In comparison to NG access, PEG has been shown to be a more reliable enteral access tube, allowing patients to receive more calories per day because of a reduction in tube dysfunction.[31]

PEG was developed by Ponsky Gauderer in the early 1980s.[32] The procedure involves the placement of a percutaneous gastrostomy tube after endoscopic transillumination of the stomach for appropriate PEG access position. The use of prophylactic antibiotics before the procedure is important for the prevention of postprocedure infections.[33] Placement of a PEG may be by either the Sachs-Vine (push) or Ponsky (pull) techniques. A decision to use either technique is simply a matter of physician preference. Prospective evaluations of PEG placement have found this procedure to be associated with few procedure-related complications.[34]

PEG kits are commercially available from multiple manufacturers (Figure 41-1). The most common sizes are 16 to 24 Fr. Most tubes are made of silicone, although there are some tubes constructed out of polyurethane. In general, these tubes start to degrade in 1 to 2 years, usually from yeast implantation and degradation of the PEG tube wall.[35] PEG tubes are less likely to clog as compared to nasoenteric tubes because of their larger size. Obstructed PEG tubes may be cleared with warm water and a syringe. In some cases, pancreatic enzymes mixed in a bicarbonate solution can also be effective.[36] There is no data to support the use of juices, soft drinks, or meat tenderizers to unclog a PEG tube. Commercially available PEG tube cleaning brushes are also useful.

Once a PEG tube malfunctions, degrades, or is no longer needed, it can be removed at the bedside with a traction pull force of 7 to 10 lbs. These PEG tubes are labeled "traction removal."[37] Some PEG tubes have a stiff internal bolster and can be removed only with an endoscope. They are labeled as "endoscopic removal." Although there is an associated increase in cost with these PEG tubes because of the need for an endoscopy at removal, they may be safer in patients who are confused or combative and at risk for pulling their PEG tube out after initial placement.

Replacement PEG tubes are broadly divided into two categories: replacement gastrostomy tubes or low-profile devices. Replacement gastrostomy tubes usually have a balloon-type internal bolster (Figure 41-2). These "balloon tubes" can be inserted blindly through the gastrostomy site into the gastric lumen. The balloon is inflated to serve as the internal bolster. An external bolster is slid down the external tube against the abdominal wall to keep the PEG tube from migrating. There are also PEG tubes with a distendible internal bolster (Figure 41-3). The internal bolster is stretched with a stylet and pushed blindly through the gastrostomy site. The stylet is removed and the internal bolster assumes its previous shape. One must be careful to know the direction of the gastrostomy tract so that damage or rupture of the gastrostomy tract does not occur with the use of the stylet.

PEG tubes may also be replaced with low profile gastrostomy devices (Figure 41-4). These devices provide skin level access to the gastric lumen. The internal bolster may be a balloon inflatable design or a distendible internal bolster that requires a stylet for placement. These devices come in predetermined lengths. The gastrostomy tract length must be measured so the physician can choose the correct length low profile device. To access the device for feeding or gastric decompression, an access tube must be used to engage a valve in the top of the low profile device. Although these tubes are cosmetically appealing, the small internal diameter of the access tubing and the valve make them more prone to valve and access tube occlusion.

After replacement of a PEG tube with a bedside replacement PEG tube, appropriate placement within the gastric lumen must be confirmed. This can be done by a combination of auscultation of the stomach for air rapidly infused through the PEG tube and visualization of gastric contents by an attached syringe. In questions of tube misplacement, a contrast fluoroscopic study through the PEG tube should be obtained. This is especially important when the originally placed PEG tube has been in place for 1 month or less. Early PEG tube removal may result in the stomach separating from the abdominal wall because the PEG tube tract has not completely formed. Bedside blind PEG tube replacement may result in the replacement PEG tube being placed into the peritoneal cavity.

In those patients in whom small bowel feedings are desired, endoscopic, percutaneous, small bowel access

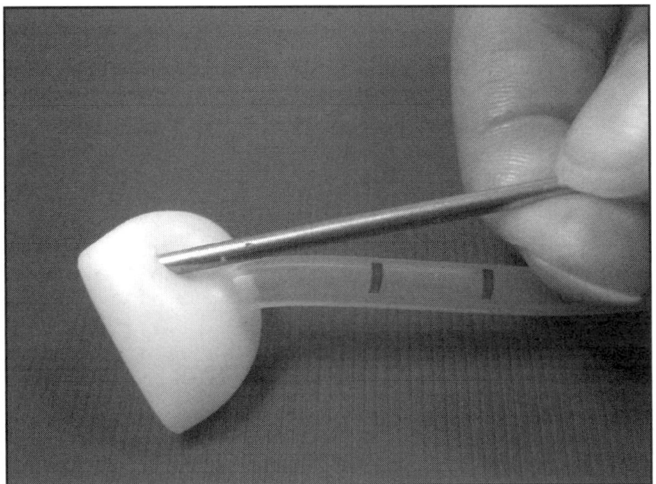

Figure 41-3. Stylet drive gastrostomy replacement tube.

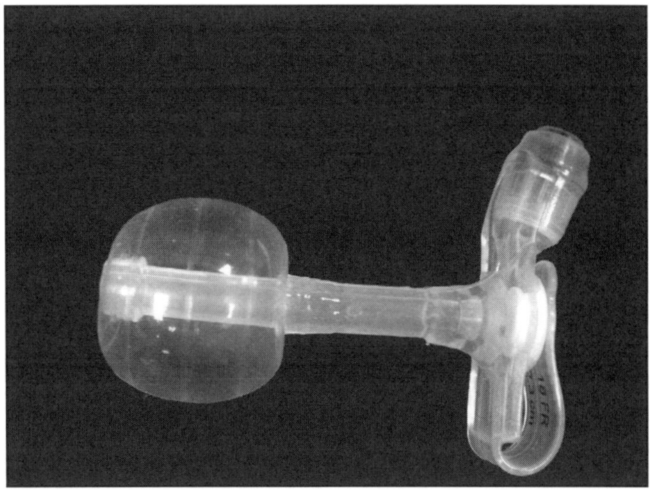

Figure 41-4. Low profile gastrostomy tube.

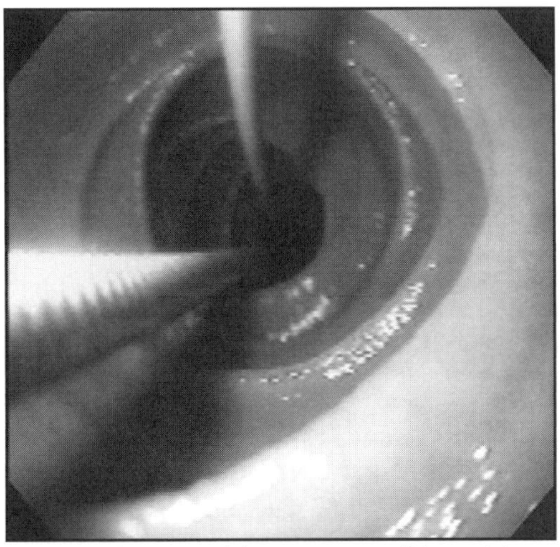

Figure 41-5. Guidewire and forceps in small bowel for jejunal tube placement through a gastrostomy tube.

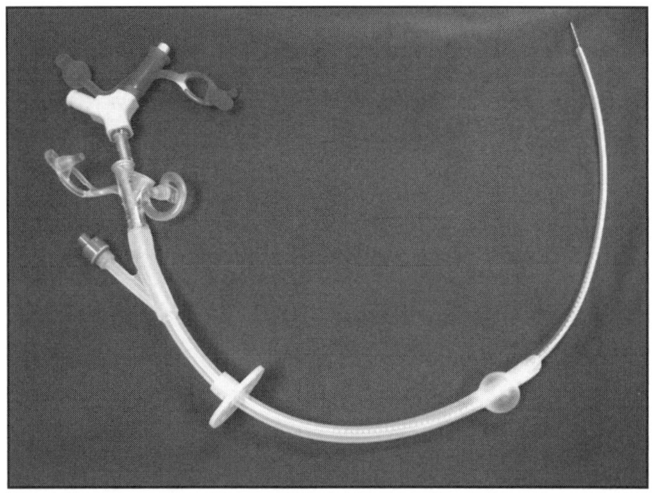

Figure 41-6. Balloon gastro-jejunostomy tube.

may be obtained by two methods. The first method, PEG/J, places a jejunal feeding tube through an existing PEG into the small bowel using an over-the-guidewire method. In this procedure, a pediatric colonoscope is used. After PEG placement, the patient is re-endoscoped and an alligator forceps is passed up through the PEG to the outside of the patient. A guidewire is grasped and the colonoscope, forceps, and guidewire are advanced to the distal duodenum or proximal jejunum. A 9 or 12 Fr J-tube is passed over the guidewire, through the existing PEG, and into position in the small bowel (Figure 41-5). The colonoscope is subsequently removed. DeLegge et al reported a 100% success rate using this technique for PEG/J placement with a procedure time of approximately 26 minutes. There were no major complications.[38] This PEG/J system allowed for both gastric decompression and small bowel feeding concurrently. The average longevity of this tube system was approximately 120 days when patients who died were excluded from the analysis of tube system longevity. Other methods have also been reported for PEG/J system placement. Taylor et al described using an ultrathin endoscope passed through an existing PEG into the small intestine. A guidewire is passed through the endoscope into position in the small bowel and the ultrathin endoscope removed. The J-tube is passed over the guidewire, through the PEG, and into position.[39] Adler et al described removing the existing PEG tube after the PEG tube tract had healed (generally 3 to 4 weeks). An endoscope is passed through the existing gastrostomy site into the small bowel. A guidewire is left in place and the endoscope is removed. A combination G/J tube is passed over the guidewire and the jejunal portion of the tube is pushed into position in the small bowel.[40] The gastric portion of the tube remains in the stomach. A balloon internal bolster serves as the anchoring device for the system (Figure 41-6).

The second method, DPEJ, directly places a J-tube into the small bowel using an endoscope. This procedure requires the use of an enteroscope or a pediatric colonoscope to reach a puncture position beyond the ligament of Treitz. Good success with this procedure has been reported by both Mellert and Shike.[41,42] There were some minor complications, including local site infection, but no reported cases of peritonitis nor bowel infarction. One of the difficulties with DPEJ was the frequent migration of

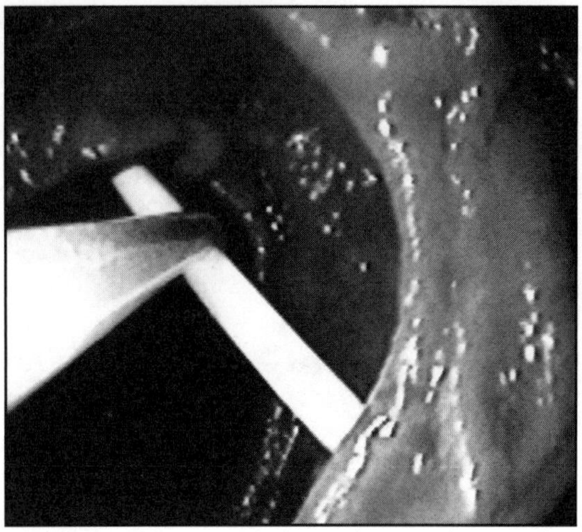

Figure 41-7. Snare around introducer catheter in the small intestine.

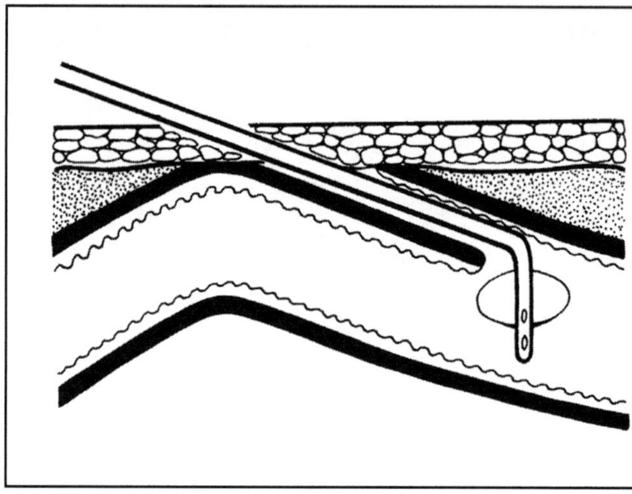

Figure 41-8. Witzel jejunostomy.

the small bowel away from the introducer trochar needle once an adequate site was located. Varadarajula resolved this problem with the use of a "2 needle stick" technique (Figure 41-7). In this procedure, a small sharp 19-gauge needle is first passed through an adequate abdominal site into the small intestine.[43] This needle is grasped by a snare, thus anchoring the small bowel against the abdominal wall. The larger introducer catheter is passed alongside the needle into the small bowel without pushing the small bowel into the abdominal cavity. The snare is removed from the 19-gauge needle and placed around the introducer catheter. A guidewire is passed through the introducer catheter into the small bowel, where it is grasped by the snare and pulled out of the oral cavity. A J-tube is attached to the guidewire and pulled into place in the small bowel in a manner similar to that used for PEG placement. Adequate positioning of the internal bolster of the J-tube is confirmed with endoscopic visualization.

Percutaneous endoscopic procedures are reliable methods for obtaining enteral access. PEG should be performed in patients who can tolerate gastric feedings and in whom gastric enteral access is required for >1 month. PEG/J allows both gastric decompression and jejunal feeding and should be used in patients who will need jejunal feedings for >1 month but <6 months, as the jejunal feeding tube component of this system may fail secondary to tube occlusion or tube displacement if left in place long term.

A retrospective study by Fan et al compared physician reinterventions for J-tube complications in a group of patients who received PEG/J as compared to another group of patients who received DPEJ. The DPEJ patients had significantly fewer reinterventions.[44] DPEJ should be performed in patients who will require long-term jejunal feedings (>6 months) or in whom gastric access for decompression or medication instillation is not necessary.

Surgical Enteral Access

Surgical enteral access was the standard of care for many years. These procedures include gastrostomy, gastrojejunostomy, and jejunostomy. These procedures may be performed via a standard open technique or with laparoscopic guidance. In recent years, the advent of PEG, PEG/J, and DPEJ has relegated the surgical access techniques to patients who are in the operating room for another surgical procedure or in patients for whom endoscopic or radiologic enteral access is technically impossible. Multiple studies have compared surgical gastrostomy to PEG. These studies have shown either a cost savings, an operative time savings, or a reduction in morbidity with PEG.[45,46]

In the standard surgical gastrostomy tube placement, an enterotomy is formed and a gastric tube is placed into the gastric lumen. The gastric wall is then fixed to the abdominal wall. The surgical gastrostomy was first described by Seidillot in 1849 and has not changed significantly in the following years.[47]

Jejunostomy is a surgical procedure in which a tube is placed into the lumen of the proximal jejunum. The first person to accomplish this procedure was Bush in 1858 in a patient with a nonoperable cancer.[48] In 1878, Surmay de Havre developed an enterostomy technique in which a J-tube was introduced into the bowel through an enterostomy.[49] In 1891, Witzel first described the most well-known technique for jejunostomy, which has subsequently undergone a number of modifications[50] (Figure 41-8).

The decision to place an operative jejunostomy follows the same decision analysis as the decision to place any small bowel feeding tube. Typically, patients who are intolerant to gastric feedings or patients in whom the stomach is either diseased or surgically absent will receive a surgical jejunostomy. Surgical jejunostomy is also a common procedure in trauma patients who also have associated gastroparesis. In a review by Meyers et al, patients received surgical jejunostomies as an additional technique during major abdominal surgery in 95% of cases and as the sole surgical technique in 5% of cases.[51] Approximately 20% of the major abdominal surgical cases were trauma-related.

In the standard jejunostomy, a transverse celiotomy is performed and a jejunal loop is identified. A purse-string suture is placed in the jejunal loop and a small enter-

TABLE 41-3.

Complications of Needle Catheter Jejunostomy

Author	Number of Patients	Complications, Incidence
Gottardi et al[53]	100	Tube occlusion, 5% Tube breakage, 2% Mortality, 0%
Myers et al[51]	2022	Catheter dislodgment or occlusion, 1% Re-operation, 1% Mortality, 0.15%
Haun et al[54]	120	Tube occlusion, 9% Tube dislodgment, 7% Mortality, 0%

ostomy is made. This enterostomy purse-string suture is subsequently attached to the abdominal wall and an 8 to 12 Fr. silicone or rubber catheter is inserted through the abdominal wall and into the jejunum. Complications with this standard technique include wound infection, wound breakdown, tube occlusion, and tube dislodgment. Holmes et al reported a complication rate of 10% and a mortality rate of 1.4% in trauma patients receiving a surgical jejunostomy directly related to the procedure.[52]

Needle catheter jejunostomy (NCJ) involves the placement of a 5 or 7 Fr catheter into the jejunum via a submucosal tunnel. It was hypothesized that this technique would have fewer complications compared with standard jejunostomy as the entrance to the jejunum was much smaller in comparison. Multiple studies have reported reduced complications of NCJ when reported either historically or directly to the standard surgical jejunostomy (Table 41-3). There is a significant percentage of tube occlusions secondary to its small size.

One needs to be careful in reviewing outcome studies comparing the technique of Witzel jejunostomy placement and its patient outcomes against NCJ. Techniques for the Witzel jejunostomy vary among many institutions. Kudsk et al recommends that the standard Witzel jejunostomy be created with a lax enterostomy tunnel to prevent tract disruption associated with bowel edema.[55] Kudsk also recommends attaching at least 5 cm of jejunum to the anterior abdominal wall to prevent torsion of the small bowel. The jejunostomy exit site on the abdominal wall should be lateral to the rectus sheath to avoid the risk of small bowel volvulus.

Laparoscopic placement of J- and gastrojejunostomy tubes was developed in the early 1990s. Initially, it was proposed that these procedures were associated with less morbidity and operative stress than were standard surgical jejunostomy and gastrostomy. Shortly, it was experienced that these laparoscopic techniques did not significantly add any advantage compared with standard surgical gastrostomy or jejunostomy with relation to operative time nor associated procedure morbidity. Rosser et al reported on the use of special suturing devices to be used with laparoscopic gastrostomy and J-tube placement.[56] These devices, however, did not significantly impact on either surgical time nor associated morbidity. More recently, Gedaly et al reported on the use of mini laparoscopic instrumentation (18 mm).[57] They reported an operative time of 44 minutes in the placement of J-tubes in nine patients. One patient developed a postoperative, peritubular leakage. Additional comparative trials of laparoscopic versus standard jejunostomy will need to be performed to determine if laparoscopic J- or gastrojejunostomy- tube placement techniques offer a clear advantage over current, open operative techniques.

The use of surgical jejunostomies has been thought of as the standard of care in trauma patients for providing enteral access. However, there is some concern of the effect of feeding into the jejunum on mesenteric blood flow, especially in hypotensive patients. Smith-Choban and Max noted a 4% incidence of bowel necrosis in 103 patients receiving tube feeding through a surgical jejunostomy.[58] The postmortem examination in these patients did not show any evidence of bowel torsion or mesenteric artery occlusion, suggesting that the jejunal feedings may have worsened a preexisting mesenteric, low blood flow state. Worthington et al and Ferrara et al demonstrated the release of proteolytic enzymes and serotonin from rat jejunum infused with hyperosmolar substances.[59,60] These released substances can affect small bowel blood flow, especially in times of physiologic stress. Thus, the decision to proceed with small bowel feedings in a patient requires not only a decision on the appropriate enteral access technique and device, but also a decision on the stability of the patient and their ability to tolerate enteral feedings.

Fluoroscopic Percutaneous Enteral Access

Placement of percutaneous gastrostomy and gastrojejunostomies with fluoroscopic guidance has continued

TABLE 41-4.

Complications of Percutaneous Fluoroscopic Enteral Access

Author	Number of Patients	Complications, Incidence	T Fastener
Halkier et al[65]	262	Peritonitis, 3.2% Death, 0.35%	No
McLoughlin et al[66]	38	Intraperitoneal leakage, 10% Death, 2.6%	No
Debarre et al[67]	500	Peritonitis, 1% Puncture artery, 0.2% Death, 0.2%	Yes
DeWald et al[68]	615	Peritonitis, 0.3% Death, 0%	Yes

to gain acceptance since their introduction in the early 1980s.[61,62] These procedures are usually performed by radiologists in the fluoroscopy suite. After topical anesthesia to the abdominal wall and occasional conscious sedation, the inferior margin of the liver is identified by ultrasound and marked on the patient's abdominal skin surface. A nasogastric tube is passed into the stomach for insufflation. After gastric insufflation, the stomach is punctured with an introducer catheter. Some radiologist will attach the stomach to the anterior abdominal wall with T-fasteners, whereas others will not. A guidewire is placed into the stomach through the introducer. The puncture site is serially dilated over a guidewire to a size of 10 to 14 Fr. A gastrostomy tube is passed over the guidewire into the stomach or into the small intestine if a gastrojejunostomy tube is desired.

This fluoroscopic approach to enteral access has excellent reported technical success.[63] These procedures can be performed with minimal sedation. The major criticism of these procedures focuses on related complications. The majority of these complications involve either inadvertent puncture of contiguous abdominal organs or separation of the abdominal and gastric wall during gastrostomy tract dilation. This separation of the abdominal and gastric walls may lead to peritonitis, intraperitoneal leakage, and even death. Many radiologists support the use of T-fasteners to attach the gastric wall to the abdominal wall to prevent tract disruption during dilation with its associated significant complications (Table 41-4). In addition, frequent occlusion of these feeding tubes because of their smaller size has been shown to be avoidable if larger gastrostomy tubes (18 to 22 Fr.) are used. The placement of these larger tubes may take some modification of the standard fluoroscopic gastrostomy tube placement technique.[64]

Conclusions

The provision of early, targeted enteral feedings is the subject of much research. To provide this therapy, enteral access needs to be established. Enteral access placement techniques may involve the nurse, the internist, the radiologist, the endoscopist, or the surgeon. The patient's current disease state, comorbidities, medical therapy, life expectancy, and expected time of need of their enteral access device and route will help determine the appropriate enteral access technique for tube placement (Table 41-5). Knowledge of all enteral access devices and techniques for placement is imperative to provide the safest and most effective route for EN.

Table 41-5.

Endoscopic Enteral Access Methods

Type of Access	*Used for*	*Length of Need*
Surgical or percutaneous access	Gastric feeding	>1 month
Gastrostomy	Gastric decompression	
Gastrojejunostomy	Gastric decompression Gastric feeding Jejunal feeding	>l month to <6 months
Jejunostomy	Jejunal feeding	>1 month
Nasal/Oral access	Gastric feeding	<1 month
Nasal/Oral Gastric Tube	Gastric decompression	
Nasal/Oral Gastrojejunal Tube	Gastric decompression Gastric feeding Jejunal feeding	<1 month
Nasal/Oral Small Bowel Tube	Jejunal feeding	<1 month

References

1. Daly JM, Lieberman MD, Goldfine J, et al. Enteral nutrition with supplemental arginine, RNA and omega 3 fatty acids in patients after operation: immunologic, metabolic and clinical outcome. *Surgery.* 1992;112:56-67.
2. Kudsk KA, Croce MA, Fabian TC, et al. Enteral vs parenteral feeding: effects on septic morbidity after blunt and penetrating abdominal trauma. *Ann Surg.* 1992;216:172-183.
3. Dewitt RC, Kudsk KA. The gut's role in metabolism, mucosal barrier function, and gut immunology. *Infect Dis Clin North Am.* 1999;13:465-481.
4. Duszak R, Mabry MA. National trends in gastrointestinal access procedures: an anlysis of Medicare services provided by radilologists and other specialists. *J Vasc Interv Radiol.* 2003;14:1031-1036.
5. Burtch CD, Shatney CH. Feeding jejunostomy (versus gastrostomy) passes the test of time. *Am Surg.* 1987;53:54-57.
6. Ho CS, Yee ACV, McPherson K. Complications of surgical and percutaneous non endoscopic gastrostomy: review of 233 patients. *Gastroenterology.* 1988;95:206-210.
7. Neumann DA, DeLegge MH. Gastric versus small bowel feeding in the ICU: a prospective comparison of efficacy [abstract]. *Gastroenterology.* 2000;118:A774.
8. McClave SA, DeMeo MT, DeLegge MH, et al. North American summit on aspiration in the critically ill patient: consensus statement. *JPEN.* 2002;26:S80-S85.
9. Caulfield KA, Page CP, Pestana C. Technique for intraduodenal placement of transnasal enteral feeding catheters. *NCP.* 1991;6:23-26.
10. McWrey RE, Curry NS, Schabel SI, et al. Complications of nasoenteric feeding tubes. *Am J Surg.* 1988;155:253-257.
11. Cataldi Belcher EI, Selzer MH, Slocumb BA, et al. Complications during enteral nutrition therapy: a prospective study. *JPEN.* 1983;7:546-552.
12. Thurlow PM. Bedside enteral feeding tube placement into duodenum and jejunum. *JPEN.* 1986;10:104-105.
13. Zaloga GP. Bedside method for placing small bowel feeding tubes in critically ill patients. *Chest.* 1991;100:1643-1646.
14. Ugo PJ, Mohler PA, Wilson GL. Bedside postpyloric placement of weighted feeding tubes. *NCP.* 1992;7:284-287.
15. Lord LM, Weiser Mamone A, Pulhamus M, et al. Comparison of weighted vs unweighted enteral feeding tubes for efficacy or transpyloric passage. *JPEN.* 1993;17:271-273.
16. Berger MM, Bollmann MD, Revelly JP, et al. Progression rates of self-propelled feeding tubes. *Int Care Med.* 2002;28:1768-1774.
17. Guitierrez ED, Balfe DM. Fluoroscopically guided nasoenteric feeding tube placement: results of a 1 year study. *Radiology.* 1991;178:759-762.
18. Roubenoff R, Ravich WJ. The technique of avoiding feeding tube misplacement. *J Crit Illness.* 1989;4:75-79.
19. Whatley K, Turner WW Jr, Dey M, et al. When does metoclopramide facilitate transpyloric intubation? *JPEN.* 1984;8:679-681.
20. Kalafarentzos F, Alivizatos V, Panagopoulos K, et al. Nasoduodenal intubation with the use of metoclopramide. *Nutr Supp Sev.* 1987;7:33-34.
21. Kittinger JM, Sandler RS, Heizer WD. Efficacy of metoclopramide as an adjunct to duodenal placement of small bore feeding tubes: A randomized, placebo controlled, double blind study. *JPEN.* 1987;11:33-37.
22. Selfert CS, Cuddy PG, Pemberton B, et al. A randomized trial of metoclopramide's effects on the transpyloric intubation of weighted feeding tubes. *Nutr Supp Serv.* 1987;11:11-13.
23. Silva CC, Saconato H, Attalah AN. Metocloramide for migration of naso-enteral tube (Cochrane Review). In: the cochrane Library, Issue 1, 2004,1-15. Chester, UK: John Wiley & Sons, Ltd.
24. Griffith DP, McNally AT, Battey CH, et al. Intravenous erythromycin facilitates bedside placement of postpyloric feeding tubes in critically ill adults: a double-blind, placebo-controlled study. *Crit Care Med.* 2003;31:39-44.
25. Baskin WN, Johansen JF. An improved approach to the delivery of enteral nutrition in the intensive care unit. *Gastrointest Endosc.* 1995;42:161-165.
26. Lovell MA, Mudaliar MY, Klineberg PL. Intrahospital transport of critically ill patients: complications and difficulties. *Anaesth Inten Care.* 2001;29;400-405.
27. Patrick PG, Marulenmdra S, Kirby DF, et al. Endoscopic nasogastric jejunal feeding tube placement in critically ill patients. *Gastrointest Endosc.* 1997;45:72-76.
28. Kulling D, Bauerfeind P, Fried M. Transnasal versus transoral endoscopy for the placement of nasoenteral feeding tubes in critically ill patients. *Gastrointest Endosc.* 2000;52:506-510.
29. Collier P, Kudsk KA, Glezer J. Fiber containing formula and the needle catheter jejunostomies: Clinical evaluation. *NCP.* 1994;9:101-103.
30. Chang B-S, Hsu P-I, Lo G-H, et al. Clip-assisted endoscopic method for placement of a nasoenteric feeding tube into the distal duodenum. *J Formos Med Assoc.* 2003;102:514-516.

31. Park HRH, Allison MC, Long J, et al. Randomized comparison of percutaneous endoscopic gastrostomy vs nasogastric feedings in patients with persistent neurological dysphagia. *Br Med J.* 1992;304:1406-1409.
32. Gauderer MWL, Ponsky J, Izant RJ Jr. Gastrostomy without laparotomy: a percutaneous endoscopic approach. *J Pediatr Surg.* 1980;15:872-875.
33. Jain NK, Larson DE, Schroeder KW, et al. Antibiotic prophylaxis for percutaneous, endoscopic gastrostomy: a prospective randomized, double blind clinical trial. *Ann Intern Med.* 1987;107:824-828.
34. Hogan RB, DeMarco DC, Hamilton JK, et al. Percutaneous endoscopic gastrostomy to push or to pull: a prospective, randomized trial. *Gastrointest Endosc.* 1986;32:253-258.
35. Marcuard SP, Finley JL, MacDonald KG. Large-bore feeding tube occlusion by yeast colonies. *JPEN.* 1993;17:187-190.
36. Marcuard SP, Stegall KS. Unclogging feeding tubes with pancreatic enzymes. *JPEN.* 1990;14:198-200.
37. Kobak GE, McClenathan DT, Schjurman SJ. Complications of removing percutaneous endoscopic gastrostomy tubes in children. *J Ped Gastro Nutr.* 2000;30:404-407.
38. DeLegge MH, Patrick PG, Gibbs R. Percutaneous endoscopic gastrojejunostomy with a tapered tip, unweighted jejunal feeding tube: improved placement success. *Am J Gastro.* 1996;91:1130-1134.
39. Taylor SJ, Przemioslom R, Manara AR. Microendoscopic nasointestinal feeding tube placement in mechanically ventilated patients with gastroparesis. *Dig Dis Sci.* 2003;48:713-716.
40. Adler DG, Gostout CJ, Baron TH. Percutaneous transgastric placement of jejunal feeding tubes with an ultrathin endoscope. *Gastrointest Endosc.* 2002;55:106-110.
41. Shike M, Berner YN, Gerdes H, et al: Percutaneous endoscopic gastrostomy and jejunostomy for long term feeding in patients with head and neck cancer. *Otolaryngol, Head Neck Surg.* 1989;101:549-554.
42. Mellert J, Naruhn MB, Grand KE, et al. Direct percutaneous jejunostomy (EPJ). Clinical results. *Surg Endosc.* 1994;8;867-869.
43. Varadarajulu S, DeLegge MH. Use of a 19-gauge needle as a direct guide for direct percutaneous endoscopic jejunostomy (DPEJ) tube placement. *Gastrointest Endosco.* 2003;57:942-945.
44. Fan AC, Baron TH, Rumalla A, et al. Comparison of direct percutaneous endoscopic jejunostomy and PEG with jejunal extension. *Gastrointest Endosco.* 2002;56:890-894.
45. Steigman GV, Goff JS, Silas D, et al: Endoscopic versus operative gastrostomy: Final results of a prospective, randomized trial. *Gastrointest Endosco.* 1990;36:1-5.
46. Scott JS, De La Torre RA, Unger SW. Comparison of operative versus percutaneous endoscopic gastrostomy tube placement in the elderly. *Am Surg.* 1991;57:338-340.
47. Munro JC. Abdominal surgery. In: Keen WW (ed). *Keen's Surgery.* London:WB Saunders; 1908:937-938.
48. Gerndt SJ, Orringer MB. Tube jejunostomy as an adjunct to esophagectomy. *Surgery.* 1994;115:164-169.
49. Rombeau JL, Carnilo J. Feeding by tube enterostomy. In: Rombeau JL, Caldwell MD, eds. *Enteral and Tube Feeding.* 2nd ed. Philadelphia: WB Saunders; 1990: 230-249.
50. Rombeau JL, Caldwell MD, Forlaw L, et al. *Atlas of Nutrition Support Techniques.* Boston: Little Brown; 1989: 167-174.
51. Meyers JG, Page CP, Stewart RM, et al. Complications of needle catheter jejunostomy in 2022 consecutive applications. *Am J Surg.* 1995;170:547-550.
52. Holmes JH, Brundage SI, Yeun PC, et al. Complications of surgical feeding jejunostomy in trauma patients. *J Trauma Infec Crit Care.* 1999;47:1009-1012.
53. Gottardi AD, Krahenbuhl L, Farhadi J, et al. Clinical experience of feeding through a needle catheter jejunostomy after major abdominal operations. *Eur J Surg.* 1999;165:1055-1060.
54. Haun JL, Thompson JS. Comparison of needle catheter versus standard jejunostomy. *Am Surg.* 1985;55:466-469.
55. Kirby DF, Kudsk KA. Obtaining and maintaining access for nutrition support. In: Kudsk KA, Pritchard C, eds. *From Nutrition Support to Pharmacologic Nutrition.* Berlin: Springer Verlag; 2000: 125-137.
56. Rosser JC, Rodas EB, Blancaflor J, et al. A simplified technique for laparoscopic jejunostomy and gastrostomy tube placement. *Am J Surg.* 1999;177:61-64.
57. Gedaly R, Briceno P, Ravelo R, et al. Laparoscopic jejunostomy with an 18 mm tracar. *Surg Lap Endo Percut Tech.* 1997;7:420-422.
58. Smith-Choban P, Max MH. Feeding jejunostomy: a small bowel stress test? *Am J Surg.* 1988;155:112-117.
59. Worthington KJ, Cuschieri A. Activation and release of proteolytic kinin forming enzymes from rat jejunum perfused with hypernsmolar solutions. *Gut.* 1977;18:279-283.
60. Ferra A, Zinner MJ, Jaffee BM. Intraluminal content affects intraluminal release of serotonin in canine small intestine. *Surg Forum.* 1985;36:173-174.
61. Preshaw RM. A percutaneous method for inserting a feeding gastrostomy tube. *Surg Gynecol Obstet.* 1981;152:659-660.
62. Ho CS. Percutaneous gastrostomy for jejunal feeding. *Radiology.* 1983;149:595-596.
63. Ho CS, Young EY. Percutaneous gastrostomy and transgastric jejunostomy. *AJR.* 1992;158:251-257.
64. Laasch H-U, Wilbraham L, Bullen K, et al. Gastrostomy insertion: comparing the options—PEG, RIG or PIG? *Clin Radiol.* 2003;58;398-405.
65. Halkier BY, Ho CS, Allan CNY. Percutaneous feeding gastrostomy with the Seldinger technique: review of 252 patients. *Radiology.* 1989;17:359-363.
66. McLoughlin RF, Gibney RG. Fluoroscopically guided percutaneous gastrostomy: tube function and malfunction. *Abd Imag.* 1994;19:195-200.
67. DeBarre T, Chapot R, Kuoch V, et al: Percutaneous gastrostomy with fluoroscopic guidance: Single center experience in 500 consecutive cancer patients. Radiology 210:651 654, 1999
68. DeWald CL, O'Heitte CO, Sewall LE, et al. Percutaneous gastrostomy and gastrojejunostomy with gastroplexy: experience in 701 procedures. *Radiology.* 1999;211:651-656.

Chapter 42

Adult Enteral Nutrition: Formulas and Supplements

Michele M. Gottschlich, PhD, RD

Introduction

Enteral nutrition (EN) therapy has advanced significantly since ancient Egyptians first utilized rectal feedings of milk, whey, and grain broths in an effort to preserve health.[1] We have entered the era whereby a broad range of medical food formulas have been created for use in a variety of conditions. Today, choices for adult EN support span from over 150 products. These substrates can vary considerably with respect to composition, cost, and efficacy. On the other hand, even subtle differences in the amounts of nutrients supplied or the sources of those nutrients may be important. It can be overwhelming for the healthcare practitioner intent on selecting therapeutic, cost-effective products for patients or hospital formularies. Furthermore, the science of EN has frequently lagged behind the marketplace, often making appropriate formula selection difficult to discern. It is, therefore, important to be familiar with the biochemical, physical, and physiological properties of enteral substrates to understand the significance of these variances pertinent to their application.

This chapter first reviews the various sources of nutrients and substrates used in the formulation of enteral products. Considerable attention will be given to clinical indications, evidence-based rationale, and emerging controversies surrounding their use, with emphasis on both the enteral (as opposed to parenteral) literature and human data. Next, the various categories of available products will be examined in an effort to aid the clinician in formula selection. Rather than reviewing specific products, general characteristics will be presented according to classification of products. Because of frequency in changes in the precise nutrient composition of commercial products and the persistent introduction of new products, the reader is referred to product labels or company websites (Table 42-1) for careful analysis of up-to-date nutrient details and market information.

Sources of Nutrients for Enteral Substrates

Nutrients that the human body requires are discussed in Chapter 8, which addresses macronutrient absorption and metabolism. The following section addresses EN-specific details regarding these nutrients.

Carbohydrate

Carbohydrate is an important ingredient in enteral formulas, largely because of its important roles in providing energy and protein sparing actions. Commonly used carbohydrate sources inherent in enteral products include corn syrup solids, maltodextrin, and intact or hydrolyzed corn starch (Table 42-2). Simple sugars (monosaccharides and disaccharides such as glucose, fructose, and sucrose) are selected to enhance the palatability of oral supplements but increase hypertonicity as well. The disaccharides require specific enzyme activity in the intestinal mucosa for hydrolysis. Disaccharidase production can be decreased during illness. Oligosaccharides contain 2 to 10 glucose moieties, and polysaccharides have more than 10 glucose units. Contributing less to osmolality than to the monosaccharides but requiring more digestion, they are more soluble than is starch.

Commercial products range in carbohydrate content between 71 to 290 g/L. The percentage of total calories

Table 42-1.

Websites Detailing Composition of Enteral Products

ajinomoto.com
bbraunusa.com
cambridgenutra.com
fresenius-kabi.com
nestleclinicalnutrition.com
novartisnutrition.com
ross.com

from carbohydrate varies from 30% to 90%, depending on the condition for which the product was designed. Pulmonary and diabetic products typically contain low amounts of carbohydrate, whereas chemically defined formulas are rich in carbohydrate. The majority of enteral products do not contain lactose, so that should not be a concern in lactose-intolerant persons.

Protein

Because the body is dependent upon the supply of exogenous amino acids and nitrogen, the protein component is of major nutritional importance in product development. The protein content of enteral formulas ranges from approximately 4% to 32% of total calories. Low protein products (<15 g/L) have been designed for clinical situations that warrant protein restriction (eg, renal disease), whereas standard products average approximately 36 g/L. Stress and immune-enhancing formulas can contain up to 94 g/L. Provision of high protein supplements is common in the acute care setting and has been shown to contribute to shortened length of stay and improved clinical outcomes in patients requiring anabolic conditions, such as those recovering from hip fractures,[2] pressure ulcers,[3] or burns.[4]

The selection of a particular medical food needs to include evaluation of the patient's quantitative and qualitative protein requirements and his or her ability to absorb the protein. Protein sources can differ widely in their composition, taste, function, digestibility, and therapeutic effectiveness. The protein component of enteral products may originate from intact protein, partially hydrolyzed protein, di- and tri-peptides, or free amino acids (see Table 42-2). How each of these forms of protein affects efficacy and tolerance has been controversial for many years.

Intact proteins are in their original natural form. Some examples are eggs, milk, and meat proteins. Intact proteins separated from the original food are termed "isolates" and include soy protein isolate, lactalbumin, casein, and whey. Because of their size, they have little impact on product osmolality, but they require normal levels of pancreatic enzymes for complete digestion.

The form of protein is important when a patient's digestive or absorptive capacity is compromised. Protein digestion is initiated by acid proteases in the stomach. These partially digested protein products are acted upon by pancreatic enzymes and are broken down to smaller peptide fragments (eg oligopeptides, tripeptides and dipeptides) and free amino acids. Peptides larger than three amino acids are hydrolyzed by brush border enzymes in the small intestine. The smaller particles increase the formula's osmolality. Although larger peptides must be hydrolyzed to smaller peptides or individual amino acids before absorption, dipeptides and tripeptides have specific carrier systems and can be absorbed intact.[5] Free amino acids, on the other hand, are absorbed by multiple transport systems that are sodium dependent.

Peptides

The promotion of peptide-containing formulas for patients with impaired digestion or absorption is largely based on research that suggests a more rapid and efficient absorption of nitrogen from di- and tri-peptide moieties rather than free amino acid sources. Although clinical studies have demonstrated increased absorption of di- and tri-peptide solutions,[6] much of the comparative data merely confirm superiority of peptides over free amino acids, intravenous nutrition, or starvation.[5,7-10] There exist several studies of small groups of critically ill patients[11-13] that demonstrate improved visceral protein response with a peptide versus a whole protein regimen. Data presented, however, does not confirm improved absorption. To date, the initial promise of enteral support with peptides has not been realized,[14-19] and it is possible that hydrolysate-based diets are unnecessary in an optimally managed enteral feeding regimen. It is important to recognize that chemically defined diets offer less trophic stimulation to the bowel and may be immunosuppressive,[20,21] consequently their use should be reserved for conditions that clearly warrant predigested products.

Enteral supplementation with specific amino acids is an exciting area of investigation. Specialized enteral formulas may be enhanced with specific amino acids such as arginine, glutamine, or branched chain amino acids (BCAA). However, crystalline amino acids are rather medicinal or metallic in taste, considerably more expensive than their equivalent protein counterparts, and contribute significantly to increased osmolality.

Arginine

Arginine is a conditionally essential amino acid (eg, a nutrient that the body normally produces in adequate amounts, but needs to be supplemented during conditions of metabolic stress). It has become a popular additive to select enteral formulas because of recognized properties such as its ability to enhance immune function, nitrogen retention, wound healing, and collagen synthesis.

TABLE 42-2.

Categories and Macronutrient Sources for Various Types of Defined Formulas

Type of Formula	Protein Sources	Carbohydrate Sources	Fat Sources	Kcal/mL	Protein Content	Nonprotein Calorie: Nitrogen Ratio
Intact (polymeric)	Calcium and magnesium caseinates Sodium and calcium caseinates Soy protein isolate Whey protein- Delactosed lactalbumin Egg white solids Beef Nonfat milk	Corn syrup solids Sucrose Cornstarch Glucose polymers Vegetables Fruit Nonfat milk Fructooligosaccharides	Medium-chain triglycerides Canola oil Corn oil Lecithin Soybean oil Fish oil Palm kernel oil Partially hydrogenated soybean oil High-oleic safflower oil Beef fat	0.53-2	30-94 g/L	67-300:1
Hydrolyzed (oligomeric or monomeric)	Enzymatically hydrolyzed whey or casein Soybean or lactalbumin hydrolysate Free amino acids Soy protein hydrolysate	Hydrolyzed cornstarch Sucrose Fructose Maltodextrin Tapioca starch Glucose oligosaccharide	Medium-chain triglycerides Sunflower oil Lecithin Soybean oil Safflower oil Corn oil Coconut oil Canola oil Sardine oil	1-1.33	15-52.5 g/L	67-282:1
Modular Protein	Low-lactose whey and casein Soy Calcium caseinate Free amino acids			Per 100 g 370-424	Per 100 g 75-88.5	
Modular Carbohydrates		Maltodextrin Hydrolized cornstarch		380-386		
Modular Fat			Safflower oil Polyglycerol esters of fatty acids Soybean oil Lecithin Medium-chain triglycerides	Per 1 Tbsp 67.5-115		

Adapted with permission from Gottschlich MM, Shronts EP, Hutchins AM. Defined formula diets. In: Rombeau JL, Rolandelli RH, eds. *Enteral and Tube Feeding*. 3rd ed. Philadelphia: WB Saunders Co.; 1997:210-211.

It also has secretagogue activities on several endocrine glands; administration of arginine promotes the secretion of growth hormone, prolactin, insulin, and glucagon. A number of animal studies using models of sepsis, trauma, and burns have demonstrated that survival was increased with arginine enrichment of enteral feeding regimens.[22-25] Improvement in outcomes have likewise been associated in patient studies of enteral arginine;[22,23,25-35] however, many of these studies contain extraneous variables (such as concomitant enrichment with n-3 fatty acids, glutamine, beta-hydroxy-beta-methylbutyrate, and nucleotides) that make effectors difficult to discern. Hence, clinical benefit from enteral arginine has been suggested but not precisely demonstrated.

Enteral formulas have always contained small amounts of arginine (approximately 1 to 2 g/L), although recently several arginine-enriched products (containing up to 18.7 g/L) have become available. The effects of enteral arginine supplementation show exciting promise; however, beneficial outcomes are lost when high doses are administered.[25,36] In addition, some think that arginine is harmful for patients with infection or uncontrolled inflammation.[26,37-39] Sufficient studies delineating optimal intake guidelines are still lacking and arginine's mechanism of action remains only partially defined; therefore, selection of a product based solely on its arginine content is unwarranted at this time.

Glutamine

Glutamine is another conditionally essential amino acid. It is the most abundant amino acid in plasma and skeletal muscle. It has several properties that theoretically make it a desirable additive to enteral substrates. Glutamine is the principal carrier of nitrogen from skeletal muscle to visceral organs. It is a regulator of protein synthesis and acid-base homeostasis and is a major fuel and substrate for the intestinal mucosa and other rapidly dividing cells. Glutamine also directly supports the immune system by fueling lymphocytes and macrophages, thus helping to fight illness-causing microbes. Some studies indicate that supplemental glutamine can prevent deterioration in gut permeability and preserve mucosal structure and function.[40-43] This may help limit bacterial translocation,[42-44] although this notion remains controversial.[45]

There exist conflicting and certainly inadequate reports of the effects of enteral glutamine supplementation in humans. Clinical studies in burns[42,43] have demonstrated enteral glutamine to improve wound healing and reduce hospital stay. Glutamine is reported by some as ineffective in altering indexes of nitrogen balance, albumin, or prealbumin in critically ill patients,[46-48] whereas Wischemeyer et al[49] found significant improvements in prealbumin and transferrin in burn patients supplemented with glutamine. Houdijk et al[50] and Garrel et al[51] showed a significantly decreased incidence of pneumonia, bacteremia, and sepsis in critically ill patients receiving glutamine. They also described a high preponderance of Gram-negative sepsis in the control group, a finding consistent with other studies[46,49] that demonstrates that enteral glutamine supplementation significantly reduces incidence of Gram-negative bacteremia. Overall, there appears to be benefit of enteral glutamine supplementation in burns and critical care;[42,43,46,49-51] however, several days of supplementation is likely to be required.[52] On the other hand, clinical results in humans are equivocal at best during conditions such as short bowel syndrome, acute pancreatitis, inflammatory bowel disease, bone marrow transplantation, radiation and chemotherapy, and AIDS.[45]

Part of the controversy may center on the fact that optimal levels of glutamine supplementation are yet to be established during various disease states. Commercial products contain up to 16.4 g glutamine/L. In enterally fed rats after small bowel resection, the maximal effect of glutamine supplementation occurred when glutamine was 25% of the total amino acids.[53] Glutamine supplementation of 20 to 40 g/day (23% to 44% of total amino acids or 0.29 to 0.57 g/kg of body weight/day) in healthy subjects and postsurgery patients has been well tolerated without evidence of toxicity, such as abnormalities in hepatic function, mental status, or blood ammonia levels.[54] Administration of glutamine may be contraindicated in patients with hyperammonemia, hepatic encephalopathy, and renal failure because of its high ammoniagenic potential.[55]

Branched Chain Amino Acids

BCAA—valine, leucine and isoleucine—are essential amino acids (EAA) that are mobilized from skeletal muscle during metabolic stress. It has been proposed that delivering formulas with high concentrations of BCAA to severely catabolic, traumatized, or septic patients may help preserve muscle,[56-59] thus possibly improving outcome. In addition, providing solutions with high ratios of BCAA to aromatic amino acids has been suggested as a method to improve advanced cirrhosis and hepatic encephalopathy.[15,60-64]

In both the critically ill or liver failure patient, a number of studies have evaluated enteral BCAA therapy. Several enteral investigations have suggested that supplemental BCAA decreases endogenous breakdown of protein, resulting in improved nitrogen retention and metabolic management.[56,57,60,63,64] On the other hand, the use of products fortified with BCAA has not consistently demonstrated clinical benefit.[15,37,61,65-67] Of particular concern is a study in burned guinea pigs by Mochizuki et al[68] whereby no benefit of enteral BCAA on protein metabolism was apparent; however, animal survival worsened. Decisive research supporting the routine use of liquids high in BCAA in critically ill or liver failure patients is lacking.

Nucleotides

Some products contain added nucleotides. These compounds are integral parts of all proteins. They are needed for the transfer of genetic information and in energy transfer, and they may also enhance immune function.[69] Outside the research setting, however, it is nearly impossible to develop a dietary nucleotide deficiency if adequate protein is consumed because diets that contain protein also provide nucleotides. Therefore, supplementing a protein-containing enteral formula with nucleotides would not likely yield additional benefit.

Fat

Fat has long been recognized to be an isotonic, calorically dense energy source that provides essential fatty acids and carries fat-soluble vitamins. It also enhances substrate flavor and palatability.[70] More recently, dietary lipids have been found to be capable of modulating the host response to disease, injury and infection as well as modifying gene expression.[70-78] This has generated enormous research interest directed towards investigating both fat metabolism and disease-specific dietary fat requirements. It is apparent that these findings have already been translated into the reformulation of the fat content of many enteral products in an effort to improve health.

The lipid content of enteral formulas varies widely from 1% to 55% of total calories (1.5 to 104 g/L); however, the vast majority of products (primarily those with intact protein) contain significant amounts of fat and linoleic acid. Chemically defined products contain the least amount of fat. Higher fat products are frequently promoted for pulmonary, diabetic, or trauma patients; however, this practice is often without scientific justification. Corn, canola, soy, safflower, coconut, palm kernel, medium chain triglycerides (MCT), and fish oil are commonly used lipid sources in enteral products (see Table 42-2). Lecithin is usually incorporated into liquid supplements to homogenize the nutrient mixture. Clinicians interested in using specialized medical foods require an understanding of the structural and biochemical differences that are inherent among the various enteral fat sources to maximize their therapeutic nutritional benefits. (Dietary lipids are discussed in Chapter 8.)

Short Chain Fatty Acids

In addition to their other roles,[70] SCFA are trophic to both the large and small bowel,[79] and they enhance water and electrolyte absorption.[80] Their reported role in reducing the frequency of tube-feeding–related diarrhea may derive from this feature. Potential clinical applications are only beginning to be recognized. Conditions such as short-bowel syndrome, colitis, and disuse atrophy may benefit from the stimulatory effects of SCFA. Enteral formulas containing SCFA appear to be promising; however, more research is needed concerning the potential utility of SCFA in nutrition support and intestinal dysfunction.

Medium Chain Fatty Acids

Medium chain fatty acids are saturated fatty acids of 6 to 12 linear carbon units. MCT oil, derived from palm kernel or coconut oil, was one of the first medical foods developed as an alternative to conventional fats. Because of its greater solubility in water, MCT can be hydrolyzed and absorbed in the presence of minimal amounts of pancreatic lipase or bile salts. It is rapidly absorbed by the intestinal mucosa and will appear in the portal bloodstream (rather than lymphatic circulation) without requiring re-esterification to triglycerides. They are readily oxidized, making them an important energy source.

MCT oil does not provide a source of essential fatty acids. MCT does, however, command an important niche in the armament of enteral products, particularly in conditions in which dietary fat digestion, absorption, or transport is impaired, such as defects in fat hydrolysis due to a lack of pancreatic enzymes and bile, inadequate mucosal fat absorption, and defective lymphatic transport of fat.[70,81,82]

Long Chain and Essential Fatty Acids

Long chain fatty acids (LCFA) include saturated, monounsaturated, or polyunsaturated fats. Four percent to 5% of enteral calories should originate from the polyunsaturated essential fatty acids to prevent deficiency.

Many enteral products are rich in the essential fatty acid linoleic (n-6). In view of the known detrimental effects of the metabolism of large quantities of n-6 fatty acids,[34,70,76,77] its excessive presence in many formulas should be reassessed.In early work, n-3 fatty acids were found to improve many physiological parameters and clinical outcomes in patients with cardiovascular disease,[82] burns,[27] critical care[31,32,84] and gastrointestinal (GI) malignancies.[28,29,85] Omega-3 fatty acids have subsequently been associated with improvement during autoimmune diseases and respiratory failure.[74,86,87] As a consequence, there is increasing interest in the inclusion of n-3 lipids in enteral formulas. It is noteworthy that a number of enteral products do not provide significant amounts of n-3 fatty acids.[70] These formula may cause alpha linolenic acid deficiency, perturb eicosanoid synthesis, and exacerbate pathophysiological conditions.

Structured Lipids

A new type of lipid is the tailor-made structured lipids.[70,88-91] Structured lipids are characterized by having a medium chain fatty acid at the sn-1 and 3 positions of the glycerol molecule and a LCFA at the sn-2 position. Clinical advances include enhanced absorption of fatty acyl chains esterified at the glycerol 2-position as well as reduced protein catabolism.[88,89,91-94] Incorporating fish-oil–structured lipids into a polymeric formula was found to improve clinical outcomes in patients with upper GI cancer, with a 50% reduction in postoperative complications and infection compared to those receiving a standard polymeric formula.[85] These results are promising; however, safety and efficacy must be documented by further research to clarify their usefulness in enteral support.

Fiber

(Dietary fiber and its role in nutrition is discussed in Chapter 11.)

A number of fiber sources have been used to enrich commercial tube-feeding products. Soy polysaccharide is one of the most frequently selected fiber additives in the manufacture of enteral products. Its constituents are mainly cellulose and hemicellulose. Soy polysaccharide has minimal effect on formula viscosity. Some other options in the design of tube feeding substrates include pea fiber, oat fiber, inulin, pectin, gum arabic and guar, all of which influence bowel function to varying degrees. However, a number of dietary fibers can increase the viscosity of liquid formulas or settle to the bottom of containers and can clog feeding tubes. The amount of fiber is highly variable across the spectrum of available products. Silk[95] recommends that multiple rather than single fiber sources be used and the quantity of fiber be restricted to 15g/L to minimize deleterious effect of fiber on mineral and trace element absorption. Currently, the dietary fiber content of tube feeding formulas ranges from 0 to 22 g/L. Quantitative and qualitative analysis of the fiber additive requires careful consideration prior to product selection.

More recently, nondigestible oligosaccharides in general and fructooligosaccharides in particular have become popular tube-feeding ingredients. Often referred to as prebiotics (Chapter 11), fructooligosaccharides are rapidly fermented in the large intestine by bacteria into SCFA. Unlike traditional sources of dietary fiber, oligofructose as a tube-feeding component is believed to possess many of the physiological advantages of fiber without increasing product viscosity or clogging feeding tubes.[96] Fructooligosaccharide does not contribute to residue in the stool. It also has the notoriety of improving bowel function, promoting cell proliferation in both small and large intestine, maintaining and restoring the healthy balance of gut flora, and also stimulating the absorption of water, calcium, magnesium, and iron.[96-101] However, fructooligosaccharide research has primarily involved animal or normal humans. Extrapolating such findings to critically ill tube-fed patients may not be appropriate because the effect of disease and antibiotics could negate benefits derived. Optimal dosage must also be examined because flatulence, abdominal distention, pain, and diarrhea have been associated with high doses of fructooligosaccharides.[102-104]

While the value of fiber in normal nutrition is well established, its utility in enteral formulas for hospitalized patients is by no means clear.[105] In tube-fed patients, products containing dietary fiber are often prescribed because of purported benefit such as ability to alleviate constipation and diarrhea,[106-109] preserve the intestinal barrier to bacteria,[110-112] and possibly improve glycemic response[113,114] and lower serum cholesterol levels, although the strength of these claims has not yet been conclusively demonstrated.[115-124]

Vitamins and Minerals

Carbohydrate, protein, fat, and energy cannot be efficiently used if essential cofactors and coenzymes are inadequate. Vitamin, mineral, and trace-element supplementation should take into consideration the patient's condition and nutritional status;[125] however, the effect of disease and injury on micronutrient requirements is not precisely understood. In general, when provided in adequate volume, most nutritionally complete products meet 100% of the recommended dietary intakes (RDI) (Chapter 6) for vitamins and minerals. However, a number of disease-specific products are intentionally not complete (eg, formulas designed for renal or hepatic insufficiency tend to have lowered amounts of vitamins, minerals and electrolytes due to retention of these elements in the body) or formulations may simply not account for the heightened needs or losses associated with illness. In addition, deficient intake may result with low-calorie or diluted formulas. Lastly, it should be recognized that enrichment with certain micronutrients including the antioxidants may help boost immune function, accelerate wound healing, and minimize some of the negative metabolic effects associated with disease and injury.[125-127] Unfortunately, other than the RDI guidelines, it is not possible to recommend optimal ranges for micronutrient intake for specific patient subgroups receiving enteral support pending the need for additional data on dose responses.

Water

The caloric density of a formula is dictated by the amount of water contained in the product. Most tube-feeding formulas provide 1 kcal/mL, which is approximately 85% water. A 2-kcal/mL product is composed of approximately 70% water. Concentrated products are appropriate for conditions that require fluid restriction such as fluid overload, renal insufficiency, respiratory distress, and congestive heart failure.

Osmolality

Osmolality or tonicity refers to the number of osmoles of ions or particles (solutes) per kilogram of water. Any dietary component that is soluble in water contributes to the osmolality of a solution. Osmolality is inversely related to the molecular size of the nutrients in solution. The smaller the particle size, the more significant the effect on osmolality. Caloric density and the presence of amino acids, small peptides, simple carbohydrates, vitamins, and minerals are connected to osmolality.[55] The osmolality of enteral formulas currently ranges from 200 to 790 mOsm/L. An isotonic solution has an osmolality of 300 mOsm/L. Although the osmolality of a product may affect patient tolerance, hypertonic formulas are generally well tolerated and other factors—such as appropriate product selection; early enteral feeding practices; and the utilization of antibiotics, fiber, and other nutrients—are more likely to be significant effectors of GI intolerance.[71,128-130]

Other Constituents

Less frequent components of enteral solutions include lutein, taurine, carnitine, and antimicrobials. Lutein supports eye health. Taurine is essential for infants and children, and conditionally essential for injured patients.[131-133] Taurine is important for normal retinal development. It is also involved in a number of metabolic processes such as conjugation of bile acids and platelet aggregation and functions as an antioxidant and neuromodulator. All LCFA supplied in the diet must be transported into the mitochondria before they can be oxidized to produce energy. Carnitine is required in the transport of LCFA across the mitochondrial membrane. Carnitine excretion increases after injury,[134] and deficiency may arise with antibiotic therapy.[135] Many enteral formulas now contain taurine and carnitine. Lastly, antimicrobials may be added to enteral products in an effort to reduce the growth of bacteria in the formula.

Categories of Formulas

The selection of an enteral formula should be patient specific. Age, GI function, underlying medical condition, nutrient requirements, and patient tolerance must be assessed along with considerations given to evidence-based research and cost in order to determine which product(s) are appropriate (Table 42-3).

Table 42-3.

Factors to Consider in Formula Selection

Assessment of Patient	Assessment of Formula
Past medical history and present problems	Composition of carbohydrate, protein, and fat
Age	Calorie:nitrogen ratio
Calorie and nutrient requirements	Electrolyte, vitamin, mineral, and trace element content
Hydration status	Osmolality
Gastrointestinal function	Renal solute load
Hepatic function	pH
Renal function	Residue/fiber content
Pulmonary status	Digestibility
	Viscosity
	Caloric density
	Convenience of administration
	Bacteriologic safety
	Cost
	Availability of evidence-based research

Adapted with permission from Gottschlich MM, Shronts EP, Hutchins AM. Defined formula diets. In: Rombeau JL, Rolandelli RH, eds. *Enteral and Tube Feeding*. 3rd ed. Philadelphia: WB Saunders Co.; 1997:226.

With recognition that a vast array of commercial formulas exists (primarily from three major nutrition corporations--Ross Nutrition, Novartis, and Nestle) and, in an effort to simplify decision-making, a number of different classification systems of enteral substrates have been generated based on various criteria.[55,61,105,136,137] Categorization and definitions have not always been consistent and the groupings often overlap, thus bringing about confusion. One term frequently used is that of "medical foods," which was coined in 1989 by the Food and Drug Administration to characterize enteral formulas in general. Medical foods are subject to governmental regulation for quality control, nutrient labeling, formula recall, and reimbursement. Detailed reviews of medical foods exist elsewhere.[61,136-140]

Three basic classification systems exist. The simplest way to group formulas is to classify them as either "complete" or "incomplete," depending on their essential nutrient profile. Complete formulas have all the necessary nutrients in sufficient quantities to maintain the nutritional status of an individual receiving no other source of nourishment. Incomplete solutions lack one or more essential nutrients and may need supplementation, particularly if used for prolonged support. Some disease-specific formulas, for example, may not be nutritionally complete.

Another way of grouping products is according to the molecular form of the nutrients they contain (eg, polymeric, oligomeric, or monomeric). Polymeric formulas contain carbohydrate, protein, and fat in intact or large molecular form. They require intact digestive and absorption processes and supply all the necessary nutrients for complete nutrition when a total daily prescription is administered. Oligomeric formulas have been referred to as semi-elemental, ie, they have macronutrients that have been hydrolyzed by enzymatic action to varying degrees. Peptide-based products would be classified under the oligomeric group. Monomeric formulas imply that all the nutrients are in their monomeric or elemental form such as simple sugars and amino acids.

For the purpose of this chapter, a third means of grouping, the descriptive method, will be employed. This type of classification is based on the formula's overall characteristics. Using this system, products can be categorized as standard, concentrated, blenderized, chemically defined, disease specific, or modules.

Standard

Products in this category are most often considered to represent "standard," over-the-counter oral supplements or general-purpose tube-feeding regimens because they are nutritionally complete and low in cost, create few osmolar problems, and meet the needs of many patients. They are composed of adequate carbohydrate, protein, fat, vitamins, and minerals sufficient to sustain normal nutritional requirements in a variety of clinical conditions. Most are lactose free and provide 1 kcal/mL. Some are enriched with fiber.

Concentrated

Formulas with higher caloric density (1.5 to 2.0 kcal/mL) exist for use in patients who are fluid restricted. Concentrated products may be necessary for patients with renal failure, pulmonary edema, liver failure, congestive heart failure, or other conditions in which fluid intake must be restricted. Higher protein formulas are also available for use when a patient's metabolic needs are great. Increased electrolytes and protein can result in a high renal solute load, which can lead to dehydration. Therefore, particular attention must be paid to the patient's hydration status with provision of additional free water, if necessary.

Blenderized

Blenderized formulas are prepared from natural foods either commercially or in the kitchen. Commercial liquids are nutritionally complete, contain high-quality protein (usually meat or milk), and have moderate to high residue. Advantages of commercial, blenderized products are that they require no preparation, and they include micronutrients, fiber, and undefined nutrients normally found in regular table food. Home or hospital-prepared formulas can be labor intensive and are associated with an increased risk of bacterial contamination. Other disadvantages include a high viscosity, which makes passage through small bore feeding tubes problematic.

Chemically Defined

Chemically defined formulas are generally high in carbohydrate, are variable in protein content, (most) are moderately low in fat and residue, are fiber free, and require minimal or no digestion for their absorption. They are hyperosmolar, although some are only minimally hyperosmolar. Dilution is unnecessary for gastric, duodenal, or jejunal feeding. A few of these products are extremely low in fat and their exclusive use can lead to essential fatty acid deficiency over an extended period of time. They are frequently referred to as "elemental," a term that was originally used to describe the original prototype product in this class, which consisted of monomeric elements of food (eg, free amino acids, oligosaccharides, glucose) and a very small amount of safflower oil. Later on, chemically defined diets began to accrue longer carbohydrate moieties and peptides. Then short chain polypeptides, hydrolyzed starches or maltodextrin, and moderate quantities of fat were included, usually with substantial proportions of MCT. Today, products containing a high proportion of dipeptides and tripeptides as the protein source have become popular. Theoretically, intestinal absorption of formulas containing di- and tripeptides may be facilitated over those containing crystalline amino acids, although this has not been conclusively demonstrated. In addition, improved absorption does not necessarily equate to increased nitrogen synthesis or better outcome.[141]

All chemically defined formulas are expensive and should be limited to those patients with impaired ability to digest or absorb intact nutrients. Routine use in patients with a normal GI tract, even in the hypoalbuminemic patient, is unwarranted.[14,105,142,143] In fact, use of intact protein formulas may actually lead to a lower incidence of diarrhea.[144]

Disease Specific

Disease-specific specialty formulas have been designed for patients with a variety of clinical conditions including GI, pulmonary, diabetes mellitus, renal and hepatic insufficiency, cancer, immunocompromise, or wound-healing states. They are usually significantly more expensive than standard products. The nutrient composition of specialty products is tailored beyond that of normal requirements in an effort to address the unique needs of specific diseases and/or conditions in an effort to maximize recovery. There exists some literature describing the use of these products; however, inadequate efficacy data exists for many of these relatively expensive products. Manufacturer claims for a product's intended use and unique features may not always equate with sound scientific principles. Therefore, careful consideration should be given when contemplating the use of any of these formulas outside of a research setting.

Gastrointestinal Dysfunction

Patients with GI tract dysfunction causing maldigestion may benefit from modified nutrient components that are easily digested and absorbed. Chemically defined products are commonly prescribed for patients with malabsorption due to critical illness, impaired digestion, extremely short bowel syndrome, refractory sprue, chronic intractable diarrhea, pancreatitis, inflammatory bowel disease, or human immunodeficiency virus (HIV)/acquired immunodeficiency syndrome (AIDS);[6-8,14,82,145-147] conditions for which randomized, prospective clinical trials providing evidence of superiority of these products have not been adequate.[15,18] In addition, GI recovery and gut health may be improved by providing glutamine,[114,118,122] SCFA,[80,148] fructooligosaccharides,[96] or fiber.[149,150] Quantity of fat, MCT, and the fatty acid composition of the enteral formula have also been postulated as being important effectors in the nutritional therapy of patients with GI disease.[82,151] There could be a number of disorders for which these various substrates may be important, but their applications require closer scrutiny.

Pulmonary

Patients with pulmonary insufficiency characteristically retain CO_2 and experience O_2 depletion. When these patients receive nutrition support, calories of any type are associated with an increase in total CO_2 production and O_2 consumption, placing an increased demand on the compromised respiratory system. The premise for initial attempts at pulmonary product development was based upon biochemistry centered at diminishing this metabolic stress. Two theoretical nutritional means for producing the least CO_2 for the oxygen consumed exist—decreasing energy intake or altering the proportions of carbohydrate and fat intake. In both cases, oxidation of fat calories produces less carbon dioxide than did other energy-generating nutrients. Decreasing carbohydrate calories while increasing fat calories should theoretically result in a decreased respiratory quotient and improved gas exchange. Extrapolation of this concept to clinical practice has led to marketing of enteral formulas with a high fat content for patients with respiratory failure.[152] These products usually contain a high caloric density for volume restriction and lower sodium content as added features.

Much of the early work promoting lower carbohydrate, higher fat feedings to pulmonary compromised patients were case reports or poorly controlled studies whereby patients were fed very high caloric loads.[153-156] Recent investigations that more carefully control caloric intake have questioned the efficacy of high-fat, low-carbohydrate enteral products on ventilation when caloric load is not excessive.[157-159] Rather, it appears that caloric intake is actually more important in order to avoid increased VCO_2 than is the ratio of carbohydrate and fat. Furthermore, disadvantages to high-fat diets include immune suppression and GI side effects such as abdominal discomfort and diarrhea.[70,71,73,156] Because studies do not reveal a clear benefit to low-carbohydrate, high-fat regimens, it is always important to first ensure that overfeeding is not the cause of excess CO_2 production and heightened ventilatory demand before substrate modifications are implemented.[15,105]

New research suggests that the usual inflammatory response in acute respiratory distress syndrome can be modulated by providing specific enteral nutrients. Substrates such as gamma-linolenic acid, eicosapentaenoic acid, and antioxidants have been shown to elicit beneficial effects by altering the phospholipid content of alveolar membranes, which leads to less production of inflammatory mediators in animals.[160-164] In clinical studies, adult patients with respiratory distress syndrome fed these nutrients showed improvements in gas exchange and spent fewer days on the ventilator compared to those receiving an isocaloric, isonitrogenous diet. Other findings included reduced ventilator time, length of stay, and incidence of new organ failure.[87,165] These nutrients also appear to facilitate remarkable recovery from acute lung injury in the treatment of pediatric burn patients, as evidenced by significant improvements in oxygenation and survival.[86]

Diabetes Mellitus

Disease-specific liquids designed to enhance blood glucose control typically contain a reduced proportion of carbohydrate. For non-critically ill diabetics requiring chronic tube feeding, the American Diabetic Association[166] recommends standard enteral formulas (which contain approximately 50% carbohydrate). Limiting carbohydrate intake to <50% of total calories may facilitate glycemic control in hospitalized patients with conditions associated with hyperglycemia who require tube feeding on a more acute basis. Lower carbohydrate products (typically 36% to 40% carbohydrate) exist to address carbohydrate intolerance associated with these high acuity conditions. Another important issue is the total amount of fat, monounsaturated fat, and omega-3 fatty acids present in supplements. Products designated for diabetics typically contain approximately 42% to 49% fat with an increased percentage of total fat comprised by monounsaturated sources. A number of studies have shown a lower glucose response with enteral diets high in monounsaturated fat versus high carbohydrate.[167,168] With regard to omega-3 fatty acids, there has been little work specific to enteral liquids; however, the findings from oral dietary studies in diabetes have been applied to the manufacture of commercial products enriched with fish oil in an effort to reduce triglycerides. In addition, a fiber source or fructose may also be included in diabetic products in an attempt to further assist in glycemic management. Modified enteral diets for diabetics reportedly improve measures of glucose control[113,114,167,169-176] and reduce infections[167] and pressure ulcers[167] in type 1 and type 2 diabetes as well as in hyperglycemia associated with critical care, although these findings have not been consistent.[116-122] More research is necessary to determine the appropriate usage of specialized enteral formulas in patients with diabetes. (Nutrition and diabetes is discussed in detail in Chapter 16.)

Immune Enhancing

Immunonutrition is an emerging form of diet therapy and various enteral products specifically formulated with nutrients believed to modulate the immune system (such as arginine, glutamine, BCAA, nucleotides, omega-3 fatty acids, and antioxidants) are in widespread use. Benefits in outcome have been described by many.[27-29,31,32,34,84,126,127,177-187] Nevertheless, immune-enhancing formulas continue to be the subject of considerable controversy as well.[15,26,37,188-194]

In intensive-care–unit (ICU) patients, those managed with one particular tube feeding containing arginine, omega-3 fatty acids, and nucleotides demonstrates improved immune function and lower incidence of the systemic inflammatory response syndrome and multiple organ failure.[31,32,34] Another commercial product consisting of glutamine, arginine, fish oil, nucleotides, and BCAA has been associated with enhanced immune function, fewer infectious complications, reduced incidence of multiple organ failure, and shortened length of hospital stay in trauma patients.[20,183] Gottschlich et al[27] reported significantly lower rates of wound infection and length of hospital stay for burn patients given a modular tube feeding enriched with arginine and fish oil. Despite rather consistent overall trends of reduced morbidity with immunonutrition, most trials have been negative for differences in mortality.

Animal research has generated much of the data supporting each of the immune modulating nutrients as single entities,[22-25,77,91,195,196] whereas clinical studies have primarily focused on investigating outcomes resulting from the use of enteral regimens that combine many of the nutrients. Recent meta analyses of randomized controlled trials using immune enhancing enteral formulas have concluded from aggregated results of elective surgical, trauma, ICU, and burn patients that immunomodulation is associated with a reduction in infectious complications and with a shorter hospital stay.[26,37,180-182,197] In critically ill patients with shock, sepsis, or organ failure, however, the benefits are less clear.[26,37] Furthermore, in certain subgroups, these formulas may be deleterious.[26,31,194] Proceedings of a consensus conference on the use of immune-enhancing products suggest that caution should be applied in patients with sepsis, in whom mortality may be increased because of an overwhelming systemic inflammatory response.[188] Hence, despite the optimistic results reported from these investigations, insufficient experimental data exist to permit firm conclusions that such formulas reduce morbidity and mortality.[193,194] Nevertheless, the concept of immunonutrition continues to be welcomed by clinicians. Certainly, results are promising enough to warrant further research, but more understanding is needed regarding the mechanism of action of various individual nutrients so that optimized ratios and concentration of the various elements are ultimately used that best promote safety and efficacy.

Cancer

Less sweet and calorically and protein dense products and also the immune products have been promoted as helpful in cancer,[198] although benefit is extremely controversial. There exist generally positive outcomes of post-surgical EN.[28,29,85,180,187,199] Preoperative delivery of immunonutrition appears to be particularly beneficial in counteracting the surgery-induced alterations of immune and inflammatory responses, including decreased infection and length of hospital stay.[184-186] One attempt, however, to improve preoperatively the status of patients with GI cancers was less encouraging. In a controlled double-blinded trial, the infusion of oral liquid supplements containing arginine plus omega-3 fatty acids before major surgery did not improve the immunological markers in patients with cancer.[177] Nor is there any clear benefit of EN as an adjunct to chemotherapy or radiation therapy.[15]

Human Immunodeficiency Virus and Acquired Immunodeficiency Syndrome

GI symptoms, weight loss, malnutrition, and infection are common components of the clinical syndrome in HIV-infected patients. Formulas containing MCT and hydrolyzed protein have been effective in treated AIDS-associated malabsorption.[81,147] Immune-enhancing formulas have also been utilized in the care of persons with HIV/AIDS with mixed results. Some research documents significant weight gain in outpatients receiving an hydrolyzed protein enteral formula containing immune-modulating nutrients such as arginine, omega-3 fatty acids, fiber, and vitamins E, C, and beta-carotene.[200,201] Chlebowski and colleagues[201] showed that nutritional status was strongly associated with survival and reported significantly reduced hospitalizations concurrent with specialized enteral support. In contrast, others[202-204] have not observed any difference in weight or fat-free mass. Investigators have likewise not identified improvement in CD4+ and CD8+ T lymphocytes when immune enhancing formulas are utilized.[200,202,205]

Renal

The aim of specialty formulas designed for use in patients with renal failure is to minimize the accumulation of nitrogenous compounds, electrolytes, and fluids. Early formulas were designed to provide just EAA. Today, enteral renal solutions vary in composition. All products are unpalatable for oral consumption and all are calorically dense (they provide 2.0 kcal/mL of formula), thus enabling caloric needs to be met with relatively small volumes of formula. Some of these products are low in protein and high in essential amino acids (or their ketoanalogues) whereas other products supply a more moderate protein load. Vitamin, mineral, and electrolyte content also vary among formulas. In deciding which formula to use, it is necessary to define the specific fluid, protein, energy, and electrolyte needs of the patient being treated. For example, those with nondialyzed chronic renal failure will have different needs than will patients with acute renal failure. Specialized renal products often become unnecessary once dialysis is initiated.

Investigations are needed to substantiate benefit of enteral products designated specifically for the renal patient in comparison to standard solutions.[61] Most studies to date involve parenteral delivery of amino acids rather than enteral. The preference of EAA versus a mixture of EAA and nonessential amino acids (NEAA) is particularly controversial. The rationale for an exclusive EAA regimen is based on the physiological theory that EAA decrease urea production and enhance recycling of the abundant urea nitrogen present for use in the endogenous synthesis of NEAA. There is no certainty, however, that this in fact happens. Recent studies have shown that nitrogen derived from urea does not appear sufficient to support nitrogen balance and fails to confirm any significant advantage to the use of strictly EAA as the nitrogen source.[205] Additionally, the use of EAA alone may disrupt the urea cycle and lead to hyperammonemia and altered mental status.[206,207] Because of the lack of demonstrable clinical efficacy coupled with the high cost of these formulas, it is recommended that patients receive a balanced mixture of both EAA and NEAA when attempting to avoid dialysis.[15]

Hepatic

Specialized formulas for patients with hepatic encephalopathy contain high quantities of BCAA and low amounts of aromatic amino acids. There is some clinical efficacy data indicating that patients who would otherwise be unable to ingest sufficient protein without precipitating a worsening of the encephalopathy seem to demonstrate some benefit from supplementation with hepatic products.[60,61,63,64,208] Other studies fail to demonstrate efficacy and evidence is often conflicting,[209-213] undoubtedly because of differences in study design and outcome measures. Meta-analyses have been difficult and fail to produce unequivocal results.[37] Recently published clinical guidelines of the American Society for Parenteral and Enteral Nutrition[15] and others[62,105] suggest that BCAA-enriched enteral formulas, which are significantly more expensive than are regular products, should be used in patients with hepatic encephalopathy only when standard medical care is ineffective in permitting adequate protein intake.

Wound Healing

Several supplements have been promoted to prevent pressure ulcers and enhance wound healing by providing higher levels of nutrients implicated in the wound-healing process such as protein, arginine, beta-hydroxy-beta-methylbutyrate (HMB), zinc, and vitamins A, beta-carotene, and C.[3,33,35] While inadequate protein, vitamins, and minerals will delay wound healing, data supporting the use of such products in the absence of deficiency are rather limited. One investigation, however, studied healthy volunteers randomized to receive daily supplementation of 14 g arginine, 3 g HMB, and 14 g glutamine, which led to a significant increase in collagen deposition.[33] Another investigation found that a formula enriched with arginine, zinc, and antioxidants was useful in pressure ulcer treatment.[35]

Modular Products and Additives

Despite the availability of a wide variety of nutritionally complete products, there are some patients for whom fixed ratio formulas may not be optimal. Utilization of modular supplements, which can supply a single nutrient or a combination of nutrients, may allow for the creation of a care plan that best meets the unique nutritional requirements of an individual patient. Modules such as carbohydrate, protein, fat, fiber, or micronutrients can be added to standard enteral products to alter the fixed ratio of nutrients inherent in a particular product or used as a supplement to enhance an oral diet. Another application of modules is the ability to design a completely new recipe, creating a unique modular tube feeding.[27,71,211] De novo production permits custom compounding of a formula, which is useful in patients with highly specialized nutritional requirements. However, the complexity of calculating and ordering a specific nutrient composition and the increased cost of labor involved may preclude some facilities from using modular systems. De novo production also carries the potential risk of microbial contamination from improper handling of ingredients, mixing errors, and potential physical incompatibilities with insoluble components.

Blue dye, used as a method for detecting early evidence of pulmonary aspiration, has been a popular enteral additive for nearly two decades. The safety of this practice, however, has been recently questioned, especially for patients with increased gut permeability.[214] Modules can also be used as a separate entity. For example, various fiber modules (dried banana flakes or liquid pectin) can be mixed with water and infused down a feeding tube (followed by water flushes) while the tube feeding formula is off.[116]

Conclusion

The evolution of enteral formulas and supplements has been dramatic. Insights into the potential health and disease modulating benefits of novel nutrients have prompted the commercial availability of a broad range of simple as well as sophisticated enteral products. Formulas vary considerably in terms of nutrient sources, complexity of the various constituents, amounts of nutrients present, digestibility, caloric density, caloric distribution among carbohydrate, fat and protein, viscosity, osmolality, cost, and scientific justification—all of which represent important considerations when selecting a product.

For enteral specialty solutions to be used most effectively, great scrutiny in evaluating their alleged efficacy is required. However, in the case of many formulations, proven effects on morbidity and mortality have not been adequately studied in prospective, randomized trials.[15,61,188] Furthermore, the popularity of key nutrients known to modulate immune, inflammatory, GI barrier function, and other metabolic responses often transcend scientific basis and thus are marketed largely based on theory. Investigations to date have provided limited but promising data, yet also bring to mind uncertainties in the scientific literature and leave clinicians pondering decisions of best practice. The nutrition support practitioner is encouraged to rely on evidence based clinical guidelines for direction. Further study is needed to ascertain the nutritional effects and pharmacologic actions of various substrates and formulas on outcomes. Dogma will likely require reinterpretation as more facts become available.

References

1. Harkness L. The history of enteral nutrition therapy: From raw eggs and nasal tubes to purified amino acids and early postoperative jejunal delivery. *J Am Diet Assoc.* 2002;102:399-404.
2. Neumann M, Friedmann J, Roy MA, Jensen GL. Provision of high protein supplement for patients recovering from hip fracture. *Nutrition.* 2004;20:415-419.
3. Bourdel-Marchasson I, Barateau M, Rondeau V, et al. A multi-center trial of the effects of oral nutritional supplementation in critically ill older patients. *Nutrition.* 2000;16:1-5.
4. Alexander JW, MacMillan BG, Stinnett JD, et al. Beneficial effect of aggressive protein feeding in severely burned children. *Ann Surg.* 1980;192:505-517.
5. Silk DBA, Fairclough PD, Clark ML, et al. Use of peptide rather than free amino acid nitrogen source in chemically defined elemental diets. *JPEN J Parenter Enteral Nutr.* 1980;4:548-553.
6. Matthews DM. Protein absorption: then and now. *Gastroenterology.* 1977;73:1267-1279.
7. Adibi SA, Fogel MR, Agrawal RM. Comparison of free amino acid and dipeptide absorption in the jejunum of sprue patients. *Gastroenterology.* 1974;67:586-591.
8. Vazquez JA, Morse EL, Adibi SA. Effect of starvation on amino acid and peptide transport and peptide by hydrolysis in humans. *Am J Physiol.* 1985;249:G563-G566.
9. Brinson RR, Hanumantha SK, Pitts WM. A reappraisal of the peptide-based enteral formulas: clinical applications. *NCP.* 1989;4:221-217.
10. Craft IL, Geddes D, Hyde CW. Absorption and malabsorption of glycine and glycine peptides in man. *Gut.* 1968;9:425-437.
11. Meredith JW, Ditesheim JA, Zaloga GP. Visceral protein levels in trauma patients are greater with peptide diet than with intact protein diet. *J Trauma.* 1990;30:825-829.
12. Ziegler F, Ollivier JM, Cynober L, et al. Efficiency of enteral nitrogen support in surgical patients: small peptides vs non-degraded proteins. *Gut.* 1990;31:1277-1283.
13. Heimburger DC, Geels WJ, Bilbrey J, Redden DT, Keeney C. Effects of small-peptide and whole-protein enteral feedings on serum proteins and diarrhea in critically ill patients: a randomized trial. *JPEN J Parenter Enteral Nutr.* 1997;21:162-167.
14. Mowatt-Larssen CA, Brown RO, Wojtysiak SL, Kudsk KA. Comparison of tolerance and nutritional outcome between a peptide and a standard enteral formula in critically ill, hypoalbuminemic patients. *JPEN J Parenter Enteral Nutr.* 1992;16:20-24.
15. Board of Directors, American Society for Parenteral and Enteral Nutrition. Guidelines for the use of parenteral and enteral nutrition in adult and pediatric patients. *JPEN J Parenter Enteral Nutr.* 2002;26:1SA-138A.
16. Ksiazyk J, Piena M, Kierkus J, Lyszkowska M. Hydrolyzed versus nonhydrolyzed protein diet in short bowel syndrome in children. *J Pediatr Gastroenterol Nutr.* 2002;35:615-618.
17. McIntyre PB, Fitchew M, Lennard-Jones JE. Patients with a high ileostomy do not need a special diet. *Gastroenterology.* 1986;91:25-33.
18. Mowatt-Larssen CA, Brown RO, Wojtysiak SL, Kudsk KA. Comparison of tolerance and nutritional outcome between a peptide and a standard enteral formula in critically ill, hypoalbuminemic patients. *JPEN J Parenter Enteral Nutr.* 1992;16:20-24.
19. Grimble GK, Silk DBA. The nitrogen source of elemental diets. An unresolved issue. *NCP.* 1990;5:227-230.

20. Deitch EA, Xu D, Qi L, Berg R. Elemental diet-induced immune suppression is caused by both bacterial and dietary factors. *JPEN J Parenter Enteral Nutr.* 1993;17:332-336.
21. Serizawa H, Miura S, Tashiro H, et al. Alteration of mucosal immunity after long-term ingestion of an elemental diet in rats. *JPEN J Parenter Enteral Nutr.* 1994;18:141-147.
22. Gianotti L, Alexander JW, Pyles T, Fukushima R. Arginine-supplemented diets improve survival in gut-derived sepsis and peritonitis by modulating bacterial clearance-the role of nitric oxide. *Ann Surg.* 1993;217:644-654.
23. Kirk SK, Barbul A. Role of arginine in trauma, sepsis and immunity. *JPEN J Parenter Enteral Nutr.* 1990;14:226S-229S.
24. Adjei AA, Yamauchi K, Nakasone Y, Konishi M, Yamamoto S. Arginine-supplemented diets inhibit endotoxin-induced bacterial translocation in mice. *Nutrition.* 1995;11:371-374.
25. Saito H, Trocki O, Wang SL, Gonce SJ, Joffe SN, Alexander JW. Metabolic and immune effects of dietary arginine supplementation after burn. *Arch Surg.* 1987;122:784-789.
26. Heyland DK, Novak F, Drover JW, Jain M, Su X, Suchner U. Should immunonutrition become routine in critically ill patients? A systematic review of the evidence. *JAMA.* 2001;286:944-953.
27. Gottschlich MM, Jenkins M, Warden GD, et al. Differential effects of three enteral regimens on selected outcome parameters in burn patients. *JPEN J Parenter Enteral Nutr.* 1990;14:225-236.
28. Daly JM, Lieberman MD, Goldfine J, et al Enteral nutrition with supplemental arginine, RNA, and omega-3 fatty acids in patients after operation: immunologic, metabolic, and clinical outcome. *Surgery.* 1992;112:56-67.
29. Senkal M, Kemen M, Homann HH, et al. Modulation of postoperative immune response by enteral nutrition with a diet enriched with arginine, RNA, and omega-3 fatty acids in patients with upper gastrointestinal cancer. *Eur J Surg.* 1995;161:115-122.
30. Barbul A, Lazarou S, Efron DT, Wasserkrug HL, Efron G. Arginine enhances wound healing in humans. *Surgery.* 1990;108:331-337.
31. Bower RH, Cerra FB, Bershadsky B, et al. Early enteral administration of a formula (Impact) supplemented with arginine, nucleotides, and fish oil in intensive care patients: results of a multicenter, prospective, randomized, clinical trial. *Crit Care Med.* 1995;23:436-449.
32. Atkinson S, Sieffert E, Bihari D. A prospective, double-blind, controlled clinical trial of enteral immunonutrition in the critically ill. *Crit Care Med.* 1998;26:1164-1172.
33. Williams JZ, Abumrad N, Barbul A. Effect of a specialized amino acid mixture on human collagen deposition. *Ann Surg.* 2002;236:369-374.
34. Kemen M, Senkal M, Homann HH, et al. Early postoperative enteral nutrition with arginine, omega-3 fatty acids and ribonucleic acid-supplemented diet versus placebo in cancer patients: an immunologic evaluation of Impact. *Crit Care Med.* 1995;23:652-659.
35. Benati G, Delvecchio S, Cilla D, Pedone V. Impact on pressure ulcer healing of an arginine-enriched nutritional solution in patients with severe cognitive impairment. *Arch Gerontol Geriatr.* 2001;7(Suppl):43-47.
36. Peck MD. High doses of dietary arginine during repletion impair weight gain and increase infectious mortality in protein-malnourished mice. *Brit J Nutr.* 1995;74:787-795.
37. Heyland DK, Cook DJ, Guyatt GH. Does the formulation of enteral feeding products influence infectious morbidity and mortality rates in critically ill patients? A critical review of the evidence. *Crit Care Med.* 1994;22:1192-1202.
38. Ochoa JB, Makarenkova V, Bansal V. A rational use of immune enhancing diets: when should we use dietary arginine supplementation? *NCP.* 2004;19:216-225.
39. Heyland DK, Dhaliwal R, Drover JW. Nutrition support in mechanically ventilated, critically ill adult patients: are we ready for evidence-based clinical practice guidelines. *NCP.* 2004;19:193-200.
40. Souba W, Smith RJ, Wilmore DW. Glutamine metabolism by the intestinal tract. *JPEN J Parenter Enteral Nutr.* 1985;9:608-617.
41. van der Hulst RR, van Kreel BK, von Meyenfeldt MF, et al. Glutamine and the preservation of gut integrity. *Lancet.* 1993;341:1363-1365.
42. Peng X, You Z, Wang P, Wang S. Effects of enteral supplementation with glutamine granules on intestinal mucosal barrier function in severe burned patients. *Burns.* 2004;30:135-139.
43. Zhou YP, Jiang ZM, Sun YH, Wang XR, Ma EL, Wilmore D. The effects of supplemental enteral glutamine on plasma levels, gut function, and outcome in severe burns: a randomized, double-blind, controlled clinical trial. *JPEN J Parenter Enteral Nutr.* 2003;27:241-245.
44. Tenenhaus M, Hansbrough JF, Zapata-Sirvent RL, et al. Supplementation of an elemental enteral diet with alanyl-glutamine decreases bacterial translocation in burned mice. Burns. 1994;20:220-225.
45. Buchman AL. Glutamine: commercially essential or conditionally essential? A critical appraisal of the human data. *Am J Clin Nutr.* 2001;74:25-32.
46. Gottschlich MM, Mayes T, Khoury J, Warden GD. Effect of enteral glutamine supplementation on selected outcome variables in burned children. *J Burn Care Rehabil.* 2004;25:S72
47. Jensen GL, Miller RH, Talabiska DG, Fish J, Gianferante L. A double-blind, prospective, randomized study of glutamine-enriched compared with standard peptide-based feeding in critically ill patients. *Am J Clin Nutr.* 1996;64:615-621.
48. Long CL, Nelson KM, DiRienzo DB, et al. Glutamine supplementation of enteral nutrition: impact on whole body protein kinetics and glucose metabolism in critically ill patients. *JPEN J Parenter Enteral Nutr.* 1995;19:470-476.
49. Wischmeyer PE, Lynch J, Liedel J, et al. Glutamine administration reduces gram-negative bacteremia in severely burned patients: A prospective, randomized, double-blind trial versus isonitrogenous control. *Crit Care Med.* 2001;29:2075-2080.
50. Houdijk APJ, Rijnsburger ER, Jansen J, et al. Randomized trial of glutamine-enriched enteral nutrition on infectious morbidity in patients with multiple trauma. *Lancet.* 1998;352:772-776.
51. Garrel D, Patenaude J, Nedelec B, et al. Decreased mortality and infectious morbidity in adult burn patients given enteral glutamine supplements: a prospective, controlled, randomized clinical trial. *Crit Care Med.* 2003;31:2444-2449.
52. Sheridan RL, Prelack K, Yu YM, et al. Short-term enteral glutamine does not enhance protein accretion in burned children: a stable isotope study. *Surgery.* 2004;135:671-678.
53. Smith RJ, Wilmore DW. Glutamine nutrition and requirements. *JPEN J Parenter Enteral Nutr.* 1990;14:94S-99S.
54. Ziegler TR, Benfell K, Smith RJ, et al. Safety and metabolic effects of L-glutamine administration in humans. *JPEN J Parenter Enteral Nutr.* 1990;14:137S-146S.
55. Gottschlich MM, Shronts EP, Hutchins AM. Defined formula diets. In: Rombeau JL, Rolandelli RH, eds. *Enteral and Tube Feeding.* 3rd ed. Philadelphia, Pa: WB Saunders, Co; 1997:207-239.
56. Cerra FB, Mazuski J, Teasley K, et al. Nitrogen retention in critically ill patients is proportional to the branched chain amino acid load. *Crit Care Med.* 1983;11:775-778.
57. Cerra FB, Shronts EP, Konstantinides NN, et al. Enteral feeding in sepsis. A prospective, randomized, double-blind trial. *Surgery.* 1985:98:632-639.
58. Kern KA, Bower RH, Atamian S, Matarese LE, Ghory MJ, Fischer JE. The effect of a new branched-chain enriched amino acid solution on post-operative catabolism. *Surgery.* 1982;92:780-785.
59. Bower RH, Muggia-Sullam M, Vallgren S, et al. Branched chain amino acid-enriched solutions in the septic patient: a randomized, prospective trial. *Ann Surg.* 1986:203:13-20.
60. Horst D, Grace ND, Conn HO, et al. Comparison of dietary protein with an oral, branched chain-enriched amino acid supplement on chronic portal-systemic encephalopathy. *Hepatology.* 1984;4:279-287.
61. Talbot JM. Guidelines for the scientific review of enteral food products for medical purposes. *JPEN J Parenter Enteral Nutr.* 1991;15:99S-174S.

62. Marchesini G, Bianchi G, Rossi B, Brizi M, Melchionda N. Nutritional treatment with branched-chain amino acids in advanced liver cirrhosis. *Gastroenterology.* 2000;35:2:7S-12S.
63. McGhee A, Henderson JM, Millikan WJ, et al. Comparison of the effects of Hepatic-Aid and a casein modular diet on encephalopathy, plasma amino acids and nitrogen balance in cirrhotic patients. *Ann Surg.* 1983;197:288-293.
64. Marchesini G, Bianchi G, Merli M, et al. Nutritional supplementation with branched-chain amino acids in advanced cirrhosis: a double-blind, randomized trial. *Gastroenterology.* 2003;124:1792-1801.
65. Brennan MF, Cerra F, Daly JM, et al. Report of a research workshop: branched-chain amino acids in stress and injury. *JPEN J Parenter Enteral Nutr.* 1986;10:446-452.
66. Eriksson LS, Persson A, Wahren J. Branched-chain amino acids in the treatment of chronic hepatic encephalopathy. *Gut.* 1982;23:801-806.
67. Christie ML, Sack DM, Pomposelli J, Horst D. Enriched branched-chain amino acid formula versus a casein-based supplement in the treatment of cirrhosis. *JPEN J Parenter Enteral Nutr.* 1985;9:671-678.
68. Mochizuki H, Trocki O, Dominioni L, Alexander JW. Effect of a diet rich in branched chain amino acids on severely burned guinea pigs. *J Trauma.* 1986;26:1077-1085.
69. Carver JD. Dietary nucleotides: Cellular, immune, intestinal and hepatic system effects. *J Nutr.* 1994;124:144S-148S.
70. Gottschlich MM. Selection of optimal lipid sources in enteral and parenteral nutrition. *Nutr Clin Pract.* 1992;7:152-165.
71. Gottschlich MM, Warden GD, Michel MA, et al. Diarrhea in tube-fed burn patients: incidence, etiology, nutritional impact and prevention. *JPEN J Parenter Enteral Nutr.* 1988;12:338-345.
72. Calder PC. N-3 Polyunsaturated fatty acids and inflammation: from molecular biology to the clinic. *Lipids.* 2003;38:343-352.
73. Bulger EM, Maier RV. Lipid mediators in the pathophysiology of critical illness. *Crit Care Med.* 2000;28(S):N27-N36.
74. Harbige LS. Fatty acids, the immune response, and autoimmunity: a question of n-6 essentiality and the balance between n-6 and n-3. *Lipids.* 2003;38:323-341.
75. Trocki O, Heyd TJ, Waymack JP, Alexander JW. Effects of fish oil on postburn metabolism and immunity. *JPEN J Parenter Enteral Nutr.* 1987;11:521-528.
76. Mochizuki H, Trocki O, Dominioni L, Ray MB, Alexander JW. Optimal lipid content for enteral diets following thermal injury. *JPEN J Parenter Enteral Nutr.* 1984;8:638-646.
77. Alexander JW, Saito H, Trocki O, Ogle CK. The importance of lipid type in the diet after burn injury. Ann Surg. 1986;204:1-8.
78. Luyer MDP, Jacobs JA, Vreugdenhil ACE, et al. Enteral administration of high-fat nutrition before and directly after hemorrhagic shock reduces endotoxemia and bacterial translocation. *Ann Surg.* 2004;239:257-264.
79. Frankel WL, Zhang W, Singh A, et al. Mediation of the trophic effects of short chain fatty acids in the rat jejunum and colon. *Gastroenterology.* 1994;106:375-380.
80. Bowling TE, Raimundo AH, Grimble GK, Silk DB. Reversal by short-chain fatty acids of colonic fluid secretion induced by enteral feeding. *Lancet.* 1993;342:1266-1268.
81. Craig CB, Darnell BE, Weinsier RL, et al. Decreased fat and nitrogen losses in patients with AIDS receiving medium-chain-triglyceride-enriched formula vs those receiving long-chain-triglyceride-containing formula. *J Am Diet Assoc.* 1997;97:605-611.
82. Shea JC, Bishop MD, Parker EM, Gelrud A, Freedman SD. An enteral therapy containing medium-chain triglycerides and hydrolyzed peptides reduces postprandial pain associated with chronic pancreatitis. *Pancreatology.* 2003;3:36-40.
83. Kromhout D, Bosschieter EB, Coulaner CDL. The inverse relationship between fish oil consumption and 20-year mortality from coronary heart disease. *N Engl J Med.* 1985;312:1205-1209.
84. Weinmann A, Bastian L, Bischoff WE, et al. Influence of arginine, n-3 fatty acids and nucleotide-supplemented enteral support on systemic inflammatory response syndrome and multiple organ failure in patients after severe trauma. *Nutrition.* 1998;14:165-172.
85. Kenler AS, Swails WS, Driscoll DF, et al. Early enteral feeding in postsurgical cancer patients. Fish oil structured lipid-based polymeric formula versus a standard polymeric formula. *Ann Surg.* 1996;223:316-333.
86. Mayes T, Gottschlich M, Carman B, Kagan R. An evaluation of the safety and efficacy of an anti-inflammatory, pulmonary enteral formula in the treatment of pediatric burn patients with respiratory failure. *JPEN J Parenter Enteral Nutr.* submitted.
87. Nelson JL, DeMichele SJ, Pacht ER, Wennberg AK. Enteral nutrition in ARDS study group: effect of enteral feeding with eicosapentaenoic acid, gamma linolenic acid, and antioxidants on antioxidant status in patients with acute respiratory distress syndrome. *JPEN J Parenter Enteral Nutr.* 2003;27:98-104.
88. Tso P, Karlstad MD, Bistrian BR, DeMichele SJ. Intestinal digestion, absorption and transport of structured triglycerides and cholesterol in rats. *Am J Physiol.* 1995;31:G568-577.
89. Christenses MS, Hoy CE, Becker CC, Redgrave TG. Intestinal absorption and lymphatic transport of eicosapentaenoic (EPA), docosahexaenoic (DHA), and decanoic acids: dependence on intramolecular triacylglycerol structure. *Am J Clin Nutr.* 1995;61:56-61.
90. Bell SJ, Bradley D, Forse RA, Bistrian BR. The new dietary fats in health and disease. *J Am Diet Assoc.* 1997;97:280-286.
91. Selleck KJ, Wan JMF, Gollaher CJ, Babayan VK, Bistrian BR. Effect of low and high amounts of a structured lipid containing fish oil on protein metabolism in enterally fed burned rats. *Am J Clin Nutr.* 1994;60:216-222.
92. McKenna MC, Hubbard VS, Bieri JG. Linoleic acid absorption from lipid supplements in patients with cystic fibrosis with pancreatic insufficiency and in control subjects. *J Pediatr Gastroenterol Nutr.* 1985;4:45-51.
93. DeMichele SJ, Karlstad MD, Babayan VK, et al. Enhanced skeletal muscle and liver protein synthesis with structured lipid in enterally fed burned rats. *Metabolism.* 1988;37:787-795.
94. DeMichele SJ, Karlstad MD, Bistrian BR, Istfan N, Babayan VK. Enteral nutrition with structured lipid: Effect on protein metabolism in thermal injury. *Am J Clin Nutr.* 1989;50:1295-1302.
95. Silk DBA. Formulation of enteral diets. *Nutrition.* 1999;15:626-632.
96. Garleb KA, Snowden MK, Wolf BW, Chow J. Application of fructooligosaccharides to medical foods as a fermentable dietary fiber. *Bioscience Microflora.* 2002;21:43-54.
97. Ohta A, Sakai K, Takasaki M, Tokunaga T. The advantages of calcium supplement tablet containing fructooligosaccharides for the healthy human being. *J Nutr Food.* 1999;2:37-43.
98. Campbell JM, Fahey GC, Wolf BW. Selected indigestible oligosaccharides affect large bowel mass, cecal and fecal short-chain fatty acids, pH and microflora in rats. *J Nutr.* 1997;127:130-136.
99. Howard MD, Gordon DT, Pace LW, Garleb KA, Kerley MS. Effect of dietary supplementation with fructooligosaccharides on colonic microbiota populations and epithelial cell proliferation in neonatal pigs. *J Pediatr Gastroenterol Nutr.* 1995;21:297-303.
100. Wang X, Gibson GR. Effects of the in vitro fermentation of oligofructose and inulin by bacteria growing in the human intestine. *J Appl Bacteriol.* 1993;75:373-380.
101. Niness KR. Inulin and oligofructose: what are they? *J Nutr.* 1999;129:1402S-1406S.
102. Olesen M, Gudmand-Hoyer E. Efficacy, safety and tolerability of fructooligosaccharides in the treatment of irritable bowel syndrome. *Am J Clin Nutr.* 2000;72:1570-1575.
103. Clausen MR, Jorgensen J, Mortensen PB. Comparison of diarrhea induced by ingestion of fructooligosaccharide Idolax and disaccharide lactulose: role of osmolarity versus fermentation of malabsorbed carbohydrate. *Dig Dis Sci.* 1998;43:2696-2707.
104. Stone-Dorshow T, Levitt MD. Gaseous response to ingestion of a poorly absorbed fructooligosaccharide sweetener. *Am J Clin Nutr.* 1987;46:61-65.
105. Kirby DF, DeLegge MH, Fleming CR. American Gastroenterological Association technical review on tube feeding for enteral nutrition. *Gastroenterology.* 1995;108:1282-1301.

106. Homann HH, Kemen M, Fuessenich C, Senkal M, Zumtobel V. Reduction in diarrhea incidence by soluble fiber in patients receiving total or supplemental enteral nutrition. *JPEN J Parenter Enteral Nutr.* 1994;18:486-490.
107. Scheppach W, Burghardt W, Bartram P, Kasper H. Addition of dietary fiber to liquid formula diets: the pros and cons. *JPEN J Parenter Enteral Nutr.* 1990;14:204-209.
108. Nakao M, Ogura Y, Satake S, et al. Usefulness of soluble dietary fiber for the treatment of diarrhea during enteral nutrition in elderly patients. *Nutrition.* 2002;18:35-39.
109. Spapen H, Diltoer M, VanMalderen C, et al. Soluble fiber reduces the incidence of diarrhea in septic patients receiving total enteral nutrition: a prospective, double-blind, randomized, and controlled trial. *Clin Nutr.* 2001;20:301-305.
110. Spaeth G, Berg RD, Specian RD, Deitch EA. Food without fiber promotes bacterial translocation from the gut. *Surgery.* 1990;108:240-247.
111. Wells CL, Barton RG, Jechorek RP, Gillingham KJ, Cerra FB. Effect of fiber supplementation of liquid diet on cecal bacteria and bacterial translocation in mice. *Nutrition.* 1992;8:266-271.
112. Nettelbladt CG, Katouli M, Bark T, et al. Bulking fiber prevents translocation to mesenteric lymph nodes of an efficiently translocating Escherichia coli strain in rats. *Clin Nutr.* 1998;17:185-190.
113. del Carmen Crespillo M, Olveira G, de Adana MS, et al. Metabolic effects of an enteral nutrition formula for diabetes: comparison with standard formulas in patients with type 1 diabetes. *Clin Nutr.* 2003;5:483-487.
114. Sturmer W, Kramer E, Kasper H, Schrezenmeir J. Favourable glycaemic effects of a new balanced liquid diet for enteral nutrition: results of a short term study in 30 type II diabetic patients. *Clin Nutr.* 1994;13:221-227.
115. Dobb GJ, Towler SC. Diarrhea during enteral feeding in the critically ill: a comparison of feeds with and without fiber. *Intens Care Med.* 1990;16:252-255.
116. Frankenfield DC, Beyer PL. Dietary fiber and bowel function in tube-fed patients. *J Am Diet Assoc.* 1991;91:590-596.
117. Frankenfield DC, Beyer PL. Soy-polysaccharide fiber: effect on diarrhea in tube-fed, head-injured patients. *Am J Clin Nutr.* 1989;50:533-538.
118. Fussell ST, Garmhausen L, Koruda MJ. The influence of guar gum on diarrhea in critically ill tube-fed patients. *JPEN J Parenter Enteral Nutr.* 1996;20:26S.
119. Hart GK, Dobb GJ. Effect of fecal bulking agent on diarrhea during enteral feeding in the critically ill. *JPEN J Parenter Enteral Nutr.* 1988;12:465-468.
120. Heymsfield SB, Roongspisuthipong C, Evert M. Fiber supplementation of enteral formulas: effects on the bioavailability of major nutrients and gastrointestinal tolerance. *JPEN J Parenter Enteral Nutr.* 1988;12:265-273.
121. Patil DH, Grimble GK, Keohane P, Attrill H, Love M, Silk DBA. Do fibre containing enteral diets have advantages over existing low residue diets? *Clin Nutr.* 1985;4:67-71.
122. Thomas BL, Laine DC, Goetz FC. Glucose and insulin response in diabetic subjects: acute effect of carbohydrate level and the addition of soy polysaccharide in defined-formula diets. *Am J Clin Nutr.* 1988;48:1048-1052.
123. Guenter PA, Settle R, Perlmutter S, et al. Tube feeding-related diarrhea in acutely ill patients. *JPEN J Parenter Enteral Nutr.* 1991;15:277-280.
124. Fisher M, Adkins W, Hail L, Seaman P, His S, Marlett J. The effect of dietary fiber in a liquid diet on bowel function of mentally retarded individuals. *J Ment Defic Res.* 1985;29:373-381.
125. Prelack K, Sheridan RL. Micronutrient supplementation in the critically ill patient: strategies for clinical practice. *J Trauma.* 2001;51:601-620.
126. Maderazo EG, Woronick Cl, Hickingbotham N, Jacopbs L, Bhagavan HN. Randomized trial of replacement antioxidant vitamin therapy for neutrophil locomotory dysfunction in blunt trauma. *J Trauma.* 1991;31:1142-1150.
127. Horton JW, White J, Maass DL, et al. Antioxidant vitamin therapy alters burn trauma-mediated cardiac NF-B activation and cardiomyocyte cytokine secretion. *J Trauma.* 2001;50:397-408.
128. Keohane PP, Attrill H, Love M, Frost P, Silk DB. Relation between osmolality of diet and gastrointestinal side effects in enteral nutrition. *Br Med J.* 1984;288:678-680.
129. Zarling EJ, Parmar JR, Mobarhan S, Clapper M. Effect of enteral formula infusion rate, osmolality, and chemical composition upon clinical tolerance and carbohydrate absorption in normal subjects. *JPEN J Parenter Enteral Nutr.* 1986;10:588-590.
130. Pesola GR, Hogg JE, Eissa N, Matthews DE, Carlon GC. Hypertonic nasogastric tube feedings: do they cause diarrhea? *Crit Care Med.* 1990;18:1378-1382.
131. Paauw JD, Davis AT. Taurine concentrations in serum of critically injured patients and age- and sex-matched healthy control subjects. *Am J Clin Nutr.* 1990;52:657-660.
132. Desai TK, Maliakkal J, Kinzie JL, et al Taurine deficiency after intensive chemotherapy and/or radiation. *Am J Clin Nutr.* 1992;55:708-711.
133. Martensson J, Larsson J, Nordstrom H. Amino acid metabolism during the anabolic phase of severely burned patients. With special reference to sulfur amino acids. *Eur J Clin Invest.* 1987;17:130-135.
134. Iapichino G, Radrizzani D, Colombo A, Ronzoni G. Carnitine excretion: A catabolic index of injury. *JPEN J Parenter Enteral Nutr.* 1988;12:35-36.
135. Holme E, Jacobson CE, Nordin I, Kristiansson B, Jodal U. Carnitine deficiency induced by pivampicillin and pivmecillinam therapy. *Lancet.* 1989;2:469-473.
136. FDA. *Compliance Program Guidance Manual.* Chapter 21. Program No. 7321.002, Washington, DC: Food and Drug Administration; 1989.
137. Heimburger DC, Weinsier RL. Guidelines for evaluating and categorizing enteral feeding formulas according to therapeutic equivalence. *JPEN J Parenter Enteral Nutr.* 1985;9:61-67.
138. Mueller C, Nestle M. Regulation of medical foods: toward a rational policy. *NCP.* 1995;10:8-15.
139. Heymsfield SB. Enteral solutions: is there a solution? *NCP.* 1995;10:4-7.
140. Mueller C. The regulatory status of medical foods and dietary supplements in the United States. *Nutrition.* 1999;15:249-251.
141. Steinhardt HJ, Wolf A, Jakober B, et al. Protein assimilation in pancreatectomized patients: efficiency of absorption from whole versus hydrolyzed protein. *Gastroenterology.* 1986;90:1648.
142. Koretz RL, Meyer JH. Elemental diets-facts and fantasies. *Gastroenterology.* 1980;78:393-410.
143. Silk DB. Diet formulation and choice of enteral diet. *Gut.* 1986;27:40-46.
144. Kemen M, Homann HH, Mumme A, Zumtobel V. Is intact protein similar for postoperative enteral nutrition than hydrolyzed protein? *Clin Nutr.* 1991;10:37S.
145. Ford EG, Hull SF, Jennings LM, Andrassy RJ. Clinical comparison of tolerance to elemental or polymeric enteral feedings in the postoperative patient. *Am J Clin Nutr.* 1992;11:11-16.
146. Rees RG, Hare WR, Grimble GK, Frost PG, Silk DB. Do patients with moderately impaired gastrointestinal function requiring enteral nutrition need a predigested nitrogen source? *Gut.* 1992;33:877-881.
147. Salomon SB, Jung J, Voss T, et al. An elemental diet containing medium-chain triglycerides and enzymatically hydrolyzed protein can improve gastrointestinal tolerance in people infected with HIV. *J Am Diet Assoc.* 1998;98:460-462.
148. Lynch JW, Miles JM, Bailey JW. Effects of the short-chain triglyceride triacetin on intestinal mucosa and metabolic substrates in rats. *JPEN J Parenter Enteral Nutr.* 1994;18:208-213.
149. Koruda MJ, Rolandelli RH, Settle RG, Saul SH, Rombeau JL. The effect of a pectin-supplemented elemental diet on intestinal adaptation to massive small intestinal resection. *JPEN J Parenter Enteral Nutr.* 1986;10:343-350.

150. Rayes N, Hansen S, Seehofer D, et al. Early enteral supply of fiber and lactobacilli versus conventional nutrition: a controlled trial in patients with major abdominal surgery. *Nutrition.* 2002;18:609-615.
151. Aldhous MC, Meister D, Ghosh S. Modification of enteral diets in inflammatory bowel disease. *Proceedings of the Nutrition Society.* 2001;60:457-461.
152. Heymsfield SB, Head CA, McManus CB, et al. Respiratory, cardiovascular and metabolic effects of enteral hyperalimentation: influence of formula dose and composition. *Am J Clin Nutr.* 1984;40:116-130.
153. Al-Saady NM, Blackmore CM, Bennet ED. High fat, low carbohydrate, enteral feeding lowers pCO_2 and reduces the period of ventilation in artificially ventilated patients. *Intensive Care Med.* 1989;15:290-295.
154. Askanazi J, Elwyn DH, Silverberg P, Rosenbaum SH, Kinney JM. Respiratory distress secondary to a high carbohydrate load: a case report. *Surgery.* 1980;87:596-598.
155. Angelillo VA, Sukhdarshan B, Durfee S, et al. Effects of low and high carbohydrate feedings in ambulatory patients with chronic obstructive pulmonary disease and chronic hypercapnia. *Ann Intern Med.* 1985;103:883-885.
156. Kuo CD, Shiao GM, Lee JD. The effects of high fat and high carbohydrate loads on gas exchange and ventilation in COPD patients and normal subjects. *Chest.* 1993;104:189-196.
157. Talpers SS, Romberger DJ, Bunce SB, Pinkerton SK. Nutritionally associated increase in carbon dioxide production. Excess total calories vs high proportion of carbohydrate calories. *Chest.* 1992;102:551-555.
158. Malone AM. Is a pulmonary enteral formula warranted for patients with pulmonary dysfunction? *NCP.* 1997;12:168-171.
159. van den Berg B, Bogaard JM, Hop WC. High fat, low carbohydrate, enteral feeding in patients weaning from the ventilator. *Intensive Care Med.* 1994;20:470-475.
160. Murray MJ, Kumar M, Gregory TJ, et al. Select dietary fatty acids attenuate cardiopulmonary dysfunction during acute lung injury in pigs. *Am J Physiol.* 1995;269:H2090-H2099.
161. Mancuso P, Whelan J, DeMichele SJ, et al. Effects of eicosapentaenoic and gamma-linolenic acid on lung permeability and alveolar macrophage eicosanoid synthesis in endotoxemic rats. *Crit Care Med.* 1997;25:523-532.
162. Mancuso P, Whelan J, DeMichele SJ, et al. Dietary fish oil and fish and borage oil suppress intrapulmonary proinflammatory eicosanoid biosynthesis and attenuate pulmonary neutrophil accumulation in endotoxic rats. *Crit Care Med.* 1997;25:1198-1206.
163. Palombo JD, DeMichele SJ, Lydon EE, et al. Rapid modulation of lung and liver macrophage phospholipid fatty acids in endotoxemic rats by continuous enteral feeding with n-3 and gamma-linolenic fatty acids. *Am J Clin Nutr.* 1996;63:208-219.
164. Palombo JD, DeMichele SJ, Boyce PJ, et al. Effect of short-term enteral feeding with eicosapentaenoic and gamma-linolenic acid on alveolar macrophage eicosanoid synthesis and bactericidal function in rats. *Crit Care Med.* 1999;27:1908-1915.
165. Gadek JE, DeMichele SJ, Karlstad MD, et al. Effect of enteral feeding with eicosaentaenoic acid, gamma-linolenic acid, and antioxidants in patient with acute respiratory distress syndrome. *Crit Care Med.* 1999;27:1409-1420.
166. American Diabetes Association. Translation of diabetes nutrition recommendations for health care institutions. Position statement. *Diabetes Care.* 2003;26:S70-S72.
167. Craig LD, Nicholson S, Silverstone FA, Kennedy RD. Use of a reduced-carbohydrate, modified-fat enteral formula for improving metabolic control and clinical outcomes in long-term care residents with type 2 diabetes: results of a pilot study. *Nutrition.* 1998;14:529-534.
168. Garg A. High-MUFA diets for patients with DM: a meta-analysis. *Am J Clin Nutr.* 1998;67:577S-582S.
169. Grahm TW, Harrington TR, Isaac RM. Low carbohydrate with fiber enteral formula impedes development of hyperglycemia in patients with acute head injury. *Clin Res.* 1989;37:138A.
170. Galkowski J, Silverstone FA, Brad M. Use of a low-carbohydrate with fiber formula as a snack for elderly patients with type II diabetes. *Clin Res.* 1989;37:89A.
171. Otto C, Sonnichsen AC, Ritter MM, Richter WO, Schwandt P. Influence of fiber, xylitol and fructose in enteral formulas on glucose and lipid metabolism in normal subjects. *Clin Invest.* 1993;71:290-293.
172. Peters AL, Davidson MB, Isaac RM. Lack of glucose elevation after simulated tube feeding with a low-carbohydrate, high-fat enteral formula in patients with type I diabetes. *Am J Med.* 1989;87:178-182.
173. Hofman Z, Van Drunen JD, De Later C, Kuipers H. The effect of different nutritional feeds on the postprandial glucose response in healthy volunteers and patients with type II diabetes. *Eur J Clin Nutr.* 2004;58(11):1553-1556.
174. Kipnes M, Shade S, Geraghty M, Craig L, Bossetti B. Effect of a liquid nutritional designed for oral supplementation on glucose tolerance in subjects with type 2 diabetes. *Diabetes.* 1998;47:A90.
175. Sanz-Paris A, Calvo L, Guallard A, Salazar I, Albero R. High-fat versus high-carbohydrate enteral formulae: effect on blood glucose, c-peptide, and ketones in patients with type 2 diabetes treated with insulin or sulfonylurea. *Nutrition.* 1998;14:840-845.
176. Peters AL, Davidson MB. Effects of various enteral feeding products on postprandial blood glucose response in patients with type I diabetes. *JPEN J Parenter Enteral Nutr.* 1992;16:69-74.
177. McCarter MD, Gentilini OD, Gomez ME, Daly JM. Preoperative oral supplement with immunonutrients in cancer patients. *JPEN J Parenter Enteral Nutr.* 1998;22:206-211.
178. Moore FA, Moore EE, Kudsk KA, et al. Clinical benefits of an immune-enhancing diet for early postinjury enteral feeding. *J Trauma.* 1994;37:607-615.
179. Cerra FB, Lehmann S, Konstantinides N, et al. Improvement in immune function in ICU patients by enteral nutrition supplemented with arginine, RNA, and menhaden oil is independent of nitrogen balance. *Nutrition.* 1991;7:193-199.
180. Heys SD, Walker LG, Smith I, Eremin O. Enteral nutritional supplementation with key nutrients in patients with critical illness and cancer. A meta-analysis of randomized controlled clinical trials. *Ann Surg.* 1999;229:467-477.
181. Zaloga GP. Immune-enhancing enteral diets. Where's the beef? Crit Care Med. 1998;25:66-72.
182. Beale R, Bryg D, Bihari D. Immunonutrition in the critically ill: a systematic review of clinical outcomes. *Crit Care Med.* 1999;27:2799-2805.
183. Kudsk KA, Minard G, Croce MA, et al. A randomized trial of isonitrogenous enteral diets after severe trauma. An immune-enhancing diet reduces septic complications. *Ann Surg.* 1996;224:531-543.
184. Gianotti L, Braga M, Fortis C, et al. A prospective, randomized clinical trial on perioperative feeding with arginine, omega-3 fatty acid and RNA-enriched enteral diet: effect on host response and nutritional status. *JPEN J Parenter Enteral Nutr.* 1999;23:314-320.
185. Gianotti L, Braga M, Nespoli L, et al. A randomized controlled trial of preoperative oral supplementation with a specialized diet in patients with gastrointestinal cancer. *Gastroenterology.* 2002:122:1763-1770.
186. Braga M, Gianotti L, Nespoli L, Radaelli G, Di Carlo V. Nutritional approach in malnourished surgical patients: A prospective randomized study. *Arch Surg.* 2002;137:174-180.
187. Wu GH, Zhang YW, Wu ZH. Modulation of postoperative immune and inflammatory response by immune-enhancing enteral diet in gastrointestinal cancer patients. *World J Gastroenterol.* 2001;7:357-362.
188. Consensus recommendations from the U.S. summit on immune-enhancing enteral therapy. *JPEN J Parenter Enteral Nutr.* 2001:25: S61-S63.
189. Roth E, Kudsk KA. Immunonutrition: back to science. *JPEN J Parenter Enteral Nutr.*2004;28:278.
190. Dickerson RN. Immune-enhancing enteral formulas in critically ill patients. *NCP.* 1997;12:49-50.

191. Barton RG. Immune-enhancing enteral formulas: Are they beneficial in critically ill patients? *NCP.* 1997;12:51-62.
192. Saffle JR, Wiebke G, Jennings K, Morris SE, Barton RG. Randomized trial of immune-enhancing enteral nutrition in burn patients. *J Trauma.* 1997;42:793-802.
193. Heyland DK. In search of the magic nutraceutical: Problems with current approaches. *J Nutr.* 2001;131:2591S-2595S.
194. Heyland DK. Immunonutrition in the critically ill patient. Putting the cart before the horse. *NCP.* 2002;17:267-272.
195. Tsai HJ, Shang HF, Yeh CL, Yeh SL. Effects of arginine supplementation on antioxidant enzyme activity and macrophage response in burned mice. *Burns.* 2002;28:258-263.
196. Boucher JL, Farges MC, Minet R, Vasson MP, Cynober L. Modulation of immune response with ornithine alpha-ketoglutarate in burn injury: An arginine or glutamine dependency. *Nutrition.* 1999;15:773-777.
197. Montejo JC, Zarazaga A, Lopez-Martinez J, et al. Immunonutrition in the intensive care unit. A systematic review and consensus statement. *Clin Nutr.* 2003;22:221-233.
198. Senkal M, Haaker R, Deska T, et al. Early enteral gut feeding with conditionally indispensable pharmaconutrients is metabolically safe and is well tolerated in postoperative cancer patients. *Clin Nutr.* 2004;23:1193-1198.
199. DeLuis DA, Izaolo O, Cuellar L, Terroba MC, Aller R. Randomized clinical trial with an enteral arginine-enhanced formula in early postsurgical head and neck cancer patients. *Eur J Clin Nutr.* 2004.
200. Suttman U, Ockenga J, Schneider H, et al. Weight gain and increased concentrations of receptor protein for tumor necrosis factor after patients with symptomatic HIV-infection received fortified nutrition support. *J Am Diet Assoc.* 1996;96:565-569.
201. Chlebowski RT, Beall G, Grosvenor M, et al. Long-term effects of early nutritional support with new enterotropic peptide-based formula vs standard enteral formula in HIV-infected patients: Randomized prospective trial. *Nutrition.* 1993;9:507-512.
202. Keithley JK, Swanson B, Zeller JM, et al. Comparison of standard and immune-enhancing oral formulas in asymptomatic HIV-infected persons: A multicenter randomized controlled clinical trial. *JPEN J Parenter Enteral Nutr.* 2002;26:6-14.
203. Hoh R, Pelfini A, Neese RA, et al. De novo lipogenesis predicts short-term body-composition response by bioelectrical impedance analysis to oral nutritional supplements in HIV-associated wasting. Am J Clin Nutr. 1998;68:154-163.
204. Pichard C, Sudre P, Karsegard V, et al. A randomized double-blind controlled study of 6 months of oral nutritional supplementation with arginine and omega-3 fatty acids in HIV-infected patients. *AIDS.* 1998;12:53-63.
205. Mirtallo JM, Schneider PJ, Mavko K, Ruberg RL, Fabri PJ. A comparison of essential and general amino acid infusions in the nutritional support of patients with compromised renal function. *JPEN J Parenter Enteral Nutr.* 1982;6:109-113.
206. Nakasaki H, Katayama T, Yokoyama S, et al. Complication of parenteral nutrition composed of essential amino acids and histidine in adults with renal failure. *JPEN J Parenter Enteral Nutr.* 1993;17:86-90.
207. Lamiell JJ, Ducey JP, Freese-Kepczyk BJ, Musio F, Hansberry KL. Essential amino acid-induced adult hyperammonemic encephalopathy and hypophosphatemia. *Crit Care Med.* 1990;18:451-452.
208. Marchesini G, Dioguardi GP, Bianchi GP, et al. Long-term oral branched chain amino acid treatment in chronic hepatic encephalopathy. *J Hepatol.* 1990;11:92-101.
209. Kondrup J, Nielsen K, Hamberg O. Nutritional therapy in patients with liver cirrhosis. *Eur J Clin Nutr.* 1992;46:239-246.
210. Fischer JE. Branched chain-enriched amino acid solutions in patients with liver failure: an early example of nutritional pharmacology. *JPEN J Parenter Enteral Nutr.* 1990;14:249S-256S.
211. McGhee A, Henderson JM, Millikan WJ, et al. Comparison of the effects of Hepatic Aid and a case in modular diet on encephalopathy, plasma amino acids and nitrogen balance in cirrhotic patients. *Ann Surg.* 1983;197:288-293.
212. Schafer K, Winther MB, Ukida M, et al. Influence of an orally administered protein mixture enriched with branched chain amino acids on the chronic hepatic encephalopathy (CHE) of proteins with liver cirrhosis. *Gastroenterology.* 1981;19:356-362.
213. Calvey N, Davis M, Williams R. Controlled trial of nutritional supplementation, with and without branched chain amino acid enrichment in treatment of acute alcoholic hepatitis. *J Hepatol.* 1985;1:141-151.
214. Maloney JP, Ryan TA, Brasel KJ, et al. Food dye use in enteral feedings: a review and a call for a moratorium. *NCP.* 2002;17:169-181.

Chapter 43

Pediatric Enteral Formulas

Timothy Sentongo, MD

Introduction

Growth in infants and children is a function of genetic potential and environmental influences, of which nutrition is the most important determinant.[1] Normal growth and nutritional status in childhood is associated with health, function, and longevity in adulthood. Human milk is the ideal food for healthy and sick infants (ages birth to 1 year);[2] therefore, the composition of commercial infant formulas is based on comparisons with breast milk. On the contrary, formulas used in pre-term and low-birthweight infants are specially constituted to a caloric density and micronutrient composition that supports growth and mineral and tissue accretion at intrauterine rates while minimizing risk for feeding intolerance and excessive solute load.[3]

Human milk and commercial infant formulas are the standard diet in infants younger than 1 year of age. Beyond infancy (age >12 months), growth in healthy children is sustained through consumption of regular table foods supplemented by milk. Therefore, the term 'enteral formula' generally applies to nutritional solutions given to children who are older than 1 year. Enteral formulas are refined mixtures of macro- and micronutrients solutions used to provide alternative or supplementary nutrition when oral feeding is absent or inadequate to meet the nutrient needs of normal-, catch-up-growth, weight maintenance, and disease modulation. The proteins, dipeptides, amino acids, vitamins, and fatty acid contents of enteral formulas impart a sour and/or bitter taste[4] that generally decreases their palatability and voluntary acceptance in many children.[5] Flavoring improves oral acceptance of enteral formulas; nonetheless, successful administration frequently involves the use of feeding tubes.[6] Progress in nutrition support over the past several years has inspired a paradigm shift in the goals of nutrition from mere provision of calories to provision of growth factors, nutrients with immune-modulating effects, and alteration of intestinal microflora.[7]

This chapter discusses the classification, composition and clinical application of old and newer enteral formulas used in pediatrics. The methodology for assessing nutritional status and caloric requirements in children and adolescents is also presented.

Classification of Enteral Formulas for Pediatric Patients

When used as the sole source of nutrition, enteral formulas are designed to provide the recommended dietary allowance (RDA) of vitamins and micronutrients. (RDAs are discussed in Chapter 6.) Therefore, this chapter focuses on the macronutrient composition of enteral formulas for infants and children.

Classifications for enteral formulas for pediatric consumers are similar to those for EN formulas for adult consumers. The descriptive classification of solutions for pediatric enteral feeding are: 1) hydration solutions, 2) blenderized diets, 3) polymeric formulas, 4) monomeric (protein hydrolysate and amino acid) formulas, 5) modular solutions, and 6) formulas for specific metabolic needs. Other classifications for formulas and the specific details regarding the formulas addressed below are discussed in detail in Chapter 42.

Hydration Solutions

The primary role of oral hydration salt (ORS) solutions in children is prevention and treatment of dehydration from acute vomiting and diarrheal illnesses.[8] Regardless

TABLE 43-1.

Composition of Common ORS Solutions and Household Beverages

Solution	CHO Mmol/l (gm/L)	Na Mmol/L	K Mmol/L	Cl Mmol/L	Base Mmol/L	Osmolarity mOsm/L	Glucose: Na molar ratio
WHO - standard (1975)	111 (90)	90	20	80	30	311	1:1.2
WHO - Hyposmolar (2002)	75 (13.5)	75	20	65	30	245	1:1
ESPGHN	90 (16)	60	20	60	30	240	1.5:1
Infalyte (formally Ricelyte)/Mead Johnson	165 (30)	50	25	45	34	200	3.3:1
Pedialyte/ Ross Laboratories	139 (25)	45	20	35	30	250	3:1
Rehydralyte/ Ross Laboratories	139 (25)	75	20	65	30	305	1.8:1
EquaLyte/ Ross Laboratories	(30)	78.2	22.3	67.7	30.1	–	–
CeraLyte	40	50-90	20	–	30	220	–
Common household beverages not appropriate for use as primary oral rehydration fluids:							
Apple juice	120	<1	44	45	–	730	–
Colas	50 – 150	1.6	<1	–	13.4	550 - 750	–
Sports drinks	45	23.5	<1	17	3	330	62.5:1
Orange juice	120	<1	50	–	50		–
Chicken broth	–	250	8	–	–	500	–

of the etiology or pathogenesis of vomiting and diarrhea, dehydration is the main cause of morbidity and mortality in children. The composition of commonly used ORS solutions is presented in Table 43-1. The World Health Organization (WHO) standard solution was among the first ORS solutions formulated to meet the criteria for optimal fluid and electrolyte absorption. Increased use of ORS has been accompanied by a reduction in morbidity and mortality in children from acute gastroenteritis, particularly in developing countries where the prevalence was considerably high.[11]

Blenderized Diets

Blenderized diets are semi-liquid food solutions that may be prepared in the home or commercially by pureeing mixtures of traditional foods such as milk, beef, oils, fruits, vegetables, and fiber. These formulas have the advantages of being "natural foods" and are less costly when prepared at home. The caloric density ranges from 0.7 to 1.0 kcal/ml. The main indication for use of blenderized diets is for nutrition support in patients with normal gastrointestinal (GI) function but compromised or absent ability to adequately feed by mouth.

Polymeric Formulas

Polymeric formulas are made of intact protein and fat mainly in the form of long chain triglycerides. They are effective for complete or supplemental nutrition in patients who require nutrition support and have no significant GI dysfunction.

Hydrolysate and Elemental Formulas

The protein source in hydrolysate and elemental formulas is partially or completely hydrolyzed peptides and or crystalline amino acids. Protein hydrolysate formulas are indicated in infants with milk-soy protein intolerance and colicky symptoms secondary to protein sensitivity.[25] Protein hydrolysates are the recommended diet for infants who cannot tolerate formulas with intact protein or in formula fed infants with a positive family history of atopy.[26] Onset of allergy manifestations in infants at-risk for atopy and food allergies may be prevented, ameliorated, or delayed by feeding protein hydrolysate formula during infancy.[27] Elemental formulas are exclusively indicated as therapy and nutrition in patients with milk-soy protein enterocolitis syndrome, eosinophilic esophagitis, and other more severe allergies or GI disorders.[28-30] Intestinal brush border hydrolysis and uptake of protein is more efficient with di- and tripeptides compared to a longer chain hydrolysates.[31] Therefore, dipeptide hydrolysate and elemental formulas are also preferred during nutrition support in infants and children with compromised GI function, eg, short gut syndrome, impaired digestion, and malabsorption. Acceptance of hydrolysate and elemental formulas is best during early infancy, before children develop the discriminatory perception of taste.[32-33] Nutritional therapy and support with protein hydrolysate- and elemental formulas in older children often necessitates administration through a feeding tube. Infant protein hydrolysate formulas are readily available over the counter. However, elemental and protein hydrolysate enteral formulas used in children aged older than 1 year are only available by prescription.

Modulars

Modular solutions are components of protein, carbohydrate, fat, and fiber alone or in combination designed for use as supplements or mixed with other enteral products to meet specific nutritional or metabolic requirements (eg, protein or caloric supplementation in malnutrition and immune modulation and during nutritional management of inborn errors of metabolism). The composition of commonly used modules is presented in Table 43-2. The protein and carbohydrate components increase osmolarity, which sometimes limits their tolerance. In the absence of contraindications related to increased renal solute load or osmolarity, concentrating infant formula is preferred over modular supplements during management of malnutrition in infants because this approach maintains a normal nutrient distribution.

Formulas for Patients With Inborn Errors in Metabolism

Special metabolic modules are designed for nutritional management of patients with inborn errors in metabolism (eg, phenylketonuria, tyrosinemia, maple syrup urine disease, and other disorders of branched chain amino acids). These formulas primarily differ in content, variety, and amount of amino acids. Use of these formulas must always be closely supervised by a certified dietician. The carbohydrate, fat, mineral and vitamin contents are similar to those of standard polymeric formulas. Because of the variable protein content, metabolic formulas are not nutritionally complete, and minimum amounts of the restricted amino acid(s) must be added to meet the requirements for normal growth. Therefore, they offer a high degree of flexibility in meeting nutritional requirements of patients with amino acid metabolic disorders. See Tables 43-3, 43-4, and 43-5 for lists of the metabolic modules and formulas.

Composition of Pediatric Formulas—Age-Appropriate Formulas

Infant Nutrition

Human milk is the perfect food for healthy and sick infants. In addition to nutrition, human milk promotes maternal-child bonding and conveys digestive enzymes and immunological factors that contribute positively to infant health and development.[3,19] Breastfed infants self-regulate their energy intake; this may be associated with metabolic programming early in life that reduces risk for overweight and obesity during later childhood.[20] The WHO recommends human milk as the exclusive nutrient source for feeding full-term infants during the first months after birth.[2] When breastfeeding is only partially successful or not possible, commercial infant formulas are appropriate alternatives. The indications for using commercial infant formulas are substitution for (or supplement to) human milk in: 1) infants whose mothers choose not to breastfeed (or not to do so exclusively), 2) in infants for whom breastfeeding is medically contraindicated, and 3) supplementing breastfed infants who do not gain weight adequately.[21]

Formulas Used in Term Infants

Human milk is the standard for comparison of commercial infant formulas. The main categories of commercial infant formulas are: 1) milk-based formulas, 2) soy formulas, 3) protein hydrolysate formulas, and 4) amino-acid–based (elemental) formulas (see Appendix). The caloric content of the standard infant formulas is similar to that of human milk—20 kcal/oz—and the average protein content of commercial infant formula is approximately 50% higher than that of human milk. The protein source varies from cow, soy, protein hydrolysate, and crystalline amino acids. The carbohydrate source of cow-milk–based infant formulas is lactose; however, lacto-free alternatives made up of cornstarch syrups are also available. All soy, protein hydrolysate, and elemental formulas are lactose-free. The fat source of cow- and soy-protein–based infant formula is mostly long chain triglycerides (LCT) from vegetable oils or a mixture of vegetable and animal fats with appropriate amounts of essential fatty acids. The fat in protein hydrolysate and elemental infant formulas is made up of a mixture of LCT and medium chain triglycerides (MCT). Figure 43-1 is an algorithm for selection of infant formulas during clinical care.

Table 43-2.

Modulars

Carbohydrate Modules

Product (Manufacturer)	Polycose Liquid 100 ml (Ross)	Polycose Powder 100 g (Ross)	Moducal Powder (Mead-Johnson)
Calories /ml (/g)	2	(3.8)	(3.8)
Protein (g/100g)	-		-
Protein source	-		-
CHO (g/100	50		
CHO source	Glucose polymer	Glucose polymer	Malto-dextrin
Fat (g/100g)			-
Fat source			-

Lipid Modules

Product (Manufacturer)	Corn Oil	Microlipid analysis per 89ml bottle (Mead Johnson)	MCT Oil (Mead Johnson)	Duocal (SHS)
Calories /ml (/g)	8.4/ml	4.5	7.7 (8.3)	(4.9)
Protein (g/100g)	--	--	--	--
Protein source	--	--	--	--
CHO (g/100	--	--	--	73
CHO source	--	--	--	-
Fat (g/100g)	15g/Tbsp.	45	8.3	22
Fat source	Corn	Safflower Oil	MCT	Blend of fats

Protein Modules

Product (Manufacturer)	Casec Powder per Tbsp= 4.4 gm (Mead Johnson)	Promod Powder one 6.6gm scoop (Ross)	Complete Amino Acid Mix (SHS)	Essential Amino Acid Mix (SHS)	Arginaid (Novartis)	Glutasolve (Novartis)
Calories /ml (/g)	(3.8)	(4.2)	(3.2)	(3.2)	(3.8)	(4)
Protein (g/100g)	90	55	98	94.5	49	66
Protein source	Calcium caseinate	Whey protein concentrate	Essential and nonessential amino acids	Essential amino acids	L-Arginine	L-Glutamine
CHO (g/100	--	0.67	--	--	0.4/g	0.31/g
CHO source	--		--	--	--	--
Fat (g/100g)	0.09	0.60	--	--	--	--
Fat source	Soy lecithin	Soy Lecithin	--	--	--	--

Table 43-3.

Pediatric Metabolic Formulas: PKU

Product (manufacturer)	Lofenalac (Mead Johnson) per 100 gm	Phenyl-Free 1 (Mead Johnson) per 100 gm	Phenyl-Free 2 (Mead Johnson) per 100 gm	Phenyl-Free 2HP (Mead Johnson) per 100 gm	Phenex-1 (Ross) per 100 gm	Xphe Analog (SHS) per 100 gm	XP Maxamaid (SHS) per 100 gm
Calories	462	500	410	390	480	475	350
Protein	15	16.2	22	40	15	13	25
Protein source	Specially treated hydrolysates & L-amino acids	L-amino acids	L-amino acids	L-amino acids	L-amino acids	L-amino acids	L-amino acids
CHO	60	51	60	44	53	59	62
CHO source	Corn syrup solids & modified tapioca starch	Corn syrup solids, modified corn starch & sucrose	Sucrose, corn syrup solids & modified corn starch	Sucrose, corn syrup solids & modified corn starch	Corn syrup solids	Corn syrup solids	Corn syrup solids
Fat	18	26	8.6	6.3	21.7	20.9	–
Fat source	Corn oil	Palm-olein, soy, coconut & high-oleic sunflower oils	Soy oil	Soy oil	High-oleic safflower, coconut & soy oils	Refined animal fat, peanut & coconut oil	–
Sodium mEq(mg)	9.5 (220)	10.4 (240)	27 (610)	18 (410)	8 (190)	5.2 (120)	25 (580)
Potassium mEq (mg)	12 (470)	14.3 (560)	28 (1100)	30 (1180)	17 (675)	10.8 (420)	22 (840)
Calcium mg	430	660	980	730	575	600	810
Phosphorus mg	320	440	980	730	400	500	810
Iron mg	8.7	9.6	12.2	15.7	9	10	12
Notes:	Low phenylalanine diet powder for infants and children w/hyperphenylalaninemia including PKU Phe = 75 gm per 100 gm powder.	Phenylalanine-free diet powder for mgt. of infants and toddlers with PKU. Important to provide enough Phe using other foods to support growth.	Phenylalanine-free powder for children and adults with PKU.	Phenylalanine-free powder for children and adults with PKU. High protein levels for maternal PKU or individuals with calorie and volume restriction.	Phenylalanine-free powder for infants and toddlers with PKU. Must be supplemented with intact protein to meet Phe requirements and support growth.	Unflavored, phenylalanine-free powdered infant formula. Must be consumed in conjunction w/ whole protein source (breast milk or infant formula) to meet phenylalanine requirements and ensure normal growth.	Phenylalanine-free powdered formula used in mgt. of PKU in children 1-8 yrs. Available in orange and unflavored. Fat, CHO, and low protein sources may be used to supply the remainder of calories and to fulfill the EFA.

Table 43-4.

Pediatric Metabolic Formulas: Maple Syrup Urine Disease (MSUD) and Urea Cycle Disorders

Product (manufacturer)	BCAD 2 (Mead Johnson) per 100 gm	Cyclinex-1 (Ross) per 100 gm	Cyclinex-2 (Ross) per 100 gm	Ketonex 1 (Ross) per 100 gm	Ketonex 2 (Ross) per 100 gm	MSUD Analog (SHS) per 100 gm	MSUD Maxamaid (SHS) per 100 gm	MSUD Diet Powder (Mead Johnson) per 100 gm
Calories	410	510	440	480	410	475	350	464
Protein	24	7.5	15	15	30	13	25	8.1
Protein source	L-amino acids	L-amino acids	L-amino acids	L-amino acids	L-amino acids	L-amino acids	L-amino acids	L-amino acids
CHO	57	57	45	53	35	59	62	63
CHO source	Corn syrup solids, sugar & modified corn starch	Corn syrup solids	Corn syrup solids	Corn syrup solids	Corn syrup solids	Corn syrup solids	Sucrose & corn syrup solids	Corn syrup solids & modified tapioca starch
Fat	8.5	24.6	17	21.7	14	20.9	<0.5	20
Fat source	Soy oil	High-oleic safflower, coconut & soy oils	High-oleic safflower, coconut & soy oils	High-oleic safflower, coconut & soy oils	High-oleic safflower, coconut & soy oils	Peanut, coconut & refined animal fat (pork)	–	Corn oil
Sodium mEq (mg)	26.5 (610)	9 (215)	51 (1175)	8 (190)	38 (880)	5.2 (120)	25 (580)	8 (184)
Potassium mEq (mg)	31.2 (1220)	20 (760	46 (1800)	17 (675)	35 (1370)	10.8 (420)	22 (840)	12.5 (490)
Calcium mg	730	650	1150	575	880	600	810	490
Phosphorus mg	730	455	1020	400	760	500	810	260
Iron mg	12.2	17	17	9	13	10	12	8.9
Notes:	Diet powder used for the dietary mgt of children and adults with Maple Syrup Urine disease (MSUD) or other inborn errors of branched chain amino acid metabolism. BCAD = branched chain amino acid disorder.	Amino acid-modified medical food. Nutrition support of infants and toddlers with a urea cycle disorder, gyrate atrophy of the choroids and retina, or HHH syndrome.	Amino acid-modified medical food. Nutrition support of children and adults with a urea cycle disorder, gyrate atrophy of the choroids and retina. Or HHH syndrome.	Amino acid-modified medical food. For infants and toddlers with MSUD & B-keto-thiolase deficiency.	Amino acid-modified medical food. For children and adults with MSUD or beta-keto-thiolase deficiency.	Unflavored, isoleucine-, leucine- & valine-free. Must be used with a whole protein source (breast milk or infant formula) in quantities to meet isoleucine, leucine & valine requirements and ensure normal growth.	Orange flavored, valine-leucine-, & isoleucine-free powdered food used in the mgt. of MSUD in children aged 1 to 8 years.	Diet powder with no leucine, isoleucine, or valine. For the mgt. of infants and children with disorders of branched chain amino acid metabolism including (MSUD).

TABLE 43-5.

Pediatric Metabolic Formulas: Organic Acidemia

Product (manufacturer)	OS 1 (Mead Johnson) per 100 gm	OS 2 (Mead Johnson) per 100 gm	Propimex-1 (Ross) per 100 gm	Propimex-2 (Ross) per 100 gm	Xphe, Xtyr (SHS) per 100 gm	Xphe Tyr (SHS) per 100 gm	Tyrosinemia Type 1 XPTM (SHS) per 100 gm	Tyros 2 (Mead Johnson) per 100 gm
Calories	280	300	480	410	475	350	475	410
Protein	42	56	15	30	13	25	13	22
Protein source	L-amino acids	L-amino acids	L-amino acids	L-amino acids	L-amino acids	L-amino acids	l-amino acids	Amino acids
CHO	27	19	53	35	59	62	59	60
CHO source	Sucrose	Sucrose	Corn syrup solids	Corn syrup solids	Corn Syrup solids	Corn syrup solids & sucrose	Corn syrup solids	Corn syrup solids, sugar & modified corn starch
Fat	0	0	21.7	13	20.9	<0.5	20.9	8.5
Fat source	–	–	High-oleic safflower, coconut & soy oils	High-oleic safflower, coconut & soy oils	Safflower, coconut & soy oils	–	Safflower, coconut & soy oils	Soy oil
Sodium mEq (mg)	47(1070)	28(640)	8(190)	38(880)	5.2(120)	25(580)	5.2(120)	27(610)
Potassium mEq (mg)	59(2300)	34(1330)	17(675)	35(1370)	10.8(420)	22(840)	10.8(420)	28(1100)
Calcium mg	2400	1310	575	880	600	810	600	730
Phosphorus mg	1860	1010	400	760	500	810	500	730
Iron mg	34	15	9	13	10	12	8	12.2
Notes:	Amino acid modified powder. Used for infants with propionic or methylmalonic academia. Isoleucine-, methionine- threonine- and valine-free. May contain 100mg ILE/ 100gm.	Amino acid-modified powder. Used for children with propionic or methylmalonic academia. Isoleucine-, methionine- threonine- and valine-free.	Amino acid-modified medical food. Nutrition support of infants and toddlers with propionic or methylmalonic academia. Methionine- and valine-free and low in isoleucine, threonine and tryptophan.	Amino acid-modified medical food. Nutrition support of children and adults with propionic or methylmalonic acidemia. Methionine- and valine-free. Low in isoleucine, threonine and tryptophan.	Unflavored phenylalanine- & tyrosine-free powdered infant formula for mgt. of tyrosinemia when plasma methionine levels are normal.	Orange flavored phenylalanine- & tyrosine-free powdered medical food. For children with tyrosinemia aged 1 to 8 years.	Unflavored, phenylalanine-, tyrosine- & methionine-free powdered infant formula. For infants with tyrosinemia type 1.	Used for dietary mgt. of children and adults with tyrosinemia type II or other inborn errors of tyrosine metabolism. Tyrosine-free.

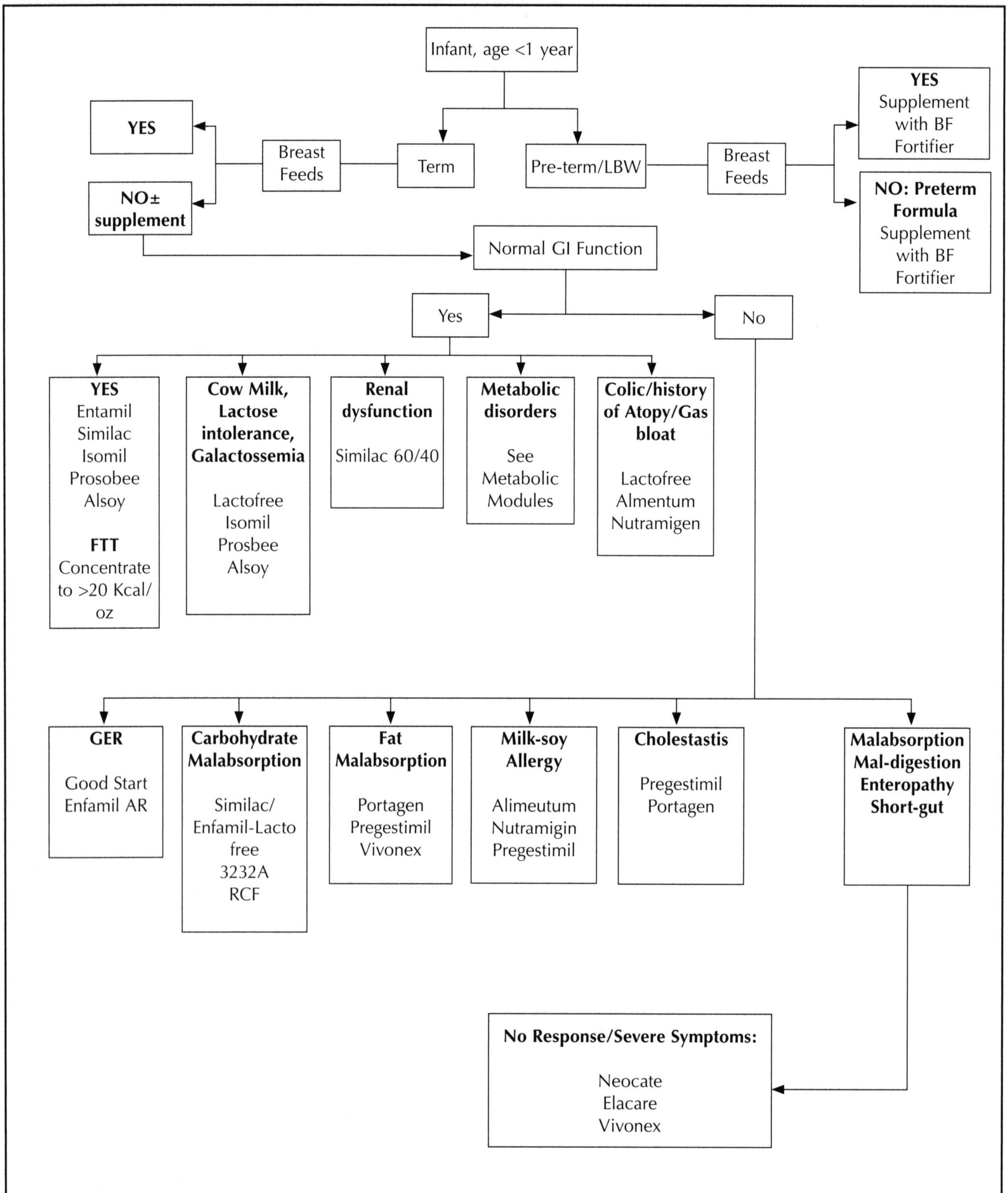

Figure 43-1. Algorithm for selection of infant formula.

Formulas for Preterm and Low Birthweight Infants

Formulas used in preterm and low birthweight (LBW) infants are designed to provide energy, protein, and micronutrients in quantities that support growth and mineral and tissue accretion at intrauterine rates while minimizing risk for excessive solute load. This is accomplished by providing an upper caloric density of 24 kcal/oz, higher protein content of 1.8 to 2.3 g/dl, and twice as much calcium and phosphorus as included in formulas for term infants. The protein source has a higher proportion of whey protein, and the fat source has an MCT content ranging from 30% to 50%. Table 43-6 shows composition of several preterm and term infant formulas.

Nutrition Support in Children Older Than 1 Year of Age—Enteral Formulas

Enteral formulas are solutions to provide supplemental or full nutrition when the nutritional requirements for growth, weight maintenance, and/or disease modulation cannot be met by regular food or oral feeding. Human milk and commercial infant formulas are the standard diet in infants, and the use of enteral formulas generally applies to children older than 1 year.

More than 100 commercial enteral products are currently available for indications and use in adult patients; however, a lack of studies that demonstrate tolerance, safety, and efficacy in young children limits indiscriminate use in pediatrics. Most adult enteral formulas meet the RDA at volumes and solute loads much higher than is practical or tolerated in younger children. Nonetheless, some adult enteral formulas can be safely and effectively used in children older than 12 years and/or after pubertal growth. The composition of pediatric enteral formulas is, therefore, designed to provide macro- and micronutrients in quantities similar to the RDA when used as full feeds. The classification and general indications of several enteral formulas is presented in Table 43-7.

Specific Nutrient Composition of Pediatric Formulas

Modular solutions are specific nutrient mixtures that can be used together or in combination to meet the consumer's specific, individualized nutrition needs. Other EN formulas for pediatric patients include many of these nutrients together.

Fat

Fat modules have the advantage of high caloric density with low osmolarity. The caloric content of a unit gram of fat is twice that of carbohydrate and protein. Therefore fat modules are commonly used to achieve high-energy diets in patients with malnutrition and inadequate caloric intake and who are on protein- and electrolyte-restricted diets.

Medium Chain Triglycerides

Intestinal absorption of MCT is less dependent on bile concentration, pancreatic enzymes, or intact villous lacteals. Therefore, MCT modules have traditionally been used in nutritional disorders associated with impaired LCT digestion (eg, cystic fibrosis, chronic cholestatic liver diseases) or transport (eg, intestinal lymphangiectasia and abetalipoproteinemia). MCT are more rapidly metabolized to ketones; therefore, their use is discouraged in diabetics.[24] Also, the finding of increased blood levels of medium- and short-chain fatty acids in patients with hepatic encephalopathy has prompted avoidance of MCT supplementation in patients with cirrhosis and/or portal-caval shunts.[24,34] The same is true with pediatric patients who have these disorders.

Symptoms of intolerance to MCT include nausea, vomiting, and diarrhea. Furthermore when mixed with aqueous formula and left to stand the MCT and LCT may separate out and float in a lipid phase that gets retained in the formula bag or delivery tubing and, therefore, not be delivered to the patient. The problem of insolubility is overcome with microlipid emulsions. Duocal powder, an energy enhancer, is also soluble in water and many liquids, and can be sprinkled on food without significantly altering the taste for the child with selective tastes or added to enteral formulas.

Protein

Protein modules contain intact protein, hydrolyzed protein, or crystalline amino acids by themselves or in a mixture (Table 43-8). The intended use is protein source or supplementation in patients with restricted or increased protein requirements—eg, inborn errors in protein metabolism, renal disease, malnutrition, burns, protein loosing enteropathy, short bowel syndrome, and other chronic intestinal diseases including Crohn's disease. Complete crystalline amino-acid mix may be used for supplementation in children with milk-soy protein intolerance. Essential amino acid mix is used during dietary management of urea cycle disorders. Glutamine and arginine are nonessential amino acids with trophic and immune-modulating effects that attain 'conditionally essential' status during severe trauma, critical illness and other situations of acute metabolic stress.

Components in Newer Formulas

Table 43-7 presents data on enteral formulas for children 1 year of age or older. More recently developed pediatric enteral formulas include additions that complete a number of roles. These added components—long chain polyunsaturated fatty acids (LC-PUFAs), omega-3 and omega-6 fatty acids, glutamine, arginine, transforming growth factor-ß (TGF-ß), probiotics, and prebiotics. (The latter two are also discussed in detail in Chapter 11.)

TABLE 43-6.

Formulas for Preterm and Low Birthweight Infants

Product (manufacturer)	Preterm Human Milk	Enfamil Human Milk Fortifier (Mead)	Similac Human Milk Fortifier (Ross)	Enfamil Premature W/iron 20*(Mead Johnson)	Enfamil Premature W/iron 24(Mead Johnson)	Similac Special Care W/iron 20*(Ross)	Similac Special Care W/iron 24(Ross)	Enfamil EnfaCare (Mead Johnson)	Similac NeoSure (Ross)
Calories	67	14	14	67	80	67	81	74	74
Protein gm/100 ml	1.4	1.1	1.0	2.0	2.3	1.8	2.1	2.0	1.9
Protein source	Preterm Human Milk	Whey Protein concentrate (WPC)	Nonfat Milk & WPC	Nonfat Milk & WPC (60:40)	Nonfat Milk & WPC (60:40)	Nonfat Milk & WPC	Nonfat Milk & WPC	Whey & Nonfat Milk Protein concentrate (60:40)	Nonfat Milk & WPC
CHO gm/100ml	6.6	1.1	1.8	7.4	8.8	7.0	8.5	7.9	7.6
CHO source	lactose	Corn syrup solids & lactose	Corn syrup solids	Corn syrup solids & lactose	Corn syrup solids & lactose	Corn syrup solids & lactose (50:50)	Corn syrup solids & lactose (50:50)	Corn syrup solids & lactose (60:40)	Maltodextrin & lactose (50:50)
Fat gm/100 ml	3.8	.65	.36	3.4	4.0	3.6	4.3	3.9	4.1
Fat source	Preterm Human Milk	20% MCT	MCT & soy lecithin oils	MCT, Soy & Coconut oils	MCT, Soy & Coconut oils (40:40:20)	MCT, Soy & Coconut oils	MCT, Soy & Coconut oils	High-Oleic Sunflower, soy, MCT, & Coconut oils	Soy, Coconut & MCT oils (45:30:25)
Osmolality mOsm/kg	290	63	90	260	310	235	280	260	250
Sodium mEq(mg)/ 100ml	1.0(24)	.47(11)	.65(15)	1.1(26)	1.3(30)	1.2(28)	1.5(34)	1.1(25)	1.0(24)
Potassium mEq (mg)/ 100ml	1.4(56)	.5(20)	1.6(63)	1.7(68)	2.0(81)	2.2(86)	2.6(104)	1.9(77)	2.6(105)
Calcium mEq (mg)/ 100ml	1.2(24)	4.5(90)	5.8(117)	5.5(110)	6.5(130)	6(120)	7.2(145)	4.4(88)	3.8(78)
Phosphorous mEq (mg)/100 ml	.8(12)	2.9(45)	4.3(63)	3.5(55)	4.2(65)	4.3(66)	5.2(80)	3.1(48)	1.1(46)
Iron mg/100ml	.12	1.4	.35	1.2 *low iron=.16	1.4	1.2 *low iron=.2	1.4	1.2	1.2
Notes:		4 packets of fortifier (.81g/pkt)	4 packets of fortifier (.9g/pkt)						

Table 43-7.
Enteral Formulas for Children Aged >1 Year

Product (manufacturer)	Compleat Pediatric (Novartis)	Pediasure (Ross)	Kindercal (Mead Johnson)	Pepdite One+(SHS)	Resource Just for Kids (Novartis)	Peptamen Jr. (Nestle)	Nutren Jr. (Nestle)	Peptamen Prebio 1* (Nestle)	Peptamen 1.5 (Nestle)	Nutren 1.5 (Nestle)
Calories/ 100 ml	100	100	106	100	100	100	100	100	150	150
Protein gm/100 ml	3.7	3.0	3.4	3.1	3.0	3.0	3.0	4.0	6.7	6.0
Protein source	Beef, Sodium caseinates	Sodium caseinate & whey protein concentrate	Sodium and calcium caseinate & milk protein concentrate (90:10)	L-Amino acids & hydrolyzed protein (44:56)	Sodium and calcium caseinates & whey protein concentrate	Enzymatically hydrolyzed whey	Milk and whey protein	Enzymatically hydrolyzed whey	Enzymatically hydrolyzed whey	Calcium-potassium caseinate
CHO gm/100ml	12.6	11	13.5	10.6	11.0	13.7	12.7	12.4	18.7	16.9
CHO source	Hydrolyzed cornstarch, apple juice. vegetables, fruits	Hydrolyzed Corn starch & sucrose(62:38)	Maltodextrin & sucrose (62:38)	Corn Syrup Solids*	Hydrolyzed Corn starch & Sucrose*	Maltodextrin & Corn starch*		Maltodextrin & Corn starch	Maltodextrin & Corn starch*	Maltodextrin*
Fat gm/100 ml	3.8	5.0	4.4	5.0	5.0	3.8	4.2	3.9	5.5	6.7
Fat source	High-oleic sunflower oil, soy bean oil, MCT	High-oleic safflower, soy & MCT oils (50:30:20)	Canola, High-oleic sunflower, corn & MCT	MCT, canola, high-oleic safflower oils (35:65)	High-oleic sunflower, soy & MCT oils	MCT, soy, canola & soy lecithin oils MCT:LCT60:40	Soybean, MCT, canola & soy lecithin	MCT, soy & soy lecithin oils MCT:LCT70:30	MCT, soy & soy lecithin oils MCT:LCT70:30	MCT, canola, corn & soy lecithin oils MCT: LCT50:50
Osmolality	380	335*345 w/ fiber	310	430	390 (440*)	260-360	25:75	290	550	510
Sodium mEq(mg)/ 100ml	2.9(68)	1.65(38)	1.6(37)	1.78(41)	2.6(59)	2.0(46)	350	2.4(56)	4.3(102)	5.0(116)
Potassium mEq (mg)/ 100ml	3.8(152)	3.3(131)	3.3(131)	3.4(136)	2.9(114)	3.3(132)	2.0(46)	3.8(150)	4.8(186)	4.8(187)

TABLE 43-7, CONTINUED

Enteral Formulas for Children Aged >1 year

Product (manufacturer)	Compleat Pediatric (Novartis)	Pediasure (Ross)	Kindercal (Mead Johnson)	Pepdite One+(SHS)	Resource Just for Kids	Peptamen Jr. (Nestle)	Nutren Jr. (Nestle)	Peptamen Prebio 1* (Nestle)	Peptamen 1.5 (Nestle)	Nutren 1.5 (Nestle)
Calcium mEq(mg)/ 100ml	(100)	4.8(97)	4.2(85)	5.6(113)	5.7(114)	5.0(100)	3.3(132)	4.0(80)	5.0(100)	5.0(100)
Phosphorous MEq (mg)/ 100 ml	(100)	5.3(80)	5.4(85)	6.0(94)	5.1(80)	5.3(80)	5.0(100)	4.5(70)	6.4(100)	6.4(100)
Iron mg/100ml	0.01	1.39	1.0	1.4	1.4	1.4	5.1(80)	1.8	2.7	1.8
Notes:	Blendarized diet	*w/fiber=.5g/ 100ml		Flavored product contains Surcrose	French Vanilla	*Flavored oral products contain sucrose	1.4	*Fiber source FOS Inulin 4gm/1000ml	*Flavored product contains sucrose	*Flavored product contains sucrose

TABLE 43-8.

Specialized Formula

Specialized Formula		**Protein Hydrolysate**				**Elemental Formula: Crystalline amino acid based**						
	Intact protein ↓LCT & ↑MCT	High MCT										Low fat, high MCT
Product (manufacturer)	Portagen (Mead Johnson)	Pregestimil (Mead Johnson)	Pregestimil 24 (Mead Johnson)	Alimentum (Ross)	Nutramigen (Mead)	Neocate (SHS)	EleCare(Ross)	Neocate 1+ (SHS)	Pediatric EO28 (SHS)	EO28 EXTRA SHS	Vivonex Pediatric (Novartis)	Tolerex (Novartis)
Calories/100 ml	67	67	81	67	67	67	100	100	100	88.6	80	100
Protein gm/100 ml	2.3	1.8	2.2	1.8	1.8	2.0	3.01	2.5	2.5	2.5	2.4	2.06
Protein source	Sodium caseinate	Hydrolyzed casein w/added L-cystine,L-tyrosine & L-tryptophan	Hydrolyzed casein w/added L-cystine, L-tyrosine &L-tryptophan	Hydrolyzed casein w/added L-cystine, L-tyrosine &L-tryptophan	Hydrolyzed casein w/added L-cystine L-tryosine & L-tryptophan	L-amino acids	L-amino acids	L-amino acids	L-amino acids	L-amino acids	L-amino acids	L-amino acids
CHO gm/100ml	7.6	6.8	8.0	6.8	7.3	7.8	10.7	14.6	14.6	11.8	13.0	22.6
CHO source	Corn syrup solids & sucrose	Corn syrup solids, dextrose & modified corn starch	Corn syrup solids, dextrose & modified corn starch	Sucrose & modified tapioca starch	Corn syrup solids & modified corn starch	Corn syrup solids	Corn syrup solids	Corn syrup solids & sucrose	Maltodextrin & sucrose	Dried glucose syrup*	Maltodextrin & modified corn starch	Maltodextrin & modified corn starch
Fat gm/100 ml	3.2	3.7	4.4	3.6	3.3	3.0	4.7	3.5	3.5	3.49	2.4	0.145
Fat source	MCT & corn oils (86% MCT)	MCT, soy, corn & high-oleic safflower	MCT, soy, corn & high-oleic safflower oils	MCT, soy & safflower oils	Palm olein, soy, coconut & high –oleic sunflower	Refined vegetable, hybrid safflower, coconut & soy oils	High-oleic safflower, soy & MCT oils	Safflower, MCT & canola oils	MCT, coconut, canola & high-oleic safflower oils	Fractionated coconut, canola & hybrid safflower oils	MCT & soy oils	Safflower oil
Osmolality mOsm/kg	230	320	380	370	320	353	596	820 610*	820	636	360	550
Sodium mEq(mg)/100ml	1.5(36)	1.3(31)	1.6(37)	1.2(29)	1.3(31)	1.0(24)	2.0(45)	.86(20)	.9(20)	2.6(61)	1.7(40)	2.0(46.8)
Potassium mEq (mg)/100ml	2.1(83)	1.8(73)	2.2(87)	2.0(78)	1.8(73)	2.6(103)	3.8(151)	2.3(93)	3.3(131)		3.1(120)	3.0(117)
Calcium mEq(mg)/100ml	3.1(62)	3.8(76)	4.5(91)	3.5(70)	3.1(62)	4.1(82)	5.4(108)	3.1(62)	3.1(62)	37.5	4.8(97)	55.6
Phosphorus mEq (mg)/100ml	3.0(46)	3.2(50)	3.8(59)	3.2(50)	2.7(42)	4.0(62)	5.2(81)	4.0(62)	4(62)	40	5.1(80)	55
Iron mg/100ml	1.2	1.2	1.4	1.2	1.2	1.2	1.8	.77	.8	.84	1.0	1.0

Long Chain Polyunsaturated Fatty Acids

The fatty acid composition of commercial standard infant formulas has evolved to include arachidonic acid and docohexanoic acid, which are LC-PUFAs that are naturally present in human milk.[35] Arachidonic acid and docohexanoic acid play major roles as structural components of cell membranes in neural tissues and retinal photo-receptor membranes.[36] Both fatty acids are accumulated in the brain and retina tissue during fetal and early infant development.[37] Improved short-term scores in visual and cognitive function have been demonstrated in preterm and term infants who were fed formula supplemented with arachidonic acid and docohexanoic acid.[38-41] These results may be influenced by several confounding factors and have not been demonstrated by all investigators;[42] furthermore, the long-term nutritional and cognitive advantage from supplementing infant formula with these LC-PUFAs is yet to be demonstrated. The beneficial effects from docohexanoic acid and arachidonic acid supplementation appear more convincing in preterm infants. A maximum, but no minimum, level of arachidonic acid and docohexanoic acid supplementation for preterm infant formulas has been specified by the Life Sciences Research Office Panel on infant formulas.[43]

Omega-3 and 6 Fatty Acids

The omega-3 and 6 families of fatty acid are also referred to as essential fatty acids because of absent de novo synthesis in humans. The omega-6 series are the precursors for arachidonic acid, which has several biological roles including structural component of cell membranes and precursor for prostaglandins and leukotrines. Omega-3 series are also popularly known as fish oils.

Increased dietary consumption of omega-3 fatty acids is associated with prolonged bleeding time, decreased platelet aggregation, increased erythrocyte deformability, and decreased tendency to forming thrombus.[44] Omega-3 fatty acids also have anti-inflammatory effects presumably mediated through competitive inhibition of arachidonic acid utilization for synthesis of prostaglandins. This competitive inhibition results in synthesis of an alternate group of prostaglandins and leukotrienes with considerably less pro-inflammatory effects. Dietary supplementation with omega-3 fatty acids was associated with decreased inflammation and improved clinical symptoms in patients with psoriasis,[44] rheumatoid arthritis,[45] chronic inflammatory bowel disease,[46,47] and acute respiratory distress syndrome.[48] The clinical response to omega-3 fatty acid supplementation is variable, depends on dose, and occurs over time.[49]

Glutamine

Glutamine is a conditionally essential amino acid with numerous metabolic roles including nitrogen shuttle, protein and nucleic acid synthesis, gluconeogenesis, glutathione precursor, and primary oxidative fuel for enterocytes. It is the most abundant amino acid in the body, accounting for more than 60% of the free amino acid pool in skeletal muscle and 20% of the free amino acid pool in plasma.[50,51] Enterally administered glutamine is mostly metabolized in the gut,[52] and was associated with reduced risk for sepsis in small infants.[53] During the metabolic response to severe trauma and critical illness, glutamine attains 'conditionally essential' status. Pilot data from patients with severe trauma suggest that glutamine supplementation enhanced gut barrier function and decreased sepsis. Adults with short gut syndrome had improved nutrient absorption when fed a modified diet combined with glutamine supplements and growth hormone.[54-55] However, it is unproven whether these effects are primarily from glutamine or an overall positive nitrogen balance.[56] Therefore, more research is needed to define the superiority of glutamine supplementation over regular isonitrogenous nutrition in at-risk patients. Additionally, although glutamine is being added to pediatric enteral formulas, further studies focusing on pediatric populations are also necessary. Glutamine is available in modular form and as a constituent in some newer enteral formulas (see Table 43-7). The main limitation of the module supplement is osmotic diarrhea.

Arginine

Arginine is the sole substrate for synthesis of nitric oxide, which is essential in mediating macrophage bactericidal activity.[57] Uncontrolled sepsis is an important cause of morbidity and mortality in patients with surgical trauma.[58] Decreased T-lymphocyte function is one of the components of altered immunity in patients after severe surgical trauma.[59] Improved function of T-lymphocytes was demonstrated in critically ill surgical trauma patients fed with an arginine-enriched diet.[60] Arginine is available as a modular supplement and nutrient component is some newer enteral formula specifically used for nutritional therapy in critically ill patients (see Table 43-7). The main limitation of arginine modules is dose-dependent osmotic diarrhea.

Transforming Growth Factor-Beta

TGF-β is an endogenous polypeptide growth factor with immune-modulating effects.[61] It is produced by leukocytes and promotes their differentiation while inhibiting proliferation and activation.[62] TGF-β1–deficient mice die from cardiac, pulmonary, and gastric inflammation, thereby suggesting the growth factor's vital role in suppressing activation and proliferation of cells.[63] TGF-β is naturally present in human and bovine milk[64] and exerts an immune-modulatory effect of inhibiting expression of class II MHC molecules in neonatal enterocytes.[65]

The immune-modulating effects of TGF-β have been applied in dietary therapy of Crohn's disease (Chapter 18). Pediatric patients with Crohn's disease exclusively fed enteral formula enriched with TGF-β had downregulated pro-inflammatory cytokines (IL-1β, IFNϒ, and IL-8) accompanied by mucosal healing.[66] However, remission in clinical symptoms, mucosal healing and improved growth in patients with chronic inflammatory bowel disease have also been achieved using monomeric and polymeric enteral formulas without TGF-β.[67] Therefore, there is currently no data demonstrating superiority of TGF-β–enriched formula over regular enteral formulas in nutritional therapy of Crohn's disease.

Probiotics

Probiotics are dietary supplements that contain one or more cultures of living organisms that play a beneficial role in "improving" the host's endogenous microflora.[68] Consumption of sour milk, yogurt, and other food preparations based on live bacteria has been practiced for centuries. The intestinal microbial flora has a vital impact on immune development, tolerance, and overall health. The most commonly studied probiotic organisms are *Lactobacillus (L.) casei, L. acidophiluus, L. rhamonsum, L. planatarum 299V, Bifidobacteria (B.) bifidum, B. longum, Streptococcus thermophilus, Enterococcus faecium SF68,* and *Saccharomyces boulardii.*

Ingestion of probiotic organism alters intestinal microbial flora, affects intestinal permeability, stimulates the nonimmunologic gut defense barrier and mucosal IgA response, and influences the balance between pro- and anti-inflammatory cytokines. These effects vary with the different probiotics.[69,70] Probiotics have been effectively used to shorten duration of infectious diarrhea and the management of antibiotic-associated diarrhea, *Clostridium difficile* colitis, traveler's diarrhea, radiation-induced diarrhea, pouchitis, atopic dermatitis, and cow's milk allergy.[71-74]

Infant formula supplemented with probiotic organisms was safe and well tolerated, resulted in normal growth, and was associated with less colic and antibiotic use in healthy infants.[75] Infants fed formula supplemented with probiotics were also less likely to develop diarrhea.[76] Infectious complications in association with probiotic therapy have been seen in high-risk and immune-compromised patients;[77-79] however, the overall impression is that these occurrences are rare in comparison with the widespread use of probiotics as well as uncontrolled natural exposure to live bacteria through ingestion of fermented foods.[80] The potential for benefit in supplementing formula with probiotics is undisputed; however, more data about safety is needed.

Prebiotics

Prebiotics are complex indigestible carbohydrates that promote the growth of probiotic organisms in the host's GI tract. Fructo-oligosaccharides and inulin are common dietary components that exert a prebiotic effect.[81] Fructo-oligosaccharides are present in a variety of common foods including tomatoes, wheat, and bananas. They are neither digested nor absorbed; therefore, they pass into the colon where they are fermented into short chain fatty acids (SCFA) by bifidobacteria and other intestinal microbial flora. SCFA are the primary fuel for colonocytes and also promote absorption of sodium and water in the colon. Saavedra et al studied the effect of oligofructose-supplemented standard infant cereal in a group of non-breastfed infants and observed good tolerance, normal growth, and decreased severity of diarrhea.[82] Other clinical applications for use of prebiotics are short bowel syndrome and chronic inflammatory bowel disease. Ingestion of prebiotics is considered very safe, despite an isolated report of anaphylaxis to inulin in vegetables and processed foods.[83] Supplementing formula with prebiotics is more readily accepted than is supplementation with probiotics. When prebiotics are used with probiotics, the combination is called a symbiotic.

Assessing Nutritional Status And Caloric Requirements of Pediatric Patients

Nutritional Assessment

A nutritional assessment is an overview of the patient's current physical status with consideration of his or her medical history. The process of obtaining a nutritional assessment is discussed in Chapter 1 but is not pediatric specific. This section specifically addresses pediatric issues in regard to assessing the patient's nutrition status.

In assessing the pediatric patient's nutritional status, it is imperative to obtain a careful history about the chronology of onset of growth problems—ie, acute versus chronic. Inquiries should also be made into the patient's prenatal and birth history, feeding patterns, intercurrent illness, chronic medications, family medical history, and social structure. A review of systems should be performed to screen for syndromes associated with impaired growth.

In addition, a good attempt should be made to obtain all previous growth records. Accurate growth measurements (weight, length/height, and head circumference) should be obtained and plotted on the updated CDC 2000 growth charts (see www.cdc.gov/growthcharts). The child's (2 to 20 years) height percentile should be within the calculated target height based on mid-parent height determined by the calculation in Sidebar 43-1. The genetic contribution of parental stature on the child's height may also be separated from the effects of malnutrition and disease using the parent-specific adjustments of Himes et al.[84] Disease-specific growth references may help minimize the severity of perceived malnutrition in children with disorders associated with impaired growth patterns (eg, cerebral palsy).[85-86] Growth reference data are also available of alternate growth measurements including upper-arm and lower-leg lengths[87] and skin-fold anthropometry.[88] These are particularly useful in situations in which measurement of length and stature would be inaccurate (eg, of children who are bed ridden or who have kypho-scoliosis, contractures, and other musculoskeletal deformities). Pubertal stage should always be assessed because of it significant impact on interpretation of weight and height gain in females >8 to 9 years and males >12 to 13 years.

In children with inadequate caloric intake and malabsorption disorders, the rate of weight gain decreases before length/height and head circumference percentiles decrease. Infants with disproportionately small heads are suspect for primary neurological problems affecting brain growth because head growth is the last to be affected by primary malnutrition and is not characteristic of primary skeletal or growth problems.[89]

Sidebar 43-1.

Male (2-20 years):

[Father's height (cm) + mother's height (cm) + 13-cm] divided by 2

Females (2-20 years):

[Father's height (cm) + mother's height (cm) – 13-cm] divided by 2

Overweight or underweight status is assessed by determining the percentiles for weight-for-length, body mass index (BMI) (Chapter 47), and/or comparing actual weight with the ideal body weight (IBW). (Overweight in children is discussed in Chapter 52.) The IBW is the median (50th percentile) weight for the patient's measured length/height. The percentage ideal body weight (IBW%) is then calculated by dividing the measured weight by the IBW and multiplying by 100. A value within 10% of IBW is considered within the normal range. An IBW% of less than 70% to 80% indicates moderate to severe wasting (marasmus) and, when associated with edema and hypoalbuminemia, constitutes Kwashiorkor.[90] Weight-for-length percentile charts are available of infants and children aged birth to 36 months. Gender based weight-for-length percentile charts for infants aged birth to 36 months and BMI percentiles for children aged 2 to 20 years are available and can be downloaded from the CDC growth charts website (see www.cdc.gov/growthcharts). A weight-for-length or BMI percentile ≤5th percentile indicates severe underweight for stature or wasting that is very suggestive of inadequate caloric intake, deprivation, or malabsorption. (Undernutrition is discussed in Chapter 4, and malabsorption is discussed in Chapter 5.)

Calculation of Energy (Calorie) Requirements

Level of energy intake from food will balance expenditure when the individual has a body size and composition and level of physical activity that are consistent with long-term good health and that allow for the maintenance of economically necessary and socially acceptable activity. In children and pregnant or lactating women, the energy requirement includes the energy needs associated with the deposition of tissues or secretion of milk at rates consistent with good health.[91] Energy requirements per kilogram of body weight are highest during the neonatal period and decline progressively until adult age. Individual children may require more or less energy depending on many factors such as activity, body composition, and disease state. The low birthweight infant may require 150 kcal/kg while normal birth weight infants require 100 to 120 kcal/kg. The caloric requirements in healthy non-stressed infants aged birth to 1 year are approximately 100 to 115 kcal/kg/day.

Resting Energy Expenditure

The components of total daily energy expenditure in children are: 1) basal metabolism (approximate REE), 2) physical activity, 3) energy cost of growth, 4) thermic effect of food (~5 kcal/kg/day), 5) thermoregulation, and 6) losses (~5 kcal/kg/day).[92] Resting energy expenditure (REE) is fairly stable; it is the largest contributor (50% to 70%) and most easily measurable component of the total energy expenditure (TEE). Therefore, determining REE provides the basis for predicting TEE.

There are three mostly commonly used REE prediction equations are: the WHO equation, the Schofield equations, and the Harris Benedict equations. The Harris Benedict equations are not recommended for use in pediatrics because they were derived mostly from REE measurements obtained in adults, and have poor accuracy in children.[93]

The WHO[91] and Schofield REE prediction equations[94] are the most appropriate and widely used in infants, children, and adolescents. Both equations are age and gender specific and have proven reliable in healthy children aged >1 year. The WHO equations predict REE based on age, gender, and weight. The Schofield equations predict REE based on age, gender, weight, and length/height (Table 43-9). The inclusion of length/height provides for better accuracy when there is altered body composition (eg, children with failure to thrive).

Reliability and accuracy of prediction equations declines in children with altered body composition (eg, FTT, obesity, and chronic disease).[93,95] In these situations, REE should be measured using indirect calorimetry. The predicted or measured REE is then multiplied by an activity/stress adjustment factor that depends on nutritional status, disease stress, and need or requirement for catch-up growth[96] (Table 43-10).

An example of calculated caloric requirements is presented in Sidebar 43-2. Note that these measurements provide a basis for initiating goal-oriented nutritional support. Other factors, such as risk for refeeding syndrome (Chapter 45), may necessitate gradual increment of caloric intake. Successful nutritional support involves monitoring the response to intervention. For children with severe malnutrition, REE calculations may be based on the IBW.[91]

Conclusion

Nutrition is the most influential environmental factor affecting growth in infants and children. There is a large array of commercial enteral products is currently available; however, a good understanding of the composition is necessary for appropriate clinical indication and application. Progress in nutrition support has inspired a paradigm shift in the goals of nutritional care from mere provision of calories to provision of growth factors, nutrients with immune-modulating effects, and alteration of intestinal microflora. Assessment of nutritional status is prerequisite to determining the protein-calorie needs in pediatrics and successful nutrition support.

Table 43-9.

REE Prediction Equations

Gender	Age, y	WHO Equations REE, Kcal/d	Schofield Equations REE, Kcal/d
Male	1 – 3	60.9W – 54	0.167W + 1517.4H – 617.6
	3 – 10	22.7W + 495	19.59W + 1303H + 414.9
	10 – 18	17.5W + 651	16.25W + 137.2H – 515.5
Female	1 – 3	61W – 51	16.252W + 1023.2H – 413.5
	3 – 10	22.5W + 499	16.969W + 161.8H + 371.2
	10 – 18	12.2W + 746	8.365W + 465H + 200

W = weight, kg
H = Length/height, m

Table 43-10.

Activity/Stress Adjustment Factors

REE x 1.3	For a well-nourished child at bed rest with mild to moderate stress (minor surgery)
REE x 1.5	For a normally active child with mild to moderate stress; an inactive child with severe stress (trauma, sepsis, cancer, extensive surgery), or child with minimal activity and malnutrition requiring catch-up growth
REE x 1.7	For active child requiring catch-up growth or an active child with sever stress

114% of predicted (mildly increased)

References

1. Binns CW. Infant-feeding and growth. In: SJ Ulijasgek, FE Johnston, MA Preece (eds). *Cambridge Encyclopedia of Human Growth and Development*. New York, NY: Cambridge University Press; 1998: 320-325.
2. WHO Expert Consultation. The optimal duration of exclusive breast feeding. Available at: http://www.who.int/child-adolescent-health/New_Publications/NUTRITION/WHO_CAH_01_24.pdf. Accessed October 20, 2005.
3. American Academy of Pediatrics. *Pediatric Nutrition Handbook*. 5th Ed. Elk Grover Village, Ill: Author; 2004:23-46.
4. Schiffman SS, Dackis C. Taste of nutrients: amino acids, vitamins, and fatty acids. *Percept Psychophys*. 1975;17:140-6
5. Vazquez M, Pearson PB, Beauchamp GK. Flavor preferences in malnourished Mexican infants. *Physiol Behav*. 1982;28:513-9
6. Access for administration of nutrition support. In: Guidelines for the use of parenteral and enteral nutrition in adults and pediatric patients. *JPEN*. 2002;26(1):33SA-35SA.
7. Sentongo TAS, Mascarenhas M. Newer components of enteral formulas. *Pediatr Clin N Amer*. 2002;49(1):113-25.
8. King CK, Glass R, Bresee JS, Duggan C. Managing acute gastroenteritis among children. *MMWR*. 2003;52(RR16):1-16.
9. Sentongo TA. The use of oral rehydration solutions in children and adults. *Curr Gastroenterol Rep*. 2004;6(4):307-13
10. Hirshhorn N. The treatment of acute diarrhea in children. An historical and physiological perspective. *Am J Clin Nutr*. 1980;33:637-63
11. Bern C, Martines J, de Zoysa I, Glass RI. The magnitude of the global problem of diarrhoel disease: a ten year update. *Bull World Health Org*. 1992;70:705-14
12. Expert Consultation of Oral Rehydration. Reduced osmolarity oral rehydration salts (ORS) formulation. Available at: http://www.who.int/child-adolescent-health/New_Publications/NEWS/Expert_consultation. Accessed September 7, 2004.
13. CHOICE Study Group. Multicenter, randomized, double blind clinical trial to evaluate the efficacy and safety of a reduced osmolarity oral rehydration salts solution in children with acute watery diarrhea. *Pediatrics*. 2001;107:613-18.
14. Dutta D, Bhattacharya MK, Deb AK, Sarkar D, et al. Evaluation of oral hypo-osmolar glucose-based and rice-based oral rehydration solutions in the treatment of cholera in children. *Acta Pædiatr*. 2000;89:787-90.

Sidebar 43-2. Example Calculation of Caloric Requirements[97–101]

A 15-kg, 5-year-old girl is hospitalized with chronic diarrhea and malnutrition. REE is measured to determine metabolic rate and to serve as a basis to determine total energy requirements.

Measured REE:

950 Kcal/d

Activity factor:

1.3 (bed rest)

1.3 x 950 = 1,235 kcal/d

Weight gain goal:

1 kg over 1-month; 1-kg ≡ ~7,700 kcal/30-day = 257 kcal/d

257 kcal/d (1 kg over 1-month) + 1,235 = 1,492 kcal/d

Stool fat losses:

CoFA 80% (nl >93%) ~15% Kcal loss

1.15 (15% Kcal loss) x 1,492 = 1,716 kcal/d

Therefore total caloric needs for meeting daily nutritional needs and achieving 1-kg weight gain in 1-month is: 1,716 kcal/day

Comparison of measured REE with predicted REE using WHO prediction equation: (22.5 x 15 [wt, kg]) + 499 = 836 kcal/day. Therefore the measured REE (950 kcal/day) was 114% of predicted (mildly increased).[102]

15. Ramkrishna BS, Venkatraman S, Srinvasan P, et al. Amylase-resistant starch plus oral rehydration solution for cholera. *N Eng J Med.* 2000;342:308-13.
16. Wingertzahn MA, Rehman KU, Altaf W, Wapnir RA. Zinc as a potential enteroprotector in oral rehydration solutions: its role in nitric oxide metabolism. *Pediatr Res.* 2003;53:434-39.
17. Altaf W, Perveen S, Rehman KU, et al. Zinc supplementation in oral rehydration solutions: Experimental assessment and mechanisms of action. *J Amer Coll Nutr.* 2002;21(1):26-32.
18. Silva AC, Santos-Neto MS, Soares AM, et al. Efficacy of a glutamine-based oral rehydration solution on the electrolyte and water absorption in a rabbit model of secretory diarrhea induced by cholera toxin. *J Pediatr Gastroenterol Nutr.* 1998;26:513-19.
19. Schanler RJ, Hurst NM, Lau C. The use of human milk and breast feeding in premature infants. *Clin Perinatol.* 1999;26:379-398.
20. Dewey KG. Is breastfeeding protective against child obesity? *J Hum Lact.* 2003;19(1):9-18
21. American Academy of Pediatrics. *Pediatric Nutrition Handbook.* 5th Ed. Elk Grover Village, Ill: Author; 2004:87-97.
22. Randall HT. Enteral nutrition: Tube feeding in acute and chronic illness. *JPEN.* 1984;8(2):113-136.
23. Keighley MR, Mogg B, Bently S, Allan C. "Home brew" compared with commercial preparation for enteral feeding. *BMJ Clin Res Ed.* 1982(6310):163.
24. Bach AC, Ingenbleek Y, Frey A. The usefulness of dietary medium-chain triglycerides in body weight control: fact or fancy. *J Lipid Res.* 1996;37:708-26
25. Jakobsson I, Lothe L, Ley D, Borschel MW. Effectiveness of casein hydrolysate feedings in infants with colic. *Acta Pædiatr.* 2000; 89:18-21
26. Menella JA, Beauchamp GK. Developmental changes in the acceptance of protein hydrolysate formula. *J Dev Behav Pediatr.* 1996;17:386-391
27. Beauchamp GK, Menella JA. Early feeding and the acquisition of flavor preferences. In: Boulton J, Laron Z, Rey J, eds. Long term consequences of early feeding. *Nestlé Nutrition Workshop Series.* Book 36. Philadelphia: Lippincott-Raven; 1996.
28. Businco L, Bruno G, Giampietro PG. Prevention and management of food allergy. *Acta Pædiatr Suppl,* 1999;430:104-109.
29. Von Berg A, Koletzko S, Gr bl A, Filipiak-Pittroff B, et al. The effect of hydrolyzed cow's milk formula for allergy prevention in the first year of life. The German Infant Nutritional Intervention Study, a randomized double-blind trial. *J Allergy Clin Immunol.* 2003; 111:533-40
30. Kelly KJ, Lazenby AJ, Rowe PC, et al. Eosinophilic esophagitis attributed to gastroesophageal reflux improvement with an amino acid-based formula. *Gastroenterology.* 1995;109:1503-1512.
31. Markowitz JE, Spergel JM, Ruchelli E, Liacouras CA. Elemental diet is an effective treatment of eosinophilic esophagitis in children and adolescents. *Am J Gastroenterol.* 2003;98(4):777-82
32. Spergel JM, Pawlowski NA. Food allergy. Mechanisms, diagnosis, and management in children. *Pediatr Clin N Amer.* 2002;49(1):73-96.
33. Grimble GK, Rees PP, Keohane T, et al. Effect of peptide chain length on absorption of egg protein hydrolysates in the normal human jejunum. *Gastroenterology.* 1987;92:136-142.
34. Bach AC, Babayan VK. Medium-chain triglycerides: an update. *Am J Clin Nutr.* 1982;36:950-962.
35. Jensen RG. Lipids in human milk. *Lipids.* 1999;34:1243-1271
36. Martinez M. Tissue levels of polyunsaturated fatty acids during early human development. *J Pediatr.* 1992;120:S129-S138.
37. Innis SM. Perinatal biochemistry and physiology of long-chain polyunsaturated fatty acids. *J Pediatr.* 2003;143:S1-S8.
38. SanGiovanni JP, Parra-Cabrera S, Colditz GA, et al. Meta-analysis of dietary essential fatty acids and long-chain polyunsaturated fatty acids as they relate to visual resolution acuity in healthy preterm infants. *Pediatrics.* 2000;105:1929-1298.
39. O'Connor DL, Hall R, Adamkin D, et al. Growth and development in preterm infants fed long-chain polyunsaturated fatty acids: A prospective, randomized controlled trial. *Pediatrics.* 2001;108:359-71.
40. Hoffman DR, Birch EE, Castañeda YS, Fawcett SL, et al. Visual function in breast term infants weaned to formula with or without long-chain polyunsaturates at 4 to 6 months: a randomized controlled trial. *J Pediatr.* 2003;142:669-677.
41. Uauy R, Hoffman DR, Mena P, Llanos A, et al. Term infant studies of DHA and ARA supplementation of neurodevelopment: results of randomized controlled trials. *J Pediatr.* 2003;143:S17-S25.
42. Auestad N, Halter R, Halla RT, et al. Growth and development in term infants fed long-chain polyunsaturated fatty acids: A double-masked, randomized, parallel, prospective, multivariate study. *Pediatrics.* 2001;108:372-381.
43. Life Sciences Research Office, American Society for Nutritional Sciences for the Center For Food Safety and Applied Nutrition, Food and Drug Administration, Department of Health and Human Services, Washington, DC 20204 under Contract No. 223-92-2185. Assessment of Nutrient Requirements for Infant Formulas. *J Nutr.* 1998;128(suppl 11S).
44. Simopoulos AP. Omega-3 fatty acids in health and disease and in growth and development. *Am J Clin Nutr.* 1991;54(3):438-63.
45. Kremer JM, Bigauotte J, Michalek AV, et al. Effects of manipulation of dietary fatty acids on clinical manifestations of rheumatoid arthritis. *Lancet.* 1985;1(8422):184-187.
46. Belluzzi A, Brignola C, Campieri M, et al. Effect of an enteric-coated fish-oil preparation on relapses in Crohn's disease. *N Engl J Med.* 1996;334(24):1557-1560.
47. Salomon P, Kornbluth AA, Janowitz HD. Treatment of ulcerative colitis with fish oil n-3-omega-fatty acid: an open trial. *J Clin Gastroenterol.* 1990;12(2):157-161.

48. Gadek JE, DeMichele SJ, Karlstad MD, et al. Effect of enteral feeding with eicosapentaenoic acid, gamma-linolenic acid, antioxidants in patients with acute respiratory distress syndrome. Enteral Nutrition in ARDS Study Group. *Crit Care Med.* 1999;27(8):1409-20.
49. Galperin C, German BJ, Gershwin ME: Nutrition and diet in rheumatic diseases. In Shils ME, Olson JA, Shike M, Ross AC, (eds). *Modern Nutrition in Health and Disease.* 9th ed. Baltimore, Md: Williams & Wilkins;1999:1139-1151.
50. van der Hulst RRWJ, von Meyenfeldt MF, Soeters PB. Glutamine: an essential aminoacid for the gut. *Nutrition.* 1996;12:S78-81.
51. Ziegler TR, Szeszycki EE, Estivariz CF, et al. Glutamine: from basic science to clinical applications. *Nutrition.* 1996;12:S68-70.
52. Parimi PS, Devapatla S, Gruca LL, et al. Effect of enteral glutamine or glycine on whole-body nitrogen kinetics in very-low-birth-weight infants. *Am J Clin Nutr.* 2004;79:402-409.
53. Neu J, Roig JC, Meetze WH, et al. Enteral glutamine supplementation for very low birth weight infants decreases morbidity. *J Pediatr.* 1997;131:691-699.
54. Houdjik AP, Rijnsburger ER, Jansen J, et al. Randomized trial of glutamine-enriched enteral nutrition on infectious morbidity in patients with multiple trauma. *Lancet.* 1998;352:772-776.
55. Byrne TA, Morrissey TB, Nattakom TV, Ziegler TR, Wilmore DW. Growth hormone, glutamine and a modified diet enhance nutrient absorption in patients with the severe short bowel syndrome. *J Parenter Enter Nutr.* 1995;19:296-302.
56. Buchman AL. Glutamine: commercially essential or conditionally essential? A critical appraisal of the human data. *Am J Clin Nutr.* 2001;74(1):25-32
57. Green SJ, Nacy CA. Antimicrobial and immunopathologic effects of cytokine-induced NO synthesis. *Curr Opinion Infect Dis.* 1993; 6:384-396
58. Bone RC. The sepsis syndrome. Definition and general approach to management. *Clin Chest Med.* 1996;17:175-181.
59. Berguer R, Bravo N, Bowyer M, et al. Major surgical suppresses maximal production of T-helper type 1 cytokines without potentiating the release of helper T-cell type 2 cytokines. *Arch Surg.* 1999; 134:540-44
60. Daly JM, Reynolds J, Thom A et al. Immune and metabolic effects of arginine in the surgical patient. *Ann Surg.* 1988;208:512-523.
61. Blobe GC, Schiemann WP, Lodish HF. Mechanisms of disease: role of transforming growth factor (beta) in human disease. *N Eng J Med.* 2000;342(18):1350-1358.
62. Lettterio JJ, Roberts AB. Regulation of immune responses by TGF-(beta). *Annu Rev Immunol.* 1998;16:137-161.
63. Shull MM, Ormsby I, Kier AB, et al. Targeted disruption of the mouse transforming growth factor-(beta) 1 gene results in multifocal inflammatory disease. Nature, 1992;359:693-9
64. Cox DA, Bürk RR. Isolation and characterization of milk growth factor, a transforming-growth-factor-β2-related polypeptide, from bovine milk. *Eur J Biochem.* 1991;197(2):353-358.
65. Donnet-Hughes A, Schiffrin EJ, Huggett AC: Expression of MHC antigens by intestinal epithelial cells. Effect of transforming growth factor-beta 2 (TGF-β2). *Clin Exp Immunol.* 1995;99(2):240-244.
66. Fell JM, Paintin M, Arnaud-Battandier F, et al: Mucosal healing and a fall in mucosal pro-inflammatory cytokine mRNA induced by a specific oral polymeric diet in paediatric Crohn's disease. *Aliment Pharmacol Ther.* 2000;14(3):281-289.
67. Zachos M, Tondeur M, Griffiths AM. Enteral nutritional therapy for induction of remission in Crohn's disease. *Cochrane Library.* 2004;2:1-33.
68. Holzapfel WH, Haberer P, Snel J, et al. Overview of gut flora and probiotics. *Int J Food Microbiol.* 1998;41(2):85-101.
69. Isolauri E, Arvola T, Sutas Y, Moilanen W, Salminem S. Probiotics in the management of atopic eczema. *Clin Exp Allergy.* 2000;30:1604-1610.
70. Vanderhoof JA. Probiotics and intestinal inflammatory disorders in infants and children. *J Pediatr Gastroenterol Nutr.* 2000;30(Suppl 2):S34-38.
71. Marteau PR, Vrese M, Cellier CJ et al: Protection from gastrointestinal diseases with the use of probiotics. *Am J Clin Nutr.* 2001;73(2 Suppl):430S-436S.
72. Majamaa H, Isolauri E. Probiotics: a novel approach in the management of food allergy. *J Allergy Clin Immunol.* 1997;99:179-185.
73. Isolauri E, Sutas Y, Kankaanpaa P, et al. Probiotics: effects on immunity. *Am J Clin Nutr.* 2001;73(2 Suppl):444S-450S.
74. Kalliomäki M, Salminem S, Arvilommi H, et al. Probiotics in primary prevention of atopic disease: a randomized placebo-controlled trial. *Lancet.* 2001;357:1076-1079.
75. Saavedra JM, Abi-Hanna A, Moore N, Yolken RH. Long-term consumption of infant formulas containing probiotics bacteria: tolerance and safety. *Am J Clin Nutr.* 2004;79:261-267.
76. Chouraqui JP, Van Egroo LD, Fichot MC: Does a probiotic added to an infant acidifies formula prevent diarrhoea? A multicenter controlled trial. *Gastroenterology.* 2000;118(4[Suppl 2 Pt 1]):A852 (4762).
77. Gasser F. Safety of lactic acid bacteria and their occurrence in human clinical infections. *Bull Inst Pasteur/* 1994;92:45-67.
78. Sussman JI, Baron EJ, Goldberg SM, Kaplan MH, Pizzarello RA. Clinical manifestation and therapy of Lactobacillus endocarditis: report of a case and review of the literature. *Rev Infect Dis.* 1986; 8:771-776.
79. MacFarland L, Bernasconi P: Saccharomyces boulardii: A review of an innovative therapeutic agent. *Microbiol Ecol Health Dis.* 1993; 6:157-71.
80. Saliminen SJ, Donohue DC. Safety assessment of Lactobacillus strain GG (ATCC 53103). *Nutr Today.* 1996;31(Suppl 1):12S-15S.
81. Roberfroid MB: Prebiotics: preferential substrates for specific germs. *Am J Clin Nutr.* 2001;73(2 Suppl):406S-409S.
82. Saavedra J, Tscherina A, Moore N, et al. Gastro-intestinal function in infants consuming a weaning food supplemented with oligofructose, a prebiotic. *J Pediatr Gastroenterol Nutr.* 1999; 29(4):513(95A).
83. Gay-Crosier F, Schreiber G, Hauser G. Anaphylaxis from inulin in vegetables and processed food. *N Eng J Med.* 2000;342(18):1372.
84. Himes JH, Roche AF, Thissen D, Moore WM. Parent-specific adjustments for evaluation of recumbent length and stature of children. *Pediatrics.* 1985;75(2):304-313.
85. Krick J, Murphy-Miller P, Zeger S, Wright E. Patterns of growth in children with cerebral palsy. *J Am Diet Assoc.* 1996;96(7):680-685.
86. Zemel BS, Stallings V. Developmental disabilities. In: Walker WA, Watkins JB, Duggan C (eds). *Nutrition in Pediatrics. Basic Science and Clinical Applications.* 3rd ed. Hamilton ON: BC Decker; 2003: 580-590.
87. Zemel BS, Stallings VA. Alternative measure for assessing linear growth. In SJ Ulijasgek, FE Johnston, MA Preece (eds). *Cambridge Encyclopedia of Human Growth and Development.* New York, NY: Cambridge University Press; 1998:74-75.
88. Frisancho A. New norms of upper limb fat and muscle areas for assessment of nutritional status. *Am J Clin Nutr.* 1981;34:2540-45.
89. Kerr DS. Failure to thrive and malnutrition. In Kleigman RM, Nieder ML, Super DM (eds). *Practical Strategies in Pediatric Diagnosis and Therapy.* Philadelphia, Pa: WB Saunders; 1996:243-257.

90. Waterlow JC. Classification and definition of protein-energy malnutrition. *Monograph Series/World Health Organization.* 1976;(62):530-55.
91. World Health Organization. Energy and protein requirements. *Report of a joint FAO/WHO/UNU Expert Consultation. (WHO Technical Report Series No. 724).* Geneva: World Health Organization; 1985.
92. Wells JCK, Davies PSW. The composition of energy metabolism in 12 week old infants [abstract]. *Ann Human Biol.* 1995;127:269-271.
93. Kaplan AS, Zemel BS, Neiswender KM, Stallings VA. Resting energy expenditure in clinical pediatrics: measured versus prediction equations. *J Pediatr.* 1995;127:200-5.
94. Schofield WN, Schofield C, James WPT. Basal metabolic rate-review and prediction, together with annotated bibliography of source material. *Hum Nutr: Clin Nutr.* 1985;39C(Suppl):5-41.
95. Sentongo TA, Tershakovec AM, Mascarenhas MR, et al. Resting energy expenditure and prediction equations in young children with failure to thrive. *J Pediatr.* 2000;136:345-350.
96. National Academy of Sciences. *Recommended Dietary Allowances.* Washington DC: National Academy Press; 1989:24-38.

Chapter 44

HOME ENTERAL NUTRITION

Lyn Howard, MD, FRCP,
and Christopher C. Ashley, MD, MPH

Historical Perspective

Provision of enteral nutrition (EN) through a tube at home has a long history[1,2] and goes back to ancient Egypt.[3] By the mid-twentieth century patients with severe swallowing disorders were quite often managed at home, fed bolus meals through large-bore rubber nasogastric (NG) or surgical gastrostomy tubes using homemade blenderized diets. But this approach tended to be uncomfortable and unsightly and was frequently refused by many stroke or cancer dysphagic persons, preferring the shorter course of aspiration pneumonia, the so-called "poor man's friend."

In the latter part of the 20th century, a number of technical advances radically changed the acceptability of tube EN to patients and their families. As a result, the use of this technology expanded rapidly. The technical advances involved all aspects of tube enteral feeding. Smaller, softer tubes became available; these were made from less biologically reactive materials, often with a valve and low-profile surface-access port suitable for active persons on intermittent feeding schedules. Industry produced an array of premade liquid diets, tailored to different age groups and different medical conditions. Small portable infusion pumps became available with shoulder packs or hip packs for mobile patients needing easy conveyance of the pump and tube feed. Tube placement methodology was revolutionized and most feeding tubes are now placed percutaneously by endoscopic or radiologic techniques. Surgical placement is typically reserved for either patients with extensive adhesions that prevent endoscopic or radiographic mobilization of the stomach or jejunum to the anterior abdominal wall or for patients in whom placement is part of an extensive operation. Home-infusion companies developed to service persons on various high-tech home therapies, ranging from parenteral nutrition (PN) and EN to home antibiotic and chemotherapy infusions. These companies not only supply the patient with the nutrient formula and infusion equipment, but also provide pharmacists and nurses to help with clinical management and financial experts to help patients and their families deal with complex reimbursement issues.

Medical advances frequently trigger ethical issues. While modern home enteral nutrition (HEN) allows many dysphagic patients to lead an active near-normal life, in less optimistic settings—such as severe dementia, head and neck cancer, or bed-ridden stroke patients—questions arise about prolonging the dying process and poor quality of life.[4] All these issues need to be considered.

Disease Spectrum of Patients on Home Enteral Nutrition

Table 44-1 summarizes the clinical diagnosis of persons receiving home enteral feeding in North America and Europe. In these countries, the four main diagnostic groups are cancer, neuromuscular disorders, small bowel malabsorption, and nutritional depletion from other causes.

The use of HEN in adult cancer patients is quite variable and country specific, reflecting different philosophic approaches. The 1998 European Survey[9] described low cancer use in Denmark, Poland, and the UK (3.6% to 12.6% of HEN use); medium use in Italy, Belgium, and France (25.3% to 33.6%); and high use in Germany (57%). In children, cancer is the underlying disease in 11% of HEN patients.[10]

TABLE 44-1.

Clinical Diagnosis of Patients Receiving Long-Term Enteral Feeding From International Studies and Registries

	North America*(%)	VA PEG Study† (%)	UK Study‡ (%)	Spanish HEN Registry§ (%)	European Survey‖ (%)
Cancer:	**42**	**32**	**14**	**33**	**30**
Head and neck	15	16			
Esophageal	8	5	13		
Gastric	5	—	—		
Other GI tumors	5	—	1		
Leukemia, lymphoma	2	—	—		
Other tumors	7	11	—		
Neuromuscular disorder:	**29**	**48**	**54**	**41**	**44**
Cerebrovascular disease	—	19	9		
Other neurologic disorders	—	29	45		
Small bowel malabsorption	**8**	**—**	**4**	**—**	**11**
Nutritional depletion, other causes¶	**21**	**21**	**15**	**—**	**15**
Total number of patients studied	**3931**	**7369**	**191**	**2986**	**1397**

*North American Home Parenteral and Enteral Nutrition Patient Registry, 1985-1992[5]
†Veterans Administration Hospital Percutaneous Endoscopic Gastrostomy Study, 1990-1992[6]
‡East Anglia U.K. Prospective Home Enteral Tube Feeding Study, November 1992-November 1993[7]
§Spanish National Registry, 2000[8]
‖Europe Multi-Center Survey, 1998[9]
¶A heterogeneous group of dementia, metabolic, cardiorespiratory, and congenital disorders

Neuromuscular disorders of swallowing are the largest group of HEN patients (29% to 54% of HEN use). In adults, cerebrovascular accidents are the commonest etiology, followed by multiple sclerosis and central nervous system trauma.[6,7] In children, neuromuscular disorders account for 50% of the underlying HEN diagnoses, and cerebral palsy is the most frequent etiology.[10]

Small bowel malabsorption is the underlying diagnosis for about 10% of HEN patients. Many of these patients initially require PN for short bowel syndrome, but after a period of adaptation are able to graduate to tube enteral support, infusing overnight and eating during the day. Not infrequently, short bowel children receive both home parenteral nutrition (HPN) and HEN. The enteral component is to stimulate bowel adaptation and to reduce parenteral support to avoid PN-induced hepatic disease.

The category of nutritional depletion is a heterogeneous group of dementia, metabolic, cardio-respiratory, and congenital disorders. In most series, this describes 15% to 20% of both adult and pediatric HEN patients.

In nursing-home patients, the same spectrum of underlying diseases are present; however, there is a major shift towards tube feeding in patients with dementia (52%).[11]

Prevalence and Growth of Home Enteral Nutrition

UNITED STATES

Because there is no national mechanism for the central collection of medical service information, the prevalence of HEN in the United States in not precisely known. Several efforts have been made, however, to estimate the prevalence of this therapy. In 1988, Bergstrom et al did a population-based study of feeding enterostomies in non-hospitalized patients in rural Minnesota.[12] They found 550 enterostomy feeding tubes were placed either endoscopically or surgically per million population. The majority of these patients were managed at home, but some were admitted to long-term care facilities, thereby overestimating the HEN prevalence.

Howard et al calculated HEN prevalence between 1989 and 1992,[13] from a combination of the Medicare Common Working File and the North American Home Parenteral and Enteral Nutrition (HPEN) Patient Registry. The registry collected outcome data on 9288 HPEN patients between 1985 and 1992 from 217 home nutrition-support programs nationwide. Figure 44-1 shows that there were 34,000 Medicare HEN beneficiaries in 1989, and this doubled

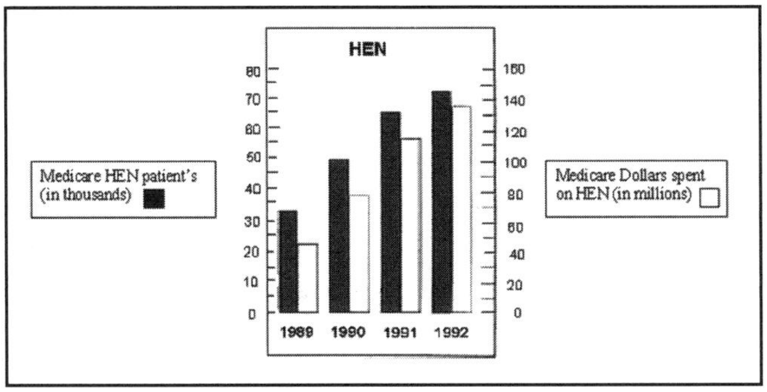

Figure 44-1. An estimate of the number of Medicare patients receiving HEN in thousand (left) and the dollars paid in millions (right) beween 1989 and 1992. These estimates were derived from Medicare part B PEN workload statistics compiled by BC/BS of South Caroline (David Denny, personal communication, February 1993). This carrier processed approximated 75% of all Medicare PEN claims. Their workload statistics have been increased to provide an estimate of national Medicare activity.

TABLE 44-2.

Primary Insurance Coverage by Percent of Home Enteral Nutrition Patients in the North American HPEN Registry[5] (1986-1992)

Insurance for HEN Patients	*1986*	*1987*	*1988*	*1989*	*1990*	*1991*	*1992*	*1986-1992*
Medicare (%)	42.0	39.1	39.8	47.7	52.9	51.3	48.3	45.8
Medicaid (%)	13.0	13.9	17.7	16.6	15.6	18.7	20.9	16.6
Private insurance (%)*	44.0	43.8	38.1	33.2	27.4	26.8	28.6	34.6
Other insurance (%)†	1.0	3.2	4.5	4.0	4.1	3.2	3.4	3.3

*All private insurances combined

†Other insurance included Veterans Affairs service-connected, self pay, Crippled Children's Fund, Workers' Compensation, etc.

to 73,000 by 1992, a growth rate of approximately 25% per year. Medicare was the primary HEN payer in 47.7% of the registry sample in 1989 and 48.3% in 1992. This implies a total US HEN population of 71,000 in 1989 and 151,000 in 1992. The US general population was 248 million in 1989 and 256 million in 1992.[14] Thus, overall, US HEN prevalence was 286 per million in 1989 and rose to 590 per million in 1992. This prevalence estimate is in the same ball park as that described for rural Minnesota.

More recently, a commercial estimate of US HEN users was quoted by Ireton Jones.[15] A corporate consulting firm estimated the prevalence by statistical extrapolation of the frequency of diseases requiring nutrition support and their prevalence in different-sized hospitals. The validation for these estimates in not known. The figure derived was 344,000 HEN patients in 2002. This is double the estimate made by Howard et al[13] a decade earlier and may include persons discharged to nursing homes.

In 1999, there were 1.6 million nursing-home residents in the United States.[16] New York State Long-Term Care Bureau describes 8% of the New York nursing-home patients as currently taking enteral feeding (Michael Lindsey, personal communication). This suggests a national figure of about 128,000 nursing-home enteral patients, a figure that has remained fairly constant for the past 10 years.[13]

UNITED KINGDOM AND EUROPE

In the United Kingdom, Parker's study described a prevalence of HEN use of 110 per million in 1992, which is roughly one-fifth of the US prevalence in the same year.[7] However, a further study by Parker et al[17] found that, during 1988 to 1993, there was a three-fold expansion of the use of HEN. In 1997, Elia confirmed that this U.K. expansion was continuing[18] and was associated with a modest decrease in length of hospital stay. As is discussed below in the section on HEN cost, transferring patients from hospital to home has cost-saving implications for the healthcare system.

The 1998 European survey of 1397 HEN patients managed in 23 nutrition support specialty centers in 8 countries (Belgium, Denmark, France, German, Italy, Poland, Spain, and the United Kingdom) described an overall European prevalence of 163 per million population.[9] This is considerably lower than that in the United States, but higher than earlier data, suggesting a trend to increased HEN utilization in Europe.

Cost

Who bears the cost of HEN? In the United States, 44% is paid by private insurance, 42% by Medicare, 13% by Medicaid, and 1% by other sources (Table 44-2). This changes dramatically for tube-fed patients in nursing homes in which 75% are part B Medicare funded. The large HEN contribution from public funding in part reflects the bi-model age distribution of HEN patients (Figure 44-2); disproportionately, HEN therapy peaks in the geriatric and pediatric age groups.[5]

In Europe, most HEN costs are absorbed by state-funded national health programs.[9]

The specific costs associated with HEN are shown in Table 44-3, which describes the Medicare allowable charge. Over the past 20 years, Medicare has tended to

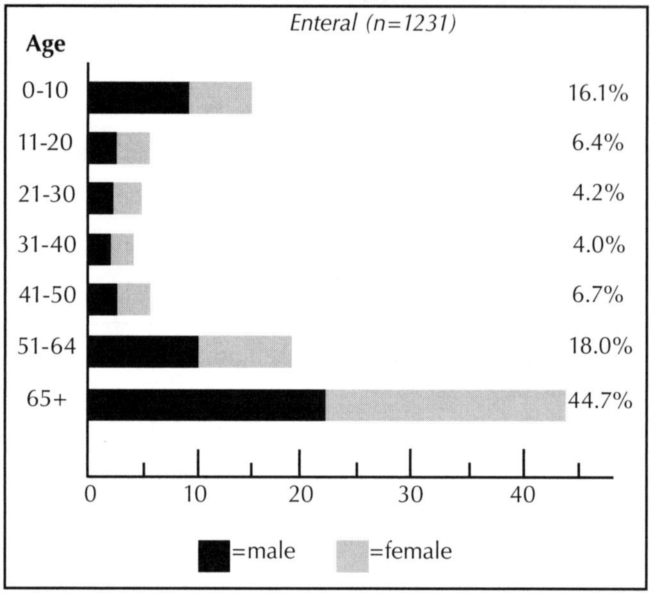

Figure 44-2. Patient age and gender distribution within HEN therapy. Reprinted from North American Home Parenteral and Enteral Nutrition Patient Registry. *Annual Reports 1985-1992*. Albany, NY: Oley Foundation; 1987-1994.

TABLE 44-3.

Medicare-Allowable Charges for Home Enteral Nutrition Therapy in 1992 and 2004

Item	*1992 ($/day)*	*2004 ($/day)*
Nutrient formula	$10.00 to $35.00	$11.00 to $31.00
Dressing kit	$0.50 to $2.00	$7.40
Administration set	$11.00	$11.00
Pump loan	$3.60	$3.60
Mean (range)	$22.00 ($25.00 to $50.00)	$38.00 ($33.00 to $53.00)

Note: Medicare pays 80% of the allowable charge. The remaining 20% is paid by a secondary insurance policy, if available, or by the patient if secondary insurance is not available. If an indigent patient submits evidence of financial inability to pay the 20% to their commercial supplier, this amount may be forgiven.

lead the field in terms of the medical indications and reimbursement for HPN and HEN in the United States. It should be noted (see Figure 44-1) that, between 1989 and 1992, there was an increase in Medicare HEN reimbursement per beneficiary served, perhaps reflecting recognition of the more costly modern techniques. Between 1992 and 2004 (see Table 44-3), HEN reimbursement changed very little. Because supplier service and marketing costs must be covered by the per diem allowable charge, HEN is becoming a less profitable therapy for the home-infusion industry. Most infusion companies accept HEN patients only if the referrals are counter balanced with HPN patient referrals, a therapy that is reimbursed with a more substantial profit margin.[13] The reimbursed HEN dollars cover only the nutrient formula, dressing kit, administration set, and pump loan. Other expenses (eg, nursing care, physician and laboratory charges, rehospitalization for therapy complications) are not included in this per-diem figure.

Cost utility analyses indicate substantial cost savings to the healthcare system when patients dependant on EN are transferred from hospital to home.[21] This reflects in part the shift of the cost onto the family. There are no studies estimating these family costs, such as loss of income when family members stop working to support the patient or lose work transporting their relative to medical follow-up appointments. In view of the bimodal peaks of HEN therapy in children and older persons, home care by a family member is common.

Clinical Outcome on Home Enteral Nutrition

The underlying disease is the most important determinant of survival and quality of life on HEN. Most HEN deaths (95%) in the first year of therapy are due to the primary disease or some other medical illness; very few (5%) are due to an HEN complication.[13] For this reason, HEN clinical outcome is best described in terms of a specific disease category. Table 44-4 summarizes the 12-month outcome for HEN patients with cancer, neuromuscular disorders of swallowing, and small bowel malabsorption.

TABLE 44-4.

Home Enteral Nutrition Clinical Outcome by Underlying Diagnosis at 12 Months

Diagnosis	Cancer (all ages)	Neuro (all ages)*	(<25 y)	(>65 y)	Short Gut (all ages)
Sample size	1644	1134	146	787	329
Average age (SD)	61(17)	65(26)	6(6)	79(8)	36(17)
12-m survival	25%	54%	89%	46%	82%
Rehabilitation†					
Complete	21%	4%	15%	2%	43%
Partial	59%	20%	39%	12%	42%
Minimal	21%	6%	46%	86%	15%
Full oral intake	30%	19%	23%	17%	45%
Continue HEN	6%	27%	59%	21%	28%
Complications‡					
HEN related	0.4	0.29	0.27	0.34	0.4
Non-HEN	2.7	0.91	0.95	0.94	2.7

Adapted from the North American Home Parenteral and Enteral Nutrition Patient Registry. *Annual Reports 1985-1992.* Albany, NY, Oley Foundation; 1987-1994.

SD = standard deviation.

* Neuro refers to neuromuscular disorders of swallowing. Separate groups are those <25 years, who commonly have stable cerebral palsy, and those >65 years, who commonly have progressive cerebrovascular disease.

† Complete, partial, or minimal in relation to the patient's ability to sustain normal age-appropriate activities, such as attending school or working.

‡ Complication rates per year refers to those that led to hospital readmission.

CANCER

The mortality rate is high in cancer patients on HEN; this is due to the low efficacy of treatment available for the sort of cancers that require HEN. In the North American HPEN Registry, of the 1644 HEN patients with cancer, 50% were dead in 4 months and 75% in 1 year[5] (Figure 44-3). The Veterans Administration (VA) follow-up of 1157 head and neck cancer patients receiving EN via percutaneous endoscopic gastrostomies (PEGs) showed a similar survival outcome: 50% were dead in 5 months and 70% in 1 year.[6] Only about one-half of the VA patients lived at home; the others either never left the hospital or were discharged to institutional settings. In the VA study, age did not influence survival; survival was equally poor in those under 65 years and those 75 years or older. Smaller studies also confirm this short survival. Stellato and Gauderer found 80% of 35 HEN cancer patients were dead in 1 year,[23] and Campos et al noted a median survival of only 176 days in 29 patients.[24]

While most HEN cancer patients have head, neck, and upper gastrointestinal (GI) cancers (see Table 44-1), a few have other cancers, some of which do have effective treatment. This is particularly true for leukemia/lymphoma patients.[25] These patients may receive EN during bone-marrow transplantation or aggressive chemotherapy regimens that are directed toward cure of the underlying disease, and a certain proportion continue the nutrition support for a few months while they recover at home. Szeluga's analysis of EN versus PN support of bone-marrow–transplant patients showed both therapies were equally helpful.[26]

In the North American Registry, HEN cancer patients were readmitted to hospital for a complication on average 3 times in the first 12 months.[13] Very few of these readmissions, however, were related to the HEN therapy (0.4 per year); most were due to the cancer itself or some other medical disorder (2.7 per year). This implies that the HEN therapy was relatively safe in these patients. It is worth noting that in cancer patients the HEN-therapy complication rate was one-third of the HPN therapy complication rate.[13]

There are no detailed quality-of-life studies in HEN cancer patients. In the North American Registry data, the level of rehabilitation was assessed by the clinician caring for the patient; such data is less informative than data provided by the patient or their family.[27] The clinicians felt most HEN cancer patients experienced partial rehabilitation (59%), at least initially and for a few months.[3]

The decision process of offering artificial nutrition support to a cancer patient is similar for both HEN and HPN therapies.[28] It depends on the clinician's judgment of how terminally ill the patient is and how active (Karnofsky performance score >50) and free of pain the patient is. An important study evaluated the role of nutrition and hydration in 32 patients predicted to have a life expectancy of 3 months or less (definition of a terminal illness); all 32 patients did, in fact, die in that period. These dying patients rarely experienced hunger or thirst, and there was no evidence that food and fluid, beyond that requested by the patient, contributed to the patient's comfort.[29] However, these patients were able to take food and water by mouth, and this is not true of many dysphagic or bowel-obstructed cancer patients. In the United States, bowel-obstructed patients with advanced malignant disease are usually given intravenous hydration and an endoscopic, radiologic, or surgical gastrostomy for distal feeding or decompression. In the United Kingdom, bowel-obstructed patients with terminal cancer are usually not treated with artificial nutrition.[30]

Neuromuscular Disorders of Swallowing

This group is heavily weighted towards older patients. In the North American Registry, 69% of persons were 65 years or older, 19% were 26 to 64 years, and 12% were 25 years or younger.[5] In the VA PEG study, 68% were 65 years or older.[6]

In the Registry analysis, because age reflects a difference in the underlying diagnosis (which in turn strongly influences clinical outcome) two age subgroups were separately evaluated (see Table 44-4). These were young persons—25 years and under—and older persons—65 years and older. The younger persons chiefly had cerebral palsy, a relatively stable condition; the older individuals had cerebrovascular disease, multiple sclerosis, motor neuron disease, and central nervous system trauma—disorders that are usually progressive. As shown in Table 45-4, 89% of the younger group survived 1 year (expected survival for a sex- and age-matched cohort of general US population is 99%) and 54% experienced complete or partial rehabilitation. Patients 65 years and older had only a 46% chance of surviving 1 year on HEN (expected survival 93%) and 86% experienced minimal rehabilitation.[5] This poor rehabilitation in the older patients probably reflects their more extensive neurological impairment. However, because it is common practice to initiate tube EN in patients who suffer a cerebrovascular accident, this poor outcome suggests quality-of-life studies are urgently needed. Not many patients with neuromuscular disorders, either young or old, graduate off HEN to full oral nutrition in the first 12 months. As with the HEN cancer patients, HEN therapy complications leading to rehospitalization are infrequent in neuromuscular disorders of swallowing.

The VA PEG study found no difference in survival between veterans discharged home on tube feeding compared to those discharged to an extended care facility. This is surprising as it would seem likely that those with a more positive prognosis were encouraged to go home.[9]

The British Artificial Nutrition Survey (1996 to 1999) looked specifically at stroke patients. The study found 1.7% of all stroke patients in the U.K. receive HEN.[21] One-year mortality was 30%, and 13% returned to oral feeding. Mortality was related to age and, for those in nursing homes, mortality was double the rate of those living at home. Among patients at home, 21% were independent, 30% were house bound, 42% were bed bound, and 2% were unconscious. Only 2% resumed full or part-time work, partly because 85% were retired or were children and partly because only one-third had normal speech and only one-fourth could leave home unaided. This group of patients spent only 0.6% of their time back in hospital. HEN represents an enormous cost saving to the hospital

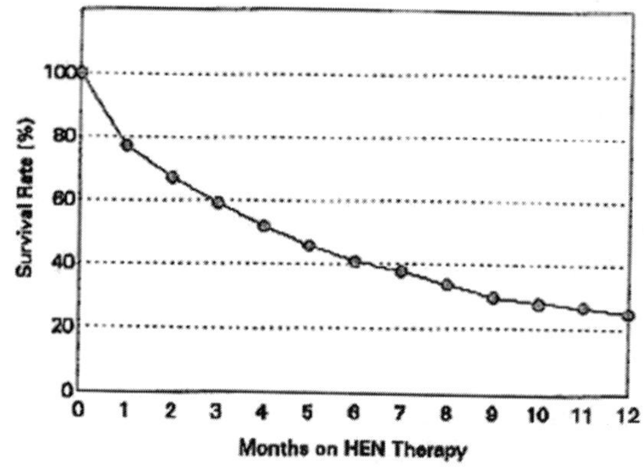

Figure 44-3. Survival rates on HEN for patients reported with active cancer to the North American HPEN Registry. The expected survival rate at 12 months for age and sex-matched individuals in the general US population is 97%.

system, but a large care burden shifted to home-care nurses and families. A study of nutrient intake in the frail, homebound, elderly population found that two-thirds of these subjects had a full-time caregiver.[31]

In most studies, tube removal has been possible in only 20% to 30% of these patients;[21,32,33] however, this points to the importance of intermittent assessment of a patient's swallowing function.[21] How to recognize the stroke patient with a good prognosis is clearly an important challenge, for in these patients, good nutrition support may speed recovery of speech and swallowing. This aspect is well described in the personal account of recovery from a stroke by Rick Davis.[34]

For stroke patients who do not regain independence (about 70%) some authors have concluded that PEG tubes serve chiefly to facilitate the patient's discharge from an expensive hospital bed to a less-expensive home or nursing-home setting.[32] This conclusion obviously raises serious ethical questions from a patient- and family-centered standpoint.

Small Bowel Malabsorption

HEN patients with small bowel malabsorption were about 10% of the North American HPEN Registry and European multicenter HEN sample. This may be an overestimate of prevalence because both of these databases obtained their information from specialized nutrition support programs. Such programs largely supervise HPN patients and only a minority of HEN patients. Most dysphagic HEN patients are cared for by other specialists: oncologists; neurologists; ear, nose, and throat surgeons; generalists; and geriatricians.

The majority of small bowel malabsorption HEN patients start out on HPN and graduate to HEN. Because their prognosis is good, they deserve special mention. The small bowel disease causing the severe malabsorption in the 329 patients reported to the North American Registry was a motility disorder in 36%, congenital bowel defect in 19%, Crohn's disease in 16%, ischemic bowel disease in 11%, and other nonmalignant causes of short bowel syndrome in 9%. The average age of these patients was 36 years and 82% survived 1 year on therapy (see Table 44-4). After a year, 45% of these patients resumed full oral nutrition, which indicates that, for many of these patients, HEN was a weaning step between HPN and the return to full oral nutrition.

Patients making this switch often experience initial problems with nausea, cramping, and diarrhea; they need strong encouragement to return to "eating" because HPN seemed easier. Most patients eventually consider the switch beneficial, recognizing they have moved away from a high-risk, high-cost therapy. Managing a short bowel patient enterally is challenging for the supervising physician, who must monitor hydration, fat-soluble vitamins, B12, and divalent cation status.

Other Disorders Leading to Nutritional Depletion

Dementia

HEN has been used in patients with Alzheimer's disease and other forms of dementia. However, the majority of tube-fed severe-dementia patients are in nursing homes. A study by Kaw and Kekas[11] found no evidence that such tube feeding improved the functional status or nutritional status of these patients. Mitchell et al[35] also found no survival benefit to nursing home residents with severe cognitive impairment compared to similar residents who were not tube fed. They emphasize that tube feeding does not prevent aspiration of pharyngeal secretions and may, in fact, increase the risk of regurgitation and aspiration.

Cystic Fibrosis

This disorder is often associated with failure to thrive due to the metabolic cost of chronic infection, increased work of breathing, and impaired absorption due to pancreatic insufficiency. The chronic malnutrition leads to growth failure, depression, impaired immunocompetence, and reduced muscle mass compromising breathing and clearance of secretions. Several reports have described improved outcome with supplemental HEN feeding in this population.[36-39] However, it is important to remember that cystic fibrosis is also associated with impaired GI motility and an increased incidence of esophageal reflux (Chapter 25). For this reason, safe tube feeding may necessitate a fundal plication or jejunal feeding.

Chronic Renal Failure

Severe nutritional depletion occurs in 15% of patients on chronic dialysis. This malnutrition chiefly reflects anorexia resulting from the uremic state; some patients also have a motility disturbance due to an autonomic neuropathy from underlying diabetes or gut muscle dysfunction from scleraderma. HEN is one of several strategies used to improve nutritional depletion in patients with chronic renal failure. The reports are mostly of children, in whom growth failure is readily recognized.[40] HEN has been delivered via NG feeding tubes or via PEGs in both hemodialysis and peritoneal dialysis patients and has been shown to restore growth,[41,42] reduce the incidence of peritonitis,[43] and improve post-transplant outcome.[44] There have also been case reports of complications.[45,46] The published reports of HEN in adults with chronic renal failure are few. Holley et al[47] described HEN in 10 dysphagic adults with renal failure. Hypophosphatemia was a common complication. Serum albumin increased and 1 patient improved sufficiently enough that he could return to full oral nutrition. Mortality rate was high at 1 year (50%). Use of HEN in malnourished adult chronic renal failure patients needs further study.

Human Immunodeficiency Virus and Acquired Immune Deficiency Syndrome

Now that therapy for human immunodeficiency virus (HIV) has improved, the problems of wasting have become less common. There are reports of HIV patients increasing their weight, function, and survival on HEN compared to nontreated controls.[48-52] However, when the HEN was delivered via a PEG,[48-51] there was an increased incidence of PEG infection and complications.

Preoperative Malnutrition

There are a few preoperative enteral studies showing substantial benefit in malnourished surgical patients. To date none of these studies have been true home tube enteral studies, but their results point in that direction. In a report from India, 110 malnourished patients awaiting surgery were randomized to 10 days of NG feeding or the routine hospital diet. The tube-fed patients showed significant improvement in body weight and serum protein levels and their postoperative mortality was reduced by 50% compared to mortality in the control group.[53] Foschi et al randomized preoperative patients with obstructive jaundice and transhepatic biliary drainage to EN or the routine hospital diet, and postoperative mortality was reduced 75% in the tube-fed group.[54] Both these early studies were preoperative in-patient studies. Flynn and Leightty conducted an outpatient study in patients with squamous cell carcinoma of the head and neck.[55] Patients were randomized to receive a nocturnal supplement or the routine diet for 10 to 20 days prior to surgery. Postoperative complications were reduced by 50% in the supplemented group. Von Meyenfeldt et al[56] randomized 151 patients with gastric or colorectal cancer to 10 days of either preoperative EN (n=50) or preoperative PN (n=51). Fifty controls went to surgery without delay. Stratification for weight loss allowed subset analysis. In the severely depleted patients, there was a significant decrease in intra-abdominal abscesses in both groups who received nutritional intervention compared to those in depleted controls.

Preoperative enteral immune-enhancing diets providing arginine, omega-3 fatty acids, and nucleotides have been shown to provide superior outcome compared to a standard isocaloric, isonitrogenous formula.[57,58] (Immune-enhancing EN formulas are discussed in detail in Chapter 42.)

These studies suggest substantial benefit from preoperative EN; to deliver this therapy by the most cost-saving approach would mean providing it to the preoperative patient at home, before their surgical admission. To date, most insurance carriers are not willing to cover such therapy at home. Under the legislated prosthetic device benefit, Medicare cannot currently cover preoperative build-up at home. This suggests that more studies are needed to demonstrate the cost effectiveness of preoperative HEN. (Perioperative nutritional support is discussed in greater detail in Chapter 29.)

Living With Home Enteral Nutrition

Because there are few quality-of-life studies published on HEN, this section is written with input from several experienced HEN patients, or "consumers," as they prefer to be called.

Physical Adjustments

All patients agree that it takes several months for their bodies to get used to HEN therapy, especially if they infuse overnight. There is interference with sleep because of some nausea, cramping, and diarrhea and the need for frequent trips to the bathroom. Eventually, with the right formula, adjustment of the feeding rate, and patient's use of medications, these difficulties generally subside.

For daytime mobility, small infusion pumps and back packs are available. These make daytime tube feeding relatively inconspicuous. Bolus infusion at several hour intervals is an option with intragastric feeding, but this is poorly tolerated with intrajejunal feeding.

Skin irritation around the feeding tube insertion site is common and may reflect increased intragastric pressure due to poor gastric emptying, too small a catheter in too large a hole, or the need to obstruct the escape of irritating digestive secretions, by "snugging up" the tube. Irritation is especially likely if the enterostomy tube is close to the consumer's waistline. After 3 to 6 months of use, the tube stem may be coated with dried secretions, which aggravate exit-site irritation. This is relieved by changing the tube. Long-term consumers with well-established enterocutaneous tracts can make this exchange themselves when the internal securing device is a balloon, readily deflated and inflated.

Figure 44-4 is an HEN complication chart developed for consumers and their caregivers by the Oley Foundation. It is available free of charge from the Foundation or copies can be downloaded from the Foundation's website.[59]

Home Parenteral Nutrition Versus Home Enteral Nutrition

Consumers with short bowel and malabsorption sometimes achieve enough bowel adaption to switch from HPN to HEN. Preference for one therapy over the other is mixed. Some people find HPN easier because of the lack of GI distress but they fear the constant risk of sepsis. Others note that, while HEN does cause more GI discomfort, it can be safely interrupted and a serious complication is rare. Both therapies are intrusive and all consumers stress the importance of having a supportive family.

Psychosocial Adjustments

Body Image

Although some HEN consumers use NG tubes and thus avoid the irritation of an enterostomy site, such tubes are conspicuous and interfere with socialization unless the consumer learns to insert their tube at night and remove it in the morning. A number of individuals have done this successfully over many years; however, percutaneous enterostomy tubes are far more common. Most consumers prefer low profile devices that are more discreet under light clothing and less often pulled on when dressing and undressing. The newly available gastro-jejunal button is an important development for persons who have to feed beyond the pylorus.

Intimacy

Experienced consumers stress the barriers to recovering an active sex life. Poor physical health, reduced self image because of tubes and ostomies, and the distress to the sexual partner all compound the situation. These consumers recommend frank discussion about sexual issues with their partner and planning intimate moments when they are off their infusion and not attached to tubes and pumps. Professionals can help by raising the topic, adjusting hormone levels to boost libido, and working out solutions to impotence.

Maintaining Compliance

Consumers describe the difficulty of maintaining the artificial feeding schedule every day. This requires determination from the patient that is similar to that required to comply with a rigid low-fat or gluten-free diet. For the consumer who has restored normal body composition and strength, a night off is usually preferred to just reducing each night's formula volume. Unfortunately, on occasion, one night off leads to skipping other nights until finally substantial weakness and weight loss recur. If the physician suspects poor compliance and the home nurse finds large amounts of unused formula, a frank discussion between the physician and the consumer is important, sometimes accepting the consumers preference to live a borderline situation. It seldom works to make the spouse a "policeman," but they can help by setting up the infusion equipment when the consumer is in an "undisciplined funk."

Not Eating

Dysphagic HEN consumers become acutely aware of how much family and social activity centers around food. Some start to avoid cooking and shopping for food and find it distressing to sit at a table and watch others eat. Experienced consumers recommend staying with a normal family role as much as possible and participating to maintain balance and sociability in the family, even when the consumer cannot eat. Some individuals choose to taste, chew, and discretely spit out. If guests are present, most consumers develop a simple way to explain that they are not eating, and they find that, when they are comfortable with their own situation, other parties accept them and their HEN.

Finding Help

With support from family and friends, most HEN consumers are better able to regain their independence and self confidence. Consumers say it takes 6 months to 1 year to adjust to their new life. They describe family support as best when help is given when they are experiencing a setback, but the family stands back when they are well again. Many HEN consumers feel they have built stronger interpersonal relationships with their family as a result of HEN and their underlying diagnosis.

HEN Complication Chart

The Oley Foundation
214 Hun Memorial, A-28
Albany Medical Ctr • Albany, NY 12208
(800) 776-OLEY/(518) 262-5079
www.oley.org bishopj@mail.amc.edu

Users are strongly advised to review this chart with their MD, noting any differences in protocols/procedures, prior to taking any actions recommended by this chart. The chart is intended as a helpful reference, and should not replace the advise of your MD. Users should read the entire chart, (at least briefly,) comparing symptoms listed in each section with those actually experienced by the consumer, before taking any action. "Prevention" steps are numbered to correspond with the "causes" listed in each section.

1- Nausea/Vomiting†

Symptoms:

* Nausea, vomiting
* Abdominal distress, distention, feeling bloated, cramping.
* Dry heaves/retching, cold sweat.

Immediate Action:

* Stop feeding.
* As per MD instruction, drain gastric contents through G-tube into a drainage bag/container or using a large syringe. If there is no return, flush with 10 cc water to make sure the tube is not blocked. Some tubes have valves (such as buttons) which make drainage difficult. If unable to vent button, call MD.
* If vomiting persists, call MD for appropriate intervention to avoid dehydration/fluid or electrolyte depletion (see Rare Complications #3 "Fluid/Electrolyte Depletion").

Causes:

1. Formula intolerance:
   A. High administration rate
   B. High formula concentration, allergy/intolerance of formula components
   C. Formula contaminated
2. Mechanical problems:
   A. Tube displaced (Improper tube placement; tube migration)
   B. Patient improperly positioned for feeding
3. Side effect of medication or other treatments such as chemotherapy
4. GI dysfunction:
   A. Poor gastric emptying, reflux, ulcer
   B. Bowel obstruction
   C. Constipation
5. Psycho-social stressors:
   A. Anxiety concerning tube feeding procedure
   B. Offensive odors, sight and smell of food
6. Coughing, post nasal drip, upper respiratory infection, sore throat
7. Intolerance to oral diet (i.e. high sugar, lactose content)

Prevention:

1 A. When feeding, build up rate and volume slowly. If nausea develops, decrease rate of HEN feeding until nausea subsides; gradually increase rate, then volume to previous level as tolerated, as per MD instruction.
   B. Discuss with MD the possibility of switching formulas.
   C. Use good handwashing and clean technique when handling HEN formula/equipment. Wash all equipment with hot water after each use. It is generally recommended to use 1 bag for feedings within a 24 to 48 hour period. Before reusing, thoroughly clean bags with warm water and place in a clean container in fridge to retard bacterial growth. Do not store or wash equipment in the bathroom. Check expiration date of formula. Inspect can for bulging/evidence of contamination before opening. Cover and store any open formula in refrigerator and discard after 24 hours. Maximum hang time for formula at room temp. is 8 to 12 hours. If possible hang cold formula to slow bacterial growth.
2. A. Examine tube for possible migration or dislodgment (See Complication #4 "Tube Displacement").
   B. Elevate head of bed or sit up with feedings. Position self onto right side after feedings.
3. When starting new medications, check with MD if nausea/vomiting is a possible side effect. If MD prescribes antiemetics, take at least 30 - 60 minutes prior to HEN feedings.
4 A. Take dysmotility/antireflux/ulcer medications as prescribed.
   B. If bowel obstruction is suspected, seek medical attention.
   C. See Complication #7 "Constipation"
5. A. Use stress reduction/relaxation techniques/antianxiety medication prior to HEN feedings. Seek out support/encouragement.
   B. Remove offensive sights/smells (bedpan/commode/smell of cooking/food aversion)
6. Notify MD of persistent cough/nasal drip/infection/sore throat for evaluation.
7. Review oral diet with RD to see if it contains elements that lead to nausea/vomiting.

† Early morning nausea/vomiting can be common when first starting tube feeds as the body adjusts to feeding overnight and waking with a "full stomach."

2 - Diarrhea

Symptoms:

* Abdominal pain or cramping with frequent loose watery stool (color may vary)

Immediate Action:

* Decrease volume/administration rate of HEN formula.
* Call MD if diarrhea is excessive (a noticeable increase in watery bowel movements for 24+ hours) to avoid fluid/electrolyte depletion (see rare complications #3).
* Call MD immediately if there is evidence of bleeding or if you are experiencing severe abdominal pain.

Causes:

1. Formula intolerance:
   A. High administration rate
   B. High formula concentration, allergy/intolerance of formula components
   C. Formula contaminated.
2. GI Dysfunction
   A. Short bowel syndrome
   B. Gastric Intestinal Colonization
   C. Bowel inflammation
3. Adverse side effects of medications, especially antibiotics
4. Intolerance to oral diet (i.e. high sugar, lactose content)

Prevention:

1 A. Use appropriate feeding method (bolus, gravity or pump). Build up feeding rate and volume slowly until you reach prescribed rate. If diarrhea develops, decrease rate of HEN feeding until diarrhea subsides; gradually increase rate, then volume to previous level as tolerated, as per MD instruction.
   B. Discuss with MD the possibility of switching formula (such as to one with fiber), and the possible need for pancreatic enzyme replacement or lactase enzyme.
   C. Use clean technique when handling and storing HEN formula/equipment. (see #1 Nausea/Vomiting - Prevention 1C.)
2. A. Discuss with MD the possible use of H2 blockers or bowel slowing medication.
   B. Report to MD any recent course of antibiotics. A stool culture may be needed.
   C. Seek MD input on controlling bowel inflammation.
3. Evaluate prescribed medications with RPh for possible sorbitol, magnesium, or phosphorus content. Take proper amount of medication as prescribed. Inform MD of any over the counter medications, herbals or supplements you may be taking.
4. Review oral diet (if any) with RD to see if it contains elements that lead to diarrhea (i.e. sugar, fat or lactose).

3 - Tube Obstruction / Blockage

Symptoms:

* Inability to flush with water, infuse tube feeding or administer medication.
* Bulging of tube when feeding by bolus.

Immediate Action:

* Make sure tube clamp is open.
* Do not force feeding or medication into clogged tube.
* Try to flush tube with large syringe (60 ml if possible) filled with warm water. Pull plunger back on syringe; try flushing again with warm water. If flushing doesn't work, call MD re: trying Viokase (see below). Viokase may not be as effective with a PEJ tube.

Causes:

1. Improper administration of medications or other non-formula additions with feeding. Medications not adequately crushed and dissolved before put into tube.
2. Inadequate flushing of tube.
3. Tube clamp is closed.
4. Defective tubing (such as valves leaking with buttons)
5. Infusion rate too low.

Prevention:

1. Consult with RPh/MD/RN regarding proper administration of medications. (Medications like Prevacid may require special attention.) When possible use liquid medications and dilute in 30 cc water; otherwise dissolve crushed or powder medications in 30 cc water. Administer each medication separately from food, flushing before and after with water: ask MD for appropriate volume to keep tube unclogged and meet your hydration needs. Never mix meds with formula.
2. Flush tube with water (ask MD for appropriate volume to keep tube unclogged and meet your hydration needs) after each feeding, administration of medication, and between administrations of medication and formula, so medications and formula never come in contact with each other in the feeding tube. Flush tube at least once a day if not in use.
3. Open clamp when flushing, feeding or administering medications.
4. Discuss tube replacement with MD.
5. Evaluate feeding rate and regimen with MD. Flush tube with water (ask MD for appropriate volume to keep tube unclogged and meet your hydration needs) every 6-8 hours with continuous feeds.

Suggested Protocol for Administering Viokase FOR MD USE ONLY:
Withdraw any EN formula or medication from tube. Attempt to flush tube with warm water. If unable to flush: **1.** Write order to obtain one Viokase® tab and one 300 mg sodium bicarbonate tablet for EN tube unclogging. **2.** Crush Viokase® tab and place in 15 ml warm water to disperse. **3.** Crush bicarbonate tablet and add to Viokase®/water mixture. **4.** Instill water/Viokase®/sodium bicarbonate mixture into tube. **5.** Allow to remain in tube for 30 minutes. **6.** Flush tube with 30 ml warm water. **7.** If tube is still clogged, consider repeating once.

4 - Tube Displacement

Symptoms:

* Tube out of body or otherwise obviously dislodged/displaced
* Choking /difficulty breathing.
* Nausea/vomiting; abdominal pain

Immediate Action:

* Discontinue feeding.
* If NG/NJ tube curled in the back of the throat, pull tube out of the entry site (not through throat). Do not remove percutaneously placed G/J/G-J tube without MD instruction: if one of these tubes falls out, reinsert if possible so the tract doesn't close, and call MD.
* Contact MD for instructions.

Causes:

1. Tube not adequately secured.
2. Accidental or excessive pulling of tube. Tubes with gastric balloon may be treated by the stomach as a piece of food and be pulled into the small bowel.
3. With G/G-J/NG/ NJ tube, persistent vomiting.
4. Balloon deflates/bursts.

Prevention:

1-3. Check external length of tube before each feeding. Mark feeding tube 1" from where it enters the body (so you can tell later if it's moved). Use a tube attachment device (catheter/tube holder) or careful taping of external tube to nose/cheek/abdomen/clothing to avoid pulling or migration. Specially-designed under garments that helps secure tubes can be purchased for active consumers.
3. See Complication #1 "Nausea/Vomiting."
4. Be sure balloon is intact (you should be able to aspirate a few cc's of water or air). If balloon has burst, wash tube, reinsert, secure position with tape, and call MD. If balloon is intact, deflate balloon, wash, reinsert and reinflate. Report to MD if problem persists.

Special thanks to the authors of this chart:
Kerry Stone, MS, RD, CNSD and Pat Brown, RN, CNSN, OCN

Figure 44-4. HEN complication chart, page 1.

5 - Skin/Site Irritation and/or Tube Leaking

Symptoms:

* Irritated skin, rash around tube; burning pain; foul odor; local infection. NG/NJ tube users may have developed sinus or ear infection.
* Leakage from the feeding tube itself (hole in tube, malfunctioning anti-reflux valve or cap) or from around the feeding tube.
* Need to change dressing more than once a day.

Immediate Action:

* If possible, clamp tube above defect.
* Stop feeding.
* Wash skin; apply dry dressing.
* Call MD.

Causes:

1. Poorly fitting tube. (Tube is too small for tube tract, stem of button is too long or internal bumper is not snug against anterior stomach wall.)
2. Tube tugging at exit site. (Excessive movement or tension at exit site causing enlargement of tube tract/ irritation/ulceration.) "Buried bumper syndrome" when an external bolster migrates into the stoma site.
3. Mechanical tube problem:
   A. Defective or deteriorated tubing or cap; or defective or clogged anti-reflux valve.
   B. Repeated clamping at same site, accidental cutting of the tube.

Prevention:

1. Discuss with MD/ET nurse tube sizing, tips to keep tube fitting snuggly to avoid skin infection. Check tube for possible migration (see #4 "Tube Displacement - Prevention 1-3."). Consult an ET nurse/MD re: skin care. The ET nurse/MD may apply/prescribe a steriod creme or silver nitrate if granulation tissue is a problem.
2. Secure tube as directed with tape or tube holder (see #4 "Tube Displacement - Prevention 1-3").
3. A. Discuss regarding tube/cap/button replacement with MD.
   B. Move clamp to a different site daily. Avoid using scissors or sharp objects near tube.

6 - Aspiration††

Symptoms:

* Vomiting, heartburn
* Coughing or choking with difficulty breathing; chest pain
* Possible fever, shortness of breath, indicating pneumonia

Immediate Action:

* Stop feeding.
* As per MD instruction, drain gastric contents through G-tube into a drainage bag/container or by a large syringe, if possible. Some tubes have valves (such as buttons) which make drainage difficult. If unable to vent button, call MD.
* Call MD for appropriate intervention.

Causes:

1. Diminished gag reflex, gastroesophageal reflux (GER), swallowing disorder
2. Delayed gastric emptying
3. Tube migration

††More likely to occur in patients whose are tube fed into their stomach (vs. small intestine)

Prevention:

1. Put head of the bed on 6" blocks for night time feedings. Feeding while sitting up or using wedge pillows increases abdominal pressure and can aggravate GER. Do not feed if stomach feels full or distended, or if individual is vomiting. Take prescribed medication for GER.
2. Position self on right side after feedings. Take prescribed medication for dysmotility. Do not feed if stomach feels full or distended, or if individual is vomiting.
3. Anchor tube with tube holder/tape to avoid pulling or dislodging. Check tube for possible migration before feeding (See Complication #4 "Tube Displacement - Prevention 1-3").

7 - Constipation

Symptoms:

* Infrequent hard stool, stool impaction. (Liquid stool may leak around impacted stool.)
* Abdominal bloating, cramping/pain.

Immediate Action:

* Increase fluid intake, use stool softener or laxative as per MD instruction.
* Call MD if no bowel movement in several days and/or are experiencing vomiting, or severe abdominal distention or cramping.

Causes:

1. Inadequate fluid or fiber intake
2. Side effect of medications (i.e. narcotics, high dose calcium or antacids containing calcium)
3. Inactivity
4. Gastrointestinal dysmotility
5. Bowel obstruction

Prevention:

1. Discuss prophylactic bowel regimen with MD/RD (i.e. increasing fluid and fiber intake, and/or use of a stool softener or laxative).
2. Discuss medications and possible side effects with MD.
3. Maintain regular exercise program, if able.
4. Take medication for dysmotility as prescribed by MD.
5. Call MD if you suspect bowel obstruction.

8 - GI Bleeding

Symptoms:

* Bright red blood on outside of stool or per rectum
* Black, tarry stool or diarrhea
* Black/brown blood in vomit (looks like coffee grounds)
* Vomiting bright red blood
* Bright red blood coming from and/or around tube

Immediate Action:

* Discuss all GI bleeding with MD. If large amounts of blood are visible, seek treatment immediately.

Cause:

1. Bright red blood on outside of stool or per rectum is likely caused by irritated hemorrhoids, fissure or an anal tear commonly linked to excessive diarrhea or constipation.
2. Black, tarry stool or diarrhea; black/brown blood in vomit; or >1 Tablespoon bright red blood in vomit likely indicates upper GI bleeding
3. Vomiting small amounts (< 1 Tablespoon) bright red blood when associated with frequent vomiting is likely caused by burst blood vessel in throat.
4. Bright red blood coming from tube or around the tube may be caused by:
   A. Gastric ulcer/irritation
   B. Erosion of stomach lining from excessive tube movement
   C. External granulation tissue.

Prevention:

1. Reduce diarrhea (see Complication #2 "Diarrhea") or avoid constipation (see Complication #7 "Constipation"). Discuss symptoms with MD.
2. Discuss with MD use of medications that block acid production.
3. Reduce vomiting (see Complication #1 "Nausea/Vomiting"). Discuss symptoms with MD.
4 A. Discuss with MD use of medications that block acid production.
   B. Secure tube as directed with tape or tube holder (see #4 "Tube Displacement - Prevention 1-3").
   C. Discuss granulation tissue with MD/ET nurse. (May be related to tube leakage and/or improper skin care. See Complication #5 "Skin/Site Irritation.")

9 - Pump or Power Failure

Symptoms:

* Unable to start pump.
* Repeated alarms without obvious cause.

Immediate Action:

* Check to see if pump is plugged into wall and that wall socket is functioning; or check that battery is charged.
* Stop pump. Consult pump user manual "trouble shooting" section for possible cause. Call home care company for replacement.
* If pump will not work and replacement pump is not available, convert to gravity drip and administer at same or lower rate. If tube is located at the jejunum, flow should not exceed a constant drip to avoid dumping syndrome.

Causes:

1. Power failure/low battery. Pump not plugged into wall outlet.
2. Pump malfunction.

Prevention:

1. Check electrical outlet. Notify local power company of durable medical equipment at home for emergency power outages. Keep pump plugged into electrical source whenever possible, even when infusing, if not ambulating to conserve battery charge.
2. Follow manufacturer/home care company recommendation for routine service/maintenance.

Rare Complications ...

1. Hyperglycemia

Symptoms: Nausea, weakness, excessive thirst or hunger, headache, anxiety, nightmares, frequent urination; Glucose levels greater than 1/2% (or other level set by your MD).

Action: Call your MD immediately for specific instructions.

Causes: Diabetes; body under a lot stress (due to illness, medications, steroids etc.)

Prevention: Discuss diabetes management with MD. Maintain prescribed volume and rate of HEN feedings.

2. Hypoglycemia

Symptoms: Shaking, nausea, pale facial color, heart palpitations, sweating, anxiety, dizziness, blurred vision, weakness, fatigue, headache, blood sugar below 50-60 mg/dl.

Action: Instill 2-4 ounces of orange juice, regular soda pop, or sugar water (1 tablespoon sugar to 4 ounces water) through feeding tube. (If you are unable to swallow, and if not contraindicated, place hard candy or cake decorating gel under tongue, or let 1-2 teaspoons of sugar dissolve in mouth.) Then call MD immediately for specific instructions.

Causes: Diabetes, Stopping a feeding suddenly for patients on insulin.

Prevention: Discuss diabetes management with MD. Maintain prescribed volume and rate of HEN feedings.

3. Fluid or Electrolyte Imbalances

Symptoms: Rapid weight loss or weight gain; thirst, weakness; edema, shortness of breath; shakiness; fine tremors; muscle cramping; numbness; tingling of hands or around mouth; palpitations; fatigue; taste changes; skin changes; loss of coordination

Causes: Increased losses from vomiting, diarrhea, fistulae/ostomy output, urine output. Decreased urine output.

Action: If you suspect a fluid overloaded or are extremely short of breath, stop HEN feedings and notify your MD immediately. Call MD regarding signs and symptoms and describe any change in weight, fluid intake or urine/stool output. MD may recommend taking more or less fluid via feeding tube.

Prevention: Take complete volume of HEN formula and fluids as ordered by MD. Discuss with MD indications for taking more or less fluid. Keep daily log of fluid intake, weight and urine/stool output — noting any significant fluctuations.

Revised 10/01

Figure 44-4. HEN complication chart, page 2.

TABLE 44-5.

Sample Articles on Enteral Nutrition Published in the Oley Foundation's Newsletter, Lifeline Letter

Article title	*Author(s)*	*Issue*
Home Enteral Nutrition	C. Ireton-Jones, PhD, RD	Nov/Dec 2003
On Top of the World	R. Davis	Nov/Dec 2003
Tube-Feeding–Associated Diarrhea	H.D. Duncan, MD, MRCP, and D.B. Silk, MD, FRCS	March/April 2003
Affiliation with Oley Foundation Improves Patient Outcome	C. Smith, RN, PhD	Sept/Oct 2002
ANCHOR: A Framework for Coping with Chronic Illness	N. Groat	March/April 2002
Tips for Traveling with Home PEN	R. Dahl	May/June 2001
There's an Elephant in Your Living Room	L. Howard	Sept/Oct 1999
Living with HEN	R. Dahl	Nov/Dec 1997

The articles listed are available, free of charge, from the Oley Foundation, (518) 262-5079. Copies can also be downloaded from the Foundation's website at www.oley.org.

Help outside the immediate circle of family and friends may come from specialists such as psychologists, who can help with body image, over dependence, or compliance problems; enterostomal therapists, who can help with tube-insertion–site problems or ostomies; and nutritionists, who can help maximize any oral intake.

National support is available through the Oley Foundation, which helps HEN and HPN consumers and their families through peer support and education. The Foundation publishes a bi-monthly newsletter that provides articles pertinent to the HEN consumer (Table 44-5). Many consumers are better able to participate in their own care if they learn more about their therapy and underlying disease. The Foundation's regional coordinator network, "toll-free hotline," and annual consumer conference provide peer support and keeps consumers abreast of new technical breakthroughs. Studies have shown the importance of peer support in fighting depression and avoiding complications.[60] Experienced consumers agree that peer support is most valuable in the first year or two, during the adjustment phase. However, many consumers stay involved with the Foundation and later play a vital mentoring role.

References

1. Bonsmann M, Hardt W, Lorber CG. The historical development of artificial enteral alimentation. Part 1. *Anasthesiol Intensivmed Notfallmed Schmerzther.* 1993;34:207-11.
2. Pariera MD. *Therapeutic Nutrition with Tube Feeding.* Springfield, IL, Charles C. Thomas; 1959.
3. Harkness L. The history of enteral nutrition therapy; from raw eggs and nasal tubes to purified amino acids and early post-operative jejunal delivery. *J Am Diet Assoc.* 2002;102(3):399-404.
4. Young-In Kim. To feed or not to feed: tube feeding in patients with advanced dementia. *Nutr Rev.* 2001;59:86-89.
5. North American Home Parenteral and Enteral Nutrition Patient Registry. *Annual Reports 1985-1992.* Albany, NY, Oley Foundation; 1987-1994.
6. Rabineck L, Wray NP, Petersen NJ, et al. Long term outcomes of patients receiving percutaneous endoscopic gastrostomy tubes. *J Gen Intern Med.* 1996;11:287-293.
7. Parker T, Neale G, Elia M. Home enteral tube feeding in East Anglia. *Eur J Clin Nutr.* 1996;50:47-53.
8. Planas M, Castell M, Garcia-Luna P, et al. Enteral nutrition at home. National Register for the year 2000. *Nutr Hosp.* 2003;18:34.
9. Hebuterne X, Bozzetti F, Moreno Villares JM, et al. ESPEN Home artificial nutrition working group. Home enteral nutrition in adults: a European multicenter survey. *Clin Nutr.* 2003;22(3):261-266.
10. Gramlich L. Home enteral nutrition in Canada: the Albertan experience. Presented at the Canadian Society for Clinical Nutrition. April, 2004; Toronto, Ontario.
11. Kaw M, Sekas G. Long term follow-up of consequences of percutaneous endoscopic gastrostomy (PEG) tubes in nursing home patients. *Dig Dis Sci.* 1994;39(4):738-743.
12. Bergstrom LR, Larson DE, Zinsmeister AR, et al. Utilization and outcomes of surgical gastrostomies and jejunostomies in an era of percutaneous endoscopic gastrostomy. A population based study of outcome (abstra). *J Parenter Enteral Nutr.* 1995;19 (Suppl):23S.
13. Howard L, Ament M, Fleming RC, et al. Current use and clinical outcome of home parenteral and enteral nutrition therapies in the U.S. *Gastroenterology.* 1995;109:355-365.
14. US Bureau of the Census. *Statistical Abstract of the United States 1994, ed 114.* Washington, DC, U.S. Government Printing Office, 1994.
15. Ireton-Jones C. Home enteral nutrition. Lifeline Letter Vol XXIV no 6. The Oley Foundation for home parenteral and Enteral Nutrition. 214 Hun Memorial, MC 28, Albany Medical College, Albany, NY 12208.
16. Health, United States, 2001, National Center for Health Statistics.
17. Parker T, Neale G, Cottee S, et al. Management of artificial nutrition in East Anglia: A community study. *J R Coll Physicians Lond.* 1996;30:27-32.

18. Elia M. Developing aspects of artificial nutrition in the community. Presented at the British Association for Parenteral and Enteral Nutrition Blackpool Conference, December 2, 1997.
19. Moreno JM, Shaffer J, Staun M, et al. Home artificial nutrition working group—ESPEN. Survey on legislation and funding of home artificial nutrition in different European countries. *Clin Nutr.* 2001;20(2):117-123.
20. Health Care Financing Administration. Medicare carriers manual: part 3 claims processs. Published 14-3, Transmittal 1036, July 1984.
21. Elia M, Stratton RJ, Holden C, et al. Committee of the British Artificial Nutrition Survey (BANS). Home enteral tube feeding following cerebrovascular accident. *Clin Nutr.* 2001;20(1):27-30.
22. Reddy P, Malone M. Cost and outcome analysis of home parenteral and enteral nutrition. *J Parenter Enteral Nutr.* 1998;22(5):302-10.
23. Stellato TA, Gauderer ML. Percutaneous endoscopic gastrostomy in the cancer patient. *Am Surg.* 1988;54:412-22.
24. Campos ACL, Butters M, Meguid MM. Home enteral nutrition via gastrostomy in advanced head and neck cancer patients. *Head Neck.* 1990;12:137-42.
25. Howard L. Home parenteral and enteral nutrition in cancer patients. *Cancer.* 1993;72:3531-41.
26. Szeluga DJ, Stuart RK, Brookmeyer R, et al. Nutritional support of bone marrow transplant recipients: a prospective randomized clinical trial comparing total parenteral nutrition to an enteral nutrition program. *Cancer Res.* 1987;47:3309-16.
27. Richards DM, Carlson GL. Quality of life assessment and cost effectiveness. In: Nightingale J, ed. *Greenwich Medical Media Limited.* 2001:447-457.
28. Schneider S, Blanc-Vincent MP Nitenberg G, et al. Standard options and recommendations for home parenteral or enteral nutrition in adult cancer patients, Bull. *Cancer.* 2001;6:605-618.
29. McCann RM, Hall WJ, Croth-Junker A. Comfort care for terminally ill patients. *JAMA.* 1994;272:1263-1266.
30. Bains M, Oliver DJ, Carter RI. Medical management of intestinal obstruction in patients with advanced malignant disease. *Lancet.* 1985;2:990-993.
31. Gloth M, Tobin J, Smith C, et al. Nutrient intake in a frail home bound elderly population in the community vs a nursing home population. *J Am Dietetic Assoc.* 1996;96:605-607.
32. Wolfsen HC, Kozarek RA, Ball TJ, et al: Long-term survival in patients undergoing percutaneous endoscopic gastrostomy and jejunostomy. *Am J Gastroenterol.* 1990;85(9):1120-1122.
33. Moran BJ, Frost RA. Percutaneous endoscopic gastrostomy outcome in 41 patients indications and clinical outcome. *J R Sco Med.* 1992;85(6):320-321.
34. Rick Davis. On top of the world. *Lifeline Letter.* 2003; XXIV(6).
35. Mitchell SL, Kiely DK, Lipsitz LA. The risk factors and impact on survival of feeding tube placement in nursing home residents with severe cognitive impairment. *Arch Intern Med.* 1997;157(3):327-32.
36. Moore MC, Greene HL, Donald WD, et al. Enteral-tube feeding as adjunct therapy in malnourisheddd patients with cystic fibrosis: a clinical study and literature review. *Am J Clin Nutr.* 1986;44(1):33-41.
37. Richter T, Meier C, Steppberger K, et al. Experiences with enteral nutrition of patients with cystic fibrosis (CF) via a percutaneous endoscopic gastrostomy (PEG). *Klin Padiatr.* 2001;213(6): 325-8.
38. Dalzell AM, Shephert RW, Dean B, et al. Nutritional rehabilitation in cystic fibrosis: a 5 year follow-up study. *J Pediatr Gastroenterol Nutr.* 1992;15(2):141-5.
39. Steinkamp G, Rodeck B, Seidenberg J, et al. Stabilization of long function in cystic fibrosis during long-term tube feeding via a percutaneous endoscopic gastrostomy. *Pneumologie.* 1990;44(10): 1151-1153.
40. Norman LJ, Coleman JE, Madonald IA, et al. Nutrition and growth in relation to severity of renal disease in children. *Pediatr Nephrol.* 2000;15(3-4):259-265.
41. Brewer ED. Growth of small children managed with chronic peritoneal dialysis and nasogastric tube feedings: 203-month experience in 14 patients. *Adv Perit Dial.* 1900;6:269-72
42. Coleman JE, Watson AR, Rance CH, et al. Gastrostomy buttons for nutritional support on chronic dialysis. *Nephrol Dial Transplant.* 1998;13(8):2041-2046.
43. Dabbagh S, Fassinger N, Clement K, et al. The effect of aggressive nutrition on infection rates in patients maintained on peritoneal dialysis. *Adv Perit Dial.* 1991;7:161-164.
44. Jones JW, Nevins T, McHugh L, et al. Nutrition and growth in pediatric renal transplant recipients. *Transplant Proc.* 1994;26(1):62-3.
45. Murugasu B, Conley SB, Lemire JM, et al. Fungal peritonitis in children treated with peritoneal dialysis and gastrostomy feeding. *Pediatr Nephrol.* 1991;5(5):620-621.
46. Wood EG, Bunchman TE, Khurana R, et al: Complications of nasogastric and gastrostomy tube feedings in children with end stage renal disease. *Adv Perit Dial.* 1990;6:262-264.
47. Holley JL, Kirk J. Enteral tube feeding in a cohort of chronic hemodialysis patients. *J Ren Nutr.* 2002;12(3):177-182.
48. Ockenga J, Suttman U, Selberg O, et al. Percutaneous endoscopic gastrostomy in AIDS and control patients: risks and outcome. *Gastroenterol.* 1996;91(9):1817-22.
49. Crotty B, McDonald J, Mijch AM, et al. Percutaneous endoscopic gastrostomy feeding in AIDS. *J Gastroenterol Hepatol.* 1998; 13(4):371-5.
50. Cappell MS, Godil A. A multicenter case-controlled study of percutaneous endoscopic gastrostomy in HIV-seropositive patients. *Am J Gastroenterol.* 1993;88(12):2059-66.
51. Brantsman A, Kelson K, Malcom J. Percutaneous endoscopic gastrostomy feeding in HIV disease. *Aust J Adv Nurs.* 1991;8(4):36-41.
52. Kotler DP, Tierney AR, Ferraro R, et al. Enteral alimentation and repletion of body cell mass in malnourished patients with acquired immunodeficiency syndrome. *Am J Clin Nutr.* 1991;53(1):149-54.
53. Shukla HS, Rao RR, Banu N, et al. Enteral hyperalimentation in malnourished surgical patients. *Indian J Med Res.* 1984;80:339-346.
54. Foschi D, Cavagna G, Callioni F, et al. Hyperalimentation of jaundiced patients on percutaneous trans-hepatic biliary drainage. *Br J Surg.* 1986;73(9);716-719.
55. Flynn MB, Leightty FF. Preoperative outpatient nutritional support of patients with squamous cancer of the upper aerodigestive tract. *Am J Surg.* 1987;154(4);359-362.
56. von Meyenfeldt MF, Meijerink WJHJ, Rouflart MMJ, et al. Perioperative nutritional support: a randomized clinical trial. *Clin Nutr.* 1992;11:180-186.
57. Gianotti L, Braga M, Vignali A, et al. Effects of route of delivery and formulation of postoperative nutrition support in patients under going major operations for malignant neoplasms. *Arch Surg.* 1997;132(11):1222-1229.
58. Braga M, Gianotti L, Radaelli G, et al. Perioperative immunonutrition in patients undergoing cancer surgery: results of a randomized double-blind phase 3 trial. *Arch Surg.* 1999:134(4):428-433.
59. The Oley Foundation. Web site. Available at: http://c4isr.com/oley. Accessed June 28, 2005.
60. Smith CE, Curtas S, Werkonitch M, et al. Home parenteral nutrition: Does affiliation with a national support and education organization improve patient outcome? *J Parenter Enteral Nutr.* 2002; 26:159-163.

Chapter 45

Refeeding Syndrome

Le-Chu Su, MD, PhD, and Laura E. Matarese, MS, RD, LDN, FADA, CNSD

Introduction

Malnutrition has an adverse impact on morbidity and mortality in hospitalized patients. The incidence of hospital malnutrition ranges from 30% to 50%,[1-3] yet is often unrecognized by healthcare professionals. Refeeding syndrome, resulting from the overzealous resuscitation of the severely malnourished patient is also unrecognized. This can result in sudden decompensation and death that may have been attributed to electrolyte, hemodynamic, and septic derangements. The exact prevalence of refeeding syndrome is unknown because it is generally underdiagnosed. The syndrome itself has not been well studied and most of the information in the literature is in the form of case reports or case series.

The refeeding syndrome is characterized by symptoms and signs, which include general fatigue, lethargy, muscle weakness, edema, cardiac arrhythmias, and hemolysis. It had been considered to result from severe hypophosphotemia and its associated complications, which may be seen in patients being repleted with parenteral nutrition (PN) after severe weight loss. However, refeeding syndrome has been re-defined as the metabolic and physiologic consequences of depletion, repletion, compartmental shifts, and interrelationships of phosphorus, potassium, magnesium, glucose metabolism, vitamin deficiency, and fluid resuscitation.[4] It is a metabolic consequence of starvation. Refeeding syndrome is a potentially life-threatening condition that requires immediate and aggressive treatment.

Historical Perspective

Keys et al reported their results of the Minnesota Experiment during the 1940s in which healthy volunteers developed diminished cardiac reserve, while being refed after a 6-month starvation.[5] These findings were similar to reports of cardiopulmonary and neurological complications experienced by victims of World War II.[6] This refeeding phenomenon was observed again in the 1970s with the introduction of PN.[7-9] It was of particular interest because the PN solution of that time tended to be high in calories and entirely dextrose based. Refeeding syndrome has also been noted in patients receiving enteral nutrition (EN).[10-12]

Pathophysiology

Patients who have been chronically starved as a result of anorexia, maldigestion, malabsorption, or chronic illness and are then aggressively fed are at risk for refeeding syndrome. Chronic undernutrition as a result of starvation or weight loss over a few weeks causes gradual loss of skeletal muscle mass and of functional tissue from organ systems. This initial phase of depletion causes a metabolic adaptation in which there is a slowing of metabolic rate. In addition, total body stores of vitamins, and electrolytes including phosphorus, potassium, magnesium, zinc and trace elements are also eventually depleted. (The clinical consequences of undernutrition are presented in detail in Chapter 4.)

There are three potential energy substrates: glucose, protein, and fat. Carbohydrate is the primary fuel for many tissues and the obligatory fuel for the brain, red blood cells, white blood cells, and the renal medula. When the available glucose decreases, glycogen stores are mobilized and can provide fuel for approximately 12 hours.[13] Protein is not stored in the body because all proteins are utilized for nonfuel functions such as contractile, structural, and enzymatic functions. Proteins, which are ingested in excess of requirements, are converted to fat, stored, eventually metabolized, and then excreted as urea.[13] Fat is stored in the adipose tissue. Circulating triglycerides provide fuel when broken down to free fatty acids and glycerol. Nonesterified fatty acids and ketone bodies provide fuel to the heart, kidneys, and skeletal muscle.

During a brief fast, energy is derived from muscle protein stores once glycogen reserves have been depleted. The liver adapts by converting pyruvate, lactate, glycerol, and glucogenic amino acids into glucose. During prolonged starvation, the body adapts by decreasing gluconeogenesis and increasing utilization of ketones and fatty acids, which do not require phosphate to produce energy. This spares protein reserves until fat stores are depleted. Insulin, thyroid, and adrenergic endocrine systems decrease activity with starvation. When refeeding occurs, an anabolic environment is created and there is a sudden shift to glucose as a primary fuel; these endocrine systems are initiated, and the metabolic rate is accelerated. Hyperglycemia can result in further metabolic derangements of osmotic diuresis, dehydration, hypotension, hyperosmolar nonketotic coma, and metabolic acidosis. Overfeeding adds to the physiologic burden by increasing cardiac output, respirations, substrate oxidation, and synthesis of ATP and protein.

Nutrient Abnormalities

Electrolyte Abnormalities

Potassium and magnesium are intracellular cations. When a starved patient is suddenly placed in anabolism, there is an increased need for potassium, magnesium, and phosphorus. During refeeding, there is an increase in insulin levels resulting from the administration of nutrient substrates. Elevated insulin levels force potassium intracellularly by increasing the cell's permeability to sodium and activating the sodium- and potassium-dependent adenosine triphosphatase. Potassium is also required for protein and glycogen anabolism, with 3 mEq of potassium required for each gram of nitrogen and 1 mEq of potassium for every 3 g of glycogen, respectively. The magnesium level may also fall with anabolism as 0.5 mEq of magnesium is required for each gram of nitrogen.[14] The situation may be further complicated by diarrhea, which is common in malnourished individuals. This may contribute to losses of both potassium and magnesium.

Phosphorus Deficiency

The most widely recognized abnormality associated with refeeding syndrome is hypophosphatemia. Phosphate is an intracellular anion that is essential for membrane structure and energy storage and transport in all cells. In particular, phosphate is necessary to produce adenosine triphosphate (ATP), which provides energy for nearly all cell functions. Phosphate also is necessary in red blood cells for production of 2,3-diphosphoglycerate (2,3-DPG), which facilitates release of oxygen from hemoglobin. During starvation, the serum concentration of phosphorus remains constant because of adjustments in renal excretion rates. However, during refeeding, particularly with carbohydrate, insulin is secreted. The combination of carbohydrate repletion and insulin release together enhance uptake of glucose, phosphorus, water, and other components into cells, as well as stimulate anabolic protein synthesis. The combination of depleted body stores and the increased cellular uptake during anabolic refeeding results in severe extracellular hypophosphatemia, which leads to a depletion of phosphorylated intermediates and compounds such as red cell ATP; 2,3-DPG; and G-3-PD. Diuretic use and concurrent hypokalemia and hypomagnesemia can potentiate phosphate losses.

Vitamin Deficiencies

Thiamin deficiency is also believed to be a component of refeeding syndrome. Thiamin is required for intermediate carbohydrate metabolism but is not stored in appreciable amounts in the body. Thiamin deficiency can develop in patients whose intake is low (eg, those with anorexia nervosa, alcoholism or prolonged starvation). Once refeeding with carbohydrate-based solutions is initiated, the need for thiamin is increased. The most severe manifestations of thiamin deficiency are cardiac failure and Wernicke's encephalopathy.[15-17] There appears to be synergistic effect between phosphorus and thiamin. Japanese prisoners during World War II who developed edema were not responsive to the administration of thiamin.[6]

Glucose Metabolism

Refeeding with dextrose-based solutions should be approached cautiously. Exogenous administration of glucose to chronically starved patients does have some positive effects. It decreases gluconeogenesis and thus preserves protein stores. However, exceeding optimal rates of glucose administration (4 mg/kg/minute) can result in hyperglycemia, hyperosmolar non-ketotic coma, metabolic acidosis, osmotic diuresis, dehydration, and hypotension. There is also a risk of increased carbon dioxide production in some patients.[18-20]

Fluid Balance

Refeeding with carbohydrate results in a decrease in sodium and water excretion. This, combined with increase sodium intake, can lead to rapid expansion of extracellular fluid volume.[21] Expansion of the extracellular fluid volume is significant and occurs rapidly. This frequently results in edema. This is a direct result of increased sodium intake combined with the antinatriuretic effect of insulin stimulated by increased carbohydrate infusion.[19] Levels of aldosterone and antidiuretic hormone are increased in injury response, a process that further enhances retention of sodium and fluids. Additionally, hypophosphatemia causes a reduction is sodium and water excretion. The exact mechanism for this is unknown.

System Dysfunction

Cardiac Abnormalities

Significant cardiac decompensation and sudden death has occurred with the infusion of fluid, glucose, and both.[3,21] The reasons for this are multifactoral. Volume overload, with peripheral and pulmonary edema, may develop rapidly during refeeding. This can be minimized by limiting the amount of sodium during this period. Left heart failure may occur, especially in predisposed patients. This results from an abrupt increase of the intravascular volume; increased resting energy expenditure (which increases demand for cardiac output); an atrophic left ventricle with a poor stroke volume;[5] and myocardial deficiencies of potassium, phosphorus, or magnesium. Cardiac arrhythmias may occur from hypokalemia and hypomagnesemia.[22] Many fatalities associated with overzealous resuscitation of the malnourished patient may be attributed to nutritional cardiomyopathy. The starved myocardium may not have the functional reserve to handle the acute volume overload that is a complication of refeeding.

Neuromuscular Dysfunction

The neuromuscular manifestations associated with refeeding syndrome are generally a result of hypophosphatemia and the resulting red blood cell dysfunction and tissue hypoxia. These include acute areflexic paralysis, paresthesias, diffuse sensory loss, weakness numbness, confusion, coma, Gullain-Barre-like syndrome, and rhabdomyolysis.[3,7,10,23-25]

Respiratory failure has also been reported.[26-28] This may be due to a reduction in available ATP to facilitate respiratory muscle contraction. Supplementation with phosphorus has been shown to improve respiratory function.[27] Respiratory status may also be influenced by excessive carbohydrate administration leading to increased carbon dioxide production.[29-30]

Risk Groups

Recognizing individuals at risk is essential to the prevention of refeeding syndrome. Chronically malnourished patients are susceptible to refeeding syndrome. Incidence of refeeding syndrome is high in cancer patients receiving nutritional support.[31] Sudden death, heart failure, rhabdomyolysis, and delirium had been reported in patients with anorexia nervosa during the first weeks of refeeding.[32-37] In addition, lower levels of prealbumin were found to be predictors of hypophosphatemia in one study.[38] Starvation for as little as 48 hours may predispose hypoalbuminemic patients in the intensive care unit to hypophosphatemia upon refeeding.

Furthermore, individuals with possible marginal nutrition stores or depletion may overwhelm their body reserves upon rapid refeeding when there are increased nutritional needs from disease or stress. Hypophosphatemia, hypokalemia, and hypomagnesemia are common in hospitalized medical and surgical patients who are severely ill and receiving either EN or PN.[38-43] It was suggested that larger doses of phosphorus may be required to meet the high metabolic needs of critically ill patients receiving PN.[44,45] Electrolyte and fluid abnormalities are also noted when patients resume nutrition either by parenteral or oral routes after being sustained with intravenous hydration for 7 to 10 days.[38,46] Elderly patients, especially those with chronic illness or medical problems, are at risk for the complications of refeeding syndrome and require closer monitoring upon refeeding.[47,48] Obese patients with massive weight loss are also prone to refeeding syndrome.[49,50] Poorly nourished alcoholic patients commonly manifest hypophosphatemia, multiple electrolyte, and vitamin disturbances during hospitalization.[39,51-53] Serum levels of electrolytes in alcoholic patients may be normal initially but decline after admission. Rhabdomyolysis, myocardial dysfunction, hematological abnormalities, and seizure had been observed in alcoholic patients with hypophosphatemia. It is a common practice to supplement thiamin to hospitalized alcoholic patients.

Management

The pathophysiological mechanism of refeeding syndrome has not been well studied. The onset of the syndrome probably depends on the patient's degree of malnutrition and the caloric, electrolyte, and vitamin supplies in parenteral or enteral formulations and concomitant medical problems and drug therapy.[54] It can occur rapidly and usually manifests within the first few days after institution of refeeding. Therefore, after nutrition support is initiated, the patient's vital functions, body weight, fluid balance, and cardiac and pulmonary status need to be followed closely.

It should be cautioned that excessive early weight gain might be caused by fluid retention.[54] In addition, tachypnea and tachycardia might be early signs of refeeding syndrome.[47,55] Serum levels of electrolytes may drop rapidly with refeeding and the adverse consequences follow. Therefore, vigilant monitoring of the serum concentrations of phosphorus, potassium, magnesium, calcium, sodium, glucose, and urinary electrolytes is vital to the prevention of refeeding syndrome. Daily monitoring of the electrolyte for the first few days of refeeding or until patient is stable is required. PN and EN may have to be temporarily stopped when there is severe electrolyte and fluid derangements.

Currently, there is no consensus about the management of refeeding syndrome. However, several investigators had proposed treatment strategies for hypophosphatemia (Table 45-1). One of the difficulties in managing electrolyte deficits lies in the lack of quick and feasible clinical means to assess the degree of electrolyte depletion because serum levels are not always reflecting body stores of the electrolytes. There is also no set rule to predict the response of patients to phosphorus repletion. Treatment of hypophosphatemic patients is considered empiric. Besides basal requirements and degree of deficit, other factors such as renal function, disease process, stress, and

TABLE 45-1.

Treatments for Hypophosphatemia in Patients With Normal Renal Function

Study	Serum Phosphorus	Intravenous Regimen	Comments
Lentz[56]	<1 mg/dl	0.08 mmol/kg/6 h	Recent, uncomplicated
		0.16 mmol/kg/6 h	Prolonged multi-causes
		25% to 50% higher dose	If symptomatic
		25% to 50% lower dose	If hypercalcemia, maximum 0.24 mmol/kg/dose
Vannatta[65,69]	≤ 1 mg/dl	9 mmol/12 h	
		0.32 mmol/kg/12 h	Multiple causes
Kingston[64]	0.5 to 1 mg/dl	<0.25 mmol/kg/4 h	
	<0.5 mg/dl	0.5 mmol/kg/4 h	
Zazzo[40]	0.65-1.5 mg/dl	0.4 mmol/kg/30 min	
	<0.65 mg/dl	0.8 mmol/kg/30 min	
Clark[61]	2.3-3 mg/dl	0.16 mM/kg	In 100 ml normal saline or 5% dextrose water over 4 to 6 h
	1.6-2.2 mg/dl	0.32 mM/kg	As above
	<1.5 mg/dl	0.64 mM/kg	In 150 ml normal saline or 5% dextrose over 8 to 12 h
Rosen[62]	1.6-1.9 mg/dl	15 mMol/2 h	No more than 45 mMol/24 h
Miller[70]	Non-life threatening	≤ 30 mMol/day	
	Life threatening	90 mMol/day	
Terlevich[71]	<1.5 mg/dl	50 mMol (1.55 g)/24 h	Phosphates polyfusor

medications also influence the need of electrolyte repletion. Furthermore, intravenous phosphorus is not without hazard. Hyperphosphatemia can cause hypocalcemia, hypernatremia, hyperkalemia, hypotension, renal failure, shock, arrhythmia, and metastatic calcification of soft tissues and death.[56-58] Phosphate supplementation is, therefore, contraindicated in patients with renal failure, hypercalcemia, symptomatic hypocalcemia, and hyperkalemia. Data are lacking about the safe dosage and rate of infusions of phosphate repletion. This is reflected by the wide variation of dosage and infusion rate in the treatment protocols (see Table 45-1). In general, the dosage and rate of infusion depend on the level of serum phosphate and symptoms. Most important of all, initial repletion should be judicious with frequent monitoring of the electrolytes. Subsequent dosage should be adjusted based on patient's response to treatment. Repeat dosages may be required and iatrogenic hyperphosphatemia should be avoided.

There is also difference of opinion in the serum concentration of phosphorus that is considered to be threshold for treatment. Symptoms of hypophosphatemia rarely occur unless the serum levels is less than 2 mg/dl. Severe cardiovascular abnormalities, respiratory complications, and rhabdomyolysis of hypophosphatemia usually manifest when the serum phosphorous level is less than 1 mg/dl.[41,56,59] Some investigators felt that the treatment is usually not necessary unless the serum level of phosphorus drops to 1 mg/dl or the patient is symptomatic,[60] while others initiate treatment at mild or moderate levels of hypophosphatemia.[61,62] Intravenous phosphate is recommended when hypophosphatemia is severe or patient is symptomatic. A separate infusion line for the large supplemental phosphate is advised to prevent potential fatal problems of compatibility and stability of the nutrition formulations.[54] When there is concurred potassium deficiency, potassium phosphate is preferred. Frequent monitoring of phosphorus, magnesium, potassium, calcium, urinary electrolytes, and renal function is very important. When the serum concentration of phosphorus reaches 2 mg/dl, intravenous phosphate should be switched to oral supplementation in patients with functional gastrointestinal (GI) tract. Potential diarrhea may be reduced by giving the oral phosphate supplements in divided doses.[63]

Hypomagnesemia and hypophosphatemia often coexist in patients who are at risk for refeeding syndrome. Magnesium deficiency impairs the secretion and action of parathyroid hormone. It may exacerbate hypophosphatemia, hypokalemia, and hypocalcemia.[39] Phosphate and magnesium should be replaced simultaneously to avoid prolong phase of treatment.[39,64,65] Hypokalemia can become refractory to treatment without first correction of hypomagnesemia.

Adverse effects of magnesium supplementation rarely occur in patients with normal renal function. Early symptoms of hypermagnesemia include nausea, vomiting, and cutaneous flushing from rapid infusions. More serious adverse effects—eg, hypotension, bradycardia, respiratory depression, mental status depression, and electrocardiographic changes—are associated with markedly elevated serum concentration and are unlikely during repletion.[54,66] Oral magnesium salts may be used in asymptomatic hypophosphatemia; however, they can be poorly absorbed and cause GI upset. In patients with moderate to severe magnesium deficiency, intravenous administration of 25 mmol of magnesium over 12 to 24 hours is suggested.[66] In severe hypomagnesemia (<1 mg/dl) or if symptomatic, 24 mmol magnesium sulfate can be given over 6 hours.[60] When seizure or arrhythmia develops, 4 to 8 mmol bolus can be given in 5 to 10 minutes and followed by 25 mmol/day.[66] Other regimens suggest supplementation of 2 to 4 mEq/kg in severe hypomagnesemia (<1.0 mg /dl) or symptomatic hypomagnesemia.[54,64] An alternative regimen administers magnesium 6g (49 mEq) over 3 hours, followed by another 6g (49 mEq/L) of fluid over the next 21 hours.[67,68] Serum concentration of magnesium should be followed closely and subsequent dose adjusted accordingly. A maintenance dose is frequently required after correction of the hypomagnesemia.

Hypokalemia is easily recognized by common routine tests and may be corrected by intravenous or oral routes. Oral repletion is preferred unless oral intake is restricted or hypokalemia is severe. For severe hypokalemia, potassium may be given through a peripheral intravenous line. In general, it should not exceed an infusion rate of 20 mEq/hour, and the total amount of potassium in a single intravenous bag should be restricted to 20 to 40 mEq to avoid the risk of hyperkalemia, local irritation, and sclerosis of the vein. Most hospitals have established protocols for intravenous potassium therapy. Electrocardiographic monitoring is usually advised. Frequent monitoring of serum potassium is crucial.

Attention should also include acid-base status, concomitant medical problems, and drug therapy in patients who are at risk for refeeding syndrome and during management of the disorder. Acid-base disturbance exacerbates intracellular shift of phosphorus and potassium. Respiratory alkalosis may cause severe hypophosphatemia. Prolonged nasogastric suctioning, vomiting, diarrhea, and renal dysfunction contribute to electrolyte abnormalities and alter repletion requirements. Medications may need to be modified to facilitate electrolyte repletion.

The disorder of refeeding syndrome is usually corrected within 24 to 48 hours after the repletion of electrolyte is initiated. Resolution of some adverse effects, particularly neurological effects, however, may lag behind.

Avoiding Refeeding Syndrome

The first step in avoiding refeeding syndrome is awareness and recognition of the patients who are at greatest risk. It is important to avoid overzealous nutritional resuscitation. Nutrition is not an emergency. It is important to first correct any fluid, electrolyte, and mineral abnormalities prior to initiation of feeding. Once feeding is initiated, provide the patient with one-half of his or her energy requirements based on current dry body weight or approximately 20 kcal/kg/day. Energy should be supplied as mixed fuels containing both lipid and carbohydrate. Protein should be supplied at 1.0 to 1.2 g/kg actual dry body weight. Electrolytes, intake and output records, and daily weights must be monitored closely. If no untoward effects are seen, the patient can advance to their full caloric requirements over a 5- to 7-day period.

Conclusions

Refeeding syndrome can result in prolonged hospital stay, morbidity, and even death if not recognized and treated promptly. The key to avoid the metabolic, physiologic, and multi-organ complications of refeeding syndrome is prevention. Gastroenterologists frequently encounter patients at risk for refeeding syndrome and can assist in enhancing its awareness, prevention, and management.

It is important to be familiar with the syndrome and recognize individuals who are likely to develop refeeding syndrome. Electrolyte, mineral, and fluid abnormalities should be corrected before the initiation of nutrition support. An initial normal level of serum electrolytes or supplementation of electrolytes, minerals, and vitamins in nutrition formulations should not be perceived as security against the development of refeeding syndrome. Importantly, caloric goals should be given gradually and slowly, based on current body weight. Vital signs, body weight, electrolytes, and fluid status must be monitored closely. When refeeding syndrome develops, replacement of the deficits should be guided by frequent and vigilant monitoring of the serum electrolytes and by patient's response to treatment.

References

1. Bistrian BR, Blackburn GL, Vitale J, et al. Prevalence of malnutrition in general medical patients. *JAMA*. 1976;235:1567-1570.
2. Hill GL, Blackett RL, Pickford I, et al. Malnutrition in surgical patients: an unrecognized problem. *Lancet*. 1977;1:689-692.
3. Weinsier RL, Hunker EM, Krumdieck CL, et al. Hospital malnutrition: a prospective evaluation of general medical patients during the course of hospitalization. *Am J Clin Nutr*. 1979;32:418-426.
4. Solomon SKD. The refeeding syndrome: a review. *Journal of Parenteral & Enteral Nutrition*. 1990;14:90-97.
5. Keys A, Brozek J, Henschel A, et al. *The Biology of Human Starvation*, vols 1, 2. Minneapolis: University of Minnesota Press; 1950.
6. Brozek J, Chapman CB, Keys A. Drastic food restriction: effect on cardiovascular dynamics in normotensive and hypertensive conditions. *JAMA*. 1948;137:1569-1575.
7. Silvis SE, Paragas Jr PD. Parasthesias, weakness, seizures, and hypophosphatemia in patients receiving hyperalimentation. *Gastroenterology*. 1972; 62:513-520
8. Sand DW, Pastore RA. Paresthesia and hypophosphatemia occurring with parenteral alimentation. *Am J Dig Dis*. 1973;18:709-13.

9. Weinsier RL, Krundieck CL. Death resulting from overzealous total parenteral nutrition: the refeeding syndrome revisited. *Am J Clin Nutr.* 1981;34:393-399.
10. Vanneste J, Hage J. Acute severe hypophosphatemia mimicking Wernicke's encephalopathy [letter]. *Lancet.* 1986;1:44.
11. Hayek ME, Eisenberg PG. Severe hypophosphatemia following the institution of enteral feedings. *Arch Surg.* 1989;124:1325-1328.
12. Silvis SE, DiBartolomeo AG, Aaker HM. Hypophosphatemia and neurological changes secondary to oral caloric intake. *Am J Gastroenterol.* 1980;73:215-222.
13. Cahill GF. Starvation in man. *N Eng J Med.* 1970;282:668-75.
14. Rudman D, Millikan WJ, Richardson TJ, Bixler TJ, Stackhouse WJ, McGarrity WC. Elemental balances during intravenous hyperalimentation of underweight adult subjects. *J Clin Invest.* 1975; 55:94-104.
15. Reuler JB, Girard DE, Cooney TG. Wernicke's encephalopathy. *N Engl J Med.* 1985;312:1035-1039.
16. Drenick EJ, Joven CB, Swendseid ME. Occurrence of acute Wernicke's encephalopathy during prolonged starvation for the treatment of obesity. *N Engl J Med.* 1966;274:937-939.
17. Mattioli S, Miglioli M, Montagna P, et al. Wernicke's encephalopathy during total parenteral nutrition: observation in one case. *J Par Ent Nutr.* 1988;12:626-627.
18. Holroyde CP, Meyers RN, Smith RD, et al. Metabolic response to total parenteral nutrition in cancer. *Cancer Res.* 1977;37:3109-3144.
19. DeFronzo RA, Jacot E, Jequier E, et al. The effect of insulin on the disposal of intravenous glucose: results from indirect calorimetry and hepatic and femoral venous catherization. *Diabetes.* 1981;30: 1000-1007.
20. Thiebaud D, Schultz Y, Acheson K, et al. Energy cost of glucose storage in human subjects during glucose-insulin infusions. *Am J Physiol.* 1983;244,E216-221.
21. Heymsfield SB, Bethel RA, Ansley JD, Gibbs DM, Felner JM, Nutter DO. Cardiac abnormalities in cachetic patients before and during nutritional repletion. *Am Heart J.* 1978;8(95):584-594.
22. Fisler JS. Cardiac effects of starvation and semistarvation diets: safety and mechanisms of action. *Am J Clin Nutr.* 1992;56:230S-234S.
23. Furlan AJ, Hanson M, Cooperman A, et al. Acute areflexic paralysis: association with hyperalimentation and hypophosphatemia. *Arch Neurol.* 1975;32:707-707.
24. Sand DW, Pastore RA. Paresthesias and hypophosphatemia occurring with parenteral alimentation. *Am J Dig Dis.* 1973;18:709-13.
25. Weintraub MI. Hypophosphatemia mimicking acute Guillain-Barre-Strohl syndrome: a complication of parenteral hyperalimentation. *JAMA.* 1976;235:1040-1041.
26. Newman JH, Neff TA, Ziporsin P. Acute respiratory failure associated with hypophosphatemia. *N Eng J Med.* 1977;296,1101-1103.
27. Youssef HAE. Hypophosphatemic respiratory failure complicating total parental nutrition—an iatrogenic potentially lethal hazard [letter]. *Anesthesiology.* 1982;57:246.
28. Fisher J, Magid N, Kallman C, et al. Respiratory illness and hypophosphatemia. *Chest.* 1983;83,504-508.
29. Covelli HD, Black JW, Olsen MS, Beekman JF. Respiratory failure precipitated by high carbohydrate loads. *Ann Intern Med.* 1981;95:579-581.
30. Askanazi J, Rosenbaum SH, Hyman AI, Silverberg PA, Milic-Emili J, Kinney JM. Respiratory changes induced by the large glucose loads of total parenteral nutrition. *JAMA.* 1980;243:1444-1447.
31. Gonzalez AG, Fajardo-Rodriguez A, Gonzalez-Figueroa E. The incidence of refeeding syndrome in cancer patient who received artificial nutritional treatment (English abstract). *Nutr Hosp.* 1996;11:98.
32. Havala T, Shronts E. Managing the complications associated with refeeding. *Nutr Clin Prac.* 1990;5:23-29.
33. Bowling TE, Silk DB. Refeeding remembered. *Nutrition.* 1995;11:32-34.
34. Fisher M, Simpser E, Schneider M. Hypophosphatemia secondary to oral refeeding in anorexia nervosa. *International J Eating Disorders.* 2000;28:181-187.
35. Kohn MR, Golden NH, Shenker IR. Cardiac arrest and delirium: presentations of the refeeding syndrome in severely malnourished adolescents with anorexia nervosa. *J Adolescent Health.* 1998;22:239-243.
36. Wada S, Nagase T, Koike Y, Kugai N. A case of anorexia nervosa with acute renal failure induced by rhambdomyolysis: possible involvement of hypophosphatemia or phosphate depletion. *Intern Med.* 1992;31:478.
37. Mehler PS, Diagnosis and care of patients with anorexia nervosa in primary care settings. *Ann Intern Med.* 2001;134:1048-1059.
38. Marik PE, Bedigian MK. Refeeding hypophosphatemia in critically ill patients in an intensive care unit. A prospective study. *Arch Surg.* 1996;131:1043-1047.
39. Knochel JP. The pathophysiology and clinical characteristics of severe hypophosphatemia. *Arch Intern Med.* 1977;137:203-204.
40. Zazzo JF, Torche G, Ruel P, et al. High incidence of hypophosphatemia in surgical intensive care patients. *Intensive Care Med.* 1995;21:826-831.
41. Halevy J, Bulvik S. Severe hypophosphatemia in hospitalized patients. *Arch Intern Scand.* 1988;148:153-155.
42. Hayek ME, Eisenberg PG. Severe hypophosphatemia following the institution of enteral feedings. *Arch Surg.* 1989:124:1325-1328.
43. Weinsier RL, Bacon, J, Butterworth CE. Central venous alimentation: a prospective study of frequency of metabolic abnormalities among medical and surgical patients. *J Parenteral Enteral Nutr.* 1982;6:421-425.
44. Takala J, Neuvonen P, Klossner J. Hypophosphatemia in hypercatabolic patients. *Acta Anaesthesiol Scand.* 1985;29:65-67.
45. Pigon J, Lindholm M, Eklund J, et al. Phosphate supplementation in parental nutrition. *Acta Anaesthesiol Scand.* 1985;29:50-54.
46. Fisher J, Magid N, Kallman C, et al. Respiratory illness and hypophosphatemia. *Chest.* 1983;83:504-508.
47. Mallet M. Refeeding syndrome. *Age and Aging.* 2002;31:65-66.
48. Vaszar LT, Culpepper-Morgan JA, Winter SM. Refeeding syndrome induced by cautious enteral alimentation of a moderately malnourished patient. *Gastroenterologist.* 1998;6:79-81.
49. Mason EE. Starvation injury after gastric reduction for obesity. *World J Surg.* 1988;22:1002-1007.
50. Baltasar A, del Rio J, Escriva C, et al. Preliminary results of the duodenal switch. *Obesity Surgery.* 1997;1007;7:500-504.
51. Knochel JP. Hypophosphatemia in the alcoholic. *Arch Intern Med.* 1980;140:613-615.
52. Cumming AD, Farquhar JR, Bouchier IAD. Refeeding hypophosphatemia in anorexia nervosa and alcoholism. *Br Med J.* 1987;295:490-491.
53. Knochel JP. Hypophosphatemia and rhabdomyolysis. *Am J Med.* 1992;92:455-457.
54. Brooks MJ, Melnik G. The refeeding syndrome: an approach to understanding its complications and preventing its occurrence. *Pharmacotherapy.* 1995;15:713-726.
55. Alpers DH, Klein S. Refeeding the malnourished patient. *Curr Opin Gastroenterol.* 1999;15:151-153.
56. Lentz, RD, Brown, DM, Kjellstrand, CM. Treatment of severe hypophosphatemia. *Ann Intern Med.* 1978;89:941-948.
57. Young IS, Neely RDG, Lavery GG. Treatment of hypophosphatemia. *Lancet.* 1993;341:374.
58. Chernow B, Rainey TG, Georges LP, et al. Iatrogenic hyperphosphatemia metabolic consideration in critical care medicine. *Crit Care Med.* 1981;9:772-774.
59. Weinsier RL, Krumdieck CL, Death resulting from overzealous total parenteral nutrition: the refeeding syndrome revisited. *Am J Clin Nutr.* 1980;34:393-399.
60. Crook MA, Hally V, Panteli JV. The importance of the refeeding syndrome. *Nutrition.* 2001;17:632-637.
61. Clark CL, Sacks GS, Dickerson RN, et al. Treatment of hypophosphatemia in patients receiving specialized nutrition support using a graduated dosing scheme: results from a prospective clinical trial. *Crit Care Med.* 1995;23:1504-1511.
62. Rosen GH, Boullata JI, O'Rangers EA, et al. Intravenous phosphate repletion regimen for critically ill patients with moderate hypophosphatemia. *Crit Care Med.* 1995:23:1204-1210.

63. Subramanian R, Khardori R. Severe hypophosphatemia. *Medicine.* 2000;79:1-8.
64. Kingston M, Al-Siba'I MB. Treatment of severe hypophosphatemia. *Crit Care Med.* 1985;13:16-18.
65. Vannatta JB, Whang R, Papper S. Efficacy of intravenous phosphorus therapy in the severely hypophosphatemic patient. *Arch Intern Med.* 1981;141:885-887.
66. Weisinger JR, Bellorin-Font E. Magnesium and phosphorus. *Lancet.* 1998;352:391.
67. Reinhart RA. Magnesium metabolism. *Arch Intern Med.* 1988:148;2415-2420.
68. Flink EB. Therapy of magnesium deficiency. *Ann NY Acad Sci.* 1969;162:901-905.
69. Vannatta JB, Andress DL, Whang R, et al. High dose intravenous phosphorus therapy for severe complicated hypophosphatemia. *South Med J.* 1983:76:1424-1426.
70. Miller DW, Alovis CM. Hypophosphatemia in the emergency department in therapeutics. *Am J Emergency Med.* 2000;18:457-461.
71. Terlevich A, Hearing SD, Woltersdorf WW, et al. Refeeding syndrome: effective and safe treatment with phosphatespolyfusor. *Aliment Pharmacol Ther.* 2003; 17:1325-1329.

Medical, Legal, and Ethical Aspects of Nutritional Support

Albert Barrocas, MD, FACS; Barbara B. Bivona, RN, BSN; and Denise Baird Schwartz, MS, RD, FADA, CNSD

Introduction

Medical technology has created a twilight zone of suspended animation where death commences while life, in some form, continues. Some patients, however, want no part of a life sustained only by medical technology. Instead, they prefer a plan of medical treatment that allows nature to take its course and permits them to die with dignity.

William Brennan, Associate Justice
US Supreme Court in Cruzan, 1990[1]

Ethical and legal issues are two of the most emotionally charged aspects of the management of gastrointestinal (GI) diseases involving nutrition-therapy interventions. Despite years of study and numerous publications and presentations, ethical and legal dilemmas challenge the healthcare provider on a daily basis. There is heterogeneity in opinions and practices; however, there is greater consensus in the management of many of these situations. This chapter presents the basic tenets of ethical and legal principles as they relate to the nutritional management of individuals with GI diseases, particularly those requiring specialized nutrition support (SNS): enteral nutrition (EN) and parenteral nutrition (PN).

Potentially Conflicting Arenas

The explosive technological advances of the past 50 years, in many instances, have outpaced the legal and bioethical arenas. The seminal work of Wilmore and Dudrick[2] in the development of PN for individuals with compromised GI tracts and impaired nutrition status is a good example of outpacing technology. Subsequent research has led to the refinement, not only of the techniques of PN, introduced in the late 1960s, but also in the broadening and increasing applicability of the techniques of EN, using the GI tract when oral feeding is not possible or inadequate.[3]

Technology is often associated with risks, burdens, and/or complications that need to be considered prior to, or periodically after, implementation. Healthcare professionals currently have the tools to confer "technological immortality on dehumanized bodies."[4] The net value and/or appropriateness of providing SNS to comatose, severely demented, or permanently/persistent-vegetative–state patients is questioned with increasing frequency. In sum, the dilemmas encountered can be viewed as a trichotomy: a struggle between the **can** (technology), the **should** (ethics) and the **must** (law).[5]

Ethics

"Morals" and "ethics" are frequently used interchangeably. "Morals"—a value system—provide the boundaries of acceptable behavior and enable one to distinguish between right and wrong conduct.[6] "Ethics," from the Greek work "ethos," refers to establishing acceptable behavior. Another definition views "ethics" as a group-imposed standard of right and wrong to regulate the behavior of individuals.[7] Terms in the medical field that are parallel to these terms are "policies" for "morals" and "procedures" for "ethics." The procedures that govern healthcare professionals are called "bioethics."[5]

Ethical Types, Classes, Sets, Categories

A variety of ethical types and categories have evolved over the years. Religious, societal, individual (existential), professional, and organizational ethics are often an unquestioned characteristic of the healthcare professional's persona. Notwithstanding earlier ethical theories, aspects of which have remained immutable over time, ethics in practice today can be viewed as adaptable, conflicting, variable, and situational.

Thus, professional ethics is based on the medieval "master craftsman" concept, which is duty oriented and governed by professional standards and a code of ethics. In the discharge of that duty, the healthcare professional must be flexible (adaptable) and provide the care and guidance required for a particular event (situational), considering the benefits, risks, and burdens of interventions (consequential). In recent years, the imperative of healthcare professionals' ethics has translated into an increasing role for the US physicians as the patient advocate—since the advent of managed care.

Ethical Principles

In the United States at the present time, decisions regarding life-sustaining therapies, such as those related to nutrition support, are guided by four ethical principles: autonomy, nonmaleficence, beneficence, and distributive justice.[8]

Autonomy

Derived from "autos" (self) and "nemos" (law, governance), autonomy—the principle of self determination—stands in stark contrast with parentalism: the "parent-knows-best" principle of medical practice. Self governance is valued by American society, which asserts that the individual's right to choice is based on their ethical value and reasoning. Autonomy protects the individual from external influences, including the beliefs or wishes of healthcare providers. Each individual has the moral "right" to refuse food and fluid, both artificial and oral, provided the refusal is informed and voluntary and the patient has adequate decision-making capacity.[9] In the absence of competency or capacity, autonomy may prevail through tools (eg, advance directives) and proxy decision makers (eg, durable power-of-attorney) for healthcare decisions. The elderly are often the beneficiaries of such efforts. Autonomy usually trumps the other three ethical principles. While potentially uncomfortable for the healthcare provider, autonomy mandates that healthcare providers cannot unilaterally make a determination as to what is best for the patient without educated dialogue between the two.[10]

Nonmaleficence

In considering an intervention, the potential for damage needs to play an integral role in the final decision. From the deontological perspective, nonmaleficence provides that the duties will not kill, cause pain and suffering, and not cause incapacity. In discharge of the provider's duties, patients sometimes have pain and suffering, are incapacitated by medical interventions and/or die. However, our ethical drive behind those interventions is the principle of beneficence.

The negative impact or outcomes that our actions may provide under the intent of "doing good" has been referred as "the rule of double effect," by Beauchamp and Childress.[8] Four premises must be satisfied to comply with this rule: the act must be good or at least morally neutral; the healthcare professional's goal must be to relieve suffering (beneficence); the effect of hastening death, though foreseen (ie, morphine for pain) is not intended; killing is not the means of relieving suffering; and the response is proportionate.

Beneficence

Doing what is best for the greatest number of individuals has been universally advocated by ethical theorists. For healthcare professionals, preventing and removing harm are additional duties. The actions of the healthcare team should benefit the patient. It is the principle of beneficence that attracts many to the healthcare profession. Parentalism may be seen as beneficence because it can result in overriding an individual's preference with the goal of benefiting him or her or preventing harm. Once again, informed and educated consent, as discussed later in this chapter, is an integral part of beneficence.[11]

Distributive Justice

This principle calls for the obligation to be fair to all. At the same time, the right to equal treatment translates to "fairness" when scarce resources are to be allocated. Another view of this principle is the duty to ensure equal treatment when all else is equal. Conflicts arise in the presence of limited total resources and when community needs are in competition with individual needs.[12]

Futile versus Low-Yield or Medically Inappropriate Interventions

A commonly held belief or practice based on the principles of beneficence and nonmaleficence is to forgo "futile" care. Healthcare personnel are often confronted with situations where the interventions provided are clearly without potential benefit and are therefore referred to as "futile." However, there are few situations in which all concerned can agree on its futility (eg, cardiopulmonary resuscitation on a decapitated individual). Universal agreement on futile care is unlikely because definitions of "futile" care are value based.[13] In the majority of situations, what may be considered "futile" by some may not be so accepted by others, which often creates conflict and obstacles to communication.[14] As suggested by the Education for Physicians in End-of-Life Care (EPEC) program, a preferred term for questionable interventions is "low yield," which emphasizes the benefit/risk analysis in

TABLE 46-1.

Levels of Resuscitation

Level	*Threat*	*Example*	*Course*	*Intervention*
Revival	Life distantly threatened	Vasovagal syncope	Reversible, limiting	Little or no intervention required
True resuscitation	Death imminent	Cardiac arrest	May be reversible; not self limiting	Heroic measures necessary
Resurrection	Assumption that death has occurred	Decapitation	Irreversible	Futile, low yield, medically inappropriate; rare

reaching decisions. Others prefer to use the designation of "medically inappropriate" treatment/intervention.[15-18]

Establishing Goals of Therapy

To facilitate unanimity in the decision making-process, the establishment of therapeutic goals is pivotal. What is the expected outcome of proposed intervention? Younger has suggested four goals for medical intervention:[19] maintaining or restoring physiologic status; postponing death; prolonging life; and improving the quality of life. A chasm is sometimes present between the perceived therapeutic goals of the patients and their surrogates and those of the healthcare team. The definition of Younger's fourth goal is often elusive and subject to varied interpretation, despite the availability of tools for its measurement. Severely physically or mentally handicapped individuals are more vulnerable to a biased definition of quality of life and more threatened by this prejudicial attitude than by the disability.[20] Consensus between healthcare personnel and patients (or their surrogates) is often achieved to add life to years rather than adding years to life.

In more acute situations, "low-yield" considerations are suddenly thrust on the healthcare team, patients, and families. In the environment of unexpected cardiopulmonary collapse, three levels of resuscitation have been proposed (Table 46-1). In contrast, decisions regarding nutrition support are not as easily determined. The concept of nutrition support is synonymous with food, which has strong emotional and symbolic overtones that include maternal nurturing, religious, cultural, ethnic and social values. Food is considered the substance of life and to withhold food is a presumed decision to let the individual die a painful death. There is a semantic quagmire between nutrition support, nonvolitional artificial nutrition, and feeding.[11] However, these interventions require the same risk/benefit, therapeutic goals, and yield scrutiny, particularly in elderly patients. The importance of frequent open communication with patients, surrogates, and healthcare-team members in resolving conflicts in this arena cannot be over emphasized. While the risks and benefits of intervention are usually discussed, the success of the intervention in achieving the desired interventional goal is often excluded from the discussion. Where is the evidence that percutaneous endoscopic gastrostomy (PEG) tubes provide any benefit particularly in severely demented individuals? Is there evidence that they cause complications, harm, or burdens? These questions are addressed later in the chapter in discussions of evidenced-based medicine (EBM) and informed consent.[21]

Ethical Dilemmas and Conflict Resolution

Because we do not live in a perfect universe, the presence of ethical dilemmas and conflicts is not surprising. Whether between the types, categories, or principles previously discussed, these highly sensitive and emotionally laden situations can be successfully managed by following established protocols and some basic principles.[15,22-26] All healthcare providers need to be on the "same page" and not deliver conflicting information to the patient or surrogate. On occasion, despite unanimity of the healthcare team as to an inappropriateness or low yield of an intervention, the patient and/or surrogate demands that it be provided. These situations require careful deliberation based on established policies.[27-29]

Communication

The most important aspect of ethical- and legal-dilemma prevention and resolution is communication. Both verbal and written documentation in the medical record are essential. From the initial encounter, the patient's capacity, a clinical decision, and competency, a legal decision, should be assessed. The mentally capable individual should be informed as to his or her plan of care and be provided the opportunity to actively participate in the decision-making process to foster the ethical tenet of autonomy. It is imperative that factors such as attention span, educational level, and ability to comprehend are taken into account to ensure that the patient is adequately informed. Whenever possible, even with capable and competent patients, family members and/or surrogate decision makers should participate in the communications, within the boundaries of patient confidentiality. Written documents expressing the patient's wishes (needs and wants) are extremely helpful. During the admission process, the patient, family, and physician (and referring facility, if the patient is transferred) should be queried as to the existence of such documents and copies should be included as part of the current medical record.

Two of the most common types of documents are the medical-care advance directives, including living wills, and the durable power of attorney or proxy for healthcare decisions. These types of documents provide additional assistance in the decision-making process and conflict prevention when they are executed according to the specific state law; reviewed at the time of admission to assure that no updates are necessary; as explicit as possible. For those healthcare professionals charged with the responsibility for providing nutrition support, it is important to establish the patient's desires regarding artificial nutrition and hydration support (in contrast to the natural food and water orally and voluntarily ingested) early in their course of treatment. Even if documents providing directives do not fall within the legal framework of the particular state, they can be extremely valuable in ethical considerations. For those individuals designated as proxy or surrogate decision makers, it is important that they are familiar with any previous medical advance directive authorized by the patient.

Mentally competent patients, particularly the elderly, experience intermittent incapacity to make decisions in a hospital setting as a result of medications, depression, anxiety, confusion, etc. It is important for those rendering care to be able to accurately determine the patient's decision-making capacity; likewise, the healthcare team should establish and document the date and time of the patient's consent or rejection of a particular intervention when he or she was deemed capable to make the particular decision. Again, when in doubt, it is best to have the surrogate decision maker, legal proxy, or otherwise designated involved simultaneously with the patient whenever possible, even via teleconference.

Despite the fact that federal law (Patient Self Determination Act, 1990) has mandated that these types of documents be available to patients in all healthcare facilities participating in the Medicare and Medicaid programs, only 18% of patients have executed such documents. Even more interesting, it is estimated that approximately 10% of physicians have a living will, though the overwhelming majority (>70%) agree that their patients should have them. This dismal percent of "subscribers" coupled with other perceived failings of living wills have led some to question whether the policy of living wills should be abandoned.[30] The likelihood, however, is that living wills and proxies for healthcare decision are here to stay. In an effort to enhance the execution and use of these documents through education of healthcare professionals, the EPEC project has provided excellent guidelines, references, and seminars.[31]

Inasmuch as there is no universality in execution of the above-listed communication tools, how should healthcare professionals proceed in their quest for meeting the four basic ethical principles? A simple template modified from the legal decision regarding Conroy[32] in 1985, provides three progressive levels or tests that are subjective, limited objective, or purely objective. A subjective tool includes clear documented evidence of a patient's wishes, including living wills, a durable power of attorney for healthcare decisions or proxy, or oral directives given to the patient's healthcare provider, a family member or a friend. A limited objective text is acceptable in the absence of unequivocal evidence of the patient's desires and is based on the patient's best interest. This includes trustworthy evidence of the patient's desires that were presented in a way that was too vague, casual, or remote to satisfy the subjective test (ie, the patient expressed his or her desires informally as a reaction to another individual's medical circumstances. This test also requires clear evidence that the intervention's burdens outweigh the benefits to the patient. A purely objective test includes a burdens/benefit analysis in absence of documentable or trustworthy evidence but shows that the care is in patient's best interest.[32]

Healthcare caregivers are often faced with incompetent or incapable patients without clear identification of a surrogate decision maker. In the absence of documented evidence or knowledge of the individual representing him- or herself as the surrogate decision maker, an addendum to the institution's informed-consent form or a separate form or affidavit signed by the self-proclaimed surrogate decision maker is recommended (see Appendix on page 580).

Communication is not only important between the healthcare givers, the patient, and patient's family. It is equally important that all members of the healthcare team have a forum to effectively express their feeling, concerns, and ethical principles in a nonthreatening environment. Such an exercise—coupled with sound, simple-to-understand protocols—can avoid the frustrations and conflicts often experienced in these situations.

Whether amongst themselves or with their patients, healthcare professionals benefit greatly from another aspect of good communications: active (engaged), effective (doing the right thing), and efficient (doing things right) listening. Lastly, despite the emotional overlay of these situations, every effort should be made to infuse appropriate humor, the catharsis of the soul, in our communication.[5]

Information Gathering, Assimilation, and Presentation

It is incumbent upon all members of the healthcare team to provide concise and credible information regarding the patient's conditions and the pros and cons of proposed interventions. Good facts form the basis of good ethics. EBM is currently providing us with a methodology for gathering dependable data and information. The information should be presented to patient and family in easily understood language and in an environment conducive for question and answers, preferably with handouts that they can keep for future reference and review (Figure 46-1).

For patients who are candidates for nutrition support, benefit/risk analysis and evidence-based outcome data of proposed interventions should be provided (Table 46-2). This established analysis is one of the six guidelines for ethical/legal decision making in nutrition support proposed by the American Society for Parenteral and Enteral Nutrition (A.S.P.E.N.)[33,34] (Table 46-3). To the extent possible, EBM should be the benchmark for data to be presented.

Providence | Health System

Patient Information Series

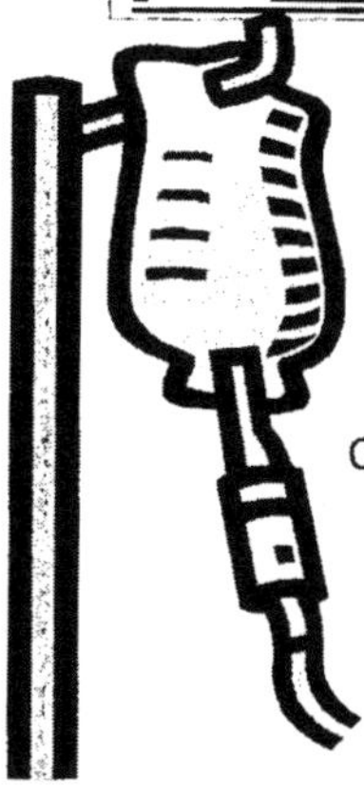

ENTERAL NUTRITION (Tube Feeding)

DID YOU KNOW?

Enteral nutrition is a specially prepared liquid formula given through a tube into the stomach or small intestine. Enteral nutrition may be given continuously through a pump, or in several small feedings per day.

Enteral nutrition is a medical therapy ordered by your doctor and given by your nurse. A dietitian calculates your individual nutrition needs. Enteral nutrition contains protein, carbohydrate, fat, vitamins, minerals and water.

FEEDING TUBES

There are three main types of feeding tubes. A nasogastric tube (NGT) is inserted into the nose to the stomach or small intestine. A more permanent type of feeding tube, a gastrostomy tube (G-Tube), is inserted by a doctor directly into your stomach through the skin. A third type of feeding tube is placed into the small intestine, bypassing the stomach. This is called a jejunostomy tube (J-Tube).

WHY DO I NEED IT?

Your doctor may recommend enteral nutrition because you can't swallow safely, or you have trouble eating enough food to maintain your nutrition status. Enteral nutrition gives you the calories and nutrients your body needs. The goal of enteral nutrition is to maintain or build up your nutrition status so you can get well.

ANY RISKS/CONCERNS?

Possible problems can occur during tube placement or if the tube becomes dislodged. Rarely, the feeding may accidentally get into your lungs and cause pneumonia. A feeding tube can cause irritation of the skin around it. The tube can develop a leak or become clogged and it may need to be replaced from time to time. You might experience some discomfort with a feeding tube, especially an NGT. Tell your nurse if you have bloating, fullness, nausea, diarrhea, or any other type of discomfort.

HOW LONG WILL I NEED IT?

Enteral nutrition is stopped when you can swallow food and liquids safely. Enteral nutrition should be stopped if it does not improve your quality of life. It should be stopped when the risks of the feeding outweigh the benefits to you. Enteral nutrition can be stopped based on your wishes. Please discuss any concerns you have with your doctor.

Figure 46-1. Patient Education Handout, page 1. Courtesy of Denise Schwartz and Providence Health System.

Providence | Health System

Patient Information Series

TOTAL PARENTERAL NUTRITION (TPN)

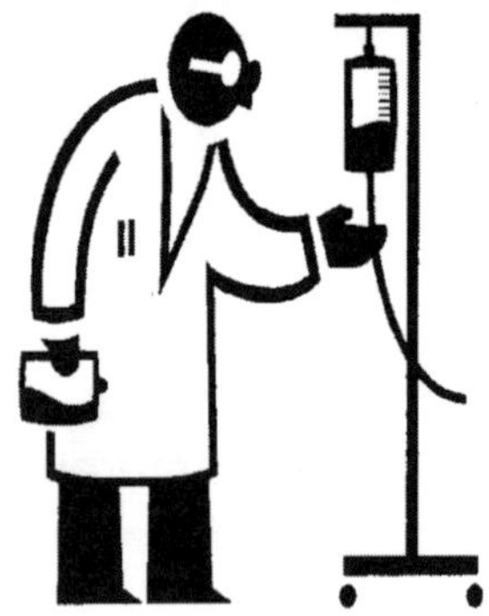

DID YOU KNOW?
TPN is a specially prepared IV formula that provides more calories and nutrients than a regular IV. It is also called IV nutrition or parenteral nutrition.

TPN is an advanced medical therapy prescribed by your doctor, prepared by a pharmacist, and given by a nurse. A dietitian calculates your individual nutrition needs. TPN contains protein, sugar, fat, vitamins, minerals and water.

WHY DO I NEED IT?
Your physician may recommend TPN because you can't eat and your digestive system doesn't work. The goal of TPN is to maintain or build up your nutrition status so you can get well.

ANY RISKS/CONCERNS?
TPN usually requires a special IV called a central line. This IV is inserted into a large, deep vein in the arm, neck, or chest. Risks with insertion of the line include bleeding and (rarely) lung problems. Other possible risks associated with central lines include infection and clotting.

Routine blood tests are necessary to monitor TPN. The nurse may prick your finger to check your blood sugar several times a day. Your doctor will adjust the TPN formula according to your test results. Sometimes nutrients in the TPN are not tolerated well when you are ill. Tell your doctor or nurse if you feel nauseated, bloated, or otherwise uncomfortable.

HOW LONG WILL I NEED TPN?
Your doctor and dietitian continually evaluate your need for TPN. TPN is stopped when you can eat enough calories safely or tolerate a tube feeding. TPN should be stopped when it does not improve your quality of life. TPN should be stopped when the risks outweigh the benefits to you. It can be stopped based on your wishes. Discuss any concerns you have with your doctor.

Figure 46-1. Patient Education Handout, page 2. Courtesy of Denise Schwartz and Providence Health System.

TABLE 46-2.

Benefits Versus Burdens of Nutrition and Nutrition Support

Benefits	*Burdens*
Oral Nutrition	
Natural	Alertness required
Easy	Aspiration
Symbolic	Feeding assistance may be required
Inexpensive	Religious/dietary restrictions
	Taste, appetite dependent
Enteral Nutrition	
Alertness not required	Requires supervision
Convenient	Aspiration
Relatively safe	Diarrhea
Mildly invasive	Metabolic complications (fluid and electrolytes)
Inexpensive	Requires access
Maintenance, restoration of mucosal integrity	Bloating, early satiety
	Mechanical (Erosion, necrosis, bleeding, sinusitis, dislodgement)
	Perforation
	Gastroesophageal reflux
Parenteral Nutrition	
Gut not required	Metabolic complications
Specific nutrients provided	Specific nutrients provided
Independent of appetite	Pneumo-/hemothorax
Precise intake	Increased monitoring required
	Requires access
	Catheter infections and thrombosis
	Relatively more expensive

TABLE 46-3.

A.S.P.E.N. Guidelines[33,34]

1. Legally and ethically, SNS should be considered a medical therapy. (A)
2. Care providers should be familiar with current evidence of the benefits and burdens of SNS. (C)
3. Patients should be encouraged to have living wills and/or advance directives and to discuss with their loved ones their wishes in the event of a serious or terminal accident or disease. (C)
4. Adult patients or their legally authorized surrogates have the right to accept or to refuse SNS. (A)
5. The benefits and burdens of SNS and the interventions required to deliver it should be considered before offering this therapy. (B)
6. Institutions should develop clear policies regarding the withdrawal or withholding of SNS and communicate these policies to patients in accordance with the patient Self-Determination Act. (A)

The strength of evidence supporting each guideline statement has been coded using a modified version of the Agency for Healthcare Research and Quality, US Department of Health and Human Services. A = strongest evidence.

Table 46-4.

Sanctions Supporting Forgoing Life-Sustaining Measures

1. President's Commission for the Study of Ethical Problems in Medicine (1983)
2. The Hastings Center (1987)
3. Society of Critical Care Medicine (1990)
4. Houston City-Wide Task Force on Medical Futility (1996)
5. EPEC (1999)
6. American Medical Association Council on Ethical and Judicial Affairs (1999, 2002)
7. American Dietetic Association guidelines (2002)
8. A.S.P.E.N. guidelines (2002)

Tube Feeding and Evidence-Based Medicine

Though counterintuitive, tube feedings do not universally benefit patients. Emotions aside, increasing number of credible studies demonstrate the low yield, medically inappropriate, or harmful aspects of tube feedings in specific subpopulations of patients. The current process of EBM and grading the strength of evidence and recommendations, as referenced by the Agency for Healthcare Research and Quality, is frequently used. While several systems have been implemented,[35] an "ABC" system is frequently preferred.[36] The "A" grade is reserved for those studies that comprise at least one randomized controlled trial of good quality addressing their topic or recommendation. In the presence of clinical studies without randomization on the topic, a "B" grade is granted. The "C" grade is reserved for evidence promulgated by respected authorities or organizations that provide recommendations based on experience or anecdotal evidence. The latter classification has been referred to as "eminence-based medicine" by D. David Thomas of St. Louis University Health Science Center (personal communication, September 2004).

In a published review of EN and enteral tube feeding, Haddad and Thomas reviewed the available evidence in these topics.[21] In their literature search, they identified the following statistics.

First, enteral feeding via PEG tube is fraught with a high complication rate—41% have a 30-day mortality (4% related to the procedure).[37] Nursing home patients (87% demented) experienced a 39.5% mortality rate.[38] Another study comprising 81,105 patients was associated with a 23.9%, 63%, and 81.3% mortality rate at 30 days, 1 year, and 3 years, respectively.[39] Thus, it is imperative that the benefit/risk ratio is objectively and critically assessed and presented to the patient and/or surrogate decision maker as part of the informed-consent proceedings. Recommendations for ethical deliberations of PEG placement were proposed during the First European Symposium on Ethics in Gastroenterology in 2002.[40]

Second, the conclusion that tube feedings should be avoided in patients with severe dementia was provided by investigators who performed a meta analysis of the literature over the past decade, looking at specific outcomes including aspiration pneumonia, pressure sores, and decline in activities of daily living, among others.[41] Other studies have arrived at similar conclusions, with no survival benefit noted in severely demented patients.[42]

Haddad and Thomas conclude that enteral feeding is associated with a high mortality and morbidity rates and associated with questionable effectiveness, with the exception of two studies—one in patients with Amyotrophic Lateral Sclerosis (ALS), also known as Lou Gehrig's disease,[43] and the other in critically ill patients. They suggest that the decision to implement tube feeding is often inappropriate and late. Furthermore, most of the guidelines currently in use are not supported by well-designed studies or available evidence. Maintaining literature surveillance to enhance our evidence-based armamentarium is a prerequisite to optimal information sharing with patients and surrogate decision makers in the informed-consent process.

Continuing Education

Regardless of their core disciplines, healthcare professionals need to incorporate bioethics and medical law into their personal program of life-long learning. As stated earlier, technological advances have elicited the need for updating our ethico-legal armamentarium. From changes in the definition of death to modified attitudes as to who, what, and when of forgoing interventions, a host of organizations and individuals have provided guidance throughout the years (Table 46-4). Keeping current with bioethical literature can often serve as an anticonvulsant to the rapid changes in the US healthcare-delivery system.[44]

The present environment of managed care has eroded the traditional patient-physician relationship. A host of new players have been introduced into the healthcare delivery drama. In some instances, the perception is that a paradigm shift has occurred from "primum non nocere" (first do no harm) to "primum pecuniae parcere (first save money), with a redefinition of the golden rule to "He who has the gold makes the rule." As third parties become more aggressive in determining the care that will be reimbursed, there is a potential for shifting towards a system of veterinarian ethics, in which the owner, master, and/or purse keeper determines the fate of his or her "pet," who has neither voice nor vote in the matter making autonomy and self-determination obsolete.[45]

Through continuing education, the healthcare team may be able to increase their role of patient advocate, thwarting the potential for transformation from the current system to one operating under the precepts of jungle ethics. The latter allows for the survival of the financially "fittest" by preferentially providing for those interventions that are denied others in precarious financial states.

Healthcare Team as Ethics Team

With the achievement of individual and collective continuing education, the healthcare team can serve as an ethics team. Every effort should be made to achieve consensus through interactive dialogue and EBM and accepted principles. Failure to establish a cohesive healthcare team adds significantly to the confusion and frustration often experienced by patients and surrogates faced with difficult situations. When dealing with issues of nutrition support, it is imperative that representatives of a nutrition support team, if one exists, and/or related disciplines serve as members or active participants of the institution's ethics committee.

Ethics Committees or Panels: Organization and Function

Despite differences among the involved parties, a consensus can generally be reached in most ethical dilemmas. There is often no "right" or "wrong" answer to a medical ethical problem. To resolve the conflict, an understanding must be negotiated. If disagreement persists, others should be involved, including, but not limited to, consultants, ethicists, chaplains, or ethics committees. In 1966, the Joint Commission on Accreditation of Healthcare Organizations began requiring that each healthcare entity have an ethics committee or a mechanism in place by which to resolve ethical conflicts. Up to that point, less than 90% of hospitals and 15% to 25% of nursing homes had ethics committees.[46]

Ethics committees help the parties involved in the dilemma identify the implications of any clinical decisions and assist them in coming to agreement. Committee members should be knowledgeable in areas of theoretical or academic ethics, clinical ethics, diversity issues that can impact decision-making, and legal consequences of ethical decisions. Ethics committees are generally multidisciplinary in structure and interdisciplinary in function, with representation by physicians, attorneys, clergy, nurses, therapists, and administrators. Included in the function of the ethics committee are the tasks of education—both of the committee members and the staff of the organization, review and development of policy regarding ethical issues, and individual-case consultation. In developing and maintaining an ethics committee, the organization should address the issues of committee purpose and goals, jurisdiction, roles, membership, record-keeping, indemnification, process of approval, institutional acceptance, policy development and modification, and annual review.[31,47]

Four Common Ethical Dilemmas in Nutrition Support

Nutrition Support as a Life-Sustaining Intervention

In contrast to food and water, artificial nutrition and hydration should be considered medical interventions subject to the same risk/benefit analysis as are other life-sustaining measures, such as ventilators and hemodialysis. Despite the emotional overlay that often accompanies it, forgoing nutrition support is ethically appropriate when the basic ethical principles are followed. In some cases, the provision of such artificial nutrition may be contraindicated. An honest, informative discussion with patient and family can outline the reason for forgoing nutrition support. On the other hand, when doubt exists about the efficacy of this or any other intervention, it is prudent to institute a time-limited trial with a similar preemptive discussion to avoid discord if and when the intervention is withdrawn after the agreed-upon time interval.[31]

"Withholding" Versus "Withdrawing"

Though removing an established intervention evokes a higher level of emotions than withholding it, almost universally, theologians and ethicists make no distinction between the two. To avoid any semantic distinction, the term "forgoing" (not "foregoing") is often used. By contrast, some states in the United States require a more stringent legal criteria for the withdrawal of an intervention by a surrogate decision maker, insisting on "clear and convincing evidence," as discussed in the Law Section of this chapter.

Nutrition Support and "Do Not Resuscitate"

"Do not resuscitate" (DNR) or "do not attempt resuscitation" (DNAR) orders are required by several states, notwithstanding the presence of advance directives and durable power-of-attorneys that are not event specific. Where the indications exist for nutrition support, it should be provided, even in a time-trial basis, regardless of the patient's DNR-order status.

Nutrition Support Therapy as a Patient's Right

Self-autonomy does not translate into interventions on demand. While patients have a right to accept or reject interventions, they do not possess the ethical imperative

TABLE 46-5.

Healthcare and Religious/Cultural Practices

Religion	Medical Treatment	Right-to-Die Issues
Catholic	Abortion and sterilization not permitted	Ordinary, not extraordinary, means to prolong life
Christian Science	Many adherents will refuse all medical treatment; may request a practitioner or reader	Will not seek medical help to prolong life
Mormon*	Individual choice	Promote a peaceful death when death inevitable
Islam	Most accepted	Efforts to shorten life not permitted
Jehovah's Witnesses	Administration of blood/blood products during surgery or at any other time is strictly forbidden	Use of extraordinary means an individual's choice
Judaism†	Most allowed	Do not believe life must be prolonged at all costs; active euthanasia prohibited

*Church of Jesus Christ of Latter Day Saints
†May differ between orthodox, conservative reform

to demand interventions that are determined low yield, harmful, and/or medically inappropriate.[13,14,27] Concerns are often raised regarding the potential for discomfort and other undesirable side effects from forgoing artificial nutrition and hydration. Evidence to the contrary has been described in the literature.[41,48] While these controversies are rare in the atmosphere of open, honest communications, they can create friction and must be handled in a careful and sensitive fashion.[49,50] The individual's insistence of a particular intervention may be rooted in his or her ethnic, cultural, and/or religious persona (Tables 46-5 and 46-6). These and other previously noted factors should comprise the basis of a stepwise deliberation outline and/or simplified, prioritized questionnaire. Clinicians need to always first address the question of should the patient received nutrition support before embarking on questions related to the appropriate route of nutrition therapy and nutrition needs. Often, this first question is omitted in the decision process and results in tremendous healthcare dilemmas for the family and healthcare team during the patient's hospitalization (Figure 46-2). If the conflict cannot be resolved and the healthcare provider's ethical principles conflict with those of the patient or surrogate, appropriate transfer of care is ethical (Figure 46-3). In summary, patients have a right to appropriate treatment but not a right to demand inappropriate treatment (Table 46-7). (A related case study is presented in Sidebar 46-1.)

Legal

The third major factor influencing the delivery of health care after technology (can) and ethics (should) is law (must). A basic primer of law is a beneficial step toward understanding legal concerns of nutrition support in GI disease. Laws—rules of conduct to manage complex interactions—reflect societal values and customs, rendering them dynamic and ever-changing. The law governing healthcare issues in the US finds its source in the federal and state constitutions, statutes, regulations, court decisions, and attorney general opinions (Table 46-8). The law is composed of two major categories: civil and criminal. Civil law comprises tort (harm) and contract law. The three basic types of tort are unintentional, intentional, and strict liability (eg, product liability). Malpractice (negligence) is an unintentional tort, as is abandonment. The latter can theoretically be part of contract law[55] (Figure 46-4).

Additionally, standards of care, which have basis in how a prudent healthcare practitioner would act in a similar situation, further assign responsibility to the practitioner for his actions. Standards of care are developed externally by laws and entities such as the Joint Commission on Accreditation of Healthcare Organizations, National Committee for Quality Assurance, A.S.P.E.N., American Medical Association, and other professional organizations.[16,24,35] Internally, standards of care are formulated by healthcare institutions and can include policies, procedures, protocols, and job descriptions.[47]

TORT

Unintentional Tort

Negligence, or unintentional tort, on the part of the practitioner in rendering care to the patient is the basis for malpractice. Palmisano's "ABCD Rule" serves as a quick reference, noting the four elements for the determination of malpractice:

TABLE 46-6.

Selected Cultural Artificial and Practice Forwards End of Life Issues*

Culture	Characteristic
Mexican-American	• Protect dying and bereaved • Difficulty accepting death • Often stay with hospital loved one (shifts of vigil) • Encourage open expression of anger and grief
African-American	• Less likely to grieve openly and publicly
Anglo-American	• Rely on friends, church members, neighbors, and nonrelatives when death of loved one occurs
Chinese-American	• Stoic and fatalistic towards terminal illness and death
Japanese-American	• May not ask questions regarding care or prognosis • Family members aware of dying, but avoid discussing situation • Request to stay with dying patient • "Ambiguous disclosure"
Armenian-American	• Designated family spoke person, decision maker • Subject of death may be avoided • Presence of family member critical • Terminal care preferred at home
Australian[12]	• Palliative care at home, but physician does not have to comply • Euthanasia not legal
Dutch (Netherlands)	• Advance directives, but physician does not have to comply • Euthanasia not legal, but decriminalized

*Characteristics not intended to be reflective of all members in each cultural group.

Adapted from: Ferrell BR, Coyle N. *Textbook of Palliative Nursing.* New York, NY: Oxford University Press; 2001; Andrews M, Boyle J. *Transcultural Concepts in Nursing Care.* 3rd ed. Philadelphia, PA: Lippincott, Williams, & Wilkins; 1999; Galanti G. *Caring for Patients from Different Cultures: Case Studies from American Hospitals.* 2nd ed. Philadelphia, PA: University of Pennsylvania Press; 1997; Lipson JG, Dibble SL, Minarik PA, eds. *Culture and Nursing Care: A Pocket Guide.* San Francisco, CA: UCSF Nursing Press; 1996.

1. Accept: The healthcare practitioner has to accept the patient. A legal relationship is established between practitioner and patient.
2. Breach: There must be a breach of duty, conduct below the reasonable standard of care, which leads to a cause.
3. Cause: A cause directly results in the specific damage.
4. Damage: damage must be alleged.[5]

Intentional Tort

Intentional torts, or those torts involving a volitional act, involve the individual intending or having knowledge that the consequences of his action would likely occur. Further, the action would be determined to be a significant cause of injury or consequence to the patient. The primary difference between intentional torts and negligence (unintentional tort) lies in the intent of the person committing the act. Intentional torts include assault, battery, defamation, invasion of privacy, misrepresentation, fraud, and false imprisonment.[47]

Assault

Assault is an attempt or threat to touch another without justification, while battery is the act of actually touching another. In regard to patient care, battery may be alleged when no consent has been given by the patient who undergoes a procedure. Lack of informed consent occurs when one or more of three things happen: consent for the specific procedure in question has not been obtained; the patient was not provided with the information necessary to give informed consent; or the patient did not consent to the particular practitioner performing the procedure. Lack of informed consent may also be grounds for negligence (malpractice).[47]

Informed Consent

Informed consent is required for all medical interventions. It must be documented. Prior to obtaining any consent for treatment, the practitioner must discuss the nature of the treatment or procedure, any risks—including special and unusual circumstances (ie, material risks, alternative procedures or treatments, expected outcome of the intervention, consequences of no treatment and of any alternative treatments)—and must answer all of

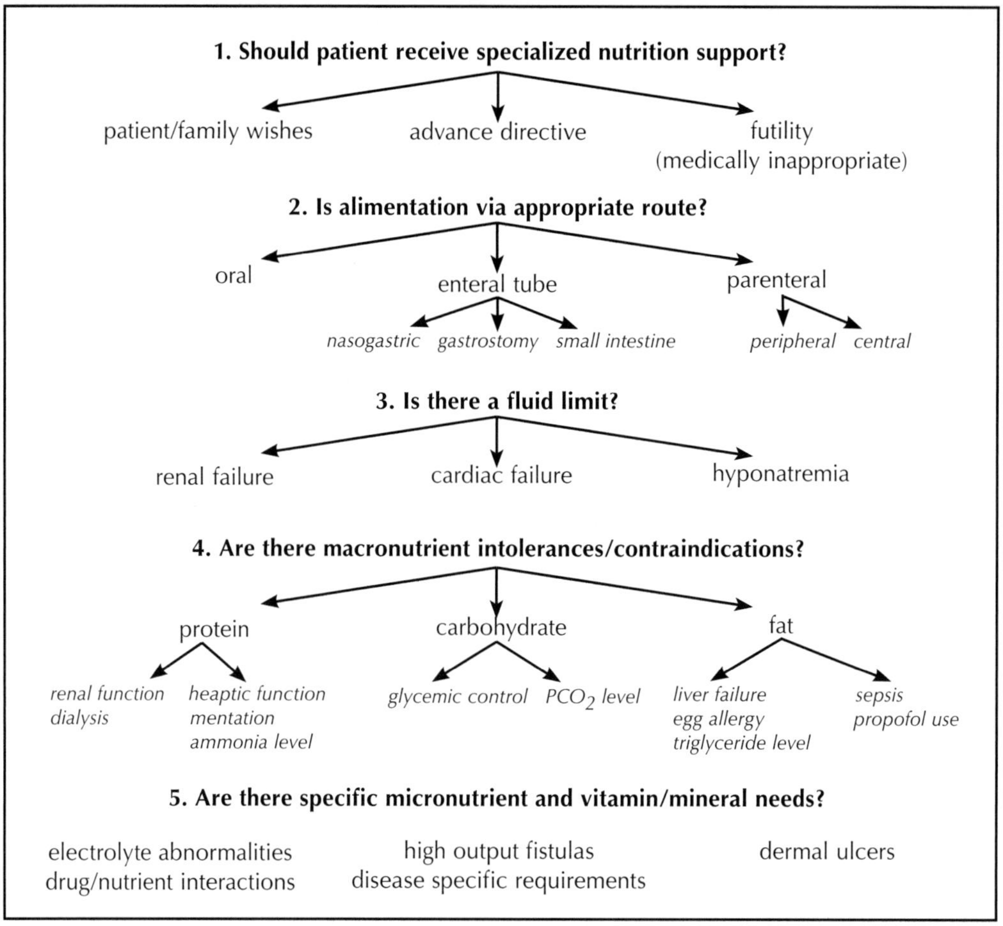

Figure 46-2. Trigger questions to optimize nutrition support recommendations in order of importance.

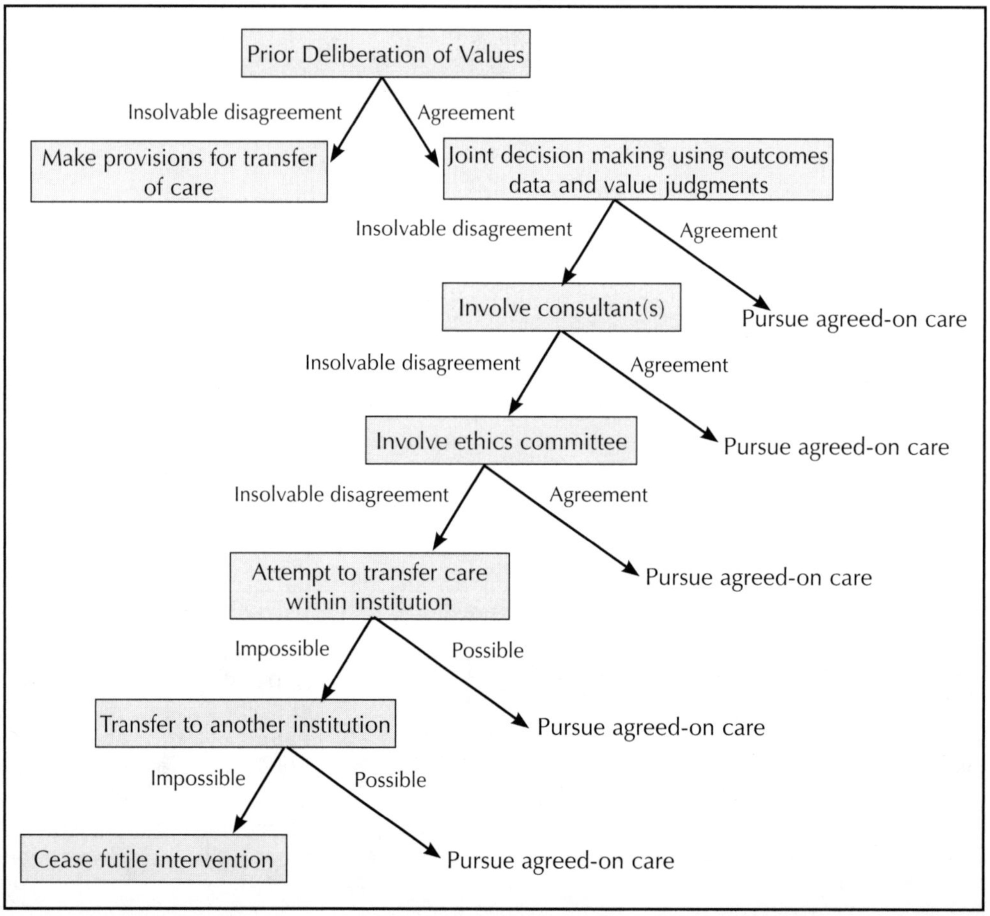

Figure 46-3. Fair process for considering futility cases. (Reprinted with permission from AMA. Medical futility in end-of-life care: report of the Council on Ethical and Judicial Affairs. *JAMA.* 1999;281(10):937-941.)

TABLE 46-7.

Suggested Ethical Deliberations About Nutrition and Hydration

1. The patient's expressed desire for extent of medical care is a primary guide for determining the level of nutrition intervention.
2. The decision to forgo hydration or nutrition should be weighed carefully because such a decision may be difficult or impossible to reverse with a period of days or weeks.
3. The expected benefits, in contrast to the potential burdens, of non-oral feeding must be evaluated by the health care team and discussed with the patient. The focus of care should include the patient's physical and psychological comfort.
4. Food and hydration are considered medical interventions.
5. Consider whether nutrient support, either oral or artificial, will improve the patient's quality of life during the final stages of life.
6. Consider whether nutrient support, either oral or artificial, can be expected to provide the patient with emotional comfort, decreased anxiety about disease cachexia, improved self-esteem with cosmetic benefits. Improve interpersonal relationships or relief from fear of abandonment.
7. If death is imminent and feeding will not alter condition consider whether nutrient support will be burdensome.
8. When oral intake is appropriate:
   a. Oral feeding should be advocated whenever possible. Food and control of food intake may give comfort, pleasure, and a sense of autonomy and dignity.
   b. Efforts should be made to enhance the patient's physical and emotional enjoyment of food by encouraging staff and family assistance in feeding the patient.
   c. Nutrition supplements, including commercial products and other alternatives, should be used to encourage intake and ameliorate symptoms associated with hunger, thirst, or malnutrition.
   d. The therapeutic rationale of previous diet prescriptions for an individual patient should be reevaluated. Many dietary restrictions can be liberalized. Coordination of medication or medication schedules with the diet should be discussed with the physician, with the objective of maximizing food choice and intake by the patient.
   e. The patient's right to self-determination must be considered in determining whether to allow the patient to consume foods that are not generally permitted within the diet prescription.
   f. Suboptimal oral feedings may be more appropriate than burdensome tube or parenteral feeding.
9. When tube feeding or parenteral feeding is being considered:
   a. The patient's informed preference for the level of nutrition intervention is primary. The patient or substitute decision maker should be advised on how to accomplish whatever feeding the patient desires.
   b. When palliative care is the agreed goal, nutritional support must be part of the palliative plan. A palliative care plan does no automatically preclude aggressive nutrition support. The decision to forgo "heroic" medical treatment does not preclude baseline nutrition support. All options for nutritional support can be considered.
   c. Feeding may not be desirable if death is expected within hours or a few days and the effects of partial dehydration or the withdrawal of nutrition support will not adversely alter patient comfort.
   d. Facilities should provide and distribute written protocols for the provision and termination of tube feedings and parenteral feedings. The protocols should be reviewed periodically, and revised if necessary, by the healthcare team. Legal and ethical counsel should be routinely sought during the development and interpretation of the guidelines. The institution's ethics com mittee, if available, should assist in establishing and implementing defined, written guidelines for nutrition support protocol. The registered dietitian should be a contributing member of or consultant to such a committee.
   e. Conflict with the family or among stakeholders can be resolved by referring to an ethics committee or consultant if available within the institution.
   f. The potential benefits versus burdens of tube or parenteral feeding should be weighed on the basis of specific facts concerning the patient's medical and mental status, as well as on the facility's options and limitations.
   g. Facility options and limitations—one should consider the following:
      i. Lack of staffing—no one to manage or monitor feeding;
      ii. Too costly without financial help; and
      iii. If a feeding strategy is started in one site, it will have to be stopped when the patient is transferred to another site, which can lead to a sense of abandonment.
10. Either short- or long-term PN should be considered only when other routes are impossible or inadequate to meet the com fort needs of the patient.
11. The physician's written diet order in the medical chart documents the decision to administer or forgo nutrition support.
    a. The registered dietitian should participate in the decision.
    b. If a decision is made that the registered dietitian does not agree with, appeal to the facility's ethics mechanism (committee or consultant) is appropriate.
    c. If the court has ordered feeding or no feeding and you do not agree with the court's decision, appealing to the facility's ethics mechanism is appropriate.

Adapted from Maillet JO, Potter RL, Heller L. Position of the American Dietetic Association: ethical and legal issues in nutrition, hydration, and feeding. *J Am Diet Assoc.* 2002;102(5):716-726.

TABLE 46-8.
The Law in Healthcare

Types of law	Civil—rights/duties of the individual (contract, labor, patent, family, tort)	Criminal (public)—right of the state in its political capacity (including criminal: conduct offensive or harmful to society)
Where created	Federal system national governance	State system cannot conflict with federal, may be more stringent, addresses issues not addressed by federal
Who creates	Common law—judges Statutory law—legislatures Regulatory law—agencies empowered by legislatures (regulations)	
Where decided	Trial court initial suit heard by judge or jury	Appellate court issue decided by judge, including interpretation of statutes or regulations
Type of enforcement and consequences	Administrative system— licensure suspension or revocation Civil system—monetary judgments or orders to act or stop action Criminal system—fines and/or incarceration	
Criteria for determining outcome (evidentiary standard)	Beyond reasonable doubt—criminal Preponderance of evidence Clear and convincing evidence—civil	

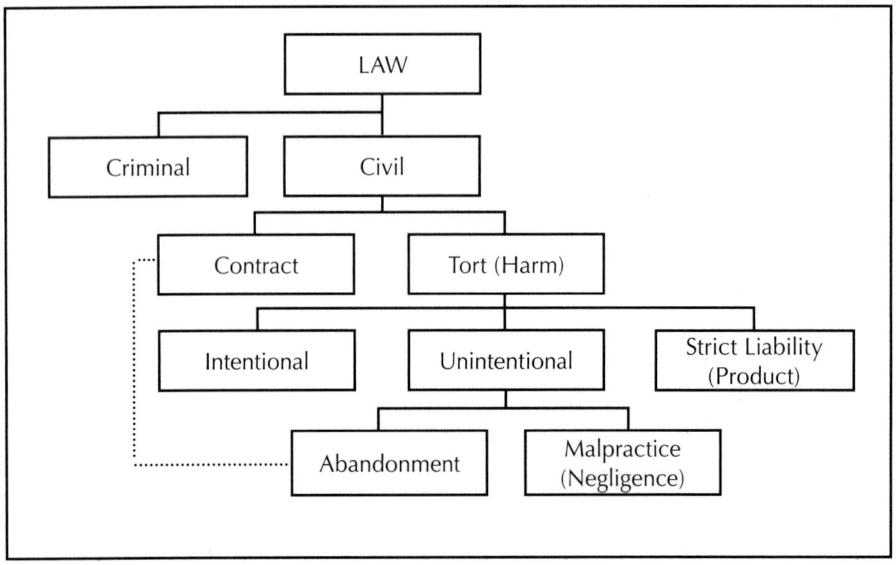

Figure 46-4. The US legal system: An overview with potential ramifications for the healthcare team.

the patient's questions. The patient must consent voluntarily and without coercion. Further, the patient should be informed that the treatment will be discontinued if it is no longer effective. In regard to what is considered adequate information, the standard for information is what is deemed "reasonable" for the patient to know to make a rational decision.[31] Problems can arise when the patient or family facing a withdrawal of treatment have not been informed of the risks/benefits at the time that treatment was initiated or that treatment would be withdrawn when or if treatment was no longer effective (time trial). Studies show that often physicians do not cover all information needed by the patient to give informed consent.[56] As previously discussed, EBM provides reliable information to incorporate in the process of informed consent.

Defamation

Defamation, another intentional tort, causes damage to an individual's reputation, in the form of libel (written) or slander (verbal). To prove defamation, actual damage must

Sidebar 46-1

Example of Multidisciplinary Involvement in Ethics Issue Case Study

Day 1: An 81-year-old female was admitted to the hospital with chest pain.

Day 2: Cardiac catheterization, which was consented for, revealed a 3-vessel disease along with left main disease. Postcatheterization, the patient developed respiratory failure and hypotension, requiring intubation. An intra-aortic balloon pump for hemodynamic stabilization was inserted. The patient was unresponsive at this point.

Day 3: In addition to the internist, cardiologist, pulmonologist, and cardiac surgeon on the case, a nephrologist consult was requested due to decreasing renal function. A gastroenterologist consult was ordered to assess the reason for bright red nasogastric output. During the GI consult, the daughter indicated that 2 years earlier the patient told her that she would never want any aggressive measures used to prolong her life. Endoscopy could be performed according to the gastroenterologist, but the risk-benefit ratio was high due to the patient's cardiac and respiratory status. The gastroenterologist documented and notified the internist and cardiologist of the daughter's concerns. The daughter discussed the situation with the family, then requested terminal extubation and indicated she would bring in documentation of the patient's wishes. However, the daughter initially indicated a timeline of 48 hours to determine if the patient would improve.

Day 4: The daughter brought in the advance directive document, indicating that her mother did not want to be kept alive by any artificial means. According to the cardiologist, the patient's clinical status appeared to be improving, based on cardiac hemodynamics, renal function, and no significant gastrointestinal bleeding. The patient was progressing in ventilatory weaning and the intra-aortic balloon pump was to be removed. The cardiologist reviewed with the daughter that the patient probably was not terminal and that he was reluctant to terminally extubate. However, the daughter was aware that if the patient survived this acute illness, she would then require cardiac surgery, which the patient would not want. The pulmonologist indicated he would wean the patient off the ventilator in the next 24 to 48 hours and that if any distress occurred with the process he would proceed with comfort measures and terminal extubation. Due to ethical concerns, the nurse manager discussed the case with the Risk Management Director and the hospital attorney to verify the ethical standpoint and legal ramifications to uphold the patient/surrogate wishes.

Day 5: The patient remained intubated, but was weaning. Tube feeding initiation was ordered by the cardiologist. During the weekly ICU multidisciplinary rounds, which included the Ethics Committee Chairman, this case was discussed. Nursing staff then asked the biomedical ethics physician to see the patient due to the conflict of the family versus a consultant. The biomedical ethics physician documented that wishes of the surrogate should prevail and that a physician unable to accede to this had the privilege of withdrawing from the case. The dietitian documented in the chart that the tube feeding initiation was being held, after discussion with the nurse. She further indicated that nutrition support should be initiated only as warranted per MD based on anticipated benefit to overall outcome in conjunction with patient/family wishes and noted the advance directive. The nurse stated that the pulmonologist was coming in to discuss with the daughter her wishes on behalf of the patient. The daughter requested that all life support and all medication be discontinued except for comfort measures. The patient was terminally extubated and died that evening.

have occurred to the individual's reputation or livelihood, the damaging information must have been communicated to a third party, and the damaging information must have been false.[47]

Right to Privacy

Violation of the patient's right to privacy, another intentional tort, involves intrusion into the patient's solitude or seclusion, publicly revealing private facts about the patient, giving false information publicly about the patient, or utilizing the patient's name or likeness for the benefit of others without his of her consent. It is not necessary to demonstrate that the patient has suffered specific damages to prove invasion of privacy. Privacy and confidentiality protection are requisites of Health Insurance Portability and Accountability Act (HIPAA), federal legislation impacting healthcare providers since 2003.

Medical Abandonment

Medical abandonment, considered a tort by the legal system, has multiple definitions. It refers to the "unilateral severance of the professional relationship without reasonable notice under the circumstance when continued attention is required."[5] Types of abandonment include inattention, nondiligence, incompetence, or delay in treatment. Abandonment can arise from the refusal to treat, insufficient treatment, delayed treatment, withdrawal without adequate notice, and premature discharge. To prove abandonment, the patient must prove that a relationship that necessitates the physician's duty to treat exists between the practitioner and the patient. The patient-practitioner relationship can be demonstrated through an appointment and examination or treatment; through communication of medical advice via telephone or the internet; through work in the emergency department; or through "taking call" for another practitioner. In providing a defense against the charge of alleged abandonment, the practitioner can demonstrate proper withdrawal with adequate time for orderly transfer of care, designation of an appropriate substitute, referral to a specialist, unreasonable patient/family demands, illness, and emergency.[47]

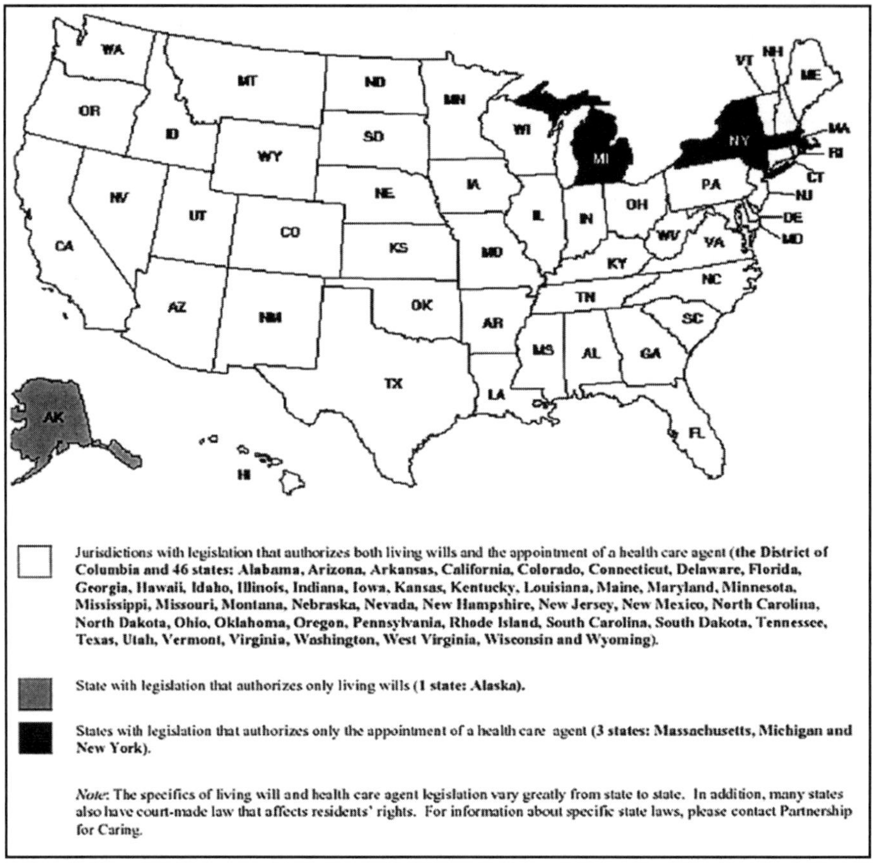

Figure 46-5. State statues governing living wills and appointment of healthcare agents.

Strict Liability

Strict liability in tort has been defined as "[l]iability that does not depend on actual negligence or intent to harm, but that is based on the breach of an absolute duty to make something safe."[57] The most common "classic" examples are in the realm of so-called "ultra-hazardous activities" or in products-liability cases, although there are numerous other areas where states have imposed liability without fault, including, for example, environmental contamination and civil liability for violation of criminal laws.

The field of products liability is perhaps the most likely to impact on medical practice, and litigation and legislation in the field are both plentiful. In general, attempts to apply product-liability principles to what would be conventional medical malpractice action against both hospitals and physicians have been unsuccessful, usually based upon the theory that the "sale" of the device or drug in question was essentially incidental, or inconsequential, to the professional services rendered. However, there have been limited exceptions.[58]

Patient Self-Determination Act of 1990

Another area of law that has impacted medical practice involves the Patient Self-Determination Act of 1990, which became effective in December 1991. This act mandates that healthcare entities who accept Medicare and Medicaid reimbursement provide written mechanisms for explaining to the patient his or her legal rights and options for accepting or declining medical treatment so the individual can make an "informed" decision. Further, the patients can formulate, while capable, an advance directive to address treatment issues or designate a surrogate to make decisions on his or her behalf, in the event that the patient lacks capacity at the time of treatment. Advance directives have been legislated in some form or another in all 50 states[59] (Figure 46-5). Advance directives can take the form of a living will and/or durable medical power-of-attorney, as previously discussed. There is some concern as to the effectiveness of the living will, as studies have shown that people are typically unable to state specifically what types of care they would actually want in various circumstances.[60] Wording of the living will can be vague or the patient may not be able to locate it to provide it to the healthcare entity. Medical (healthcare) power-of-attorney enables a patient to designate another person or surrogate to act on his or her behalf when incapacitated. It is imperative that surrogate decision makers, whether as a power-of-attorney for healthcare decisions or not, discuss the living will and other "directives" with the individual. The legislation of advance directives usually gave immunity from successful prosecution to practitioners who, in good faith, follow the directives.[31] A variety of other resources are available for individuals to express their wishes if incapacitated (Table 46-9).

"Capacity" is defined as the patient having the ability to understand information about his or her healthcare problem and the results/risks of treatment; evaluate options based upon the risk/benefit of each; make rational choices; and communicate the decision. The incapacity to form decisions can be noted in comatose patients, infants, children, mentally disabled patients, and disoriented patients.[31] The

TABLE 46-9.

Types of Advance Medical Directives and Substituted Judgment

Medical Directives

Statutory
Directive portion of natural death/living will act
Nonstatutory
Living will
Partnership for Caring
Other organizations (Hemlock)
Personalized
A more detailed matrix for establishing individual preferences for a variety of interventions in a variety of clinical situations.[61]
Ethical will[62]
Individual written document
Five wishes[63]
Other (Internet) (see other resources)

Substituted (Surrogate) Judgment

Statutory
Durable power of attorney
Proxy/agent for healthcare decisions
Non-statutory
Durable power of attorney
Proxy/agent for healthcare decisions
Organization forms, individual papers
Judicial/legal guardian, court hearing

*These options are not universally available in every state.

surrogate's goal is to arrive at the same decision for healthcare choice that the patient would make, were he or she able to do so. The surrogate, in this case, should consider the patient's past stated wishes regarding treatment, the patient's religious or cultural beliefs, what effect the decision will have on the family, likelihood of adverse effects of the treatment, and prognosis both with and without treatment. The principle of best interest involves the surrogate making decisions that will benefit the patient, including relief of suffering; quality and extent of the patient's life (quality being based on the patient's own goals and values); patient's wishes; preserving or restoring function to the patient; possibility of patient's future satisfaction with life; and the patient's possibility of regaining "capacity", even if these decisions are counter to the surrogate's personal beliefs and convictions.[47]

The patient has a legal right to refuse treatment, regardless of health condition and including life-saving and life-prolonging treatment. This affirms the basic legal tenet of autonomy and self determination as in the ethical arena, and as expressed by the New York State Supreme Court Judge Cardozo in 1914,[64] and the US Supreme Court in the Cruzan case in 1990.[1] A patient may determine that care be withdrawn or withheld, as long as the patient has "capacity" and documentation of appropriate informed, educated consent meeting previously outlined criteria. Forgoing medical treatment is considered neither suicide nor homicide. Further, there has been no legal distinction drawn between withholding and withdrawing medical treatment, though there are more stringent requirements in some states with regard to surrogate decision makers and artificial nutrition and hydration[31] (Table 46-10).

CASES IN THE UNITED STATES

Despite federal and state statues, organizational guidelines, templates, and other efforts and resources, controversies continue to emerge demonstrating the complexity and heterogeneity of issues regarding forgoing life-sustaining interventions (Figure 46-6). Several cases illustrate these points.

Precedent Setting Legal Cases

Quinlan

Karen Ann Quinlan experienced anoxic brain damage resulting in her remaining in a permanent vegetative state and requiring ventilator support and EN support. Based on earlier comments by their daughter, her parents requested removal of the ventilator. Fearing criminal repercussions, her physicians were reluctant to comply. Her parents pursued their quest in the New Jersey court system. The New Jersey Supreme Court allowed the removal of the ventilator, ruling that physicians could remove life-sustaining treatments provided a prognosis of "no reasonable possibility of a patient returning to a cognitive, sapient state"

Table 46-10.

Legal Decisions Regarding Forgoing Medical Therapies Anthology

1976—Quinlan (NJ)
1979—Spring (MA)
1980-1984—(TX)
1982—Baby Doe (IN, AZ)
1983—Barber (CA)
1984—Bartling (CA)
1984-1986—Bouvia (CA)
1984—Conroy (NJ)
1985—State Supreme Court (GA)
1985-1986—Brophy (MA)
1986—Jobes (NJ)
1986—Peters (NJ)
1986—Corbett (FL)
1990—Cruzan (MO)
1991—Wanglie (MN)
1998—Finn (VA)
1999-2000—Blouin (NY)
2001—Wendland (CA)
2003-2005—Schiavo (FL)

(State in which decision made is in parentheses.)

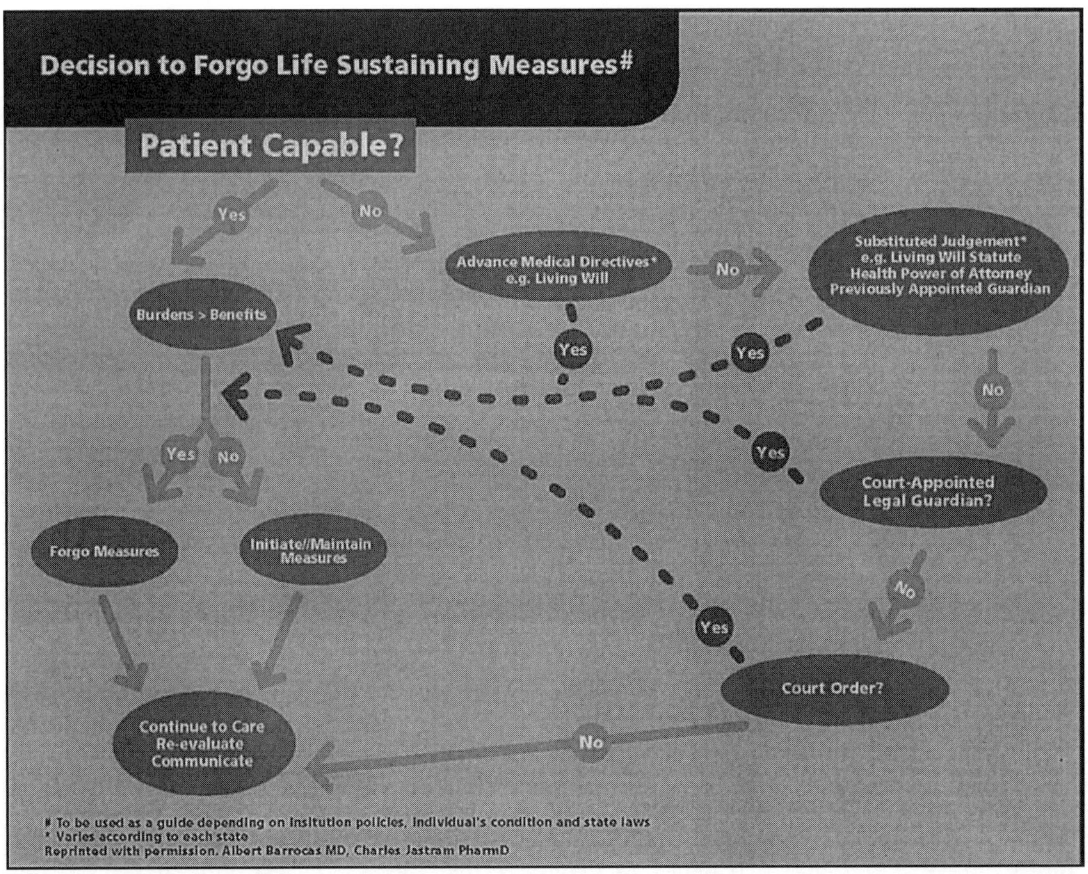

Figure 46-6. Decisions to forgo life-sustaining measures.

was confirmed by a hospital ethics committee. Criminal and civil legal protection was provided to all involved in the decision making process. Interestingly, Karen Quinlan lived for several more years without a ventilator, but with tube feedings, which were never challenged by family or physicians. The Quinlan case is credited with the impetus for the establishment of hospitals' ethics committees and the enactment of states' "living will" legislation.[65,66]

Cruzan

Despite the pivotal decision of the Quinlan case, it was limited in its legal impact to the State of New Jersey. In the case of Nancy Cruzan, the US Supreme Court asserted and clarified the current management of these issues in the United States. Like Karen Quinlan, Nancy Cruzan was in a persistent vegetative state: she experienced extensive brain damage following a motor vehicular accident. She was not on a ventilator; however, she required tube feedings to survive. She did not have a living will. At that time, the State of Missouri required such an advance directive or other "clear and convincing" evidence for the removal of life-sustaining therapies by noncapable individuals.[1,66]

In 1990, the US Supreme Court affirmed the authority of individual states to establish a higher standard of evidence if they so choose. In its deliberation, the Court, for the first time in federal history, established that artificial nutrition and hydration were life-support/sustaining interventions, no different than ventilators and hemodialysis, which could be withdrawn/withheld provided the appropriate clinical, ethical, and legal criteria are met. The decision stimulated the increased use of healthcare proxies or durable power-of-attorney for healthcare decisions and the eventual enactment of the Patient Self Determination Act of 1990 by the US Congress.[1,66]

Blouin Versus Spitzer

Sheila Pouliot, a clinically disabled 44-year-old woman with mental retardation, severe cerebral palsy, and incomplete quadriparesis was admitted to the SUNY Health Science Center in Syracuse, NY, acutely ill and near death, on December 19, 1999. Three days later—after a conference of family (sister Ms. Blouin), medical staff, institutional ethics committee, and clergy—and with the agreement of all present, a decision was made to provide palliative care, consisting mainly of intravenous morphine sulfate. The patient was to receive no antibiotics and no artificial nutrition or hydration. All other treatments that would prolong the dying process were discontinued.

Five days later, while the patient was felt to be in her last hours of life, the attending physician was ordered by the office of the State of New York Attorney General (Spitzer) to provide resuscitative measures. The order set in motion a cascade of legal activities, which included application to the State Court by the Attorney General for appointment of an attorney ad litem. The Attorney General further held the position that no one other than a competent patient could decide to withhold nutrition and hydration. Despite concurrence by all concerned, including the court-appointed guardian and the patient's continued intolerance to the attempts at artificial and hydration via a PEG tube, it was not until 3 months later (March 6, 2000) that the healthcare team was able to implement the original recommendations of the family, staff, and ethics committee and to discontinue the artificial hydration. The patient died on the same day. The perseverance of the Attorney General position in this case was based on the absence of documented expressions of her desires or a designated proxy or durable power of attorney for healthcare decisions.[65]

Arkansas Rights for the Terminally Ill and Permanently Unconscious Act

In a similar situation, the State of Arkansas, in 2003, amended the Arkansas Rights for the Terminally Ill and Permanently Unconscious Act (commonly known as "ARTIPUA") to imply a "clear and convincing evidence" standard. In addition, the legislation also requires that Advance Directive must have specific instructions regarding the withholding of nutrition and hydration for directives executed after July 2003. In 2005, the Louisiana legislature amended its statute in like fashion. The Arkansas amendment included a new section specific to long-term care.[66]

Another Potential Controversy

In his address to the International Congress of "Life Sustaining Treatments and Vegetative State: Scientific Advances and Ethical Dilemmas" on March 20, 2004, Pope John Paul II stated:

"I should like particularly to underline how the administration of water and food, even when provided by artificial means, always represents a natural means of preserving life, not a medical act. Its use, furthermore, should be considered, in principle, ordinary and proportionate, and as such morally obligatory, insofar as and until it is seen to have attained its proper finality, which in the present case consists in providing nourishment to the patient and alleviation of his suffering."[67]

The Pope's remarks have stimulated discussion by Catholic healthcare facility leaders in the United States because their hospitals (as do other US hospitals) defer to the 1990 US Supreme Court ruling in the Cruzan Case.[1] Currently, the Catholic healthcare institutions are following the Ethical and Religious Directives for Catholic Health Care.[68] The US Conference of Catholic Bishops is expected to review, and perhaps revise, the directives in the future.

It is noteworthy that on April 2, 2005, Pope John Paul II died—approximately 1 year after his remarks reaffirming the dignity of death, after his failing health was complicated by urosepsis and cardiovascular collapse. During his final days, he was fed via a nasoenteric feeding tube. When informed of the gravity of his condition, he elected to remain in his apartment in the Vatican overlooking St. Peter's Square rather than returning to the hospital. Thus, until the end, he lived as he taught: that life holds inherent dignity until the moment of death. In his case, he was able to make decisions about his own healthcare, with full acceptance of his wishes by those around him. His case is in direct contrast with that of Terri Schiavo.

Theresa "Terri" Schiavo

In the much publicized case of Theresa "Terri" Schiavo, from the state of Florida, the involved parties included the patient's parents and the husband as well as Florida's governor, legislature, and supreme court. Following a cardiac arrest on February 25, 1990, Schiavo was in a persistent vegetative state requiring artificial nutrition support. Unfortunately, Terri did not have a living will or a proxy for healthcare decisions prior to her cardiac arrest. Her husband, Michael Schiavo, was appointed by the Florida Court as her guardian, without objection from her parents, Mary and Bob Schindler. She was transferred to multiple healthcare facilities including rehabilitation centers.[69]

The Schiavos received $4 million total for three settlements; in February 1993, Michael and the Schindlers began struggling over Terri's therapy and division of the malpractice money. From that time, the adversarial relationship between Michael and the Schindlers resulted in numerous legal proceedings.[70] Michael claimed that Terri had voiced her desire to not be artificially supported if she ever became incapable of making her own healthcare decisions and he fought to have her PEG tube removed; however, the Schindlers disagreed and persisted, unsuccessfully, to have Michael removed as Terri's guardian.

On behalf of the Schindlers, the Florida State Legislature passed "Terri's Law" and Governor Jeb Bush signed it on October 21, 2003. The law gave the Governor the authority to issue a one-time stay of withholding/withdrawing feeding tube if there were no written directives; the patient was in a permanent vegetative state; she (or he) had nutrition and hydration withheld; and family members challenged the decision to forgo nutrition/hydration. Upon creation of the law, Terri's feeding tube was reinserted. (This was the third removal and reinsertion in 6 months.) Michael Schiavo's attorney challenged the constitutionality of the law, while the Schindlers' again requested termination of Michael's guardianship. After much legal activity, the Florida Supreme Court deemed "Terri's Law" unconstitutional; however, her feeding tube remained in temporarily because of numerous appeals.

The Schiavo case attracted national attention, and the federal government became involved. The US House of Representatives and the Senate passed legislation intended to move the case from state to federal court on Friday March 17, 2005. The following week was full of legal activity on behalf of both sides of the struggle.[70] In a historical maneuver, the US Senate delayed its spring recess, working on Saturday, March 19, to reach a compromise with the House bill. Subsequently, the US House of Representatives returned from spring recess on the evening of Sunday, March 20, to debate and pass S 686. President George W. Bush signed the law, which allowed the Schindlers to request a federal judge to order the reinsertion of the PEG tube while the lawsuit was litigated.

During a national frenzy supporting both sides of the issue, the courts asserted the right of Terri Schiavo, through her court-appointed guardian and husband, to withdraw life-sustaining measures on March 22. In comments concurring with the US Court of Appeals for the 11th District on March 30, 2005, Circuit Court Judge Birch stated:

"In resolving the Schiavo controversy, it is my judgment that, despite sincere and altruistic motivation, the legislative and executive branches of our government have acted in a manner demonstrably at odds with our Founding Fathers' blueprint for the governance of a free people—our Constitution."

Later that day, the US Supreme Court denied a stay of enforcement of the judgment of the US Court of Appeals. Terri Schiavo remained in the hospice, receiving other comfort measures until her death at 9:05 am EST on March 31, 2005.[70,71]

Recent International Cases

The struggle to establish unanimity in thought about this thorny decision is not limited to the US. In 1998, the first officially authorized removal of ventilator support in Israel was carried out in a 49-year-old, retired fighter pilot with ALS, who had expressed his wishes for forgoing the support much earlier. He died shortly after the removal of the ventilator support. In July of 2004, Israel's court allowed the termination of ventilator support for another individual with terminal ALS at the request of the patient's wife, but in the absence of the patient's expressed consent. This departure from previous practice drew immediate protest from many individuals who viewed the action as "active" euthanasia and feared that Israel may be following other countries down the "slippery slope" of end-of-life care decisions.[72]

Part of the controversy in Israel stems from two sources that influence the country's laws. One source, the Talmud, forbids all acts that may hasten death, based on Medieval Jewish Law. Alternatively, the Shulchan Aruch, the authoritative 16th-century code of law, states that any hindrance to the soul's departure may be removed because there is no act involved, only the removal of the impediment.[73]

The differences in opinions are not limited to the secular Israeli government. Within Judaism, debate continues between Orthodox, Conservative, and Reform Rabbinical authorities. Whereas some make the distinction between withdrawing and withholding, others differentiate between ventilators and artificial nutrition and hydration, counter to the overwhelming US position.

Professor Avinoam Reches, a neurologist at Hadassah University Hospital, has championed the cause of advance directives and has been involved in the two cases cited, in addition to several others. He was successful in having the Israel Language Hebrew Academy approve the term "mitat hesed" or "mercy dying" as in passive euthanasia, to differentiate from the term "hamatat hesed" or "mercy killing" referring to active euthanasia, or euthanasia for those who do not accept the dual classification.[5]

Summary of Recent Cases

In sum, these cases illustrate the importance of communication as stated in the ethical section of this chapter.

1. It is highly recommended that medical directives be as explicit as possible and include specific language addressing artificial and nonvolitional hydration and nutrition.
2. Serious deliberation should be undertaken in the selection of a surrogate decision maker, and, whenever possible, execute state-approved documents for the designation of a durable power of attorney for healthcare decisions.
3. The written advance directive should be discussed thoroughly with the surrogate decision maker in the presence of interested parties (eg, family members) to minimize later conflicts, within the limits of patient privacy and confidentiality.

4. These documents should be reviewed annually.
5. The location of these documents should be known by all concerned and always be accessible in case of admission to a healthcare facility.
6. Diligent updating of the documents should be undertaken to assure their compliance with the ever-changing state statutory landscape.
7. Where possible, the executed documents should be registered with the State Attorney General's Office.

Despite the practitioner's understanding of patient rights and healthcare law, this knowledge does not insulate him/her from litigation. Anyone can bring suit against a practitioner. The majority of malpractice suits arise from misunderstanding or lack of communication among the parties involved. It behooves the practitioner to maintain a current knowledge base regarding the law, and to practice, taking into consideration the impact of culture, age, religion and ethnicity on the patient's respective view of the care provided.[74,75]

Conclusion: Implementing the "Can," the "Should," and the "Must"

The complex tapestry of the trichotomy of technology, ethics, and law, as applied to nutrition support in GI disease, is interwoven with 12 very practical threads or the 12 Cs: common sense, common decency, competence, commitment, communications, consultations, collaboration, consent/consensus, concern, care, compassion, and comfort.[5]

Comfort represents the strongest and most durable fiber in dealing with the decision-making process and the interactions between patient, healthcare team, family and friends.[76] It forms the foundation of the goals of healthcare professionals: to cure rarely, to treat often, and to comfort always.

References

1. Cruzan v Director, Missouri Department of Health, 497 U.S. 261 (1990).
2. Wilmore DW, Dudrick SJ. Growth and development of an infant receiving all nutrients exclusively by vein. *JAMA*. 1968;203:860-864.
3. Barrocas A, Baumgartner TG, Jastram CW, et al. Enteral and parenteral nutrition. *Problems Crit Care*. 1991;5:411-471.
4. Levinsky NG. The doctor's master. *N Engl J Med*. 1984;311:1573-1575.
5. Barrocas A, Yarbrough G, Becnel PA III, Nelson JE. Ethical and legal issues in nutrition support of the geriatric patient: the can, should, and must of nutrition support. *Nutr Clin Pract*. 2003;18(1):37-47.
6. Webster's New Collegiate Dictionary. Springfield, MA: G. & C. Merriam Co.; 1981.
7. Hippocratic corpus. In: Reiser SJ, Dyck AJ, Curran WJ, eds. *Ethics in Medicine*. Cambridge, Mass: MIT Press; 1977.
8. Beauchamp T, Childress J. *Principles of Biomedical Ethics*. 4th ed. New York, NY: Oxford University Press; 1994.
9. Ganzini L, Volicer L, Nelson WA, Fox E, Derse AR. Ten myths about decision-making capacity. *J Am Med Dir Assoc*. 2004;5(4):263-267. Available at: www.ilcusa.org/_lib/pdf/soul0205.pdf. Accessed June 18, 2005.
10. Ganzini L, Volicer L, Nelson W, Derse A. Pitfalls in assessment of decision-making capacity. *Psychosomatics*. 2003;44:237-243. Available at: http://psy.psychiatryonline.org/cgi/content/abstract/44/3/237. Accessed June 18, 2005.
11. Lipman TO. Ethical issues in nutrition support and cancer. *Nutrition Week Program Handbook*. 2004;812-814.
12. Ferrell BR, Coyle N. *Textbook of Palliative Nursing*. New York, NY: Oxford University Press; 2001.
13. E-2.035 Futile care. [AMA Web site]. June 1994. Available at: http://www.ama-assn.org/ama/pub/category/8389.html. Accessed June 18, 2005.
14. E-2.037 Medical futility in end-of-life-care. [AMA Web site]. June 1997. Available at: http://www.ama-assn.org/ama/pub/category/8390.html. Accessed June 18, 2005.
15. Halevy A, Brody BA. A multi-institution collaborative policy on medical futility. *JAMA*. 1996;276(7):571-574.
16. The Ethics Committee of the Society of Critical Care Medicine. Consensus statement of the Society of Critical Care Medicine's Ethics Committee regarding futile and other possible inadvisable treatment. *Crit Care Med*. 1997;25(5):887-892.
17. Engelhardt HT. Rethinking concepts of futility in critical care. Center for Medical Ethics and Health Policy. Baylor College of Medicine. October 1996. Available at: http://www.mediscene.com/medpub/futile.htm. Accessed June 18, 2005.
18. Cohen NH. Assessing futility of medical interventions. *Crit Care Med*. 2003;31(2):646-648.
19. Youngner SJ. Who defines futility? *JAMA*. 1988;260(14):2094-2095.
20. NCCB Committee for Pro-Life Activities. Nutrition and hydration: moral and pastoral reflections (1992). [United States Confederacy of Catholic Bishops Web site]. Available at: http://www.usccb.org/prolife/issues/euthanas/nutindex.htm. Accessed June 18, 2005.
21. Haddad RY, Thomas DR. Enteral nutrition and enteral tube feeding. Review of the evidence. *Clin Geriatr Med*. 2002;18(4):867-881.
22. Medical futility in end-of-life care: report of the Council on Ethical and Judicial Affairs. *JAMA*. 1999;281(10):937-941.
23. Hinshaw DB, Pawlik T, Mosenthal AC, Civetta JM, Hallenbeck J. When do we stop and how do we do it? Medical futility and withdrawal of care. *J Am Coll Surg*. 2003;196(4):621-651.
24. American College of Physicians Ethics Manual. 4th ed. *Ann Intern Med*. 1998;128(7):576-594.
25. Schneiderman LJ, Jecker NS, Jonsen AR. Medical futility: its meaning and ethical implications. *Ann Intern Med*. 1990;112(12):949-954.
26. Fine RL, Mayo TW. The rise and fall of the futility movement. *N Engl J Med*. 2000;343(21):1575-1576.
27. Luce JM. Physicians do not have a responsibility to provide futile or unreasonable care if a patient or family insists. *Crit Care Med*. 1995;23:760-766.
28. Weijer C, Singer PA, Dickens BM, Workman S. Bioethics for clinicians: 16. Dealing with demands for inappropriate treatment. *CMAJ*. 1998;159(7):817-821.
29. Turner L. Recognizing the persistence of an ethical conflict: disputes concerning what constitutes appropriate levels of care: part 1. *Ann Long Term Care*. 2004;12(2):15-20. Available at: http://www.mmhc.com/altc/displayArticle.cfm?articleID=altcac1932. Accessed June 18, 2005.
30. Fagerlin A, Schneider CE. Enough: the failure of the living will. Hastings Center Report. 2004 March-April; 34(2):30-42. Available at: http://www.thehastingscenter.org/pdf/publications/hcr_mar_apr_2004_enough.pdf. Accessed June 18, 2005.

CERTIFICATION OF AUTHORITY
TO
CONSENT ON BEHALF OF A PATIENT TO MEDICAL TREATMENT

I/we have discussed the condition of ______________________, my/our

______________________ (relationship), with the attending physician, ________________, M.D.

I/we are hereby agree that the patient is now unable to consent. I/we are hereby being advised and understand that when consent to medical treatment is needed on behalf of a minor (under 18) or an adult who is unable to consent, the person or persons specified in the next paragraph may consent under Louisiana Law (L.R.S. 40:1299.53)

I/we represent that I/we am/are, in the following order of priority if there is no individual in a prior class who is reasonably available, willing, and competent to act:

(1) Any judicially appointed guardian (tutor or curator). Present if requested and attach copy of court order;
(2) Any appointee under a power of attorney specifically authorizing healthcare decisions. Present if requested and attach copy of power of attorney;
(3) The husband or wife if not legally separated;
(4) A majority of the adult children available for consultation;
(5) Both parents, whether adult or minor, or one parent if the other parent is not available for consultation;
(6) A majority of brothers and sisters available for consultation;
(7) A majority of grandparents, grandchildren, and other ascendants or descendants available for consultation.

This document is being executed in the presence of the undersigned witness(es).

SIGNATURE	NAME PRINTED	RELATIONSHIP	DATE	WITNESS

Appendix. Documentation of Authority to Consent (compatible with Louisiana law).

31. Emanuel LL, von Gunten CF, Ferris FD, eds. *Education for Physicians on End-of-Life Care.* Module 9:1-13. Chicago, IL: EPEC Project, The Robert Wood Johnson Foundation, 1999.
32. In Conroy RE. 98 NJ 321 486A. 2d, 1209, 1985.
33. A.S.P.E.N. Board of Directors and Clinical Guidelines Task Force. Guidelines for the use of parenteral and enteral nutrition in adult and pediatric patients. *JPEN J Parenter Enteral Nutr.* 2002;26(2):144.
34. A.S.P.E.N. *Clinical Guidelines Handbook 2002.* Silver Springs, MD: A.S.P.E.N.; 2002.
35. Agency for Healthcare Research and Quality. [AHRQ Web site]. Available at: http://www.ahcpr.gov Accessed June 25, 2005.
36. Ebell MH, Siwek J, Weiss BD, et al. Strength of recommendation taxonomy (SORT): a patient-centered approach to grading evidence in the medical literature. *Am Fam Physician.* 2004;69(3):548-556.
37. Oyogoa S, Schein M, Gardezi S, Wise L. Surgical feeding gastrostomy: are we overdoing it? *J Gastrointest Surg.* 1999;3(2):152-155.
38. Abuksis G, Mor M, Segal N, et al. Percutaneous endoscopic gastrostomy: high mortality rates in hospitalized patients. *Am J Gastroenterol.* 2000;95(1):128-132.
39. Grant MD, Rudberg MA, Brody JA. Gastrostomy placement and mortality among hospitalized Medicare beneficiaries. *JAMA.* 1998;279(24):1973-1976.

40. Kruse A, Misiewicz JJ, Rokkas, et al. Recommendations of the ESGE workshop on the ethics of percutaneous endoscopic gastrostomy (PEG) placement for nutrition support. First European Symposium on Ethics in Gastroenterology and Digestive Endoscopy. *Endoscopy.* 2003;35(9):778-780.
41. Finucane TE, Christmas C, Travis K. Tube feeding in patients with advanced dementia: a review of the evidence. *JAMA.* 1999;282(14):1365-1370.
42. Murphy LM, Lipman TO. Percutaneous endoscopic gastrostomy does not prolong survival in patients with dementia. *Arch Intern Med.* 2003;163(11):1351-1353.
43. Mazzini L, Corra T, Zaccala M, Mora G, Del Piano M, Galante M. Percutaneous endoscopic gastrostomy and enteral nutrition in amyotrophic lateral sclerosis. *J Neurol.* 1995;242(10):695-698.
44. Barrocas A, Barrocas N. Health care in the 1990s: old wine in new bottles. *South Med J.* 1988;81(2):243-246.
45. Barrocas A, Barrocas NY, Griver YM. Health care in transition: the physician and the OWAs. *J La State Med Soc.* 1988;140(1):37-44.
46. Fletcher JC, Lombardo PA, Marshall MF, Miller FG, eds. *Introduction to Clinical Ethics.* Frederick, MD: University Publishing Group; 1997.
47. Feutz-Harter S. *Nursing and the Law.* 6th ed. Madison, WI: Professional Educations Systems, Inc.; 1997.
48. Mion LC, O'Connell A. Parenteral hydration and nutrition in the geriatric patient: clinical and ethical issues. *J Infusion Nursing.* 2003;26(3):144-152.
49. Sheehan MN. Feeding tubes: sorting out the issues. Several clinical factors determine the efficacy of artificial nutrition and hydration. Health Progress: *Official J Catholic Health Association* [serial online]. Nov-Dec 2001;82(6). Available at: http://www.chausa.org/PUBS/PUBSCONT.ASP?ISSUE=HP0111. Accessed June 25, 2005.
50. Winter SM. Terminal nutrition: framing the debate for the withdrawal of nutritional support in terminally ill patients. *Am J Med.* 2000;109(9):723-726.
51. Andrews M, Boyle J. *Transcultural Concepts in Nursing Care.* 3rd ed. Philadelphia, PA: Lippincott, Williams, & Wilkins; 1999.
52. Galanti G. *Caring for Patients from Different Cultures: Case Studies from American Hospitals.* 2nd ed. Philadelphia, PA: University of Pennsylvania Press; 1997.
53. Lipson JG, Dibble SL, Minarik PA, eds. *Culture and Nursing Care: A Pocket Guide.* San Francisco, CA: UCSF Nursing Press; 1996.
54. Maillet JO, Potter RL, Heller L. Position of the American Dietetic Association: ethical and legal issues in nutrition, hydration, and feeding. *J Am Diet Assoc.* 2002;102(5):716-726.
55. Barrocas A, Faquharson J, Fernandez M. Legal considerations in nutritional support. *Nutr Support Serv.* 1986;(6):13-15.
56. Braddock CH 3rd, Edwards KA, Hasenberg NM, Laidley TL, Levinson W. Informed decision making in outpatient practice: time to get back to basics. *JAMA.* 1999;282(24):2313-2320.
57. Garner BA, ed. *Black's Law Dictionary.* 8th ed. Eagan, MN: West Group; 2004.
58. Annot., 65 A.L.R.5th 357 (2005).
59. State statutes governing living wills and appointment of health care agents. *Partnership for Caring 2000* [serial online]. Available at: http://www.partnershipforcaring.org/Resources/map.html Accessed October 10, 2004.
60. Ruffenach G. Rethinking living wills. *The Times-Picayune.* June 27, 2004:F10.
61. Emanuel LL, Emanuel EJ. Decisions at the end of life: guided by communities of patients. *Hastings Cent Rep.* 1993;23:6.
62. Baines BK. *Ethical Wills: Putting Your Values on Paper.* Cambridge, MA: Peseus Publishing; 2002.
63. Five Wishes [Aging with Dignity Web site]. Available at: http://www.agingwithdignity.org/5wishes.html. Accessed June 26, 2005.
64. Schloendorff v Society of New York Hospital, 211 NY 125, 105 NE 92, 93 (1914).
65. Blouin v Spitzer, 356 F.3d. 348, 356. n.8 (2d. Cir. 2004)
66. Ark. Code. Ann. 20-17-02 (f and g).
67. Address of John Paul II to the participants in the International Congress on "Life-Sustaining Treatments and Vegetative State: Scientific Advances and Ethical Dilemmas". Sat. March 20, 2004. Available at: http://www.vatican.va/holy_father/john_paul_ii/speeches/2004/march/documents/hf_jp-ii_spe_20040320_congress-fiamc_en.html. Accessed June 25, 2005.
68. *Ethical and Religious Directives for Catholic Health Services.* 4th ed. Washington, DC: USCCB Publishing, United States Conference of Catholic Bishop; 2001.
69. Documents in the Schiavo Case. Supreme Court of Florida. Available at: http://www.flcourts.org/pubinfo/Schiavo/index.html. Accessed June 18, 2005.
70. Cerminara K, Goodman K. Key events in the case of Theresa Marie Schiavo. http://www.miami.edu/ethics2/schiavo/timeline.htm. Accessed: June 18, 2005.
71. Barrocas A. Letter to the editor: the last word on Terri Schiavo. *The Jewish Times.* April 29, 2005;20:7.
72. Elliman W. To die without suffering—Israel's first euthanasia. *The Jewish Post of New York Online* [serial online]. May 1999. Available at: http://www.jewishpost.com/jp0505/jpn0505k.htm. Accessed June 18, 2005.
73. Neeman Y, Sacks E. Euthanasia: the approach of the courts in Israel and the application of the Jewish Law Principles. Jewish Virtual Library: A Division of the American-Israeli Cooperative Enterprise. Available at: http://www.jewishvirtuallibrary.org/jsource/Judaism/euth.html. Accessed June 25, 2005.
74. Hallenbeck JL Palliative care: intercultural differences and communication at the end of life. *Primary Care: Clinics in Office Practice.* 2001;28(2).
75. Last Acts Diversity and End of Life Care Literature Review. Annotated Bibliography- Center to Advance Palliative Care; 2004. Available at: http://old.capc.org/content/105/?topic=11. Accessed October 10, 2004.
76. Quill TE. Terri Schiavo–A tragedy compounded. *N Engl J Med.* 2005;352(16):1630-1033.

Section VII

Obesity

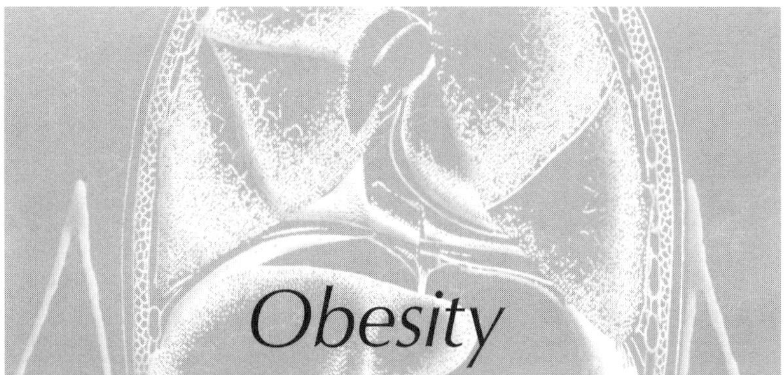

Chapter 47

Medical Management of Obesity

Robert F. Kushner, MD

Introduction

Overweight and obesity is the most common medical problem seen in primary care practice, affecting over 60% of adults and 15% of adolescents.[1,2] Obesity, along with diet and physical inactivity, is estimated to be responsible for approximately 400,000 preventable deaths per year and is expected to soon rival cigarette smoking as the most important public health concern.[3] The etiology of obesity is multifactorial, brought about by an interaction between predisposing genetic and metabolic factors and a rapidly changing environment. Interactive influences include social, behavioral, physiological, metabolic, cellular, and molecular factors. The most exciting breakthroughs in obesity research over the past decade have come from our understanding of the metabolic processes that control body-weight regulation. It appears that multiple feedback loops exist between the central and autonomic nervous systems, the endocrine glands, and adipose tissue, which operate to adjust hunger, satiety, and energy expenditure. Weight maintenance is now considered to be governed by a combination of short-term mechanisms originating in the gastrointestinal (GI) tract and longer-term processes, which monitor total adipose mass involving feedback to the central nervous system (CNS).[4] Signals that provide short-term information about hunger and satiety include gut hormones, such as cholecystokinin (CCK), ghrelin, and peptide $YY_{3\text{-}36}$ (PYY), and signals from the vagus afferent neurons within the GI tract that respond to mechanical deformation, macronutrients, pH, tonicity, and hormones.[5] Whereas ghrelin stimulates food intake, PYY produces satiety. Several recent reviews on the metabolic regulation of body weight and appetite control have been published.[6-8]

From a clinical perspective, weight gain and obesity occur when there is an imbalance in energy (calories), where $\text{energy}_{\text{in}}$ exceeds $\text{energy}_{\text{out}}$. The societal pressures that expose individuals to high-calorie and large-portion convenience foods along with technical advances that promote sedentary behavior have led to unintentional obesity. Regardless of its underlying cause, obesity is a major risk factor for increased morbidity and mortality from type 2 diabetes mellitus, hypertension, the metabolic syndrome, coronary heart disease, sleep apnea, and some forms of cancer, among other diseases. As overweight and obesity affect nine organ systems including the GI system, it is appropriate and imperative that the gastroenterologist address this highly prevalent and serious medical condition. This chapter reviews the identification, evaluation, and medical management of the adult obese patient. A recently published 10-booklet primer from the American Medical Association that reviews the assessment and treatment of obesity will be helpful to interested readers who want further information about the implementation of obesity care into their office practice.[9]

Assessment of the Overweight and Obese Patient and Identification of Risk

In 1998, the National Heart, Lung, and Blood Institute (NHLBI) published the "Clinical Guidelines on the Identification, Evaluation, and Treatment of Overweight and Obesity in Adults".[10] The Expert Panel used evidence-based methodology to develop key recommendations for assessing and treating overweight and obese patients. "A Practical Guide to the Identification, Evaluation, and Treatment of Overweight and Obesity in Adults" was subsequently developed cooperatively by the NHLBI and North American Association for the Study of Obesity (NAASO) and published in 2000.[11] Both guidelines recommend proactive obesity care, beginning with identification, classification, and categorization of risk. Recently, the US Preventive Services Task Force reinforced this recommendation by concluding that clinicians should screen all adult patients for obesity and offer intensive counseling and behavioral interventions to promote sustained weight loss for obese adults.[12]

A thorough obesity-focused history, physical examination, and laboratory evaluation based on the patient's risk factors should be completed prior to discussing and initiating treatment.[13] Assessment of the patient should include the evaluation of body mass index (BMI), waist circumference (for BMI <35 kg/m^2), and overall medical risk. BMI is calculated as weight (kg)/height (m^2), or more conveniently as weight (lb)/height $(in)^2$ x 703. For easy reference, Table 47-1 shows the corresponding BMI based on height and weight. Table 47-2 is used to define classification of weight status and risk of disease. A desirable or healthy BMI is 18.5 to 25 kg/m^2, overweight is 25 to 29.9 kg/m^2, and obesity is ≥30 kg/m^2. Obesity is further subdefined into class I (30.0 to 34.9 kg/m^2), class II (35.0 to 39.9 kg/m^2), and class III (≥40 kg/m^2). Although "morbid obesity" is still listed in the IDC9 CM for coding purposes, it is currently being replaced by other descriptive terms including class III obesity, extreme obesity, or clinically severe obesity. According to the Practical Guide, patients at very high absolute risk that trigger the need for intense risk-factor modification and management include the following: established coronary heart disease; presence of other atherosclerotic diseases such as peripheral arterial disease, abdominal aortic aneurysm, or symptomatic carotid artery disease; type 2 diabetes; and sleep apnea. Other symptoms and diseases listed by organ system that are directly or indirectly related to obesity are displayed in Table 47-3.[13]

Overall risk is independently associated with excess abdominal fat, which can be clinically defined as a waist circumference ≥102 cm (≥40 in) in men and ≥88 cm (≥35 in) in women. According to the Practical Guide,[11] "To measure waist circumference, locate the upper hip bone and the top of the right iliac crest. Place a measuring tape in a horizontal plane around the abdomen at the level of the iliac crest. Before reading the tape measure, ensure that the tape is snug, but does not compress the skin, and is parallel to the floor. The measurement is made at the end of a normal expiration." Overweight persons with waist circumferences exceeding these limits should be urged more strongly to pursue weight reduction. The importance of measuring and documenting waist circumference in patients with a BMI <35kg/m^2 is due to the independent contribution of abdominal fat to the development of comorbid diseases, particularly the metabolic syndrome. The National Cholesterol Education Program's Adult Treatment Panel III report (ATP III), released in 2001, identified the metabolic syndrome as a multiplex risk factor for cardiovascular disease with clinically defined criteria (Table 47-4).[14] According to the ATP III criteria, factors characteristic of this syndrome are abdominal obesity, elevated triglycerides, low high-density–lipoprotein (HDL) cholesterol, raised blood pressure, and impaired fasting glucose. Using this definition, it is estimated that approximately 24% of US adults have the metabolic syndrome with higher prevalence rates among older individuals and Mexican Americans.[15] Although the components and cutoff values selected to define the metabolic syndrome are useful for clinical practice, the constellation of abnormalities associated with insulin resistance are much broader. These include increased atherogenic lipoproteins (small dense low-density–lipoprotein particles, apolipoprotein B), biomarkers of chronic inflammation (C reactive protein, tumor necrosis factor-α, interleukin-6), a prothrombotic state (increased plasma plasminogen activator inhibitor (PAI)-1 and fibrinogen), endothelial dysfunction (decreased endothelium-dependent vasodilatation), hemodynamic changes (increased sympathetic nervous activity and renal sodium retention), hyperuricemia, and nonalcoholic fatty liver disease (NAFLD).[16-18] When viewed in this context, it is clear that the metabolic syndrome is "more than the sum of its parts" and may explain the diversity of conditions associated with abdominal obesity.

As seen in Table 47-3, obesity is a risk factor for several GI diseases. These include gastroesophageal reflux disease (GERD),[19-24] NAFLD,[25-30] cholelithiasis,[31,32] umbilical and incisional hernias, and colon cancer.[33-36] Although not identified as a diagnostic criterion, NAFLD is now thought to be part of the metabolic syndrome that is related to insulin resistance.[37-39] Most patients with NAFLD present with a constellation of other components of the metabolic syndrome, including abdominal obesity, type 2 diabetes, and hyperlipidemia. Although not all patients with NAFLD are obese, obesity is considered the most important risk factor, both for its occurrence and for its progression to fibrosis and cirrhosis.[40] Data from the Third National Health and Nutrition Examination Survey (NHANES III) showed that 69% of cases of aminotransferase elevations are unexplained and strongly associated with central adiposity and related features, including dyslipidemia and higher insulin levels, as well as diabetes and hypertension.[41] Obesity is also considered an independent risk factor for nonresponse to antiviral treatment in chronic hepatitis C.[42,43]

Medical Management of the Overweight and Obese Patient

The Goal of Therapy

Information obtained from the history, physical examination and diagnostic tests is used to determine risk and develop a treatment plan. The primary goal of treatment is to improve obesity-related comorbid conditions and reduce the risk of developing future comorbidities. The physician's decision of how aggressively to treat the patient and which modalities to use is determined by the patient's risk status, his or her expectations, and what resources are available. Table 47-5 provides a guide to selecting adjunc-

TABLE 47-1.
BMI Table

BMI	19	20	21	22	23	24	25	26	27	28	29	30	31	32	33	34	35
Height (inches)								Body Weight (pounds)									
58	91	96	100	105	110	115	119	124	129	134	138	143	148	153	158	162	167
59	94	99	104	109	114	119	124	128	133	138	143	148	153	158	163	168	173
60	97	102	107	112	118	123	128	133	138	143	148	153	158	163	168	174	179
61	100	106	111	116	122	127	132	137	143	148	153	158	164	169	174	180	185
62	104	109	115	120	126	131	136	142	147	153	158	164	169	175	180	186	191
63	107	113	118	124	130	135	141	146	152	158	163	169	175	180	186	191	197
64	110	116	122	128	134	140	145	151	157	163	169	174	180	186	192	197	204
65	114	120	126	132	138	144	150	156	162	168	174	180	186	192	198	204	210
66	118	124	130	136	142	148	155	161	167	173	179	186	192	198	204	210	216
67	121	127	134	140	146	153	159	166	172	178	185	191	198	204	211	217	223
68	125	131	138	144	151	158	164	171	177	184	190	197	203	210	216	223	230
69	128	135	142	149	155	162	169	176	182	189	196	203	209	216	223	230	236
70	132	139	146	153	160	167	174	181	188	195	202	209	216	222	229	236	243
71	136	143	150	157	165	172	179	186	193	200	208	215	222	229	236	243	250
72	140	147	154	162	169	177	184	191	199	206	213	221	228	235	242	250	258
73	144	151	159	166	174	182	189	197	204	212	219	227	235	242	250	257	265
74	148	155	163	171	179	186	194	202	210	218	225	233	241	249	256	264	272
75	152	160	168	176	184	192	200	208	216	224	232	240	248	256	264	272	279
76	156	164	172	180	189	197	205	213	221	230	238	246	254	263	271	279	287

BMI	36	37	38	39	40	41	42	43	44	45	46	47	48	49	50	51	52	53	54
58	172	177	181	186	191	196	201	205	210	215	220	224	229	234	239	244	248	253	258
59	178	183	188	193	198	203	208	212	217	222	227	232	237	242	247	252	257	262	267
60	184	189	194	199	204	209	215	220	225	230	235	240	245	250	255	261	266	271	276
61	190	195	201	206	211	217	222	227	232	238	243	248	254	259	264	269	275	280	285
62	196	202	207	213	218	224	229	235	240	246	251	256	262	267	273	278	284	289	295
63	203	208	214	220	225	231	237	242	248	254	259	265	270	278	282	287	293	299	304
64	209	215	221	227	232	238	244	250	256	262	267	273	279	285	291	296	302	308	314
65	216	222	228	234	240	246	252	258	264	270	276	282	288	294	300	306	312	318	324
66	223	229	235	241	247	253	260	266	272	278	284	291	297	303	309	315	322	328	334
67	230	236	242	249	255	261	268	274	280	287	293	299	306	312	319	325	331	338	344
68	236	243	249	256	262	269	276	282	289	295	302	308	315	322	328	335	341	348	354
69	243	250	257	263	270	277	284	291	297	304	311	318	324	331	338	345	351	358	365
70	250	257	264	271	278	285	292	299	306	313	320	327	334	341	348	355	362	369	376
71	257	265	272	279	286	293	301	308	315	322	329	338	343	351	358	365	372	379	386
72	265	272	279	287	294	302	309	316	324	331	338	346	353	361	368	375	383	390	397
73	272	280	288	295	302	310	318	325	333	340	348	355	363	371	378	386	393	401	408
74	280	287	295	303	311	319	326	334	342	350	358	365	373	381	389	396	404	412	420
75	287	295	303	311	319	327	335	343	351	359	367	375	383	391	399	407	415	423	431
76	295	304	312	320	328	336	344	353	361	369	377	385	394	402	410	418	426	435	443

TABLE 47-2.

Classification of Weight Status and Risk of Disease

		Risk of Disease (relative to having a healthy weight and waist size) Waist circumference:* 35″ or less (women) 40″ or less (men)	Waist circumference:* More than 35″ (women) More than 40″ (men)
Underweight	BMI below 18.5		
Healthy weight	BMI 18.5 – 24.9		
Overweight	BMI 25.0 – 29.9	Increased	High
Obesity	BMI 30.0 – 34.9	High	Very High
Obesity	BMI 35.0 – 39.9	Very High	Very High
Extreme Obesity	BMI 40 or more	Extremely High	Extremely High

* Measure waist circumference just above the iliac crest. An increased waist circumference may indicate increased disease risk even at a normal weight.

Adapted from National Institutes of Health, National Heart, Lung, and Blood Institute. Clinical Guidelines on the Identification, Evaluation, and Treatment of Overweight and Obesity in Adults. US Department of Health and Human Services, Public Health Service; 1998.

TABLE 47-3.

Obesity-Related Organ Systems Review

Cardiovascular

Hypertension
Congestive Heart Failure
Cor Pulmonale
Varicose Veins
Pulmonary Embolism
Coronary Artery Disease

Respiratory

Dyspnea
Obstructive sleep apnea
Hypoventilation syndrome
Pickwickian syndrome
Asthma

Endocrine

Metabolic syndrome
Type 2 diabetes
Dyslipidemia
Polycystic ovarian syndrome (PCOS)/angrogenicity
Amenorrhea/infertility/menstrual disorders

Gastrointestinal

GERD NAFLD
Cholelithiasis
Hernias
Colon cancer

Musculoskeletal

Hyperuricemia and gout
Immobility
Osteoarthritis (knees and hips)
Low back pain

Genitourinary

Urinary stress incontinence
Obesity-related glomerulopathy
Hypogonadism (male)
Breast and uterine cancer
Pregnancy complications

Psychological

Depression/low self-esteem
Body image disturbance
Social stigmatization

Neurologic

Stroke
Idiopathic intracranial hypertension
Meralgia paresthetica

TABLE 47-3, CONTINUED

Obesity-Related Organ Systems Review

Integument

Striae distensae (stretch marks)
Stasis pigmentation of legs
Lymphedema
Cellulitis
Intertrigo, carbuncles
Acanthosis nigricans/skin tags

Adapted from Kushner RF, Roth JL. Assessment of the obese patient. *Endocrinol Metab Clin N Am.* 2003; 32(4):915-934.

TABLE 47-4.

Clinical Identification of the Metabolic Syndrome

Risk Factor	*Defining Level*
Abdominal Obesity	Waist Circumference
Men	>102 cm (>40 in)
Women	>88 cm (>35 in)
Triglycerides	≥150 mg/dl
HDL cholesterol	
Men	<40 mg/dl
Women	<50 mg/dl
Blood pressure	≥130/85 mmHg
Fasting glucose	≥110 mg/dl

Adapted from National Institutes of Health. Third report of the national cholesterol education program expert panel on detection, evaluation, and treatment of high blood cholesterol in adults (Adult treatment panel III).

tive treatments based on BMI category. Therapy for obesity always begins with lifestyle management and may include pharmacotherapy or surgery. Setting an initial weight loss goal of 10% over 6 months is reasonable, achievable, and clinically significant.[10]

LIFESTYLE MANAGEMENT

Lifestyle management incorporates the three essential components of obesity care: dietary therapy, physical activity, and behavior therapy. Because obesity is fundamentally a disease of energy imbalance, all patients must learn how and when energy is consumed (diet), how and when energy is expended (physical activity), and how to incorporate this information into their daily life (behavior therapy). Referral to a registered dietitian or enrollment in a commercial weight-loss program is useful to provide the education, skills, encouragement, and accountability needed for success.

Diet Therapy

The NHLBI Guidelines recommend initiating treatment with a diet producing a calorie deficit of 500 to 1000 kcal/day. Although the guidelines suggest prescribing a diet containing 1000 to 1200 kcal/day for most women and between 1200 and 1600 kcal/day for men, there is little value in calculating the patient's current dietary caloric intake because dietary records and the recall method are typically inaccurate and underestimate actual intake.[44] Rather, the focus should be on where and how the patient will reduce daily calories. In practice, it is more therapeutic to emphasize what patients should eat, drink, or do more often rather than admonishing them on what they should limit, avoid, or restrict. For example, simple targeted messages to choose more fruits and vegetables, include 25 to 30 grams of dietary fiber per day, consume more whole grain cereals, select learner cuts of meat and skimmed dairy products, and drink more water are positive recommendations. Advising a reduction in portion sizes and moderation in added fats and oils can follow.

The primary focus of diet therapy is on reducing overall consumption of calories and dietary sources of excessive fat and simple sugars. The macronutrient composition of the diet will vary depending on the patient's preference and medical condition. The Institute of Medicine (IOM) Report, published in 2002, recommends a broad range of acceptable macronutrient levels consisting of 45% to 65% of total calories from carbohydrates, 20% to 35% of total calories from fat, and 10% to 35% of total calories from protein.[45] Portion control is one of the most difficult

Table 47-5.
A Guide to Selecting Treatment

	BMI Category				
	25 to 26.9	27 to 29.9	30 to 35	35 to 39.9	>40
Treatment					
Diet, Exercise, Behavior Therapy	With co-morbidities	With co-morbidities	+	+	+
Pharmacotherapy		With co-morbidities	+	+	+
Surgery				With co-morbidities	+

Adapted from *The Practical Guide: Identification, Evaluation, and Treatment of Overweight and Obesity in Adults.* US Department of Health and Human Services, Public Health Service, National Institutes of Health, National Heart, Lung, and Blood Institute. NIH Publication No. 00-4084, October, 2000.

strategies for patients to manage; therefore, use of pre-prepared products, called meal replacements, is a simple and convenient suggestion. Meal replacements are foods that are designed to take the place of a meal while at the same time providing nutrients and good taste within a known caloric limit.[46] Examples include frozen entrees, canned beverages, and bars. In a meta-analysis of six studies with a study duration ranging from 3 to 51 months, use of partial meal replacements resulted in a 7% to 8% weight loss.[47]

Occasionally, very-low calorie diets (VLCD) are prescribed as a form of more aggressive dietary therapy. The primary purpose of prescribing a VLCD is to promote a rapid and significant (13 to 23 kg) short-term weight loss over a 3- to 6-month period. These propriety formulas typically supply ≤800 kcal, 50 to 80 gm protein, and 100% of the recommended daily intake (Chapter 6) for vitamins and minerals. A recent meta-analysis[48] found that after a weight loss of ≥20 kg, individuals maintained significantly more weight loss than patients after low-calorie diets or weight loss of <10 kg. In contrast, others studies have found no difference in long-term weight loss between VLCD and low-calorie diets.[49] According to a review by the National Task Force on the Prevention and Treatment of Obesity,[50] indications for initiating a VLCD include well-motivated individuals who are moderately to severely obese (BMI >30), have failed at more conservative approaches to weight loss, and have a medical condition that would be immediately improved with rapid weight loss. Conditions include poorly controlled type 2 diabetes, hypertriglyceridemia, obstructive sleep apnea, and symptomatic peripheral edema. The risk for gallstone formation increases exponentially at rates of weight loss above 1.5 kg/week.[51] Prophylaxis against gallstone formation with ursodeoxycholic acid, 600 mg/day, is effective in reducing this risk.[52] Because of the need for close metabolic monitoring, these diets are usually prescribed by physicians specializing in obesity care.

Physical Activity Therapy

Although exercise alone is only moderately effective for weight loss, the combination of dietary modification and exercise is the most effective behavioral approach for treatment of obesity. In contrast, the most important role of exercise appears to be in the maintenance of the weight loss.[53] Physical activity is beneficial for improved cardiorespiratory fitness, cardiovascular disease and cancer risk reduction, and improved mood and self-esteem. Currently, the minimum public health recommendation for physical activity is 30 minutes of moderate intensity physical activity on most, preferably all, days of the week.[54] Focusing on simple ways to add physical activity into the normal daily routine—such as walking, using the stairs, doing home and yard work, and increasing recreational activity—is a useful first step in counseling. Our group routinely recommends that patients purchase and wear a pedometer to monitor total accumulation of steps as part of the activities of daily living, or ADLs. Step counts are highly correlated with inactivity (low number of steps) as well as with activity (high number of steps).[55] Studies have demonstrated that lifestyle activities are as effective as structured exercise programs in improving cardiorespiratory fitness[56] and weight loss.[57] The American College of Sports Medicine (ACSM) recommends that overweight and obese individuals progressively increase to a minimum of 150 minutes of moderate intensity physical activity per week as a first goal.[58] However, for long-term weight loss, higher amounts of exercise (eg, 200 to 300 minutes/week or ≥2000 kcal/week) is needed. The ACSM also recommends that resistance exercise supplement the endurance exercise program. Many patients would benefit from consultation with an exercise physiologist or personal trainer.

Behavioral Therapy

Cognitive behavioral therapy (CBT) incorporates various strategies intended to help change and reinforce new dietary and physical activity behaviors.[59,60] Strategies include self-monitoring techniques (eg, journaling, weighing, and measuring food and activity), stress management, stimulus control (eg, using smaller plates and not eating in front of the television or in the car), social support, problem solving, and cognitive restructuring (ie, helping patients develop more positive and realistic thoughts about themselves). These techniques can be learned and used by physicians, but they do take time. In the setting of a busy practice, they are probably more reasonably applied by ancillary office staff such as a nurse clinician or registered dietitian. Nonetheless, a few key behavioral principles should be utilized when possible. When recommending any behavioral lifestyle change, have the patient identify what, when, where, and how the behavioral change will be performed; have the patient and yourself keep a record of the anticipated behavioral change; and follow-up progress at the next office visit. Rollnick, Mason, and Butler have written an excellent guide for practitioners on a method to use when helping patients make decisions about health behavior change in both the hospital and office setting.[61]

An instructive exercise in evaluating the relative importance of implementing various lifestyle management strategies for weight control is to query individuals who are successful at long-term maintenance. This innovational approach forms the basis for the National Weight Control Registry (NWCR).[62] To enroll, participants must have lost ≥13.6 kg (30 lb) and have maintained the loss for ≥1 year. Currently, over 3000 subjects are in the NWCR; average age 45 years and 80% are women. Overall, the participants lost an average of 30 kg (76 lb) and maintained for an average of 5.5 years. The most commonly reported strategies for long-term success were eating a diet low in fat and high in carbohydrate, frequent self-monitoring of weight, and regular physical activity expending an average of 2545 kcal/week. The lesson learned from the NWCR is that there are no easy solutions or magic cures; patients need to adopt and sustain healthy lifestyle habits.

Pharmacotherapy

Adjuvant pharmacological treatments should be considered for patients with a BMI >30 kg/m^2 or with a BMI >27 kg/m^2 who also have concomitant obesity-related risk factors or diseases and for whom dietary and physical activity therapy has not been successful (see Table 47-5). With the exception of the BMI cut points, these indications are identical to starting cholesterol-lowering agents, anti-hypertensives, or anti-diabetic drugs. Similar to these other drugs, the patient must have realistic expectations regarding what the medication can accomplish and how to use it properly. What makes the use of anti-obesity drugs different is the absolute need to utilize lifestyle modification as a foundation for drug action because of the importance of a drug-behavior interaction. Whether the medication acts centrally to suppress appetite or peripherally to block the absorption of fat, patients must deliberately and consciously alter their behavior for weight loss to occur. In other words, for all anti-obesity drugs, the pharmacological action must be translated into behavior change. For anorexiants, a reduced sense of hunger and/or increased satiety must be translated into choosing smaller, healthier meals and reducing snacking. Failure to sense and act upon these inhibitory internal signals will result in modest or no weight loss. Similarly, if a patient takes an intestinal fat-blocking agent and does not limit the consumption of dietary fat to 30% or less, she will discontinue the medication because of intolerable side effects. Moreover, failure to incorporate physical activity as part of the lifestyle change will seriously hinder maintenance of the initial weight loss. Thus, there is a bi-directional, mutually beneficial relationship between anti-obesity drugs and lifestyle management, each therapy enhancing the efficacy of the other.

In a randomized trial by Wadden et al[63] evaluating the benefits of lifestyle modification in the pharmacologic treatment of obesity, investigators showed that the efficacy of sibutramine-induced mean weight loss at 1 year was significantly enhanced when subjects also attended a lifestyle support group (-10.8%) or lifestyle support group plus portion controlled diet (-16.5%) versus sibutramine alone (-4.1%). Thus, when prescribing an anti-obesity medication, patients must be actively engaged in a lifestyle program that provides the strategies and skills needed to effectively use the drug.

There are several potential targets of pharmacological therapy for obesity, all based on the concept of producing a sustained negative-energy (calorie) balance. The earliest and most thoroughly explored treatment has been suppression of appetite via centrally active medications that alter monoamine neurotransmitters. A second strategy is to reduce the absorption of selective macronutrients from the GI tract, such as fat. These two mechanisms form the basis for all currently prescribed anti-obesity agents. A profile of sibutramine and orlistat, the only two medications approved for long-term use, is shown in Table 47-6. Readers are referred to recent comprehensive review articles on the pharmacological treatment of obesity.[64-70]

Centrally Acting Anorexiant Medications

Appetite suppressing drugs, or anorexiants, effect *satiation*—the processes involved in the termination of a meal, *satiety*—the absence of hunger after eating, and *hunger*—a biological sensation that initiates eating. By increasing satiation and satiety and decreasing hunger, these agents help patients reduce caloric intake while providing a greater sense of control, more contentment with food intake, and reduced feelings of deprivation. The target site for the actions of anorexiants is the ventromedial and lateral hypothalamic regions in the central nervous system. Their biological effect on appetite regulation is produced by variably augmenting the neurotransmission of three monoamines: norepinephrine, serotonin (5-hydroxytryptamine, 5-HT), and to a lesser degree, dopamine. The classical sympathomimetic adrenergic agents function by either stimulating norepinephrine release or blocking its reuptake. The classical sympathomimetic adrenergic agents (benzphetamine, phendimetrazine, diethylpropion, mazindol, and phentermine) function by either stimulating norepinephrine release or blocking its reuptake. In contrast, sibutramine (Meridia) functions as a serotonin and norepinephrine reuptake inhibitor (SNRI). Furthermore, unlike other previously FDA-approved anorexiants, sibutramine is not pharmacologically related to amphetamine and has

TABLE 47-6.

Antiobesity Drugs Approved for Long-Term Use

Sibutramine (Meridia)	*Orlistat (Xenical)*
FDA approved 1997	FDA approved 1999
Acts centrally: Anorexiant (SNRI)	Acts peripherally: lipase inhibitor
Induces feeling of satiety	Reduces absorption of 30% dietary fat
Once daily with or without food	Three times daily with meals and a vitamin supplement recommended
Dosage: 5, 10, and 15 mg capsules	Dosage: 120 mg capsules
Side effects: dry mouth, headache, elevations in blood pressure and heart rate	Side effects: oily/fatty stool, increased defecation
Two year clinical data	Four year clinical data

no addictive potential. Sibutramine is the only drug in this class that is approved for long-term use. It produces a dose-dependent weight loss (available doses are 5, 10, and 15 mg capsules), with an average loss of about 5% to 9% of initial body weight at 12 months.[71] The medication has been demonstrated to be useful in maintenance of weight loss for up to 2 years.[72]

The most commonly reported adverse events of sibutramine are headache, dry mouth, insomnia, and constipation. These are generally mild and well tolerated. The principal concern is a dose-related increase in blood pressure and heart rate that may require discontinuation of the medication. A dose of 10 to 15 mg/day causes an average increase in systolic and diastolic blood pressure of 2 to 4 mmHg and an increase in heart rate of 4 to 6 beats/minute. For this reason, all patients should be monitored closely and seen back in the office within 1 month after initiating therapy. The risk of adverse effects on blood pressure are no greater in patients with controlled hypertension than in those who do not have hypertension[73] and the drug does not appear to cause cardiac valve dysfunction.[74] Contraindications to sibutramine use include uncontrolled hypertension, congestive heart failure, symptomatic coronary heart disease, arrhythmias, or history of stroke. Similar to other anti-obesity medications, weight reduction is enhanced when the drug is used along with behavioral therapy, and body weight increases once the medication is discontinued.[75]

Peripherally Acting Medication

Orlistat (Xenical) is a synthetic hydrogenated derivative of a naturally occurring lipase inhibitor, lipostatin, produced by the mold *Streptomyces toxytricini.* Orlistat is a potent, slowly reversible inhibitor of pancreatic, gastric, and carboxylester lipases and phospholipase A_2, which are required for the hydrolysis of dietary fat in the GI tract into fatty acids and monoacylglycerols. The drug's activity takes place in the lumen of the stomach and small intestine by forming a covalent bond with the active serine residue site of these lipases. Taken at a therapeutic dose of 120 mg tid, orlistat blocks the digestion and absorption of about 30% of dietary fat. On discontinuation of the drug, fecal fat usually returns to normal concentrations within 48 to 72 hours.[76]

Multiple randomized, 1- to 2-year, double-blind, placebo-controlled studies have shown that after 1 year, orlistat produces a weight loss of about 9 to 10% compared with a 4 to 6% weight loss in the placebo-treated groups.[77-79] When categorized by percent weight loss, more subjects randomized to orlistat compared to placebo lost >5% (average 55% versus 33%) and >10% (average 34% versus 16%) of body weight. Pooled data has also shown that early weight loss (>5% of initial weight after 3 months) predicts weight loss at 18 months. Since orlistat is minimally (<1%) absorbed from the GI tract, it has no systemic side effects. Tolerability to the drug is related to the malabsorption of dietary fat and subsequent passage of fat in the feces. Six GI tract adverse effects have been reported to occur in at least 10% of orlistat-treated patients; oily spotting, flatus with discharge, fecal urgency, fatty/oily stool, oily evacuation, and increased defecation. The events are generally experienced early, diminish as patients control their dietary fat intake, and infrequently cause patients to withdraw from clinical trials. Psyllium mucilloid is helpful in controlling the orlistat-induced GI side effects when taken concomitantly with the medication.[80] Serum concentrations of the fat-soluble vitamins D and E and β–carotene have been found to be significantly lower in some of the trials although generally remain within normal ranges. The manufacturer's package insert for orlistat recommends that patients take a vitamin supplement along with the drug to prevent potential deficiencies.

One additional caveat regarding orlistat is necessary. There are four sources of calories in the diet: fat, carbohydrate, protein, and alcohol. Orlistat partially blocks the absorption of only one of these sources. If patients increase the consumption of nonfat foods in place of the fatty foods they have to eliminate, they may actually increase total caloric intake and gain weight. Thus, attention to the whole diet, including reduction of total calories, must be carefully maintained for the medication to be effective.

Conclusion

Obesity is a serious and highly prevalent disease associated with increased morbidity and mortality. Assessment and evaluation of obesity by BMI and risk classification should be part of the patient encounter. Treatment modalities should include diet, physical activity, and behavior therapy for all patients and use of pharmacotherapy in those selected as reasonable candidates. Primary treatment should be directed at preventing further weight gain for overweight patients and achieving a modest 10% weight loss for obese patients.

References

1. Must A, Spadano J, Coakley E, Field AE, Colditz G, Dietz WH. The disease burden associated with overweight and obesity. *JAMA*. 1999;282:1523-1529.
2. Mokdad AH, Serdula MK, Dietz WH, et al: The continuing epidemics of obesity and diabetes in the United States. *JAMA*. 2001;286:1195-1200.
3. Makdad AH, Marks JS, Stroup DF, Gerberding JL. Actual causes of death in the United States, 2000. *JAMA*. 2004;291:1238-1245.
4. Korner J, Leibel RL. To eat or not to eat—how the gut talks to the brain. *N Engl J Med*. 2003;349:926-928.
5. Korner J, Aronne LJ. The emerging science of body weight regulation and its impact on obesity treatment. *J Clin Invest*. 2003;111:565-570.
6. Marx J. Cellular warriors at the battle of the bulge. *Science*. 2003;299:846-849.
7. Schwartz MW, Woods SC, Seeley RJ, Barsh GS, Baskin DG, Leibel RL. Is the energy homeostasis system inherently biased toward weight gain? *Diabetes*. 2003;52:232-238.
8. List JF, Habener JF. Defective melanocortin 4 receptors in hyperphagia and morbid obesity. *N Engl J Med*. 2003;348:1160-1163.
9. Kushner RF. Roadmaps for Clinical Practice: Case Studies in Disease Prevention and Health Promotion—Assessment and Management of Adult Obesity: A Primer for Physicians. Chicago, Illinois: American Medical Association; 2003. Available at: www.ama-assn.org/ama/pub/category/10931.html). Accessed May 18, 2004.
10. National Heart, Lung, and Blood Institute (NHLBI). Clinical guidelines on the identification, evaluation, and treatment of overweight and obesity in adults. The evidence report. *Obes Res*. 1998;6(Suppl 2):51S-210S.
11. National Heart, Lung, and Blood Institute (NHLBI) and North American Association for the Study of Obesity (NAASO). Practical guide to the identification, evaluation, and treatment of overweight and obesity in adults. Bethesda, MD: National Institutes of Health, NIH Publ number 00-4084, Oct. 2000.
12. U.S. Preventive Services Task Force. Screening for obesity in adults: recommendations and rationale. *Ann Intern Med*. 2003;139:930-932.
13. Kushner RF, Roth JL. Assessment of the obese patient. *Endocrinol Metab Clin N Am*. 2003; 32(4):915-934.
14. National Institutes of Health. Third report of the national cholesterol education program expert panel on detection, evaluation, and treatment of high blood cholesterol in adults (Adult treatment panel III). Bethesda, MD: National Institutes of Health; 2001. NIH Publication 01-3670.
15. Ford ES, Giles WH, Dietz WH. Prevalence of the metabolic syndrome among US adults: Findings from the third national health and nutrition examination survey. *JAMA*. 2002;287:356-359.
16. Grundy SM, Brewer B, Cleeman JI, Smith SC, Lenfant C. Definition of metabolic syndrome. Report of the National Heart, Lung, and Blood Institute/American Heart Association conference on scientific issues related to definition. *Circ*. 2004;109:433-438.
17. Isomaa B. A major health hazard: the metabolic syndrome. *Life Sciences*. 2003;73:2395-2411.
18. Reaven G. Metabolic syndrome. Pathophysiology and implications for management of cardiovascular disease. *Circ*. 2002:106:286-288.
19. Fisher BL, Pennathur A, Mutnick JL, Little AG. Obesity correlates with gastroesophageal reflux. *Dig Dis Sci*. 1999;44:2290-2294.
20. Locke GR, Talley NJ, Fett SL, Zinsmeister AR, Melton J: Risk factors associated with symptoms of gastroesophageal reflux. *Am J Med*. 1999;106:642-649.
21. Wajed SA, Streets CG, Bremner CG, DeMeester TR. Elevated body mass disrupts the barrier to gastroesophageal reflux. *Arch Surg*. 2001;136:1014-1019.
22. Kiljander T, Salomaa ER, Helenius H, Liippo K, Terho EO. Asthma and gastro-oesopheal reflux: can the response to anti-reflux therapy be predicted? *Respiratory Medicine*. 2001;95:387-392.
23. Mayne ST, Navarro SA. Diet, obesity and reflux in the etiology of adenocarcinoma of the esophagus and gastric cardia in humans. *J Nutr*. 2002;132:3467S-3470S.
24. Nilsson M, Johnsen R, Ye W, Hveem K, Lagergren J. Obesity and estrogen as risk factors for gastroesophageal reflux symptoms. *JAMA*. 2003;290:66-72.
25. Sheth SG, Gordon FD, Chopra S. Nonalcoholic steatohepatitis. *Ann Intern Med*. 1997;126:137-145.
26. Diehl AM. Nonalcoholic steatohepatitis. *Sem Liver Dis*. 1999;19:221-229.
27. Kumar KS, Malet PF. Nonalcoholic steatohepatitis. *Mayo Clin Proc*. 2000;75:733-739.
28. Clinical Practice Committee. American Gastroenterological Association Medical Position Statement: nonalcoholic fatty liver disease. *Gastro*. 2002;123:1702-1704.
29. Angulo P. Nonalcoholic fatty liver disease. *N Engl J Med*. 2002;346:1221-1231.
30. Clark JM, Diehl AM. Nonalcoholic fatty liver disease. An under-recognized cause of cryptogenic cirrhosis. *JAMA*. 2003;289:3000-3004.
31. Syngal S, Coakley EH, Willet WC, et al. Long-term weight patterns and risk for cholecystectomy in women. *Ann Intern Med*. 1999;130:471-477.
32. Erlinger S. Gallstones in obesity and weight loss. *European J Gastro Hepatol*. 2000;12:1347-1352.
33. Shike M. Body weight and colon cancer. *Am J Clin Nutr*. 1996;63(3 Suppl):442S-444S.
34. Giacosa A, Franceschi S, La Vecchia C, Favero A, Andreatta R. Energy intake, overweight, physical exercise an colorectal cancer risk. *European J Cancer Prev*. 1999;8(Suppl 1):S53-S60.
35. Calle EE, Radriguez C, Walker-Thurmond K, Thun MJ. Overweight, obesity, and mortality from cancer in a prospectively studied cohort of U.S. adults. *N Engl J Med*. 2003;348:1625-1638.
36. Moore LL, Bradlee ML, Singer MR, et al. BMI and waist circumference as predictors of lifetime colon cancer risk in Framingham study adults. *Int J Obesity*. 2004;28:559-567.
37. Marceau P, Biron S, Hould FS, et al. Liver pathology and the metabolic syndrome X in severe obesity. *J Clin Endocrinol Metab*. 1999;84:1513-1517.
38. Ratziu V, Giral P, Charlotte F, et al. Liver fibrosis in overweight patients. *Gastro*. 2000;118:1117-1123.
39. Chitturi S, Abeygunasekera S, Farrell GC, et al. NASH and insulin resistance: insulin hypersecretion and specific association with the insulin resistance syndrome. *Hepatology*. 2002;35:373-379.
40. Ruhl CE, Everhart JE. Determinants of the association of overweight with elevated serum alanine aminotransferase activity in the United States. *Gastro*. 2003;124:71-79.
41. Clark JM, Branacati FL, Diehl AM. The prevalence and etiology of elevated aminotransferase levels in the United States. *Am J Gastro*. 2003;98:960-967.
42. Bressler BL, Guindi M, Tomlinson G, Heathcote J. High body mass index is an independent risk factor for nonresponse to antiviral treatment in chronic hepatitis C. *Hepatology*. 2003;38:639-644.

43. Lonardo A, Adinolfi LE, Loria P, Carulli N, Ruggiero G, Day CP. Steatosis and hepatitis C virus: mechansims and significance for hepatic and extrahepatic disease. *Gastro.* 2004;126:586-597.
44. Black AE, Prentice AM, Goldberg GR, et al. Measurements of total energy expenditure provide insights into validity of dietary measurements of energy intake. *J Am Diet Assoc.* 1993;93:572-579.
45. National Research Council. *Dietary reference intakes for energy, carbohydrate, fiber, fat, fatty acids, cholesterol, protein, and amino acids.* Washington, DC: National Academy Press; 2002.
46. Bowerman S. The role of meal replacements in weight control. In Bessesen DH, Kushner R (eds). *Evaluation & Management of Obesity.* Philadelphia, PA: Hanley & Belfus, Inc; 2002:53-58.
47. Heymsfield SB, van Mierlo CAJ, van der Knaap HCM, Frier HI. Weight management using meal replacement strategy: meta and pooling analysis from six studies. *Int J Obesity.* 2003;27:537-549.
48. Anderson JW, Kontz EC, Frederich RC, et al. Long-term weight-loss maintenance: a meta-analysis of US studies. *Am J Clin Nutr.* 2001;74:579-584.
49. Wadden TA, Osei S. The treatment of obesity: an overview. In: Wadden TA, Stunkard AJ, eds. *Handbook of Obesity Treatment.* New York: The Guilford Press; 2002:229-248.
50. National task force on the prevention and treatment of obesity. Very low-calorie diets. *JAMA.* 1993;270:967-974.
51. Weinsier RL, Wilson LJ, Lee J. Medically safe rate of weight loss for the treatment of obesity: a guidelines based on risk of gallstone formation. *Am J Med.* 1995;98:115-117.
52. Shifman ML, Kaplan GD, Brinkman-Kaplan V, et al. Prophylaxis against gallstone formation with urodeoxycholic acid in patients participating in a very-low-calorie diet program. *Ann Intern Med.* 1995;122:899-905.
53. Votrubo SB, Horvitz MA, Schoeller DA. The role of exercise in the treatment of obesity. *Nutrition.* 2000;16:179-188.
54. Pate RR, Pratt M, Blair SN, et al. Physical activity and public health: a recommendation from the Centers for Disease Control and Prevention and the American College of Sports Medicine. *JAMA.* 1995;273:402-407.
55. Welk GJ, Differding JA, Thompson RW, et al. The utility of the Digi-Walker step counter to assess daily physical activity patterns. *Med Sci Sports Exerc.* 2000;32(Suppl):S481-S488.
56. Dunn AL, Marcus BH, Kampert JB, Garcia ME, Kohl HW, Blair SN. Comparison of lifestyle an structured interventions to increase physical activity and cardiorespiratory fitness. A randomized trial. *JAMA.* 1999;281:327-334.
57. Anderson RE, Wadden TA, Bartlett SJ, Zemel B, Verde TJ, Franckowiak SC. Effects of lifestyle activity vs structured aerobic exercise in obese women: a randomized trial. *JAMA.* 1999;281:335-340.
58. Jakacic JM, Clark K, Coleman E, et al. Appropriate intervention strategies for weight loss and prevention of weight regain for adults. *Med Sci Sports Exerc.* 2001;33:2145-2156.
59. Foreyt JP, Poston WSC. What is the role of cognitive-behavior therapy in patient management? *Obesity Res.* 1998;6(Suppl 1):18S-22S.
60. Wadden TA, Foster GD. Behavioral treatment of obesity. *Med Clinics North America.* 2000;84:441-462.
61. Rollnick S, Mason P, Butler C, Eds. *Health Behavior Change: A Guide for Practitioners.* Philadelphia, PA: Churchill Livingstone; 2000.
62. Wing RR, Hill JO. Successful weight loss maintenance. *Ann Rev Nutr.* 2001;21:323-341.
63. Wadden TA, Berkowitz RI, Sarwer DB, et al. Benefits of lifestyle modification in the pharmacologic treatment of obesity. A randomized trial. *Arch Intern Med.* 2001;161:218-227.
64. Hensrud DD. Pharmacotherapy for obesity. *Med Clin North Am.* 2000;84:463-476.
65. Glazer G. Long-term pharmacotherapy of obesity 2000: a review of efficacy and safety. *Arch Intern Med.* 2001;161:1814-1824.
66. Bray GA, Tartaglia LA. Medicinal strategies in the treatment of obesity. *Nature.* 2001;404:672-677.
67. Yanovski S, Yanovski JA. Obesity. *N Engl J Med.* 2002;346:591-602.
68. Kushner RF, Manzano H. Obesity pharmacology: past, present, and future. *Curr Opin Gastroenterol.* 2002;18:213-220.
69. Haddock CK, Poston WSC, Dill PL, Foreyt JP, Ericsson M. Pharmacotherapy for obesity: a quantitative analysis of four decades of published randomized clinical trials. *Int J Obesity.* 2002;26:262-273.
70. Padwal R, Li SK, Lau DCW. Long-term pharmacotherapy for overweight and obesity: a systematic review and meta-analysis of randomized controlled trials. *Int J Obesity.* 2003;27:1437-1446.
71. Arterburn DE, Crane PK, Veenstra DL. The efficacy and safety of sibutramine for weight loss: a systematic review. *Arch Intern Med.* 2004;164:994-1003.
72. James WPT, Astrup A, Finer N, et al. Effect of sibutramine on weight maintenance after weight loss: a randomized trial. *Lancet.* 2000;356:2119-2125.
73. Hazenberg BP. Randomized, double-blind, placebo-controlled, multicenter study of sibutramine in obese hypertensive patients. *Cardiology.* 2000;94:152-158.
74. Bach DS, Rissanen AM, Mendel CM, et al. Absence of cardiac valve dysfunction in obese patients treated with sibutramine. *Obes Res.* 1999;4:363-369.
75. Fanghanel G, Cortinas L, Sachez-Reyes L, et al. Second phase of a double-blind study clinical trial on sibutramine for the treatment of patients suffering essential obesity: 6 months after treatment cross-over. *Int J Obes.* 2001;25:741-747.
76. Lucas KH, Kaplan-Machlis B. Orlistat—a novel weight loss therapy. *Ann Pharmacother.* 2001;35:314-328.
77. Sjostrom L, Rissanen A, Anderson T, et al. Randomised placebo-controlled trial of orlistat for weight loss and prevention of weight regain in obese patients. *Lancet.* 1998;352:167-173.
78. Davidson MH, Hauptman J, DiGirolamo M, et al. Weight control and risk factor reduction in obese subjects treated for 2 years with orlistat: a randomized trial. *JAMA.* 1999;281:235-242.
79. Finer N, James WPT, Kopelman PG, Lean MEJ, Williams G. One-year treatment of obesity: a randomized double-blind, placebo-controlled, multicentre study of orlistat, a gastrointestinal lipase inhibitor. *Int J Obes.* 2000;24:306-313.
80. Cavaliere H, Floriano I, Medeiros-Neto G. Gastrointestinal side effects of orlistat may be prevented by concomitant prescription of natural fibers (psyllium mucilloid). *Int J Obes.* 2001;25:1095-1099.

Chapter 48

Control of Food Intake

Allen S. Levine, PhD; Pawel K. Olszewski, PhD; Charles J. Billington, MD; and Catherine M. Kotz, PhD

Introduction

Eating is essential and, for most individuals, pleasant. Clinicians deal with the consequences of eating in their daily practice. The manner in which humans eat and the amount of food people ingest changes from birth to late years. Individuals have eating disorders, are allergic to foods, overeat (which leads to a series of obesity-related comorbidities), and need surgical procedures to stop them from eating or to help them receive the needed nutrients when there are assaults on their gastrointestinal (GI) tract.

As is true of other behaviors, eating is primarily regulated by the brain. Regulatory functions within the brain are complex, involving a network of brain nodes. Eating must satisfy a variety of goals including those related to energy needs, pleasure, taste, time of the day, stress, and boredom, all of which involve neural networks. Integrative functions within the brain are informed, not only by the senses that convey information about the outside world, but also by afferent nerve traffic from the stomach, gut, liver, and other peripherals sites, as well as by an expanding corps of hormonal signals originating in stomach, gut, adipose tissue, and other sites.

Brain Sites Involved in Appetite

Critical sites within the brain that participate in regulation of eating have been identified by a substantial database generated in animal and human studies. Foremost among these brain sites is the hypothalamus.[1] Damage to specific areas within the hypothalamus can create insatiable hunger or almost total lack of hunger.[2] For example, damage to the ventromedial hypothalamus or paraventricular hypothalamus results in greatly heightened appetite, which, if left unrestrained, can encourage consequent obesity. Lateral hypothalamic damage can leave affected individuals so lacking in appetite that nutrition support is required. Such observations led to the view, still current today, that eating results from a balance between neural signals driving or suppressing food intake. Originally, this balance was understood as a balance between the hypothalamic divisions, but now a host of neurotransmitters and neuropeptides, which are considered below, are seen as the players exerting the competitive drives toward either eating or not eating.

Other brain sites outside the hypothalamus have also been linked to aspects of appetite. The brainstem clearly plays an important role, in that structures within the brainstem are the first to receive signals from the body relating to energy status and gut function.[3,4] In addition, neurons that directly sense glucose and possibly other macronutrient levels are found within the brainstem, as well as within the hypothalamus. Some crucial feeding-related behaviors can be produced by the brainstem itself; evidence shows that supported intake can occur in animals whose connection to the forebrain has been cut. At the same time, reciprocal projections exist between brainstem and hypothalamus and between brainstem and several other feeding-related brain sites.

Limbic brain structures, such as the amygdala and nucleus accumbens, have also been linked to aspects of eating behavior. Considerable evidence now supports the idea that dopamine within the nucleus accumbens is responsive to food intake and probably particularly responsive to the rewarding aspects of eating.[5,6] In addition, the amygdala is also likely involved in aspects of food reward or the affective quality of foods.[7,8]

Several other brain sites have also been implicated in regulation of food intake, with lesser specificity regarding concrete function. Each of the above brain structures communicates with many of the rest, thus forming the basis for a network that can integrate the various inputs about energy needs, gut function, results of external sensing, and so on, which then organizes the behavioral output that is seen as eating behavior.

Much of what has been learned involves the action of the various neurotransmitters and neuropeptides on elements of this appetite regulatory network. Attempts at simplifying the feeding network often leads to attributing one function to one molecule. However, it is apparent that this approach is too simplistic for the study of human physiology, including the study of brain networks mediating feeding behavior. Different portions of the feeding network act in an integrative fashion to influence the behavioral outcome of feeding.

The actions of these signal molecules are reviewed below. In many cases, the peptides involved are also gut peptides and recognition that regulatory peptides within the gut also act within the brain has become widespread. This chapter first considers neuromodulators of appetite that are produced in and exert their action primarily in the brain, then addresses hormones that originate in adipose tissue and influence the brain, and finally presents gut peptide hormones that participate in appetite regulation (Table 48-1).

Signals in the Brain

MONOAMINES

Among the first neurotransmitters whose role in appetite was identified are norepinephrine and serotonin.[6,9] Each of these monoamines is widely distributed in the brain, and norepinephrine is widely present throughout the neuraxis. Pharmacologic studies indicate that both of these factors can reduce food intake in many different settings among humans and animals. Norepinephrine decreases intake via the alpha-1 adrenergic receptor but increases food when injected into selected brain sites via the alpha-2 adrenergic receptors.[10] Serotonin decreases the size of the meal, and overall food consumption over 24 hours is diminished.[11,12] The mechanism by which the reductions take place has been attributed to enhanced satiety. However, particularly in the case of norepinephrine type drugs, there is a significant possibility that food intake is reduced by displacement of feeding behavior by some other behavior. Further, what is meant by satiety with respect to specific brain mechanisms is not yet completely understood and thus refers simply to the cessation of eating. Norepinephrine and serotonin are active within the hypothalamus, and the hypothalamus may contain important sites of action for these stimuli. These neurotransmitters continue to be highly significant in the clinical application of appetite science because they form the pharmacological basis for sibutramine, one of the few appetite suppressant drugs that have been used clinically.[13]

Amphetamines, which stimulate norepinephrine pathways, were among the very first drugs used in treatment of obesity, and while clinical effectiveness was quite potent the drugs are not now used because of addictive adverse effects. Attenuated amphetamines, such as phentermine, have continued to be used for appetite suppression with modest success and no known addiction.[14] Fenfluramine was the most potent serotonin-based obesity medication and significant weight loss, on order of 10% of initial body weight, was observed during treatment. Fenfluramines have been withdrawn from worldwide markets because of cardiac-valve side effects.[15,16] One currently available drug, sibutramine, stimulates both norepinephrine and serotonin pathways by inhibiting presynaptic reuptake of those neurotransmitters. Sibutramine produces approximately 8 to 10% of initial body weight loss with side effects including possible blood pressure increases, gut disturbance, and some central nervous and mood effects.[13]

NEUROPEPTIDE Y

In addition to the monoamines, several neuropeptides have been shown to influence feeding behavior. Perhaps the most studied to date is neuropeptide Y (NPY). NPY was discovered in 1982 by Tatemoto et al and is a member of the pancreatic polypeptide family.[17] Two years later, Clark and colleagues demonstrated that intracerebroventricular injection of NPY or pancreatic polypeptide induced vigorous feeding in rats.[18] Several other laboratories confirmed the marked orexigenic effect of centrally administered NPY in rats.[19,20] NPY did not seem to affect other behaviors including grooming, rearing, sleeping, resting, or activity when food was present. This led investigators to conclude that NPY had selective effects on feeding behavior. When food was not present, NPY resulted in food-seeking behaviors.

NPY clearly acts as a central regulator of feeding because it has no effects on feeding behavior when injected peripherally. It induces feeding after injection into a number of brain areas but seems to be most effective after injection in the perifornical area or paraventricular nucleus (PVN) of the hypothalamus.[21] The idea that the primary site of NPY stimulus in the brain is the PVN is further supported by data from Kalra et al, which indicates that the level of NPY in the PVN rises before a meal and then falls after a meal.[22] However, neuroregulators of feeding do not act alone nor does the behavioral output of feeding rely solely on one brain region. For example, blockade of opioid receptors in the hindbrain of the rat (nucleus of the solitary tract) results in a decrease in eating stimulated by NPY injection into the PVN, suggesting that NPY-driven feeding is dependant on functional opioid receptor activity in the hindbrain.[23] NPY-induced feeding is also decreased by central injection of alpha-melanocyte-stimulating hormone (alpha-MSH) or its synthetic receptor analogue MTII.[24] Other peptides that decrease NPY-induced feeding include corticotropin-releasing factor, urocortin, cocaine and amphetamine regulated transcript, and leptin, anorectic peptides that are discussed below. Thus, although NPY appears to act in the PVN to

TABLE 48-1.

Peptides Regulating Feeding

Central Peptides	Peripheral Peptides
Agouti related protein (O)	Amylin (A)
Alpha melanocyte-stimulating hormone (A)	Apolipoprotein AIV (A)
Amylin (A)	Bombesin (A)
Apolipoprotein AIV (A)	Calcitonin gene-related peptide (A)
Calcitonin gene-related peptide (A)	Cholecystokinin (A)
Cholecystokinin (A)	Enterostatin (A)
Cocaine and amphetamine regulated transcript (A/O)	Ghrelin (O)
Corticotropin-releasing factor (A)	Glucagon (A)
Endogenous opioids (O)	Glucagon-like peptide-1 (A)
Enterostatin (A)	Insulin (O)
Galanin (O)	Leptin (A)
Glucagon-like peptide (A)	Neurotensin (A)
Insulin (A)	Peptide YY3-36 (A)
Leptin (A)	Somatostatin (A)
Melanin concentrating hormone (O)	Tumor necrosis factor (A)
Neuropeptide W (O)	
Neuropeptide Y (O)	
Neurotensin (A)	
Nociceptin (A)	
Orexins (O)	
Somatostatin (A)	
Tumor necrosis factor beta (A)	
Thyrotropin-releasing hormone (A)	
Urocortin (A)	

Key: A=anorectic; O=orexigenic

stimulate feeding, it is apparent from these data that this action is sensitive to signals from other neurotransmitters acting in multiple brain sites, data which supports a network model of feeding behavior.

There has been a great deal of discussion about macronutrients and body weight regulation. Many investigators have suggested that neuropeptides can have selective effects on intake of carbohydrate, fat, and protein. NPY was first reported to increase intake of carbohydrate-rich diets more effectively than of high-fat diets. In addition to solid diets, Lynch et al demonstrated that NPY markedly increased ingestion of sucrose solutions.[25] However, while NPY increased intake of starches and sugars, it also increased intake of fat.[26] Like other peptides, NPY may have a more marked effect on intake of one macronutrient, but it also influences intake of other macronutrients.

Another approach to understanding links between consumption of specific macronutrients and regulators of appetite is to do the converse of injection studies and to determine the effect of specific macronutrient consumption on brain activity of the neuroregulator(s) in question. In the case of NPY, it was found that a high fat diet resulted in a decrease of NPY gene expression in the arcuate nucleus (ARC) of the hypothalamus (primary site of NPY synthesis in the brain and origin of NPY released in the PVN).[27] If, as the injection studies suggest, the role of NPY is to ensure sufficient intake of carbohydrate, then one might have predicted that ingestion of a high fat diet would increase gene expression of NPY to stimulate carbohydrate intake. However, these data are inconclusive because diet-sensitive neural elements that regulate NPY synthesis and release have not been identified, and macronutrient feeding studies are difficult to interpret for the following study-design issue: altering percent intake of one macronutrient changes the percent intake of the other macronutrient by default, and it is thus difficult to determine whether the effect observed was due to the result of an increase in one macronutrient or to a decrease in another. Thus, with the possible exception of enterostatin, a peptide that inhibits fat intake, the current available dataset does not yet support a strong case for links between specific macronutrients and specific neuroregulators of feeding.[28]

As mentioned above, there are several reasons or "drives" behind eating behavior. NPY appears to be an important regulator of "hunger"-induced feeding. For example, satiated rats injected intracerebroventricularly with NPY will work (as determined in lever-pressing behavioral studies) as hard for food as a rat that has been deprived of food for over 36 hours.[29] If NPY is a "hunger"-related neuropeptide, then it would be expected to sense and attempt to correct energy deficits. In agreement with this idea, NPY gene expression in the ARC of the hypothalamus increases during food deprivation, food restriction, exercise, and in diabetic rats—conditions that may be perceived by the brain as states of negative energy balance.[30] These data suggest that rats needing energy to maintain body weight synthesize more NPY, resulting in food-seeking behavior and increased intake.

NPY also has important effects on energy expenditure. Bray has suggested that there is a reciprocal relationship between sympathetic nervous system activity and food intake.[31] Thus, one would predict that NPY, which increases food intake, would decrease sympathetic induced changes in energy expenditure. In rodents, central administration of NPY decreases sympathetic nerve activity to interscapular brown adipose tissue—a tissue thought to be important in thermogenesis and energy expenditure—independent of food intake, suggesting that decreasing energy expenditure is another primary function of NPY stimulus.[32] This peptide also decreases GDP-binding, a measure of brown fat thermogenic activity.[33] Uncoupling protein 1 is a mitochondrial protein found solely in brown adipose tissue that functions to collapse the electrochemical gradient regulating ATP formation, which in effect results in the dissipation of energy as heat, rather than in the storage of energy as ATP. As one might predict based on these results, NPY decreases brown fat uncoupling protein gene expression. Furthermore, NPY increases lipoprotein lipase activity in white fat in both ad libitum fed and food-restricted rats, which suggests that not only does NPY inhibit the dissipation of energy as heat, but it also increases the propensity to store fat by increasing the activity of the enzyme necessary for bringing fat into cells. In concordance with the above data, NPY injection decreases energy expenditure measured by calorimetry.[34] Together, the above results suggest that NPY represents a powerful orexigenic stimulus: increasing energy intake and storage, and decreasing mechanisms that waste energy. However, as will become apparent, NPY is only one player in a group of neuroregulators acting to regulate energy balance.

Melanocortins

More recent data have highlighted the importance of the melanocortin system in regulating ingestive behavior. Proopiomelanocortin (POMC) is a gene that serves as the precursor for alpha-MSH, an agonist of melanocortin receptors 3 and 4 (MCR3/4). Agonists of these receptors decrease feeding and body weight, whereas antagonists increase feeding and body weight.[35] A unique aspect of melanocortin signaling is that an endogenous antagonist for the MC receptors exists. This antagonist is Agouti-related protein (AgRP), produced in the ARC and with projections containing this peptide terminating in the PVN and lateral hypothalamus.[36] An animal model of overexpression of AgRP exists and is referred to as the "Agouti mouse". This mouse produces an excess amount of the Agouti-protein and is hyperphagic and obese, indicating that blocking endogenous "satiety" (MCR3/4-expressing) pathways is an effective means of producing obesity. Like most of the neuroregulators we discuss, gene expression of the ligands for the MCR3/4 are affected by energy status. An energy-deficient rodent expresses less POMC and more AgRP, whereas the opposite is true for animals in a positive energy state. Also, alpha-MSH neurons in the ARC are activated at the time of meal termination, suggesting that these neurons play an importation role in signals conveying information important to the cessation of eating.[38]

The melanocortin system interacts with various other neuroregulators of food intake. Low doses of the opioid antagonist naltrexone decrease food intake stimulated by ventricular injection of AgRP, and peripheral injection of naltrexone induces c-Fos immunoreactivity (an indirect measure of neural activation) in alpha-MSH neurons present in the ARC.[39] Interestingly, both NPY and AgRP receptor stimulation, which are considered agonist and antagonist binding respectively, results in a signal that requires functional opioid pathways. These data provide evidence that opioid signaling represents an important component of the feeding network, necessary for several different mechanisms that produce changes in feeding behavior (discussed in the next section). In addition to opioids, the anorectic effects of both leptin and insulin involve the melanocortins,[40,41] and MTII, an agonist of the MCR3/4 receptors, decreases feeding induced by ghrelin.[42]

Opioids

As mentioned earlier, opioids appear to be an important component of the feeding network, interacting with several other neuroregulators of feeding, and may be implicated in the propensity for palatable food ingestion.[43] Some investigators suggest that opioids increase the intake of high fat diets more effectively than do high carbohydrate diets, whereas others suggest that opioids are involved in intake of preferred foods rather than a specific macronutrient rich diet. Most agree that intake of preferred palatable foods involve opioid peptides and that palatable foods affect opioidergic circuitry.[43] Several groups have noted that blocking opioid receptors with naloxone or naltrexone after feeding sugar solutions for 1 to 3 weeks to rats alters neuronal activity in several brain regions and changes release of dopamine and acetylcholine.[44-46] Also, naloxone-precipitated withdrawal has been observed following chronic ingestion of glucose solutions given for 12 hours/day. Rats and humans can easily discriminate sweet taste following naltrexone administration; however, the pleasure associated with the taste is diminished.[43] Furthermore, gene expression of opioid peptides is increased by ingestion of highly palatable foods, supporting the notion that opioid circuitry is involved in reward-related feeding.[47]

The difficulty in studying this issue is that palatability is not static and changes with the energy status of an individual. For example, a hungry individual will find fairly bland foods to be highly desirable. This may be one example of the network "at work". Increased value of previously uninteresting food may be a result of "energy deficit" signals intersecting with signals related to "reward", the end result being that an uninteresting food becomes more palatable, thus increasing the propensity for food consumption. On the other hand, at the end of a large meal, unadorned toast would not be chosen by most, perhaps reflecting a dissociation of "energy" signals from "reward" signals. However, sweet and fat combinations, such as candy and cake, would be considered pleasant at the end of a feast.

Blockade of opioid receptors decreases nocturnal feeding and intake stimulated by food restriction or deprivation and by a variety of orexigenic peptides.[43] This has led to suggestions that opioids act downstream in feeding pathways and may be one of the final gatekeepers of eating behavior. Opioids and their receptors are widely distributed from the hindbrain to the forebrain, in brain sites identified to be involved in consummatory behavior. Unfortunately, none of the opioid ligands have been found to be useful in the treatment of eating disorders or obesity.

CANNABINOIDS

During the past decade, it has become clear that there are endogenous receptors and ligands related to marijuana, a drug that results in food cravings. The endocannabinoids and cannabinoid receptors are now known to be involved in consummatory behavior.[48] The cannabinoid 1 receptor (CB1) antagonist SR141716 (a Sanofi compound) has provided a means to study cannabinoid-induced changes in intake.[49] This antagonist decreases intake in rats and in humans. The endocannabinoids and the active compound in marijuana (delta9-THC) both stimulate feeding and bind to the CB1 receptor. The levels of the endocannabinoids also change with food restriction/deprivation and are also higher in rodents with leptin deficiency or leptin-receptor insensitivity.[50,51] As is true for opioids, it appears that endocannabinoids affect the rewarding properties of foods. They influence motivation to eat and intake of palatable foods. SR141716 not only decreases intake but also sustains weight loss in animals given a high fat diet.[52] Studies are beginning to demonstrate interactions between cannabinoids and other neuroregulators of feeding behavior. For example, the CB1 receptor antagonist SR141716 decreases feeding induced by ghrelin.[53] Also, Kirkham demonstrated synergistic anorectic effects of the opioid antagonist naltrexone and SR141716.[54]

OREXIN

Orexins are a recently identified class of neuropeptides first described by de Lecea, who termed them "hypocretins".[55] Sakurai et al independently identified the same compounds and named these peptides orexin A and B, in reference to their orexigenic effect. Both peptides are coded from the same prepro-mRNA. Prepro-orexin is limited to the lateral hypothalamus, perifornical hypothalamus, dorsomedial hypothalamus, and posterior hypothalamus.[55-57] These orexin-containing neurons project throughout the hypothalamus—including the PVN, the ARC, the lateral hypothalamus, the perifornical hypothalamus, and the ventromedial hypothalamus—as well as to several extrahypothalamic sites.[57] The locus coeruleus receives the densest extra-hypothalamic innervation,[57] which may have implications for mechanisms supporting wakefulness. Elevated wakefulness may be part of a normal feeding sequence (discussed below). Other extra-hypothalamic projection sites include lateral septal nuclei, dorsal raphe nuclei, and the nucleus of the solitary tract. Many of these sites have well-established roles in feeding regulation and wakefulness.[58-64]

Orexin A increases feeding after injection into specific sites, including the lateral hypothalamus and PVN, whereas orexin B has not been shown to stimulate feeding after injection into specific central areas.[65,66] Meal pattern analysis by the Rodgers and Blundell group indicate that orexin A delays the transition period between eating and resting. The overall effect is to increase the length of the meal, rather than the number of meals. This indicates that orexin A maintains and prolongs rather than initiates feeding behavior,[67-69] which is similar to the pattern observed after opioid injections.

Several studies have shown that orexin neurons are activated by orexigenic neuropeptides and the activity of orexin neurons and receptors are responsive to changes in energy balance. Orexin neurons are stimulated by food restriction and low blood glucose and are inhibited by high blood glucose.[70,71] However, food restriction has also been shown to decrease expression of orexin receptor OX2R gene in the parvocellular division of the PVN.[71] Robust physical activity response after orexin injection into this part of the PVN suggest that the OX2R in this region regulates activity,[72] which is known to be decreased during chronic food restriction, likely in an effort to conserve energy.[73] Several neuropeptides with established roles in feeding behavior also activate orexin neurons. Ghrelin given into the ventricles or the rostral lateral hypothalamic area activates orexin-containing neurons in the more caudal lateral hypothalamus.[74,75] The stimulation of orexin neurons (as measured by cFos-ir), coincident with the delayed feeding response to central Agouti-related protein injection, was demonstrated by the Berthoud laboratory.[76] This important finding makes a strong case for orexin participation in the maintenance of feeding.

Orexins are also implicated in the sleep/wake cycle in both animals and humans, where deficiency of prepro-orexin or the OX2R receptor is associated with narcolepsy.[77-81] Rats infused with antisense to orexin have increased REM sleep[82] and activity of orexin-containing neurons,[83] and levels of orexin A peptide in CSF[84] are correlated with wakefulness. Work by Berridge et al indicate that ventricular orexin infusion at different times of the day increase wakefulness; the increased amount of time awake results in increased feeding behavior,[85] and enhanced orexin neurotransmission is associated with increased wakefulness.[86]

It is likely that elevated feeding and arousal due to stimulation with orexin A is an integrated response. As discussed above, feeding behavior occurs for many reasons and it is possible that enhanced arousal is one route by which this feeding occurs. A large amount of evidence suggests that wakefulness and feeding behavior are linked. A word commonly used for snacks—"refreshments"—indicates the association between food ingestion and feelings of wakefulness. Sleep deprivation results in lower leptin levels, with restoration of normal circulating leptin upon return of normal sleeping patterns.[87] Likewise, narcoleptic patients, who lack orexin transmission and tend to become obese, have significantly reduced leptin levels.[88,89] Although the parallel animal model suggests that the obesity results from inactivity associated with narcolepsy,[90] at least one human study suggests that elevated BMI in narcolepsy may have a more direct relationship to the lack of orexin neurotransmission.[91] Feeding patterns have not been reported for narcoleptic patients, but decreased leptin could be related to the increased number of meals consumed by sleep-deprived individuals, which can result in obesity. In children, sleep loss is dose-dependently correlated to level of obesity.[92] It is often reported that when dieting, good sleeping patterns are helpful in succeeding on the diet, the implication being that feelings of sleepiness can lead one to eat, perhaps in an effort to refresh or awaken oneself. Although problems such as sleep apnea, which result in sleep deprivation, are thought to be a consequence of obesity, it is clear that sleep loss itself may be the cause of some forms of obesity. It is well known that obesity increases risk of mortality,[93] but the effect of insomnia on mortality risk is controversial. One study reports an increased risk, and another study reports increased mortality risk with either too much (>8.5 hours nightly) or too little sleep (<4 hours nightly).[94,95] In current society, which is relatively sleep-deprived and obese compared to just 20 years ago, it is important to understand the neurobiological underpinnings linking sleep, wakefulness, and feeding behavior. As discussed earlier, a distributed network exists in which many neurochemicals in different brain regions communicate with each other in a dynamic model of feeding regulation; orexin stimulation of wakefulness may be one component of that model.

Melanin Concentrating Hormone

Melanin concentrating hormone is present in the lateral hypothalamic area in neurons distinct from those containing orexin A,[96] and ventricular injections of melanin concentrating hormone have been shown to stimulate feeding.[97] The lateral hypothalamic area has historically been regarded as a central feeding center. Chronic injections of melanin concentrating hormone induce obesity, and mice lacking the gene for melanin concentrating hormone are lean. Thus, it appears that melanin concentrating hormone may provide an orexigenic stimulus to the feeding network. However, no study to date has demonstrated activation of melanin concentrating hormone neurons (as measured by cFos-ir) in situations of elevated feeding behavior, diminishing the impact of the data suggesting that melanin concentrating hormone is part of the orexigenic feeding network.

Corticotropin-Releasing Factor and Urocortin

Corticotropin-releasing factor, produced primarily in the hypothalamic PVN, has been shown to be related to "stress"-induced changes in feeding behavior. Stress can have opposite effects on feeding, with animal studies indicating that chronic low-level stress induces overeating, whereas acute high-level stress results in undereating. CRF may be involved in both processes, with underexpression occurring in the first stress model and overexpression occurring in the latter model.

Urocortin is a recently identified neuropeptide related to corticotropin-releasing factor that has a dense fiber network in the intermediate portion of the lateral septum,[98-100] which is part of the limbic system. Urocortin has 45% sequence identity with corticotropin-releasing factor[98] and binds to all three corticotropin-releasing factor receptors with higher affinity than corticotropin-releasing factor, but binds with particular avidity to CRF-R2.[98] Urocortin peptide and CRF-R2 coexist within the intermediate lateral septum[98,100-102] and it is thought that urocortin may be the endogenous ligand for CRF-R2.[98,100] Although there are reports of corticotropin-releasing factor immunoreactivity in fibers in the lateral septal area,[103] urocortin is highly concentrated in the intermediate lateral septum, whereas corticotropin-releasing factor is predominant in the medial septum,[104] which is distinct from the lateral septum. Ventricular administration of urocortin promotes c-fos expression (an indicator of cellular activation) in CRF-R2 containing cell bodies within the intermediate lateral septum.[98]

These neuroanatomic data provide a basis for urocortin action within the intermediate lateral septum. A recent report indicates that ventricular urocortin inhibits feeding without inducing a conditioned taste aversion, whereas corticotropin-releasing factor's feeding inhibition is accompanied by conditioned taste-aversion induction, suggesting that corticotropin-releasing factor inhibition of feeding may be due to aversive consequences of this peptide's administration.[105] CRF-R2 has been further implicated in feeding behavior by use of knockout and antisense technology. Both CRF-R2 knockout mice and rats treated with antisense to CRF-R2 display alterations in feeding behavior.[106-109] Recent data indicate that ventricular administration of urocortin and corticotropin-releasing factor results in elevated thresholds for lateral hypothalamic area self-stimulation suggesting that urocortin/corticotropin-releasing factor may modulate lateral hypothalamic area reward processes.[110] Two additional peptides related to urocortin and corticotropin-releasing factor, urocortin II,[111] and urocortin III[112] have recently been identified. These peptides bind exclusively to CRF-R2, and urocortin II has been shown to inhibit feeding after central injection.[111,113]

Adiposity Signals: Leptin and Insulin

There is a variety of adiposity signals that have been identified over the past decade. Leptin and insulin have been widely studied and it is generally agreed that these peptides are important signals involved in energy metabolism.[41] Leptin and insulin levels are correlated with adiposity and body weight, both enter the brain, both decrease feeding when injected into the brain, and both affect similar neuropeptidergic pathways. Leptin received a good deal of attention after its initial cloning in 1994.[114] It was hoped, as was true for many other regulators, that it would be a useful means of weight reduction in the obese patient. Unfortunately, its only major effect was in humans that were missing the leptin gene. However, the role of adiposity signals in energy metabolism are still of great interest.

Woods and colleagues have emphasized the importance of insulin as an adiposity signal.[115] They and others have found that insulin levels correlate with body adiposity and body weight, that obese individuals (both rats and humans) have relatively high basal insulin levels and also secrete more insulin following a meal than do lean individuals, that insulin levels increase during a meal and decrease during fasting, and that obese individuals are resistant to insulin's effects.[41] Insulin receptors have been mapped to brain areas known to be involved in food-intake regulation, such as the ARC of the hypothalamus. Central administration of insulin decreases food intake and increases energy expenditure. Injection of insulin antibodies into the brain increases body weight and food intake.[41]

The theme of a widely distributed network is also apparent in insulin-related changes in food intake. Central injection of insulin enhances the anorectic effects of peripherally injected CCK.[116] Intracerebroventricular injection of insulin increases the expression of corticotropin-releasing factor in the PVN and decreases expression of NPY in the ARC.[117,118] Thus, insulin effectively increases and decreases activity of anorectic and orexigenic pathways, respectively, a dual mode of interaction with other feeding neuroregulators that renders central insulin a powerful anorectic signal.

As is true for insulin, plasma leptin levels are positively correlated with adipose cell mass. Leptin receptors are present in the brain, and leptin is transported into the brain.[119] Leptin also decreases food intake and increases energy expenditure. While leptin levels correlate with adipose mass, they fall rapidly with food restriction or deprivation.[120] Leptin has been said to reflect the overall energy status of an individual. Knockout of leptin or its receptor results in an obese animal.[114] The ob/ob mouse is missing leptin whereas the db/db mouse has an ineffective leptin receptor, both models having an obese phenotype. Leptin is known to stimulate pro-opiomelanocortin (POMC) synthesis and to decrease synthesis of NPY.[41] POMC is the precursor of alpha-melanocyte–stimulating hormone, a peptide that decreases food intake. Clearly, leptin arriving in the brain does not work alone in regulating intake.

Gut Signals

Cholecystokinin

The laboratory of Smith and Gibbs reported that the gut-peptide cholecystokinin had a profound anorectic effect in rats, in a manner that resembled normal satiety.[121] This effect was subsequently found to extend to chickens, rabbits, pigs, sheep, rhesus monkeys, lean mice, genetically and neurologically obese mice and rats, lean men and women, and obese men.[122] There are two receptors for cholecystokinin, known as CCK1R and CCK2R (also referred to as CCK-A and CCK-B), and cholecystokinin-binding sites have been localized throughout the periphery and in the brain in both animals and humans.[123-130] Peripheral injections of cholecystokinin in animals and humans decrease feeding, whereas cholecystokinin-receptor antagonists increase feeding. Additional satiety signals derived from the intestine and pancreas include peptide YY, pancreatic polypeptide, glucagon-like peptide 1; and oxyntomodulin; cholecystokinin is the most studied to date.

Cholecystokinin is predominately expressed and released in the upper small intestine in response to a gastric load,[131] but there also exists a separate pool of CCK that is produced in the brain.[132] Vagotomy inhibits the effect of CCK on satiety, indicating that CCK activates afferent vagal fibers innervating the brain.[133] Peripheral and specific site-brain injection of cholecystokinin reduces feeding, indicating that cholecystokinin from either central or peripheral reservoirs may interact with receptors in the brain to modulate feeding behavior.

CCK "interacts" with several other neuropeptides involved in feeding. Peripheral injections of cholecystokinin and/or analogues of cholecystokinin result in decreased hypothalamic neuropeptide Y concentrations, which indicates that a reciprocal relationship exists between these two peptides with opposing actions on feeding.[134,135] Leptin and cholecystokinin interact synergistically to inhibit feeding, and recent data suggests that this requires activation (as measured by cFos-like immunoreactivity) of the hypothalamic PVN.[136] This finding was reversed by pretreatment with a cholecystokinin-receptor antagonist, providing further evidence that the hypothalamic PVN is an important site mediating an interaction between leptin and cholecystokinin in reducing food intake.[136] Further highlighting the importance of the hypothalamic PVN in mediating satiety induced by cholecystokinin is the finding that lesioning this brain region abolishes the inhibition of feeding induced by cholecystokinin, whereas lesions of the bed nucleus of the stria terminalis or the central nucleus of the amygdala had no effect on cholecystokinin-induced satiety.[132] Cholecystokinin released from endocrine intestinal cells acts either on afferent nerves or directly on ARC neurons. This results in inhibition of expression of neuropeptide Y and Agouti-related peptide in the ARC and consequently decreases release of these same peptides in the PVN.[137] Thus, it appears that these orexigenic peptides are important targets of cholecystokinin, and the suppression of their orexigenic activity is part of the cholecystokinin-induced satiety sequence. It has also been shown that pro-opiomelanocortin neurons in the nucleus of the solitary tract are activated by cholecystokinin in mice.[138] Furthermore, activation of the melanocortin-4 receptor is necessary for cholecystokinin-induced suppression of feeding, as blockade of this receptor reverses cholecystokinin-induced satiety.[138]

A useful animal model for elucidating the role of cholecystokinin in satiety is the Otsuka Long-Evans Tokushima Fatty (OLETF) rat, which lacks CCKA (CCK1R) receptors. These animals are hyperphagic, obese, and diabetic. Moran and colleagues have determined that OLETF rats have increased meal size[139,140] and have further determined that overexpression of neuropeptide-Y in the dorsomedial hypothalamus may be important in the obese phenotype. These investigators found that characteristics of OLETF rats, including increased body weight, elevated plasma insulin and leptin, increased proopiomelanocortin and decreased neuropeptide-Y gene expression in the hypothalamic ARC, could all be reversed by restricting food intake to levels observed in control animals. Yet surprisingly, OLETF rats also display elevated neuropeptide-Y gene expression in the dorsomedial hypothalamus, a phenotype not reversed by pair-feeding. Furthermore, elevated neuropeptide-Y gene expression in the dorsomedial hypothalamus was also observed in 5-week-old pre-obese OLETF rats. These findings present a strong case for the suggestion that upregulated neuropeptide Y in the dorsomedial hypothalamus mediates the hyperphagia and obesity in these animals.[141,142] Of note is the finding that NPY gene expression in this animal model varies, depending on brain site of measurement, which emphasizes the notion that brain location of feeding neuroregulators has an important influence on the behavioral effects of that particular neuroregulator.

Peptide YY

Another member of the pancreatic polypeptide family is peptide YY. In the 1980s, central injection of this peptide was found to increase feeding in a fashion similar to that of NPY.[143] However, another form of PYY_{3-36} that is produced in the L cells of the GI tract appears to have anorectic effects.[144] PYY_{3-36} is produced by processing of PYY by the enzyme dipeptidyl peptidase-IV. PYY_{3-36} levels increase after eating and appears to be correlated with the amount of calories ingested. Either peripheral or central injection of PYY_{3-36} decreases food intake. Also, in humans, peripheral injections of PYY_{3-36} reduced food intake and appetite over a 24-hour period.[145] It should be noted that Tschop et al have not been able to repeat the rodent work demonstrating that PYY_{3-36} decreases food intake.[146]

Ghrelin

Ghrelin is a 28-amino–acid acetylated peptide discovered recently[147] and was found to be the agonist for the growth hormone secretagogue receptor (GHSr). It is the first identified endogenous ligand of the G-protein-coupled GHSr, although synthetic analogs displaying affinity for this receptor have been known for more than two decades. Ghrelin is found in a variety of tissue types including, among others, the brain, kidney, testis, ovary, and pancreas. The majority of this peptide is synthesized by enteroendocrine–A–like cells in the oxyntic glands of the stomach and within the intestine, and it reaches the general circulation.[148] As anticipated, this GHSr ligand was initially shown to stimulate the release of growth hormone (GH) from the anterior pituitary in a manner independent from the counter-balancing mechanism provided by GH-releasing hormone and somatostatin.[147]

Based on a proposed connection between feeding status and the concentration of plasma GH, a hypothesis was put forth that ghrelin, which stimulates GH release, may be involved in the control of some aspects of consummatory behavior. Indeed, substantial evidence gathered over the past several years, has strongly supported this speculation.

Injection studies have shown that ghrelin acts as one of the most powerful orexigenic substances known to date.[149] The magnitude of the observed hyperphagic effect appears to be comparable to that induced by NPY, and like NPY, ghrelin-generated overfeeding is also relatively short, lasting several hours post-injection. Long-term infusions of this peptide lead to an increase in body weight, which, in addition to elevated food consumption, has been attributed to altered metabolism and energy expenditure.[150] Interestingly, both peripheral and central routes of administration are effective at stimulating food intake and at promoting body-weight gain. One should note that ghrelin can cross the blood-brain barrier bidirectionally in a highly regulated process. However, only the form of this peptide acylated at Ser3, which appears to be of endocrine importance contrary to non-acetylated ghrelin, is capable of being transported across the barrier.[151] It has been shown that over 95% of GHSr ligand molecules found in the circulation do not contain the acyl group, yet changes in the energy/feeding state of the organism modify plasma levels of the two forms. It is very likely that both of them serve a unique function in feeding control; however, the acetylated one seems to be able to act via peripheral and central mechanisms. Some authors have suggested that the non-acetylated form may bind to certain subtypes of the GHSr.

The ability of ghrelin to cross the blood-brain barrier suggests a dual (ie, peripheral and central) mode of action. Also, the distribution of the GHSr in the brain and in peripheral tissues (notably, in the adipose tissue) indicates that ghrelin affects energy homeostasis via complex mechanisms. For example, it has been shown to increase fat mass by decreasing fat oxidation (152). In addition, motility and gastric emptying induced by ghrelin may involve a local effect, although a central influence has also been suggested.

As mentioned above, circulating ghrelin levels are sensitive to the feeding state of the organism. For example, a 48-hour fasting period causes an increase in the plasma profile of this substance,[153] whereas an infusion of glucose into the stomach, hyperinsulinemia, or food ingestion reduces intestinal ghrelin concentration.[154] Levels of mRNA of the GHSr ligand in the stomach are reduced as a result of food intake or hyperglycemia and are higher after fasting. Similarly, a surge in peripheral ghrelin secretion can be observed shortly before a meal in schedule-fed humans and laboratory animals.[155] Interestingly, the actual presence of food is not necessary to elevate the concentration of this peptide in a scheduled-feeding paradigm; it appears that anticipation of a consummatory activity is sufficient to cause such response.

In addition, scenarios and diseases associated with starvation and negative energy balance—such as aging, anorexia nervosa, cancer-dependent anorexia, dieting, or chronic physical exercise—are associated with high levels of circulating ghrelin.[156,157] On the other end of the spectrum, in obese and overeating adult humans, plasma concentration of the GHSr ligand is generally low, which probably reflects a vigorous and frequent intake of high-calorie foods by these subjects.[158] Proper dietary interventions in anorexic and overweight patients modify their ghrelin profile. Surprisingly, in patients who have undergone stomach-bypass procedure, ghrelin levels in the blood are low, which suggests that the size of the stomach may contribute to the concentration of this peptide in the plasma.[155]

Ghrelin appears to be a peptide that serves as an endocrine link between the periphery and the brain (in particular, the hypothalamus); its ability to cross the blood-brain barrier in a bidirectional manner supports this theory. The pathways through which the circulating peptide conveys its signal to the hypothalamus are not clearly understood. However, the hypothalamic ARC, the site where the GHSr is located, has been proposed as a

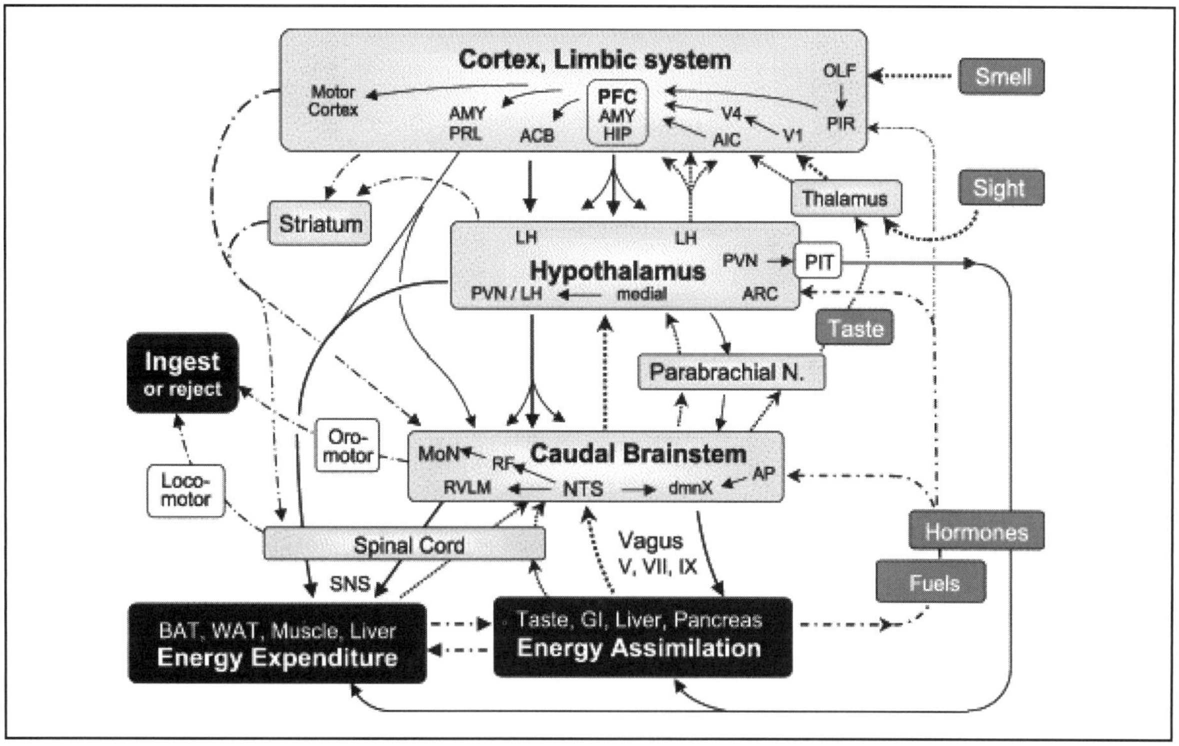

Figure 48-1. Representation of the distribution network involved in control of food intake. (From Berthoud HR. Brain, appetite and obesity. *Physiology and Behavior.* 2004;81:781-793. Reprinted with permission from Elsevier.)

target area for gut-derived ghrelin. The ARC hosts several populations of neurons that affect ingestive behavior, including NPY and AgRP. Studies employing functional neuroanatomy or antagonist injections indicate that ARC cells containing these two particular peptides seem to play a crucial role in mediating ghrelin-dependent hyperphagia.[159,160] For example, it has been shown that AgRP and NPY cells express the GHSr. Furthermore, injection of ghrelin upregulates NPY and AgRP mRNA expression in the ARC.[159] In addition, antagonism of the Y1 receptor for NPY inhibits intracerebroventricular-ghrelin–generated consumption.[74,161]

A question that needs to be brought up is whether it is only circulating or also central (ARC-derived) ghrelin that affects consummatory behavior. It appears that both pools of the peptide influence feeding. In the brain, the GHSr and fiber terminals containing this receptor's ligand are distributed in sites responsible for food-intake control. A vigorous feeding response has been observed following administration of this substance into the PVN[162] and lateral hypothalamic[75] nuclei of sated animals. Furthermore, intracerebroventricular injection of ghrelin at a dose that causes a powerful orexigenic effect, increases the presence of the immediate-early gene product, c-Fos, in the regions mentioned above as well as in the nucleus of the solitary tract and area postrema, the brainstem sites that provide the hypothalamus with a strong input.[74] It has been found that an infusion of ghrelin into the lateral hypothalamus activates orexin-containing neurons localized in this region, which indicates that orexin cells may be sensitive to ghrelin.[75]

In sum, ghrelin—a powerful orexigenic substance—constitutes a part of the distributed feeding network that encompasses both peripheral and central elements. Those elements appear to be engaged in a "cross-talk" with each other and ghrelin may, to some degree, serve as a facilitator of these interactions. Such a prominent role of the ghrelin peptide/receptor system places it as a possible target for pharmacological interventions in the treatment of eating disorders.

Network Integration

Within the appetite network (Figure 48-1), the influences of many neuromodulators and other signals sketched above must be processed and integrated, thus producing eating behavior. However, it must be re-emphasized that the network is multilayered and complex. The signals work their effect on the substrate of brain sites reviewed briefly at the beginning of this section. Each signal may exert its influence at one or several sites and may affect more than one neurally mediated motivation for eating. Studies of brain sites and neurochemicals in 'isolation', or without concurrent measurement of activity of other neurochemicals at different brain sites, gives information on just one portion of the network. As each positive and negative stimulation is received within each relevant brain site, those brain sites also communicate with one another, therefore allowing the integration of many positives and negatives relating to several different reasons to eat.

The complexity and interdependence of the network is likely a major stabilizing force, restricting the possibility of variation in appetite, particularly over long-term. Attempts to modify appetite, particularly the clinical motivation of suppressing appetite for treatment of obesity, is likely to be limited and frustrated when only a single point in the network is being changed. This phenomenon is often referred to as "redundancy" in the appetite system, but a more nuanced view is that there are several appetites that are being integrated and that the ambition to reduce overall appetite by affecting only a single type of appetite is unlikely to be very successful. It should be possible in the future to exploit the developing knowledge of brain networks and the systems that underlie them to find a multi-point intervention strategy that may be more effective both for suppressing appetite in the context of obesity and stimulating it in the context of anorexia.

References

1. Schwartz MW, Woods SC, Porte D, Jr., Seeley RJ, Baskin DG. Central nervous system control of food intake. *Nature.* 2000;404(6778):661-71.
2. Anand B, Brobeck J. Hypothalamic control of food intake in rats and cats. *Yale J Biol Med.* 1951;24:123-140.
3. Norgren R, Leonard CM. Taste pathways in rat brainstem. *Science.* 1971;173(2):1136-9.
4. Kirchgessner AL, Sclafani A, Nilaver G. Histochemical identification of a PVN-hindbrain feeding pathway. *Physiol Behav.* 1988;42(6):529-43.
5. MacDonald AF, Billington CJ, Levine AS. Alterations in food intake by opioid and dopamine signaling pathways between the ventral tegmental area and the shell of the nucleus accumbens. *Brain Res.* 2004;1018(1):78-85.
6. Hoebel BG. Brain neurotransmitters in food and drug reward. *Am J Clin Nutr.* 1985;42(5 Suppl):1133-50.
7. Glass MJ, Billington CJ, Levine AS. Opioids and food intake: distributed functional neural pathways? *Neuropeptides.* 1999;33(5):360-8.
8. Rolls ET. The neurophysiology of feeding. *Int J Obes.* 1984;(8 Suppl)1:139-50.
9. Hoebel BG. Pharmacologic control of feeding. *Ann Rev Pharmacol Toxicol.* 1977;17:605-21.
10. Wellman PJ. Norepinephrine and the control of food intake. *Nutrition.* 2000;16(10):837-42.
11. Shor-Posner G, Grinker JA, Marinescu C, Brown O, Leibowitz SF. Hypothalamic serotonin in the control of meal patterns and macronutrient selection. *Brain Res Bull.* 1986;17(5):663-71.
12. Blundell JE. Serotonin manipulations and the structure of feeding behaviour. *Appetite.* 1986;(7 Suppl):39-56.
13. Ryan DH. Clinical use of sibutramine. *Drugs Today* (Barc). 2004;40(1):41-54.
14. Bray GA. Drug treatment of obesity. *Baillieres Best Pract Res Clin Endocrinol Metab.* 1999;13(1):131-48.
15. Cannistra LB, Davis SM, Bauman AG. Valvular heart disease associated with dexfenfluramine. *N Engl J Med.* 1997;337(9):636.
16. Connolly HM, Crary JL, McGoon MD, et al. Valvular heart disease associated with fenfluramine-phentermine. *N Engl J Med.* 1997;337(9):581-8.
17. Tatemoto K. Neuropeptide Y: complete amino acid sequence of the brain peptide. *Proc Natl Acad Sci U S A.* 1982;79(18):5485-9.
18. Clark JT, Kalra PS, Crowley WR, Kalra SP. Neuropeptide Y and human pancreatic polypeptide stimulate feeding behavior in rats. *Endocrinology.* 1984;115(1):427-9.
19. Stanley BG, Leibowitz SF. Neuropeptide Y: stimulation of feeding and drinking by injection into the paraventricular nucleus. *Life Sci.* 1984;35(26):2635-42.
20. Levine AS, Morley JE. Neuropeptide Y: a potent inducer of consummatory behavior in rats. *Peptides.* 1984;5(6):1025-9.
21. Stanley BG, Daniel DR, Chin AS, Leibowitz SF. Paraventricular nucleus injections of peptide YY and neuropeptide Y preferentially enhance carbohydrate ingestion. *Peptides.* 1985;6(6):1205-11.
22. Kalra SP, Dube MG, Sahu A, Phelps CP, Kalra PS. Neuropeptide Y secretion increases in the paraventricular nucleus in association with increased appetite for food. *Proc Natl Acad Sci U S A.* 1991;88(23):10931-5.
23. Kotz CM, Grace MK, Briggs J, Levine AS, Billington CJ. Effects of opioid antagonists naloxone and naltrexone on neuropeptide Y-induced feeding and brown fat thermogenesis in the rat. Neural site of action. *J Clin Invest.* 1995;96(1):163-70.
24. Wirth MM, Olszewski PK, Yu C, Levine AS, Giraudo SQ. Paraventricular hypothalamic alpha-melanocyte-stimulating hormone and MTII reduce feeding without causing aversive effects. *Peptides.* 2001;22(1):129-34.
25. Lynch WC, Grace M, Billington CJ, Levine AS. Effects of neuropeptide Y on ingestion of flavored solutions in nondeprived rats. *Physiol Behav.* 1993;54(5):877-80.
26. Glass MJ, Cleary JP, Billington CJ, Levine AS. Role of carbohydrate type on diet selection in neuropeptide Y-stimulated rats. *Am J Physiol.* 1997;273(6 Pt 2):R2040-5.
27. Giraudo SQ, Kotz CM, Grace MK, Levine AS, Billington CJ. Rat hypothalamic NPY mRNA and brown fat uncoupling protein mRNA after high-carbohydrate or high-fat diets. *Am J Physiol.* 1994;266(5 Pt 2):R1578-83.
28. Erlanson-Albertsson C, Mei J, Okada S, York D, Bray GA. Pancreatic procolipase propeptide, enterostatin, specifically inhibits fat intake. *Physiol Behav.* 1991;49(6):1191-4.
29. Jewett DC, Cleary J, Levine AS, Schaal DW, Thompson T. Effects of neuropeptide Y on food-reinforced behavior in satiated rats. *Pharmacol Biochem Behav.* 1992;42(2):207-12.
30. Brady LS, Smith MA, Gold PW, Herkenham M. Altered expression of hypothalamic neuropeptide mRNAs in food-restricted and food-deprived rats. *Neuroendocrinology.* 1990;52(5):441-7.
31. Bray GA. Reciprocal relation of food intake and sympathetic activity: experimental observations and clinical implications. *Int J Obes Relat Metab Disord.* 2000;24 (Suppl 2):S8-17.
32. Egawa M, Yoshimatsu H, Bray GA. Neuropeptide Y suppresses sympathetic activity to interscapular brown adipose tissue in rats. *Am J Physiol.* 1991;260(2 Pt 2):R328-34.
33. Billington CJ, Briggs JE, Grace M, Levine AS. Effects of intracerebroventricular injection of neuropeptide Y on energy metabolism. *Am J Physiol.* 1991;260(2 Pt 2):R321-7.
34. Hwa JJ, Witten MB, Williams P, et al. Activation of the NPY Y5 receptor regulates both feeding and energy expenditure. *Am J Physiol.* 1999;277(5 Pt 2):R1428-34.
35. Voisey J, Carroll L, van Daal A. Melanocortins and their receptors and antagonists. *Curr Drug Targets.* 2003;4(7):586-97.
36. Broberger C, Johansen J, Johansson C, Schalling M, Hokfelt T. The neuropeptide Y/agouti gene-related protein (AGRP) brain circuitry in normal, anorectic, and monosodium glutamate-treated mice. *Proc Natl Acad Sci U S A.* 1998;95(25):15043-8.
37. Morton GJ, Schwartz MW. The NPY/AgRP neuron and energy homeostasis. *Int J Obes Relat Metab Disord.* 2001;25(Suppl 5): S56-62.
38. Olszewski PK, Wirth MM, Shaw TJ, et al. Role of alpha-MSH in the regulation of consummatory behavior: immunohistochemical evidence. *Am J Physiol Regul Integr Comp Physiol.* 2001;281(2): R673-80.
39. Olszewski PK, Wirth MM, Grace MK, Levine AS, Giraudo SQ. Evidence of interactions between melanocortin and opioid systems in regulation of feeding. *Neuroreport.* 2001;12(8):1727-30.
40. Trayhurn P, Hoggard N, Mercer JG, Rayner DV. Leptin: fundamental aspects. *Int J Obes Relat Metab Disord.* 1999;23(Suppl 1):22-8.
41. Benoit SC, Clegg DJ, Seeley RJ, Woods SC. Insulin and leptin as adiposity signals. *Recent Prog Horm Res.* 2004;59:267-85.

42. Shrestha YB, Wickwire K, Giraudo SQ. Action of MT-II on ghrelin-induced feeding in the paraventricular nucleus of the hypothalamus. *Neuroreport.* 2004;15(8):1365-7.
43. Levine AS, Billington CJ. Opioids as agents of reward-related feeding: a consideration of the evidence. *Physiol Behav.* 2004;82(1):57-61.
44. Colantuoni C, Rada P, McCarthy J, et al. Evidence that intermittent, excessive sugar intake causes endogenous opioid dependence. *Obes Res.* 2002;10(6):478-88.
45. Colantuoni C, Schwenker J, McCarthy J, et al. Excessive sugar intake alters binding to dopamine and mu-opioid receptors in the brain. *Neuroreport.* 2001;12(16):3549-52.
46. Pomonis JD, Jewett DC, Kotz CM, Briggs JE, Billington CJ, Levine AS. Sucrose consumption increases naloxone-induced c-Fos immunoreactivity in limbic forebrain. *Am J Physiol Regul Integr Comp Physiol.* 2000;278(3):R712-9.
47. Welch CC, Kim EM, Grace MK, Billington CJ, Levine AS. Palatability-induced hyperphagia increases hypothalamic Dynorphin peptide and mRNA levels. *Brain Res.* 1996;721(1-2):126-31.
48. Cooper SJ. Endocannabinoids and food consumption: comparisons with benzodiazepine and opioid palatability-dependent appetite. *Eur J Pharmacol.* 2004;500(1-3):37-49.
49. McLaughlin PJ, Winston K, Swezey L, et al. The cannabinoid CB1 antagonists SR 141716A and AM 251 suppress food intake and food-reinforced behavior in a variety of tasks in rats. *Behav Pharmacol.* 2003;14(8):583-8.
50. Di Marzo V, Goparaju SK, Wang L, et al. Leptin-regulated endocannabinoids are involved in maintaining food intake. *Nature.* 2001;410(6830):822-5.
51. Gomez R, Navarro M, Ferrer B, et al. A peripheral mechanism for CB1 cannabinoid receptor-dependent modulation of feeding. *J Neurosci.* 2002;22(21):9612-7.
52. Black SC. Cannabinoid receptor antagonists and obesity. *Curr Opin Investig Drugs.* 2004;5(4):389-94.
53. Tucci SA, Rogers EK, Korbonits M, Kirkham TC. The cannabinoid CB1 receptor antagonist SR141716 blocks the orexigenic effects of intrahypothalamic ghrelin. *Br J Pharmacol.* 2004.
54. Kirkham TC, Williams CM. Synergistic efects of opioid and cannabinoid antagonists on food intake. *Psychopharmacology* (Berl). 2001;153(2):267-70.
55. de Lecea L, Kilduff TS, Peyron C, et al. The hypocretins: hypothalamus-specific peptides with neuroexcitatory activity. *Proc Nat Acad Sci USA.* 1998;95(1):322-7.
56. Sakurai T, Amemiya A, Ishii M, et al. Orexins and orexin receptors: a family of hypothalamic neuropeptides and G protein-coupled receptors that regulate feeding behavior [see comments]. *Cell.* 1998;92(4):573-85.
57. Peyron C, Tighe DK, van den Pol AN, et al. Neurons containing hypocretin (orexin) project to multiple neuronal systems. *J Neurosci.* 1998;18(23):9996-10015.
58. Leibowitz SF, Hoebel BG. Behavioral neuroscience of obesity. In: James WPJ, ed. *Handbook of Obesity.* New York, NY: Marcell Dekker, Inc; 1998:313-358.
59. Brown RE, Sergeeva OA, Eriksson KS, Haas HL. Convergent excitation of dorsal raphe serotonin neurons by multiple arousal systems (orexin/hypocretin, histamine and noradrenaline). *J Neurosci.* 2002;22(20):8850-9.
60. Bernard R, Lydic R, Baghdoyan HA. Hypocretin-1 activates G proteins in arousal-related brainstem nuclei of rat. *Neuroreport.* 2002;13(4):447-50.
61. Greco MA, Shiromani PJ. Hypocretin receptor protein and mRNA expression in the dorsolateral pons of rats. *Brain Res Mol Brain Res.* 2001;88(1-2):176-82.
62. van den Pol AN, Ghosh PK, Liu RJ, Li Y, Aghajanian GK, Gao XB. Hypocretin (orexin) enhances neuron activity and cell synchrony in developing mouse GFP-expressing locus coeruleus. *J Physiol.* 2002;541(Pt 1):169-85.
63. Sunter D, Morgan I, Edwards CM, et al. Orexins: effects on behavior and localisation of orexin receptor 2 messenger ribonucleic acid in the rat brainstem. *Brain Res.* 2001;907(1-2):27-34.
64. Hervieu GJ, Cluderay JE, Harrison DC, Roberts JC, Leslie RA. Gene expression and protein distribution of the orexin-1 receptor in the rat brain and spinal cord. *Neuroscience.* 2001;103(3):777-97.
65. Dube MG, Kalra SP, Kalra PS. Food intake elicited by central administration of orexins/hypocretins: identification of hypothalamic sites of action. *Brain Res.* 1999;842(2):473-7.
66. Sweet DC, Levine AS, Billington CJ, Kotz CM. Feeding response to central orexins. *Brain Res.* 1999;821(2):535-8.
67. Rodgers RJ, Halford JC, Nunes de Souza RL, et al. Dose-response effects of orexin-A on food intake and the behavioural satiety sequence in rats. *Regul Pept.* 2000;96(1-2):71-84.
68. Rodgers RJ, Halford JC, Nunes de Souza RL, et al. SB-334867, a selective orexin-1 receptor antagonist, enhances behavioural satiety and blocks the hyperphagic effect of orexin-A in rats. *Eur J Neurosci.* 2001;13(7):1444-52.
69. Rodgers RJ, Ishii Y, Halford JC, Blundell JE. Orexins and appetite regulation. *Neuropeptides.* 2002;36(5):303-25.
70. Cai XJ, Evans ML, Lister CA, et al. Hypoglycemia activates orexin neurons and selectively increases hypothalamic orexin-B levels: responses inhibited by feeding and possibly mediated by the nucleus of the solitary tract. *Diabetes.* 2001;50(1):105-12.
71. Kurose T, Ueta Y, Yamamoto Y, et al. Effects of restricted feeding on the activity of hypothalamic Orexin (OX)-A containing neurons and OX2 receptor mRNA level in the paraventricular nucleus of rats. *Regul Pept.* 2002;104(1-3):145-51.
72. Kiwaki K, Kotz CM, Wang C, Lanningham-Foster L, Levine JA. Orexin A (hypocretin 1) injected into hypothalamic paraventricular nucleus and spontaneous physical activity in rats. *Am J Physiol Endocrinol Metab.* 2004;286(4):E551-9.
73. Zaki MS, Katayama T, Murata T, Konishi H, Shiota K, Takahashi M. The regulation of food intake and correlated energy balance in mice. *J Vet Med Sci.* 1991;53(2):249-54.
74. Lawrence CB, Snape AC, Baudoin FM, Luckman SM. Acute central ghrelin and GH secretagogues induce feeding and activate brain appetite centers. *Endocrinology.* 2002;143(1):155-62.
75. Olszewski PK, Li D, Grace MK, Billington CJ, Kotz CM, Levine AS. Neural basis of orexigenic effects of ghrelin acting within lateral hypothalamus. *Peptides.* 2003;24(4):597-602.
76. Zheng H, Corkern MM, Crousillac SM, Patterson LM, Phifer CB, Berthoud HR. Neurochemical phenotype of hypothalamic neurons showing Fos expression 23 h after intracranial AgRP. *Am J Physiol Regul Integr Comp Physiol.* 2002;282(6):R1773-81.
77. Chemelli RM, Willie JT, Sinton CM, et al. Narcolepsy in orexin knockout mice: molecular genetics of sleep regulation. *Cell.* 1999;98(4):437-51.
78. Lin L, Faraco J, Li R, et al. The sleep disorder canine narcolepsy is caused by a mutation in the hypocretin (orexin) receptor 2 gene. *Cell.* 1999;98(3):365-76.
79. Nishino S, Ripley B, Overeem S, Lammers GJ, Mignot E. Hypocretin (orexin) deficiency in human narcolepsy. *Lancet.* 2000;355(9197):39-40.
80. Reilly CE. I. Mutation in the hypocretin (orexin) receptor 2 gene causes canine narcolepsy. *J Neurol.* 1999;246(10):985-6.
81. Siegel JM. Narcolepsy: a key role for hypocretins (orexins). *Cell.* 1999;98(4):409-12.
82. Thakkar MM, Ramesh V, Cape EG, Winston S, Strecker RE, McCarley RW. REM sleep enhancement and behavioral cataplexy following orexin (hypocretin)-II receptor antisense perfusion in the pontine reticular formation. *Sleep Res Online.* 1999;2(4):112-20.
83. Estabrooke IV, McCarthy MT, Ko E, et al. Fos expression in orexin neurons varies with behavioral state. *J Neurosci.* 2001;21(5):1656-62.
84. Fujiki N, Yoshida Y, Ripley B, Honda K, Mignot E, Nishino S. Changes in CSF hypocretin-1 (orexin A) levels in rats across 24 hours and in response to food deprivation. *Neuroreport.* 2001;12(5):993-7.
85. Espana RA, Plahn S, Berridge CW. Circadian-dependent and circadian-independent behavioral actions of hypocretin/orexin. *Brain Res.* 2002;943(2):224-36.

86. Espana RA, Valentino RJ, Berridge CW. Fos immunoreactivity in hypocretin-synthesizing and hypocretin-1 receptor-expressing neurons: effects of diurnal and nocturnal spontaneous waking, stress and hypocretin-1 administration. *Neuroscience.* 2003;121(1):201-17.
87. Mullington JM, Chan JL, Van Dongen HP, et al. Sleep loss reduces diurnal rhythm amplitude of leptin in healthy men. *J Neuroendocrinol.* 2003;15(9):851-4.
88. Overeem S, Mignot E, van Dijk JG, Lammers GJ. Narcolepsy: clinical features, new pathophysiologic insights, and future perspectives. *J Clin Neurophysiol.* 2001;18(2):78-105.
89. Kok SW, Meinders AE, Overeem S, et al. Reduction of plasma leptin levels and loss of its circadian rhythmicity in hypocretin (orexin)-deficient narcoleptic humans. *J Clin Endocrinol Metab.* 2002;87(2):805-9.
90. Hara J, Beuckmann CT, Nambu T, et al. Genetic ablation of orexin neurons in mice results in narcolepsy, hypophagia, and obesity. *Neuron.* 2001;30(2):345-54.
91. Dahmen N, Bierbrauer J, Kasten M. Increased prevalence of obesity in narcoleptic patients and relatives. *Eur Arch Psychiatry Clin Neurosci.* 2001;251(2):85-9.
92. Sekine M, Yamagami T, Handa K, et al. A dose-response relationship between short sleeping hours and childhood obesity: results of the Toyama Birth Cohort Study. *Child Care Health Dev.* 2002;28(2):163-70.
93. Mokdad AH, Ford ES, Bowman BA, et al. Prevalence of obesity, diabetes, and obesity-related health risk factors, 2001. *JAMA.* 2003;289(1):76-9.
94. Nilsson PM, Nilsson JA, Hedblad B, Berglund G. Sleep disturbance in association with elevated pulse rate for prediction of mortality--consequences of mental strain? *J Intern Med.* 2001;250(6):521-9.
95. Kripke DF, Garfinkel L, Wingard DL, Klauber MR, Marler MR. Mortality associated with sleep duration and insomnia. *Arch Gen Psychiatry.* 2002;59(2):131-6.
96. Broberger C, De Lecea L, Sutcliffe JG, Hokfelt T. Hypocretin/orexin- and melanin-concentrating hormone-expressing cells form distinct populations in the rodent lateral hypothalamus: relationship to the neuropeptide Y and agouti gene-related protein systems. *J Comp Neurol.* 1998;402(4):460-74.
97. Qu D, Ludwig DS, Gammeltoft S, et al. A role for melanin-concentrating hormone in the central regulation of feeding behaviour. *Nature.* 1996;380(6571):243-7.
98. Vaughan J, Donaldson C, Bittencourt J, et al. Urocortin, a mammalian neuropeptide related to fish urotensin I and to corticotropin-releasing factor. *Nature.* 1995;378(6554):287-92.
99. Bittencourt JC, Vaughan J, Arias C, Rissman RA, Vale WW, Sawchenko PE. Urocortin expression in rat brain: evidence against a pervasive relationship of urocortin-containing projections with targets bearing type 2 CRF receptors. *J Comp Neurol.* 1999;415(3):285-312.
100. Kozicz T, Yanaihara H, Arimura A. Distribution of urocortin-like immunoreactivity in the central nervous system of the rat. *J Comp Neurol.* 1988;391(1):1-10.
101. Primus RJ, Yevich E, Baltazar C, Gallager DW. Autoradiographic localization of CRF1 and CRF2 binding sites in adult rat brain. *Neuropsychopharmacology.* 1997;17(5):308-16.
102. Eckart K, Radulovic J, Radulovic M, et al. Actions of CRF and its analogs. *Curr Med Chem.* 1999;6(11):1035-53.
103. Sakanaka M, Magari S, Shibasaki T, Lederis K. Corticotropin releasing factor-containing afferents to the lateral septum of the rat brain. *J Comp Neurol.* 1988;270(3):404-15, 396-7.
104. Morin SM, Ling N, Liu XJ, Kahl SD, Gehlert DR. Differential distribution of urocortin- and corticotropin-releasing factor-like immunoreactivities in the rat brain. *Neuroscience.* 1999;92(1):281-91.
105. Benoit SC, Thiele TE, Heinrichs SC, Rushing PA, Blake KA, Steeley RJ. Comparison of central administration of corticotropin-releasing hormone and urocortin on food intake, conditioned taste aversion, and c-Fos expression. *Peptides.* 2000;21(3):345-51.
106. Kishimoto T, Radulovic J, Radulovic M, et al. Deletion of crhr2 reveals an anxiolytic role for corticotropin-releasing hormone receptor-2. *Nat Genet.* 2000;24(4):415-9.
107. Bale TL, Contarino A, Smith GW, et al. Mice deficient for corticotropin-releasing hormone receptor-2 display anxiety-like behaviour and are hypersensitive to stress. *Nat Genet.* 2000;24(4):410-4.
108. Coste SC, Kesterson RA, Heldwein KA, et al. Abnormal adaptations to stress and impaired cardiovascular function in mice lacking corticotropin-releasing hormone receptor-2. *Nat Genet.* 2000;24(4):403-9.
109. Smagin GN, Howell LA, Ryan DH, De Souza EB, Harris RB. The role of CRF2 receptors in corticotropin-releasing factor- and urocortin-induced anorexia. *Neuroreport.* 1998;9(7):1601-6.
110. Macey DJ, Koob GF, Markou A. CRF and urocortin decreased brain stimulation reward in the rat: reversal by a CRF receptor antagonist. *Brain Res.* 2000;866(1-2):82-91.
111. Reyes TM, Lewis K, Perrin MH, et al. Urocortin II: a member of the corticotropin-releasing factor (CRF) neuropeptide family that is selectively bound by type 2 CRF receptors. *Proc Natl Acad Sci U S A.* 2001;98(5):2843-8.
112. Lewis K, Li C, Perrin MH, et al. Identification of urocortin III, an additional member of the corticotropin-releasing factor (CRF) family with high affinity for the CRF2 receptor. *Proc Natl Acad Sci U S A.* 2001;98(13):7570-5.
113. Inoue K, Valdez GR, Reyes TM, et al. Human urocortin II, a selective agonist for the type 2 corticotropin-releasing factor receptor, decreases feeding and drinking in the Rat. *J Pharmacol Exp Ther.* 2003;305(1):385-93.
114. Zhang Y, Proenca R, Maffei M, Barone M, Leopold L, Friedman JM. Positional cloning of the mouse obese gene and its human homologue. *Nature.* 1994;372(6505):425-32.
115. Woods SC. Lessons in the interactions of hormones and ingestive behavior. *Physiol Behav.* 2004;82(1):187-90.
116. Figlewicz DP, Sipols AJ, Seeley RJ, Chavez M, Woods SC, Porte D, Jr. Intraventricular insulin enhances the meal-suppressive efficacy of intraventricular cholecystokinin octapeptide in the baboon. *Behav Neurosci.* 1995;109(3):567-9.
117. Schwartz MW, Seeley RJ, Campfield LA, Burn P, Baskin DG. Identification of targets of leptin action in rat hypothalamus. *J Clin Invest.* 1996;98(5):1101-6.
118. Schwartz MW, Sipols AJ, Marks JL, et al. Inhibition of hypothalamic neuropeptide Y gene expression by insulin. *Endocrinology.* 1992;130(6):3608-16.
119. Banks WA, Kastin AJ, Huang W, Jaspan JB, Maness LM. Leptin enters the brain by a saturable system independent of insulin. *Peptides.* 1996;17(2):305-11.
120. Levine AS, Billington CJ. Do circulating leptin concentrations reflect body adiposity or energy flux? *Am J Clin Nutr.* 1998;68(4):761-2.
121. Antin J, Gibbs J, Holt J, Young RC, Smith GP. Cholecystokinin elicits the complete behavioral sequence of satiety in rats. *J Comp Physiol Psychol.* 1975;89(7):784-90.
122. Smith GP, Gibbs J, Jerome C, Pi-Sunyer FX, Kissileff HR, Thornton J. The satiety effect of cholecystokinin: a progress report. *Peptides.* 1981;2 Suppl 2:57-9.
123. Carlberg M, Gundlach AL, Mercer LD, Beart PM. Autoradiographic Localization of Cholecystokinin A and B Receptors in Rat Brain Using [125I]d-Tyr25 (Nle28,31)-CCK 25 - 33S. *Eur J Neurosci.* 1992;4(6):563-573.
124. Hill DR, Shaw TM, Woodruff GN. Species differences in the localization of 'peripheral' type cholecystokinin receptors in rodent brain. *Neurosci Lett.* 1987;79(3):286-9.
125. Kritzer MF, Innis RB, Goldman-Rakic PS. Regional distribution of cholecystokinin receptors in primate cerebral cortex determined by in vitro receptor autoradiography. *J Comp Neurol.* 1987;263(3):418-35.
126. Kohler C, Chan-Palay V. Cholecystokinin-octapeptide (CCK-8) receptors in the hippocampal region: a comparative in vitro autoradiographic study in the rat, monkey and the postmortem human brain. *Neurosci Lett.* 1988;90(1-2):51-6.

127. Morency MA, Quirion R, Nair NP, Mishra RK. Localization of cholecystokinin binding sites in canine brain using quantitative autoradiography. *Prog Neuropsychopharmacol Biol Psychiatry.* 1991;15(2):291-6.
128. Reubi JC, Waser B, Laderach U, et al. Localization of cholecystokinin A and cholecystokinin B-gastrin receptors in the human stomach. *Gastroenterology.* 1997;112(4):1197-205.
129. de Weerth A, Jonas L, Schade R, et al. Gastrin/cholecystokinin type B receptors in the kidney: molecular, pharmacological, functional characterization, and localization. *Eur J Clin Invest.* 1998;28(7):592-601.
130. Dietl MM, Probst A, Palacios JM. On the distribution of cholecystokinin receptor binding sites in the human brain: an autoradiographic study. *Synapse.* 1987;1(2):169-83.
131. Gibbs J, Smith GP. Gut peptides and food in the gut produce similar satiety effects. *Peptides.* 1982;3(3):553-7.
132. Crawley JN, Kiss JZ. Paraventricular nucleus lesions abolish the inhibition of feeding induced by systemic cholecystokinin. *Peptides.* 1985;6(5):927-35.
133. Smith GP, Gibbs J. The satiety effect of cholecystokinin. Recent progress and current problems. *Ann N Y Acad Sci.* 1985;448:417-23.
134. Gourch A, Orosco M, Pages N, et al. Changes in hypothalamic neuropeptide Y concentrations induced by cholecystokinin analogues. *Eur J Pharmacol.* 1990;187(1):117-22.
135. Pages N, Gourch A, Orosco M, et al. Changes in brain neuropeptide Y induced by cholecystokinin peptides. *Neuropeptides.* 1990;17(3):141-5.
136. Wang L, Martinez V, Barrachina MD, Tache Y. Fos expression in the brain induced by peripheral injection of CCK or leptin plus CCK in fasted lean mice. *Brain Res.* 1998;791(1-2):157-66.
137. Konturek SJ, Konturek JW, Pawlik T, Brzozowski T. Brain-gut axis and its role in the control of food intake. *J Physiol Pharmacol.* 2004;55(1 Pt 2):137-54.
138. Fan W, Ellacott KL, Halatchev IG, Takahashi K, Yu P, Cone RD. Cholecystokinin-mediated suppression of feeding involves the brainstem melanocortin system. *Nat Neurosci.* 2004;7(4):335-6.
139. Moran TH. Cholecystokinin and satiety: current perspectives. *Nutrition.* 2000;16(10):858-65.
140. Bi S, Moran TH. Actions of CCK in the controls of food intake and body weight: lessons from the CCK-A receptor deficient OLETF rat. *Neuropeptides.* 2002;36(2-3):171-81.
141. Bi S, Ladenheim EE, Schwartz GJ, Moran TH. A role for NPY overexpression in the dorsomedial hypothalamus in hyperphagia and obesity of OLETF rats. *Am J Physiol Regul Integr Comp Physiol.* 2001;281(1):R254-60.
142. Bi S, Moran TH. Response to acute food deprivation in OLETF rats lacking CCK-A receptors. *Physiol Behav.* 2003;79(4-5):655-61.
143. Morley JE, Levine AS, Grace M, Kneip J. Peptide YY (PYY), a potent orexigenic agent. *Brain Res.* 1985;341(1):200-3.
144. Batterham RL, Cowley MA, Small CJ, et al. Gut hormone PYY(3-36) physiologically inhibits food intake. *Nature.* 2002;418(6898):650-4.
145. Batterham RL, Bloom SR. The gut hormone peptide YY regulates appetite. *Ann N Y Acad Sci.* 2003;994:162-8.
146. Tschop M, Castaneda TR, Joost HG, et al. Physiology: does gut hormone PYY3-36 decrease food intake in rodents? *Nature.* 2004;430(6996):1 p following 165; discussion 2 p following 165.
147. Kojima M, Hosoda H, Date Y, Nakazato M, Matsuo H, Kangawa K. Ghrelin is a growth-hormone-releasing acylated peptide from stomach. *Nature.* 1999;402(6762):656-60.
148. Date Y, Kojima M, Hosoda H, et al. Ghrelin, a novel growth hormone-releasing acylated peptide, is synthesized in a distinct endocrine cell type in the gastrointestinal tracts of rats and humans. *Endocrinology.* 2000;141(11):4255-61.
149. Wren AM, Small CJ, Ward HL, et al. The novel hypothalamic peptide ghrelin stimulates food intake and growth hormone secretion. *Endocrinology.* 2000;141(11):4325-8.
150. Wren AM, Small CJ, Abbott CR, et al. Ghrelin causes hyperphagia and obesity in rats. *Diabetes.* 2001;50(11):2540-7.
151. Kojima M, Kangawa K. Ghrelin, an orexigenic signaling molecule from the gastrointestinal tract. *Curr Opin Pharmacol.* 2002;2(6):665-8.
152. Horvath TL, Castaneda T, Tang-Christensen M, Pagotto U, Tschop MH. Ghrelin as a potential anti-obesity target. *Curr Pharm Des.* 2003;9(17):1383-95.
153. Kim MS, Yoon CY, Park KH, et al. Changes in ghrelin and ghrelin receptor expression according to feeding status. *Neuroreport.* 2003;14(10):1317-20.
154. McCowen KC, Maykel JA, Bistrian BR, Ling PR. Circulating ghrelin concentrations are lowered by intravenous glucose or hyperinsulinemic euglycemic conditions in rodents. *J Endocrinol.* 2002;175(2):R7-11.
155. Cummings DE, Weigle DS, Frayo RS, et al. Plasma ghrelin levels after diet-induced weight loss or gastric bypass surgery. *N Engl J Med.* 2002;346(21):1623-30.
156. Shimizu Y, Nagaya N, Isobe T, et al. Increased plasma ghrelin level in lung cancer cachexia. *Clin Cancer Res.* 2003;9(2):774-8.
157. Rigamonti AE, Pincelli AI, Corra B, et al. Plasma ghrelin concentrations in elderly subjects: comparison with anorexic and obese patients. *J Endocrinol.* 2002;175(1):R1-5.
158. English PJ, Ghatei MA, Malik IA, Bloom SR, Wilding JP. Food fails to suppress ghrelin levels in obese humans. *J Clin Endocrinol Metab.* 2002;87(6):2984.
159. Kamegai J, Tamura H, Shimizu T, Ishii S, Sugihara H, Wakabayashi I. Chronic central infusion of ghrelin increases hypothalamic neuropeptide Y and Agouti-related protein mRNA levels and body weight in rats. *Diabetes.* 2001;50(11):2438-43.
160. Kohno D, Gao HZ, Muroya S, Kikuyama S, Yada T. Ghrelin directly interacts with neuropeptide-Y-containing neurons in the rat arcuate nucleus: Ca2+ signaling via protein kinase A and N-type channel-dependent mechanisms and cross-talk with leptin and orexin. *Diabetes.* 2003;52(4):948-56.
161. Shintani M, Ogawa Y, Ebihara K, et al. Ghrelin, an endogenous growth hormone secretagogue, is a novel orexigenic peptide that antagonizes leptin action through the activation of hypothalamic neuropeptide Y/Y1 receptor pathway. *Diabetes.* 2001;50(2):227-32.
162. Olszewski PK, Grace MK, Billington CJ, Levine AS. Hypothalamic paraventricular injections of ghrelin: effect on feeding and c-Fos immunoreactivity. *Peptides.* 2003;24(6):919-23.

Chapter 49

Surgical Management of Obesity

Alexander P. Nagle, MD; Jay B. Prystowsky, MD;
Brintha Enestvedt, MD; and John E. Pandolfino, MD

Introduction

Obesity may be defined as an abnormal state of health in which there is an excess of body fat. Morbid obesity is the most serious form of obesity and generally correlates with a body weight that is more than 70% above ideal body or a body mass index (BMI) greater than 40 kg/m^2. BMI represents the relationship between height and weight and is calculated as weight (kg) divided by height squared (m^2). Based on US 1999-2000 population data, 64.5% of US adults are overweight (BMI >25), 30.5% are obese (BMI >30), and 4.7% are morbidly obese (BMI >40).[1] The prevalence of obesity has increased steadily over the past several decades and obesity has become an important public health problem. From 1960 to 2000, the prevalence of obesity has increased from 13.4% to 30.5%—a relative increase of more than 50%.[1] In the 21st century, obesity is predicted to surpass cigarette smoking as the number one cause of preventable death in the United States. The Centers for Disease Control and Prevention (CDC) reported that tobacco was responsible for 435,00 deaths and poor diet and physical inactivity were responsible for 400,000 deaths in the year 2000. Healthcare costs associated with obesity are astronomical. Annual direct costs for treating obesity-related illnesses have been estimated at nearly $51.6 billion and indirect costs are estimated at $47.6 billion.[2] Furthermore, the annual US expenditure on weight reduction products and services exceeds $30 billion.[3]

Obesity: A Complex Disease

There is general agreement that clinically severe obesity is a complex disease with multiple causes. A simple explanation of obesity is that caloric intake exceeds the expenditure of calories to maintain body function and perform physical activity. Excess calories are stored as fat in the adipose tissue. However, there is significant variability in the energy requirements of individuals. Obesity does not ensue simply because an individual either eats more or exercises less than do normal-weight individuals. In short, there is individual variation in susceptibility to develop obesity.[4] There is a strong familial factor in the development of obesity. Children of two obese parents have a 50% likelihood of becoming overweight themselves.[5] Twin studies have suggested that genetic factors predominate environmental influences in predicting the development of obesity.[6]

The development of obesity is strongly influenced by social, economic, racial, and ethnic factors.[7] Women are more likely than are men to be obese. In developed countries, both children and adults from lower socioeconomic classes are more likely to be overweight.[8] African American women are at higher risk for obesity than are Caucasian women, while the reverse is true for men. Cultural factors may have a role in that different ethnic groups have different ideals regarding body size and appearance. Pregnancy is a precursor to obesity, especially in women with multiple pregnancies.[9]

There is significant evidence that obesity is associated with increased mortality.[10-15] In a 14-year prospective study of more than 1 million adults in the United States, the risk of death increased with an increasing BMI for both men and women in all age groups.[10] A recent study demonstrated that race and gender affect the estimated years of life lost (YLL) associated with obesity.[11] The maximum YLL for young white men with a BMI >45 was 13 years and was 8 years for white women.[11] Young blacks with severe levels of obesity had a maximum YLL of 20 years for men and 5 years for women.[11] In short, it appears that obese individuals die at a younger age than do normal-weight individuals.[10-15]

Obesity is related to a significant number of comorbid illnesses. There is a strong association between obesity and the prevalence of type 2 diabetes mellitus.[16,17] A Scandinavian study demonstrated that moderate obesity was associated with a 10-fold increase in the risk of diabetes.[18] There is an increased prevalence of other cardiovascular comorbidities in obese patients. These include hypertension, hypertriglyceridemia, hyperlipidemia, hyperinsulinemia, and low levels of high-density lipoprotein (HDL) cholesterol.[19] Other obesity-related illnesses include osteoarthritis of weight-bearing joints, gastroesophageal reflux disease (GERD), cholelithiasis, hepatic steatosis, obstructive sleep apnea, obesity hypoventilation syndrome, stress urinary incontinence, migraine headaches, lower extremity venous insufficiency, deep venous thrombosis, pulmonary emboli, and hernias.[20-25] Menstrual irregularities and infertility are common in women with clinically severe obesity.[26] Dermatitides, notably fungal infections, commonly occur in the intertriginous regions of obese patients.[27]

Perhaps the most significant impact of obesity is the social effects on these individuals.[28] Obesity carries a stigma in our society, which places a high value on thinness. Obesity is often associated with a lack of self-control or other character disorders. Obese children frequently have a reduced self-esteem due to the consistent ridicule by their peers.[29] There are many daily activities that are taken for granted by normal-weight individuals that are challenging for obese individuals[30] (Table 49-1).

In summary, obesity is a complex disorder with a multifactorial etiology. Clinically severe obesity is generally defined as a BMI ≥40 kg/m2. These individuals experience significant medical comorbidities, reduced life expectancy, and impaired social function.

Indications for Surgery

Severe obesity has been notoriously refractory to virtually every method of nonsurgical treatment. The failure rate of diet and behavior modification treatment at 2 years in the morbidly obese approaches 100%.[31] Likewise, the results of drug therapy and jaw-wiring in this group of patients have been disappointing. Surgery has been shown to be the most effective treatment for achieving sustained weight loss with subsequent control of obesity-related comorbidities. However, the primary justification for surgical treatment of morbid obesity is the overwhelming evidence that severe obesity is associated with a poor quality of life, serious medical problems, and a shortened lifespan.

The National Institutes of Health (NIH) Consensus Development Conference of 1985 determined that weight reduction should be recommended to obese persons, defined as a body weight of 200% or more above ideal body as defined by the 1983 Metropolitan Life Insurance Company's Height/Weight Tables.[32] Weight reduction was also recommended to patients with lesser degrees of obesity if they suffered from comorbid illnesses such as diabetes, hypertension, hyperlipidemia, coronary artery disease, or gout. The 1991 NIH Consensus Development Conference also affirmed the benefits of treating such patients by surgical means given the ineffectiveness of all non-operative methods to achieve and sustain significant weight loss for clinically severe obesity.[21,33] These NIH consensus statements, along with guidelines recommended by the American Society for Clinical Nutrition, have helped to form the basis of the indications for the surgical treatment of obesity that includes the following five conditions:

1. The patient should be >100 lb above desirable weight, according to the 1983 Metropolitan Life Insurance Company Height/Weight Tables, or have a BMI ≥40 kg/m^2.
2. Significant obesity-related illnesses must be present with a BMI ≥35 kg/m^2.
3. The patient has experienced failure of sustained weight loss on supervised dietary and/or medical regimens.
4. The patient shows understanding of the risks and benefits of surgery and understands the lifestyle changes subsequent to the operation.
5. The operative risk is acceptable.

Some patients may not meet the weight criteria for operation but may still be candidates for a surgical procedure. If their medical complications are severe and progressive, then surgery may be considered on an individual basis. Bariatric surgery has typically been reserved for patients ages 18 to 60 years. The results and expected benefits of surgery in teenagers and in the elderly are less clear. Again, each patient needs to be addressed individually.

Patient Selection

Bariatric surgery is an appropriate treatment option for well-informed patients with acceptable operative risks whose BMI is >40 or >35 with obesity-related illnesses such as type 2 diabetes or hypertension. Optimal results are obtained with a highly motivated patient and the involvement of a multidisciplinary team (including physician/surgeon, nutritionist, dietitian, psychologist and/or psychiatrist).[34]

A thorough history and physical examination should be supplemented by routine blood tests, chest radiographs, and electrocardiogram. Pulmonary function tests and cardiac stress tests are frequently useful for accurate risk stratification. Polysomnography to detect sleep apnea is

TABLE 49-1.

Specific Problems Associated With Massive Obesity

	% of Patients (n = 1,549)
Unable to:	
Cut toenails*	73
Cross legs (ie, thighs)	85
Buckle normal belt	27
Fit in fixed booth at McDonald's	33
Fit in theatre seat†	36
Wipe self	21
Urinate accurately (men)	52
Walk down stairs, unless backwards	16
Will not:	
Undress in front of spouse	73
Wear short sleeves in summer	68
Sleep in room with significant other (snores)	81

* Usually accompanied by inability to tie own shoelaces, put on socks, fit winter boots.
† Problems in bus, airplanes, turnstiles.

Reprinted with permission from Deitel N, Camilleri A. Overlooked problems in morbidly obese patients. *Obes Surg*. 2000;10:125.

indicated when the diagnosis is suspected. Patients who suffer from obstructive sleep apnea may benefit from continuous positive airway pressure (CPAP) prior to surgery and during the perioperative period. As for any major operation, other consultations and/or tests may be needed for optimal preoperative preparation and perioperative care.

A thorough discussion of the operations and subsequent lifestyle changes with the surgeon and healthcare team are mandatory for each patient. A complete explanation of the risks of surgery including mortality and major morbidity is indicated. Patients need to be aware that the operation itself is only one aspect of the entire weight-loss process. The behavioral and lifestyle adjustments that will occur subsequent to the operation are difficult and challenging. It is often helpful for prospective patients to speak with those who have already undergone the operation to learn more about the changes they will encounter.

Patients also meet with a dietitian and psychologist preoperatively. These individuals are often critical in helping a patient manage the lifestyle and dietary changes subsequent to the operation. Their inclusion as part of the multidisciplinary team caring for the bariatric surgical patient cannot be underestimated. Patients who have developed a bond with these healthcare providers prior to surgery benefit greatly, in terms of achieving significant and sustained weight loss postoperatively.

Behavioral modification is critical to the long-term success of most bariatric surgical procedures. Accordingly, although there are few medical conditions that absolutely contraindicate performance of surgery, there are behavioral or psychological considerations that might disqualify patients as candidates for surgery. These may include significant psychiatric disorders such as psychosis or schizophrenia, substance abuse, self-destructive mental behavior, or medical retardation. Even with a technically successful operation, these patients are unlikely to have a satisfactory long-term result. This point emphasizes the value of a comprehensive preoperative psychological evaluation.

In summary, preoperative evaluation of patients for bariatric surgery is an important step in the surgical care of these patients. It is important, both for the purpose of patient selection and for patient education. Patients need to understand the risks of surgery and the dramatic lifestyle changes they will encounter. The healthcare team needs to complete both medical and psychological assessments of each patient to be confident the individual can withstand the operative procedure and successfully adapt to the behavioral changes that the operation intends to stimulate. Patient selection and patient education are critical to achieve optimal long-term outcomes.

Operative Procedures

A successful bariatric operation has two major goals: significant magnitude and duration of weight loss and a reasonably low perioperative and long-term complication rate. In general, operations leading to the greatest amount of weight loss also have higher short-term and long-term complications. Thus, the risk/benefit ratio must be considered when the surgeon assigns bariatric operations. Bariatric surgical procedures are categorized into four main types: malabsorptive, purely restrictive, combined restrictive and malabsorptive, and experimental procedures. The Roux-en-Y gastric bypass (RYGB) is currently the most common bariatric procedure in the United States and is a combined restrictive and malabsorptive procedure. The most popular malabsorptive procedures are the biliopancreatic diversion (BPD) and the duodenal switch

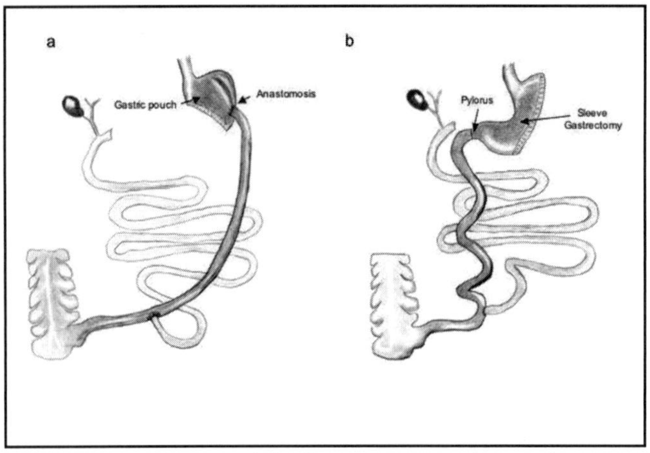

Figure 49-1. (a) BPD and (b) the DS. Drawing by Brintha Enestvedt, MD.

(DS). Purely restrictive procedures include the vertical banded gastroplasty (VBG) and adjustable silastic gastric band (ASGB). Gastric pacing is an experimental bariatric procedure. A membership survey of the American Society for Bariatric surgery revealed that RYGB constitutes 70% of the bariatric procedures performed each year; the VBG and ASGB constitute 16%; and the BPD constitutes 10% of operations performed.[35] All of these operations can be performed by an open or laparoscopic approach.

Malabsorptive Procedures

Malabsorptive operations limit or bypass small intestinal length to create a significantly reduced surface area for calorie and nutrient absorption.

Jejunoileal Bypass

The first popular operation for clinically severe obesity was the jejunoileal bypass (JIB), a malabsorptive procedure.[36] A short length of proximal jejunum was connected to the distal ileum and created an obligatory malabsorptive state. Significant weight-loss was achieved, but the JIB was associated with serious short-term and long-term complications. Perhaps the most serious postoperative complication was the development of cirrhosis. Nephrolithiasis, intractable diarrhea with associated hypokalemia and hypomagnesemia, vitamin B12 deficiency, and severe malnutrition were common sequelae of this operation. The metabolic complications of this operation resulted in significant late morbidity and mortality. The JIB has been largely abandoned.

Biliopancreatic Diversion and Duodenal Switch

The BPD, as described by Scopinaro et al, is a bariatric surgical procedure that aims for selective malabsorption of fat and also provides some restriction of caloric intake.[37] (Figure 49-1.) A BPD involves creating a 200-ml gastric pouch, distal gastrectomy, and a gastroileostomy 250-cm proximal to the ileocecal valve. The biliopancreatic limb is anastomosed to the intestinal limb 50-cm proximal to the ileocecal valve. Fat absorption, therefore, is restricted to the short 50-cm common channel.

BPD results in significant weight loss, especially in the first postoperative year, through a decrease in oral intake and primarily, induction of a significant amount of malabsorption. Critics of this procedure are concerned about the malabsorptive effects of the operation and the potential for deleterious nutritional consequences. The most serious potential complication is protein malnutrition, which is associated with hypoalbuminemia, anemia, edema, ascites, alopecia, and may even require revision surgery to correct the malabsorptive effects of their original operation. BPD patients require life-long supplementation with calcium and vitamins. Perhaps most importantly, meticulous follow-up of the patient's nutritional status is critical to a successful long-term result. (Nutrient deficiency is discussed in Chapter 3.)

The DS, as described by Marceau et al, is a variant of the BPD.[38] The primary differences of the DS[39,40] include a greater curve "sleeve" gastrectomy and preservation of the pylorus with anastomosis of the intestinal limb to the first portion of the duodenum.

Compared to the JIB, these modern malabsorptive operations are associated with less long-term postoperative complications. In particular, there is reduced protein malabsorption and reduced hepatic dysfunction. In addition, there is no blind loop so that the complications related to "blind-loop syndrome" are avoided. The short-term morbidity and mortality rates appear to be slightly higher than those associated with gastric bypass. The BPD and DS have yet to be accepted widely, primarily because of the complexity of the operation and potential for severe protein-calorie malabsorption. Nonetheless, they are effective weight-loss procedures and have gained popularity at several centers around the world.

Purely Restrictive Operations

Purely restrictive procedures rely on mechanical restriction of food passage through the stomach; resulting in significantly decreased caloric intake. These procedures are attractive in that there is no gastrointestinal (GI) anastomosis. Also, the stomach is not excluded from the alimentary stream so that the nutritional consequences of bypassing the stomach are avoided.

Vertical Banded Gastroplasty

The VBG is a gastric-restrictive operation that was introduced by Mason in 1980.[41] A "window" is cut into the body of the stomach using a specialized stapling device approximately 5 cm from the gastroesophageal junction. A second stapling device is then used to partition the stomach into a small gastric pouch (about 15 ml) and the excluded stomach. A stoma is created between the small gastric pouch and the remainder of the stomach, which is 12 mm in diameter and reinforced with a collar of synthetic material such as Marlex (C.R. Bard, Inc, Murray Hill, NJ), GoreTex (W.L. Gore, Ltd., Flagstaff, AZ), or Silastic (Dow Corning, Midland, MI) (Figure 49-2).

The VBG was very popular in the late 1980s and early 1990s. The results are acceptable although this method is not as effect in long-term reduction of excess weight (25% to 45%).[42-44] Also, there are numerous problems with the VBG. Up to 38% of patients develop reflux symptoms, which generally require conversion to a gastric

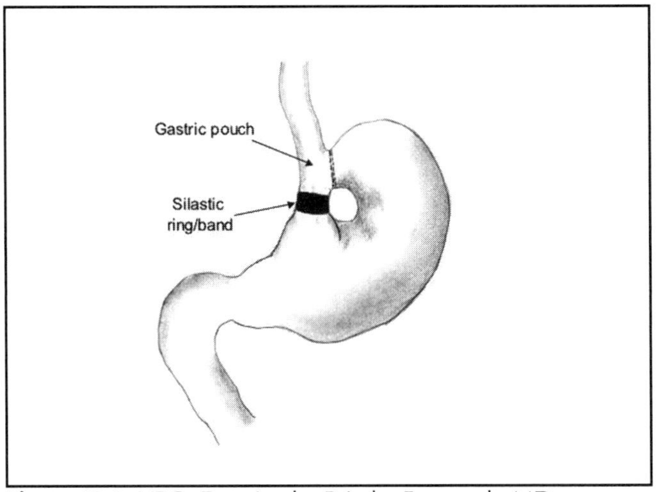

Figure 49-2. VBG. Drawing by Brintha Enestvedt, MD.

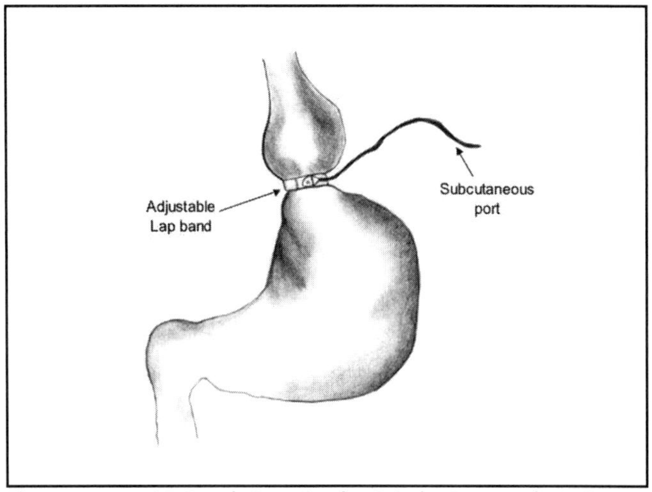

Figure 49-3. LAP-Band. Drawing by Brintha Enestvedt, MD.

bypass. The operation is highly dependent on the staple-line integrity: the most frequent cause of VBG failure is staple-line break down, with subsequent development of a gastro-gastric fistula. Stomal stenosis is also a frequent complication following VBG. Response to endoscopic dilation is poor because of the rigid extraluminal ring and reoperation is almost always necessary. Furthermore, in a prospective, randomized trial, Sugerman et al reported less weight loss following VBG compared to RYGB.[42] Accordingly, gastric bypass has become more popular in North America in recent years.

Gastric Banding

The ASGB is placed around the stomach just below the gastro-esophageal junction to create a small (15-ml) gastric pouch with an adjustable stoma through which food can enter the distal stomach. The stomach is not cut or stapled and no anastomosis is made (Figure 49-3). The diameter of the band can be adjusted by infusion of saline through a subcutaneous reservoir. Advantages of the band include ease of insertion, highly amenable to a laparoscopic or minimally invasive approach, adjustability, reversibility, and low rates of morbidity and mortality.

Excellent results with the ASGB have been reported in Mexico, Europe, and Australia.[45-59] O'Brien et al reported 57% excess weight loss (EWL) at 6 years, which is comparable to that of the gastric bypass.[57] Several international groups have demonstrated a low complication and a very low mortality rate.[45-59] A systematic review of all the published literature comparing the safety and efficacy of the ASGB with that of gastric stapling procedures showed the mortality rate to be 10 times greater for the RYGB and 6 times greater for VBG.[60] However, the initial American experience in the FDA clinical trial resulted in lower-than-expected weight loss (38% EWL) and higher-than-expected rate of complications (>40%). This included serious complications such as band slippage (23%) and esophageal dilation. Follow-up from one center demonstrated that the device required removal in 41% of the cases.[61]

The discrepancy between the results of the FDA trial and the international results may be partially explained by the learning curve and differences in surgical technique. In particular, employment of the "pars flaccida" technique appears to minimize many of the device-related complications. As this approach becomes increasingly established,[59] it is likely that US results will mimic those obtained elsewhere.

Combined Restrictive/ Malabsorptive Operations

Mason and Ito performed the first gastric bypass operation for clinically severe obesity using a loop gastrojejunostomy.[62,63] They defined the anatomic parameters of gastric restriction to include a 12-mm diameter gastrojejunostomy stoma and a small (less than 50 ml) upper gastric pouch.[64] Griffen et al modified Mason and Ito's loop gastrojejunostomy by performing a retrocolic Roux-en-Y gastrojejunostomy.[65] The construction of a Roux-en-Y or alimentary limb permits diversion of bile and pancreatic juices from the gastrojejunostomy and thereby prevents bile reflux gastritis or esophagitis. It also facilitates technically the mobilization of the jejunum to the upper portion of the abdomen (Figure 49-4).

Roux-en-Y Gastric Bypass

Over the past two decades, the RYGB has undergone many technical modifications. Surgeons may choose to partition the stomach or actually divide it. The gastrojejunostomy may be stapled or hand sewn. The Roux limb may be brought up to the gastric pouch in an antecolic or retrocolic fashion. The length of the Roux limb may vary, although the conventional procedure calls for a length of approximately 75 to 150 cm. Despite these technical choices, most surgeons would agree that Mason and Ito's admonition to create a small gastric pouch and a calibrated gastrojejunostomy along with a Roux limb for ingested food to bypass the excluded stomach comprise the critical elements of the operation. The combination of a small gastric pouch and a small outlet stimulates significant caloric restriction and the body's satiety mechanism. The RYGB does cause malabsorption of certain mineral and vitamins, but there is no significant malabsorption of

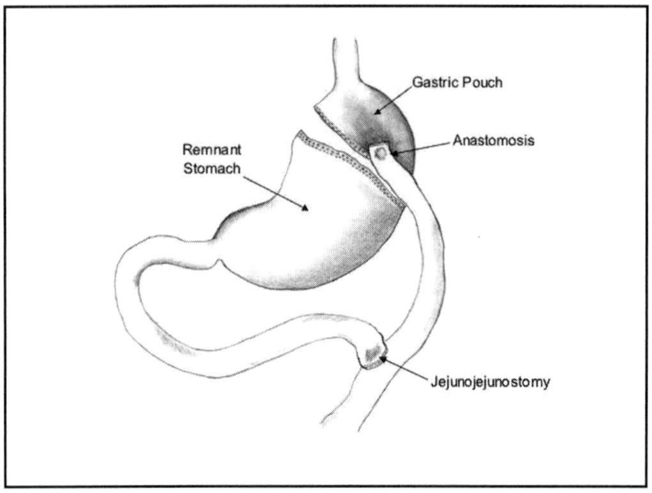

Figure 49-4. RYGB. Drawing by Brintha Enestvedt, MD.

protein or fat. Protein malnutrition can develop, however, if protein intake is not adequate or if the surgeon creates a very lengthy roux limb.

The RYGB operation is the most popular choice for weight-reduction surgery in the United States. Thus far, it has proven to be the best operation in achieving sustained and significant weight-loss. The short-term complication rates are acceptable for a major operation and the long-term nutritional consequences can be easily treated. Both surgeon and patient satisfaction are high with this operation.

Laparoscopic Bariatric Surgery

Two major events characterize the current era of bariatric surgery. The first event is the accumulation of numerous outcome-based studies that provide reliable information on both short-term and long-term results of bariatric operations that have been proven relatively safe and effective. The second event is the development, maturation, and application of laparoscopic techniques to the field of bariatric surgery. Laparoscopic bariatric surgery was first performed in the early 1990s. Since that time, multiple series have confirmed that laparoscopic RYGB, laparoscopic VBG, laparoscopic BPD and DS, and laparoscopic ASGB can all be performed with acceptable results. There is clearly a need for advanced laparoscopic skills with all bariatric procedures, and there is a steep learning curve associated with their performance.[66] Schauer et al showed that operative time decreased significantly and that technical complications decreased by 50% after an experience of 100 laparoscopic RYGB cases.[66] Hand-assisted techniques have been developed with the intention of proving benefits similar to those seen with completely laparoscopic procedures.[67,68] Technical difficulty increases with an android body habitus and as the BMI increases.

The benefits of laparoscopic surgery are related to minimizing the length of the incision. Cardiopulmonary complications have been shown to occur less commonly after laparoscopic procedures compared to laparotomy. Preserved pulmonary function is the most well-documented benefit of laparoscopic surgery, with comparatively less impairment in postoperative ventilation, total lung capacity, and oxygen saturation.[69] Nguyen et al, in a prospective randomized study, showed that laparoscopic compared with open RYGB resulted in less blood loss, reduced pulmonary complications, shorter hospital stay, faster recovery, and reduced need for intensive care.[70,71] Furthermore, wound complications such as hernia formation, seroma, infection, hematoma, and dehiscence are minimized after laparoscopic surgery.[72-76] Overall, operative morbidity and mortality appear to be comparable to an open approach.[72-76] There appears to be no significant difference in weight loss between open and laparoscopic approaches.[72-76] In summary, laparoscopic bariatric surgery is an excellent approach for many patients. Its use in any given patient depends largely on surgeon experience and the patient's BMI.

Outcomes

Weight Loss

Successful weight loss is defined as a loss of at least 25% of the preoperative weight or at least 50% of the excess weight. Excess weight is the calculated difference between the ideal body weight and the preoperative weight. Following RYGB, the mean percent EWL range is 50% to 75% at 5 years.[77-80] Pories et al reported a series of 608 patients with 14-year follow-up after RYGB. Patient follow-up was an extraordinary 97%. These patients experienced a maximum weight loss at 24 months (73% EWL) and at 14-year follow-up the mean percent EWL exceeded 50%.[81]

As mentioned previously, weight loss following ASGB is very good with EWL, typically in the range of 50 to 60%. Weight loss tends to occur more gradually than with RYGB, but most investigators have found that after 2 to 3 years, weight loss from ASGB approaches or equals weight loss from RYGB.

The reported weight loss after the BPD and the DS exceeds that of the RYGB. In a series of 2241 patients operated on over a 21-year period, the BPD provided a mean percent EWL of about 75%.[37] However, the BPD is the bariatric operation with the greatest amount of anatomical reconstruction and obligatory nutrient malabsorption. Close monitoring is needed because of the potential adverse metabolic effects of the BPD.

Amelioration of Medical Comorbidities

Most obesity-related illnesses improve substantially after weight-reduction surgery. Multiple studies have shown improvement or even resolution of diabetes, sleep apnea, GERD, hypertension, and serum lipid abnormalities.[81-86] Peripheral edema, arthralgia, easy fatigability, and dyspnea are also usually improved after weight-reduction surgery.

Diabetes Mellitus

A strong association exists between type 2 diabetes and obesity. Both disorders respond poorly to dietary measures alone. Gastric bypass has proven to be very effective in sustained weight loss and control of type 2 diabetes. Sustained normal concentrations of plasma glucose, insulin, and glycosylated hemoglobin have been reported in 80% to 100% of morbidly obese diabetics managed by RYGB or BPD. Pories et al reported that 82% of obese patients with type 2 diabetes were cured (euglycemic and normal levels of glycosylated hemoglobin) by RYGB with 14-years follow-up.[81] Reduced caloric intake contributes to improvement in diabetes, but the exact mechanism for cure is not known. Interestingly, improved glucose control with concomitant reduced serum insulin levels occurs immediately following surgery, prior to any postoperative weight loss. Patients regain normal glucose-insulin homeostasis despite continuing to have relatively high proportions of body fat, suggesting that the effect of gastric bypass on diabetes may be mediated by a change in the pattern of secretion of GI hormones. Bypass of the duodenum and jejunum allows early presentation of undigested or incompletely digested food to ileum, which leads to the production of hormones such as glucagons like peptide 1, which improves insulin action. Following gastric bypass, the enteroglucagon and gastro-inhibitory peptide response to oral glucose is increased. Furthermore, there are increased levels of insulin-like growth factor 1 and decreased levels of plasma leptin. Although significant changes in GI hormones have been documented, the exact mechanism of action is not completely understood. Importantly, the duration of diabetes is a predictor of outcome, which indicates the importance of early treatment of obesity in a patient with newly diagnosed diabetes.

Sleep Apnea

Gastric bypass surgery resulting in significant weight loss very effectively controls sleep apnea. Obstructive sleep apnea is defined as having breathing cessation exceeding 10 seconds during sleep, occurring more than five times per hour and having a concomitant ≥4% decrease in oxygen saturation. The magnitude of sleep apnea is determined by the apnea index, which is the number of apneic episodes observed per hour by polysomnography. The apnea index is directly related to the amount of excess weight. Patients with sleep apnea will have as many as 400 to 500 apnea events per night. In addition, there is potential for cardiovascular collapse during the apnea episodes. Atrial and ventricular arrhythmias are frequently observed in association with apnea episodes and these are ameliorated after gastric bypass surgery.[87] Long-term follow-up after gastric bypass demonstrated that 93% of patients had improved sleep quality and apneic indices.[88,89]

Gastroesophageal Reflux Disease

The mechanism of obesity-induced GERD is not clearly understood. One likely hypothesis is that severe obesity causes chronically increased intra-abdominal pressure that promotes the reflux of gastric contents through an ineffective lower esophageal sphincter. The relative pressure gradient from the abdomen to the chest is therefore exaggerated, promoting gastroesophageal reflux. Bariatric surgery and subsequent weight loss have been demonstrated to be very effective therapy for GERD. Schauer et al reported improvement of GERD symptoms in 24% of patients and resolution of GERD symptoms in 72% of patients after RYGB.[90]

Following RYGB, there is very little (if any) acid in the gastric pouch. Smith et al reported that basal and stimulated gastric acid secretion to be virtually absent from the gastric pouch following RYGB.[91] Bile reflux is also eliminated because of bile diversion into the Roux-limb distal to the gastrojejunal anastomosis. Furthermore, the small pouch minimizes any reservoir capacity to promote regurgitation.

Hypertension

The etiology for obesity-related hypertension is unclear but may be related to increased tubular reabsorption of sodium in the kidney. Other proposed mechanisms include intrinsically high levels of leptin and chronic hyperinsulinemia. Surgical treatment of obesity improves both hypertension and cardiac function. Alpert et al reported that surgically induced weight loss was associated with improvement of left ventricular ejection fraction, mean blood pressure, cardiac chamber size, and ventricular wall thickness.[92] Successful treatment of hypertension following bariatric surgery correlates with the amount of weight loss and not the final weight. Hypertension is improved or eliminated, even though patients never approached ideal body weight. This data reinforces the concept that an important goal for surgical treatment of obesity should be control of comorbidities.

Serum Lipid Abnormalities

Obese patients frequently have elevated serum lipid levels, which increases their risk for cardiovascular disease. Gastric bypass has been demonstrated to be very effective in lowering triglycerides and low-density lipoprotein (LDL), with a concomitant increase in the high-density lipoprotein (HDL).[93] Gonen et al showed a favorable increase in the HDL/LDL ratio following RYGB, which suggests that the risk of arteriosclerosis may be decreased by postoperative weight loss.[93] The mechanism by which serum lipids are altered in not clear, but it is partially explained by the decreased caloric intake following bariatric surgery.

Quality of Life

The physical and psychosocial limitation of obesity adds considerably to the morbidity of the disease. A number of studies have clearly demonstrated major improvement in quality of life after bariatric surgery. Many patients report improved self-esteem and lessened self-consciousness.[94] Bariatric patients are delighted to be able to buy clothes at major department stores, sit comfortably in an airplane seat, or even climb a flight of stairs.[95] Employment opportunities also increase. One study showed that 75% of patients who were receiving public assistance before gastric bypass surgery were able to find full-time jobs at 2

TABLE 49-2.

Perioperative Deaths and Complications Within 30 Days of Operations (N=14,641)

Adverse Event	Incidence (%)
Death	0.17
Respiratory	2.35
Wound infection	1.02
Hepatic or cardiac	0.25
Splenic injury	0.21
Pulmonary embolism	0.21
Subphrenic abscess	0.19
Gastrointestinal leak	0.16
Evisceration, dehiscence	0.13
Gastrointestinal bleeding	0.13
Deep venous thrombosis	0.11
Neurologic	0.11
Renal	0.11
Wound seroma	0.04

Reprinted with permission from Mason EE, Tang S, Renquist KE, et al. A decade of change in obesity surgery. *Obes Surg*. 1997;7:189-197.

years postoperatively.[96] An improved quality of life is one of the most gratifying outcomes of bariatric surgery.

LIFE EXPECTANCY

As mentioned previously, obesity is associated with a reduced life expectancy. After a successful bariatric operation, life expectancy is significantly improved. MacLean et al reported in a well-matched cohort study, over a 19-year period, that the mortality rate was 0.68% in the bariatric surgery group and 6.17% in the no surgery (control) group. Bariatric surgery reduced the relative risk of death by 89% with an absolute mortality reduction of 5.59%.[97]

Complications

Complications of bariatric surgery can be separated into complications associated with alterations in the GI anatomy and those associated with surgery. GI complications (ie, leaks, distention, strictures, ulcers, obstruction) that are associated with changes in the patient's anatomy because of bariatric procedures are discussed at length in Chapter 50 of this book. Surgery-related complications are discussed below.

Operative complications include death, pulmonary embolus, hemorrhage, and wound infection. Obese patients have a high risk of complications after any operation; however, bariatric operations are associated with relatively low morbidity and mortality. Most series report operative death rates of approximately 0.5% to 1%, with pulmonary embolus and sepsis due to anastomotic leak as the most common causes of mortality. The major complication rate ranges from 2% to 8%. A partial listing of these complications and their incidence are listed in Table 49-2.

Pulmonary complications are a significant concern in the perioperative period. Pneumonia occurs in approximately 1.9% of cases, and pulmonary emboli occur in 0.8% to 2.0% of cases.[98,99] Respiratory insufficiency with polycythemia, inactivity, and having undergone abdominal surgery in the supine position for several hours all contribute to the classic Virchow's triad for the development of thromboembolic disease in these patients. Additionally, the presence of pulmonary hypertension with obesity hypoventilation can further increase the risk of fatal pulmonary embolism.[100] In this subset of patients, the placement of a prophylactic vena cava filter is frequently considered.[101]

Wound infections are also a concern, as they occur in approximately 6% of cases and have been found to be associated with decreased tissue perfusion and oxygenation[102] and with the chronic inflammatory state of obesity.[103] Additional wound complications, such as impaired healing and incisional hernia (a late complication), tend to occur in the obese more frequently as well and are likely secondary to the panniculus and the higher incidence of diabetes.[104,105]

Pregnancy After Bariatric Surgery

As more and more obese women of childbearing age consider bariatric surgery, the issue of safety of pregnancy after bariatric surgery has surfaced—is it safer to become pregnant while morbidly obese, or safer to become pregnant once the patient has lost weight after a bariatric operation? Obese pregnant women are considered to be high-risk for pregnancy-related complications. Obese pregnant women have an increased incidence of gestational diabetes and hypertension, spontaneous abortion, pre-eclampsia, Cesarean section, and deep venous thrombosis. Infants of obese women are more likely to have fetal growth abnormalities, macrosomia, and intrauterine growth retardation. There are no prospective or large series reported in the literature of women who have become pregnant after bariatric surgery. Wittgrove et al, in a retrospective study of 41 women who become pregnant after bariatric surgery, found a decreased incidence of gestational diabetes, gestational hypertension, macrosomia, and Cesarean section, compared to incidence in a control group of obese women.[106] There were no patients with clinically significant anemia and there was no increased risk of spontaneous abortion, intrauterine growth retardation, congenital anomalies, or maternal nutritional deficiencies. Based on this series and other reports, pregnancy after bariatric surgery is not only safe but is associated with fewer complications than is pregnancy while a woman is obese.[106-108]

Women who are pregnant after bariatric surgery require intense counseling and frequent follow-up. This requires close coordination between the obstetrician and the bariatric surgeon. These patients are at risk for iron deficiency and vitamin B12 anemias. Adequate calcium intake or supplementation is important for mineralization of the fetal skeleton and folic acid must be supplemented to avoid neural tube abnormalities. Pregnancy after bariatric surgery should be delayed until after the phase of rapid weight loss and once the weight loss has stabilized, generally after 12 to 18 months. It is important to educate women that their fertility may be increased, and it may be necessary for them to take birth control pills. Following bariatric surgery, the pregnant women should be under close surveillance to assure proper weight gain for the development of a healthy fetus. If adequate weight is not gained during the pregnancy, the fetus risks intrauterine growth retardation and fetal abnormalities.

Conclusion

The field of bariatric surgery has undergone significant evolution over the past 40 years. Over the past 15 to 20 years, it has been increasingly recognized that the VBG and the RYGB procedures are highly viable options in terms of short-term and long-term safety and weight loss that is superior to medical alternatives.

Patient selection remains an important and challenging aspect of the surgical care of these patients. For appropriate patients, sustained weight loss of greater than 50% of the patient's excess weight can be anticipated, as shown by multiple studies with 5- to 14-year follow-ups. Resolution or improvement in obesity-related illnesses and improvement in patient's activity and lifestyle are frequent outcomes from these operations. Laparoscopic approaches to weight-reduction surgery are likely to be more available in the future, thereby minimizing the morbidity and recovery time for patients.

In summary, bariatric surgery has undergone a virtual renaissance over the past 10 to 15 years and is now a reliable treatment for selected patients with clinically severe obesity.

References

1. Flegal KM, Carroll MD, Odgen CL, et al. Prevalence and trends in obesity among US adults, 1999 – 2000. *JAMA*. 2002;288:1723-1727.
2. Wolf AM, Colditz GA. Current estimates of the economic cost of obesity in the United States. *Obes Res*. 1998;6:97-106.
3. Colditz GA. Economic costs of obesity. *Am J Clin Nutr*. 1992;55(suppl 2):503S-507S.
4. Sims EA. Experimental obesity, dietary-induced thermogenesis, and their clinical implications. *Clin Endocrinol Metab*. 1976;5:377-395.
5. Mayer J. Correlation between metabolism and feeding behavior in multiple etiology of obesity. *Bull NY Acad Med*. 1957;33:744-761.
6. Borneson M. The etiology of obesity in children: a study of 101 twin pairs. *Acta Pediatr Scand*. 1976;65:279-287.
7. Goldblatt PB, Moore ME, Stunkard AJ. Social factors in obesity. *JAMA*. 1965;192:1039-1044.
8. Garn SN, Clark DC. Trends in fatness and the origins of obesity, Ad Hoc Committee to review the ten-state nutrition survey. *Pediatrics*. 1976;57:443-456.
9. McKeown T, Record RG: The influence of reproduction on body weight in women. *J Endocrinol*. 1957;15:393-409.
10. Calle EE, Thun MJ, Petrelli JM, et al. Body mass index and mortality in a prospective cohort of US adults. *N Eng J Med*. 1999;341:1097-1105.
11. Fontaine KR, Redden DT, Wang C, et al. Years of life lost due to obesity. *JAMA*. 2003;289:187-193.
12. Blair DF, Haines LW. Mortality experience according to build at higher durations. *Society of Actuaries*. 1966;18:35-46.
13. Stevens J, Cai H, Pamuk ER, et al. The effect of age on the association between body-mass index and mortality. *N Engl J Med*. 1998;338:1-7.
14. Lew EA, Garfinkel L. Variation in mortality by weight among 750,000 men and women. *J Chronic Dis*. 1979;32:563-576.
15. Drenick EJ, Bale GS, Seltzer F, et al. Excessive mortality in causes of death in morbidly obese men. *JAMA*. 1980;243:433-445.
16. Rimm A, Werner LH, Burnstein R, et al. Disease and obesity in 73,532 women. *Obes Bariat Med*. 1972;1:77-84.
17. Report of the United States National Commission on Diabetes to the Congress of the United States. U.S. Department of Health, Education, and Welfare, 1975.
18. Westlund K, Nickolaysen R. Ten-year mortality and morbidity related to serum cholesterol. A follow-up of 3,751 men aged 40-49. *Scand J Clin Lab Invest*. 1992;30:1-24.
19. Kannel WE. Health and obesity: an overview. In Kuo PT, Conn HL, Jr, DeFelice EA (eds). *Health and Obesity*. New York: Raven Press; 1983: 1-19.
20. Van Itallie TB. Morbid obesity: a hazardous disorder that resists conservative treatment. *Am J Clin Nutr*. 1980;33:358-363.
21. Freemen JB, Deitel M, Anand SA, et al. Symposium: morbid obesity. *Contemp Surg*. 1986;26:71-118.
22. White F, Pereira I. In search of the ideal body weight. *Ann Roy Coll Phys Surg Can*. 1987;20:129-132.
23. Adler M, Schaffner F. Fatty liver hepatitis and cirrhosis in obese patients. *Am J Med*. 1979;67:811-816.
24. Maybee TM, Myer P, DenBesten I, et al. The mechanism of increased gallstone formation in obese human subjects. *Surgery*. *19796*;79:460-468.
25. Hagen J, Deitel M, Khanna RK, et al. Gastroesophageal reflux in the massively obese. *Int Surg*. 1987;72:1-3.
26. Garner P. Management of female hyperandrogenic states. *Ann R Coll Phys Surg Can*. 1985;18:458-489.
27. Angel A, Winocur JT, Roncari D. Morbid obesity: the problem and its consequences. In Deitel M (ed). *Surgery for the Morbidly Obese Patient*. Toronto: FD Communications, Inc; 1998: 19-26.

28. Cahnman WJ. The stigma of obesity. *Social Q.* 1968;9:283-299.
29. Tobias AL, Gordon JB. Social consequences of obesity. *J Am Diet Assoc.* 1980;76:338-342.
30. Deitel N, Camilleri A. Overlooked problems in morbidly obese patients. *Obes Surg.* 2000;10:125.
31. Van Itallie TB. Health implications of overweight and obesity in the United States. *Ann Intern Med.* 1985;103:983-988.
32. Reisin E, Frohlich ED, Messerli FH, et al. Cardiovascular changes after weight reduction in obesity hypertension. Ann Intern Med. 1983;98:315-319.
33. Gastrointestinal surgery for severe obesity: National Institutes of Health Consensus Development Conference Statement. *Am J Clin Nutr.* 1992;55:615S-619S.
34. Balsiger BM, Murr MM, Poggio JL, Sarr MG. Bariatric surgery. Surgery for weight control in patients with morbid obesity. *Med Clin N Am.* 2000;84(2):477-489.
35. American Society for Bariatric Surgery. Membership survey. Presented at 18th Annual Meeting of the American Society for Bariatric Surgery; May 2000; Gainesville, Fla.
36. Deitel M. Jejunocolic and jejunoileal bypass: an historical perspective. In Deitel M (ed). *Surgery for the Morbidly Obese Patient.* Philadelphia, PA: Lea & Febiger; 1989: 81-90.
37. Scopinaro N, Adami GF, Marinari GM, et al. Biliopancreatic diversion. *World J Surg.* 1998;22:936-946.
38. Marceau P, Hould FS, Simard S, et al. Bilopancreatic diversion with duodenal switch. *World J Surg.* 1998;22:947-54.
39. Hess DS, Hess DW. Biliopancreatic diversion with a duodenal switch. Obes Surg. 1998 Jun;8(3):267-282.
40. Rabkin RA. Distal gastric bypass/duodenal switch procedure. Roux-en-Y gastric bypass and biliopancreatic diversion in a community practice. *Obes Surg.* 1998;8(1):53-59.
41. Mason EE. Vertical banded gastroplasty. *Arch Surg.* 1982;117:701-706.
42. Sugerman HJ, Starky JV, Birkenhauer R. A randomized prospective trial of gastric bypass versus vertical-band gastroplasty for morbid obesity and their effects on sweets versus non-sweets eaters. *Ann Surg.* 1987;205:613-624.
43. Balsiger BM, Poggio JL, Mai J, Kelly KA, Sarr MG. Ten and more years after vertical banded gastroplasty as primary operation for morbid obesity. *J Gastrointest Surg.* 2000;4(6):598-605.
44. MacGregor A. The Story of Surgery for Obesity. American Society for Bariatric Surgery website. 2002; http://www.asbs.org/html/story/chapter1.html.
45. Fielding GA, Rhodes M, Nathanson LK. Laparoscopic gastric banding for morbid obesity: surgical outcome in 335 cases. *Surg Endosc.* 1999;13:550-554.
46. O'Brien PE, Brown WA, Smith A, McMurrick PJ, Stephens M. Prospective study of a laparoscopically placed, adjustable gastric band in the treatment of morbid obesity. *Br J Surg.* 1999;86:113-118.
47. Zimmermann JM, Mashoyan Ph, Michel G, et al. Laparoscopic adjustable silicon gastric banding: Une etude preliminaire personnelle concernant 900 cas operas entres juillet 1995 et Decembre 1998. *J Coelio-Chir.* 1999;29:77-80.
48. Dargent J. Laparoscopic adjustable gastric banding: lesson from 500 patients in a single institution. *Obes Surg.* 1999;9:446-452.
49. Doldi SB, Micheletto G, Lattuada E, Zappa MA, Bona D, Sonvico U. Adjustable gastric banding: 5-year experience. *Obes Surg.* 2000;10:171-173.
50. Blanco ER, Gascon M, Weiner R, et al. Video laparoscopic placement of adjustable gastric banding in the treatment of morbid obesity: preliminary results after 407 interventions. *Gastroenterol Hepatol.* 2001;24:381-386.
51. Angrisani L, Alkilani M, Basso N, et al. Laparoscopic Italian experience with the Lap-Band. *Obes Surg.* 2001;11:307-10.
52. Szold A, Abu-Abeid S. Laparoscopic adjustable silicone gastric banding for morbid obesity: results and complications in 715 patients. *Surg Endosc.* 2002;16:230-233.
53. Nowara HA. Egyptian experience in laparoscopic adjustable gastric banding (technique, complications and intermediate results). *Obes Surg.* 2001;11:70-75.
54. Chevallier JM, Zinzindohoue F, Elian N, et al. Adjustable gastric banding in a public university hospital: prospective analysis of 400 patients. *Obes Surg.* 2002;12:93-99.
55. Belachew M, Belva PH, Desaive C. Long-term results of laparoscopic adjustable gastric banding for the treatment of morbid obesity. *Obes Surg.* 2002;12:564-568.
56. Favretti F, Cadiere GM, Segato G, et al. Laparoscopic banding: selection and technique in 830 patients. *Obes Surg.* 2002;12:385-390.
57. O'Brien PE, Dixon JB, Brown W, et al. The laparoscopic adjustable gastric band (Lap-Band): a prospective study of medium-term effects on weight, health and quality of life. *Obes Surg.* 2002;12:652-660.
58. Fielding G. Laparoscopic adjustable gastric banding for massive super obesity. *Obes Surg.* 2002;12:203.
59. O'Brien PE, Dixon JB. Weight loss and early and late complications – the international experience. *Am J Surg.* 2002;184:42S-45S.
60. Chapman A, Kiroff G, Game P, et al. Systemic review of laparoscopic adjustable gastric banding in the treatment of obesity. Adelaide, South Australia: ASERNIP-S Report No. 31, 2002.
61. DeMaria EJ, Sugerman HJ, Meador JG, et al. High failure rate after laparoscopic adjustable silicone gastric banding for treatment of morbid obesity. *Ann Surg.* 2001;233:809-18.
62. Mason EE, Ito C. Gastric bypass and obesity. *Surg Clin N Am.* 1967;47:1345-1352.
63. Mason EE, Ito C. Gastric bypass. *Ann Surg.* 1969;170:329-339.
64. Mason EE, Printen KJ, Hartford CE, et al. Optimizing results of gastric bypass. *Ann Surg.* 1975;182:405-413.
65. Griffen WO Jr, Young VL, Stevenson CC. A perspective comparison of gastric and jejunal ileal bypass procedures for morbid obesity. *Ann Surg.* 1977;186:500-509.
66. Schauer PR, Ikramuddin S, Hamad G, et al. The learning curve for laparoscopic Roux-en-Y gastric bypass in 100 cases. *Surg Endosc.* 2003;17:212-215.
67. Sundbom M, Gustavsson S. Hand-assisted laparoscopic Roux-en-Y gastric bypass: aspects of surgical technique and early results. *Obes Surg.* 2000;10:420-427.
68. Bleier JI, Krupnick AS, Kreisel D, Song HK, Rosato EF, Williams NN. Hand-assisted laparoscopic vertical banded gastroplasty: early results. *Surg Endosc.* 2000;14:902-907.
69. Shauer PR, Luna J, Ghiatas AA, et al : Pulmonary function after laparoscopic cholecystectomy. *Surgery.* 1993;114:389-399.
70. Nguyen NT, Lee SL, Goldman, et al. Comparison of pulmonary function and postoperative pain after laparoscopic vs open gastric bypass: a randomized trail. *J Am Coll Surg.* 2001;192:469-476.
71. Nguyen NY, Goldman C, Rosenquist CJ et al.: Laparoscopic versus open gastric bypass: A randomized study of outcome, quality of life and costs. *Ann Surg.* 234: 279-291, 2001.
72. Schauer PR, Ikramuddin S, Gourash W, et al. Outcomes after laparoscopic Roux-en- Y gastric bypass for morbid obesity. *Ann Surg.* 2000;232:515-529.
73. Wittgrove AC, Clark GW, Schubert KR. Laparoscopic gastric bypass, Roux-en-Y: technique and results in 75 patients with 3-30 months follow-up. *Obes Surg.* 1996;6:500-504.
74. Wittgrove AC, Clark GW. Laparoscopic gastric bypass: a five-year prospective study of 500 patients followed from 3 to 60 months. *Obes Surg.* 1999;9:123-143, .
75. Higa KD, Ho T, Boone KB. Laparoscopic Roux-en-Y gastric bypass: technique and 3-year follow-up. *J Laparoendosc Adv Surg Tech A.* 2001;11:377-382.
76. DeMaria EJ, Sugerman HJ, Kellum JM, et al. Results of 281 consecutive total laparoscopic Roux-en-Y gastric bypasses to treat morbid obesity. *Ann Surg.* 2002;235:640-647.
77. Benotti PN, Hollingshead J, Mascioli EA, et al. Gastric restrictive operations for morbid obesity. *Am J Surg.* 1989;157:150-155.
78. Yale CE. Gastric surgery for morbid obesity. Complications and long-term weight control. *Arch Surg.* 1989;124:941-946.
79. Linner JH, Drew RL. Why the operation we prefer is the Roux-en-Y gastric bypass. *Obes Surg.* 1:305-306, 1991.
80. Hall JC, Watts JM, Pe OB, et al. Gastric surgery for morbid obesity. The Adelaide Study. *Ann Surg.* 1990;211:419-427.

81. Pories WJ, Swanson MS, McDonald KG, et al. Who would have thought it? An operation proved to be the most effective therapy for adult onset diabetes malitous. *Ann Surg.* 1995;222:339-350.
82. Charuzi I, Lavie P, Peiser J, et al. Bariatric surgery in morbidly obese sleep-apnea patients: Short- and long- term follow-up. *Am J Clin Nutr.* 1992;55:594S-596S.
83. Sugerman HJ, Fairman RP, Sood RK, et al. Long-term effects of gastric surgery for treating respiratory insufficiency of obesity. *Am J Clin Nutr.* 1992;55:597S-60lS.
84. Benotti PN, Bistrain B, Benotti JR, et al. Heart disease and hypertension in morbid obesity: The benefits of weight reduction. *Am J Clin Nutr.* 1992;55:586S-590S.
85. Brolin RE. Results of obesity surgery. *Gastroenterol Clin North Am.* 1987;16:317-338.
86. Glysteen JJ. Results of surgery: long-term effects on hyperlipidemia. *Am J Clin Nutr.* 1992;55:59lS-594S.
87. Peiser J, Ovnat A, Uwyyed K, et al. Cardiac arrhythmias during sleep in morbidly obese sleep-apneic patients before and after gastric bypass surgery. *Clin Cardiol.* 1985;8:519-21.
88. Charuzi I, Ovnat A, Peiser J, et al. The effect of surgical weight reduction on sleep quality in obesity-related sleep apnea syndrome. *Surgery.* 1985;97:535-8.
89. Charuzi I, Lavie P, Peiser J, Peled R. Bariatric surgery in morbidly obese sleep-apnea patients: short- and long term follow-up. *Am J Clin Nutr.* 1992;55:594S-596S.
90. Biertho L, Steffen R, Richlin T, et al. Laparoscopic gastric bypass versus laparoscopic adjustable gastric banding: a comparative study of 1,200 cases. *J Am Coll Surg.* 2003;197(4):536-544; discussion 544-545.
91. Smith CD, Herkes SB, Behrm KE, et al. Gastric acid secretion and vitamin B12 absorption after vertical Roux en Y gastric bypass for morbid obesity *Ann Surg.* 1993;218:91-96.
92. Alpert MA, Terry BE, Kelly DL. Effect of weight loss on cardiac chamber size, wall thickness and left ventricular function in morbid obesity. *Am J Cardiol.* 1985;56:783-786.
93. Gonen B, Halverson JD, Schonfeld G. Lipoprotein levels in morbidly obese patients with massive surgically induced weight loss. *Metabolism.* 1990;32:774-778.
94. Rand CS, Macgregor A, Hankins G. Gastric bypass surgery for obesity: weight loss, psychosocial outcome, and morbidity one and three years later. *South Med J.* 1986;79:1511-1514.
95. Brolin RE. Gastrointestinal surgery for obesity. *Semin Gastrointest Dis.* 1998;9:163-175.
96. Brolin RE. Results of obesity surgery. *Gastroenterol Clin N Am.* 1987;16:317-338.
97. Christou NV, Sampalis JS, MacLean LD, et al. Surgery Decreases Long-Term Mortality in Morbidly Obese Patients. Presented at: 124th Annual Meeting of the American Surgical Association; April 2004; San Francisco, CA.
98. Mason EE, Tang S, Renquist KE, et al. A decade of change in obesity surgery. *Obes Surg.* 1997;7:189-197.
99. Sugerman HJ, Kellum JM, Engle KM, et al. Gastric bypass for treating severe obesity. *Am J Clin Nutr.* 1992;55(2 Suppl):560S-566S.
100. MacGregor MI, Block AJ, Ball WC, Jr. Topics in clinical medicine: serious complications and sudden death in the Pickwickian syndrome. *Johns Hopkins Med J.* 1970;126(5):279-295.
101. Sapala JA, Wood MH, Schuhknecht MP, Sapala MA. Fatal pulmonary embolism after bariatric operations for morbid obesity: a 24-year retrospective analysis. *Obes Surg.* 2003;13(6):819-825.
102. Kabon B, Nagele A, Reddy D, et al. Obesity Decreases Perioperative Tissue Oxygenation. Anesthesiology. Feb 2004;100(2):274-280.
103. Levi D, Goodman ER, Patel M, Savransky Y. Critical care of the obese and bariatric surgical patient. *Crit Care Clin.* 2003;19(1):11-32.
104. Byrne TK. Complications of surgery for obesity. *Surg Clin North Am.* 2001;81(5):1181-1193, vii-viii.
105. Wilson JA, Clark JJ. Obesity: impediment to wound healing. *Crit Care Nurs Q.* 2003;26(2):119-132.
106. Wittgrove AC, Jester L, Wittgrove P, et al.: Pregnancy following gastric bypass for morbid obesity. *Obes Surg.* 1998;8:461-464.
107. Dixon JB, Dixon ME, O'Brien PE. Pregnancy after LAP-BAND surgery: management of the band to achieve healthy weight outcomes. *Obes Surg.* 2001;11:59-65.
108. Martin LF, Finigan KM, Nolan TE. Pregnancy after adjustable gastric band. *Obstetric & Gynecology.* 2000;95: 927-930.

Chapter 50

Gastrointestinal Complications of Bariatric Surgery

Brintha Enestvedt, MD; John E. Pandolfino, MD; Alexander P. Nagle, MD; and Jay B. Prystowsky, MD

Introduction

Bariatric surgery, a collective term for operations that involve reducing the size of the gastric reservoir with or without associated induced malabsorption, has achieved impressive results, with approximately a 50% or more reduction in excess body weight by 18 to 24 months post operation.[1] Although most patients achieve successful outcomes, many patients develop postoperative gastrointestinal (GI) symptoms. Whether these symptoms represent necessary evils (adverse events related to dietary indiscretion) or unnecessary evils (true postoperative complications) is difficult to interpret clinically and frequently will require gastroenterology consultation. Gastroenterologists, therefore, are and will continue to be an integral component to the successful outcomes of bariatric surgery. The aim of this chapter is to describe the role of the gastroenterologist in the management of the various GI complications that may occur. (Bariatric surgeries are discussed in detail—with descriptions of the procedures, comparison of the outcomes, and a discussion of outcomes—in Chapter 49.)

Gastrointestinal Complications of Bariatric Surgery

Given the alteration in the upper GI anatomy, certain side effects of bariatric surgery are to be expected and can be ameliorated through patient education and postoperative treatment. Symptoms may arise secondary to dietary noncompliance with a bariatric diet or may be related to a more serious medical and surgical complication. The challenge for the gastroenterologist and referring physician lies in delineating between necessary evils (side effects of the procedure arising from dietary noncompliance) and unnecessary evils (true operative complications). Gastroenterologists should remain aware of common GI problems in this population. However, their work up and management may be complicated by the patients' altered anatomy.

Adverse Events

Adverse events represent the expected side effects of an operation that has significantly altered the anatomy of the GI tract. The most common adverse events are nausea and vomiting, dumping syndrome and diarrhea, and nutrient deficiency. One must remember that these adverse events are expected with inappropriate diet and thus act to deter excessive food intake. However, a balance between expecting specific symptoms and being cognizant of more ominous signs is imperative.

Nausea/Vomiting

The majority of bariatric surgery patients will complain of nausea and vomiting at some point in their postoperative care. Because of the size limitations of the gastric pouch, patients are often unable to tolerate certain quantities of food or liquid. They are typically advised to eat along the rules of a gastroplasty diet: eat undisturbed, chew meticulously, never drink with meals, and wait 2 hours before drinking after solid food is consumed. As these patients adjust to their new diets, they may challenge the amount of food they are recommended to eat or they may revert to previous habits of overeating, which result in abdominal pain, nausea, and vomiting related to food. Patient education in motivation and specific dietary restrictions, along with emotional support, help to decrease instances of these symptoms.

It is not appropriate to simply attribute nausea and vomiting to dietary indiscretion. Doing so may result in overlooking an overt complication. Such symptoms in combination with abdominal pain are also associated with anastomotic complications such as ulcers, strictures, leaks, or even internal hernias, all of which require further evaluation. If a patient's symptoms do not respond to a fasting period or if he or she is unable to tolerate a liquid challenge, further evaluation is required with either upper endoscopy or an upper GI contrast study. (While barium may provide superior mucosal detail, gastrograffin is preferred if a leak or perforation is suspected.)

Dumping/Diarrhea

The symptoms of the dumping syndrome are nausea, bloating, abdominal pain, flushing, tachycardia, lightheadedness, and diarrhea. These are the result of the direct transit of ingested food directly into the jejunum from the gastric pouch. Dumping-syndrome symptoms increase with the ingestion of food with a high sugar, fat, or carbohydrate content or high osmotic activity. These symptoms often serve as a deterrent to overeating or dietary indiscretions and may partially explain the difference in excess-weight loss between VBG (no dumping syndrome) and gastric bypass.[2]

The pathophysiology of dumping syndrome includes a postprandial peripheral and splanchnic vasodilation resulting in hypovolemia. Additionally, the reactive hypoglycemia, as a result of an exaggerated insulin release, may also be responsible for the experienced symptoms.[3] Dumping symptoms should improve with a period of fasting. However, if they do not, alternative diagnoses must be considered.

Diarrhea is a component of dumping syndrome that can be used to elucidate whether these symptoms are indeed due to dumping physiology or due to some other medical concern. Diarrhea secondary to bariatric surgery anatomic changes is osmotic and will generally cease with fasting. If a patient has more than three watery stools a day despite fasting and dietary restriction, microbial stool studies are warranted. Because gastric bypass patients may be predisposed to bacterial overgrowth and the blind-loop syndrome, empiric antibiotics may be considered in patients who show no improvement with fasting and who have negative stool studies.

Nutrient Deficiency

Many patients have difficulty adjusting to their new, small gastric pouch after a gastric restrictive procedure. Protein or caloric malnutrition, and even dehydration, may result in the first few weeks or months after surgery. Hospitalization may be required for rehydration. A general recommendation is for a patient to ingest at least 60 g of protein daily, but this is an elusive goal for many patients in the early months after surgery. Some patients will develop intolerance to some foods including red meat, certain vegetables, fruit, or dairy products. Intensive collaboration with a dietitian is critical to ensure that the patient is following a satisfactory dietary program. In general, restrictive bariatric operations are devoid of long-term metabolic complications. However, patients who undergo procedures that induce a selective malabsorption or maldigestion (biliopancreatic diversion [BPD], Roux-en-Y gastric bypass [RYGB]) should be monitored for nutritional deficiencies, as many important nutrients are absorbed in the proximal small bowel. BPD, in particular, has been associated with an incidence of protein malnutrition in 11.9% of the cases.[4] However, the duodenal switch (DS), a modification of BPD, has significantly decreased concerns of this specific nutritional problem.

Iron, calcium, folate, and vitamin B12 are the most common nutrients that are affected by bariatric procedures secondary to impaired absorption and decreased intake.[5-8] Vitamin A and other B vitamins are also affected. Vitamin-B12 deficiency is predictable;[9] it occurs in up to 50% of patients after RYGB if they do not take supplements, but it rarely becomes clinically relevant.[7] It is most likely the consequence of an insufficient acidic environment necessary to release B12 from food and thus the Schilling test is normal.[2] Folate deficiency, due to inadequate intake, is also a rare complication.

Conversely, many patients experience symptoms of iron deficiency and anemia; these are potentially serious problems after gastric bypass, particularly in women who are menstruating. Combined with blood loss during menses, duodenal bypass and surgery-induced iron malabsorption make these women particularly susceptible to iron-deficiency anemia. Prophylactic oral iron supplementation is recommended for these patients.[8] Although calcium malabsorption is significant, serum levels are usually normal because it can be mobilized from bone; however, osteoporosis is a significant concern and patients require careful follow-up.

Amaral et al observed significant vitamin and mineral deficiencies up to 6 years after surgery in gastric-bypass patients who were not taking supplements.[10] Deficiencies of iron, folate, and vitamin B12 were most pronounced. Avinoah et al observed a similar finding up to 7 years after gastric-bypass surgery and observed that these micronutrients were independent of protein and caloric deficiencies.[11]

Nutrient deficiencies can be prevented and managed with supplementation and prompt recognition and treatment. These measures have prevented the development of clinical deficiency syndromes in most patients. To prevent selective micronutrient deficiencies that may jeopardize the long-term health status of postbariatric surgery patients, all should receive daily supplemental calcium and a multivitamin containing folate and vitamin B12, with supplementation being for life.[6,12] Menstruating women should also take supplemental iron with meals.

True Complications: Early Complications (Within 30 days of Operation)

Morbidly obese patients are considered surgically high-risk, given the comorbidities associated with obesity, such as diabetes mellitus, cardiovascular disease, thromboembolic disease, and hypertension. They are susceptible to all the same postoperative complications as are non-obese patients; however, it is believed that these complications tend to occur at slightly higher rates.[13]

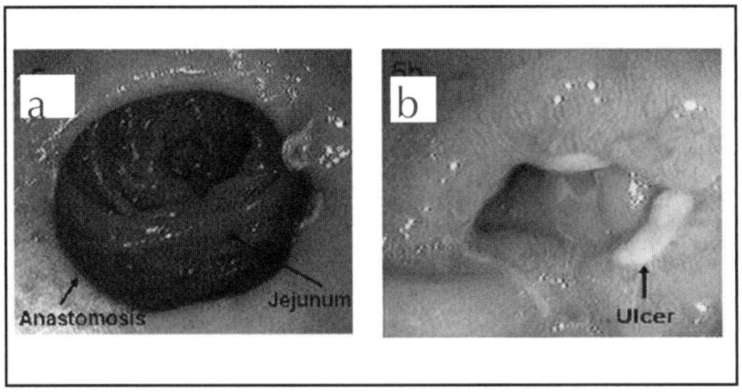

Figure 50-1. (a) Normal gastrojejunal anastomosis. (b) Gastric ulcer.

Additionally, complications may be more difficult to diagnose in the morbidly obese patient, a difficulty that can lead to delayed diagnosis and treatment.[14]

Complications caused by the reconstruction of the GI tract are discussed below. General surgery-related complications—eg, morbidity, pulmonary embolism and pneumonia, and wound infection—are discussed in Chapter 49.

Anastomatic Leak

A devastating complication of bariatric surgery is anastomotic leak, which occurs in 1.2% of open gastric-bypass cases.[15] This potentially disastrous complication occurs in BPD and gastric bypass but does not occur in VBG (because there is not true anastomosis in VBG). The difficulty in this complication lies in its diagnosis: symptoms and signs are most often vague without the presence of frank peritoneal signs. If a leak is present, most patients complain of mild abdominal pain, shoulder pain, back pain, or alteration in urination and bowel-movement frequency and have unexplained tachycardia or fever.

Given the variety in presenting symptoms and the devastating outcome of anastomotic leaks, there should be a low threshold for evaluation with water-soluble contrast agents (gastrograffin) and surgical exploration. If a leak is suspected, the safest course of action is surgery, rather than endoscopy which is contraindicated in the case of suspected perforation.[2] Failure to recognize and intervene if an abdominal catastrophe is suspected will most certainly lead to sepsis and possibly death.

Distention

Acute gastric distention is a rare but fatal complication of gastric-bypass procedures. It is caused by edema and obstruction at the enteroenterostomy that causes the bypassed stomach to develop massive gaseous distention. The distention may become so severe that it can cause a staple line disruption or a gastroenterostomy leak. The patient may complain of abdominal discomfort with bloating or hiccups. Plain abdominal films will demonstrate an excluded stomach that is distended with air-fluid levels. Radiographically guided percutaneous decompression with tube gastrostomy is the treatment of choice. The cause of the obstruction should be identified, as surgical revision may be necessary.

Late Complications (More Than 30 Days Post Surgery)

When a patient follows the recommended dietary program and continues to have complaints, the physician must take an aggressive approach to find the source of the patient's symptoms. Assessment of the patient's collaboration with a dietitian and adherence to a dietary program will often provide a clue as to the nature of his or her symptoms. Patients who are not following a prescribed program carefully will often have a variety of GI complaints. Strict monitoring of their diet by a dietitian is often helpful to find the source of their difficulty, whether it is eating too fast, too much, or the wrong foods. Dietary modification may provide a solution to the patient's GI complaints.

Anastomotic Complications

"Anastomotic complications" is an umbrella term for ulcers and strictures that occur at the gastrojejunostomy. They are a common cause of nausea and vomiting postoperatively and are typically diagnosed on endoscopy by the gastroenterologist. In the literature, the naming of ulcers at the anastomotic site has become an issue of semantics. Some authorities choose to differentiate anastomotic ulcers into marginal and stomal ulcers based on location and possible etiology. We here will refer to ulcers based on their mucosal location: gastric or jejunal.

Gastric Ulcers

Gastric ulcers, also referred to as stomal ulcers, occur in approximately 5% to 15% of undivided gastric bypass or VBG patients and are typically found on the gastric side of the anastomosis (Figure 50-1).[16-18] Most patients will present with symptoms of nausea, vomiting, severe dyspepsia, and retrosternal pain within 3 months of their operations.[15] Upon upper endoscopy, the diagnosis is made; however, upper GI contrast studies may also reveal abnormalities at the gastrojejunostomy.

Although no unifying explanation for the etiology of gastric ulcers exists, most agree that the pathogenesis is likely multifactorial. It is thought to be because of a combination of preserved acid secretion in the pouch, tension from the Roux limb, ischemia from the operation, non-steroidal anti-inflammatory drug (NSAID) use, and possibly *Helicobacter pylori* (*H. pylori*) infection.[19] Although studies assessing acid exposure in the pouch reveal low acid levels,[20-22] these ulcers typically respond to proton pump inhibitor therapy, carafate, or sucralfate.[15,23] In addition to antisecretory therapy, the presence of *H. pylori* infection should be evaluated and treated (if positive) and all NSAID therapy should be discontinued indefinitely. Although rare, these ulcers may become refractory to therapy and may require surgical intervention.

Jejunal Ulcers

Jejunal ulcers, also called marginal ulcers, occur in 5% to 15% of all cases of gastric bypass and typically extend from the jejunal side of the anastomosis. Occasionally, these ulcers may not involve the anastomosis and can be

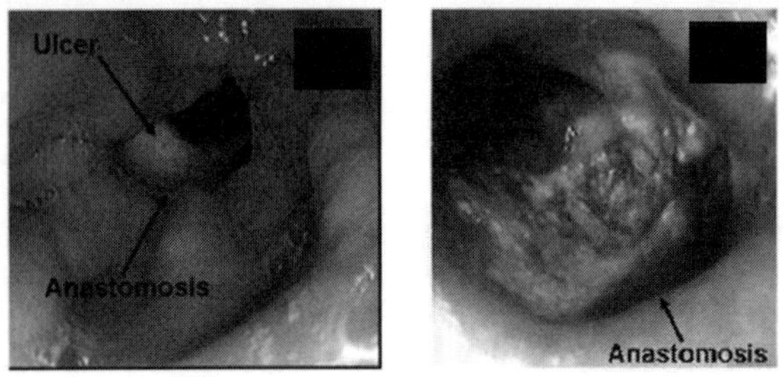

Figure 50-2. Jejunal ulcers beyond the anastomosis.

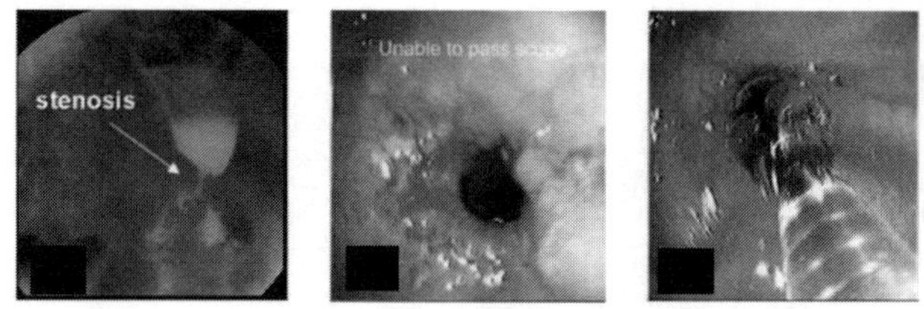

Figure 50-3. (a) Gastrograffin evidence of stricture. (b) Endoscopic evidence of anastomotic stricture. (c) TTS balloon inflated in anastomosis.

found further down the Roux limb (Figure 50-2).[16] These ulcers are also likely secondary to multiple insults.

Their predominant pathophysiologic abnormality is thought to be related to small bowel exposure to acid. This may result from preserved acid secretion in the gastric pouch or staple line dehiscence, which results in the continuous bathing of the anastomosis in acid from the remnant stomach.[2] Proponents of the divided gastric bypass approach (in which the remnant stomach is completely transected from the pouch) argue that acid production in the bypassed stomach can lead to staple line disruptions and gastro-gastric fistulas. Therefore, dividing the gastric pouch from the main stomach may decrease the incidence of these ulcers.[23-25]

These patients present similarly to those with gastric ulcers. Marginal ulcers, which can cause GI bleeding, have been recognized at anastomotic sites; the presence of hemorrhage or other indications of the complication in bariatric patients should prompt endoscopy so the provider can assess these potential bleeding sites. Treatment of jejunal ulcers consists of proton pump inhibitor therapy and/or sucralfate; unfortunately, the data with respect to treatment outcomes is limited.

Anastomotic Stenosis

Stenosis is a relatively common complication (12%) of bariatric surgery that presents with obstructive symptoms.[16] Anastomotic stenosis can exist with or without an accompanying ulcer; it may even develop as a consequence of an ulcer. Patients usually present with nausea, vomiting and post-prandial epigastric pain. The pouch outlet in bariatric surgery is generally created to be 1 to 1.5 cm in diameter, and a stenosis is defined by the inability to cannulate the gastrojejunostomy with a 9 to 9.8 mm endoscope.[26,27] The etiology of the stenosis is unclear; however, it is believed that they are secondary to ischemia or tension at the anastomosis.

Diagnosis can be made through an upper GI gastrograffin or upper endoscopy and treatment is dilation through the scope (TTS) with balloon dilators (Figure 50-3). Some patients may require multiple dilations and others, who do not respond to sequential dilation, may require surgical revision. Recognizing symptoms and seeking treatment is vitally important to prevent protein-calorie malnutrition and thiamine deficiency which can develop within weeks.[15]

Obstructive Complications in Vertical Banded Gastroplasty and LAP-Band

Patients who have had VBG have higher rates of outlet obstruction (20%) than do RYGB patients.[28] Obstruction is typically related to a band or ring complication at the end of the gastroplasty. Prolonged outlet obstruction may lead to GERD and esophagitis, potentially requiring another operation. Attempts to dilate the narrowing by endoscopic balloon dilation have been largely unsuccessful because of the stiff silastic ring or bands. These complications are better managed with surgical conversion to gastric bypass.[16] LAP-band and VBG patients also uniquely experience band erosion, in which the external band erodes into the wall of the stomach, requiring surgical removal and suturing of the stomach.[29] This late complication occurs with an incidence of 1.0% to 5.6%[29-31] and may jeopardize the aim of long-term weight reduction. This is a rare but extremely serious complication of restrictive procedures.

Weight Gain

Approximately 1 to 2 years after gastric bypass surgery, most patients lose up to two-thirds of their excess weight.[2] However, about 15% of patients will not lose 40% of their excess weight after gastric bypass.[32] The primary cause for failure to lose weight or regaining weight after surgery is noncompliance with the recommended bariatric diet. Patients will often continue to eat foods high in fat or calories. These patients need to be identified early and be provided with both educational and emotional support. Post surgery, a multidisciplinary team is essential to a patient's success in maintaining long-term weight loss.

If a patient continues to eat large volumes and their intake exceeds the capacity of their pouch stomach, staple-line disruption may occur. This, in turn, enables them to eat much larger quantities of food. In fact, the ability of a patient to consume large amounts of food and experience rapid weight gain should encourage the evaluation of staple-line disruption. This occurs in up to 1% of gastric bypass patients.[15] However, this figure is likely to decrease, as surgeons are now placing several rows of superimposed staples. Treatment involves surgical re-stapling and dividing the stomach. VBG patients, in general, are most susceptible to staple-line disruption[28] if a single vertical staple line is employed. Once again, conversion to gastric bypass is an appropriate option when this occurs.

In restrictive operations that utilize an external band (VBG and LAP-band), band slippage can lead to an increased ability to consume food and gain weight. Band slippage is probably caused by initial malpositioning of the band, which allows the pouch to dilate. In these cases, laparoscopic-band repositioning can be performed, but a better option for these patients may be revisional gastric bypass.[33]

The most serious cause of weight gain postoperatively is the formation of a fistula. Gastro-gastric fistulas occur when the pouch is not divided from the stomach, allowing consumed food to enter the bypassed stomach and to access the duodenum where the majority of absorption takes place. This leads to weight gain by removal of the functional bypass. Transection of the stomach with interposition of the jejunum prevents gastro-gastric fistula formation[34] and subsequent weight gain.

Internal Hernia

Internal hernias occur when the Roux limb passes through the transverse mesocolon or at a mesenteric defect at the enteroenterostomy. This results in a mechanical obstruction of the bowel. This problem is extremely difficult to diagnose clinically; symptoms are usually nonspecific (cramping, periumbilical pain with or without nausea, vomiting) and often times, radiographic studies are normal.[35] If symptoms persist or become severe, surgical exploration is necessary to rule out internal hernia and prevent intestinal necrosis from a closed-limb obstruction.[2] The decision to proceed to surgery is a clinical one.

Incisional or trocar hernias may also occur after bariatric procedures and can lead to both abdominal pain and obstructive symptoms. GI hemorrhage may occur in patients with intestinal anastomoses. The presence of hemorrhage in any bariatric patient requires endoscopy for the assessment of these problematic sites.

Cholelithiasis

Morbid obesity is a major risk factor for gallbladder disease, and this risk increases with rapid weight loss. Gallstones are a very common problem in the morbidly obese and form in at least one-third of patients within 6 months of their operation.[2] Not all patients who develop gallstones will develop symptoms of biliary colic or cholecystitis. A double-blind, placebo controlled, randomized clinical trial showed that the prophylactic use of 600 mg ursodiol reduced gallstone formation to 2% as compared with 32% in the placebo group.[36] However, not all patients can afford or tolerate this drug.

Some surgeons routinely remove the gallbladder during the bariatric operation, while others believe that this may introduce unnecessary complications to the procedure. In the hands of experienced surgeons, cholecystectomy is associated with little morbidity[37] and would eliminate gallbladder disease as a diagnostic entity in patients with pain symptoms postoperatively. However, simultaneous gastric bypass and cholecystectomy will increase operative time and may increase a patient's hospital stay.[38] These factors must be weighed against the prevention of the formation of gallstones.

Some have suggested the use of intraoperative ultrasound as a screening mechanism to help determine if a cholecystectomy should also be performed.[39] Others suggest a cholecystectomy if symptoms of biliary disease are present preoperatively. Despite such debates, no consensus exists on what should be done. Currently, the choice of concomitant cholecystectomy in the asymptomatic patient is left to the discretion of the surgeon.[40]

Endoscopic Management Issues

Upper endoscopy has become an important tool in the evaluation of postbariatric complications. In fact, a recent retrospective review of 540 consecutive RYGB patients revealed that almost 20% (101) of these patients required endoscopic evaluation for various complaints, such as intractable nausea and vomiting, abdominal pain, dysphagia and hematemesis.[41] Given this endoscopic burden, it is imperative that all gastroenterologists have some familiarity with these surgical procedures and the challenges that may present given the alteration in upper GI tract anatomy. Recently, Stellato et al presented an outline of basic management principles to guide the endoscopist in the evaluation of postbariatric patients.[42] These guidelines were modified from previous work by Feitoza et al, which focused on endoscopic evaluation and treatment in patients with previous upper GI surgery.[43] The guidelines are summarized here and should be followed to ensure an efficient and safe exam. They stress communication between the surgical staff and the gastroenterologist, once again illustrating the multidisciplinary aspect of care involved in gastric-bypass patients.

1. Know your anatomy. Prior to endoscopy, speak with the bariatric surgeon to thoroughly understand the patient's new anatomy. If the surgeon is unavailable, be sure to review the operative report in detail, including any records that may contain figures or diagrams. Any questions or concerns should be addressed to another bariatric surgeon.
2. Know the patient's postoperative course. This is especially relevant if a GI procedure is being contemplated in the early postoperative period. All imaging studies should be reviewed and additional contrast studies should be considered, if relevant.
3. Prepare for your procedure. Select the appropriate type of endoscope, dilators, or other special accessories beforehand.

Indications for Upper Endoscopy

Nausea/Vomiting

When an obvious cause for nausea and vomiting is not clear and/or the symptoms are associated with abdominal pain, one should suspect an anastomotic complication such as ulceration or stricture in RYGB patients or outlet obstruction or band erosion in VBG patients. These diagnoses are easily identified using a standard videoendoscope, which also allows anastomotic strictures to be treated simultaneously during the diagnostic procedure. Anastomotic ulceration may occur with and without overt stricturing and are usually treated medically if obstruction is absent. Band erosion in VBG patients and LAP-Band patients may require surgical removal of the band.

Currently, there is no absolute threshold diameter that defines critical obstruction of the anastomosis in gastric-bypass patients. Most published experience define an obstruction based on the endoscopist's inability to pass a 9-10 mm scope without resistance. This appears logical, as this is similar to the target surgical diameter. Therefore, small-caliber 27 Fr (9 mm) endoscopes are preferred because symptomatic stricture or obstructions are typically less than 12 mm. Both TTS balloon dilators[27,42,44-46] and Savary dilators[47] have been used to dilate anastomotic strictures in gastric-bypass patients. Most studies report using TTS balloon dilators, which is considered the preferred procedure. Dilation of an anastomotic stricture presents different challenges than do esophageal strictures. The luminal area behind the anastomotic stricture is short and composed of jejunum. In contrast, the luminal area beyond an esophageal stricture is large and composed of a thick-walled stomach, which accommodates more to distal movement during dilation than does the jejunum. Theoretically, it is possible that the tip of the rigid guide wire or Savary dilator could potentially become lodged behind the anastomosis in the blind pouch or Roux limb and cause a perforation. Care must be taken to avoid such a complication.

Unlike esophageal dilation, there are no set guidelines regarding technique for anastomotic dilation.[48] Decisions regarding the size of balloon to use during the procedure and the number of dilations depend on the degree of narrowing, presence of ulceration, postoperative time period, and symptoms. Fluoroscopy should be used when visualization through the anastomosis is not adequate to ensure proper and safe placement of the balloon dilator across the stricture into the Roux limb. The presence of ulceration may increase the risk of perforation and dilation should typically not be performed in this circumstance. Similarly, a "fresh anastomosis"—less than 4 weeks postoperatively—may also increase the risk of perforation. Careful assessment of the risks and benefits should be discussed with both the patient and the surgeon if endoscopy is performed within 4 to 6 weeks of the operation.

GI Bleeding

GI bleeding is an uncommon complication of bariatric surgery,[46,49] but anatomical considerations pose both diagnostic and therapeutic dilemmas. Upper GI bleeding in patients with gastric bypass may occur in the esophagus, gastric pouch, or Roux limb just distal to the anastomosis. These areas are readily accessible to standard upper endoscopy and therapy. GI bleeding may also occur in the distal stomach (remnant) and proximal duodenum; however, these areas are not readily available to standard upper endoscopy. The bypassed stomach may be accessed with a pediatric colonoscope or enteroscope of adequate length[50,51] or via a gastrostomy obtained by radiographic guidance or surgery.[52] Given these difficulties and the fact that NSAIDs are associated with anastomotic complications including GI bleeding from ulceration, it is prudent to advise all patients to avoid NSAIDs and other ulcerogenic medications. Whether or not *H. pylori* is an important risk factor for anastomotic ulceration is somewhat controversial. Given the increased lifetime risk for peptic ulceration, it is not unreasonable to test patients preoperatively and institute treatment (if positive) to avoid future complications.

Cancer Screening

Obesity surgery should not alter GI-cancer–screening recommendations. Colonoscopy is uncomplicated in postbariatric surgical patients and consideration of tolerable bowel preparations is the only issue that deserves special attention. Large-volume preparations may be difficult to tolerate and patients may require low-volume preparations. Similarly, there should be no differences in surveillance regimens for bariatric patients with Barrett's esophagus. However, the finding of high-grade dysplasia or adenocarcinoma will create additional technical problems concerning operative treatment. Esophagectomy may be technically challenging or impossible depending on the type of bariatric surgery performed. It is currently unclear whether the presence of Barrett's esophagus should alter bariatric operative choice.

Conclusion

Obesity is one of the most striking public health problems in America today. Despite increased public awareness and aggressive education measures, the prevalence of obesity continues to increase. Because early data support that bariatric surgery and its consequent weight loss can significantly relieve the comorbidities of obesity, surgery has become an essential part of the treatment of morbid obesity, notwithstanding the necessary evils that accompany it. The adverse events and true complications often call for a gastroenterology consultation, requiring the endoscopist to be well versed in the care of postbariatric patients. For the gastroenterologist, successful management of these patients necessitates communication with the bariatric surgeon, knowledge of postoperative anatomy, an understanding of the potential complications and implementation of appropriate treatment.

Acknowledgment

This work was supported by grant K23 DK62170-01 (JEP) from the Public Health Service.

References

1. Balsiger BM, Murr MM, Poggio JL, Sarr MG. Bariatric surgery. Surgery for weight control in patients with morbid obesity. *Med Clin North Am.* 2000;84(2):477-489.
2. Klein S, Wadden TA, Sugerman HJ. AGA Technical review on obesity. *Gastroenterology.* 2002;123:882-932.
3. Vecht J, Masclee AA, Lamers CB. The dumping syndrome. Current insights into pathophysiology, diagnosis and treatment. *Scand J Gastroenterol Suppl.* 1997;223:21-27.
4. MacGregor A. The story of surgery for obesity. American Society for Bariatric Surgery. 2002; http://www.asbs.org/html/story/chapter1.html.
5. Halverson JD. Vitamin and mineral deficiencies following obesity surgery. *Gastroenterol Clin North Am.* 1987;16(2):307-315.
6. Rhode BM, Arseneau P, Cooper BA, Katz M, Gilfix BM, MacLean LD. Vitamin B-12 deficiency after gastric surgery for obesity. *Am J Clin Nutr.* 1996;63(1):103-109.

7. Brolin RE, Gorman JH, Gorman RC, et al. Are vitamin B12 and folate deficiency clinically important after roux-en-Y gastric bypass? *J Gastrointest Surg.* 1998;2(5):436-442.
8. Brolin RE, Gorman JH, Gorman RC, et al. Prophylactic iron supplementation after Roux-en-Y gastric bypass: a prospective, double-blind, randomized study. *Arch Surg.* 1998;133(7):740-744.
9. Nanji AA, Freeman JB. Gastric by-pass surgery in morbidly obese patients markedly decreases serum levels of vitamins A and C and iron in the peri-operative period. *Int J Obes.* 1985;9:177-179.
10. Amaral JF, Thompson WR, Caldwell MD, et al. Prospective hematologic evaluation of gastric exclusion surgery for morbid obesity. *Ann Surg.* 1985;201:186-193.
11. Avinoah E, Ovnat A, Charuzi I: Nutritional status seven years after Roux-en-Y gastric bypass surgery. *Surgery.* 1992;111:137-142.
12. Brolin RE, Gorman RC, Milgrim LM, et al: Multivitamin prophylaxis in prevention of post-gastric bypass vitamin and mineral deficiencies. *Int J Obes.* 1991;15:661-667.
13. Senagore AJ, Delaney CP, Madboulay K, Brady KM, Fazio VW, Fazio CV. Laparoscopic colectomy in obese and nonobese patients. *J Gastrointest Surg.* 2003;7(4):558-561.
14. Mehran A, Liberman M, Rosenthal R, Szomstein S. Ruptured appendicitis after laparoscopic roux-en-y gastric bypass: pitfalls in diagnosing a surgical abdomen in the morbidly obese. *Obes Surg.* 2003;13(6):938-940.
15. Byrne TK. Complications of surgery for obesity. *Surg Clin North Am.* 2001;81(5):1181-1193, vii-viii.
16. Sanyal AJ, Sugerman HJ, Kellum JM, Engle KM, Wolfe L. Stomal complications of gastric bypass: incidence and outcome of therapy. *Am J Gastroenterol.* 1992;87(9):1165-1169.
17. Schauer PR, Ikramuddin S, Gourash W, Ramanathan R, Luketich J. Outcomes after laparoscopic Roux-en-Y gastric bypass for morbid obesity. *Ann Surg.* 2000;232(4):515-529.
18. Pope GD, Goodney PP, Burchard KW, et al. Peptic ulcer/stricture after gastric bypass: a comparison of technique and acid suppression variables. *Obes Surg.* 2002;12(1):30-33.
19. Sapala JA, Wood MH, Sapala MA, Flake TM, Jr. Marginal ulcer after gastric bypass: a prospective 3-year study of 173 patients. *Obes Surg.* 1998;8(5):505-516.
20. Mason EE, Munns JR, Kealey GP, et al. Effect of gastric bypass on gastric secretion. *Am J Surg.* 1976;131(2):162-168.
21. Behrns KE, Smith CD, Sarr MG. Prospective evaluation of gastric acid secretion and cobalamin absorption following gastric bypass for clinically severe obesity. *Dig Dis Sci.* 1994;39(2):315-320.
22. Smith CD, Herkes SB, Behrns KE, Fairbanks VF, Kelly KA, Sarr MG. Gastric acid secretion and vitamin B12 absorption after vertical Roux-en-Y gastric bypass for morbid obesity. *Ann Surg.* 1993;218(1):91-96.
23. MacLean LD, Rhode BM, Nohr C, Katz S, McLean AP. Stomal ulcer after gastric bypass. *J Am Coll Surg.* 1997;185(1):1-7.
24. Capella JF, Capella RF. Staple disruption and marginal ulceration in gastric bypass procedures for weight reduction. *Obes Surg.* 1996;6(1):44-49.
25. Fobi MA, Lee H, Igwe D, Jr., Stanczyk M, Tambi JN. Prospective comparative evaluation of stapled versus transected silastic ring gastric bypass: 6-year follow-up. *Obes Surg.* 2001;11(1):18-24.
26. Huang CS, Forse RA, Jacobson BC, Farraye FA. Endoscopic findings and their clinical correlations in patients with symptoms after gastric bypass surgery. *Gastrointest Endosc.* 2003;58(6):859-866.
27. Ahmad J, Martin J, Ikramuddin S, Schauer P, Slivka A. Endoscopic balloon dilation of gastroenteric anastomotic stricture after laparoscopic gastric bypass. *Endoscopy.* 2003;35(9):725-728.
28. MacLean LD, Rhode BM, Forse RA. Late results of vertical banded gastroplasty for morbid and super obesity. *Surgery.* 1990;107(1):20-27.
29. Abu-Abeid S, Keidar A, Gavert N, Blanc A, Szold A. The clinical spectrum of band erosion following laparoscopic adjustable silicone gastric banding for morbid obesity. *Surg Endosc.* 2003;17(6):861-863.
30. Suter M, Giusti V, Heraief E, Zysset F, Calmes JM. Laparoscopic gastric banding. *Surg Endosc.* 2003;17(9):1418-1425.
31. Fobi M, Lee H, Igwe D, et al. Band erosion: incidence, etiology, management and outcome after banded vertical gastric bypass. *Obes Surg.* 2001;11(6):699-707.
32. Sugerman HJ, Kellum JM, Engle KM, et al. Gastric bypass for treating severe obesity. *Am J Clin Nutr.* 1992;55(2 Suppl):560S-566S.
33. Suter M. Laparoscopic band repositioning for pouch dilatation/slippage after gastric banding: disappointing results. *Obes Surg.* 2001;11(4):507-512.
34. Capella JF, Capella RF. Gastro-gastric fistulas and marginal ulcers in gastric bypass procedures for weight reduction. *Obes Surg.* 1999;9(1):22-27; discussion 28.
35. Blachar A, Federle MP, Pealer KM, Ikramuddin S, Schauer PR. Gastrointestinal complications of laparoscopic Roux-en-Y gastric bypass surgery: clinical and imaging findings. *Radiology.* 2002;223(3):625-632.
36. Sugerman HJ, Brewer WH, Shiffman ML, et al. A multicenter, placebo-controlled, randomized, double-blind, prospective trial of prophylactic ursodiol for the prevention of gallstone formation following gastric-bypass-induced rapid weight loss. *Am J Surg.* 1995;169(1):91-96; discussion 96-97.
37. Fobi M, Lee H, Igwe D, et al. Prophylactic cholecystectomy with gastric bypass operation: incidence of gallbladder disease. *Obes Surg.* 2002;12(3):350-353.
38. Hamad GG, Ikramuddin S, Gourash WF, Schauer PR. Elective cholecystectomy during laparoscopic Roux-en-Y gastric bypass: is it worth the wait? *Obes Surg.* 2003;13(1):76-81.
39. Scott DJ, Villegas L, Sims TL, Hamilton EC, Provost DA, Jones DB. Intraoperative ultrasound and prophylactic ursodiol for gallstone prevention following laparoscopic gastric bypass. *Surg Endosc.* 2003;17(11):1796-1802.
40. Mason EE, Renquist KE. Gallbladder management in obesity surgery. *Obes Surg.* 2002;12(2):222-229.
41. Krishnamoorthy B, Kuwada TS, Denham E, et al. Endoscopic burden of anastomotic ulceration and stricture after Roux-en-Y gastric bypass. *Digestive Diseases Week.* 2004; *Gastroenterology.* 2004;126(4): Suppl 2.
42. Stellato TA, Crouse C, Hallowell PT. Bariatric surgery: creating new challenges for the endoscopist. *Gastrointest Endosc.* 2003;57(1):86-94.
43. Feitoza AB, Baron TH. Endoscopy and ERCP in the setting of previous upper GI tract surgery. Part I: reconstruction without alteration of pancreaticobiliary anatomy. *Gastrointest Endosc.* 2001;54(6):743-749.
44. Nguyen NT, Stevens CM, Wolfe BM. Incidence and outcome of anastomotic stricture after laparoscopic gastric bypass. *J Gastrointest Surg.* 2003;7(8):997-1003.
45. Barba CA, Butensky MS, Lorenzo M, Newman R. Endoscopic dilation of gastroesophageal anastomosis stricture after gastric bypass. *Surg Endosc.* 2003;17(3):416-420.
46. Huang CS, de las Morenas A, Farraye FA. Focal intestinal lymphangiectasia. *Gastrointest Endosc.* 2004;59(1):74.
47. Bell RL, Reinhardt KE, Flowers JL. Surgeon-performed endoscopic dilatation of symptomatic gastrojejunal anastomotic strictures following laparoscopic Roux-en-Y gastric bypass. *Obes Surg.* 2003;13(5):728-733.
48. Spechler SJ. AGA technical review on treatment of patients with dysphagia caused by benign disorders of the distal esophagus. *Gastroenterology.* 1999;117(1):233-254.
49. Braley SC, Nguyen NT, Wolfe BM. Late gastrointestinal hemorrhage after gastric bypass. *Obes Surg.* 2002;12(3):404-407.
50. Flickinger EG, Sinar DR, Pories WJ, Sloss RR, Park HK, Gibson JH. The bypassed stomach. *Am J Surg.* 1985;149(1):151-156.
51. Park HK, Sinar DR, Sloss RR, Whitley TW, Silverman JF. Histologic and endoscopic studies before and after gastric bypass surgery. *Arch Pathol Lab Med.* 1986;110(12):1164-1167.
52. Sundbom M, Nyman R, Hedenstrom H, Gustavsson S. Investigation of the excluded stomach after Roux-en-Y gastric bypass. *Obes Surg.* 2001;11(1):25-27.

Chapter 51

Hyperlipidemia: Genetic and Nutritional Considerations for the Gastroenterologist

Neil J. Stone, MD

Introduction

This chapter will discuss lipid physiology and an approach to clinical lipid problems with a view towards emphasizing those areas that are pertinent to the gastroenterologist. It begins with a review of lipid and lipoprotein physiology that is critical to understanding alterations in lipids and lipoproteins that are observed in clinic practice.[1] After a detailed consideration of the National Cholesterol Education Program's Adult Treatment Panel (ATP) III report[2] and its approach to the patient with hypercholesterolemia, this chapter will focus on secondary disorders that cause lipid abnormalities and will review lipid treatment issues that particularly bear on the gastrointestinal (GI) tract and nutrition.

Physiology

Lipid physiology is focused on the GI tract, the circulation, the liver, and peripheral tissues. Dietary lipid loads are absorbed in the intestine in the form of micelles that bind to the brush border membrane of intestinal enterocytes. Two transport mechanisms have proved to be pivotal for efficient sterol transport. First, cholesterol is transported from the micelles into duodenal and jejunal enterocytes via the Neiman Pick-1 Like-1 (NPC1L1) sterol transporter.[3] Second, intestinal cholesterol and nearly all of the absorbed plant sterols are exported back from the enterocyte into the intestinal lumen by the ATP-binding cassette (ABC) transporters ABCG5 and ABCG8.[4] Most of the bile salts are reabsorbed farther down in the distal ileum through the intestinal bile acid transporter and are transported back to the liver via the hepatic portal circulation. (The partial ileal bypass operation takes advantage of this to provide obligatory bile salt loss and lower cholesterol levels). Unabsorbed cholesterol and other sterols are excreted in the feces.

Lipid transport in the circulation requires large macromolecules with an outer solubilizing coat of phospholipids and apolipoproteins and an inner oily core of triglycerides and cholesterol ester. These lipoproteins may be distinguished by their size and their density. Nuclear magnetic resonance can determine the total low-density lipoproteins (LDL) particle number as well as the LDL and high-density lipoproteins (HDL) subclasses. Five major lipoproteins classes are summarized in Table 51-1.

Cholesterol that remains in the intestinal cells is esterified and packaged into chylomicrons, which are released into the lymphatic circulation. Chylomicrons are the largest of the lipoproteins particles and carry a predominant triglyceride load. They are metabolized by lipoprotein lipase, an enzyme that acts on the triglyceride-laden chylomicrons at the endothelial surface of extrahepatic capillaries and provides cells with fatty acids for either storage or energy purposes. It requires thyroid hormone and insulin for its effective action. The chylomicron remnants so produced are taken up by a specific hepatic receptor called LDL-related proteins (LRP).

In the postprandial state, blood that is drawn and spun down and refrigerated shows a typical white creamy supranatant. This should not be present in the fasting state. For those with genetic defects in lipoprotein lipase action, the fasting triglyceride levels usually exceed 1000 mg/dl and a creamy supranatant layer is seen despite the fasting condition.

Very low-density lipoproteins (VLDL) transport cholesterol to the periphery. These are large, triglyceride-rich particles whose outer coat carries apolipoprotein

TABLE 51-1.

*Five Major Lipoprotein Classes**

Lipoprotein Classes	*% Fasting Total Chol. (approx)*	*Density, g/dL*	*Chol. %*	*TG %*	*Major Apolipoproteins*
LDL	60 to 70%	1.019 to 1.063	40 to 50	5 to 15	Apo B 100
VLDL	10 to 15%	0.95 to 1.006	5 to 15	55 to 80	Apo B100, CI, CII, CIII, E
IDL	If LDL-c is by calculation, included in LDL-c*	1.006 to 1.019	20t o 40	20 to 50	Apo B100, E
Chylomicrons	None	0.95	2 to 7	80 to 95	Same as for VLDL except has Apo B 48
HDL	20 to 30%	1.063 to 1.210	15 to 25	5 to 10	Apo A1, A2

Chol. = cholesterol, TG = triglycerides, LDL= low density lipoproteins, VLDL= very low density lipoproteins; IDL = intermediate density lipoproteins, HDL = high density lipoproteins; apo= apolipoproteins.

This is a simplified scheme. There are subclasses of LDL, VLDL, and HDL that are particularly well-appreciated by nuclear magnetic resonance.

*LDL-c is calculated by LDL-c = Total cholesterol – HDL-c – (TG/5) where total cholesterol, triglycerides, and HDL-c are determined on fasting plasma and TG.

(apo) B as well as apo CII, apo CIII, and apo E. They have a half-life measured in hours. The triglyceride concentration carried on VLDL is approximately five times that of the cholesterol concentration. Thus, an approximation of VLDL cholesterol is obtained by dividing the triglycerides by five. LDL is formed in the circulation from VLDL. Cholesterol on VLDL is either recycled to HDL through cholesterol-ester transport proteins (CETP) or metabolized to remnant lipoproteins that are further metabolized to LDL or removed by hepatic cell-surface receptors called LDL receptors (LDLR). Indeed, chylomicron remnants, VLDL, and LDL are all internalized in the liver through these cell-surface hepatic receptors. The synthesis of VLDL is increased in states of increased free fatty acid flux, acute increases in carbohydrates, obesity, and estrogen administration. The catabolism of VLDL is impaired in diabetes mellitus and chronic renal disease.

Intermediate-density lipoproteins (IDL) are formed from the catabolism of VLDL. They are atherogenic particles that, as do VLDL and LDL, have one molecule of apo B on each particle.

LDL with a mean life span of 2.5 days carry approximately 70% of the plasma cholesterol. (5) The apo B100 on LDL binds to the LDLR and then is internalized by receptor-mediated endocytosis in coated pits. Once in the liver cell, LDL is degraded in lysosomes, freeing its cholesterol load to enter the hepatic cholesterol pool. As the hepatic cholesterol level rises, the transcription of the LDLR gene is suppressed, and plasma LDL cholesterol (LDL-c) levels remain high. Conversely, when hepatic cholesterol levels fall, transcription of the LDLR gene is induced and plasma LDL-c falls as LDL is avidly taken up by the hepatocyte. Saturated fatty and dietary cholesterol downregulate the LDLR and, when weight is held constant, increase levels of LDL-c.

The gene for the LDLR is located on chromosome 19. Those with an inherited defect in the genes controlling receptor action are either heterozygous or homozygous for this condition, depending on the severity of the defect. The statins, HMG Coa Reductase inhibitors, have altered the natural history of this condition because of their ability to markedly lower LDL-c (and other apo B containing lipoproteins) in these patients by causing a reduced hepatocyte cholesterol synthesis, a decreased hepatic cholesterol pool, and an increased expression of LDLR.

Genetics

Genetic considerations are important because they can determine the basis for the response to diet of abnormal lipid levels. For example, those with familial hypercholesterolemia (FH) are diet-resistant and require drug therapy to achieve goal levels of LDL-c. On the other hand, those with familial dysbeta-lipoproteinemia (Type III) are diet-sensitive and respond to carbohydrate restriction, whereas those with severe hypertriglyceridemia (triglycerides >1000 mg/dL) that is due to accumulation of chylomicrons that is due to a genetic absence/deficiency of lipoprotein lipase (and often an acquired cause) require fat restriction initially to aid in clearing the chylomicron excess.

An understanding of the impaired functioning of LDLR underlies the genetic basis for four disorders that elevate LDL-c (Table 51-2). These were recently reviewed by Goldstein and Brown, who won the Nobel prize for their discovery of the key role of the LDLR in cholesterol metabolism.[6] The disorders range in frequency from 1 in 500 for a heterozygous person with FH (although the frequency is higher in places such as Quebec, Canada, where 11 mutations account for more than 90% of the cases)[7] and 1 per 1000 in familial ligand defective apo B-100 to less than 1 in 10 million for autosomal recessive hypercholesterolemia or sitosterolemia.

In FH, heterozygote have high LDL-c that lead, if untreated, to xanthomas and early onset of coronary heart disease (CHD) in the 4th and 5th decades of life. The homozygous state leads to xanthomas and premature

TABLE 51-2.

Genetic Disorders of Cholesterol Metabolism

Diseases Associated With Increased LDL-cholesterol	*Gene*	*Mechanism*
Familial hypercholesterolemia (FH)	LDL receptor	Absent or nonfunctional receptors
Familial ligand defective apo B-100	apo B-100	Decreased LDL binding to receptors
Autosomal recessive hypercholesterolemia	ARH	LDL receptor activity is disrupted
Sitosterolemia	ABCG5 and/or ABCG8	Suppression of receptor gene transcription

Adapted from the following sources: Third Report of the National Cholesterol Education Program (NCEP) Expert Panel on Detection, Evaluation, and Treatment of High Blood Cholesterol in Adults (Adult Treatment Panel III) final report. *Circulation*. 2002;17;106(25):3143-421; Berge KE, Tian H, Graf GA, et al. Accumulation of dietary cholesterol in sitosterolemia caused by mutations in adjacent ABC transporters. *Science*. 2000;290:1771; Rader DJ, Cohen J, Hobbs HH. Monogenic hypercholesterolemia: new insights in pathogenesis and treatment.*J Clin Invest*. 2003;111(12):1795; Goldstein JL, Brown MS. Molecular medicine. The cholesterol quartet. *Science*. 2001;292(5520):1310; Weisgraber KH, Innerarity T, Newhouse YM, et al. Familial defective apolipoprotein B-100: enhanced binding of monoclonal antibody MB47 to abnormal low density lipoproteins. *Proc Natl Acad Sci U S A*. 1988;85(24): 9758; Pullinger CR, Kane JP, Malloy MJ. Primary hypercholesterolemia: genetic causes and treatment of five monogenic disorders. *Expert Rev Cardiovasc Ther*. 2003;1(1):107; Soutar K, Naoumova RP, Traub LM. Genetics, clinical phenotype, and molecular cell biology of autosomal recessive hypercholesterolemia. *Arterioscler Thromb Vasc Biol*. 2003;23(11):1963.

atherosclerosis in the 1st and 2nd decades of life. Because of advances in combination LDL-c–lowering therapy and LDL apheresis, survival into middle age is now possible.[8]

Familial ligand-defective apo B-100 (FDB) is caused by mutations in the gene encoding apo B-100. The defective apo B is unable to bind efficiently to LDLRs, with the consequence of impaired clearance of LDL and raised LDL-c.[9]

Mutations in ABC half-transporters ABCG5 (G5) or ABCG8 (G8) cause sitosterolemia, a rare (under 50 persons identified) autosomal recessive disease characterized by sterol accumulation (plant and animal), early onset of tendon and tuberous xanthomas, and premature atherosclerosis.[4,10] Normal individuals absorb less than 5% of dietary sitosterol, the major plant sterol and, because of pairing of G5 and G8 transporters, efficiently excrete plant sterols into bile. Plasma sitosterol concentrations rarely exceed 1 mg/dl in most people, despite their high intakes of dietary plant sterols. In contrast, sitosterolemic subjects absorb about 15% to 20% of dietary sitosterol and levels range from 14 to 65 mg/dl. Moreover, affected individuals have a markedly reduced capacity to excrete sitosterol into bile. This explains the striking accumulation of sterols in the blood and body tissues of patients with this genetic disorder. These individuals also have an increased fractional absorption and reduced biliary excretion of cholesterol that (not surprisingly) results in hypercholesterolemia and premature CHD.

Finally, autosomal recessive hypercholesterolemia (ARH) also results in severely affected individuals who are homozygous for the condition.[11] They can be distinguished from FH patients by the fact that their parents, obligate heterozygotes, have normal levels of LDL-c. The molecular defect has been traced to the gene encoding a cytosolic hepatic adaptor protein. The mechanism for decreased LDL-R function is the presence of defects in this protein, which binds to the cytoplasmic tail of the LDL-R molecule.

Disorders that involve triglyceride metabolism include familial combined hyperlipidemia (FCHL), Type III hyperlipoproteinemia, familial hypertriglyceridemia (FHTG), and familial lipoprotein lipase deficiency (Table 51-3).[1]

FCHL is seen in 1% to 2% of the population; however, among survivors of myocardial infarction (MI) under age 60 years, its frequency is increased 10-fold.[12] It is the most common genetic lipid disorder in these nonelderly CHD patients. It is characterized by the presence of elevated cholesterol and triglycerides, but in affected kindreds individuals can present with elevations of LDL and VLDL, singly or alone. Because there is one molecule of apo B on each VLDL and LDL, it is not surprising that plasma apo B levels tend to be high. Both increased secretion rates and impaired clearance have been described. The precise mechanism for this disorder remains unknown, but genetic abnormalities within the apo A-I/C-III/A-IV/A-V gene locus seems important in modifying both triglyceride levels and particle size.[13] Other loci, including abnormalities in lipoprotein lipase may be involved in FCHL's pathogenesis and association with increased susceptibility to atherosclerotic events. High triglycerides, low HDL-c, and systolic hypertension can be seen with heterozygous lipoprotein lipase deficiency.[14]

In familial dysbetalipoproteinemia or familial type III hyperlipoproteinemia, the accumulation of triglyceride-rich remnants is seen. Often the patients have tubo-eruptive xanthomas and some present with a pathognomonic lipid-laden palmar crease. Premature CHD and peripheral vascular disease are seen. The characteristic lipid abnormalities are cholesterol and triglyceride values that range from 250 to 500 mg/dL and a lipoprotein pattern of cholesterol-rich VLDL. The genetic abnormality involves several different mutations of apo E that interfere with its interaction with cell-surface receptors.[15] Affected individuals have the apo E-II/E-II phenotype. This is necessary but not sufficient for the full expression of the disorder. Conditions that increase the synthesis of VLDL—such as

TABLE 51-3.

Some Genetic Disorders of Triglyceride Metabolism

Disease Associated With Increased Triglycerides	*Gene*	*Mechanism*
Familial combined hyperlipidemia	A1/C3/A4/A5 gene cluster on chromosome 11; other gene loci may contribute including those affecting Apo B	No agreement on mechanism; gene cluster modifes triglyceride concentration and LDL size.
Familial dysbetalipoproteinemia	Apo E	Defective apo E (E2/E2) and an associated condition either increasing VLDL synthesis or suppressing LDL-R.
Familial hypertriglyceridemia	LPL, other loci	Increased hepatic TG production and/or heterozygosity for LPL deficiency.
Familial lipoprotein lipase deficiency	LPL, apo CII	Deficiency of lipoprotein lipase or its co-factor, apo CII.

Adapted from Stone NJ, Blum CB. *Management of Lipids in Clinical Practice*; 4th ed. Caddo, OK: Professional Communications, Inc; 2002.

obesity, caloric excess, and alcohol use—make detection more obvious in those with the apo E-II/E-II phenotype. Hypothyroidism is an important trigger for type III hyperlipoproteinemia in patients with defective apo E because the hypothyroid state suppresses the synthesis of hepatic LDL-R, further impairing clearance. A very rare cause of accumulation of remnant lipoproteins (the type III phenotype) in patients with normal apo E is deficiency of hepatic triglyceride lipase, an enzyme involved in conversion of VLDL remnants to LDL. HDL levels are generally elevated in these patients; in typical type III patients, HDL levels are quite low.

FHTG is associated with an increased production of VLDL particles and some cases seem to result from the effects of aging and partial lipoprotein lipase (LPL) deficiency.[1] In patients with FHTG and multiple metabolic risk factors of the metabolic syndrome, there is an increased CHD risk.[16]

Severe hypertriglyceridemia with its consequence of acute pancreatitis can be seen in those born with two defective alleles for the LPL gene or its cofactor, apolipoprotein C-II. These are rare causes of acute pancreatitis, but the presentation is characteristic with onset early in life of recurrent abdominal pain and the typical eruptive xanthomatosis, lipemia retinalis, and hepatosplenomegaly that indicate marked elevations of fasting chylomicronemia. Astute clinicians can spin down plasma and note the large white creamy supranatant. Recognition can be lifesaving because therapy with a markedly fat-restricted diet, a fibric acid drug such as gemfibrozil or fenofibrate, fish oil capsules, and (in recalcitrant cases) plasma exchange with removal of the excess chylomicrons must be instituted promptly to prevent recurrent pancreatitis that can lead to fatal issue.

Familial hypoalphalipoproteinemia or HDL deficiency and the rare Tangier's disease present with very low or nearly absent HDL-c (Table 51-4).[17] Inherited mutations of the ABC1 gene that codes for the ABC1 protein are often found as the genetic defects that impair cholesterol efflux from the cell in these disorders. At least 10% of individuals with low HDL-c in the general population are heterozygous for mutations in ABC1.[18]

Common genetic variations within ABC1 are associated not only with altered plasma lipid levels but also a variable risk of CHD. One variant, the R219K variant, with a carrier frequency of 46% in European populations, is associated with a decreased severity of CAD, whereas others are associated with decreased HDL-c, increased triglycerides, and an increased risk of CHD.[19]

Patients with isolated low HDL-c (and normal triglycerides and LDL-c levels) are often resistant to lifestyle measures and medications. Many experts hold that lowering LDL-c in these patients is a useful long-term strategy, although there is a paucity of supportive data. Those whose low HDL-c is associated with features of the metabolic syndrome (high triglyceride, abdominal obesity, hypertension, glycemic abnormalities) may respond surprisingly well to a lifestyle regimen of an appropriate diet, regular exercise, weight loss, and cessation of smoking.

Clinical Approach to Patient With Hyperlipidemia

The National Cholesterol Education Program's Adult Treatment Panel (ATP) III placed primary emphasis on published, large-scale, randomized, clinical trial data when their guidelines for cholesterol management were published in May 2001.[2] The clinical algorithm involves the following features.

1. CHD risk determination; an essential initial step in cholesterol management. For those with 0-1 risk factors, the near-term CHD risk is low and lifestyle goals are emphasized. For those with 2 or more risk factors, the Framingham risk score was emphasized, as near-term CHD risk can vary from

TABLE 51-4.

Some Genetic Disorders of HDL Metabolism

Disease Associated With Low HDL	Gene	Mechanism
Familial hypoalphalipoproteinemia	ABCA1	Impaired functioning of ABCA 1 Cassette transporter.
Tangier's disease	ABCA1	Impaired functioning of ABCA 1 Cassette transporter.

Adapted from Stone NJ, Blum CB. *Management of Lipids in Clinical Practice*. 4th ed. Caddo, OK: Professional Communications, Inc; 2002; Third Report of the National Cholesterol Education Program (NCEP) Expert Panel on Detection, Evaluation, and Treatment of High Blood Cholesterol in Adults (Adult Treatment Panel III) final report. *Circulation*. 2002;106(25):3143; Frikke-Schmidt R, Nordestgaard BG, Jensen GB, Tybjaerg Hansen A. Genetic variation in ABC transporter A1 contributes to HDL cholesterol in the general population. *J Clin Invest*. 2004;114(9):1343; Clee SM, Zwinderman AH, Engert JC, et al. Common genetic variation in ABCA1 is associated with altered lipoprotein levels and a modified risk for coronary artery disease. *Circulation*. 2001;103(9):1198.

either low (<10%), intermediate (10%-20%), or high (>20%). For those with 2 or more risk factors, the LDL-c goal was <130. For those with CHD or high-risk conditions that impart a greater than 20% 10-year Framingham risk, an LDL-c goal of <100 mg/dL is assigned.

2. Emphasis on therapeutic lifestyle change (TLC) in the management of atherogenic diet, sedentary behavior, and excessive weight gain due to caloric excess. Although there is a genetic basis for insulin resistance, the recent upswing in overweight and obesity in the US population suggests that unhealthy lifestyle (too many calories and not enough exercise) is greatly to blame.
3. Focus on two secondary goals that are particularly affected by unhealthy lifestyles. The first is hypertriglyceridemia that persists despite the patient having an LDL-c at goal. (This differentiates ATP III from ATP II, which was more solely focused on LDL-c.) The presence of atherogenic triglyceride-rich particles correlates with a measurement called "non-HDL-cholesterol" (non-HDL-c). This requires no additional testing, as non-HDL-c is simply total cholesterol and the goal for non-HDL-c is set 30 mg/dL above that for LDL-c. Non-HDL-c is the sum of LDL and IDL and VLDL and lipoprotein (a) [Lp(a)] and its values correlates with apo B.
4. The second is metabolic syndrome (MetS). The initial treatment step is intensifiedTLC.

For the gastroenterologist, diagnosis of the MetS is of utmost importance because of problems such as fatty liver and related consequences of diabetes and CHD. MetS is a collection of metabolic variables that develop in response to genetics, obesity, and insulin resistance. Ginsberg has pointed out that the inability of insulin-resistant fat cells to store triglycerides is probably the initial step in the development of the dyslipidemia seen with insulin resistance.[20] This leads to the characteristic high triglyceridemia from VLDL excess, low HDL-c, and small dense LDL, which are the lipid hallmarks of the insulin-resistant state. Of interest is the face that, in overweight individuals, optimal metabolic cut-points for diagnosing the insulin-resistant state are suggested to be triglycerides of 130 mg/dL, triglyceride/HDL cholesterol of 3.0, and 109 pmol/L for insulin.[21]

The ATP III panel recommended an operational definition of MetS that required three of the five metabolic parameters for diagnosis, which are listed in Table 51-5.

It should be noted that some males can develop multiple metabolic risk factors when their waist circumferences are only marginally elevated (37 to 39 in). This can be seen in some who have a strong genetic component. Indeed, in Quebec, a waist of 35 in and a triglyceride value of 2 mmol (176 mg/dL) identified men not only likely to have elevated insulin and apo B levels but also a high likelihood of CAD.[22]

Other definitions for MetS that are beyond the scope of this chapter involve some measurement of insulin resistance that are harder to achieve in day-to-day practice. Moreover, ATP III's definition involves metabolic factors that all respond to small, achievable amounts of weight loss, improved diet, and regular exercise. A final advantage of the ATP III definition is that it can be applied to other large-scale studies that have measured the five metabolic parameters. For example, the West of Scotland Study was a prospective intervention study of pravastatin 40 mg versus placebo in men with high CHD risk.[23] Using the ATP III definition of MetS—with the substitution of body mass index (BMI) for waist circumference—the investigators showed an impressive increased CHD risk as well as risk for diabetes. Of interest, MetS continued to predict CHD events in a multivariate model that incorporated the traditional risk factors. Indeed, when 4 to 5 metabolic parameters of MetS were present, there was a 3.7-fold increase in risk for CHD and a 24.5-fold increase for diabetes compared with risk in men with none (both $P<0.0001$). The Nurses Health Study, a large prospective study of healthy female nurses, demonstrated a similar negative prognosis for those with MetS.[24] In both studies, addition of high sensitivity C-reactive protein enhanced the prognostic information seen.

The Third National Health and Nutrition Examination Survey (NHANES) showed that there is a rising incidence

Table 51-5.

Clinical Criteria for Metabolic Syndrome

1. Increased abdominal circumference
   - 40 or more inches for men (100 cm)
   - 35 or more inches for women (90 cm) (in men, may be significant 37 to 40 inches; see below)
2. Elevated Triglycerides (TG) > 150 mg/dL (> 1.7 mmol/L)
3. Low HDL-c
   - <40 mg/dL in men (<1 mmol/L)
   - <50 mg/dL in women (<1.3 mmol/L)
4. Elevated blood pressure (> 130/85 mm Hg)
5. Elevated blood glucose: > 110 mg/dL (6.1 mmol/L)

Proposed by ATP III. Three or more required for diagnosis.
Adapted from Third Report of the National Cholesterol Education Program (NCEP) Expert Panel on Detection, Evaluation, and Treatment of High Blood Cholesterol in Adults (Adult Treatment Panel III) final report. *Circulation.* 2002;106(25):3143.

of MetS with aging.[25] The unadjusted and age-adjusted prevalences are 21.8% and 23.7%, respectively, with the prevalence increasing as age increases. The prevalence was similar overall in men and women, although among African Americans and Mexican Americans, the prevalence in women exceeded that of men significantly. Many ethnic subpopulations are particularly affected by MetS. Mexican Americans had the highest prevalence: exceeding 30%.

In addition, NHANES investigators found that nonalcoholic fatty liver disease (NAFLD) is clearly linked to MetS. Indeed, their survey showed that after high alcohol consumption, hepatitis virus B, C infection, and hemochromatosis were accounted for, almost 70% of individuals with unexplained elevations of aminotransferases had features of the MetS.[26] As might be expected, the incidence of NAFLD was proportional to BMI, although multivariate analysis showed that insulin, leptin, and waist-to-hip ratio were the most important determinants. The concern, of course, is not the presence of simple steatosis (most likely not progressive) but the potential, concerning progression to nonalcoholic steatohepatitis (NASH). Although NASH has a prevalence of 2% to 3% (1/10th of NAFLD), it can advance to cirrhosis and end-stage liver disease. Not surprisingly, NASH is characterized by significant lipid abnormalities that include combined elevations of LDL-c, triglycerides, and apo B. In one controlled study of 36 subjects with NASH, as the grade of liver disease increased, lower levels of apo A1 were found.[27]

Angulo's detailed review of NAFLD noted that four factors (Table 51-6) increased the ratios for septal fibrosis or cirrhosis and these may inform the decision regarding biopsy.[28] Liver biopsy is essential for diagnosis, but may not be necessary for clinical management, especially in the early stages of MetS and low-grade transaminase abnormalities.

The primary causes of MetS are an atherogenic diet, sedentary lifestyle, and weight gain.[29] ATP III placed major emphasis on lifestyle change to help reverse the multiple metabolic risk factors. It should be emphasized that gradual and not rapid weight loss is most likely to be maintained; more importantly, some hold that rapid weight loss could aggravate the liver inflammation seen in NAFLD. Thus, two strong reasons to emphasize lifestyle change producing gradual weight loss as a primary step in the treatment of MetS is its ability to reverse all of the clinical abnormalities upon which the diagnosis made and as well as the added benefit of lowering raised aminotransferases indicative of liver steatosis.

Alcohol can cause raised aminotransferases as well as elevate levels of HDL-c. An interesting observation from a large prospective study in Kuopio, Finland indicated that a high HDL-c lost its beneficial effects in those with elevated liver enzyme activity (measured as glutamyltransferase [GGT]) in this study.[30] The risks for all cause deaths and cardiovascular and coronary events decreased with each mmol/L elevation in HDL-c in those with normal levels of GGT and decreased in those with elevated GGT levels. As expected, mean alcohol intake was higher in those with elevated GGT as compared to that of those with normal GGT levels. The author speculated that, in the presence of a raised GGT, the implication that a high HDL-c represents improved reverse cholesterol transport or anti-oxidant effects may not be justified.

Secondary Causes of High Cholesterol

A useful way to think of secondary causes of high cholesterol is to consider the "Four Ds": Diet, Diseases, Disturbances of Metabolism, and Drugs. Common causes of high cholesterol include a dietary excess of saturated fat and cholesterol, weight gain, nephrosis, diabetes, hypothyroidism, pregnancy (cholesterol goes up each trimester), and drugs such as steroids and progestins. The elevated lipids seen after transplantation can ascribed to a combination of factors including weight gain, prednisone, and diet.

The gastroenterologist should be aware that high cholesterol and planar xanthomas along with an obstructive liver pattern are characteristic of primary biliary cirrhosis (PBC). In PBC, serum cholesterol levels markedly increase with worsening of cholestasis and decrease in the late dis-

TABLE 51-6.

Factors in Nonalcoholic Fatty Liver That Increase Odds of Septal Fibrosis or Cirrhosis

- Age >45 years
- BMI >30 (wt/ht2)
- AST/ALT >1.0
- Type 2 diabetes mellitus

BMI = body mass index; AST = aspartate aminotransferase; ALT = alanine aminotransferase

Adapted from Angulo, P. Nonalcoholic fatty liver disease. *New Engl J Med.* 2002;346:1221-1231.

ease stages, despite a severe reduction in biliary secretion. A study of 400 subjects with PBC followed for a mean of 6.2 years indicated that high levels of serum cholesterol, typical of severe longstanding cholestasis, is not associated with an excess risk of cardiovascular disease, while less advanced subjects with more moderate cholesterol levels appeared to have enhanced cardiovascular risk.[31] Small studies have indicated improvements in lipids with both pravastatin[32] and simvastatin.[33] An abnormal form of LDL, identified as lipoprotein-X (Lp-X), is found in the circulation of patients with cholestatic liver disease. This is also the abnormal form found in those with lecithin-cholesterol acyl transferase deficiency. In both cases, there is an elevation in the level of circulating free cholesterol and phospholipids.

Dietary Recommendations for Patients With Dyslipidemia

An atherogenic diet and sedentary lifestyle with weight gain during the adult years underscore much of the atherogenic dyslipidemia seen. An effective approach should go beyond diet and focus on lifestyle changes that include both diet and regular exercise. ATP III called this TLC. The diet recommended by the ATP III panel was a diet that allowed total fat calories to range from 25% to 35% and was low in saturated fat,trans fatty acids, and dietary cholesterol. It emphasized higher fiber and plant stanol/sterol esters for those who needed additional LDL-c lowering from diet. The range in calories from daily fat ingestion was done to allow a lower carbohydrate and a higher unsaturated fat composition in those with MetS and diabetes. This has many of the same characteristics of the lifestyle change regimens (low in saturated fats, high in fiber, regular exercise, and calories adjusted to achieve modest weight loss) that were used successfully in the Finnish Prevention Program[34] and the Diabetes Prevention Program.[35] In both studies, the subjects were middle-aged and overweight and had impaired glucose tolerance. The results from Europe and the United States were remarkably consistent; the lifestyle regimens used in these programs reduced onset of type 2 diabetes by approximately 60%.

Trials of low carbohydrate diets show improved weight loss at 6 months, but at the end of 1 year, follow-up data do not show that they are significantly better at achieving weight loss than standard diets.[36-38] The carbohydrate restriction, however, did appear to show beneficial effects on triglycerides and HDL-c and measures of glycemia. Ornish and colleagues popularized a very low fat diet that reduced cholesterol levels and had favorable effects on coronary prevention in a small group of subjects with CHD.[39] Both of these diets may have difficulties in adherence that limit their usefulness.

A popular diet style is termed the "Mediterranean diet." This was tested in the Lyon Diet Heart Study, a randomized secondary prevention trial that compared a Mediterranean-type diet with a usual postinfarct prudent diet in 605 survivors of myocardial infarction (MI).[40,41] The striking difference in CHD events was seen at 27 months and maintained at the 46-month follow-up. This appeared to be a nonlipid effect. The intervention diet had more monounsaturated fats, more omega-3 fatty acids (there was a canola-oil based margarine rich in alpha-linolenic acid that was given), and more fiber. It was of interest that major risk factors, such as high blood cholesterol and blood pressure, continued to be independent and joint predictors of recurrence despite the beneficial effects of the Mediterranean diet.

A plant-based form of omega-3 fatty acids was utilized in the Lyon Diet Heart Study. Marine forms of omega-3 fatty acids—eicosapentanoic acid (EPA) and docosahexanoic acid (DHA)—reduce CHD mortality in survivors of MI.[42] Omega-3 fatty acids can be utilized in those with elevated triglyceride values, but only the marine forms of omega-3 fatty acids have a significant effect on lowering elevated triglyceride values.[43] In those with severe hypertriglyceridemia, the addition of fish oil to the usual therapeutic regimen can reduce excessive triglyceride levels to a safer level and reduce the risk of pancreatitis. The major GI effect from omega-3 fatty acids taken as capsules is belching and a fishy aftertaste. Keeping the fish oil refrigerated may be the best way to limit this. Those taking high concentrations of fatty acids (approximately more than 3 g/day) must be warned about an increased bleeding time and should be monitored for elevated blood sugars or a mildly increased LDL-c.

Drug Therapy for Hyperlipidemia

In brief, the major drug classes for treatment of hyperlipidemia[1,2] are HMG Coa Reductase inhibitors (statins), intestinally active drugs such as resins and cholesterol absorption inhibitors, fibric acid drugs (fibrates), and niacin (nicotinic acid). For lowering LDL-c, the statins are the drugs of choice. Statins also lower triglyceride-rich lipoproteins and raise HDL-c in variable amounts. They do not lower Lp(a).

Intestinally active drugs can augment the LDL-c lowering seen with statins and may allow attainment of LDL-c goals with moderate doses of statins for those with higher initial values of LDL-c. Resins are nonabsorbable and the toxicity of older resins such as cholestyramine and colestipol relates to significant drug interactions (eg, digoxin, diuretics, thyroid) as well as GI effects such as constipation, abdominal bloating, or aggravation of hemorrhoids especially when used in high dosages. A newer resin form, colesevelam, has fewer drug interactions than do older resins but should be taken with a large glass of water to avoid esophageal irritation. These are nonsystemic, unlike ezetimibe, a new cholesterol absorption inhibitor, that is taken up by the liver for glucuronidation but then resides in the intestine where it reduces uptake of dietary and biliary cholesterol. Side effects are usually not more likely than those seen with placebo, but a liver panel should be checked after 6 weeks, especially after it is added to a statin.

The most effective drugs for lowering high levels of triglycerides are fibrates such as gemfibrozil and fenofibrate. In a large scale clinical trial, gemfibrozil's beneficial effects on cardiovascular endpoints were much less dependent on HDL-c and triglycerides than on the presence or absence of insulin resistance.[44] Thus, fibrates are particularly useful in those with metabolic syndrome. Fenofibrate, unlike gemfibrozil, doesn't raise statin concentrations when statins and fibrates are combined, which makes fibrate-statin–induced rhabdomyolysis much less likely to occur. Niacin or nicotinic acid is the best drug for raising HDL-c. At dosages under 1500 mg/d, it is very effective in elevating HDL-c and lowering triglycerides. LDL-c is lowered as is Lp(a). In those at highest risk, combining niacin with statins or intestinally active drugs is both effective and safe.[45] Statins and niacin, however, can both cause elevated liver transaminases, and liver enzymes need to be followed more carefully in patients on either high-dose statins or lower doses of statins combined with niacin.

Since the ATP III report was published in 1991, the results from five additional large-scale, randomized trials of HMG Coa Reductase inhibitors (statins) with clinical endpoints have been reported. Important insights were gained from careful review that both confirmed and extended the current guidelines. The updated algorithm published by a writing group for the ATP III panel is summarized as follows.[46]

1. Calculate global risk to determine an overall strategy for cholesterol management.
2. Emphasize the benefits of diet, exercise, and weight control (TLC). In those with lifestyle-related risk factors such as obesity, high TG, low HDL-c, and sedentary lifestyle, a major emphasis on TLC should occur at all levels of LDL-c.
3. Use statins as first-line drugs in patients at risk to lower elevated LDL-c.
4. If used, statins should be given in doses that are lower LDL-c 30% to 40% minimally to obtain the CHD event reduction seen in clinical trials.
5. Determine in those at very high or moderately high risk if new, lower optional goals for LDL-c are reasonable.

- Very high risk defined as cardiovascular disease and either acute coronary syndrome, diabetes, metabolic syndrome or persistent, severe risk factors such as cigarette smoking.
- High risk indicates those with two or more risk factors who may merit more intensive LDL lowering; factors that inform the decision to include the lower optional LDL-c goal of < 100 mg/dL include:
    - older age
    - more than two risk factors
    - severe risk factors
    - strong family history
    - high TG/low HDL-c and MetS
    - emerging risk factors—
        - high sensitivity C-reactive protein (CRP) >3 and
        - coronary calcium score >75th percentile

6. If a high risk patient has a high TG and/or low HDL-c, consider adding a fibrate or nicotinic acid to an LDL-lowering drug. (This should be done carefully considering the increased risks of therapy when two drugs for abnormal lipids are given.)
7. Continue to treat those at low risk in similar fashion as before. This is an important point worthy of reemphasis. The only individuals for whom the clinical trial data suggested optional, lower LDL-c goals were in those at highest risk for a CHD event.

The ATP III writing group noted that several other informative large-scale trials are still on-going and look specifically at the question of lowering LDL-c to lower levels. Authoritative opinions, then, about how low to get LDL-c should await this important information that will be forthcoming over the next few years.

Conclusion

This brief chapter reviews lipid metabolism with a consideration of genetic, disease-related, lifestyle, and medication factors that are important for clinical decisions, particularly from the standpoint of the gastroenterologist.

References

1. Stone NJ, Blum CB. *Management of Lipids in Clinical Practice*. 4th ed. Caddo, OK: Professional Communications, Inc; 2002.
2. Third Report of the National Cholesterol Education Program (NCEP) Expert Panel on Detection, Evaluation, and Treatment of High Blood Cholesterol in Adults (Adult Treatment Panel III) final report. *Circulation*. 2002;106(25):3143-421.
3. Altmann SW, Davis HR Jr, Zhu LJ, et al. Niemann-Pick C1 Like 1 protein is critical for intestinal cholesterol absorption. *Science*. 2004;303(5661):1201-4.
4. Berge KE, Tian H, Graf GA, et al. Accumulation of dietary cholesterol in sitosterolemia caused by mutations in adjacent ABC transporters. *Science*. 2000;290:1771-1775.
5. Rader DJ, Cohen J, Hobbs HH. Monogenic hypercholesterolemia: new insights in pathogenesis and treatment. *J Clin Invest*. 2003;111(12):1795-803.
6. Goldstein JL, Brown MS. Molecular medicine. The cholesterol quartet. *Science*. 2001;292(5520):1310-2.
7. Couture P, Morissette J, Gaudet D, et al. Fine mapping of low-density lipoprotein receptor gene by genetic linkage on chromosome 19p13.1-p13.3 and study of the founder effect of four French Canadian low-density lipoprotein receptor gene mutations. *Atherosclerosis*. 1999;143(1):145-51.
8. Sibley C, McGann S, Stone N. Long-term survival of childhood coronary artery disease in a patient severely affected with familial hypercholesterolemia. *Am J Cardiol*. 2004;94(5):699-700.
9. Weisgraber KH, Innerarity T, Newhouse YM, et al. Familial defective apolipoprotein B-100: enhanced binding of monoclonal antibody MB47 to abnormal low density lipoproteins. *Proc Natl Acad Sci U S A*. 1988;85(24):9758–9762.
10. Pullinger CR, Kane JP, Malloy MJ. Primary hypercholesterolemia: genetic causes and treatment of five monogenic disorders. *Expert Rev Cardiovasc Ther*. 2003;1(1):107-19.
11. Soutar K, Naoumova RP, Traub LM. Genetics, clinical phenotype, and molecular cell biology of autosomal recessive hypercholesterolemia. *Arterioscler Thromb Vasc Biol*. 2003;23(11):1963-1970.
12. Hazzard WR, Goldstein JL, Schrott MG, Motulsky AG, Bierman EL. Hyperlipidemia in coronary heart disease. 3. Evaluation of lipoprotein phenotypes of 156 genetically defined survivors of myocardial infarction. *J Clin Invest*. 1973;52(7):1569-77.
13. Mar R, Pajukanta P, Allayee H, et al. Association of the APOLIPOPROTEIN A1/C3/A4/A5 gene cluster with triglyceride levels and LDL particle size in familial combined hyperlipidemia. *Circ Res*. 2004;94(7):993-9.
14. Sprecher DL, Harris BV, Stein EA, Bellet PS, Keilson LM, Simbartl LA. Higher triglycerides, lower high-density lipoprotein cholesterol, and higher systolic blood pressure in lipoprotein lipase-deficient heterozygotes. A preliminary report. *Circulation*. 1996;94(12):3239-45.
15. Mahley RW, Huang Y, Rall SC Jr. Pathogenesis of type III hyperlipoproteinemia (dysbetalipoproteinemia). Questions, quandaries, and paradoxes. *J Lipid Res*. 1999;40(11):1933-49.
16. Hopkins PN, Heiss G, Ellison RC, et al. Coronary artery disease risk in familial combined hyperlipidemia and familial hypertriglyceridemia: a case-control comparison from the National Heart, Lung, and Blood Institute Family Heart Study. *Circulation*. 2003;108(5):519-23.
17. Mott S, Yu L, Marcil M, Boucher B, Rondeau C, Genest J Jr. Decreased cellular cholesterol efflux is a common cause of familial hypoalphalipoproteinemia: role of the ABCA1 gene mutations. *Atherosclerosis*. 2000;152(2):457-68.
18. Frikke-Schmidt R, Nordestgaard BG, Jensen GB, Tybjaerg Hansen A. Genetic variation in ABC transporter A1 contributes to HDL cholesterol in the general population. *J Clin Invest*. 2004;114(9):1343-1353.
19. Clee SM, Zwinderman AH, Engert JC, et al. Common genetic variation in ABCA1 is associated with altered lipoprotein levels and a modified risk for coronary artery disease. *Circulation*. 2001;103(9):1198-205.
20. Ginsberg, H. Insulin resistance and cardiovascular disease. *J Clin Invest*. 2000;106:453-458.
21. McLaughlin T, Abbasi F, Cheal K, Chu J, Lamendola C, Reaven G. Use of metabolic markers to identify overweight individuals who are insulin resistant. *Ann Intern Med*. 2003;139(10):802-9.
22. Lemieux I, Pascot A, Couillard C, et al. Hypertriglyceridemic waist: A marker of the atherogenic metabolic triad (hyperinsulinemia; hyperapolipoprotein B; small, dense LDL) in men? *Circulation*. 2000;102(2):179-84.
23. Sattar N, Gaw A, Scherbakova O, et al. Metabolic syndrome with and without C-reactive protein as a predictor of coronary heart disease and diabetes in the West of Scotland Coronary Prevention Study. *Circulation*. 2003;108(4):414-9.
24. Ridker PM, Buring JE, Cook NR, et al. C-reactive protein, the metabolic syndrome, and risk of incident cardiovascular events: an 8-year follow-up of 14 719 initially healthy American women. *Circulation*. 2003;107:391-397.
25. Ford ES, Giles WH, Dietz WH. Prevalence of the metabolic syndrome among US adults: findings from the third National Health and Nutrition Examination Survey. *JAMA*. 2002;287(3):356-9.
26. Ruhl CE, Everhart JE. Determinants of the association of overweight with elevated serum alanine aminotransferase activity in the United States. *Gastroenterology*. 2003;124(1):71-9.
27. Koruk M, Savas MC, Yilmaz O, et al. Serum lipids, lipoproteins and apolipoproteins levels in patients with nonalcoholic steatohepatitis. *J Clin Gastroenterol*. 2003;37(2):177–182.
28. Angulo P. Nonalcoholic fatty liver disease. *New Engl J Med*. 2002;346;1221-1231.
29. Grundy SM. Atherogenic dyslipidemia: lipoprotein abnormalities and implications for therapy. *Am J Cardiol*. 1995;75 (Suppl 1):45B-52.
30. Salonen JT. Liver damage and protective lipoprotein cholesterol *BMJ*. 2003;327:1082–3.
31. Longo M, Crosignani A, Battezzati PM, et al. Hyperlipidaemic state and cardiovascular risk in primary biliary cirrhosis. *Gut*. 2002;51(2):265-9.
32. Kurihara T, Akimoto M, Abe K, et al. Experimental use of pravastatin in patients with primary biliary cirrhosis associated with hypercholesterolemia. *Clin Ther*. 1993;15(5):890-8.
33. Del Puppo M, Galli Kienle M, Crosignani A, et al. Cholesterol metabolism in primary biliary cirrhosis during simvastatin and UDCA administration. *J Lipid Res*. 2001;42:437-441.
34. Diabetes Prevention Program Research Group. Reduction in the Incidence of Type 2 Diabetes with Lifestyle Intervention or Metformin. *N Engl J Med*. 2002;346:393-403.
35. Tuomilehto J, Lindstrom J, Eriksson JG, et al. Finnish Diabetes Prevention Program Prevention of type 2 diabetes mellitus by changes in lifestyle among subjects with impaired glucose tolerance. *N Engl J Med*. 2001;344(18):1343-50.
36. Foster GD, Wyatt HR, Hill JO, et al. A randomized trial of a low-carbohydrate diet for obesity. *N Engl J Med*. 2003;348(21):2082-90.
37. Samaha FF, Iqbal N, Seshadri P, et al. A low-carbohydrate as compared with a low-fat diet in severe obesity. *N Engl J Med*. 2003;348(21):2074-81.
38. Stern L, Iqbal N, Seshadri P, et al. The effects of low-carbohydrate versus conventional weight loss diets in severely obese adults: one-year follow-up of a randomized trial. *Ann Intern Med*. 2004;140(10):778-85.
39. Ornish D, Scherwitz LW, Billings JH, et al. Intensive lifestyle changes for reversal of coronary heart disease. *JAMA*. 1998;280(23):2001.

40. de Lorgeril M, Salen P, Martin JL, Monjaud I, Delaye J, Mamelle N. Mediterranean diet, traditional risk factors, and the rate of cardiovascular complications after myocardial infarction: final report of the Lyon Diet Heart Study. *Circulation*. 1999;99(6):779-85.
41. de Lorgeril M, Salen P. Alpha-linolenic acid and coronary heart disease. *Nutr Metab Cardiovasc Dis*. 2004;14(3):162-9.
42. Marchioli R, Barzi F, Bomba E, et al. GISSI-Prevenzione Investigators. Early protection against sudden death by n-3 polyunsaturated fatty acids after myocardial infarction: time-course analysis of the results of the Gruppo Italiano per lo Studio della Sopravvivenza nell'Infarto Miocardico (GISSI)-Prevenzione. *Circulation*. 2002;105(16):1897-903.
43. Kris-Etherton PM, Harris WS, Appel LJ. American Heart Association Nutrition Committee. Fish consumption, fish oil, omega-3 fatty acids, and cardiovascular disease. *Circulation*. 2002;19;106(21):2747-57.
44. Robins SJ, Rubins HB, Faas FH, et al. Insulin resistance and cardiovascular events with low HDL cholesterol: the Veterans Affairs HDL Intervention Trial (VA-HIT). *Diabetes Care*. 2003;23(5):1513.
45. Miller, M. Niacin as a component of combination therapy for dyslipidemia. *Mayo Clin Proc*. 2003;78:735-742.
46. Grundy SM, Cleeman JI, Merz CN, et al. Implications of recent clinical trials for the National Cholesterol Education Program Adult Treatment Panel III Guidelines. *Circulation*. 2004;110(2):227-39.

Chapter 52

MANAGEMENT OF CHILDHOOD OBESITY

Robert Suskind, MD

Introduction

According to the National Health and Nutrition Survey III (NHANES III), obesity in American children ages 12 to 19 years increased from 15% in 1985 to 21% in 1995. Today, over 27% of children under 12 years of age are obese, indicating a 54% increase in obesity in the United States within the past 20 years. Of this increase, the super-obese (greater than 50% overweight) are becoming even heavier. Unless intervention is successful, these children and adolescents will contribute to the 35% of adult Americans who are currently obese. The related disease risks in children include diabetes mellitus, hypertension, heart disease, stroke, gout, arthritis, and cancer. The primary causes, experts agree, are excessive intake and decreased activity levels.

Pediatric obesity is a serious chronic disease that is associated with hypertension, hypercholesterolemia, diabetes, and an increased incidence of musculoskeletal injuries.[1-9] Recent studies suggest that obese children and adolescents are at increased risk for future cardiovascular disease.[6] Furthermore, children may be severely psychologically affected because of being obese. Obese children often have lowered self-esteem and increased depression ratings.[10]

Lifestyle Changes for Weight Loss

Traditional treatment of obesity—including changes in lifestyle through modification of behavior, nutrition, education, and increases in exercise—have resulted in limited success in adult populations.[11] However, the prevention of adult obesity by targeting children and their parents may provide the best solution to the increasing prevalence of obesity.[11] Research indicates that obese children are better able to maintain weight loss over a long-term period than are obese adults.[22] Therefore, addressing obesity in an overweight child and establishing healthy eating and exercise habits early in his or her life can affect that individual's future struggle with obesity.

Programs to treat obesity in childhood are not commonly available and, when available, are usually unsuccessful in preparing these younger patients to maintain their weight loss. This may be because lifestyles that contributed to the development of the participants' obesity were not effectively altered. With an increase in the prevalence of obesity, it will be important to develop effective treatment programs that will promote the long-term health benefits associated with achieving and maintaining one's ideal body weight (IBW).

Treatment for pediatric patients is currently through weight-loss programs. Multidisciplinary weight-loss programs integrate medical supervision, dietary restriction, nutrition education, physical activity, behavior modification, and family lifestyle-change components.[21-23] This chapter discusses these components as well as studies—with emphasis on one program in particular—that show success in addressing obesity in children. Many of the recommended lifestyle changes discussed have been established in this particular program, "Committed to Children."

MEDICAL SUPERVISION

Obesity-related lifestyle changes are a necessity for any overweight individual; however, leaving that patient on his or her own to learn and accomplish these changes does not encourage success. Supervision and accountability are necessary. No diet or exercise regimen should be induced without medical advice, be that from the child's pediatrician or from a dietician. Children and their parents must be taught why and how to make the changes discussed below and then coached through the process so that misconceptions can be corrected promptly. Additionally, follow-up after the weight loss—specifically continued contact with the clinic staff—may be a key factor in the maintenance of weight loss in obesity-treatment programs.

Dietary Restriction

The National Task Force on the Prevention and Treatment of Obesity noted that very-low–calorie diets (VLCDs) are generally safe when used under proper medical supervision in moderately and severely obese patients.[13] VLCDs are also considered safe for obese pediatric patients with medical supervision. The diets are usually effective in promoting significant short-term weight loss, with a concomitant improvement in obesity-related conditions; however, long-term maintenance of weight loss with VLCDs alone is not satisfactory and is no better than other forms of obesity treatment. The Task Force did note that the incorporation of behavioral therapy and physical activity into VLCD treatment programs appeared to improve weight-loss maintenance.[13]

Protein-sparing modified fast (PSMF) is a weight-loss diet that is also safe for children, provided they are closely monitored by a physician. The diet promotes rapid weight loss (1 kg/week), minimizes hunger, preserves lean body mass, has no adverse psychological consequences, and allows for normal growth and activity. The PSMF diet typically provides 600 to 800 kcal/day, consisting of animal protein (2 g/kg protein up to 100 g/day) with small amounts of carbohydrate and added vitamins and minerals (Table 52-1).

PSMF, used in conjunction with a multidisciplinary program, has been shown effective in the treatment of childhood and adolescent obesity. The initial studies demonstrating the safety and effectiveness of PSMF were first published by Merritt et al during 1980-1983.[24-26] They found that, within a metabolic unit, PSMF was effective, safe, and simple and provided preservation of lean body mass. Subsequent studies yielded similar results in the adolescent population.[27-29] Stallings and colleagues[30] treated 17 obese adolescents with a PSMF diet. At a 1-year follow-up examination of 12 (71%) subjects, 48% had maintained a weight loss. Brown and colleagues[31] treated 8 severely obese adolescents for 5 months with a liquid-protein diet. Initial weight loss was 20% to 25% of body weight. At 1-year follow-up, 5 of the 8 subjects (62%) were evaluated, and 2 (25%) had maintained weight loss.

Nutrition Education

While diet is important, patients and their families must understand the diet and comprehend what makes it successful. Pediatric patients must learn about the Food Guide Pyramid, a standardized guide to what foods should be consumed and in what quantity each day. They must be instructed on how to choose healthy alternatives to prepackaged and "fast" foods.

Physical Activity

Year 2000 health objectives for the United States[32] included, as a priority for youth and adults, an increase in daily physical activity and a decrease in sedentary lifestyles. These recommendations should lead to both increased cardiovascular fitness and enhanced cardiovascular risk profiles.

It is clear that physical activity is important in the prevention and treatment of obesity in children.[33,34] One rationale for promoting physical activity in childhood is to establish long-term lifestyle patterns of regular activity that can be maintained.[35] Inactivity, with decreased energy expenditure and increased diet density, plays a major role in the development of childhood obesity.[36,37]

The role of physical activity in weight-loss programs for children and adolescents has been the subject of several studies. Epstein et al[38] and Reybrouck et al[39] found greater weight loss when exercise was combined with a low-calorie diet versus dietary treatment alone. Increased physical activity has been shown to decrease adiposity in obese populations.[40] In addition, obese children were observed as typically less active than were their nonobese counterparts.[38] Taylor and Baranowski[41] concluded that children with lower adiposity had higher physical activity scores than did those with higher adiposity levels.

A structured exercise program, combined with a PSMF diet and behavior modification, has a positive impact on body composition, and exercise may positively affect the ratio of fat-free body mass (FFB) to fat.[42-44] A previous study reported resting energy expenditure (REE) and body composition in 10 children after weight loss.[45] Despite being on a VLCD, there was no significant decrease in REE. When these values were compared to normal ranges for height and weight, the REE was actually higher after 10 weeks of intervention. (This study is discussed below.) The increase in FFB is the most likely explanation for the increase in energy expenditure. Increases in height must also be taken into consideration when analyzing increases in FFB. These results are promising because they suggest an important effect of exercise on REE during severe caloric restriction.[45]

Another study, discussed below, concluded that integrating activity into the daily routine had better long-term weight-loss outcomes than did structured aerobic-activity programs.[48] In addition to a prescribed exercise program, subjects were shown different methods of increasing their level of activity on a daily basis. Brisk walking to and from their homes and schools and walking between classes were encouraged and shown to be an important means of increasing daily energy expenditure. The energy cost in calories of being seated versus standing and walking was discussed.[18] Research has suggested a need to develop effective interventions and to explore the impact of physical activity on weight reduction and body composition.[37]

Behavior Modification

Varni and Banis[49] outlined behavioral techniques currently utilized in the modification of eating, exercise, and diet patterns in childhood obesity to achieve the goal of altering antecedents and consequences of health behaviors. Applicable behavior-modification components for children have included self-monitoring of diet and activity,

Table 52-1.
Protein-Sparing Modified Fast and Foods Allowed

PSMF Requirements

600 to 800 kcal/day
1.5 to 2.0 g protein/kg IBW/day to 100 g protein/day (7 g protein/30 g of meat, fish or fowl)
Low-starch vegetables
Water or calorie-free fluids at least 2 L/day
Daily supplements: calcium—800 mg/day; potassium—25 meq/day; multivitamins with minerals

Foods Allowed

Protein

Lean beef (fat trimmed and unmarbled) such as a roast, steak, ground round (hamburger)
Chicken, turkey (remove skin)
Fish (if canned, water-packed)
Seafood, such as shrimp, lobster, oysters, clams

Vegetables—serving size, 4 oz (120 g)

okra	artichokes	cabbage	beets	radishes	sauerkraut	onion	eggplant
cauliflower	spinach	squash	chicory	carrots	mushrooms	tomato	asparagus
rhubarb	watercress	vegetable juice	brussel sprouts		bamboo shoots	broccoli	tomato juice

Vegetables—serving size, 8 oz (240 g)

lettuce	endive	chard	cabbage	spinach	dandelion greens
romaine	mushrooms	celery	turnip greens	zucchini	cucumber
hot pepper	green onions	collard greens	mustard greens	kohlrabi	Chinese cabbage

Free Food

tea	rennet	clear broth	lime	mustard	lemon	pepper	catsup*
bouillon	coffee	vinegar	diet sodas	artificial sweetener		gelatin (unsweetened)	
BBQ sauce*	salt	spices	low-cal salad dressing			dill and sour pickles	

Foods to Avoid

oil	liver	flour, cornmeal	cold cuts	fried food	nuts	sugar	sausage
eggs	avocado	peanut butter	cream	cheese	mayonnaise	cereal	pork
fruits	breads	margarine	milk	butter	wieners	olives	starchy vegetables
bacon	candy	regular chewing gum					

*limit intake to 1 Tbs/day

goal setting, stimulus control, cue examination, behavioral substitution, and the development of alternatives to overeating.[10] Coates and others have demonstrated the effectiveness of behavioral techniques, such as token economies in children.[50-52] Other investigators[21,53-55] have focused on the role of parental involvement. Booster sessions, monetary contracting, ongoing support groups, and mail and telephone contacts have also been evaluated as maintenance techniques, with mixed results.[56,57]

Family Lifestyle Changes

Epstein and others[46-48] examined the impact of parental involvement on the long-term effectiveness of a family-based treatment program for childhood obesity. They found that targeting both the parent and the child during treatment resulted in lower relative weights for those children after 5 and 10 years than those for children treated without their parents. Furthermore, a greater percentage of children in the parent-plus-child treatment group achieved or approached normal weight-for-height than did children treated without their parents.

There is some evidence that parental obesity may negatively affect children's physical activity. Family-based programs in which parents were trained to reinforce their children's physical activity have increased both activity levels and fitness in obese children.[46-48] Parental involvement at home and in education sessions improve a child's compliance and overall success.

Family intervention can assist with an obese child's success. Involving the parents by educating them on various techniques—such as cue elimination, goal setting, and limit setting—can assist parents and subjects in controlling eating patterns. In one program, patients and their parents attended weekly sessions that included discussion of positive, family lifestyle alterations that promoted the individuals' weight loss.[10]

Maintenance of Weight Loss

A major challenge faced by individuals who lose weight is maintaining their weight loss. Multifaceted maintenance programs, with continued counseling during the maintenance period to address specific problems, appear promising.[57-59] The results are difficult to interpret, however, because of different treatment regimens, sample sizes, study populations, and evaluation techniques. Evaluation of group mean weight loss can be misleading because of large individual variations in weight loss and gain.[43,48,60-62]

Recently, Figueroa-Colon et al found that weight loss (expressed as a decrease in weight/height ratio) achieved by obese children on PSMF could be maintained for 14.5 months.[63] Kayman and coworkers[61] examined exercise habits, coping skills, and social support of obese females who had maintained weight loss or relapsed after weight loss. They found that maintainers, in contrast to relapsers, exercised regularly, used social support, and developed specific problem-solving skills.

From existing literature, it is apparent that a variety of effective obesity-treatment programs for adults do exist. In a recent review, however, Brownell and Wadden calculated that, during the year following treatment, participants regained, on average, 36% of the weight they had lost.[64] The challenge remains to develop and implement a culture-specific obesity-intervention program that promotes long-term lifestyle changes, including healthy eating, exercise, and behavior modification, and create this for obese children and adolescents.

Growth

In an evaluation of growth patterns in children treated for obesity, Epstein and coworkers,[23] after 5 years of follow-up, found that no negative long-term effects on height occurred because of childhood weight control. These results took into account both parental height and the increased height of obese children.

Lipid Changes

Weight changes in children have been associated with significant reductions in serum cholesterol and triglycerides (TG) and an increase in high-density lipoprotein cholesterol (HDL-c).[58] In one study, significant reductions were observed in total cholesterol and TG. In addition, in a subgroup of 8 subjects analyzed for HDL-c and low-density lipoprotein cholesterol (LDL-c) concentrations, there were significant decreases in LDL-c and maintenance of HDL-c, probably due to the combined effects of PSMF and the modified progress exercise program (MPEP).

The "Committed to Kids" Pediatric Weight-Management Program

As stated above, there is a shortage of obesity-treatment programs for pediatric and adolescent patients. One program, however, has proven successful and is being used as a model for other institutions and similar programs.

The Program

The "Committed to Kids" Pediatric Weight-Management Program was developed over a 12-year period by members of the Department of Pediatrics, Louisiana State University, and the Children's Hospital of New Orleans. The 1-year, four-phase program is an individualized program conducted in a group setting that is structured to the specific needs of children of varying levels of obesity: mild, moderate, and severe. A medical-treatment team consisting of a pediatrician, registered dietician, exercise physiologist, and a psychologist meet once per week with obese children and their families to discuss nutrition, exercise, and overall health. The children are placed on a structured diet and exercise plan and are provided with nutrition education, fitness education, and behavior modification during each weekly session. The program has also been successfully reproduced in other clinical settings in the state of Louisiana. The Earl K. Long Hospital in Baton Rouge and the University Medical Center in Lafayette have successfully treated obese children and adolescents, with results similar to the New Orleans-based program.[14]

Related Study

A short-term, clinical-outcome trial using the "Committed to Kids" program was conducted in two locations, with repeated measurements at 10 and 36 weeks. In addition to program-specific data, investigators recorded anthropometric, metabolic, and biochemical parameters in a before and after comparison of participants in these multidisciplinary weight-management intervention programs for obese children and adolescents. Fifty subjects (17 males, 33 females) who were 7 to 17 years of age (mean age: 12.4 years) were enrolled in a weight-reduction program at Children's Hospital of New Orleans (n = 34) (cohorts 1 and 2) for 36 weeks and at the General Clinical Research Center (GCRC) at the Medical Center of Louisiana (n = 16) (cohort 3) for a 10-week, summer, weight-reduction program (Table 52-2). Subjects entered the program in cohorts of approximately 12 to 20 children quarterly over a 1-year period. Subjects and legal guardians read and signed the consent form and provided comprehensive medical histories prior to beginning the program.

Participants were stratified into three categories of obesity for differential exercise prescriptions: severely obese, >200% IBW; moderately obese, 150% to 199% IBW; and mildly obese, 120% to 149% IBW. Subjects were placed

TABLE 52-2.

Physical Characteristics of Subjects in "Committed to Kids" Program

	Children's Hospital of New Orleans	GCRC
Subjects (n)	34	16
Ages (years)	11.7±2.6	11.4±3.1
Gender	17 female, 17 male	16 female, 0 male
Ethnicity	21 white, 13 black	16 black
Height (cm)	155.5±13.1	151.5±17.6
Weight (kg)	85.4±25.4	84.2±31.7
Percent IBW	179.8±28.5	177.1±40.8

Values denoted as mean ±SD

on a PSMF diet (see Table 52-1) and were instructed to obtain morning urine samples for ketones. Ketone records were checked weekly for compliance. Dietary and behavior-modification intervention remained standard for all three groups.

Subjects were also assigned to one of three phases according to their degrees of obesity: phase I for the severely obese, phase II for the moderately obese, and phase III for the mildly obese. Each child was given a weight goal that was 120% of his or her IBW (ie, 20% above ideal weight/height ratio). Anthropometric (height and weight) and body composition (skin-fold to determine relative fat and FFB) assessments were performed at baseline, 10 weeks, and every 3 months thereafter in all of the subjects. After their baseline measurements were recorded, subjects began attending weekly outpatient education sessions that covered topics in nutrition, behavior modification, exercise/fitness, and medical issues related to obesity.

In addition to a 30- to 40-minute weekly session, subjects were given a MPEP to be performed at home, designed according to each participant's degree of obesity. This home-based program included moderate intensity (45% to 55% $V0_2$max) aerobic, strength, and flexibility exercises, which gradually increased in duration (time per session) and frequency (sessions per week) through the 10th week of the program.[17,18] Specific recommendations, however, were given for duration, frequency, and intensity of the exercise.[18] Strength and flexibility exercises, designed especially for this population, were simple and easy to execute.[17] Each subject maintained an exercise record that listed the frequency, duration, and type of exercise as well as the patient's perceived exertion and heart rates; the record was checked weekly by the exercise physiologist. Incentive awards were given for consistent reporting of ketones and exercise patterns and for overall compliance with the weight-loss program.

Each patient underwent a variety of evaluation tests at enrollment (baseline) and again after 10 weeks of participation in the program. Tests run included assessment of triglycerides (TG), total cholesterol (TC), high-density lipoprotein (HDL), and low-density lipoprotein (LDL). Complete blood count and sequential multiple analysis 12 chemical analyses were also performed to determine the impact of weight reduction on biochemical and hematological parameters. In addition, the subjects from cohort 3 (the short-term summer program at the GCRC) had samples drawn for insulin-like growth factor-1 (IGF-1), tri-iodothyronine (T3), and thyroid-stimulating hormone (TSH).

After attending for 10 weeks, a subject graduates to the next phase of the program. Phase III (mildly overweight) subjects moved into the long-term maintenance phase (phase IV) of the program. Subjects continued to attend weekly exercise sessions with bi-monthly, multi-topic meetings on nutrition and behavior modification. They were instructed to continue the home-based exercise program. Phase II (moderately overweight) subjects graduated into Phase III of the program and followed appropriate exercise guidelines. Phase I (severely overweight) subjects, likewise, graduated into Phase II. Subjects were given the option to remain on the PSMF diet at the completion of the initial 10 weeks. Twenty-two of the long-term subjects remained on PSMF for 15-, 20-, 25-, or 30-week intervals. All other subjects were instructed to adhere to a 1200-cal balanced-diet regime following the American Dietetic Association guidelines for up to 36 weeks.

The Children's Hospital study (cohorts 1 and 2) included children who were Caucasian, African-American, and Hispanic (see Table 52-2). Their socioeconomic status was middle to upper income. The GCRC (cohort 3) subjects were African-American female children who came from lower-income families. All subjects, as determined by self-reporting, were sedentary prior to entry into the program.

STUDY RESULTS

Forty of the original 50 subjects completed the initial 10-weeks of the program. At the time of the data analysis, only 20 subjects (cohorts 1 and 2) had completed 26 weeks and only 10 subjects (cohort 1) had completed 36 weeks of the study. The attendance rate for the short-term phase (10 weeks) was 90%; for the long-term phase (36 weeks), it decreased to 75%. This was partially due to transportation, school, and sport-club conflict. Attendance also decreased once the child's weight decreased to less than 120% IBW.

All subjects reported 100% compliance with the exercise program and experienced no problems with the combination of this program and the PSMF diet. In addi-

Table 52-3.

Comparison of Serum Cholesterol and Triglycerides of Study Participants

Variable (mg/dL)	n	Baseline	10 weeks
Cholesterol*	23	175.0 ± 26.0	160.0 ± 30.0
TG*	23	103.0 ± 53.0	72.0 ± 30.0
LDL-C†	8	114.0 ± 22.8	90.0 ± 25.0
HDL-C‡	8	41.4 ± 12.7	39.3 ± 13.8

Baseline and 10-week values denoted as mean ±SD
* <0.0001
† <0.05
‡ nonsignificant

Table 52-4.

Biochemical Parameters Before and After the PSMF Diet

	n	Baseline*	10 Weeks*
Hemoglobin (g%)	21	13.1 ± 1.0	13.3 ±1.1
MCV	20	83.6 ± 5.3	82.9 ± 5.1
Lymphocyte counts (cells/mm3)	20	2577.0 ± 731	2389.0 ± 704.0
Total protein (g/dL)	23	7.4 ± 0.5	7.3 ± 0.5
Albumin (g/dL)	23	4.4 ± 0.4	4.4 ± 0.4
Blood urea nitrogen (mg/dL)	23	10.4 ± 2.8	11.4 ± 3.0
Potassium (mmol/L)	23	4.2 ± 0.3	4.03 ± 0.3
Sodium (mmol/L)	23	139.8 ± 2.6	139.4 ± 1.8
Calcium (mg/dL)	23	9.6 ± 0.3	9.9 ± 0.5
Phosphate (mg/dL)	23	4.4 ± 0.6	4.3 ± 0.6
AST (u/L)	23	25.1 ± 8.6	21.7 ± 5.2
ALT (u/L)	23	26.0 ± 14	24.0 ± 12.0
LDH (u/L)	22	425.7 ± 178	391.2 ± 168.0

* Mean ± SD
IGF-1, T3, and TSH

tion, although the exercise intensity was set at a moderate level (45% to 55% $V0_2$max), it was of sufficient duration, frequency, and intensity to promote a significant increase in estimated VO_2max. This and weight-loss observations combined suggest an overall improvement in participants' physical fitness with use of the MPEP during the program.

Each participant underwent a series of tests at baseline and 10 weeks to determine the affects of participation in this program on his or her health. Group results from these tests are presented in Tables 52-3 and 52-4. Even after this short term on the PSMF diet and complying with the MPEP, the children's test results showed improvements in a number of their health assessments. Significant increases were noted in mean scores in adjusted values of estimated aerobic capacity in a group of 17 subjects tested after the 10-week intervention (Figure 52-1). There was a significant increase in mean IGF-1 values, with all subjects (Figure 52-2) experiencing an increase in their fasting IGF-1 levels after the 10-week program. T3 and the percentage of T3 resin uptake were significantly reduced after the 10-week intervention.

Growth velocity was within normal limits for cohort 3 after 10 weeks. Although cohort 2 had a reduction in height velocity at 10 weeks, this was reversed at 26 weeks with a significant increase in height velocity. There was no significant overall decrease in height velocity during the course of the study.

Statistical analysis consisted of a repeated-measures analysis of variance (ANOVA) and paired Student's t-tests.

An average weight loss of 9 kg was observed in the 40 subjects from cohorts 1, 2, and 3 who completed the initial 10-week phase of the program (Figure 52-3). Subjects from cohort 3 were not followed after 10 weeks. Weight loss was maintained at 26 weeks in cohorts 1 and 2. In cohort 1, weight loss was maintained through 36 weeks of the program. In addition, there was a significant decrease in the percentage of body fat (Figure 52-4), with significant increases reported in FFB (Figure 52-5) in the sub-group of 17 subjects. At 36 weeks, cohort 1 (n = 10) experienced no significant change in weight, percent of IBW, or relative body fat (percent of fat). Fewer subjects were available for these specific body-composition measures at 36 weeks; however, those tested were representative of the total group.

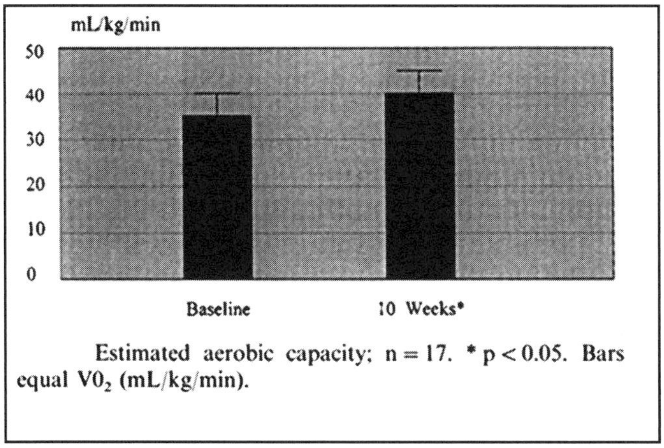

Figure 52-1. Comparison of body composition. FFB; n = 17; *p <0.05.

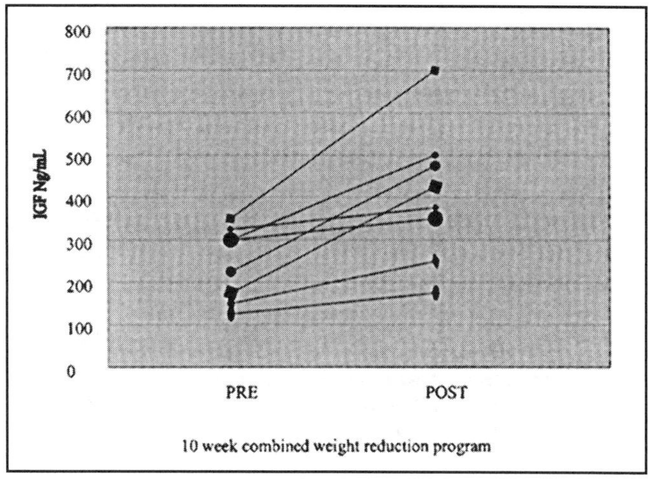

Figure 52-2. Estimated aerobic capacity; n = 17. *p <0.05. Bars equal VO_2 (mL/kg/minute).

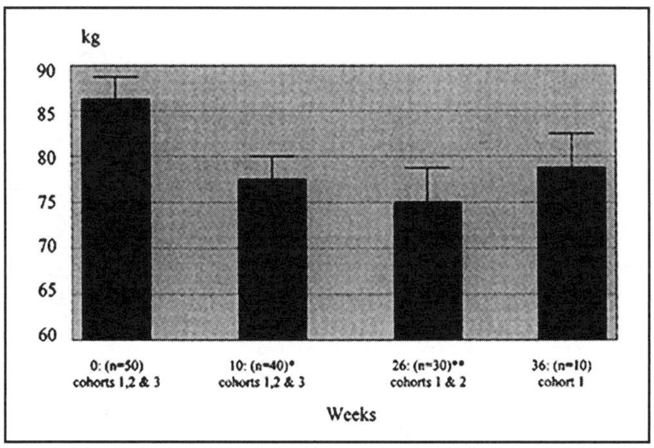

Figure 52-3. Fasting serum IGF-1. Changes after 10 weeks of PSFM, behavior modification, and MPEP.

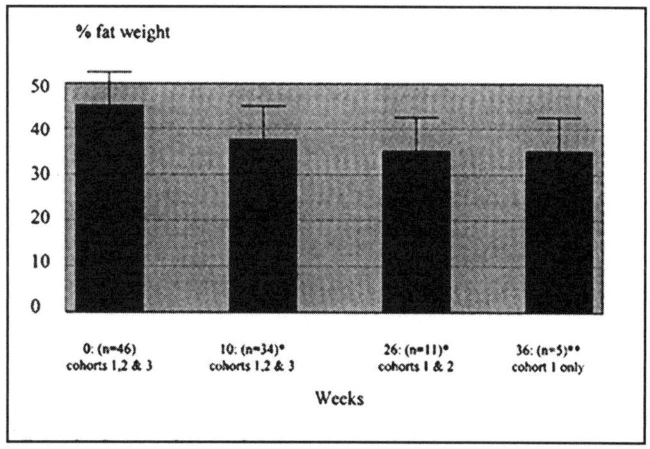

Figure 52-4. Comparison of weight changes during program. *p <0.0001; ** not significant from 10-week measurement. Cohort 3 was not followed beyond the 10-week summer weight-loss program.

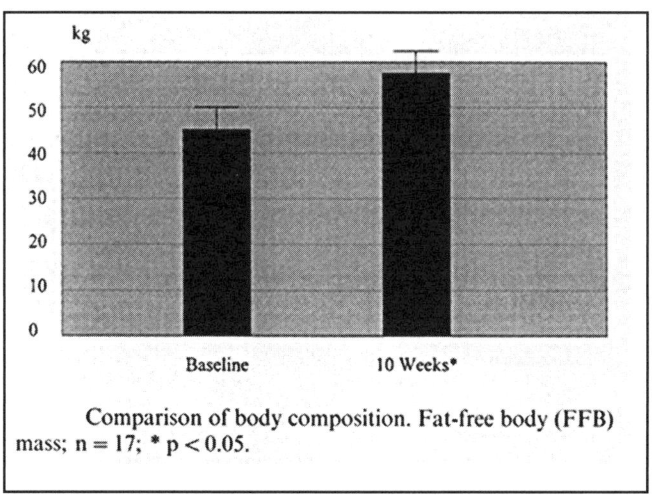

Figure 52-5. Comparison of body-composition relative fat (%). *p <0.0001; ** not significant from 26-week measurement. Cohort 3 was not followed beyond the 10-week summer weight-loss program.

In this study, 77% of the Children's Hospital subjects maintained weight loss, with a significant improvement in body composition after 36 weeks. All subjects completing the initial 10-week phase maintained weight loss at 36 weeks. Several of the subjects continued on the PSMF diet for 5 to 20 additional weeks; these subjects reported no adverse symptoms or medical problems during this extended period. The majority of the attrition was seen during the first 10 weeks of this study. Dropouts were from lower-income backgrounds where parental involvement and support were inadequate.

The approach through this program has a short-term success rate of 95% and a 1-year success rate of 70% to 75%.[14] Preliminary data in 85% of subjects reporting after 5 years indicate that participating children maintain an average weight loss of 31%.[15] In the younger children and those with mild obesity at program entry, the success rate is even higher.[16]

Conclusion

The prevalence of pediatric obesity is increasing in the United States. As a result, children and adolescents are suffering from this chronic disease and related psychological issues and comorbidities—including hypertension, hypercholesterolemia, and diabetes—and at younger ages.[6] Addressing pediatric obesity requires educating the children and their families on healthy eating and exercise habits. Programs for pediatric weight loss are not common; many more need to be established if Americans are to avoid obesity in their children. These programs need to integrate medical supervision, dietary restriction, nutrition education, physical activity, behavior modification, and family lifestyle-change components.

One program has been established, used as a model in several institutions, and is continuing to report success (long- and short-term) in pediatric patients. The multidisciplinary, four-phase approach, which includes PSMF, is successful in treating mild, moderate, and severe degrees of childhood and adolescent obesity. The program has reported success in children's weight loss and maintenance, as well as in improving participant's health as indicated by assessments of metabolic functions. Additional studies of this and other programs as well as of pediatric obesity in general are needed if the present epidemic is to be dealt with effectively.

References

1. Pongprapai S, Mo-suwan L, Leelasamran W. Physical fitness of obese school children in Hat Yai, southern Thailand. *Southeast Asian J Trop Med Public Health.* 1994:25(2):354-360.
2. Waxman M, Stunkard AJ. Caloric intake and expenditure of obese boys. *J Pediatr.* 1980:96(2):187-193.
3. Reybrouck T, Weymans M, Vinckx J, Stijns H, Vanderschueren-Lodeweyckx M. Cardiorespiratory function during exercise in obese children. *Acta Paediatr Scand.* 1987:76(2):342-348.
4. Gortmaker SL, Dietz WH Jr, Sobol AM, Wehler CA. Increasing pediatric obesity in the United States. *Am J Dis Child.* 1987:141(5): 535-540.
5. Zannolli R, Rebeggiani A, Chiarelli F, Morgese G. Hyperisulinism as a marker in obese children. *Am J Dis Child.* 1993:147(8):837-841.
6. Hubert HB, Feinleib M, McNamara PM, Castelli WP. Obesity as an independent risk factor for cardiovascular disease: a 26-year follow-up of participants in the Framingham Heart Study. *Circulation.* 1983:67(5):968-977.
7. Sullivan M, Karlson J, Sjostrom L, et al. Swedish obese subjects (SOS)—an intervention study of obesity. Baseline evaluation of health and psychosocial functioning in the first 1743 subjects examined. *Int J Obes Relat Metab Disord.* 1993:17(9):503-512.
8. Must A, Jacques PF, Dallal GE, Bajema CJ, Dietz WH. Long-term morbidity and mortality of overweight adolescents. A follow-up of the Harvard Growth Study of 1922 to 1935. *N Engl J Med.* 1992:327(19):1350-1355.
9. Dietz WH Jr. Childhood obesity: susceptibility, cause and management. *J Pediatr.* 1983:103(5):676-686.
10. von Almen TK, Figueroa-Colon R, Suskind RM. Psychosocial considerations in the treatment of childhood obesity. In: Giorgi PL, Suskind RM, Catassi C, eds. *The Obese Child* (Pediatric and Adolescent Medicine). Karger, Basel. 1992:162-171.
11. Dyer R. Traditional treatment of obesity: does it work? *Clin Endocrinol Metab.* 1994:8(3):661-688.
12. Epstein L, Valoski A, Kalarchian M, McCurley J. Do children lose and maintain weight easier than adults: a comparison of child and parent weight changes from six months to ten years. *Obes Res.* 1995:3(5):411-417.
13. National Task Force on the Prevention and Treatment of Obesity, National Institutes of Health. Very low-calorie diets. *JAMA.* 1993:270(8):967-974.
14. Sothern MS, Ewing T, Davis R, et al. Introduction of a pediatric weight management program to obese inner city African-American youth. *J Investig Med.* 1998;46:8A.
15. Blecker U, Sothern M, Udall JN, et al. Initial obesity level impact long term weight maintenance in obese youth. *Int J Obes Relat Metab Disord.* 1998:22(Suppl 4):S4.
16. Von Almen K, Sothern MS, Suskind RM, et al. Age as a factor in long term program retention and weight maintenance in obese children and adolescents. *Pediatr Res.* 1998:43(Suppl):121A.
17. Sothern MS, Loftin JM, Udall JN, et al. Inclusion of resistance exercise in a multidisciplinary outpatient treatment program for preadolescent obese children. *South Med J.* 1999:92(6):585-592.
18. Sothern MS, Hunter S, Suskind RM, Brown R, Udall JN Jr, Blecker U. Motivating the obese child to move: the role of structured exercise in pediatric weight management. *South Med J.* 1999:92(6):577-584.
19. Slaughter MH, Lohman TG, Boileau RA et al. Skinfold equations for estimation of body fatness in children and youth. *Hum Biol.* 1988:60(5):709-723.
20. Legge BJ, Banister EW. The Astrand-Rhyming nomogram revisted. *J Appl Physiol.* 1986:61(3):1203-1209.
21. Wadden TA, Stunkard AJ, Rich L, Rubin CJ, Sweidel G, Mckinney S. Obesity in black adolescent girls: a controlled clinical trial of treatment by diet, behavior modification and parental support. *Pediatrics.* 1990:85(3):345-352.
22. Merritt RJ. Treatment of pediatric and adolescent obesity. *Int J Obesity.* 1978:2(2):207-214.
23. Epstein LH, Mccurley J, Vasoski A, Wing RR. Growth in obese children treated for obesity. *Am J Dis Child.* 1990:144(12):1360-1364.
24. Merritt RJ, Bistrian BR, Blackburn GL, Suskind RM. Consequences of modified fasting in obese pediatric and adolescent patients. I. Protein sparing modified fast. *J Pediatr.* 1980:96(l):13-19.

25. Merritt RJ, Blackburn GL, Bistrian BR, Palombo J, Suskind RM. Consequences of modified fasting in obese pediatric and adolescent patients: effect of a carbohydrate-free diet on serum proteins. *Am J Clin Nutr.* 1981:34(12):2752-2755.
26. Merritt RJ, Blackburn GL, Bristrian BR, Batrus C, Suskind RM. Consequences of modified fasting in obese pediatric and adolescent patients. II. Metabolic effects of glucose compared to fat non-protein calories. *Nutr Res.* 1983: 3: 33-41.
27. Archibald EH, Harrison JE, Pencharz PB. Effect of a weight-reducing high-protein diet on the body composition of obese adolescents. *Am J Dis Child.* 1983:137(7):658-662.
28. Dietz WH Jr, Schoeller DA. Optimal dietary therapy for obese adolescents: comparison of protein plus glucose and protein plus fat. *J Pediatr.* 1982:100(4):638-644.
29. Catassi C, Ratsch I M, Rossin M, Ruggeri AG, Coppa GV, Giorgi PL. Treatment of childhood obesity by a protein sparing diet. In: Giorgi PL, Suskind RM, Catassi C, eds. *The Obese Child.* (Pediatric and Adolescent Medicine.) Karger, Basel; 1992: 197-205.
30. Stallings VA, Archibald EH, Pencharz PB, Harrison JE, Bill LE. One-year follow-up of weight, total body potassium, and total body nitrogen in obese adolescents treated with the protein-sparing modified fast. *Am J Clin Nutr.* 1988:48(1):91-94.
31. Brown MR, Klish WJ, Hollander J, Campbell MA, Forbes GB. A high protein, low calorie liquid diet in the treatment of very obese adolescents: long-term effect on lean body mass. *Am J Clin Nutr.* 1983:38(1):20-31.
32. Healthy People 2000: National Health Promotion and Disease Prevention Objectives [DHHS Pub. No. (PHS) 91-50213]. Washington, DC: US Dept Health and Human Services, Public Health Service, 2000.
33. Epstein LH, Koeske R, Wing RR. Adherence to exercise in obese children. *J Cardiac Rehab.* 1984: 4: 185-195.
34. Sothern MS, Loftin M, Suskind RM, Udall JN, Blecker U. The health benefits of physical activity in children and adolescents: implications for chronic disease prevention. *Eur J Pediatr.* 1999:158(4):271-274.
35. Corbin CB. Fitness is for children: developing lifetime fitness. *J Phys Educ Recreat Dance.* 1986:57(5):82-84.
36. Sallis JF, Simons-Morton BG, Stone EJ, et al. Determinants of physical activity and interventions in youth. *Med Sci Sports Exerc.* 1992:24(6 Suppl):S248-257.
37. Sothern MS, Loftin JM, Suskind RM, Udall JN, Blecker U. Physiologic function and childhood obesity. *Int Pediatr.* 1999;14(3):135-139.
38. Epstein LH, Wing RR, Koeski R, Ossip D, Beck S. A comparison of lifestyle change and programmed aerobic exercise on weight and fitness changes in obese children. *Behav Ther.* 1982:13:651-665.
39. Reybrouck T, Vinckx J, Van Den Berghe G, Vanderschueren-Lode-Weyckx M. Exercise therapy and hypocaloric diet in the treatment of obese children and adolescents. *Acta Pediatr Scand.* 1990:79(1):84-89.
40. Baranowski T, Bouchard C, Bar-or O, et al. Assessment, prevalence, and cardiovascular benefits of physical activity and fitness in youth. *Med Sci Sports Exerc.* 1992:24(6 Suppl):S237-247.
41. Taylor W, Baronowski T. Physical activity, cardiovascular fitness and adiposity in children. *Res Q Exerc Sport.* 1991:62(2):157-163.
42. Forbes GB. Exercise and body composition. *J Appl Physiol.* 1991:70(3):994-997.
43. Ballor DL, Tommerup LJ, Thomas DP, Smith DB, Keesey RE. Exercise training attenuates diet-induced reduction in metabolic rate. *J Appl Physiol.* 1990:68(6):2612-2617.
44. Andersson B, Xu XF, Rebuffe-Scrive M, Termy K, Krotkiewski M, Bjomtorp P. The effects of exercise, training on body composition and metabolism in men and women. *Int J Obes.* 1991:15(1):75-81.
45. Sothern MS, Loftin M, Suskind RM, Udall JN Jr, Blecker U. The impact of significant weight loss on resisting energy expenditure in obese youth. *J Investig Med.* 1999:47(5):222-226.
46. Klesges RC, Malott JM, Boschee PF, Weber JM. The effects of parental influences on children's food intake, physical activity, and relative weight. *Int J Eating Disord.* 1986:5:335-345.
47. Epstein LH, Wing RR, Koeske R, Valoski A. Long-term effects of a family-based treatment of childhood obesity. *J Consult Clin Psychol.* 1987:55(l):91-95.
48. Epstein LH, Valoski A, Wing RR, Mccurley J. Ten-year follow-up of behavioral, family-based treatment for obese children. *JAMA.* 1990:264(19):2519-2523.
49. Varni JW, Banis HT. Behavior therapy techniques applied to eating, exercise, and diet modification in childhood obesity. *J Dev Behav Pediatr.* 1985:6(6):367-372.
50. Epstein LH, Masek BJ, Marshall WR. A nutritionally based school program for control of eating in obese children. *Behav Ther.* 1978:9:766-778.
51. Stark LJ, Collins FL Jr, Osnes PG, Stokes TF. Using reinforcement and cueing to increase healthy snack food choices in preschoolers. *J Appl Behav Anal.* 1986:19(4):367-379.
52. Coates TJ, Jeffery RW, Slinkard LA, Killen JD, Dancher BG. Frequency of contact and monetary reward in weight loss, lipid change and blood pressure reduction with adolescents. *Behav Ther.* 1982:13:175-185.
53. Brownell KD, Kelman JH, Stunkard AJ. Treatment of obese children with and without their mothers: changes in weight and blood pressure. *Pediatrics.* 1983:71:515-523.
54. Epstein LH, Wing RR, Koeske R, Andrasik F, Ossip DJ. Child and parent weight loss in family-based behavior modification programs. *J Consult Clin Psychol.* 1981:49(5):674-685.
55. Israel AC, Stolmaker L, Sharp JP, Silverman WK, Simon LG. An evaluation of two methods of parental involvement in treating obese children. *Behav Ther.* 1984:15:266-272.
56. Kramer FM, Jeffrey RW, Snell MK, Forster JL. Maintenance of successful weight loss over 1 year: effects of financial contracts for weight maintenance or participation in skills training. *Behav Ther.* 1986:17:295-301.
57. Peri MG. Maintenance strategies for the management of obesity. In: Johnson WG, ed. *Advances in Eating Disorders. Treating and Preventing Obesity.* Vol 1. Greenwich, CT: JAI Press; 1987:177-194.
58. Perri MG, Mcallister DA, Gange JJ, Jordan RC, Mcadoo G, Nezu AM. Effects of four maintenance programs on the long-term management of obesity. *J Consult Clin Psychol.* 1988:56(4):529-534.
59. Lavery MA, Loewy JW, Kapadia AS, Nichaman MZ, Foreyt JP, Gee M. Long-term follow-up of weight status of subjects in a behavioral weight control program. *J Am Diet Assoc.* 1989:89(9):1259-1264.
60. Fitzwater SL, Winsier RL, Woodridge NH, Birch R, Liu C, Bartolucci AA. Evaluation of long-term weight changes after a multidisciplinary weight control program. *J Am Diet Assoc.* 1991:91(4):421-426.
61. Kayman S, Bruwold W, Stern JS. Maintenance and relapse after weight loss in women: behavioral aspects. *Am J Clin Nutr.* 1990:52 (5):800-807.
62. Harris MB, Sutton M, Kaufman EM, Carmichael CW. Correlates of success and retention in a multifaceted, long-term behavior modification program for obese adolescent girls. *Addict Behav.* 1980:5 (1):25-34.
63. Figueroa-Colon R, VonAlmen TK, Franklin FA, Schuftan C, Suskind RM. Comparison of two hypocaloric diets in obese children. *Am J Dis Child.* 1993:147(2):160-166.
64. Brownell KD, Wadden TA. Behavior therapy for obesity: modern approaches and better results. In: Brownell KD, Foreyt JP, eds. *Handbook of Eating Disorders. Physiology, Psychology, and Treatment of Obesity, Anorexia, and Bulimia.* New York: Basic Books; 1986:180-197.

Chapter 53

Nutritional Support of Obese and Bariatric Patients

Scott A. Shikora, MD, FACS,
and Phyllis Thomason, MS, RD, LDN

Introduction

Sixty-four percent of adults in the United States are obese.[1] Almost 5% or 14 to 16 million adult Americans are extremely (morbidly) obese, which is defined as a body mass index (BMI) greater than or equal to 40 kg/m^2.[2] Twenty-three million adults have a BMI ≥35 kg/m^2. Comorbid conditions that are associated with overweight and obesity are numerous and include type 2 diabetes mellitus, obstructive sleep apnea, hyperlipidemia, hypertension, degenerative joint disease, and asthma (Table 53-1). The surgical management of morbid obesity (bariatric surgery) has become the fastest growing specialty in the field of medicine. In the last decade, the number of procedures increased by 644% and was estimated to be over 100,000 this past year.[3] This dramatic increase in operative procedures can be attributed not only to the rise in extreme obesity, but also to other factors including the introduction of laparoscopic, minimally invasive surgical techniques and the publicity given to a few celebrities who undergone bariatric surgery.

Although the bariatric procedures have never been safer or more effective for achieving meaningful and sustainable weight loss, all of the currently performed operations result in dramatic changes in gastrointestinal anatomy, physiology, and/or dietary habits. Good surgical results do not ensure successful outcome. Even after excellent weight loss, patients must still be closely followed long term to guard against the development of nutritional deficiencies. In addition, operative complications can result in critical illness. Furthermore, with the high prevalence of obese in society, it is highly likely that even nonbariatric surgical patients will inhabit intensive care units at ever-greater numbers. Unfortunately, standard involutional nutritional approaches may, in fact, be harmful for this patient group. A unique feeding regimen may be preferred. This chapter will review both the standard nutritional management of the bariatric patient and the nutritional support of the critically ill obese.

Long-Term Nutritional Management of the Bariatric Patient

The long-term nutritional consequences of bariatric surgery vary according to the procedure performed. Some are common to all procedures while others may be specific to one operative procedure. For most nutritional deficiencies, the etiology may be multifactorial—ie, secondary to the dramatic reduction of macronutrient and micronutrient intake, altered dietary choices, and/or nutrient malabsorption. The degree of the deficiencies will be determined not only by the specific operative procedure but also by the dietary habits of the individual patient. Some deficiencies may develop quickly, while others slowly and in an insidious manner.

To understand the potential long-term consequences of bariatric surgery, it is important to first understand the more commonly performed procedures. The bariatric procedures that are currently performed include Roux-en-Y gastric bypass (RYGB), vertical-banded gastroplasty (VBG), biliopancreatic diversion (BPD), biliopancreatic diversion with duodenal switch (DS), and the laparoscopic adjustable gastric band (LAGB).

All of these procedures are effective for weight loss, but all achieve it by different mechanisms. The LAGB

Table 53-1.

Medical Conditions Associated With Obesity

Cardiovascular	• Cardiomyopathy • Cerebrovascular disease • Coronary artery disease • Dyslipidemia • Sudden death • Hypertension
Endocrine	• Amenorrhea • Diabetes mellitus • Hirsutism • Infertility
Hepatobiliary/Gastrointestinal	• Hepatic steatosis • Gallstones • Gastroesophageal reflux • Steatohepatitis • Venous stasis ulcers
Musculoskeletal/Skin	• Accident proneness • Chronic back pain • Degenerative joint disease • Diaphoresis • Hernia • Immobility • Infections • Intertriginous dermatitis
Psychological	• Depression • Low self-esteem • Poor quality of life • Poor relationships • Suicide
Pulmonary/Respiratory	• Dyspnea • Obesity hypoventilation • Obstructive sleep apnea
Venous	• Deep vein thrombosis • Lower limb edema • Pulmonary embolus • Venous stasis
Miscellaneous	• Chronic fatigue • Malignancies • Pseudotumor cerebri • Urinary stress incontinence

(Figure 53-1) is a procedure where an inflatable silicone band is placed around the uppermost stomach. A small gastric pouch of 15 to 30 cc is created in the process, which is partially obstructed by the narrow band. Weight loss is due exclusively to the restriction of nutrient intake created by the small gastric pouch reservoir and the narrow outlet. The RYGB (Figure 53-2) also relies on a small gastric pouch reservoir of 15 to 30 cc, which is created by surgical stapling devices. The pouch drains through a narrow anastomosis to a Roux limb of jejunum. Weight loss is due predominantly to nutrient restriction. However, the bypass of the fundus, duodenum, and proximal jejunum may contribute to the weight loss by influencing gut hormones such as ghrelin.[4] The BPD and DS (Figure 53-3) are predominantly malabsorptive procedures. A partial gastrectomy is performed and results in a large gastric pouch (200 cc), which mildly reduces gastric-reservoir volume. An anastomosis is created between the distal ileum to the stomach pouch or duodenum. Nutrients bypass the majority of the small bowel. Weight loss is mainly due to the limited intestinal absorptive capacity in the terminal ileum.

The LAGB, short-limb RYGB, BPD, and DS will be considered in this chapter. The VBG behaves nutritionally similarly to the LAGB and is also being replaced by it. (All of these procedures are discussed in Chapter 49.)

The Significance of Long-Term Follow-Up

For all of the bariatric procedures, long-term follow-up is critical for success and patient well-being. During the first year, patient monitoring is most critical. Weight loss is analyzed and patients are evaluated for overall heath, medication titration, activity level, dietary habits, bowel function, and hydrational status. After the first postoperative year, patients are seen less frequently. However, at these visits, patients should be assessed for nutritional deficiencies, appropriateness of their diet, weight maintenance, the presence of symptoms, and overall health and well-being.

Protein-Calorie Malnutrition

Unlike past experiences with the intestinal bypass (an operation no longer performed), the risk of protein deficiency with the current operative procedures is dramati-

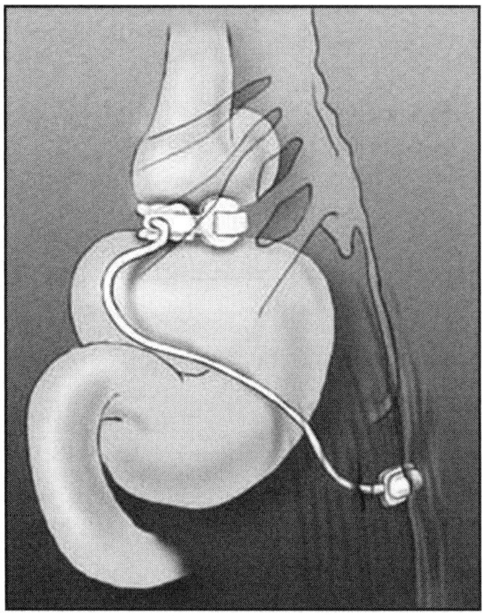

Figure 53-1. Laparoscopic adjustable gastric band. An adjustable silicone band is placed around the top of the stomach. Its diameter can be adjusted by injecting or removing saline from the reservoir. Reprinted with permission from the American Society for Bariatric Surgery (www.ASBS.org).

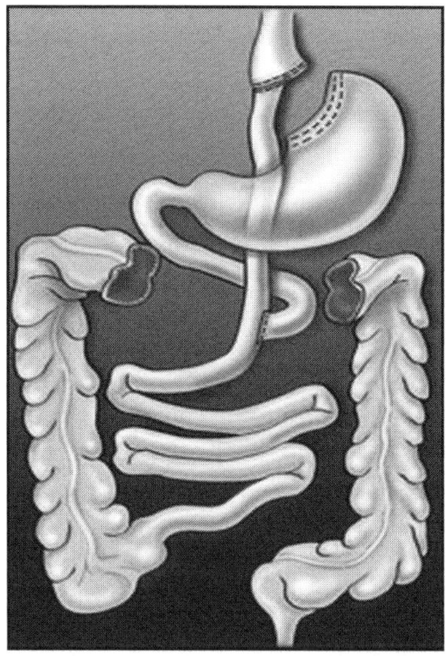

Figure 53-2. Roux-en-Y gastric bypass. A small gastric pouch is created by staple transection of the stomach. The pouch is anastomosed to the proximal jejunum. Reprinted with permission from the American Society for Bariatric Surgery (www.ASBS.org).

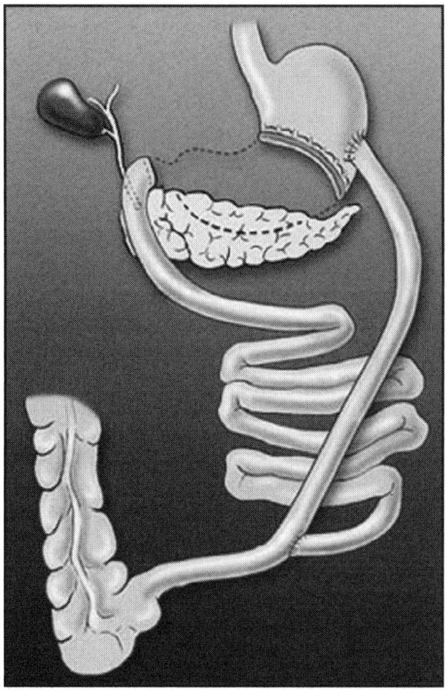

Figure 53-3A. Biliopancreatic diversion with and without duodenal switch. A. BPD without the duodenal switch. After a partial gastrectomy, the ileum is anastomosed to the stomach remnant. The intestinal limb that drains the bile and pancreatic juices is anastomosed to the terminal ileum. Reprinted with permission from the American Society for Bariatric Surgery (www.ASBS.org).

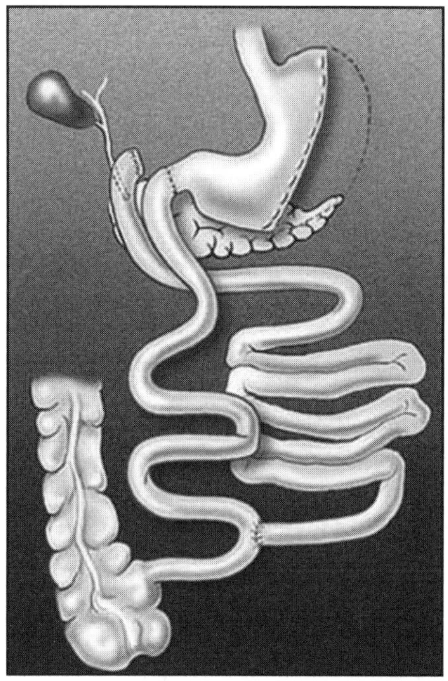

Figure 53-3B. BPD with duodenal switch. Similar to the BPD except that a sleeve gastrectomy is performed, and the ileum is anastomosed to the duodenum. Reprinted with permission from the American Society for Bariatric Surgery (www.ASBS.org).

cally less likely. The restrictive procedures, including the RYGB and LAGB, rarely cause protein-calorie malnutrition. The weight loss seen is predominantly from adipose tissue with only minor changes in lean body tissue.[5,6] However, protein malnutrition can occur in certain conditions such as dysfunctional eating habits (eg, anorexia), severe depression, or protracted vomiting. Dietary habits can also lead to protein deficiency, as some patients avoid protein-dense foods, secondary to inappropriate eating behaviors, food intolerances, and preferences.

For the malabsorptive procedures, malnutrition is more common, as ingested protein may be poorly absorbed and lost in the stool. The incidence has been reported to be approximately 7% to 21%.[7] The yearly hospitalization rate for protein deficiency after BPD is 1%. Hypoalbuminemia can be seen as early as 6 months after surgery but often will gradually return to preoperative levels. Tacchino et al studied changes in total and segmental body composition at 2, 6, 12, and 24 months after BPD and discovered that weight loss was achieved with an appropriate decline of lean body mass. After weight stabilization, all parameters were similar to weight-matched controls.[8] However, persistent hypoalbuminemia leads to revisional surgery in 1%-2% of patients after BPD.[9]

The diagnosis of protein malnutrition may not be easy. Patients lose weight rapidly and serum protein levels will often stay in the normal range until late.[10-12] Therefore, after all of the bariatric procedures, dietary monitoring is important during both active weight-loss phase and long-term weight maintenance. We recommend that most bariatric patients consume approximately 60 to 80 g of protein daily. Higher intake may be necessary for the malabsorptive procedures and should be guided by serum protein levels as well as overall health, dietary habits, and bowel-habit activity. For patients with significant deficiency who cannot replete by oral diet alone, a course of

Table 53-2.
Additional Supplementation for Diagnosed Deficiencies

At Risk Nutrient	Deficiency Syndrome/Symptoms	Assessment of Nutriture	Supplementation
Vitamin B12	Megaloblastic anemia/glossitis, peripheral neuropathy	Serum B12	1000 µg po daily or 1000 g or 1mL q monthly
Folate	Megaloblastic anemia/diarrhea, fatigue, depression, confusion	RBC folate	1 mg daily
Iron	Microcytic anemia/fatigue, listlessness, angular stomatitis	Iron, TIBC, and serum ferritin	325 mg ferrous sulfate t.id. taken with vitamin C or vitamin C food
Calcium	Metabolic bone disease/fractures	DEXA	1200-1500 mg with added vitamin D daily
Thiamin	Wernicke-Korsakoff syndrome/gait ataxia, diplopia, nystagmus	Erythrocyte transketolase	100 mg IV or IM for 7 to 10 days initiated prior to glucose infusion plus 10mg po

parenteral nutrition (PN) may be necessary. However, for long-term benefit, common channel-limb lengthening, or even reversal may be necessary.

Severe calorie deficiency (cachexia) is also unusual after bariatric surgery but may be seen in patients with protracted vomiting, diarrhea, or anorexia. Treatment includes nutritional supplementation (even involuntary if necessary), correction of any underlying anatomical abnormalities (ie, stricture, obstruction), and/or psychologic intervention as indicated. For the most extreme or intractable cases, common channel limb lengthening, or even reversal, may be necessary.

Vitamin and Mineral Deficiencies

Vitamin and/or mineral deficiencies (Table 53-2) are more likely to occur after RYGB, BPD, and DS than are protein and calorie deficiencies.[12-24] After surgery, all patients should comply with life-long supplementation. Deficiencies may develop slowly and not become evident until years after surgery supporting the requirement for lifelong surveillance (Table 53-3). In general, the gastric restrictive LAGB and VBG cause few micronutritional deficiencies.[15] Because nutrients are not diverted from the duodenum, gastric mixing is unchanged postoperatively. However, deficiencies may develop in those patients with intractable vomiting or those with suboptimal nutrient intake (reduced meal size or dietary choices). RYGP patients are at greater risk for deficiencies than are LAGB and VBG patients. Not only is nutrient intake reduced because of small meal size and dietary choices that are altered by taste and eating behaviors, but the nutrient stream is diverted away from the fundus, duodenum, and proximal jejunum, which causes deficiencies of iron, folate, calcium, and vitamin B12. The malabsorptive procedures, such as the BPD and DS, place patients at even greater risk for deficiencies of the above vitamins and calcium, as well as for the fat-soluble vitamins (A, D, E, K) and electrolytes, such as sodium, potassium, chloride, phosphorus, magnesium, and possibly even zinc.[17,19,23,24] For all bariatric patients, assessment of nutriture needs to be aggressively followed yearly, and supplementation should be prescribed judiciously. Because many bariatric programs rely on different supplementation protocols, there is no consensus as to what represents the optimal regimen. However, there is general agreement concerning the importance of life-long surveillance of patients' vitamin/mineral status. Table 53-4 presents the specific vitamin and mineral supplementation protocol for the Obesity Consult Center at Tufts-New England Medical Center in Boston.

Iron

Iron deficiency is commonly found in bariatric patients and, in particular, in premenopausal women.[12,13,15,18,21] It manifests as a microcytic anemia. The etiology for iron deficiency is multifactorial. It is partly due to the nutrient restriction that limits intake of dietary iron. In addition, after RYGB, BPD, and DS, malabsorption of iron also occurs. Iron absorption is facilitated by gastric acid. After RYGB, gastric-acid production is dramatically reduced in the small gastric pouch.[16] In addition, iron is predominantly absorbed in the duodenum and proximal jejunum. RYGB and BPD reroute the nutrient stream from the upper stomach "pouch" directly into the jejunum or ileum, thereby avoiding the duodenum altogether. Therefore, patients may not maintain normal serum levels of iron or iron saturation after these procedures. The DS keeps part of the duodenum in the nutrient circuit but bypasses all of the jejunum. Lastly, patients who do not tolerate or avoid

Table 53-3.
Theoretical Advantages of Hypocaloric Feeding

Avoidance of glucose-related complications
Avoidance of hyperglycemia
Decrease in endogenous insulin secretion
Marked decrease of or avoidance of need for exogenous insulin, even in diabetic patients
Improved ventilatory mechanics
Improved diuresis
Decreased CO_2 production
Enhanced protein anabolism
Promotion of positive nitrogen balance
Enhanced wound healing
Improved immune function

Table 53-4.
Body Composition Changes Associated With Obesity

Increased adipose tissue
Increased lean body mass
Increased total body water
Increased extracellular fluid (ECF)
Increased intracellular fluid (ICF)
Increased protein content
Increased mineral weight

meat in their diet will be more likely to be iron deficient.[11] Patients found to be deficient should be supplemented with 325 mg of $FeSO_4$ orally one to three times daily. Patients prescribed supplementation should be monitored for possible side effects of oral iron, such as constipation. If repletion is unsuccessful orally, parenteral iron infusions may be required.

Vitamin B12

Deficiencies of vitamin B12 commonly occur following bariatric surgery.[12-16] Significant deficiencies can lead to macrocytic anemia, megaloblastosis of the bone marrow, leukopenia, thrombocytopenia, glossitis, or neurologic derangements. However, despite the high incidence of low serum levels, few patients develop these sequelae. The normal absorption of vitamin B12 is a complex process. The vitamin must first be freed from the food source, particularly meat protein. This is facilitated by gastric acid. The free B12 is then bound to R-protein in the stomach. Within the duodenum, R-protein is cleaved from the vitamin, which then binds to intrinsic factor (IF). The B12-IF complex then travels intact through the intestinal tract and is absorbed into the circulation in the distal ileum.

After RYGB and BPD, B12 intake and absorption are diminished. Several studies have reported that oral crystalline B12 can be absorbed and normal serum levels maintained in RYGB patients.[14,16] Therefore, in many patients, acceptable vitamin B12 serum levels can be obtained if the vitamin is provided orally. Several of the studies recommend 500 to 600 mcg daily. If a mild or moderate deficiency is identified, some suggest oral supplementation with 1000 mcg daily. If oral supplementation does not replete the deficiency, or if it is severe, intramuscular injections (1000 mcg) can be administered monthly.

Vitamin B12 deficiency should be much less likely after LAGB procedures, in which the nutrient stream is not diverted, and after BPD and DS, in which gastric-acid production is less altered than after RYGB and the terminal ileum is kept intact. If a deficiency is identified, poor dietary choices, suboptimal intake, and/or nonadherence with vitamin supplementation may be implicated.

Folic Acid

Folic-acid deficiency is also a potential complication following bariatric surgery. It can manifest as macrocytic anemia, leukopenia, thrombocytopenia, glossitis, or megaloblastic marrow. For the most part, folate deficiency is thought to be predominantly due to decreased intake and not to malabsorption, and it is easily corrected by oral vitamin supplementation.[13] It has also been shown to be less likely in meat eaters than in meat avoiders.[11] Vitamin B12 is also necessary for the conversion of methyltetrahydrofolic acid to tetrahydrofolic acid; therefore, a B12 deficiency may result in a folate deficiency. Unfortunately, serum folate levels are more indicative of acute dietary insufficiency of folate than are more chronic tissue levels. Red-blood–cell folate levels change more gradually and are thought to be more predictive of tissue levels.

However, the significance of lower red-blood–cell folate levels is questioned because few patients actually develop megaloblastic anemia. The usual recommendation for supplementation is 1 mg of folate daily.

Calcium

Calcium deficiencies are arguably the most difficult to assess and treat after procedures that produce micronutrient malabsorption, including RYGB, BPD, and DS. Given no other underlying medical conditions, measurement of serum calcium will remain within normal limits because of the vast amount of calcium reserves in the skeletal structure. Changes in bone density may provide the only accurate assessment of long-term calcium deficits. Goode et al found that ≥3 years postoperative RYGB postmenopausal women who supplemented with 1.2 g/day elemental calcium and 8 g vitamin D for 6 months showed significant increases in bone resorption when compared with weight-matched controls. However, similarly supplemented premenopausal postoperative patients showed no significant difference when compared with matched controls.[25]

Because LAGB and VBG are restrictive procedures with no subsequent malabsorption, patients can still be at risk for calcium deficiency with inadequate calcium intake. Pugnale et al reported that 1 year after gastric banding, premenopausal women had a negative bone remodeling inversely proportional to a decrease in hip circumference and body fat.[26] These findings may reflect the impact of weight loss and a subsequent change in weight-bearing bone remodeling.

Calcium replacement therapy is somewhat controversial. Vitamin-D supplementation has been shown to either have no effect or to increase supplemental calcium absorption.[27,28] Supplemental calcium in available in a variety of compositions, the most common of which are calcium carbonate and calcium citrate. Bioavailability of the different forms was found to be similar in postmenopausal women, perhaps the population most difficult to treat, with adequate estrogen and vitamin-D stores when compared with a control population.[28] Daily recommendations for calcium supplementation are 1200 to 1500 mg calcium from a source that also contains vitamin D. To maximize absorption, supplementation with calcium carbonate, the most widely available chewable form, should be taken with food.

Other Deficiencies

Other vitamin and mineral deficiencies can occur and include vitamin A noted in 10% of patients, hypokalemia in 56%, and hypomagnesemia in 34% of patients.[12] However, these were not considered significant as no patient experienced night blindness and low potassium and magnesium levels were easily corrected with oral supplementation. Fat-soluble vitamins are at risk of deficiency, especially after the malabsorptive procedures.

Thiamine deficiency is generally uncommon after bariatric surgery. However, it must always be considered for any patient who presents with intractable vomiting and dehydration. Symptoms include gait impairment, diplopia, and nystagmus. Assessment of erythrocyte transketolase thiamine status may not reveal a deficiency.[29] Rehydration with a glucose-based intravenous fluid without the supplementation of thiamine can result in Wernicke-Korsakoff syndrome. Supplementation recommendations are 100 mg intravenously[29-33] for 7 to 10 days followed by 10 mg oral thiamine.[32]

Nutrition Support for the Critically Ill Who Are Extremely Obese

With the dramatic increase of the prevalence of obesity in the United States (and worldwide), an increasing number of extremely obese patients will require intensive care. Like other patients residing in the intensive care unit, many of these patients will be unable to adequately nourish orally. Despite their excessive adiposity, when critically ill, the severely obese are likely to require (and entitled to receive) early, aggressive, involutional feeding. Unfortunately, their comorbid conditions (see Table 53-4) and deranged body habitus negatively impacts the ability to provide care. A recent study in a surgical intensive care unit found obesity to be an independent risk factor for morbidity and mortality. Not surprising, these complex patient-care issues spill over into the field of nutritional support. Standard nutritional approaches may in fact be harmful for this patient group. Unique nutritional approaches should be considered.

The Hazards of Standard Nutritional Support

Standard nutritional support generally involves the infusion of a concentrated formulation comprised of protein, carbohydrate, and lipid. Most patients will be prescribed approximately 1.0 to 2.0 g of protein per kg of actual body weight per day. Carbohydrate is usually given as dextrose and can range from as little as 150 g to as much as 700 g daily. Lipid calories are often provided to a level of 30% to 40% of the total calories. Total calorie infusion for most patients falls within the range of 20 to 35 kcal per kg of actual body weight per day.[34] This approach may be potentially harmful for the severely overweight.

Fluid Load

The stress response of severe illness promotes the retention of salt and water. In addition, overweight patients often require more volume for fluid homeostasis. Involutional feeding relies on a volume load to serve as the vehicle for delivering the nutrients. This fluid load can rapidly expand blood volume, as many overweight patients have hyperinsulinemia. The close association of obesity with heart disease may place the critically ill overweight patient at risk for fluid overload, which may lead to myocardial infarction, pulmonary edema, or congestive heart failure.

Restricting volume to avoid fluid overload may lead to inadequate nutrition or dehydration. This is particularly true with the use of the enteral route as formulas are usually isoosmolar or mildly hyperosmolar. However, determining fluid needs is often difficult. There are no formulas in the literature that accurately predicts fluid requirements in the severely obese. Measuring central venous and/or right heart pressures may be the best determinants of volume status.

Glucose Load

The concentrated glucose solution provided by feeding may have a number of adverse effects for the severely obese. Concentrated dextrose can cause hyperglycemia in both glucose-intolerant and "normal" stressed patients. Elevated blood glucose levels have been implicated in poor wound healing[35] and immune dysfunction, leading to an increased susceptibility to infections.[36-39] Van Den Berghe et al reported that hyperglycemia significantly increased morbidity and mortality in critically ill patients.[40] As the extremely overweight patients are three times more likely to be diabetic than are nonobese patients, this can be an even greater problem than for the nonobese.[41]

Excessive glucose infusion is particularly dangerous. The administration of excess parenteral glucose can enhance lipogenesis, causing hepatic steatosis and subsequent hepatic dysfunction.[42] In addition, excess glucose can also increase the production of CO_2, which increases respiratory work. For the obese with underlying respiratory compromise, consistently elevated CO_2 levels may lead to respiratory failure.[43,44] The infusion of a concentrated glucose load will also increase the secretion of insulin. Insulin is a potent antinatriuretic hormone that stimulates salt and water retention, which can exacerbate the fluid overloaded state and place the patient at risk for cardiac failure, infarction, and/or pulmonary edema.

Lipid Load

Unlike dextrose, lipids are generally safe for obese patients. However, fats provide significant calories. Because obesity is a state of both fat and energy excess, there may be little immediate benefit to infusing lipid. In addition, estimating calorie requirements in the severely obese patient is difficult and often inaccurate. Therefore, the standard use of energy-dense lipids to meet estimated needs may lead to overfeeding in this population.

Appropriately Feeding the Critically Ill Who Are Severely Obese

Because standard nutritional practices can be harmful for the obese patient, a nutritional formulation that restricts calories—and particularly calories from glucose—may be more beneficial. This approach, often referred to as hypocaloric feeding, is based on the theory that an energy deficit caused by restricting calorie administration below actual requirements can be safely compensated for by the mobilization of endogenous fat. In addition, by providing adequate protein, nitrogen homeostasis would be maintained.

Hypocaloric Nutritional Support

A protein-sparing, hypocaloric approach to nutritional support may have several potential short-term benefits for use in the critically ill obese[45-47] (see Table 53-3). Although dextrose is the sole source for nonprotein calories, elevated blood sugars are rarely seen. Because the likelihood of hyperglycemia is reduced, many of the dextrose-associated complications are avoided. Therefore, one would anticipate less wound infections, enhanced immune function, the promotion of diuresis instead of fluid retention, and decreased carbon dioxide production. The reduction in carbon dioxide production may decrease respiratory work, potentially decreasing the need for mechanical ventilatory support. In addition, despite the deliberate restriction in energy provision, protein anabolism and successful wound healing have been reported in critically ill obese patients who are placed on this feeding regimen.[46,47] Another beneficial attribute of the hypocaloric feeding approach is that, while insulin secretion is decreased, the need for exogenous insulin administration is markedly diminished or even avoided altogether (even in diabetic patients).

Fat Oxidation

Although a hypocaloric-feeding regimen has many theoretical benefits for the severely obese patient, its success is based predominantly on the premise that the critically ill obese patient can oxidize stored fat to compensate for the calorie deficit and spare protein stores. To date, this concept has not been conclusively validated. In the non-stressed patient, decreased insulin secretion and insufficient calorie administration would favor fat oxidation. However, critical illness may alter normal metabolic pathways. Currently, only two studies have considered this issue. Jeevanandam and colleagues demonstrated poor fat oxidation in a population of fasted obese critically ill patients.[48] In contrast, using indirect calorimetry to analyze substrate utilization, Dickerson et al estimated fat oxidation at 68% of nonprotein energy expenditure in a similar population of stressed postoperative obese patients who were receiving hypocaloric PN.[46] They also reported that their patients achieved protein anabolism, increases in serum proteins and complete wound healing. Since this study did not compare a hypocaloric regimen with a standard, it could not prove superiority. It does, however, suggest that this approach seems safe.

Maximizing Protein Sparing

While the major benefits of hypocaloric feeding are secondary to the reduced glucose infusion, protein sparing is still one of the hallmarks of nutritional support. It would be attractive to postulate that completely eliminating nonprotein calories from the infusion would be even better for preventing hyperglycemia. However, the infusion of a dextrose-free amino acid solution was shown to decrease net nitrogen loss but not prevent it.[49] On the contrary, the addition of a non-protein calorie source such as glucose appears to be necessary to improve protein sparing.[50] This is thought to be due, in part, to the need for protein catabolism to fuel gluconeogenesis in a glucose-deficient state. After rapid depletion of the glycogen stores, the body relies on gluconeogenesis to provide glucose to the glucose-dependent tissues such as the immune system, the healing wound, and the peripheral nervous system.[51,52]

The amount of glucose necessary to achieve maximal protein sparing is not known. Nitrogen preservation increases with higher energy administration, but the effect is blunted as energy delivery increases above 60% of resting energy expenditure (REE).[53] Therefore, it may be postulated that to maximize the protein-sparing effect yet still limit caloric intake, the total energy provided should exceed about 50% of the energy expenditure to be effective. A severely energy-restricted diet—ie, providing less than 50% of the energy expenditure—would compromise protein sparing while a less restricted diet would risk the complications of a higher dextrose infusion.

Adverse Effects of Hypocaloric Feeding

To date, there have been no reports in the literature that have found any adverse effects with hypocaloric feeding. Despite the limited use (or absolute avoidance) of lipid, an essential fatty acid deficiency is unlikely to develop. Linoleic acid, the most important essential fatty acid, comprises approximately 10% of the stored lipid. Mobilization of fat releases more than the 2 to 3.5 g of linoleic acid required daily.[54] Even if lipolysis and fat oxidation are less efficient in the stressed obese patient, most patients would only require this form of nutritional support for a relatively limited period of time. If a patient requires longer support, an intralipid infusion can be given once weekly to prevent an essential fatty acid deficiency.

Enteral Hypocaloric Feeding

The hypocaloric protein-sparing approach was originally conceived for PN support. Because parenteral formulations are generally made to order, adjusting the macronutrient concentrations is commonplace. However, because most enteral formulations are provided "ready made" from the manufacturer, it can be more challenging. To produce a hypocaloric, protein-sparing enteral formula, one can either construct an enteral formulation entirely out of modular protein and dextrose components or modify a commercially prepared product. In the latter, there are several high-protein, low-fat formulas that can be chosen. More standard products can also be used and are usually more cost-effective.

The daily administration of a standard formulation can be based on the provision of 60% of the calculated energy requirements. Additional protein can be added to meet 100% of the protein needs. Although these formulas tend to provide approximately 30% of the total calories as lipid, with a hypocaloric regimen, the lipid contribution will be minimized and of no significance.

When using the enteral route, one must be mindful of meeting vitamin and mineral requirements. Most standard commercially available enteral products contain the sufficient vitamins and minerals to meet the FDA guidelines when 2000 kcal are administered daily. Because hypocaloric feeding generally will provide less than 2000 kcal, additional micronutrient supplementation may be required.

Estimating Energy Requirements

The estimation of energy expenditure can be difficult in this population of patients. Most current equations for calculating energy expenditure have not been derived for the extremely obese. Firstly, body composition is quite different (see Table 53-4). As compared to the nonobese, the majority of overweight patients have both an increased fat mass and increased lean body mass.[55,56] However, the proportion of lean body mass to fat mass can vary greatly.

Obesity is the state of excess adipose tissue. Adipose tissue can be divided into extracellular and intracellular components. The extracellular space contains fluid, electrolytes, protein, and blood vessels. The major cellular component is the adipocyte. The intracellular components include fluid, protein, and triglycerides.

Adipose tissue on average is approximately 80% lipid, 15% water and 5% protein.[57] In individuals of normal weight, the extracellular fluid (ECF) is 40% to 50% of total body water. Adipose tissue has an elevated ECF to intracellular fluid (ICF) ratio on the order of 3:1 or 4:1.[57] It would then follow that the obese have a higher proportion of fat-free mass as ECF.[57]

The expanded fat-free mass of obesity is in part due to excess fat-free adipose tissue (ie, adipocyte elements). Organ enlargement, increased skeletal muscle mass, and increased skeletal weight are also seen. The end result is that the obese patients have more total body water, protein content, and mineral weight than do the nonobese.[57]

Other obesity-associated factors may also affect body composition. Obesity in adults is often associated with hypertension, edema, and congestive heart failure, all of which may be secondary to overexpansion of the ECF. It has been shown that total body water, ECF, ICF, and the ratio of ECF/ICF are significantly increased in obese women compared to levels in normal-weight subjects.[58]

Therefore these derangements in body composition, and the great variability from patient to patient, makes using ideal body weight in standard energy-expenditure equations inaccurate. Given the larger lean body mass, using ideal body weight will generally underestimate caloric requirements. However, using actual body weight may massively overestimate energy expenditure, as fat is less metabolically active than is fat-free tissue, and body fluid is inactive. Using an adjusted body weight may better estimate lean body mass in the obese; however, this equation has not been validated.[59]

There are numerous formulas available to estimate energy requirements for patients. All suffer from inaccuracies that have been described elsewhere.[60-62] Most rely on weight as a gross estimate of lean body mass. Some differentiate men from women and the young from the old. Most have been criticized for lack of accuracy for the

TABLE 53-5.

Published Studies Utilizing Hypocaloric Feeding in the Obese

Study Type Patients	*Results*	
Dickerson et al[46]	Prospective 13 postoperative patients with complications	Protein anabolism Wound healing
Burge et al[47]	PRDBT 16 hospitalized patients No critically ill patients	Positive N2 balance Outcome not studied
Choban et al[69]	PRDBT 30 hospitalized patients Included critically ill	Positive N2 balance Outcome not studied

PRDBT = Prospective, randomized, double-blind trial

critically ill. Few even consider obesity as an independent variable.[63,64] Das et al found that predicted energy expenditure deviated from measured for both equations thought to be useful for the obese.[65] Unfortunately, her study was performed in non-critically ill obese patients. There is no similar work performed for the critically ill obese.

INDIRECT CALORIMETRY

Respiratory indirect calorimetry is considered the gold standard for accurately measuring energy expenditure. It does not rely on body weight, gender, age, or any other patient characteristics. Simply stated, a portable gas analyzer (CART) measures oxygen consumption and carbon dioxide production. It then converts this data into REE by utilizing the modified Weir equation.[66] This formula determines energy expenditure based solely on metabolic activity. It has been shown to be "extremely accurate" in the nonobese. To date, there are no studies that have specifically analyzed the accuracy of indirect calorimetry in the obese. However, because it only relies on gas exchange, there is no reason to doubt its potential accuracy in this unique patient population.

An alternative to respiratory indirect calorimetry is circulatory indirect calorimetry. This technique utilizes the thermodilution method from data acquired from a pulmonary artery catheter.[67] Cardiac output (CO), arterial oxygen, and mixed venous oxygen saturations are measured and then applied to the modified Fick equation. Although this technique is easy, rapid, and readily available, one study demonstrated that it suffered from unacceptable variability compared to respiratory indirect calorimetry.[68] This prospective trial was done with critically ill patients and was not limited to obese patients; however, there is no reason to suspect that a trial exclusively involving obese patients would demonstrate different results.

The Application of Hypocaloric Feeding

Although the concept of a specialized approach for nourishing the severely ill obese patient has been considered for a number of years, there are few studies in the literature evaluating this technique, and even fewer prospective randomized trials comparing it to standard feeding regimens (Table 53-5).

In a nonrandomized trial, Dickerson et al placed 13 obese patients requiring PN for postoperative complications on a hypocaloric regimen.[46] The researchers reported net protein anabolism, complete tissue healing, and lack of major complications. Burge and colleagues, in a randomized, prospective trial of non-critically ill obese patients, compared a hypocaloric parenteral formulation with a standard approach.[47] In both groups, positive nitrogen balances were achieved. However, these researchers did not report the incidence of complications or the effect on outcome. In a second prospective, randomized trial by the same group of investigators, Choban and colleagues studied hypocaloric feeding in both critically ill and non-critically ill obese patients.[69] Positive nitrogen balances were again achieved in both groups. Glucose control was better in the hypocaloric fed group but did not reach statistical significance. This may have been because of the small study size. Complication rates were equivalent and there were no untoward effects noted in the group given the lower energy formulations. Importantly, they were able to obtain these results without the need for indirect calorimetry. Unfortunately, effects on outcome were not reported.

Table 53-6.

Access Problems in the Obese Patient

Central Venous Access	
	Normal anatomical landmarks are obscured
	Patients may be unable to tolerate Trendelenberg positioning
	Needles may not be long enough to reach the vein
	Complications: hemothorax, pneumothorax, infection, hemorrhage, arrhythmias, hypoxia, respiratory failure
Enteral Access	
	Soft tissue adiposity complicates nasal placement
	Patient weight may preclude use of fluoroscopy
	Patients may not tolerate lying flat for the duration of the procedure
	Gastroesophageal reflux may lead to aspiration
	Sedatives may be contraindicated secondary to respiratory concerns
	Abdominal wall transillumination for endoscopy may be impossible
	Increased intraabdominal pressure may lead to gastric wall necrosis
	Patients are high risk for surgical tube placement
	Complications:
	Nasal placement: epistaxis, esophageal perforation, tube misplacement, aspiration, respiratory failure
	Endoscopic placement: respiratory failure, infection, tube misplacement, gastric wall necrosis, aspiration
	Surgical placement: Increased likelihood of all of the usual risks associated with surgery and anesthesia, infection, wound dehiscence, respiratory compromise

Access Issues

Although little is written in the literature that describes the possible difficulties of establishing feeding access in the severely obese, most clinicians are very familiar with them. The obese patients are probably more prone to access-related complications because of their body habitus and concomitant medical conditions (Table 53-6).

Central Venous Access

Most clinicians who place central venous access are aware of the difficulties with obtaining access in the severely obese. Their increased body size obscures the normal anatomical landmarks, which greatly increases the likelihood of unsuccessful venous cannulation and complications, such as pneumothorax, hemothorax, hemorrhage, and infection. Ultrasonography and even fluoroscopy may be necessary to "find the vein." To further complicate the situation, many severely obese patients are unable to tolerate lying flat or being placed in the Trendelenberg position (angling the bed with the legs up and head down). Unfortunately, this maneuver is extremely important for venous cannulation. Short, wide necks and large chest walls may compromise the ability to identify the typical anatomical landmarks. Standard prepackaged catheter kits may not have sufficiently long needles.

In general terms, the best recommendations for venous access placement are to have the most experienced clinician attempt to place the line with good illumination and adequate assistance. Should the patient need to go to surgery, the operating room is an excellent place for line central venous catheter placement or exchange.

Enteral Access

Enteral access can also be challenging.[70] Blind nasal-enteric placement is made more difficult by the increased adiposity of the soft tissues of the palate and pharynx. This can lead to an increase in the incidence of tube-placement complications that include epistaxis, esophageal perforation or hemorrhage, inadvertent placement into the trachea or bronchus, and pneumothorax. Fluoroscopic tube placement may be impossible for patients weighing over 400 lb, as many fluoroscopy tables are not designed for patients who weigh more than 350 lb. In addition, underlying conditions such as pulmonary insufficiency or severe degenerative joint disease may prevent the patient from being able to remain still in the supine position for the duration of the procedure. Respiratory difficulties may be compounded by the occlusion of a nostril with the tube. Gastroesophageal reflux is thought to occur more commonly in the severely obese, placing them at higher risk for aspiration pneumonia both during tube placement and while feeding.[71]

Endoscopic tube placement in this population is also risky. Lying supine and the need for sedation can compromise respiration. With most endoscopic techniques, illumination of the abdominal wall is necessary to insure that the stomach is adjacent to the abdominal wall without other viscera in between. Inability to transilluminate the skin secondary to the large layer of subcutaneous fat may increase the risk of colon injury. Once the tube is placed, increased intraabdominal pressure, common in these patients, can cause tension on the tube that can lead to gastric-wall necrosis, leakage with peritonitis, necrotizing fasciitis, or superficial infections.

Surgical tube placement carries all of the potential problems associated with surgery. These include complications associated with medical diseases (cardiac, pulmonary, thromboembolic, etc), and those associated with the actual surgery. The operative incision is more prone to infection and healing complications. The incisional discomfort will limit ambulation, cause respiratory splinting, and require treatment with analgesics. All of these issues could increase the risk of respiratory insufficiency, pneumonia, and thromboembolic events.

While laparoscopic surgery minimizes problems associated with an "incision," it is not immune to other complications. Patients still require general anesthesia for laparoscopy. The carbon dioxide gas used to create the pneumoperitoneum may lead to carbon dioxide retention in patients with pulmonary insufficiency. Standard trocars and laparoscopic instruments may be too short to be used for patients with massive abdominal walls. The increased intraabdominal pressure created by the pneumoperitoneum (necessary to elevate the anterior abdominal wall to create a work space), and the heavy abdominal wall can cause derangements in venous blood return to the heart.

Conclusion

The ongoing growth of the incidence of obesity in western society ensures that all practitioners will be exposed to severely overweight patients. Concomitant with this phenomenon is the growth of bariatric surgery. As more severely obese patients undergo these procedures, it is likely that most clinicians will be asked to care for these patients after surgery. While the operative procedures are increasingly safe and efficacious for achieving meaningful weight loss, long-term nutritional complications can occur and, therefore, must be recognized.

Additionally, critically ill severely obese patients can be extremely difficult to provide care for. This group is more prone to become severely ill and therefore to require involutional nutritional support. Unfortunately, the standard nutritional regimens intended to support these patients may be harmful. Many of the potential risks of traditional feeding regimens are secondary to the dependence upon the infusion of large quantities of glucose. The protein-sparing, hypocaloric approach is a unique feeding regimen that restricts glucose infusion and is offered as a safe alternative.

An understanding of the unique nutritional issues of the postbariatric surgery and the critically ill obese patient is vital to the provision of safe and effective nutritional care.

References

1. Flegal KM, Carroll MD, Ogden CL, et al. Prevalence and trends in obesity among US adults, 1999-2000. *JAMA*. 2002;288:1723-1727.
2. Freedman DS, Khan LK, Serdula MK, et al. Trends and correlates of class 3 obesity in the United States from 1990-2000. *JAMA*. 2002;288:1758-1761.
3. Steinbrook R. Surgery for severe obesity. *N Engl J Med*. 2004;350:1075-1079.
4. Cummings DE, Weigle DS, Frayo RS, et al. Plasma ghrelin levels after diet-induced weight loss or gastric bypass surgery. *N Engl J Med*. 2002;346:1623-1630.
5. Das SK, Roberts SB, McCrory MA, et al. Long-term changes in energy expenditure and body composition after massive weight loss induced by gastric bypass surgery. *Am J Clin Nutr*. 2003;78:22-30.
6. Bothe A, Bistrian BR, Greenberg I. Energy regulation in morbid obesity by multidisciplinary therapy. *Surg Clin North Am*. 1979;59:1017-1031.
7. Scopinaro N, Gianetta E, Adami GF, et al. Biliopancreatic diversion for obesity at eighteen years. *Surgery*. 1996;119:261-268.
8. Tacchino RM, Mancini A, Perrelli M, et al. Body composition and energy expenditure: relationship and changes in obese subjects before and after biliopancreatic diversion. *Metabolism*. 2003;52:552-558.
9. Hess DS, Hess DW. Biliopancreatic diversion with a duodenal switch. *Obes Surg*. 1998;8:267-282.
10. Pories WJ, Swanson MS, MacDonald KG, et al. Who would have thought it? An operation proves to be the most effective therapy for adult-onset a mellitus. *Ann Surg*. 1995;222:339-352.
11. Avinoah E, Ovnat A, Charuzi I. Nutritional status seven years after Roux-en-Y gastric bypass surgery. *Surgery*. 1992;111:137-142.
12. Halverson JD. Micronutrient deficiencies after gastric bypass for morbid obesity. *Am Surg*. 1986;52:594-598.
13. Amaral JF, Thompson WR, Caldwell MD, et al. Prospective hematologic evaluation of gastric exclusion surgery for morbid obesity. *Ann Surg*. 1985;201:186-192.
14. Rhode BM, Arseneau P, Cooper BA, et al. Vitamin B-12 deficiency after gastric bypass surgery for obesity. *Am J Clin Nutr*. 1996;63:103-109.
15. Printen KJ, Halverson JD. Hemic micronutrients following vertical banded gastroplasty. *Am Surg*. 1988; 54:267-268.
16. Smith CD, Herkes SB, Behrns KE, et al. Gastric acid secretion and vitamin B12 absorption after vertical Roux-en-Y gastric bypass for morbid obesity. *Ann Surg*. 1993; 218:91-96.
17. Slater GH, Ren CJ, Siegel N, et al. Serum fat-soluble vitamin deficiency and abnormal calcium metabolism after malabsorptive bariatric surgery. *J Gastrointest Surg*. 2004;8:48-55.
18. Brolin RE, La Marca LB, Kenler HA, et al. Malabsorptive gastric bypass in patients with superobesity. *J Gastrointest Surg*. 2002;6:195-203.
19. Skroubis G, Sakellaropoulos G, Pouggouras K, et al. Comparison of nutritional deficiencies after Roux-en-Y gastric bypass and after biliopancreatic diversion with Roux-en-Y gastric bypass. *Obes Surg*. 2002;12:551-558.
20. Goldner WS, O'Dorisio TM, Dillon JS, et al. Severe metabolic bone disease as a long-term complication of obesity surgery. *Obes Surg*. 2002;12:685-692.
21. Rhode BM, Shustik C, Christou NV, et al. Iron absorption and therapy after gastric bypass. *Obes Surg*. 1999;9:17-21.
22. Brolin RE, Leung M. Survey of vitamin and mineral supplementation after gastric bypass and biliopancreatic diversion for morbid obesity. *Obes Surg*. 1999;9:150-154.
23. Hatizifotis M, Dolan K, Newbury L, et al. Symptomatic vitamin A deficiency following biliopancreatic diversion. *Obes Surg*. 2003;13:655-657.
24. Newbury L, Dolan K, Hatzifotis M, et al. Calcium and vitamin D depletion and elevated parathyroid hormone following biliopancreatic diversion. *Obes Surg*. 2003;13:893-895.
25. Goode LR, Brolin RE, Chowdhury HA, et al. Bone and gastric bypass surgery: effects of dietary calcium and vitamin D. *Obes Res*. 2004;12:40-7.
26. Pugnale N, Giusti V, Suter M, et al. Bone metabolism and risk of secondary hyperparathyroidism 12 months after gastric banding in obese pre-menopausal women. *Int J Obes Relat Metab Discord*. 2003;27:110-6.
27. Heaney RP, Dowell MS, Buerman J, et al. Absorbability and cost effectiveness in calcium supplementation. *J Am Coll Nutr*. 2001;20:239-246.

28. Heller HJ, Poindexter JR, Adams-Huet B. Effect of estrogen treatment and vitamin D on differing bioavailabilities of calcium carbonate and calcium citrate. *J Clin Pharmacol.* 2002;42:1251-6.
29. Villar HV, Ranne RD. Neurologic deficit following gastric partitioning: possible role of thiamine. *JPEN.* 1984;8:575-578.
30. Cirignotta F, Manconi M, Mondini S, et al. Wernicke-Korsakoff encephalopathy and polyneuropathy after gastroplasty for morbid obesity: report of a case. *Arch Neurol.* 2000;57(9):1356-1359.
31. Chaves LCL, Faintuch J, Kahwage S, et al. A cluster of polyneuropathy and Wernicke-Korshakoff syndrome in a bariatric unit. *Obes Surg.* 2002;12:328-334.
32. Kushner R. Managing the obese patient after bariatric surgery: a case report of severe malnutrition and review of the literature. *JPEN.* 2000;24:126-132.
33. Salas-Salvado J, Garcia-Lorda P, Cuatrecasas G, et al. Wernicke's syndrome after bariatric surgery. *Clin Nutr.* 2000;19(5):371-373.
34. Hunter DC, Jaksic T, Lewis D, et al. Resting energy expenditure in the critically ill: Estimations versus measurement. *Br J Surg.* 1988,75:875-878.
35. McMurray JF. Wound healing with diabetes mellitus. Better glucose control for better wound healing in diabetes. *Surg Clin N Am.* 1984;64:769-778.
36. Bagdade JD, Stewart M, Walters E. Impaired granulocyte adherence. A reversible defect in host defense in patients with poorly controlled diabetes. *Diabetes.* 1978;27:677-681.
37. Jones RL, Peterson CM. Hematologic alterations in diabetes mellitus. *Am J Med.* 1981;70:339-352.
38. Hostetter MK. Handicaps to host defense. Effects of hyperglycemia on C3 and Candida Albicans. *Diabetes.* 1990;39:271-275.
39. Pomposelli JJ, Baxter JK 3rd, Babineau TJ, et al. Early postoperative glucose control predicts nosocomial infection rate in diabetic patients. *JPEN.* 1998;22:77-81.
40. Van Den Berghe, Wouters P, Weekers F, et al. Intensive insulin therapy in critically ill patients. *N Engl J Med.* 2001;345:1359-1367.
41. Van Itallie TB. Health implications of overweight and obesity in the United States. *Ann Intern Med.* 1985;103(6 pt 2):983-988.
42. Baker AL, Rosenberg IH. Hepatic complications of total parenteral nutrition. *Am J Med.* 1987;82:489-497.
43. McMahon MM, Benotti PN, Bistrian BR. A clinical application of exercise physiology and nutritional support for the mechanically ventilated patient. *JPEN.* 1990;14:538-542.
44. Askanazi J, Rosenbaum SH, Hyman AI, et al. Respiratory changes induced by the large glucose loads of total parenteral nutrition. *JAMA.* 1980;243:1444-1447.
45. Baxter JK and Bistrian BR. Moderate hypocaloric parenteral nutrition in the critically ill, obese patient. *Nutr Clin Pract.* 1989;4:133-135.
46. Dickerson RN, Rosato EF, Mullen JL. Net protein anabolism with hypocaloric parenteral nutrition in obese stressed patients. *Am J Clin Nutr.* 1986;44:747-755.
47. Burge JC, Goon A, Choban PS, et al. Efficacy of hypocaloric total parenteral nutrition in hospitalized obese patients: A prospective, double-blind randomized trial. *JPEN.* 1994;18:203-207.
48. Jeevanandam M, Young DH and Schiller WR. Obesity and the metabolic response to severe multiple trauma in man. *J Clin Invest.* 1991;87:262-269.
49. Greenberg GR, Marliss EB, Anderson GH, et al. Protein sparing therapy in post-operative patients. *N Engl J Med.* 1976;294:1411-1416.
50. Young GA, Hill GL. A controlled study of protein-sparing therapy after excision of the rectum. *Ann Surg.* 1980;192:183-191.
51. Hensle TW, Askanazi J. Metabolism and nutrition in the perioperative period. *J Urol.* 1988;139:229-239.
52. Douglas RG, Shaw JHF. Metabolic response to sepsis and trauma. *Br J Surg.* 1989;76:115-122.
53. Elwyn DH, Kinney JM, Askanazi J. Energy expenditure in surgical patients. *Surg Clin N Am.* 1981;61:545-556.
54. Mascioli EA, Smith MF, Trerice MS, et al. Effect of total parenteral nutrition with cycling on essential fatty acid deficiency. *JPEN.* 1979;3:171-173.
55. Benedetti G, Mingrone G, Marcoccia S, et al. Body composition and energy expenditure after weight loss following bariatric surgery. *J Am Coll Nutr.* 2000;19:270-274.
56. Das SK, Roberts SB, Kehayias JJ, et al. Body composition assessment in extreme obesity and after massive weight loss induced by gastric bypass surgery. *Am J Physiol.* 2003;284:E1080-1088.
57. Waki M, Kral JG, Mazariegos M, et al. Relative expansion of extracellular fluid in obese vs. nonobese women. *Am J Physiol.* 1991;261:E199-E203.
58. Heymsfield SB, Lichtman S, Baumgartner RN, et al. Assessment of body composition: An overview. In: Bjorntorp P, Brodoff BN, eds. *Obesity.* 1st ed. Philadelphia: J.B. Lippincott Co; 1992: 37-54.
59. Wilkens, K. Adjustment for obesity. ADA Renal Practice Group Newsletter, Winter 1984.
60. Osborne BJ, Saba AK, Wood SJ, et al. Clinical comparison of three methods to determine resting energy expenditure. *Nutr Clin Pract.* 1994;9:241-246.
61. Daly JM, Heymsfield SB, Head CA, et al. Human energy expenditure: Overestimation by widely used prediction equations. *Am J Clin Nutr.* 1985;42:1170-1174.
62. Cortes B, Nelson LD. Errors in estimating energy expenditure in critically ill surgical patients. *Arch Surg.* 1989;124:287-290.
63. Ireton-Jones CS. Evaluation of energy expenditure in obese patients. *Nutr Clin Pract.* 1989;4:127-129.
64. Bernstein RS, Thornton JC, Yang MU, et al. Prediction of the resting metabolic rate in obese patients. *Am J Clin Nutr.* 1983;37:595-602.
65. Das SK, Saltzman E, McCrory MA, et al. Energy expenditure is very high in extremely obese woman. *J Nutr.* 2004;134:1412-1416.
66. Weir JB de V. New methods for calculating metabolic rate with special reference to protein metabolism. *J Physiol.* 1941;109:1-9.
67. Ligett SB, St John RE, Lefrak SS. Determination of resting energy expenditure utilizing the thermodilution pulmonary artery catheter. *Chest.* 1987;4:562-566.
68. Ogawa AM, Shikora SA, Burke LM, et al. The thermodilution technique does not agree with indirect calorimetry for the critically ill patient. *JPEN.* 1998;22:347-351.
69. Choban PS, Burge JC, Scales D, et al. Hypoenergetic nutrition support in hospitalized obese patients: a simplified method for clinical application. *Am J Clin Nutr.* 1997;66:546-550.
70. Shikora SA. Enteral Feeding tube placement in obese patients: considerations for nutrition support. *Nutr Clin Pract.* 1997;12:S9-S13.
71. Vaughan RW, Bauer S, Wise L. Volume and pH of gastric juice in obese patients. *Anesthesiology.* 1981;55:180.

Index